White and Pharoah's

ORAL RADIOLOGY

Principles and Interpretation

White and Pharoah's

ORAL RADIOLOGY

Principles and Interpretation

9th EDITION

ERNEST W.N. LAM, DMD, MSc, PhD, FRCD(C), Dip ABOMR
Professor
Oral and Maxillofacial Radiology,
Faculty of Dentistry
The University of Toronto
Toronto, Ontario, Canada

SANJAY M. MALLYA, BDS, MDS, PhD, Dip ABOMR
Professor and Chair
Section of Oral and Maxillofacial Radiology
School of Dentistry
University of California, Los Angeles
Los Angeles, California

ELSEVIER

Elsevier
3251 Riverport Lane
St. Louis, Missouri 63043

WHITE AND PHAROAH'S ORAL RADIOLOGY:
PRINCIPLES AND INTERPRETATION, NINTH EDITION

ISBN: 978-0-443-11871-5

Senior Content Strategist: Kelly Skelton
Senior Content Development Specialist: Shilpa Kumar
Publishing Services Manager: Deepthi Unni
Senior Project Manager: Beula Christopher
Designer: Patrick Ferguson

Printed in India

Last digit is the print number: 9 8 7 6 5 4 3 2 1

PREFACE

We are encouraged by the positive feedback on the 8th edition that we received from colleagues and students. This book has an international readership, and we consider it a privilege to serve as editors of this trusted and reliable knowledge source. The book encompasses the full scope of the subject and introduces the undergraduate dental student to oral and maxillofacial radiology, while also serving as a comprehensive resource for graduate students and dental practitioners.

Diagnostic imaging is integral to the practice of dentistry. Oral and maxillofacial radiologic imaging accounts for more than a quarter of all healthcare imaging procedures done worldwide and underscores the importance of training dentists to use diagnostic imaging. Part I of the book provides foundational knowledge of radiation sciences that is essential for the safe and effective use of x-rays. Part II discusses principles, techniques and technology of radiologic imaging. Keeping with changing trends in the use of imaging, this edition includes new chapters on *Computed Tomography*, *Magnetic Resonance Imaging*, *Nuclear Medicine* and *Ultrasound*. The chapters reflect contemporary technologic enhancements and innovations and changing practices in the use of these imaging modalities in dentistry. Chapter 14, *Quality Assurance*, has been updated to reflect new standards and recommendations for equipment maintenance and quality assessment. Chapter 15, *Prescribing Diagnostic Imaging*, reflects current imaging guidelines, provides the reader with guidance to follow prescription imaging rather than protocol imaging, and encourages critical thinking in designing radiologic examinations.

Dentists must be familiar with the key radiologic features of diseases in the oral and maxillofacial region. In Part III, this book provides comprehensive coverage of the radiologic manifestations and the differential interpretation of diseases affecting the teeth, jaws, paranasal sinuses, salivary glands and temporomandibular joints. The chapters emphasize the biological foundations of disease and link these to the appearances they produce on imaging and, ultimately, image interpretation. Where appropriate, the radiologic appearances of disease are illustrated using not only conventional 2-dimensional planar imaging but also advanced imaging, providing an additional dimension of imaging to support the work of dentists in both general and specialty practice.

There is an increase in the use of digital technologies for treatment planning and for manufacture of guides and dental prosthesis. Products that use artificial and augmented intelligence (AI) for radiologic image assessment are now approved by the US Food and Drug Agency (FDA) for use in dentistry. Both these technologies are discussed in Part IV, Chapter 32—*Beyond three-dimensional imaging*.

The book also offers the following supplemental resources:

- An image collection for faculty on the Evolve Resources companion site (http://evolve.elsevier.com/White/oralradiology/)
- Videos and a test bank of review questions for students in the enhanced eBook included with every print purchase (http://ebooks.health.elsevier.com/)

We desire to make the study of oral and maxillofacial radiology stimulating and exciting.

Ernest W. N. Lam
Sanjay M. Mallya

ACKNOWLEDGMENTS

We thank our colleagues who have contributed as chapter authors. We appreciate their willingness to share their expertise and knowledge with our readers. This edition welcomes nine new authors: Drs. Mansur Ahmad, Avni Bhula, Anita Gohel, Mohammed Husain, Shumei Murakami, Kumar Shah, Hiroaki Shimamoto, Trevor Thang, and Stuart White.

We thank Mr. John Harvey and Mr. Samir Mallya for creating some of the new graphic illustrations. We thank Drs. Freny Karjodkar, Matheus Oliveira, and Nandita Shenoy for providing region-specific information that adds to the book's global reach. We are particularly thankful to our colleagues and students and our readers worldwide, who have contacted us to suggest improvements or to report that they have uncovered an error. Among these individuals are Ulkem Aydin, Rumpa Ganguly, Sung Kim, Peter Mah, Mohadeseh Markazimoghadam, and Matheus Oliviera.

We thank the staff at Elsevier whose tireless efforts supported this work and helped move the process to meet production milestones: Kristin Wilhelm, Kelly Skelton, Shilpa Kumar, Manjinder Singh, Beula Christopher, Deepthi Unni and Patrick Ferguson.

Ernest W. N. Lam
Sanjay M. Mallya

CONTENTS

1

Physics

Sanjay M. Mallya

To access the videos in this chapter, please visit ebooks.health.elsevier.com.

One atom says to a friend, "I think I lost an electron." The friend replies, "Are you sure?" "Yes," says the first atom, "I'm positive."

Radiologic examination is an integral component of the dentist's diagnostic armamentarium. Dentists often make radiographic images of patients to obtain additional information beyond that available from a clinical examination or their patient's history. The combined information is used to make a diagnosis and formulate an appropriate treatment plan. This chapter provides basic knowledge on the nature of radiation, the operation of an x-ray machine, and the interactions of x-radiation with matter, with an emphasis on diagnostic x-radiation. This foundational knowledge is important for the safe and effective use of x-rays in dentistry.

COMPOSITION OF MATTER

Matter is anything that has mass and occupies space. The atom is the basic unit of all matter and consists of a nucleus containing protons and neutrons, and electrons that are bound to the nucleus by electromagnetic force. The classic view of the atom, the **Bohr model,** considers the structure of atoms like a solar system, with negatively charged electrons that travel in discrete orbits around a central, positively charged nucleus (Fig. 1.1A). The contemporary view, the **standard model** or **quantum mechanical model,** assigns electrons into complex three-dimensional orbitals with energy sublevels (see Fig. 1.1B).

Atomic Structure

Nucleus

In all atoms except hydrogen, the nucleus consists of positively charged protons and neutral neutrons. A hydrogen nucleus contains a single proton. The number of protons in the nucleus, its **atomic number** *(Z),* is unique to each element. Each of 118 known elements has a unique atomic number. The total number of protons and neutrons in the nucleus of an atom is its **atomic mass** *(A).* The ratio of neutrons to protons determines the stability of the nucleus and is the basis of radioactive decay.

Electron Orbitals

Electrons are negatively charged particles that exist in the extranuclear space and are bound to the nucleus by electromagnetic force. The *Bohr model* considers that electrons exist in discrete orbits or "shells" denoted as K, L, M, N, O, and P, with the K-shell being closest to the nucleus (see Fig. 1.1A). The shells are also described by a quantum number 1, 2, 3, …, with 1 being the quantum number for the K-shell. Each shell can hold a maximum of $2n^2$ electrons, where n is the quantum number of the shell.

The *quantum mechanical model* describes the electrons within three-dimensional orbitals, or electron clouds (see Fig. 1.1B). The electron orbitals are described based on their distance from the nucleus (*principal quantum number*; $n = 1, 2, 3, \ldots$) and their shape (designated s, p, d, f, g, h, and i). Only two electrons may occupy an orbital. The electron orbitals in order of filling are 1s, 2s, 2p, 3s, 3p, 4s, 3d, 4p, 5s, 4d, 5p, 6s, and so forth. The Bohr model and the quantum mechanical model both provide an adequate basis to conceptually understand diagnostic x-ray production and interactions.

The energy needed to overcome the electromagnetic force that binds an electron to the nucleus is termed the **electron binding energy.** The electron binding energy is related to the atomic number and the orbital type. Elements with a large atomic number (high Z) have more protons in their nucleus and thus bind electrons in any given orbital more tightly than smaller Z elements. Within a given atom, electrons in the inner orbitals are more tightly bound than the more distant outer orbitals. Electron binding energy is the conceptual basis to understand ionization, which occurs when matter is exposed to x-rays.

Ionization

When the number of electrons in an atom is equal to the number of protons in its nucleus, the atom is electrically neutral. If a neutral atom loses an electron, it becomes a positive ion, and the free electron becomes a negative ion. This process of forming an ion pair is termed **ionization.** To ionize an atom, sufficient external energy must be provided to overcome the electromagnetic forces and free the electron from the nucleus. High-energy particles, x-rays, and ultraviolet radiation have sufficient energy to displace electrons from their orbitals and ionize atoms. Such radiations are referred to as **ionizing radiations.** In contrast, visible light, infrared and microwave radiations, and radio waves do not have sufficient energy to remove bound electrons from their orbitals and are **nonionizing radiations.**

NATURE OF RADIATION

Radiation is the transmission of energy through space and matter. It may occur in two forms: (1) electromagnetic and (2) particulate (Table 1.1). Practical applications of these radiations in healthcare are listed.

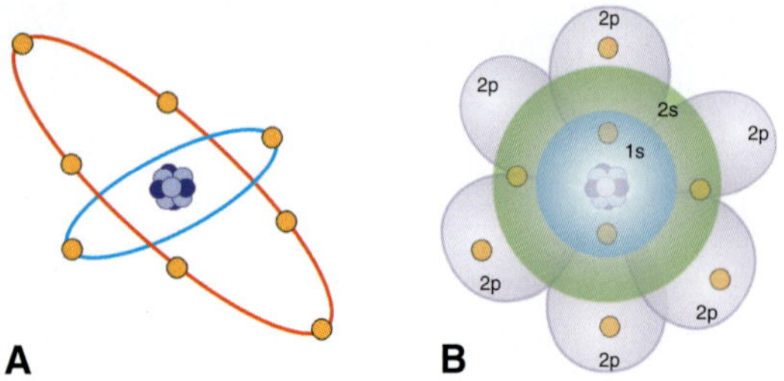

Fig. 1.1 (A) Schematic view of the Bohr model of the oxygen atom showing a nucleus with electrons that travel around the nucleus in circular orbits. (B) Schematic view of the quantum mechanical model of the oxygen atom. The central nucleus is surrounded by an electron cloud that represents probability plots of the location of the electron in a complex arrangement.

TABLE 1.1 Particulate Radiation

Particle	Symbol	Elementary Charge[a]	Rest Mass (amu)
Alpha	α	+2	4.00154
Beta$^+$ (positron)	β^+	+1	0.000549
Beta$^-$ (electron)	β^-	−1	0.000549
Electron	e^-	−1	0.000549
Neutron	n^0	0	1.008665
Proton	p	+1	1.007276

[a]Elementary charge of 1 equals that the charge of a proton or the opposite of an electron.
amu, Atomic mass units, where 1 amu = 1⁄12 the mass of a neutral carbon-12 atom.

- Diagnostic imaging with projection radiography and computed tomography (CT) use x-rays, a category of electromagnetic radiation that is ionizing in nature.
- Magnetic resonance imaging (MRI; Chapter 10) uses electromagnetic radiations of significantly lower energies than x-rays and at energies that are nonionizing.
- Some radiopharmaceuticals used in diagnostic nuclear medicine emit particulate radiation. For example, ^{18}F-fluorodeoxyglucose (^{18}F-FDG) emits positrons, a key step in imaging with **positron emission tomography** (PET; Chapter 11).
- High-energy electromagnetic radiations (gamma rays, γ) and high-energy particulate radiations (electron beams and protons) are used in cancer therapy (see Chapter 2).

Electromagnetic Radiation

Electromagnetic radiation is the movement of energy through space as a combination of electric and magnetic fields. It is generated when the velocity of an electrically charged particle is altered. γ-Rays, x-rays, ultraviolet rays, visible light, infrared radiation (heat), microwaves, and radio waves are examples of electromagnetic radiation (Fig. 1.2). γ-Rays originate in the nuclei of radioactive atoms. They have greater energy than diagnostic x-rays. In contrast, x-rays are produced outside the nucleus and result from the interaction of electrons with large atomic nuclei, as in x-ray machines. The higher-energy types of radiation in the electromagnetic spectrum—ultraviolet rays, x-rays, and γ-rays—are capable of ionizing matter. Some properties of electromagnetic radiation are best explained by quantum theory, whereas others are most successfully described by wave theory.

Quantum theory considers electromagnetic radiation as small discrete bundles of energy called **photons**, which are the carriers of electromagnetic force. Each photon travels at the speed of light and contains a specific amount of energy, expressed with the unit **electron volt** (eV).

The wave theory of electromagnetic radiation maintains that radiation is propagated in the form of waves, similar to the waves resulting from a disturbance in water. Such waves consist of electric and magnetic fields oriented in planes at right angles to one another that oscillate perpendicular to the direction of motion (Fig. 1.3). All electromagnetic waves travel at the velocity of light ($c = 3.0 \times 10^8$ m/s) in a vacuum. Waves are described in terms of their wavelength (λ, meters) and frequency (ν, cycles per second, hertz).

Both theories are used to describe properties of electromagnetic radiation. Quantum theory has been successful in correlating experimental data on the interaction of radiation with atoms, the photoelectric effect, and the production of x-rays. Wave theory is more useful for considering radiation in bulk when millions of quanta are being examined, as in experiments dealing with refraction, reflection, diffraction, interference, and polarization. Considering the value of both theories, electromagnetic radiations are described in terms of their energy, wavelength, and frequency. In practical use, high-energy photons such as x-rays and γ-rays are typically characterized by their energy (eV), medium-energy photons (e.g., visible light and ultraviolet waves) are typically characterized by their wavelength (nanometers), and low-energy photons (e.g., AM and FM radio waves) are typically characterized by their frequency (kHz and MHz).

Box 1.1 shows the relationships between photon energy, wavelength, and frequency.

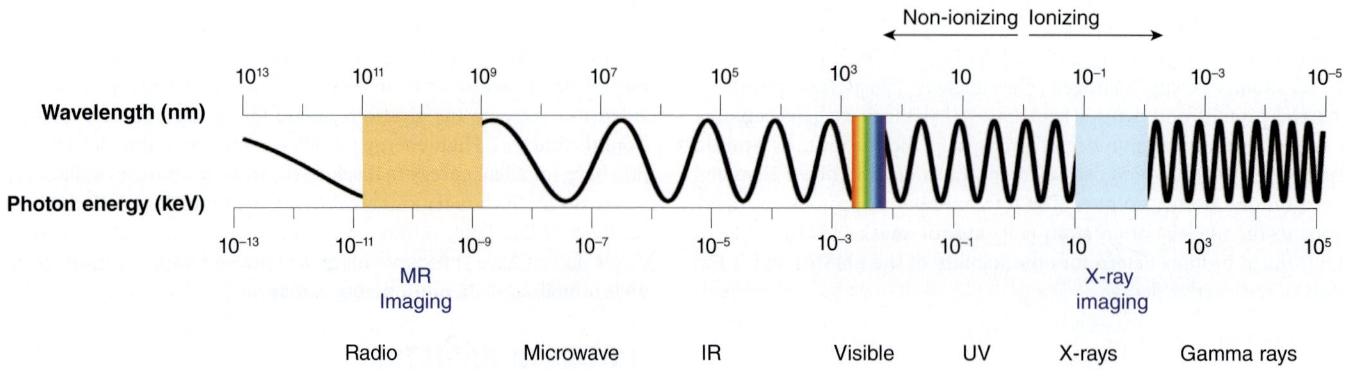

Fig. 1.2 Electromagnetic spectrum showing the relationship between photon wavelength and energy and the physical properties of various portions of the spectrum. Photons with shorter wavelengths have higher energy. Photons used in dentomaxillofacial radiography *(blue)* have energies of 10–120 keV. Magnetic resonance *(MR)* imaging uses radio waves *(orange)*. *IR,* Infrared radiation; *UV,* ultraviolet radiation.

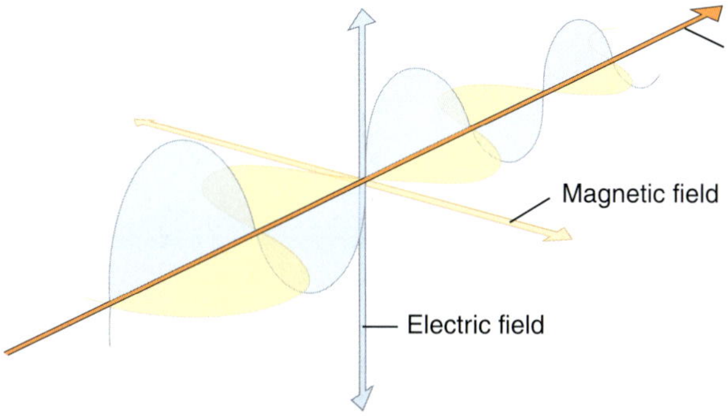

Fig. 1.3 Electric and magnetic fields associated with electromagnetic radiation.

BOX 1.1 Relationship Between Energy *(E)* and Wavelength (λ) of Electromagnetic Radiation

$$E = h \times \frac{c}{\lambda}$$

simplified as

$$E = \frac{1.24}{\lambda}$$

$$E \propto \frac{1}{\lambda}$$

E is energy (kiloelectron volts, keV)
h is the Planck constant (6.626×10^{-34} joule-seconds or 4.13×10^{-15} eV-s)
c is the velocity of light = 3×10^8 m/s
λ is wavelength (nanometers, nm)

Key point: **Inverse relationship between energy and wavelength of an electromagnetic radiation**

Particulate Radiation

Small atoms have approximately equal numbers of protons and neutrons, whereas larger atoms tend to have more neutrons than protons. Larger atoms are unstable because of the unequal distribution of protons and neutrons, and they may break up, releasing α (alpha) or β (beta) particles or γ (gamma) rays. This process is called **radioactivity.** When a radioactive atom releases an α or a β particle, the atom is transmuted into another element. Another type of radioactivity is γ decay, producing γ-rays. They result as part of a decay chain where a nucleus converts from an excited state to a lower level ground state; this often happens after a nucleus emits an α or β particle or after nuclear fission or fusion.

Examples of radioactive decay that are important in healthcare are listed.

- An unstable atom with an excess of protons may decay by converting a proton into a neutron, a β^+ particle (positron), and a neutrino. Positrons quickly annihilate with electrons to form two γ-rays. This reaction is the basis for PET imaging (see Chapter 11).
- An unstable atom with an excess of neutrons may decay by converting a neutron into a proton, a β^- particle, and a neutrino. β^- particles are identical to electrons. High-speed β^- particles are able to penetrate up to 1.5 cm in tissue. β^- particles from radioactive iodine-131 are used for treatment of some thyroid cancers.
- α particles are helium nuclei consisting of two protons and two neutrons. They result from the radioactive decay of many large atomic number elements. Because of their double positive charge and heavy mass, α particles densely ionize matter through which they pass and penetrate only a few micrometers of body tissues. This limited range has prompted use of alpha emitters such as radium-223 in targeted radiation therapy for bone metastasis.

The capacity of particulate radiation to ionize atoms depends on its mass, velocity, and charge. The rate of loss of energy from a particle as it moves along its track through matter (tissue) is its **linear energy transfer** (LET). The greater the physical size of the particle, the higher its charge, and the lower its velocity, the greater its LET. For example, α particles, with their high mass compared with an electron, high charge, and low velocity, are densely ionizing, lose their kinetic energy rapidly, and have a high LET. β^- particles are much less densely ionizing because of their lighter mass and lower charge; they have a lower LET. High-LET radiations concentrate their ionization along a short path, whereas low-LET radiations produce ion pairs much more sparsely over a longer path length (see Fig. 2.3A) The densely ionizing tracks of high LET radiation cause more closely spaced DNA damage, which is difficult to repair. Thus, high LET radiations are more effective at cell killing than low LET radiations (see Chapter 2).

X-RAY MACHINE

X-ray machines produce x-rays that pass through a patient's tissues and strike a digital receptor or film to make a radiographic image. The primary components of an x-ray machine are the x-ray tube and its power supply, positioned within the tube head. For intraoral x-ray units, the tube head is typically supported by an arm that is usually mounted on a wall (Fig. 1.4A). A control panel allows the operator to adjust the duration of the exposure, and often the energy and exposure rate, of the x-ray beam. Dental x-ray machines are also manufactured as handheld devices (Fig. 1.4B). The power supply for these devices is provided by a rechargeable battery, and the control panel is integrated into the handheld device. An electrical insulating material, usually oil, surrounds the tube and transformers. Often, the tube is recessed within the tube head to increase the source-to-object distance and minimize distortion (Fig. 1.5; also see Chapter 5).

X-Ray Tube

An x-ray tube is composed of a cathode and an anode situated within an evacuated glass envelope or tube (Fig. 1.6). To produce x-rays, electrons stream from the filament in the cathode to the target in the anode, where the energy from some of the electrons is converted into x-rays.

Cathode

The cathode (Figs. 1.7B and 1.8) in an x-ray tube consists of a filament and a focusing cup. The **filament** is the source of electrons within the x-ray tube. It is a coil of tungsten wire approximately 2 mm in diameter and 1 cm or less in length. Filaments typically contain approximately 1% thorium, which greatly increases the release of electrons from the heated wire. The filament is heated to incandescence with a

A

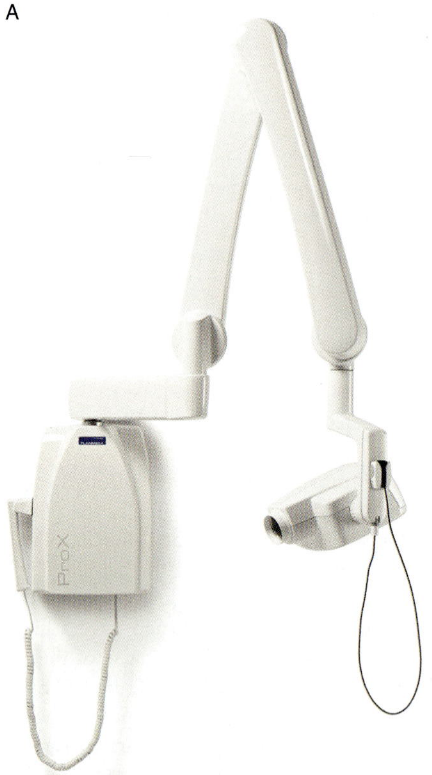

B

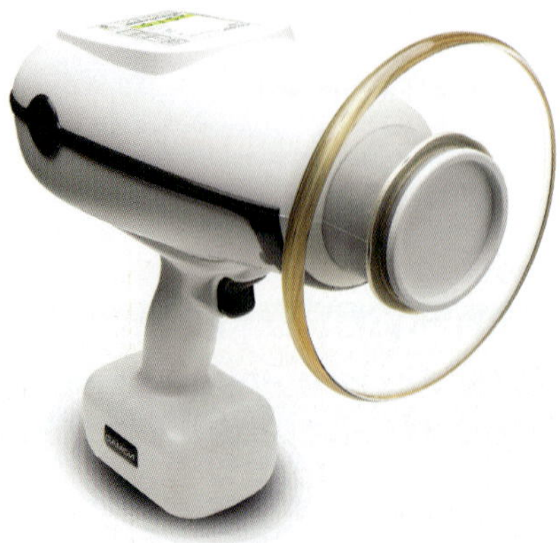

Fig. 1.4 (A) Example of an intraoral wall-mounted x-ray device, the Planmeca ProX. (B) Example of a handheld dental x-ray device, the Nomad Pro 2. (A, Courtesy Planmeca USA, Inc. Roselle, IL. B, Courtesy Dexis USA.)

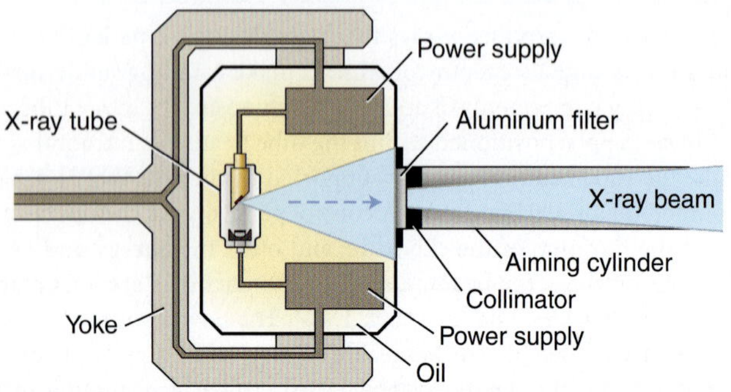

Fig. 1.5 Tube head showing a recessed x-ray tube, components of the power supply, and oil that conducts heat away from the x-ray tube. Path of useful x-ray beam *(blue)* from the anode, through the glass wall of the x-ray tube, oil, and finally an aluminum filter. The beam size is restricted by the metal tube housing and collimator. Low-energy photons are preferentially removed by the aluminum filter.

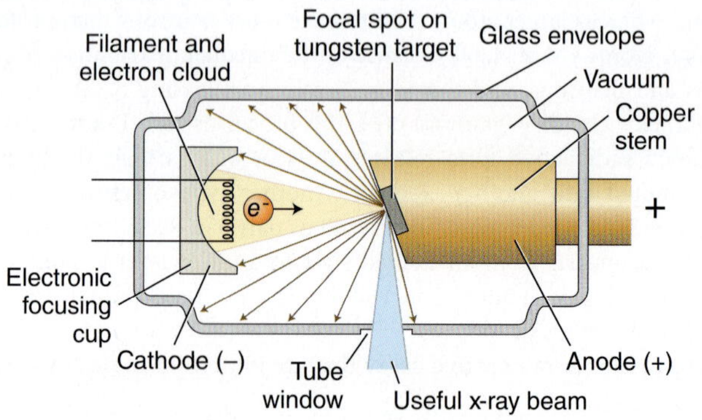

Fig. 1.6 X-ray tube with the major components labeled. The path of the electron beam is shown in *yellow*. X-rays produced at the target travel in all directions. The useful x-ray beam is shown in *blue*.

low-voltage source and emits electrons at a rate proportional to the temperature of the filament.

The filament lies in a **focusing cup** (see Fig. 1.7B; see also Fig. 1.8), a negatively charged concave molybdenum bowl. The parabolic shape of the focusing cup electrostatically focuses the electrons emitted by the filament into a narrow beam directed at a small rectangular area on the anode called the **focal spot** (see Figs. 1.7C and 1.8). The electrons move to the focal spot because they are both repelled by the negatively charged cathode and attracted to the positively charged anode. The x-ray tube is evacuated to prevent collision of the fast-moving electrons with gas molecules, which would significantly reduce their speed. The vacuum also prevents oxidation, or "burnout," of the filament.

Anode

The anode in an x-ray tube consists of a tungsten target embedded in a copper stem (see Figs. 1.6 and 1.7C). The purpose of the **target** in an x-ray tube is to convert the kinetic energy of the colliding electrons into x-ray photons. The conversion of the kinetic energy of the electrons into x-ray photons is an inefficient

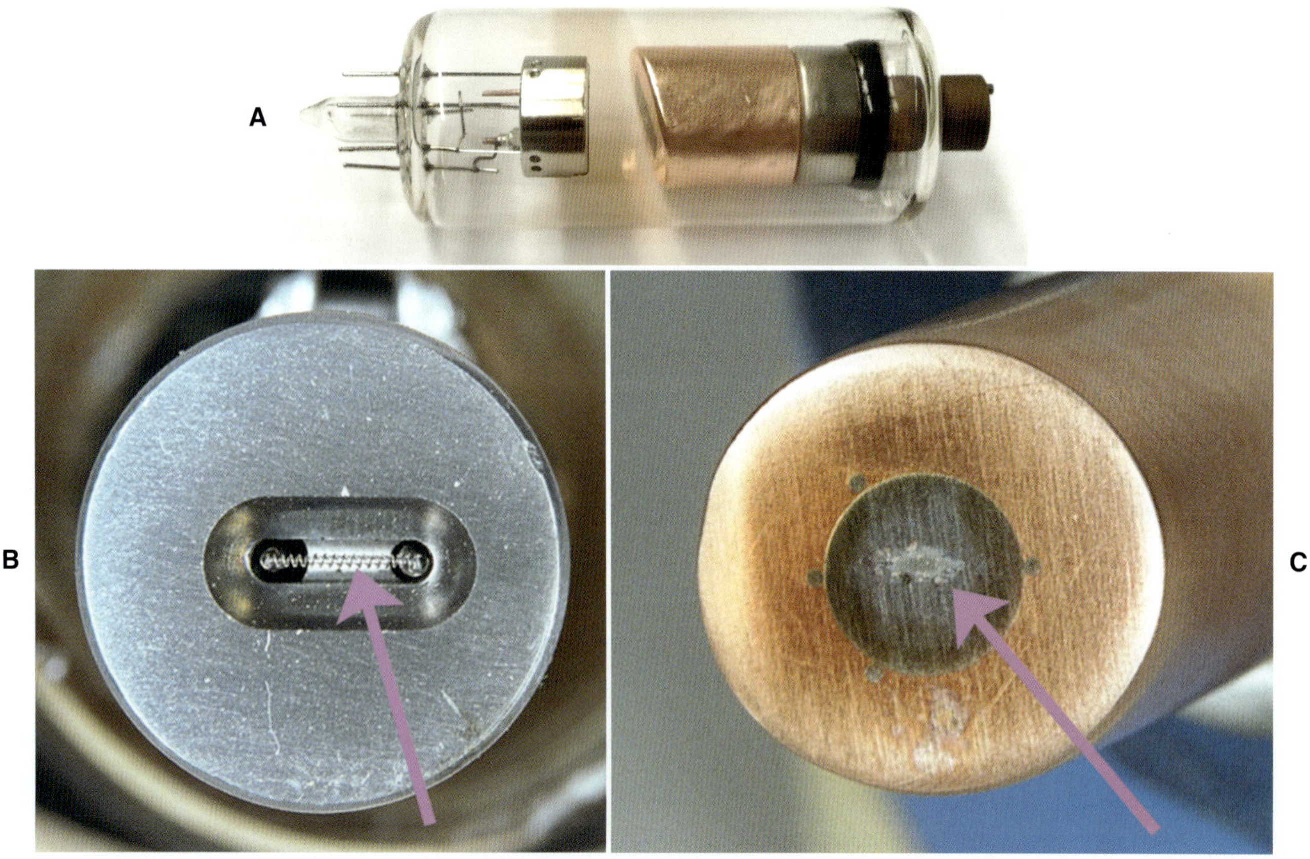

Fig. 1.7 (A) Dental stationary x-ray tube with cathode on left and copper anode on right. (B) Focusing cup containing a filament *(arrow)* in the cathode. (C) Copper anode with tungsten inset. Note the elongated actual focal spot area *(arrow)* on the tungsten target of the anode. (B and C, Courtesy John DeArmond, Tellico Plains, TN.)

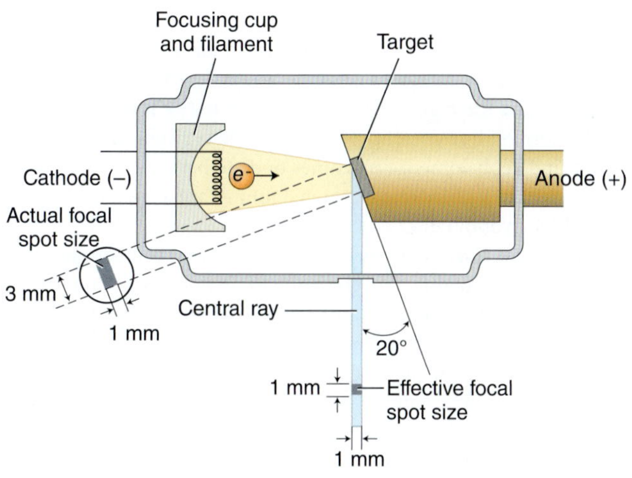

Fig. 1.8 The angle of the target to the central ray of the x-ray beam has a strong influence on the apparent size of the focal spot. The projected effective focal spot (seen below the target) is much smaller than the actual focal spot size (projected to the left). This provides a beam that has a small effective focal spot size to produce images with high resolution, while allowing for heat generated at the anode to be dissipated over the larger area.

process, with more than 99% of the electron kinetic energy converted to heat.

The target is made of tungsten, an element that has several characteristics of an ideal target material, including the following:

- **High atomic number** (74), allows for efficient x-ray production.
- **High melting point** (3422°C), to withstand heat produced during x-ray production.
- **High thermal conductivity** (173 $W{\cdot}m^{-1}{\cdot}K^{-1}$), to dissipate the heat produced away from the target.
- **Low vapor pressure** at the working temperatures of an x-ray tube, to help maintain vacuum in the tube at high operating temperatures.

The tungsten target is typically embedded in a large block of copper, which functions as a **thermal conductor** to remove heat from the tungsten target, reducing the risk of the target melting.

The **focal spot** is the area on the target to which the focusing cup directs the electrons and from which x-rays are produced. The size of the focal spot is an important technical parameter of image quality—a smaller focal spot yields a sharper image (see Chapter 5). The size of the focal spot for dental, panoramic, and cone beam CT machines ranges from 0.4 to 0.8 mm, depending on manufacturer and model. A limitation to reducing focal spot size is the heat generated. To overcome this limitation, x-ray tubes use one of the two anode configurations.

Stationary anode: In this configuration, the target is placed at an angle to the electron beam (see Fig. 1.8). Typically, the target is inclined approximately 20 degrees to the central ray of the x-ray beam. When viewed through the aiming ring, the area from which the photons of the useful x-ray beam originate appears smaller, making the **effective focal spot** smaller than the actual focal spot size. This allows production of x-rays from a larger area, allowing better heat distribution while maintaining the image quality benefits of a small focal spot. In the example shown in Fig. 1.8, the effective focal spot is approximately 1 mm × 1 mm, as opposed to the actual focal spot, which is approximately 1 mm × 3 mm. This smaller effective focal spot results in a small apparent source of x-rays and an increase in the sharpness of the image (see Figs. 5.1 and 5.2), with a larger actual focal spot size to improve heat dissipation.

Rotating anode: In this design, the tungsten target is in the form of a beveled disk that rotates during the period of x-ray production (Fig. 1.9). As a result, the electrons strike successive areas of the target disk, distributing the heat over an extended area of the disk. However, at any given time, x-rays are produced from a small spot on the target. X-ray tubes with rotating anode can be used with longer exposures and with higher tube currents of 100–500 milliamperes (mA), which is 10–50 times that possible with stationary targets. The target and rotor (armature) of the motor lie within the x-ray tube, and the stator coils (which drive the rotor at approximately 3000 revolutions per minute) lie outside the tube. Rotating anodes are not used in intraoral, panoramic, and cephalometric x-ray machines; are used in some cone beam CT machines; and are always used in multidetector CT x-ray machines, which require high radiation output for longer, sustained exposures (see Chapter 9).

Power Supply

The x-ray tube and two transformers lie within an electrically grounded metal housing called the **head** of the x-ray machine. The primary functions of the power supply transformers of an x-ray machine are to:

- Provide a low-voltage current to heat the x-ray tube filament (Fig. 1.10, filament transformer).
- Generate a high potential difference to accelerate electrons from the cathode to the focal spot on the anode (see Fig. 1.10, high-voltage transformer).

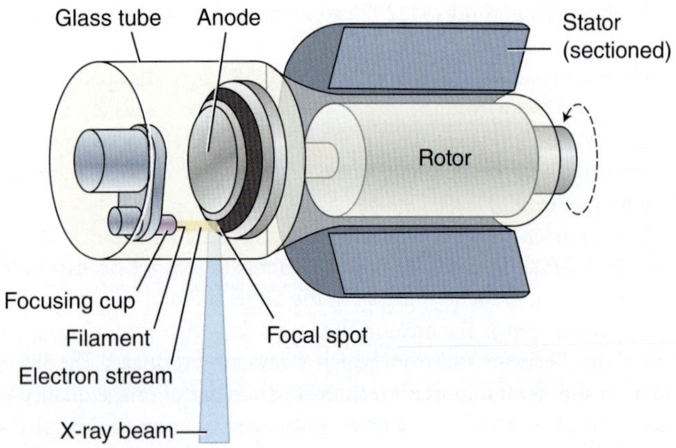

Fig. 1.9 X-ray tube with a rotating anode allows heat at the focal spot to spread out over a large surface area *(dark band)*. Current applied to the stator induces rapid rotation of the rotor and the anode. The path of the electron beam is shown in *yellow*, and the useful x-ray beam is shown in *blue*.

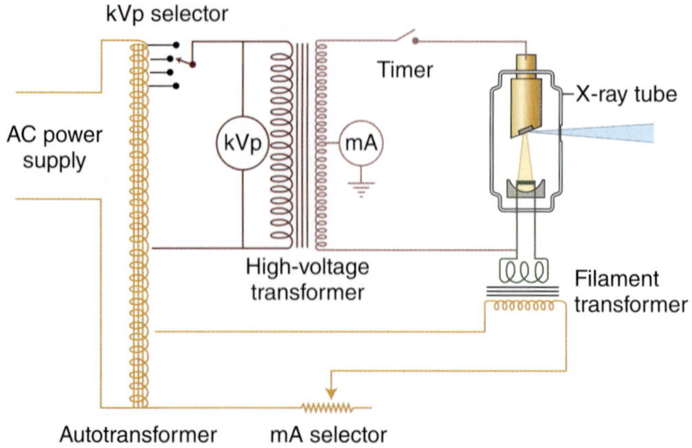

Fig. 1.10 Schematic of dental x-ray machine circuitry and x-ray tube with the major components labeled. The operator selects the desired kVp from the autotransformer. The voltage is greatly increased by the high-voltage step-up transformer and applied to the x-ray tube. The kVp dial measures the voltage on the low-voltage side of the transformer but is scaled to display the corresponding voltage in the tube circuit. The timer closes the tube circuit for the desired exposure time interval. The mA dial measures the current flowing through the tube circuit. The filament circuit heats the cathode filament and is regulated by the mA selector. *AC,* Alternate current.

X-Ray Tube Controls

Tube Current (Milliamperes, mA)

During x-ray production, electrons produced at the filament are attracted to the anode. This flow of electrons from the cathode to the anode generates a current across the x-ray tube and is called the tube current. The magnitude of this current is regulated by the milliampere control (see Fig. 1.10, mA selector), which adjusts the resistance and the current flow through the filament, thereby regulating the number of electrons produced. For many intraoral dental x-ray units, the mA setting is fixed, typically at 7–10 mA. Some units offer the flexibility of a selection of mA settings, ranging from 2 to 10 mA.

Tube Voltage (Kilovoltage, kV)

A high voltage is required between the anode and cathode to give electrons sufficient energy to generate x-rays. The kilovolt peak (kVp) selector adjusts the high-voltage transformer to boost the peak voltage of the incoming line current (110 or 220 V). Typically, intraoral, panoramic, and cephalometric machines operate between 50 and 90 kVp (50,000–90,000 V), whereas computed tomographic machines operate at 90–120 kVp and higher.

Alternating Current X-Ray Generators: For an incoming power supply with alternating current (AC), the polarity of the current alternates (60 cycles per second in North America; Fig. 1.11A), and the polarity of the x-ray tube alternates at the same frequency (see Fig. 1.11B). When the polarity of the voltage applied across the tube causes the target anode to be positive and the filament to be negative, the electrons around the filament accelerate toward the positive target, and x-rays are produced (see Fig. 1.11C). When the voltage across the cathode and anode is the highest, the efficiency of x-ray production is the highest, and thus the intensity of x-ray pulses peaks at the center of each cycle (see Fig. 1.11C).

During the following half (or negative half) of each cycle, the filament becomes positive and the target becomes negative (see Fig. 1.11B). At these times, the electrons do not flow across the gap between the two electrodes of the tube, and no x-rays are generated. When an x-ray tube is powered with 60-cycle AC, 60 pulses of x-rays

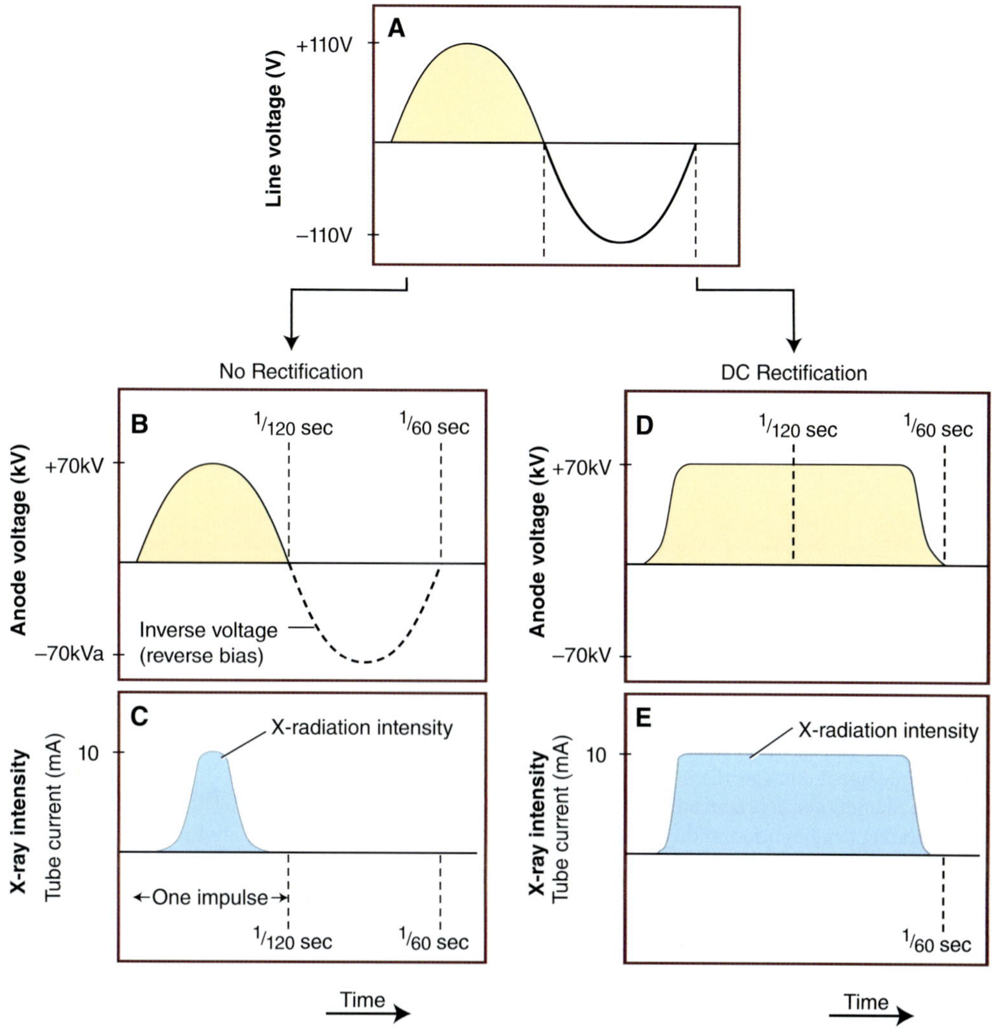

Fig. 1.11 (A) Incoming alternate current voltage (110 V, 60 cycles per second in this example). (B) Voltage at the anode varies from zero up to the kVp setting (70 kVp in this example). (C) The intensity of radiation produced at the anode *(blue)* is strongly dependent on the anode voltage and is the highest when the tube voltage is at its peak. (D) Incoming constant potential (110 V in this example) that is maintained through the operation cycle. (E) Voltage at the anode varies from zero up to the kVp setting (70 kVp in this example). Note that the increase and decrease of the potential difference at the start and end of the cycle is rapid. The intensity of radiation produced at the anode *(blue)* is higher with considerably less heterogeneity of photon energy. (Modified from Johns HE, Cunningham JR. *The Physics of Radiology.* 3rd ed. Charles C. Thomas; 1974.)

are generated each second, each having a duration of $\frac{1}{120}$ second. Thus, when using a power supply with AC, x-ray production is limited to half the AC cycle. Such x-ray units are referred to as **self-rectified** or **half-wave rectified.** Many conventional dental x-ray machines are self-rectified.

Constant Potential (Direct Current) X-Ray Generators: Some dental x-ray manufacturers produce machines that replace the conventional 60-cycle AC, half-wave-rectified power supply with a high-frequency power supply that provides an almost direct current (see Fig. 1.11D). This results in an almost constant potential between the anode and cathode (see Fig. 1.11E), and x-rays are produced through the entire cycle. The almost constant voltage yields x-rays with a narrower energy spectrum, and the mean energy of the x-ray beam produced by these x-ray machines is higher than the mean energy from a conventional half-wave-rectified machine operated at the same voltage. Handheld x-ray devices are powered using a battery and, thus, provide a constant potential.

Practical implications with the use of constant potential intraoral x-ray units are as follows:

- Because x-ray production occurs during the entire voltage cycle, constant potential units require shorter exposure times to produce the same number of x-ray photons, minimizing patient motion.
- The intensity of x-ray photons produced is more consistent, especially with short exposure times. This consistency is practically relevant when using digital receptors, which require less radiation.
- When operated at the same kVp, the x-ray beam produced by constant potential units has a higher mean energy, which decreases radiographic image contrast. To offset this effect, constant potential x-ray units are typically operated at a slightly lower kVp, typically 60 to 65 kVp.
- The narrower spectrum of energies, with fewer lower-energy photons, lowers the patient radiation dose by 35% to 40% compared with conventional AC x-ray generators.

BOX 1.2 Practical Applications of Exposure Controls

In many intraoral x-ray units, the mA setting, kVp setting, or both are fixed. If the mA setting is variable, the operator should select the highest mA value available and operate the machine at this setting; this allows the shortest exposure time and minimizes the chance of patient movement.

If tube voltage can be adjusted on an intraoral radiographic unit, the operator may choose to operate at a fixed voltage, typically 65–70 kVp. This protocol simplifies selecting the proper patient exposure settings by using just exposure time as the means to adjust for anatomic location within the mouth and patient size.

The kVp is often adjusted to compensate for patient tissue thickness, particularly for panoramic and cephalometric radiography. A rule of thumb is to vary the setting by 2 kVp/cm of tissue thickness. *A rule of thumb is to vary the setting by 2 kVp/cm of tissue thickness.*

Timer

A timer is built into the high-voltage circuit to control the duration of the x-ray exposure (see Fig. 1.10). The electronic timer controls the length of time that high voltage is applied to the tube and thus the time during which x-rays are produced. However, before the high voltage is applied across the tube, the filament must be brought to operating temperature to ensure an adequate rate of electron emission. Subjecting the filament to continuous heating at normal operating current shortens its life. To minimize filament damage, the timing circuit first sends a current through the filament for approximately half a second to bring it to the proper operating temperature and then applies power to the high-voltage circuit. In some circuit designs, a continuous low-level current passing through the filament maintains it at a safe low temperature, further shortening the delay to preheat the filament. For these reasons, an x-ray machine may be left on continuously during working hours.

Some x-ray machine timers display the exposure time in fractions of a second. In some intraoral units, the exposure times are preset for different anatomic areas of the jaws. In some units, the exposure time is expressed as number of pulses in an exposure (e.g., 3, 6, 9, 15). The number of pulses divided by 60 (the frequency of the power source) gives the exposure time in seconds. A setting of 30 pulses means that there will be 30 pulses of radiation, equivalent to a 0.5-second exposure (Box 1.2).

Tube Rating and Duty Cycle

X-ray tubes produce heat at the target while in operation. The heat buildup at the anode is measured in heat units (HU), where HU = kVp × mA × seconds. The heat storage capacity for anodes of dental diagnostic tubes is approximately 20 kHU. Heat is removed from the target by conduction to the copper anode and then to the surrounding oil and tube housing and by convection to the atmosphere.

Each x-ray machine comes with a **tube rating** chart that describes the longest exposure time the tube can be energized for a range of voltages (kVp) and tube current (mA) values without risk of damage to the target from overheating. These tube ratings generally do not restrict tube use for intraoral radiography. **Duty cycle** relates to the frequency with which successive exposures can be made without overheating the anode. The interval between successive exposures must be long enough for heat dissipation. This characteristic is a function of the size of the anode, the exposure kVp and mA, and the method used to cool the tube. A duty cycle of 1:60 indicates that one could make a 1-second exposure every 60 seconds.

PRODUCTION OF X-RAYS

Most high-speed electrons traveling from the filament to the target interact with target electrons and release their energy as heat. Occasionally, the electron's kinetic energy is converted into x-ray photons by the formation of **bremsstrahlung radiation** and **characteristic radiation.**

Bremsstrahlung Radiation

Bremsstrahlung photons are the primary source of radiation from an x-ray tube. *Bremsstrahlung* means "braking radiation" in German, and these photons are produced by the sudden stopping or slowing of high-speed electrons by tungsten nuclei in the target as follows.

Most high-speed electrons pass by tungsten nuclei with near or wide misses (Fig. 1.12A). In these interactions, the electron is attracted toward the positively charged nuclei, its path is altered toward the nucleus, and it loses some of its velocity. This deceleration causes the electron to lose kinetic energy that is given off in the form of x-ray photons. The closer the high-speed electron approaches the nuclei, the greater the electrostatic attraction between the nucleus and the electron, and the resulting bremsstrahlung photons have higher energy. The efficiency of this process is proportional to the square of the atomic number of the target; high-Z metals are more effective in

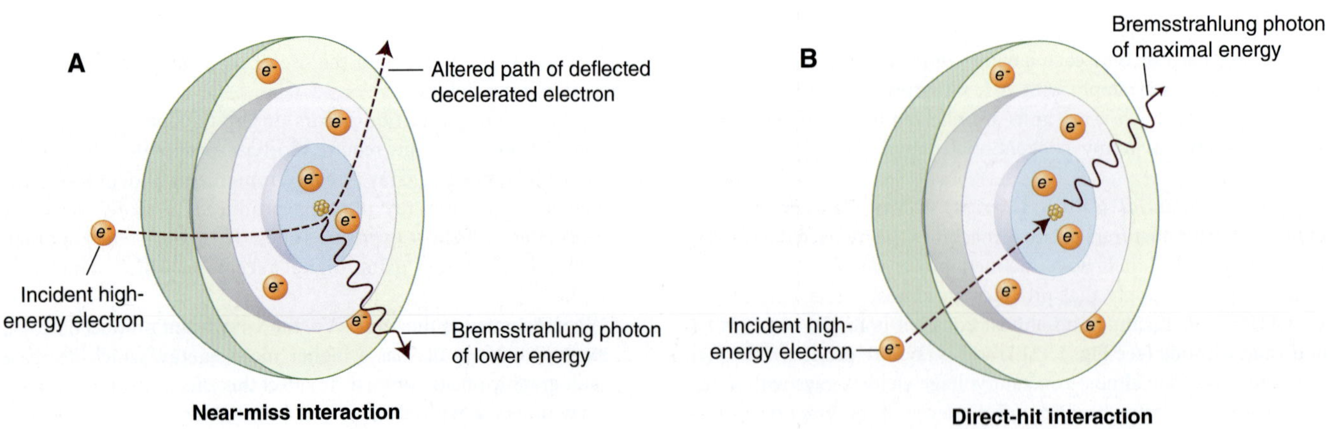

Fig. 1.12 Bremsstrahlung radiation is produced most often by the passage of an electron near a nucleus, which results in electrons being deflected and decelerated (A) or, less frequently, by the direct hit of an electron on a nucleus in the target (B). For the sake of clarity, this diagram and other similar figures in this chapter show only the 1s, 2s, and 3s orbitals.

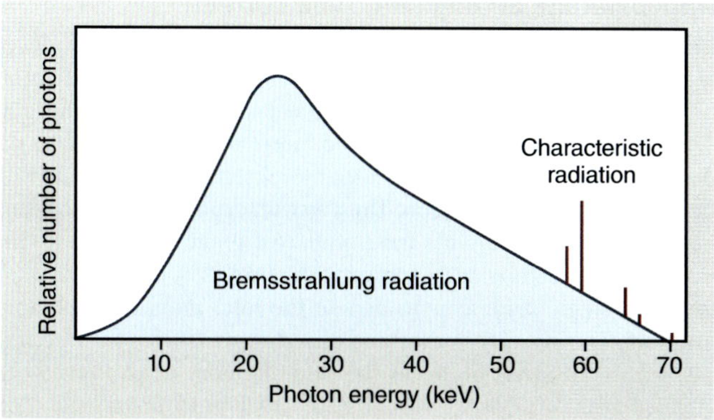

Fig. 1.13 Spectrum of photons emitted from an x-ray machine operating at 70 kVp. The vast preponderance of radiation is bremsstrahlung *(blue)*, with a minor addition of characteristic radiation.

deflecting the path of the incident electrons, and this is one reason to select tungsten ($Z = 74$) as a target material.

Occasionally, electrons from the filament directly hit the nucleus of a target atom. When this happens, all the kinetic energy of the electron is transformed into a single x-ray photon (see Fig. 1.12B). The energy of the resultant photon (in keV) is numerically equal to the energy of the electron (i.e., the voltage applied across the x-ray tube at that instant).

Bremsstrahlung interactions generate x-ray photons with a continuous spectrum of energy. The energy of an x-ray beam is usually described by identifying the peak operating voltage (in kVp). For example, a dental x-ray machine operating at a peak voltage of 70 kVp applies a voltage of up to 70 kV across the tube. This tube therefore produces a continuous spectrum of x-ray photons with energies ranging to a maximum of 70 keV (Fig. 1.13). The reasons for this continuous spectrum are as follows:

- The continuously varying voltage difference between the target and filament causes the electrons striking the target to have varying levels of kinetic energy.
- The bombarding electrons pass at varying distances around tungsten nuclei and are thus deflected to varying extents. As a result, they give up varying amounts of energy in the form of bremsstrahlung photons.
- Most electrons participate in multiple bremsstrahlung interactions in the target before losing all their kinetic energy. Consequently, an electron carries differing amounts of energy after successive interactions with tungsten nuclei.

Characteristic Radiation

Characteristic radiation contributes only a small fraction of the photons in an x-ray beam. It is made when an incident electron ejects an inner electron from the tungsten atom. When this happens, an electron from an outer orbital is quickly attracted to the void in the deficient inner orbital (Fig. 1.14). When the outer orbital electron replaces the displaced electron, a photon is emitted with energy equivalent to the difference in the binding energies of the two orbitals. The energies of characteristic photons are discrete because they represent the difference of the energy levels of specific electron orbitals and are characteristic of the target atoms. The production of characteristic radiation has no practical implications for dentomaxillofacial radiography.

FACTORS CONTROLLING THE X-RAY BEAM

An x-ray beam may be modified by altering the beam exposure duration (timer), exposure rate (mA), energy (kVp and filtration), shape (collimation), or intensity (source-patient distance).

Exposure Time (s)

Changing the exposure time—typically fractions of a second—modifies the duration of the exposure and thus the number of photons generated (Fig. 1.15). When the exposure time is doubled, the number of photons generated at all energies in the x-ray emission spectrum is doubled. The range of photon energies is unchanged. Practically, it is desirable to keep the exposure time as short as possible to minimize blurring from patient motion.

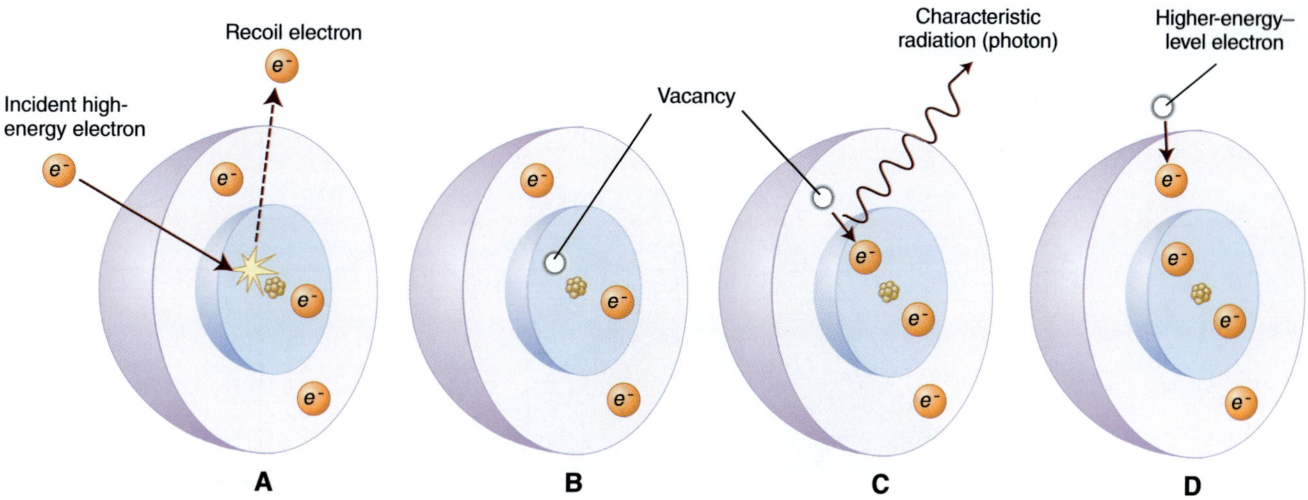

Fig. 1.14 Production of characteristic radiation. An incident electron (A) ejects an electron from an inner orbital creating an electron vacancy (B). (C) An electron from an outer orbital fills this vacancy, and a photon is emitted with energy equal to the difference in energy levels between the two orbitals. (D) Electrons from various orbitals may be involved, giving rise to other characteristic photons. The energies of the photons released are characteristic of the energy transitions for the target atom.

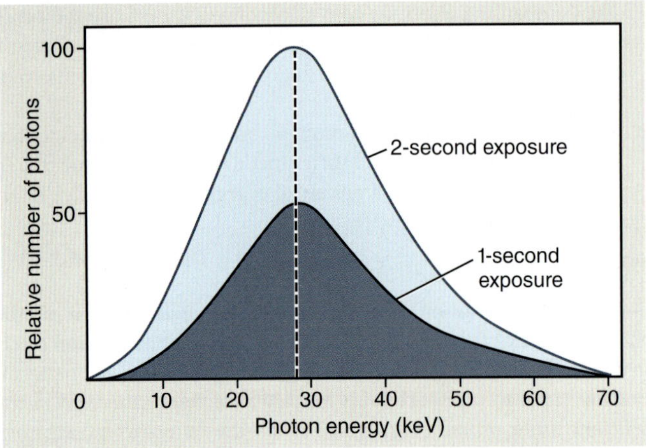

Fig. 1.15 Spectrum of photon energies generated in an x-ray machine showing that as exposure time increases (kVp and mA settings held constant), so does the total number of photons. The mean energies (*dotted line*, approximately 29 keV in this example) and maximal energies (70 keV in this example) of the beams are unchanged.

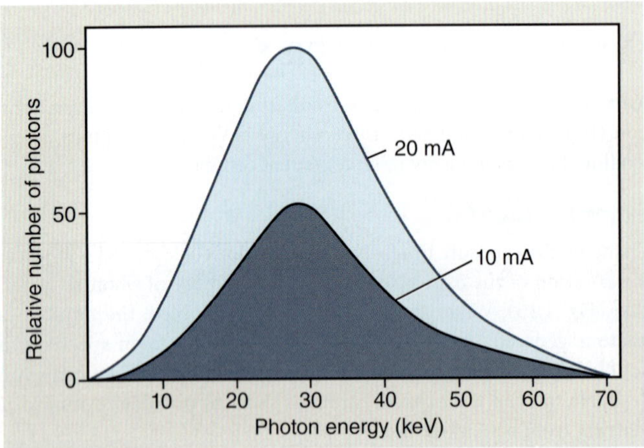

Fig. 1.16 Spectrum of photon energies generated in an x-ray machine showing that as the mA setting increases (kVp and exposure time held constant), so does the total number of photons. The mean energies and maximal energies of the beams are unchanged. Note similarity to the effect of exposure time; see Fig. 1.15.

Milliamperage Setting (mA, Tube Current)

Like the effects of exposure time, the quantity of radiation produced by an x-ray tube (i.e., the number of photons that reach the patient) is directly proportional to the milliamperage setting (mA setting; Fig. 1.16). As the mA setting is increased, more power is applied to the filament, which heats up and releases more electrons that collide with the target to produce radiation. Thus, as with exposure time, doubling the mA setting will double the number of photons produced. The product of mA setting and exposure time (**mA × s**, or **mAs**) is often used as a single parameter to denote the total number of photons produced. For instance, a machine operating at 10 mA for 1 second (**10 × 1 = 10 mAs**) produces the same number of photons when operated at 20 mA for 0.5 second (**20 × 0.5 = 10 mAs**). The term **beam quantity** refers to the number of photons in an x-ray beam. Linearity and reproducibility of the mA and s settings are often included in the quality assurance programs for x-ray units, including those used in dental and maxillofacial imaging (see Chapter 14).

Tube Voltage Peak (kVp)

Increasing the kVp increases the potential difference between the cathode and the anode, increasing the kinetic energy of the electrons as they move toward the target. The greater the energy of an electron, the greater the probability it will be converted into x-ray photons at the target. Increasing the kVp of an x-ray machine increases:

- The number of photons generated.
- The mean energy of the photons.
- The maximal energy of the photons (Fig. 1.17).

The term **beam quality** refers to the mean energy of an x-ray beam.

Filtration

Although an x-ray beam consists of a continuous spectrum of x-ray photon energies, only photons with sufficient energy to penetrate through anatomic structures and reach the image receptor (digital or film) are useful for diagnostic radiology. Low-energy photons that cannot reach the receptor contribute to patient risk but do not offer any benefit. Consequently, it is desirable to remove these low-energy photons from the beam. This removal can be accomplished in part by placing a metallic disk (filter) in the beam path. A filter preferentially removes low-energy photons from the beam but allows high-energy photons that contribute to making an image to pass through (Fig. 1.18).

Inherent filtration consists of the materials that x-ray photons encounter as they travel from the focal spot on the target to form the

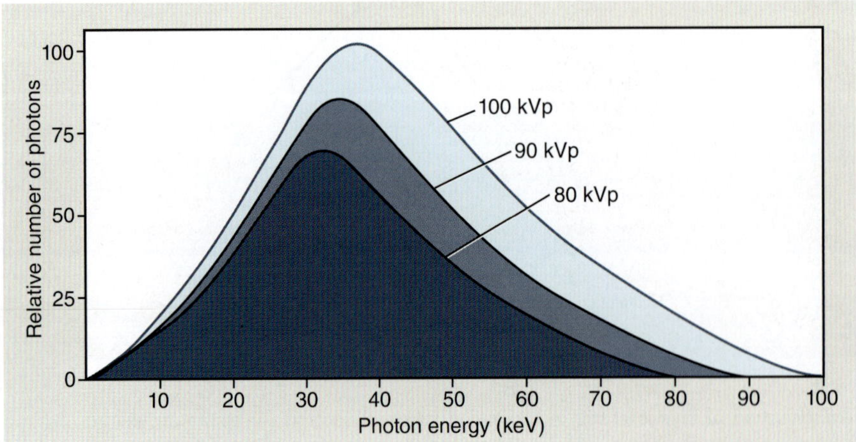

Fig. 1.17 Spectrum of photon energies generated in an x-ray machine showing that as the kVp is increased (mA and s held constant), there is a corresponding increase in the mean energy of the beam, the total number of photons emitted, and the maximal energy of the photons. Compare with Figs. 1.15 and 1.16.

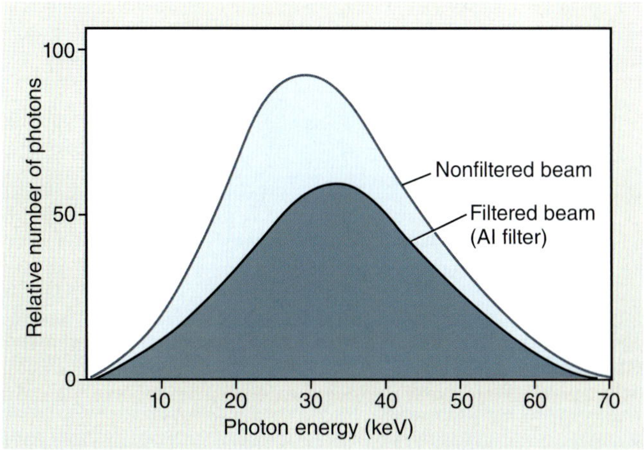

Fig. 1.18 Spectrum of filtered x-ray beam generated in an x-ray machine showing that an aluminum filter preferentially removes low-energy photons, reducing the beam intensity, while increasing the mean energy of the residual beam. Compare with Figs. 1.15–1.17.

usable beam outside the tube enclosure. These materials include the glass wall of the x-ray tube, the insulating oil that surrounds many dental tubes, and the barrier material that prevents the oil from escaping through the x-ray port. The inherent filtration of most x-ray machines ranges from the equivalent of 0.5 to 2 mm of aluminum.

Added filtration may be supplied in the form of aluminum disks placed over the port in the head of the x-ray machine. **Total filtration** is the sum of the inherent and added filtration. Federal regulations in the United States require the total filtration in the path of a dental x-ray beam to be equal to the equivalent of 1.5 mm of aluminum for a machine operating at up to 70 kVp and 2.5 mm of aluminum for machines operating at higher voltages (see Chapter 3).

Collimation

A collimator is a metallic barrier with an aperture in the middle used to shape and restrict the size of the x-ray beam and the volume of tissue irradiated (Fig. 1.19). Round and rectangular collimators are most frequently used in intraoral radiography. Dental x-ray beams are usually collimated to a circle 2.75 inches (7 cm) in diameter at the patient's face. A round collimator (see Fig. 1.19A) is a thick plate of metal with a circular opening centered over the port in the x-ray head through which the x-ray beam emerges. Typically, round collimators are built into open-ended aiming cylinders. Rectangular collimators (see Fig. 1.19B) further limit the size of the beam to just larger than the intraoral receptor, further reducing patient exposure. Some types of receptor-holding instruments also provide rectangular collimation of the x-ray beam (see Chapters 3 and 6).

Collimators also improve image quality. When an x-ray beam is directed at a patient, the hard and soft tissues absorb approximately 91% of the photons, and approximately 9% pass through the patient to reach the image receptor (film, or digital receptor; see Fig. 1.21). Many of the absorbed photons generate scattered radiation within the exposed tissues by a process called **Compton scattering** (see later in chapter). These scattered photons travel in all directions, and some reach the receptor and degrade image quality. Collimating the x-ray beam thus reduces the exposed volume and thereby the number of scattered photons reaching the image receptor, resulting in reduced patient exposure and improved images.

Inverse Square Law

The intensity of an x-ray beam (the number of photons per cross-sectional area per unit of exposure time) varies with distance from the focal spot. For a given beam, the intensity is inversely proportional to the square of the distance from the source (Fig. 1.20). The reason for this decrease in intensity is that an x-ray beam spreads out as it moves from its source. The relationship is as follows:

$$\frac{I_1}{I_2} = \frac{(D_2)^2}{(D_1)^2}$$

where I is intensity and D is distance. If a dose of 4 Gy is measured at 1 m, a dose of 1 Gy would be found at 2 m and a dose of 0.25 Gy would be found at 4 m.

Practical Applications

- Changing the distance between the x-ray tube and the patient, such as by switching from a machine with a short aiming tube to one with a long aiming tube, has a marked effect on beam intensity. Such a change requires a corresponding modification of the kVp or mA to maintain the same intensity at the image receptor.
- Increasing operator distance from the x-ray source is an effective method to minimize operator dose (see Chapter 3).

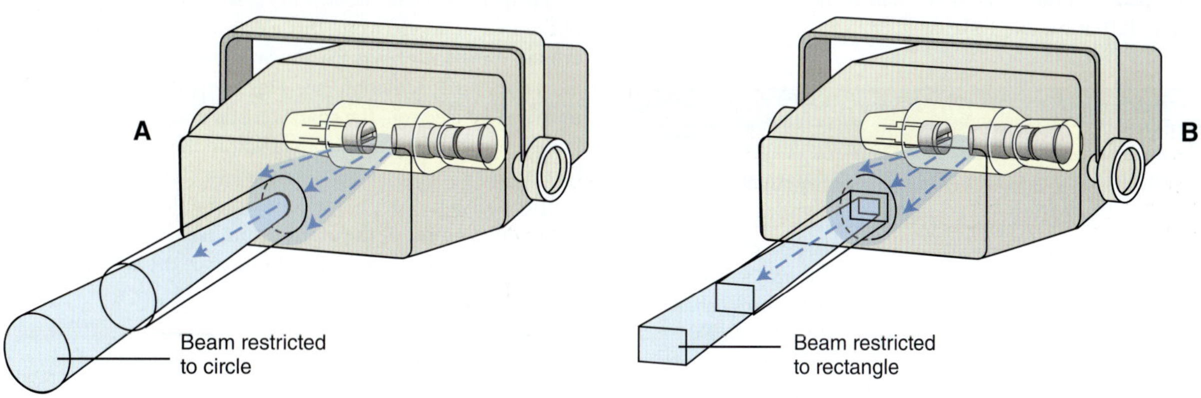

Fig. 1.19 Collimation of an x-ray beam *(blue)* is achieved by restricting its useful size. (A) Circular collimator. (B) Rectangular collimator restricts area of exposure to just larger than the detector size and thereby reduces unnecessary patient exposure.

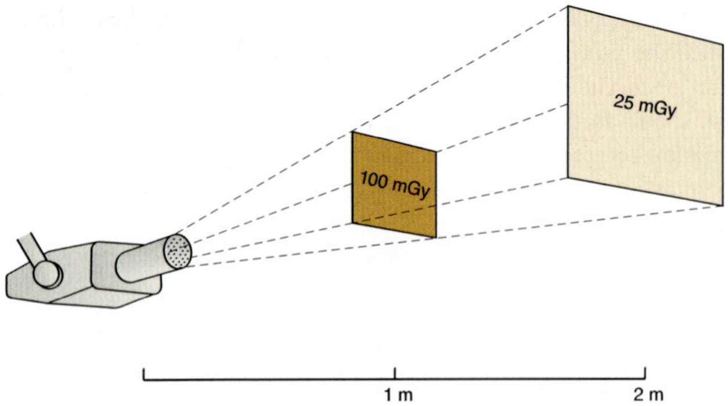

Fig. 1.20 Intensity of an x-ray beam is inversely proportional to the square of the distance between the source and the point of measure. When the distance from the focal spot is doubled, the intensity of the beam decreases to one quarter.

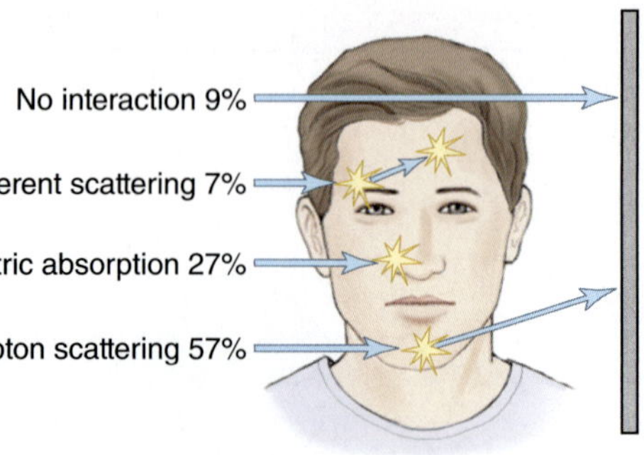

Fig. 1.21 Photons in a dental x-ray beam interact with the object primarily by Compton scattering (57% of primary interactions), in which case the scattered photon may strike the receptor and degrade the radiographic image by causing fog. The next most frequent interaction is photoelectric absorption (27%), in which the photons cease to exist. A radiographic image is produced by photons passing through low atomic number structures (soft tissue) and preferentially undergoing photoelectric absorption by high atomic number structures (bone, teeth, and metallic restorations). Relatively few photons undergo coherent scattering (7%) within the object or pass through the object without interaction (9%) and expose the image receptor.

INTERACTIONS OF X-RAYS WITH MATTER

In dental and maxillofacial imaging, the x-ray beam enters the face of a patient, interacts with hard and soft tissues, and strikes a digital sensor or film. The incident beam contains photons of many energies but is spatially homogeneous. That is, the intensity of the beam is relatively uniform from the center of the beam outward. As the beam goes through the patient, it is reduced in intensity (attenuated). This **attenuation** results from absorption of individual photons in the beam by atoms in the tissues or by photons being scattered out of the beam. In **absorption interactions,** photons interact with tissue atoms and cease to exist. In **scattering interactions,** photons also interact with tissue atoms but then move off in another direction. The frequency of these interactions depends on the type of tissue exposed (e.g., bone vs. soft tissue). Bone is more likely to absorb x-ray photons, whereas soft tissues are more likely to let them pass through. Although the incident beam striking the patient is spatially homogeneous, the remnant beam—the attenuated beam that exits the patient—is spatially heterogeneous because of differential absorption by the anatomic structures through which it has passed. This differential exposure of the film or digital sensor forms a radiographic image.

There are three means of beam attenuation in a diagnostic x-ray beam (Table 1.2):

- Photoelectric absorption
- Compton scattering
- Coherent scattering

In addition, approximately 9% of the primary photons pass through the patient's tissues without interaction and strike the sensor to form an image (Fig. 1.21 and Table 1.3).

TABLE 1.2 Interactions of Photons From a Diagnostic X-Ray Beam

Interaction	Ionization	Scatter	Practical Implications
Photoelectric absorption	Yes	No	Basis of radiographic image formation
Compton scatter	Yes	Yes	Scatter radiation can degrade image, expose personnel and patient
Coherent scatter	No	No	Minimal contribution to scatter

Photoelectric Absorption

Photoelectric absorption is critical in diagnostic imaging because it is the basis of image radiographic formation. This process occurs when an incident photon interacts with an electron in an inner orbital of an atom in the patient. The incident photon loses all its energy to the electron and ceases to exist. The energy absorbed by the electron is expended to overcome the binding energy, and the remainder energy remains as the kinetic energy of the electron as it escapes the confines of its orbital (Fig. 1.22). The kinetic energy imparted to the electron (termed **recoil electron** or **photoelectron**) is equal to the energy of the incident photon minus the binding energy of the electron. In the case of atoms with low atomic numbers (e.g., atoms in most biologic molecules), the binding energy is small and the photoelectron acquires most of the energy of the incident photon. Photoelectrons ejected during photoelectric absorption travel only short distances in the absorber before they give up their energy through secondary ionizations (see Fig. 2.3A).

Most photoelectric interactions occur in the 1s orbital because the density of the electron cloud is the greatest in this region, and there is a higher probability of interaction. Approximately 27% of primary photon interactions in a dental x-ray beam exposure involve photoelectric absorption.

The photoelectric interaction causes ionization of the atom because of the loss of an electron. This electron deficiency (usually in the 1s orbital) is instantly filled, usually by a 2s or 2p electron, with the release of characteristic radiation (see Fig. 1.14). Whatever the orbital of the replacement electron, the characteristic photons generated are of such low energy that they are absorbed within the patient and do not fog the receptor.

The probability of photoelectric interaction is directly proportional to the **third power of the atomic number** *(Z)* of the absorber, and inversely proportional to the **third power of the energy of the incident photon** *(E)*.

$$\text{Probablity of photoelectric interaction} \propto \frac{Z^3}{E^3}$$

The practical implications of photoelectric interaction are listed in Box 1.3.

TABLE 1.3 Fate of 1 Million Incident Photons in Bite-Wing Projection

Interaction	Fate of Incident Photon	Primary Photons	Scattered Photons[a]	Total[b]
Coherent scattering	Scatters from atom	74,453	78,117	152,570
Photoelectric absorption	Ejects inner electron and ceases to exist; releases characteristic photon	268,104	261,041	529,145
Compton scattering	Ejects outer electron, both scatter	565,939	549,360	1,115,300
No interaction	Passes through patient	91,504	379,350	470,855
Total		*1,000,000*	*1,267,868*	*2,267,869*

[a]The fate of scattered photons resulting from primary Compton and coherent interactions.
[b]The sum of the total number of photoelectric interactions and photons that exit the patient equals the total number of incident photons.
From S.J. Gibbs, personal communication, 1986.

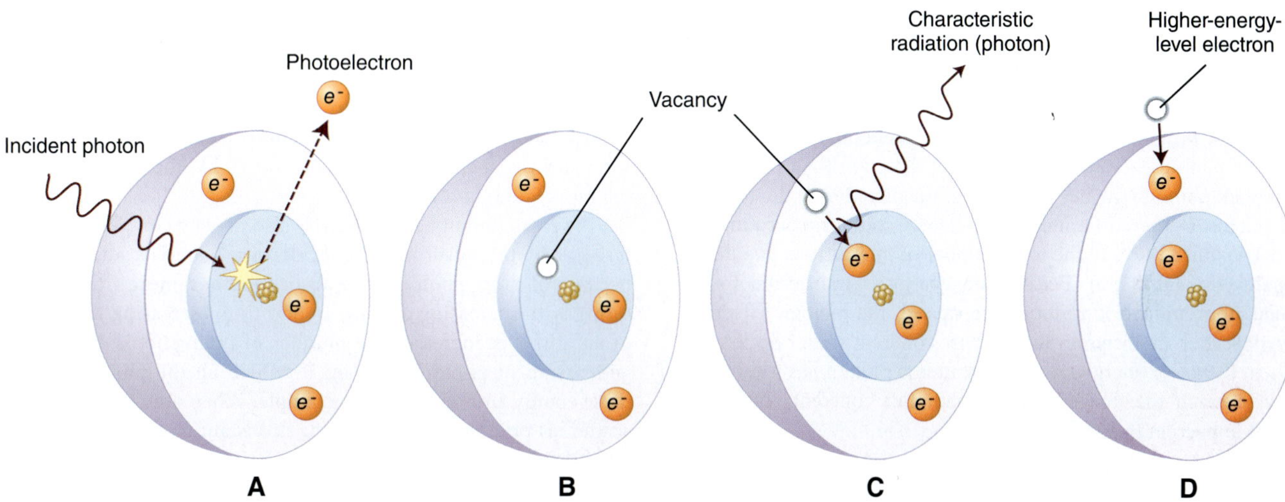

Fig. 1.22 Photoelectric absorption. (A) Photoelectric absorption occurs when an incident photon gives up all of its energy to an inner electron, which is ejected from the atom (a photoelectron). The incident electron ceases to exist at this point. (B) The ionized atom now has an electron vacancy in the inner orbital. (C) An electron from a higher energy level fills the vacancy and emits characteristic radiation. (D) All orbitals are subsequently filled, completing the energy exchange.

BOX 1.3 Practical Implications of Photoelectric Absorption

Differential absorption in various tissues and objects (restorations for example) provides radiographic contrast. Because the effective atomic number of compact bone ($Z = 13.8$) is greater than that of soft tissue ($Z = 7.4$), the probability of photoelectric interaction of x-ray photons in bone is approximately 6.5 times greater than in an equal thickness of soft tissue ($13.8^3/7.4^3 = 6.5$). This marked difference in the absorption of x-ray photons by the soft and hard tissues makes the production of a radiographic image possible. This differential photoelectric absorption of x-ray photons in enamel, dentin, pulp, bone, and soft tissue is what we observe as different degrees of radiopacity on the radiographic image.

It causes ionization and potential for biological damage.

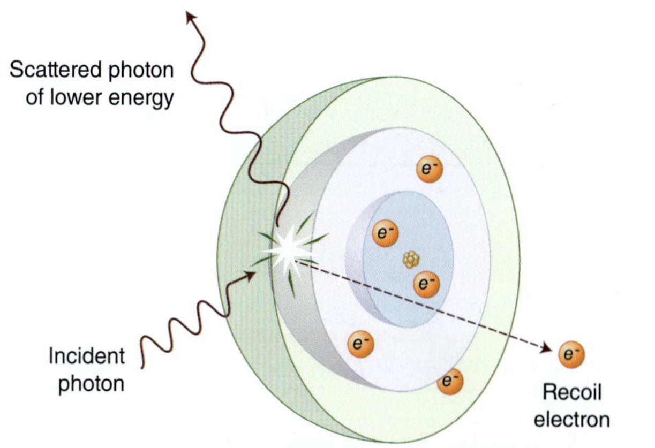

Fig. 1.23 Compton scattering occurs when an incident photon interacts with an outer electron, producing a scattered photon of lower energy than the incident photon and a recoil electron ejected from the target atom. The new scattered photon travels in a different direction from the incident photon.

Compton Scatter

Compton scatter occurs when a photon interacts with an outer orbital electron (Fig. 1.23). Approximately 57% of primary photon interactions in a dental x-ray beam exposure involve Compton scatter. In this interaction, the incident photon collides with an outer orbital electron, which receives kinetic energy and recoils from the point of impact. The path of the incident photon is deflected by this interaction and is scattered in a new direction. The energy of this scattered photon equals the energy of the incident photon minus the sum of the kinetic energy gained by the recoil electron and its binding energy. In the diagnostic energy range, most of the energy is retained by the scattered photon which can then cause additional ionizations, often at tissue sites outside the circumference of the incident beam. When these scattered photons reach the image receptor, they cause degradation of the image.

As with photoelectric absorption, Compton scatter results in the loss of an electron and ionization of the absorbing atom. Additional ionizations are caused by the scattered photons and the recoil electrons as they course through the patient's tissues. The probability of a Compton interaction is inversely proportional to the photon energy and is independent of atomic number. The probability of Compton scatter is dependent on the **electron density** of the absorber, which is relatively constant in tissue.

The practical implications of Compton scatter are listed in Box 1.4.

Coherent Scatter

Coherent scatter (also known as **Rayleigh, classical,** or **elastic scatter**) may occur when a low-energy incident photon (<10 keV) interacts with a whole atom. The incident photon causes it to become momentarily excited (Fig. 1.24). The incident photon then ceases to exist. The excited atom quickly returns to the ground state and generates another x-ray photon with the same energy as the incident photon. Usually the secondary photon is emitted in a different direction than the path of the incident photon. The net effect is that the direction of the incident x-ray photon is altered (scattered). Coherent scattering accounts for only approximately 7% of the total number of interactions in a dental exposure (see Table 1.3). Because no energy is transferred to the biologic atom and no ionizations are caused, the biologic effects of coherent scatter are insignificant. Because coherent scatter occurs primarily in the lower energy range, the scattered photon has insufficient energy to reach the image receptor, and thus coherent scatter has minimal impact on image degradation.

BOX 1.4 Practical Implications of Compton Scatter

Scattered photons travel in all directions and may exit the patient and strike the image receptor. These photons carry no useful information and degrade the image by reducing contrast.

Scattered photons that exit the patient can expose the operator.

Scattered photons travel varying distances within the patient's tissues and cause ionizations. This internal scatter increases patient radiation dose and often exposes organs and tissues outside of and distant from the path of the primary beam.

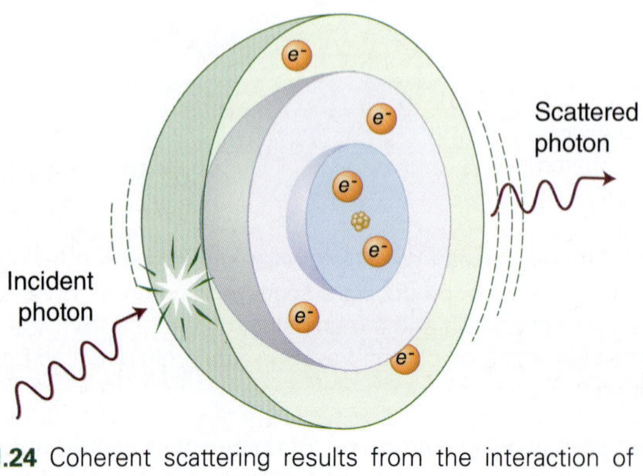

Fig. 1.24 Coherent scattering results from the interaction of a low-energy incident photon with a whole atom, causing it to be momentarily excited. After this interaction, the atom quickly returns to the ground state and emits a scattered photon of the same energy but at a different angle from the path of the incident photon.

Beam Attenuation

As an x-ray beam travels through matter, its intensity is reduced primarily through photoelectric absorption and Compton scattering. The extent of beam attenuation depends primarily on the energy of the beam and the thickness and density of the attenuating material. High-energy x-ray photons have a greater probability of penetrating matter, whereas lower-energy photons have a greater probability of being attenuated. The higher the kVp setting, the greater the penetrability of the resulting beam through matter. A useful way to characterize the penetrating quality of an x-ray beam is by its *half-value layer* (HVL). The HVL is the thickness of an absorber, such as aluminum, that reduces the number of x-ray photons by 50%. As the mean energy of an x-ray beam increases, so does the amount of material required to reduce the beam intensity by half (its HVL). The HVLs of several materials have been established for a wide range of photon energies. This allows medical physicists to calculate the thickness of shielding material required in diagnostic radiology facilities. HVL is measured as an indicator of beam quality for acceptance testing and periodic quality assurance of dental x-ray machines (see Chapter 14). For dental x-ray devices operating between 60 and 70 kV, the minimum HVL is 1.5 mm of aluminum.

The reduction of beam intensity also depends on physical characteristics of the absorber. Higher-density materials attenuate more because of more photoelectric absorption and more Compton scattering with increasing density. In addition, increasing the thickness of an absorber increases the number of interactions. A monoenergetic beam of photons, a beam in which all the photons have the same energy, provides a useful example. When only the primary (not scattered) photons are considered, a constant fraction of the beam is attenuated as the beam moves through each unit thickness of an absorber. For example, if 1.5 cm of water reduces a beam intensity by 50%, the next 1.5 cm reduces the beam intensity by another 50% (to 25% of the original intensity), and so on. This is an exponential pattern of absorption (Fig. 1.25). The HVL described earlier is a measure of beam energy describing the amount of an absorber that reduces

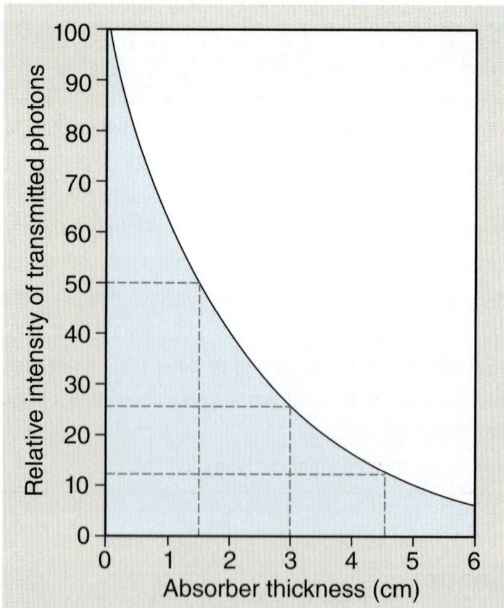

Fig. 1.25 Intensity of an energetically homogeneous x-ray beam declines exponentially as it travels through an absorber. In this instance, the half-value layer of the beam is 1.5 cm of absorber (i.e., every 1.5 cm of the absorber reduces the intensity of the beam by half). The curve for a heterogeneous x-ray beam (e.g., a dental x-ray beam) does not drop quite as precipitously because of the preferential removal of low-energy photons by the absorber and the increased mean energy of the resulting beam.

the beam intensity by half; in the preceding example, the HVL is 1.5 cm of water.

In contrast to the previous example using a monoenergetic x-ray beam, there is a wide range of photon energies in an x-ray beam. Low-energy photons are much more likely than high-energy photons to be attenuated. Thus the superficial layers of an absorber remove the low-energy photons but transmit many of the higher-energy photons. As an x-ray beam passes through this material, the intensity of the beam decreases from preferential removal of low-energy photons. Because the transmitted photons are predominantly of higher energy, the mean energy of the residual beam increases. The term **beam hardening** is used to describe this increase in the mean energy of the beam by preferential removal of lower-energy photons.

As the energy of an x-ray beam increases, so does the transmission of the beam through an absorber. However, when the energy of the incident photon is increased to match the binding energy of the 1s orbital electrons of the absorber, the probability of photoelectric absorption increases sharply and the number of absorbed photons is greatly increased. This is called **K-edge absorption.** The probability that a photon will interact with an orbital electron is the greatest when the energy of the photon equals the binding energy of the electron; it decreases as the photon energy increases. Photons with energy less than the binding energy of 1s orbital electrons interact by photoelectric absorption only with electrons in the 2s or 2p orbitals and in orbitals even farther from the nucleus. Rare earth elements are sometimes used as filters because their 1s orbital binding energies, or K edges (e.g., 50.24 keV for gadolinium), greatly increase the absorption of high-energy photons. This is desirable because these high-energy photons degrade image contrast, unlike mid-energy photons that primarily contribute to a radiographic image.

DOSIMETRY

Table 1.4 presents some frequently used units of radiation and radiation detriment. Contemporary literature uses radiation measurement units from the **SI system** *(Système International d'Unitès)*, and these will be used in this book. Traditional units and their conversion have been included for reference.

Exposure

Exposure is a measure of the capacity of x-rays or γ-rays to ionize air. It is measured as the amount of charge per mass of air—**coulombs/kg.** It is a measure of the intensity of the radiation field as opposed to the amount of radiation absorbed, although there is a direct relationship. The roentgen has been largely replaced by the SI equivalent unit of air kerma.

Traditional unit: **roentgen (R)**

1 R = 2.58×10^{-4} C/kg

One R will produce 2.08×10^{8} ion pairs in 1 cm^3 of air.

Air Kerma

When radiation interacts with matter via photoelectric absorption and Compton scattering, it transfers energy to electrons of the absorber. The **kerma,** an acronym for *k*inetic *e*nergy *r*eleased in *ma*tter, measures the kinetic energy transferred from photons to electrons and is expressed in units of dose (gray [Gy]), where 1 Gy equals 1 J/kg. Kerma is the sum of the initial kinetic energies of all the charged particles liberated by uncharged ionizing radiation (e.g., x-rays) in a sample of matter divided by the mass of the sample. Kerma values made in air are called air kerma. The kerma is rapidly replacing exposure measured in coulombs/kg or R. An exposure of 1 R results in an air kerma of approximately 8.77 mGy.

Absorbed Dose

Absorbed dose is a measure of the total energy absorbed by any type of ionizing radiation per unit of mass of any type of matter. It varies with the type and energy of radiation and the type of matter absorbing the energy.

SI unit: gray, where 1 Gy = 1 J/kg

Traditional unit: rad (radiation absorbed dose)

1 rad = 100 erg/g of absorber

1 Gy = 100 rad

Equivalent (Radiation-Weighted) Dose

The equivalent dose *(H_T)* is used to compare the biologic effects of different types of radiation on a tissue or organ. Particulate radiations have a high LET and are more damaging to cells than is radiation with low LET, such as x-rays. Thus deposition of 1 Gy of α particles causes much more biologic damage than 1 Gy of x-ray photons. The equivalent dose considers not only the absorbed dose but also this relative biologic effectiveness of the incident radiation using a radiation-weighting factor *(W_R)*. The W_R of photons, the reference, is 1. The W_R of 5-keV neutrons and high-energy protons is 5, and the W_R of α particles is 20. The equivalent dose *(H_T)* is computed as the product of the radiation-weighting factor *(W_R)* and the absorbed dose averaged over a tissue or organ *(D_T)*.

$$H_T = W_R \times D_T$$

SI unit: Sievert (Sv)

For x-rays, 1 Sv = 1 Gy

Traditional unit: rem (roentgen equivalent mammal)

1 Sv = 100 rem

Effective Dose

The effective dose *(E)* is used to estimate the risk of stochastic effects in humans. It is hard to compare the risk from a dental exposure with, for example, the risk from a radiographic chest examination because different tissues with different radiosensitivities are exposed. To allow

TABLE 1.4 Summary of Radiation Quantities and Units

Quantity	Description	SI Unit	Traditional Unit	Conversion
Exposure	Amount of ionization of air by x- or γ-rays	coulomb/kg (C/kg)	roentgen (R)	1 C/kg = 3876 R
Kerma	Kinetic energy transferred to charged particles	gray (Gy)	—	—
Absorbed dose	Total energy absorbed by a mass	gray (Gy)	rad	1 Gy = 100 rad
Equivalent dose	Absorbed dose weighted by biologic effectiveness of radiation type used	sievert (Sv)	rem	1 Sv = 100 rem
Effective dose	Sum of equivalent doses weighted by radiosensitivity of exposed tissue or organ	sievert (Sv)	—	—
Radioactivity	Rate of radioactive decay	becquerel (Bq)	curie (Ci)	1 Bq = 2.7×10^{-11} Ci

TABLE 1.5 Tissue Weighting Factors[a]

Tissue	Tissue Weighting Factor
Bone marrow, breast, colon, lung, stomach, remainder tissues[b]	0.12
Gonads	0.08
Bladder, esophagus, liver, thyroid	0.04
Bone surface, brain, salivary glands, skin	0.01

[a]ICRP Publication 103: The 2007 Recommendations of the International Commission on Radiological Protection.

[b]Adrenals, extrathoracic region, gallbladder, heart, kidneys, lymphatic nodes, muscle, oral mucosa, pancreas, prostate, small intestine, spleen, thymus, uterus/cervix.

such comparisons, the effective dose is a calculation that considers the relative biologic effectiveness of different types of radiation *and* the radiosensitivity of different tissues exposed in terms of the risk for stochastic effects of radiation (cancer induction and heritable effects). Tissue weighting factors (W_T) have been developed to factor individual tissue radiosensitivity (Table 1.5). E is the sum of the products of the equivalent dose to each organ or tissue (H_T) and the tissue weighting factor (W_T):

$$E = \sum W_T \times H_T$$

SI unit: Sievert (Sv)
Traditional unit: rem (roentgen equivalent mammal)
1 Sv = 100 rem

Radioactivity

The measurement of radioactivity (A) describes the decay rate of a sample of radioactive material. Although not directly applicable to dentomaxillofacial radiography, diagnostic nuclear medicine examinations indicate the amount of radiopharmaceutical delivered to the patient using the following units.

SI unit: becquerel (Bq)
1 Bq = 1 disintegration per second (dps)
Traditional unit: curie (Ci)
$1\ \text{Ci} = 3.7 \times 10^{10}$ dps
$1\ \text{Bq} = 2.7 \times 10^{-11}$ Ci
1 mCi = 37 MBq

BIBLIOGRAPHY

Bushberg JT, Seibert JA, Leidholdt EM, Boone JM. *The Essential Physics of Medical Imaging*. 4th ed. Lippincott Williams and Wilkins; 2020.

Bushong SC. *Radiologic Science for Technologists: Physics, Biology, and Protection*. 12th ed. Mosby; 2020.

The 2007 recommendations of the International Commission on Radiological Protection. ICRP Publication 103. *Ann ICRP*. 2007;37:1-332.

National Council on Radiation and Measurements Report No.082. *SI units in Radiation Protection and Measurements: Recommendations of the National Council on Radiation Protection and Measurements*. Bethesda, MD: National Council on Radiation Protection and Measurements; 1985.

CERN. The Standard Model. https://home.cern/science/physics/standard-model. [Accessed 10 Jun 2024].

2

Biologic Effects of Ionizing Radiation

Sanjay M. Mallya and Stuart C. White

Ionizing radiations have sufficient energy to overcome electron binding energy and form ion pairs in matter. The initial interactions between the incident photon and tissue atoms occur almost instantaneously, within 10^{-13} seconds after radiation exposure, and subsequent DNA damage is completed within 1 millisecond (Fig. 2.1A). Cell responses to DNA damage follow within seconds to days, and the consequences of these biologic responses manifest in hours, days, or years, depending on the extent and type of damage. This chapter provides the foundation to understand the biologic effects of diagnostic and therapeutic radiation, with special emphasis on oral tissues.

CHEMICAL, MOLECULAR, AND CELLULAR CONSEQUENCES OF RADIATION ABSORPTION

Ionizing radiation deposits energy in matter. The pattern of energy deposition varies with the type of radiation. High-velocity charged particles (alpha particles, beta particles, electrons, and protons) have a high *linear energy transfer* (LET) and transfer most of their energy over a short distance. These particles have *densely ionizing* tracks and penetrate short distances into tissues. In contrast, x-rays and gamma rays are *low LET* radiations. They deposit less energy per unit track length and thus penetrate deeper into tissues.

Biological manifestations of ionizing radiation damage are primarily a consequence of damage to the cell's deoxyribonucleic acid (DNA). Radiation-induced DNA damage can occur both through direct and indirect actions (Fig. 2.1B). In *direct actions,* the photon directly interacts with and ionizes DNA. The free electrons produced by the ionization interaction *(secondary electrons)* may also interact directly with DNA. In contrast, in *indirect actions,* photons and secondary electrons ionize water and yield unstable *free radicals* and oxidizing species that subsequently diffuse and damage DNA. Free radicals are atoms or molecules that have an unpaired valence electron, are extremely reactive, and have very short lives. Free radicals play a dominant role in x-radiation–caused biologic damage.

Direct Actions

In **direct actions,** DNA molecules absorb energy from the incident photon or a secondary electron to ionize its constituent bases or sugar-phosphate backbone (Fig. 2.1B) and form unstable radicals within 10^{-10} seconds. These free radicals quickly return to stable configurations by dissociation (breaking apart) or cross-linking (joining of two molecules), causing chemical and physical alterations in DNA. *Direct actions predominate over indirect actions with high LET radiations but are less frequent with low-LET radiations such as x- and gamma-rays.* With low LET radiation, approximately 30% of the DNA damage results from direct actions.

$$\textbf{x-radiation} + \textbf{DNA} \rightarrow \textbf{DNA}^{\bullet}$$

$$\textbf{DNA}^{\bullet} + \textbf{OH}^{-} \rightarrow \textbf{DNA–OH} \quad \text{(Oxidized DNA bases and strand breaks)}$$

$$\textbf{DNA}^{\bullet} + \textbf{DNA}^{\bullet} \rightarrow \textbf{DNA–DNA} \quad \text{(Cross-links)}$$

Indirect Actions

In **indirect actions,** the initial interaction of a photon or secondary electron occurs with a water molecule (Fig. 2.1B)—which constitutes approximately 70% of the mass of a mammalian cell. *Indirect actions account for approximately 70% of x-radiation–induced DNA damage.* Ionizing radiation initiates a complex series of chemical changes in water, collectively referred to as **radiolysis of water.** The initial interaction of an x-ray photon with water yields an ionized water molecule (**H_2O^+**) plus an ejected electron or an excited water molecule (**H_2O^***). Ion–water reactions produce hydronium ions (**H_3O^+**), hydroxyl (**$OH^{\bullet}$**) radicals, and aqueous electrons (**$e-_{aq}$**). Excited water molecules dissociate into hydrogen (**$H^{\bullet}$**) and hydroxyl (**$OH^{\bullet}$**) radicals.

$$\textbf{x-radiation} + H_2O \rightarrow H_2O^+ + e^- \ \textbf{(Ionization)}$$

$$H_2O^+ + H_2O \rightarrow H_3O^+ + OH^{\bullet}$$

$$e^- + H_2O \rightarrow e^-_{aq}$$

$$\textbf{x-radiation} + H_2O \rightarrow H_2O^* \ \textbf{(Excitation)} \rightarrow H^{\bullet} + OH^{\bullet}$$

The presence of dissolved oxygen, as is the case in normal tissues, significantly modifies the species of free radicals formed during water radiolysis. In the presence of oxygen, hydroperoxyl (**$HO_2^{\bullet}$**) radicals (Fig. 2.1B) and hydrogen peroxide are formed, which contribute to DNA damage.

$$H^{\bullet} + O_2 \rightarrow HO_2^{\bullet}$$

$$HO_2^{\bullet} + HO_2^{\bullet} \rightarrow H_2O_2$$

The ionic and radical products of water radiolysis are highly reactive, have short half-lives, and diffuse distances of a few molecular dimensions. Thus only radicals produced within a 4-nm diameter around the DNA double helix cause DNA damage (Fig. 2.1B). Among the radical products produced by x-rays, hydroxyl radicals cause two-thirds of the biologic damage.

$$\textbf{DNA} + OH^{\bullet} \rightarrow \textbf{DNA–OH} \quad \text{(Oxidized DNA bases and strand breaks)}$$

$$\textbf{DNA} + H^{\bullet} \rightarrow \textbf{DNA}^{\bullet}$$

$$\textbf{DNA}^{\bullet} + \textbf{DNA}^{\bullet} \rightarrow \textbf{DNA–DNA} \ \text{(Cross-links)}$$

Deoxyribonucleic Acid and Chromosomal Damage and Damage Response

Damage to a cell's DNA is the primary cause of radiation-induced cell death, carcinogenesis, and heritable mutations. The indirect and direct

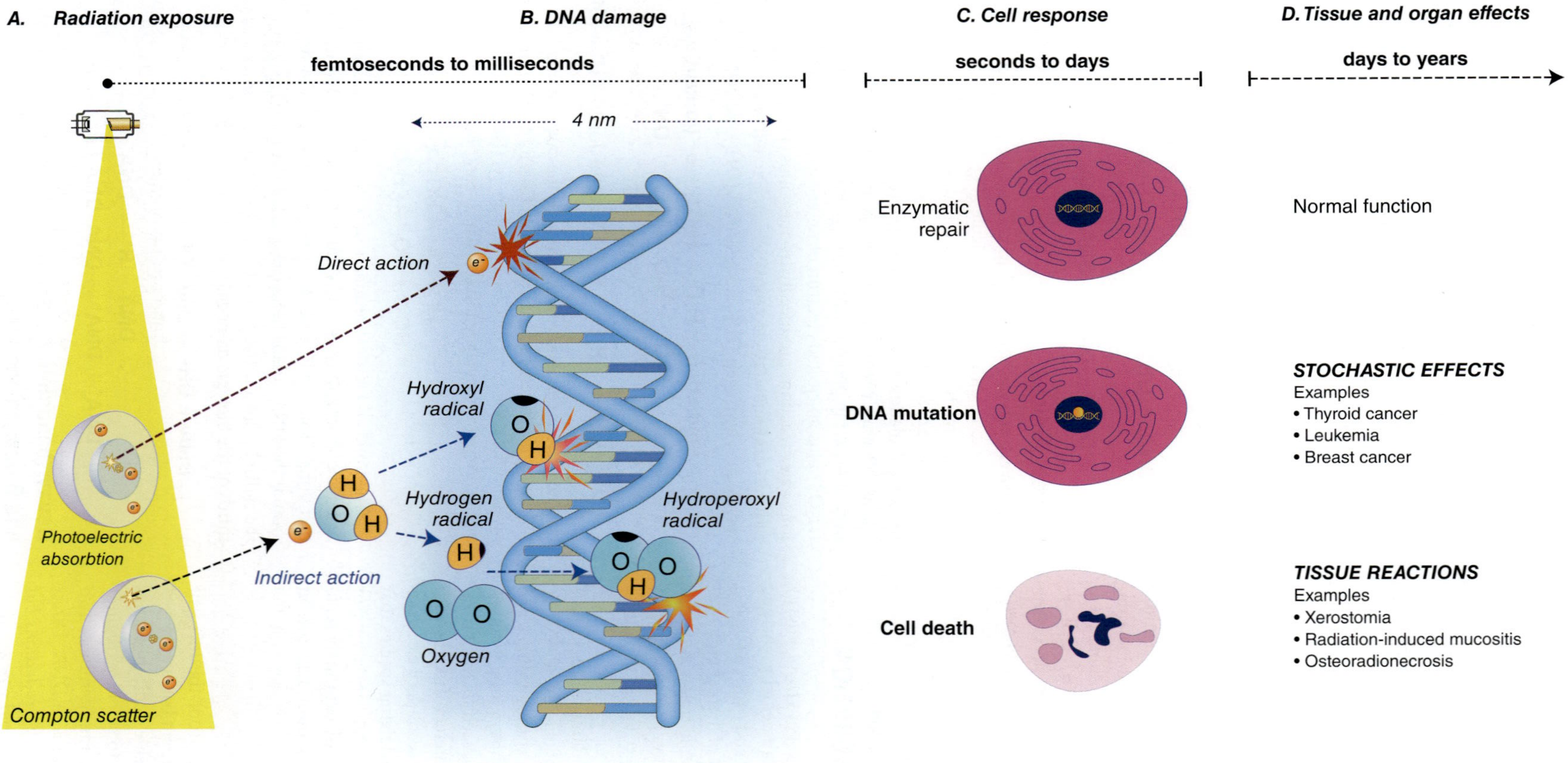

Fig. 2.1 Overview of events after exposure to ionizing radiation. (A) Radiation exposure. Electrons are ejected during the initial Compton and photoelectric interactions. (B) DNA damage. Ejected electrons can act directly on DNA or indirectly via radicals produced by radiolysis of water. In the presence of oxygen, hydroperoxyl radicals are formed. Radicals produced within a 4 nm diameter around the DNA double-helix can diffuse to and damage DNA in less than a millisecond. Damages shown in the bottom half of the DNA constitute a clustered lesion—two or more damages within two turns of the DNA double-helix. (C) Cell response. Enzymatic repair, DNA mutation, or cell death occurs in seconds to days. (D) Tissue and organ effects. DNA mutations cause stochastic effects, whereas cell death causes tissue reactions. Both effects manifest over a time scale of months to years. *DNA*, Deoxyribonucleic acid.

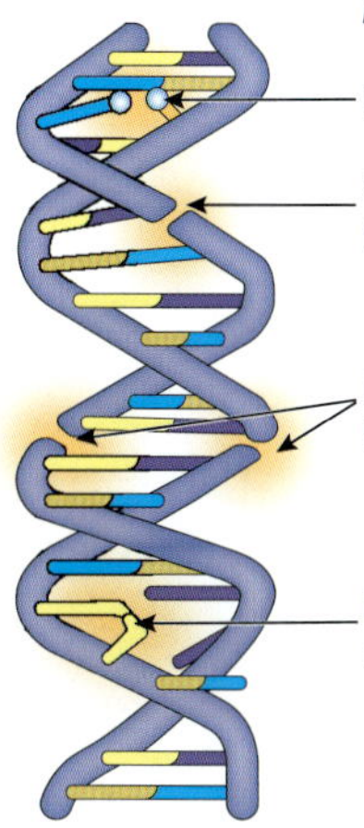

Fig. 2.2 Deoxyribonucleic acid *(DNA)* damage and repair. Damages caused by ionizing radiation are illustrated and the corresponding DNA repair pathway(s) indicated. A pyrimidine dimer is an intra-DNA cross-link between two adjacent cytosine or thymine nucleotides induced by exposure to ultraviolet radiation. *SSB*, Single-strand break; *DSB*, double-strand break.

actions of ionizing radiation on DNA result in base damage, single- and double-strand breaks, and intra-DNA and DNA-protein cross-links (Fig. 2.2). X-ray–induced DNA damages are predominantly base damage (72%) and single-strand breaks (27%). DNA double-strand breaks are 25-fold less frequent than single-strand breaks and comprise 1% of the total DNA damage from low to moderate doses of x-rays. Although infrequent, a DNA double-strand break is an extremely important form of damage as it is believed to cause both cell killing and tumorigenesis. In this situation DNA strand breaks are on opposing strands and closely spaced (Fig. 2.2). When two or more base damages or strand breaks occur within two turns of a DNA helix, the damage is termed *clustered lesion*. These DNA clustered lesions are more difficult to repair and are thought to account for most of the low LET radiation-induced mutations and chromosomal rearrangements. In contrast to low LET radiation where the damage is disributed sparsely, high LET radiations have densely ionizing tracks and cause more double-strand breaks and clustered lesions. Thus high LET radiations are more effective at cell killing than low LET radiations.

Approximately 95% of x-ray photon energy is deposited as *spurs*—deposition of 100 eV within a 4-nm diameter, yielding three ion or radical pairs. However, individual spurs are physically separated and x-rays have a *sparsely ionizing* track pattern (Fig. 2.3A). Thus DNA damage caused by x-rays are mostly base damages, and single-strand breaks and double-strand breaks are rare. However, when overlapped on the 2-nm DNA double helix, energy deposition from a single spur may cause a *clustered lesion* (Fig. 2.3B). With x-rays, such lesions are approximately threefold more frequent than double-strand breaks.

Mammalian cells have evolved elaborate mechanisms to respond to specific DNA damage types (Fig. 2.2). The *base excision repair* and *nucleotide excision repair* mechanisms efficiently repair most base damages, single-strand breaks, and DNA cross-links using the opposite strand as a template. Errors during repair can result in DNA mutations. DNA double-strand breaks are repaired by either *nonhomologous end-joining* or *homologous recombination*. Nonhomologous end-joining is an error-prone mechanism. In human cells, nonhomologous end-joining repairs 80% of the double-strand breaks. *Nucleotide excision repair* is a mechanism that repairs pyrimidine dimers and 6,4-photoproducts, damages caused by ultraviolet radiation damage.

The DNA in the nucleus of eukaryotes is distributed into chromosomes. Each chromosome is a long DNA molecule associated with proteins that fold and pack the DNA into a compact structure. Human somatic cells have 46 chromosomes. During the S phase of the cell cycle (Fig. 2.4), the chromosomes are duplicated and the two daughter **sister chromatids** are held together at a region called the centromere. During mitosis, the sister chromatids separate at the centromere and are segregated into the daughter cells. This process is tightly regulated to ensure that each daughter cell receives the appropriate chromosomal complement. A DNA double-strand break causes a breach in the integrity of the chromosome. If the breaks rejoin with fidelity to re-create the original intact chromosome, the damage will go unrecognized. However, failure to rejoin or incorrect rejoining of broken chromosomal ends will result in aberrations.

When a DNA strand break occurs prior to chromosomal duplication (G_1 and early S phase of the cell cycle; Fig. 2.4), the break is replicated and both sister chromatids will carry the damage. Resultant aberrations are termed **chromosome aberrations** (Fig. 2.4). If the cell is irradiated after chromosomal duplication, the break will occur in only one of the sister chromatids and generate a **chromatid aberration** (see Fig. 2.4). The frequency of aberrations is generally proportional to the radiation dose received. The aberrations may be deletions of chromosome regions or may result from the incorrect joining of two or more broken chromosome ends. The aberrations may be *symmetrical* (inversions, translocations) or may be *asymmetrical* (deletions). Asymmetrical aberrations produce acentric fragments that are subsequently eliminated during cell division. Some aberrations are lethal to the cell—*ring chromosome, dicentric chromosome,* and *anaphase bridge* (Fig. 2.5A–C)—and cause cell death during mitosis. Other types of aberrations are nonlethal and include *translocations* and *small deletions* (see Fig. 2.5D and E). When these nonlethal aberrations involve oncogenes and tumor suppressor genes, they may dysregulate cell growth to initiate tumorigenesis.

Cell Killing

Radiation-induced damage to DNA may result in the death of the cell. Such cell death is dose dependent, and loss of cells may impair function of the irradiated tissue or organ. Short-term effects may become apparent in hours to days and are consequent to a reduction in the number of mature cells in the tissues. The long-term effects (developing in months and years after exposure) are primarily caused by the death of replicating cells, which result in their replacement with fibrous tissue as well as damage to the fine vasculature.

Mitotic Death

The predominant mode of radiation-induced cell killing is mitotic death (or mitotic catastrophe), resulting from lethal chromosomal and chromatid aberrations (see Fig. 2.5). Irradiated cells with chromosome or chromatid aberrations may undergo cell division to yield cells with aneuploidy.

A cell's sensitivity to this mode of death is determined by its mitotic rate and degree of differentiation. This relationship is referred to as the law of Bergonié and Tribondeau, in honor of the radiobiologists that first described this principle.

$$\text{Cell radiosensitivity to killing} \propto \frac{\text{Mitotic rate}}{\text{Degree of differentiation}}$$

This rule predicts that rapidly dividing cells will be more radiosensitive, and postmitotic specialized cells will be most radioresistant; it holds true for most cell types. Building on the work of Bergonié and Tribondeau, Casarett categorized cell types based on their radiosensitivity (Table 2.1). This classification system predicts the sensitivity of most individual tissues and organs to manifest tissue reactions following radiation-induced cell killing.

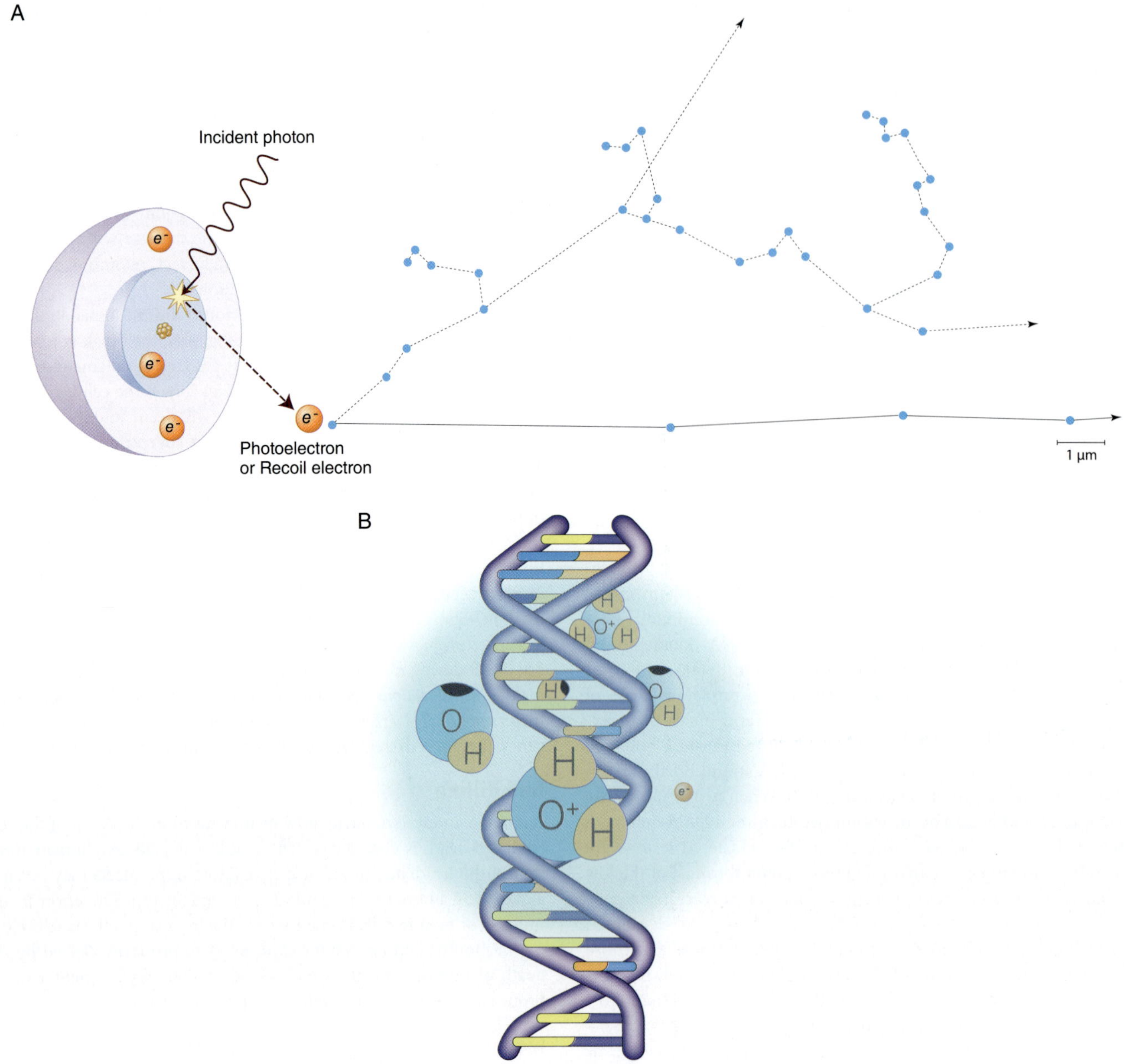

Fig. 2.3 (A) Illustration of x-ray energy deposition in tissues. Interaction of a photon with tissue atoms causes ejection of electrons, either photoelectrons from photoelectric absorption or recoil electrons from Compton scatter. The track of a primary electron *(solid line)* and secondary electron *(dashed lines)* is shown. Only a single secondary electron track is shown. The *blue dots* represent energy deposition by primary and secondary electrons. Energy deposition occurs within a 4-nm diameter and the deposition events are magnified in this illustration. Only the track length is drawn to scale. Contrast the track length to the dimension of mammalian cells (20–100 microns) to recognize the sparseness of energy deposition events in a cell. Adapted from Goodhead DT. Particle track structure and biological implications. In: Young LR, Sutton JP, eds. *Handbook of Bioastronautics*. Cham: Springer International Publishing; 2020. (B) X-ray energy deposition in the vicinity of DNA. Approximately 95% of x-ray energy is deposited as spurs, which are 4 nm in diameter and contain three ion pairs. When superimposed over the 2-nm DNA double helix, the density of ions and radicals, shown as a blue-green cloud, is sufficient to cause closely spaced damages yielding a clustered lesion. Molecules depcited with a black void represent radicals.

Apoptosis

Lymphocytes are the most radiosensitive mammalian cells and are an exception to the law of Bergonié and Tribondeau. Likewise, serous acini of the salivary glands are highly radiosensitive, although they do not divide rapidly. In these cell types, *apoptosis* is the predominant mode of radiation-induced death. In this mechanism, radiation damage induces a cascade of events that rapidly causes cell death within hours after radiation exposure. Unlike mitotic death, apoptotic death does not require the cell to undergo mitosis, and the cell dies in interphase. There is strong evidence that the initial signals for apoptosis are triggered by radiation-induced DNA damage. The tumor suppressor gene *p53* is a major regulator of the DNA damage response pathway and an important mediator of radiation-induced apoptosis.

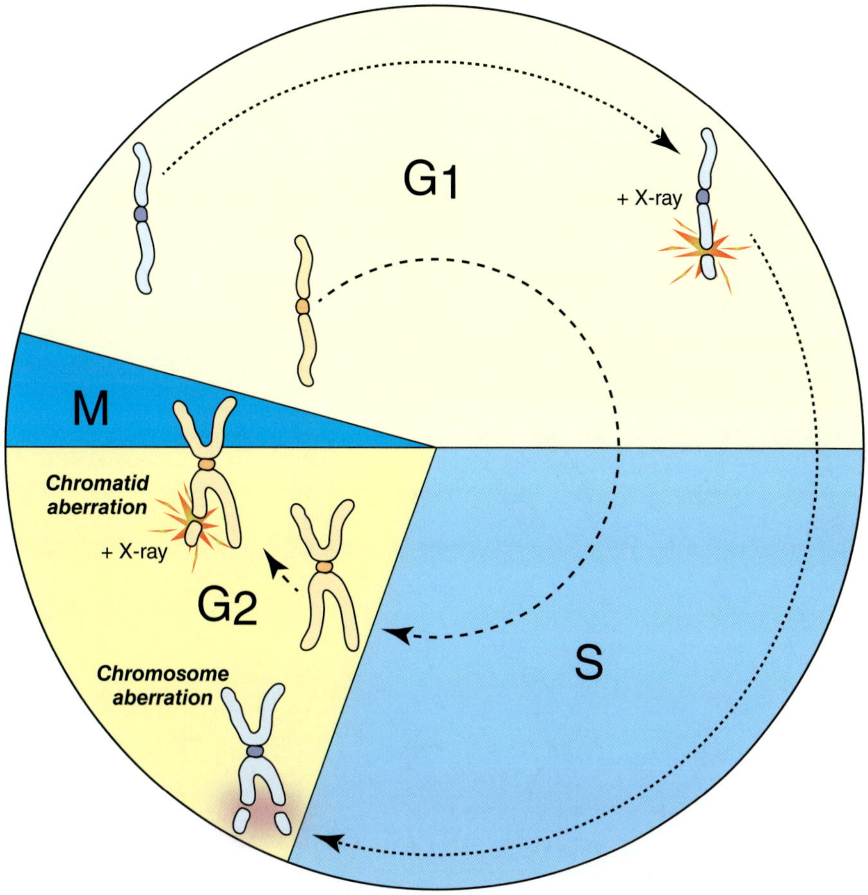

Fig. 2.4 Cell cycle and DNA aberrations. A proliferating cell alternates between periods of mitosis and deoxyribonucleic acid *(DNA)* synthesis (S), with intervening gaps (G_1 and G_2). Cells are most radiosensitive in the G_2 and mitosis phases, less sensitive in the G_1 phase, and least sensitive during the latter part of the S phase. Radiation damage before *DNA* synthesis *(outer arc)* is replicated in the next S phase and results in a chromosome (double-arm) aberration. Irradiation of a cell after DNA synthesis *(inner arc)* results in a chromatid (single-arm) aberration.

Bystander Effects

Studies of cultured cells have demonstrated a *bystander effect,* in which cells that are in the proximity of irradiated cells, but not directly exposed, exhibit radiation-induced responses and damages. These include changes in gene expression, occurrence of DNA damage, altered cell proliferation, and induction of cell death. The mechanism of this effect is not understood, but intracellular communication, responses to chromosome fragments released by dead cells, and diffusible chemokines from irradiated cells have been proposed to mediate these distant, nontarget effects. The impact of bystander effects in vivo is not known.

BIOLOGIC MANIFESTATIONS OF IONIZING RADIATION DAMAGE

There are two fundamental categories of radiation-induced biologic effects—*stochastic effects* and *tissue reactions* (previously termed deterministic effects). The differences between these effects are summarized in Table 2.2. The characterizing difference between these two categories is the dose threshold for its occurrence (Fig. 2.6). Stochastic effects do not exhibit a dose threshold, whereas tissue reactions manifest only when the radiation dose exceeds a certain threshold. *Diagnostic radiation levels are well below the threshold to cause tissue reactions but do pose a risk of causing stochastic effects.*

Stochastic Effects

One outcome of radiation-induced DNA damage is that the cell survives but with mutation of its DNA. Stochastic effects are the consequence of such sublethal DNA alterations in an individual cell. *In humans, carcinogenesis is the only relevant stochastic effect.* Causation of a stochastic effect is dependent on the specific DNA mutation created. For example, for cancer to occur, the mutation must confer that specific cell with a selective growth advantage.

Stochastic effects are considered to not have a dose threshold (Fig. 2.6). This assumption is shaped by our current understanding of the molecular mechanisms of DNA damage repair. At least in principle, a single x-ray photon has the potential to cause a DNA mutation. Thus even the smallest radiation dose could cause a cancer. When radiation dose increases, the number of radiation-induced DNA damage sites increases and the risk of subsequent cancer-causing mutation is higher. Thus *the probability of occurrence of a stochastic effect increases with dose.*

Radiation-Induced Cancer

Carcinogenesis is a multistep process in which a cell accumulates DNA mutations that provide it with a selective growth advantage. This occurs by activation of oncogenes and inactivation of tumor-suppressor genes. The mutations may occur sporadically or may be caused by exogenous insults from chemicals and ionizing radiation. There is strong

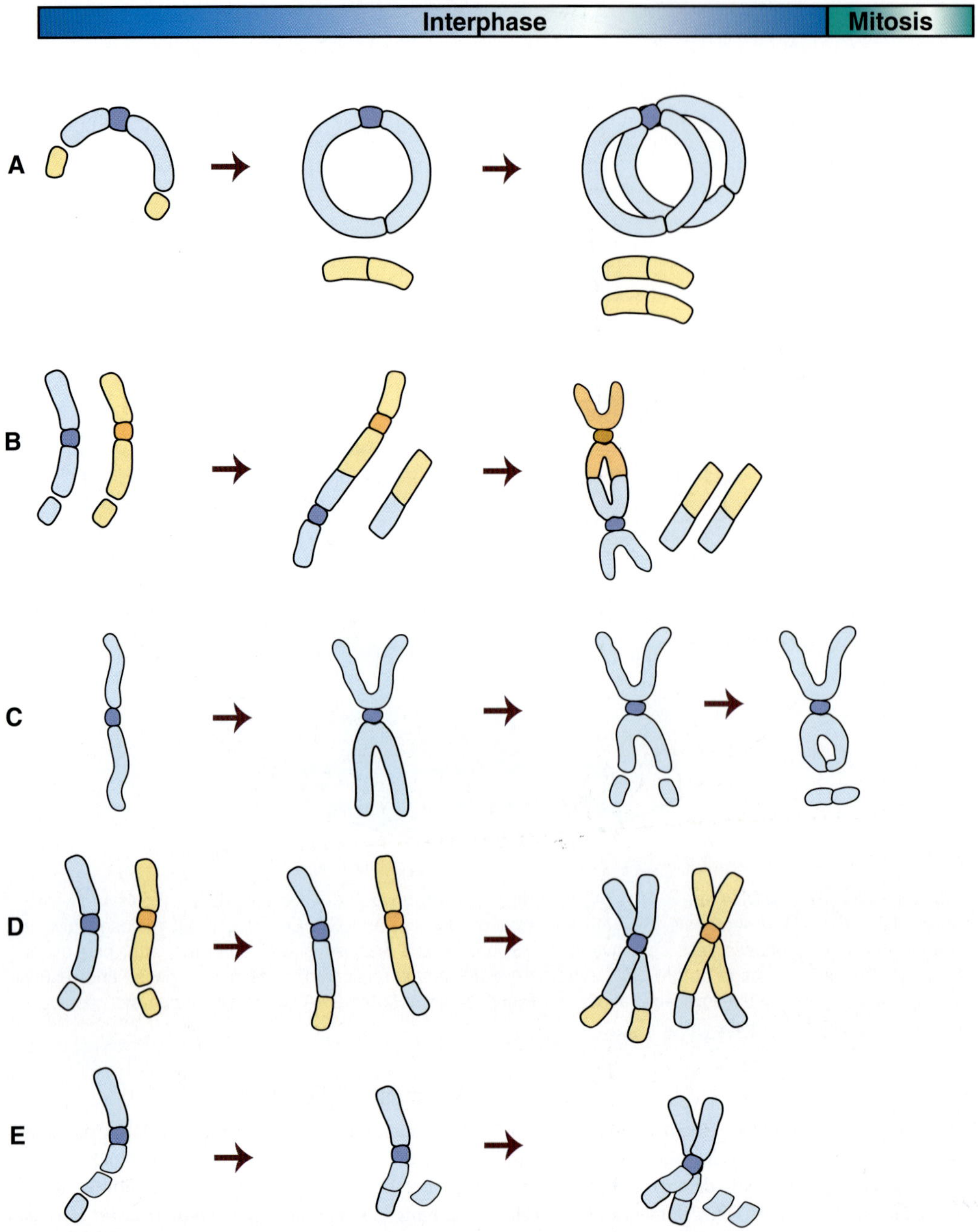

Fig. 2.5 Chromosome and chromatid aberrations. (A) Ring formation plus acentric fragment. (B) Dicentric formation. (C) Anaphase bridge formation. (D) Translocation and (E) deletion. The occurrence of the breakage and fusion events relative to the cell cycle phase is denoted by the bar on the top.

TABLE 2.1 Casarett's Categorization of Cell Types by Radiosensitivity

		Characteristics		
Radiosensitivity	**Category**	**Cell Division**	**Differentiation Status**	**Examples**
High	I. Vegetative intermitotic	Rapid	Undifferentiated	Basal cells of oral mucosa, bone marrow stem cells
↑	II. Differentiating intermitotic	Regular	Some differentiation	Myelocytes, spermatocytes
Intermediate	III. Multipotent connective tissue			Fibroblasts, endothelial cells
↑	IV. Reverting postmitotic	Not regular but can be stimulated to divide	Fully differentiated	Hepatocytes
Low	V. Fixed postmitotic	No	Highly differentiated	Neurons, muscle cells

Modified from Rubin P, Casarett GW. *Clinical Radiation Pathology*. Saunders; 1968.

TABLE 2.2 Comparison of Stochastic Effects and Tissue Reactions of Radiation

	Stochastic Effects	Tissue Reactions
Caused by	Sublethal DNA damage	Cell killing
Threshold dose	No There is no minimum threshold dose. Effect can be caused by any dose of radiation	Yes Effect occurs only when the threshold dose is exceeded
Severity of clinical effects and dose	Severity of clinical effects is independent of dose; all-or-none response—an individual either manifests effect or does not	Severity of clinical effects is proportional to dose; the higher the dose, the more severe the effect
Relationship between dose and effect	Frequency of effect proportional to dose; the higher the dose, the higher the risk of manifesting the effect	Probability of effect independent of dose; most individuals manifest effect when threshold dose is exceeded
Caused by doses used in diagnostic radiology	Yes	No
Examples	Radiation-induced cancer Heritable effects Radiation-induced skin cancer	Osteoradionecrosis Radiation-induced cataract formation Radiation-induced skin burns

DNA, Deoxyribonucleic acid.

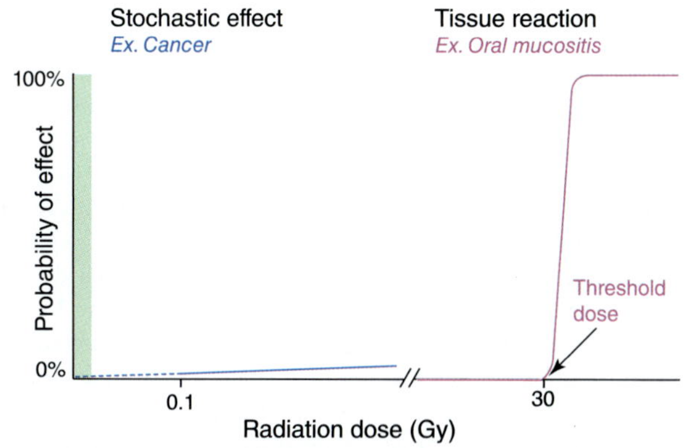

Fig. 2.6 Radiation dose-risk relationships for stochastic effects and tissue reactions. The data for radiation-induced cancer and radiation-induced mucositis are used to illustrate the differences between stochastic effects and tissue reactions. The solid blue line represents data from human populations. At doses above 0.1 Gy, the probability of cancer induction increases linearly with ionizing radiation dose. The dashed blue line represents the assumed extrapolation of radiation-induced cancer risk at lower doses. In contrast, oral mucositis following radiation therapy, a tissue reaction, occurs only when threshold dose of 30 Gy is exceeded *(solid pink line)*, and the effect probability increases rapidly to 100%. The shaded area (green) represents the dose range of diagnostic imaging.

evidence that ionizing radiation causes cancer—the *only* adverse effect of concern from diagnostic imaging. Our current understanding of the molecular basis for radiation-induced cancer builds on experimental studies of cultured cells and animals, and human populations that were exposed to ionizing radiation, either accidentally or for medical purposes. In particular, the human population studies have provided insights into tissue sensitivities and risk estimates for carcinogenesis. Such populations include the radium watch-dial painters, children irradiated to treat scalp infections, women who underwent repeated fluoroscopies to monitor tuberculosis, and survivors of the atomic bombings in Japan and the Chernobyl nuclear reactor disaster. The Radiation Effects Research Foundation, which studied survivors of the atomic bombings of Hiroshima and Nagasaki, has accumulated considerable data to advance our understanding of the relationship

BOX 2.1 General Features of Radiation-Induced Cancer

- Radiation-induced cancers are clinically and histologically indistinguishable from sporadically occurring or chemical-induced cancers.
- Certain tissues, for example, the female breast, the thyroid gland, and the red bone marrow, are more sensitive to the carcinogenic effects of ionizing radiation.
- There is a long latent period, ranging from years to decades, between radiation exposure and the occurrence of cancer.
- The risk of radiation-induced tumor induction is approximately threefold higher in children than in adults.

between radiation and cancer induction. The conclusions that emerge from these studies are listed in Box 2.1. In general, experimental evidence shows that cancer risk increases linearly with radiation exposures greater than 100 mSv. Certain tissues are more sensitive to radiation-induced carcinogenesis, and the age at exposure strongly influences risk.

However, there is great uncertainty regarding the extrapolation of these risks with exposures less than 100 mSv, the dose range of most diagnostic radiographic procedures. Scientific investigation of the uncertainties of low-dose radiation effects are challenging. Radiation-induced tumors do not have specific clinical, histologic, or molecular signatures, which complicates establishing a definitive causative role of radiation in tumor induction. Epidemiologic studies designed to address cancer risk from low-dose radiation would require huge sample sizes and are impractical to conduct. The long latent period between radiation exposure and cancer manifestation further compounds the experimental analysis of this relationship. These uncertainties have resulted in disagreements with regard to the application of this knowledge to develop radiation protection guidelines and policy.

The following tissues are at risk for radiation-induced cancer from diagnostic maxillofacial radiography.

Leukemia. The incidence of leukemia (other than chronic lymphocytic leukemia) increases after exposure of the red bone marrow to radiation. In the atomic bomb survivors, radiation exposure increased risks for acute lymphocytic and myelogenous leukemias and chronic myelogenous leukemia. The risks are the highest in children, peaking at approximately age 7 and with no demonstrable risk when exposed at age 30 years and above. Notably, the latent period for radiation-associated leukemias is much shorter than the decades-long latent period for solid tumors. Radiation-induced leukemias manifest as short as 2 years postexposure with a median latent period of 6–8 years.

Thyroid cancer. The incidence of thyroid carcinomas, predominantly papillary thyroid carcinomas, increases in humans after radiation exposure. Females and males are equally susceptible. Thyroid cancer risk is present when exposed at ages 19 years and under and is the highest when exposed before age 4 years. There is no detectable risk when exposed after age 20.

Salivary gland tumors. The incidence of salivary gland tumors, both benign and malignant, was increased both in patients treated with irradiation for diseases of the head and neck as well as in Japanese atomic bomb survivors. Most of the tumors are benign, with Warthin tumor being the most frequent. Mucoepidermoid tumor was the most frequent of the malignant tumors.

Breast cancer. The female breast is highly sensitive to radiation-induced cancer. Studies from several cohorts demonstrate a linear relationship between risk and dose in humans. The risk is present when exposed before age 20. There is no measurable radiation-associated risk in women exposed after the age of 50 years.

Brain and nervous system cancers. Studies of cancer survivors have shown that children who received therapeutic head irradiation (average midbrain dose of approximately 1 Gy) are at increased risk to brain tumors, predominantly meningiomas and gliomas. Meningiomas (benign tumors of the meninges) develop after a long latent period (17–20 years), whereas gliomas occur relatively sooner (5–9 years). The risk for developing glioma was the highest when exposed at age 5 and less.

Radiation-Induced Heritable Effects

DNA mutations that occur in germ cells could potentially manifest as disease in the offspring of the exposed individual. Such radiation-induced mutagenic, heritable effects have been well studied in *Drosophila* and in corn. However, there is no evidence of radiation-induced heritable effects in humans. Studies of progeny of the atomic bomb survivors show no evidence of any disease associated with maternal or paternal radiation exposure. *Thus there is no risk of radiation-induced heritable effects in humans,* and there is no scientific rationale to shield the gonads from radiation during diagnostic radiography.

Tissue Reactions (Deterministic Effects)

Tissue reactions of radiation (previously termed deterministic effects) are the consequences of cell death in a tissue or organ. Tissue reactions manifest only when the radiation exposure to an organ or tissue exceeds a threshold level. The magnitude of this threshold dose is dependent on the cell type. *The threshold dose is the radiation dose that produces the tissue reaction in 1% of the exposed individuals.* At doses below the threshold, the effect does not occur. Most individuals who receive doses higher than the threshold will develop the effect. The severity of this effect is proportional to the dose: the higher the dose, the more severe the effect. *Diagnostic radiologic examinations are designed to deliver doses below the threshold dose, and thus deterministic effects are not encountered in diagnostic maxillofacial radiography.* Nevertheless, it is a common misperception that diagnostic dental imaging can potentially cause tissue reactions in the fetus when imaging a pregnant patient. Likewise, it is often misunderstood that radiation exposure of the lens of the eyes during dental radiography places the patient at risk for cataract induction. Dental personnel who use radiation must be familiar with the threshold doses to cause these effects and understand that lack of scientific basis to consider these as risks from diagnostic imaging. Dentists will frequently manage patients with current or prior radiation therapy for head and neck malignancies. These therapeutic protocols do deliver doses that far exceed the threshold for various tissues reactions. However, particularly in such patients, it is important to use diagnostic imaging to detect manifestations of these radiation effects that have important implications for patient management and are discussed below.

Radiation Effects on Embryos and Fetuses

Embryos and fetuses are considerably more radiosensitive than adults because most embryonic cells are relatively undifferentiated and rapidly mitotic. The effects of radiation on embryos and fetuses have been extensively studied in animals, predominantly rodents. Data on effects on human embryos and fetuses are derived from studies of survivors of the atomic bomb, exposed in utero, and from children of women exposed to diagnostic or therapeutic radiation during pregnancy. The conclusions from these studies are summarized as follows:

- The effects are dependent on the dose and gestational age during irradiation.
- Irradiation during preimplantation (0–9 days in humans) causes embryonic death (Fig. 2.7). The threshold for this effect is estimated to be 100 mGy—approximately 10,000 times more than the fetal dose from dental radiographic examinations. In comparison, the average dose to an embryo and fetus from natural background radiation is approximately 0.5–1 mGy during the 9 months of gestation.
- In humans, fetal irradiation is associated with microcephaly, when irradiated up to 15 weeks' gestation. The threshold dose is 100 mGy—approximately 10,000 times higher than fetal doses from dentomaxillofacial radiographic examinations (Fig. 2.7). Radiation-induced microcephaly is often associated with intellectual disability.
- Fetal irradiation is strongly associated with intellectual disability, with severe intellectual disability occurring at doses above 300 mGy, when delivered at 8–25 weeks' gestation. The threshold dose is approximately 30,000 times higher than fetal doses from dentomaxillofacial radiographic examinations (Fig. 2.7).

Radiation doses that cause tissue reactions in the embryo and fetus are 10,000 to 30,000 times higher than the fetal dose from dentomaxillofacial radiography. Thus dentomaxillofacial imaging is safe during pregnancy. Chapter 3 discusses imaging of the pregnant patient.

Cataracts

Ionizing radiation damage to the lens of the eye induces cataracts—clouding or opacification of the lens. These cataracts are mostly of the posterior subcapsular or cortical type. The International Commission on Radiological Protection (ICRP) estimates the threshold for cataract induction to be 0.5 Gy for low LET radiations such as x-rays. The National Council on Radiation Protection and Measurements (NCRP) estimates of the threshold dose are slightly higher, at 1–2 Gy, for vision-impairing cataracts. The absorbed dose in the lens of the eye during dentomaxillofacial radiographic examinations ranges from 0.02 to 0.4 mGy—at least 1250 times lower than the conservative estimate from ICRP.

RADIOTHERAPY INVOLVING THE ORAL CAVITY

Dentists are likely to manage patients who are undergoing radiation therapy or have received such treatment for management of head and neck malignancies. Often, the radiotherapy approach is combined with surgery and chemotherapy.

The radiation treatment is administered as many daily small doses (fractions). Such fractionation of the total x-ray dose provides greater tumor destruction than is possible with a large single dose.

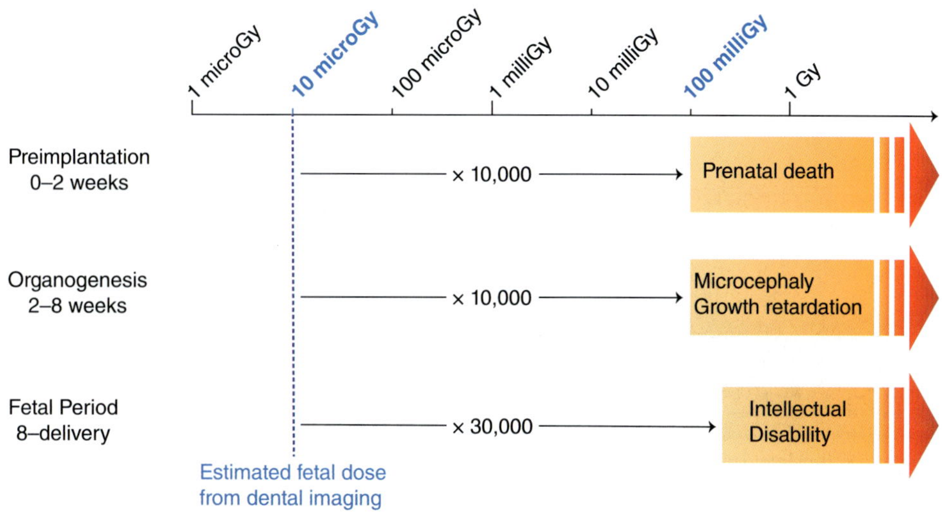

Fig. 2.7 Radiation effects on the embryo and fetus during preimplantation, organogenesis, and fetal period. The effects and threshold doses are shown. The estimated fetal dose from dentomaxillofacial imaging is indicated *(blue dashed line)*, and its relative magnitude to the threshold doses for effect causation are shown.

Fractionation also allows increased cellular repair of surrounding normal tissues that are unavoidably exposed. Fractionation also increases the mean oxygen tension in an irradiated tumor, rendering the tumor cells more radiosensitive. This results from killing rapidly dividing tumor cells and shrinking the tumor mass after the first few fractions, reducing the distance that oxygen must diffuse from the fine vasculature through the tumor to reach the remaining viable tumor cells. Typically, 2 Gy is delivered daily for a weekly exposure of 10 Gy. The radiotherapy course continues for 6–7 weeks until a total of 60–70 Gy is administered. Fig. 2.8 summarizes the temporal sequence of occurrence of oral complications from this therapy. In recent years, new three-dimensional techniques called intensity-modulated radiotherapy (IMRT) have been used to control the dose distribution with high accuracy, minimizing exposure to adjacent normal tissues.

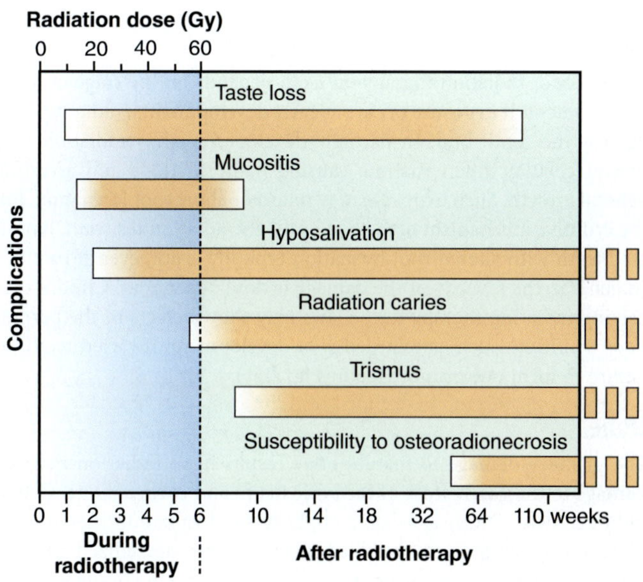

Fig. 2.8 Oral complications. Typical time course of complications seen during and after a course of radiation therapy to the head and neck. *Shaded area* in the first 6 weeks represents accumulated dose. *Shading within bars* indicates severity of complication. Note recovery of taste and healing of mucositis. Changes persisting after 2 years pose lifelong risks. (Adapted from Kielbassa AM, Hinkelbein W, Hellwig E, Meyer-Lückel H. Radiation-related damage to dentition. *Lancet Oncol.* 2006; 7:326-335.)

Oral Mucosa

The oral mucosa contains a basal layer composed of rapidly dividing, radiosensitive progenitor cells. By the end of the second week of therapy, the cell death induces an inflammatory response, and the mucous membranes begin to show areas of redness and inflammation (mucositis). During therapy, the irradiated mucous membrane separates from the underlying connective tissue and forms a white-to-yellow pseudomembrane (the desquamated epithelial layer) (Fig. 2.9). At the end of therapy, the mucositis is usually most severe, discomfort is at a maximum, and food intake is difficult. Good oral hygiene minimizes infection. Topical anesthetics may be required at mealtimes. Secondary yeast infection by *Candida albicans* is a common complication and may require treatment.

Following completion of radiotherapy, the mucosa heals rapidly. Healing is usually complete by approximately 2 months. However, fibrosis of the underlying connective tissue causes the mucosa to become atrophic, thin, and relatively avascular. These atrophic changes complicate denture wearing because they may cause oral ulcerations of the compromised tissue. Ulcers may also result from radiation necrosis or tumor recurrence. A biopsy may be required to make the differentiation.

Taste Buds

Taste buds are sensitive to radiation. Doses in the therapeutic range cause a loss of taste acuity during the second or third week of radiotherapy, and taste acuity usually decreases by a factor of 1000–10,000 during the treatment period. Bitter and acid flavors are more severely affected when the posterior two-thirds of the tongue is irradiated, and salt and sweet flavors are affected more when the anterior third of the tongue is irradiated. Alterations in the saliva may partly account for this reduction. Loss of taste combines with mucositis to adversely affect nutrition by discouraging eating. Taste loss is reversible, and recovery takes 2–4 months.

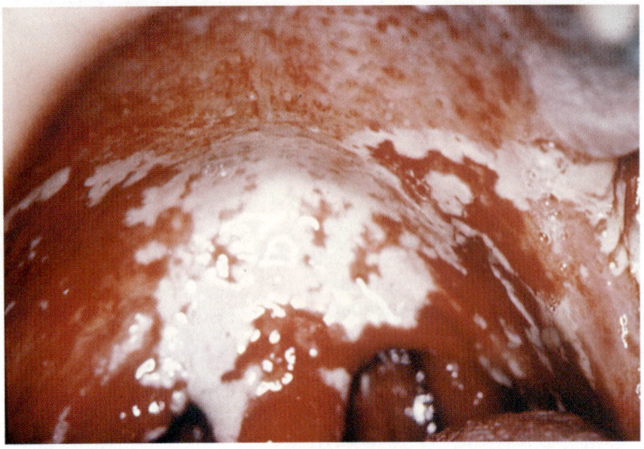

Fig. 2.9 Mucositis of hard and soft palate. This patient is at the end of a course of radiotherapy and demonstrates an inflammatory response in the oral mucosa and areas of white pseudomembrane, areas where the oral epithelium separated from the underlying connective tissue.

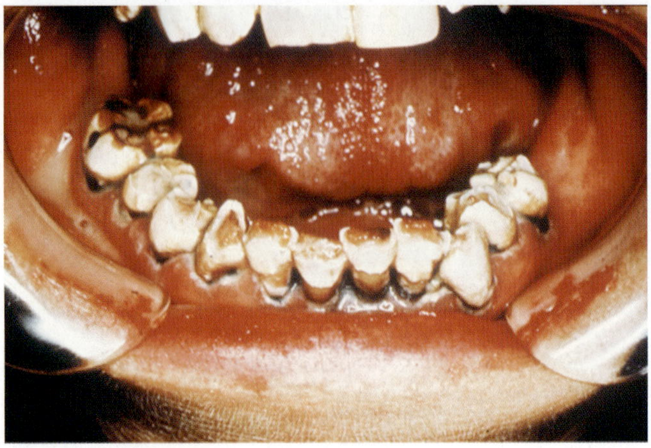

Fig. 2.10 Radiation caries. Note the extensive loss of structure on the occlusal surface of the mandibular teeth resulting from radiation-induced xerostomia.

Salivary Glands

Salivary glands are highly sensitive to radiation, despite their relatively differentiated constituent cells. Radiation therapy protocols attempt to limit the cumulative dose to the parotid to approximately 25 Gy so that salivary function can be restored posttherapy. This dose limit is 39 Gy for submandibular glands, which are more radioresistant than the parotid. Within the first week of radiation therapy, patients experience an approximately 50% decrease in salivary flow. The salivary flow gradually decreases to less than 10% within 1 year. Late changes in the gland include fibrosis and decreased vascularity, impacting regaining salivary gland function. The residual gland function is dose dependent. At doses less than 45 Gy, only 5% of patients experience permanent loss of function, determined at 5 years posttherapy. At doses of 60 Gy and greater, this fraction increases to 50%. Use of IMRT has helped to spare the contralateral salivary glands and thus minimize the loss of salivary function.

The loss of saliva production results in xerostomia, a debilitating consequence with a significant impact on quality of life. Patients with xerostomia have trouble with chewing and swallowing. The biochemical properties of the saliva produced are different—the saliva has a lower pH, an average of 5.5 in irradiated patients compared to 6.5 in unexposed individuals. This pH is low enough to initiate decalcification of normal enamel. The buffering capacity of saliva is also decreased. Various saliva substitutes are available to help restore function.

Radiation Caries

Radiation caries is a rampant form of dental decay that may occur in patients with radiation-induced xerostomia. Caries results from changes in the salivary glands and saliva, including reduced flow, decreased pH, reduced buffering capacity, increased viscosity, and an altered flora. Patients receiving radiation therapy to oral structures have increases in *Streptococcus mutans, Lactobacillus,* and *Candida.* The residual saliva in individuals with xerostomia also has a low concentration of Ca^{2+} ion; this results in greater solubility of tooth structure and reduced remineralization. Because of the reduced or absent cleansing action of normal saliva, debris accumulates quickly.

Three patterns of radiation caries are found clinically. The most common is widespread superficial lesions attacking buccal, occlusal, incisal, and palatal surfaces (Fig. 2.10). Another type involves primarily the cementum and dentin in the cervical region. These lesions may progress around the teeth circumferentially and result in loss of the crown. The third type appears as a dark pigmentation of the entire crown. The incisal edges may be markedly worn. Combinations of all these lesions develop in some patients. The location, rapid course, and widespread attack distinguish radiation caries. There is also evidence that radiation caries is more likely to lead to periapical inflammatory lesions if the periapical bone received a high dose of radiation.

The best method to reduce radiation caries is daily application of a viscous topical 1% neutral sodium fluoride gel in custom-made applicator trays. Topical fluoride should be combined with restorative dental procedures as needed, excellent oral hygiene, and a diet restricted in cariogenic foods. Patient cooperation in maintaining oral hygiene is extremely important because radiation caries is a lifelong threat. Teeth with gross caries or periodontal involvement are often extracted before irradiation.

Teeth

The effect of radiation therapy on teeth depends on the stage of tooth development. If exposure occurs at early development, irradiation may destroy the tooth bud. In partially developed teeth, irradiation may inhibit cellular differentiation, causing malformations and arresting general growth. Such exposure may retard or abort root formation, but the eruptive mechanism of teeth is relatively radiation resistant. Irradiated teeth with altered root formation typically erupt, even if rootless. In general, the severity of the damage is dose dependent. Children receiving radiation therapy to the jaws may show defects in the permanent dentition, such as retarded root development, dwarfed teeth, or failure to form one or more teeth (Fig. 2.11).

Bone

The primary damage to mature bone results from radiation-induced damage to the vasculature of the periosteum and cortical bone. Osteoradionecrosis (ORN) is a late complication of radiation therapy and occurs when an area of irradiated bone becomes devitalized. ORN is formally defined as "an area of exposed irradiated bone tissue that fails to heal over a period of three months, without residual or recurrent tumor; and when other causes of osteonecrosis have been excluded" (Fig. 2.12). A widely accepted model is that radiation-induced microvascular changes create a state of hypoxia, hypovascularity, and hypocellularity, thereby disturbing normal bone homeostasis and leading to a chronic, nonhealing wound. Radiation-induced fibrosis also contributes to ORN development. Radiation-induced cell damage triggers a

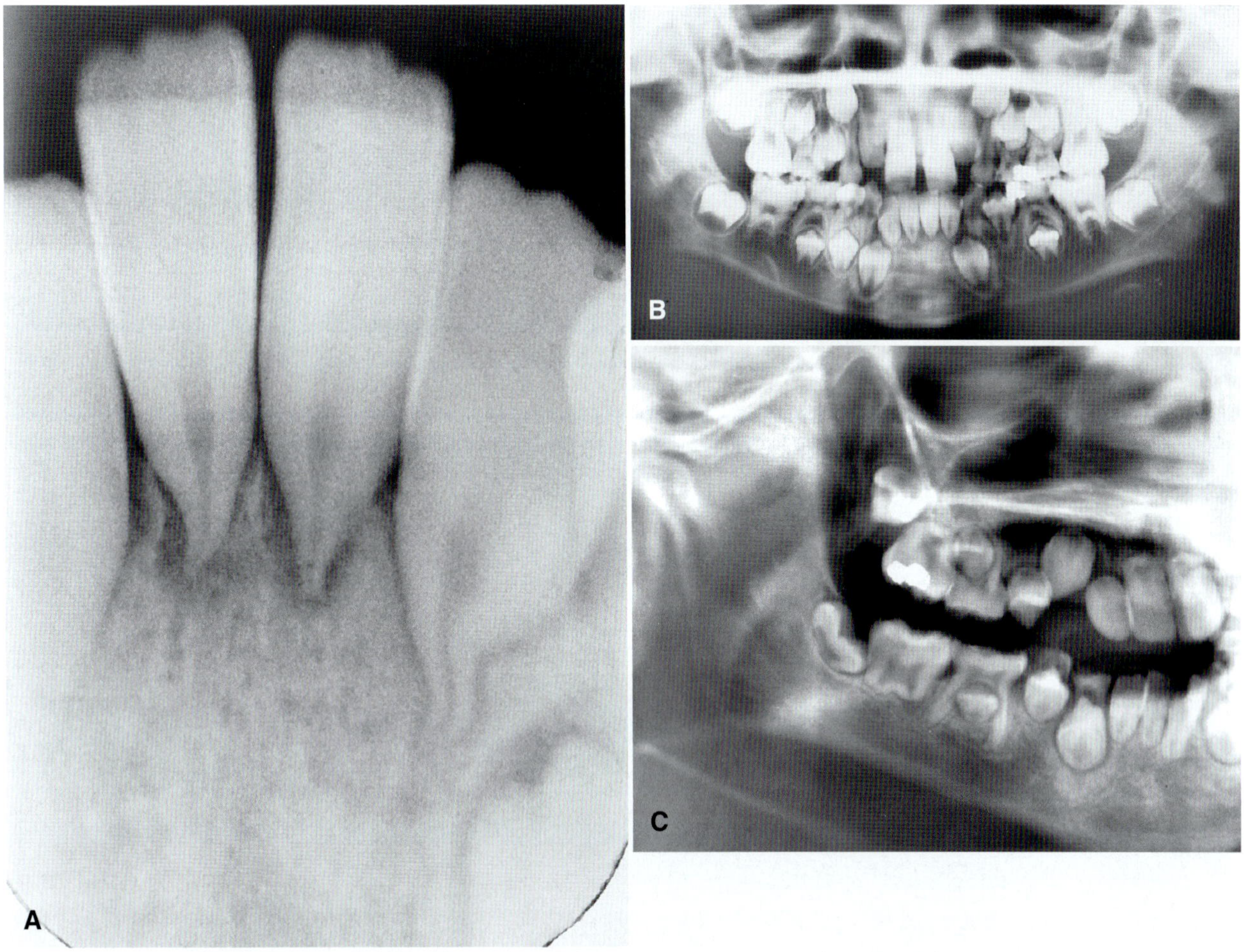

Fig. 2.11 Dental abnormalities after radiotherapy in two patients. The first patient, a 9-year-old girl who received 35 Gy at age 4 years because of Hodgkin disease, had severe stunting of the incisor roots with premature closure of the apices at 8 years (A) and retarded development of the mandibular second premolar crowns with stunting of the mandibular incisor, canine, and premolar roots at 9 years (B). The second patient (C), a 10-year-old boy who received 41 Gy to the jaws at age 4 years, had severely stunted root development of all permanent teeth with a normal primary molar. (A and B, Courtesy Mr. P. N. Hirschmann, Leeds, UK. C, Courtesy Dr. James Eischen, San Diego, California.)

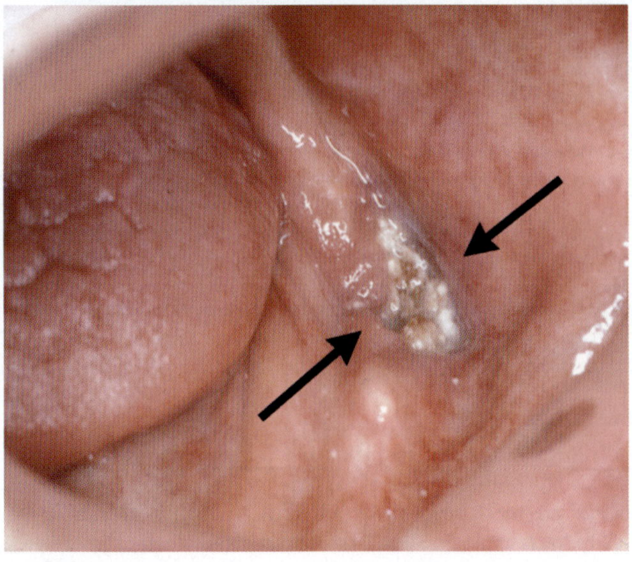

Fig. 2.12 Osteoradionecrosis presenting as an area of exposed bone in the irradiation field. Note the loss of oral mucosa *(arrows)*.

cascade of chronic inflammation and deregulated fibroblastic activity around the blood vessel walls, exacerbating a chronic fibrotic response in both the bone and the overlying mucosa.

ORN typically manifests 6–12 months following radiation treatment but can develop anytime, from months to years following radiation therapy. The incidence of ORN is approximately 5%–7% for conventional radiotherapy, IMRT, and brachytherapy (where the radioactive material is placed inside the body). ORN is more frequent in the mandible than in the maxilla, likely due to the relatively lower vascularity in the mandible. ORN is unlikely and rarely occurs if the dose is less than 50 Gy. However, the risk of ORN increases 11-fold when the dose to the bone exceeds 66 Gy. Important risk factors of clinical significance include carious teeth, periodontal disease, and trauma from dental extractions or ill-fitting dentures. Widening of the periodontal ligament space along the mandibular tooth roots is a common finding in the irradiated mandible but requires no management if the adjacent bone is intact. As the disease progresses, bone destruction becomes radiographically evident as patchy radiolucent areas with radiodense islands of necrotic bone, or sequestrum. The bone destruction may be severe enough to cause pathologic fracture (Fig. 2.13A and B).

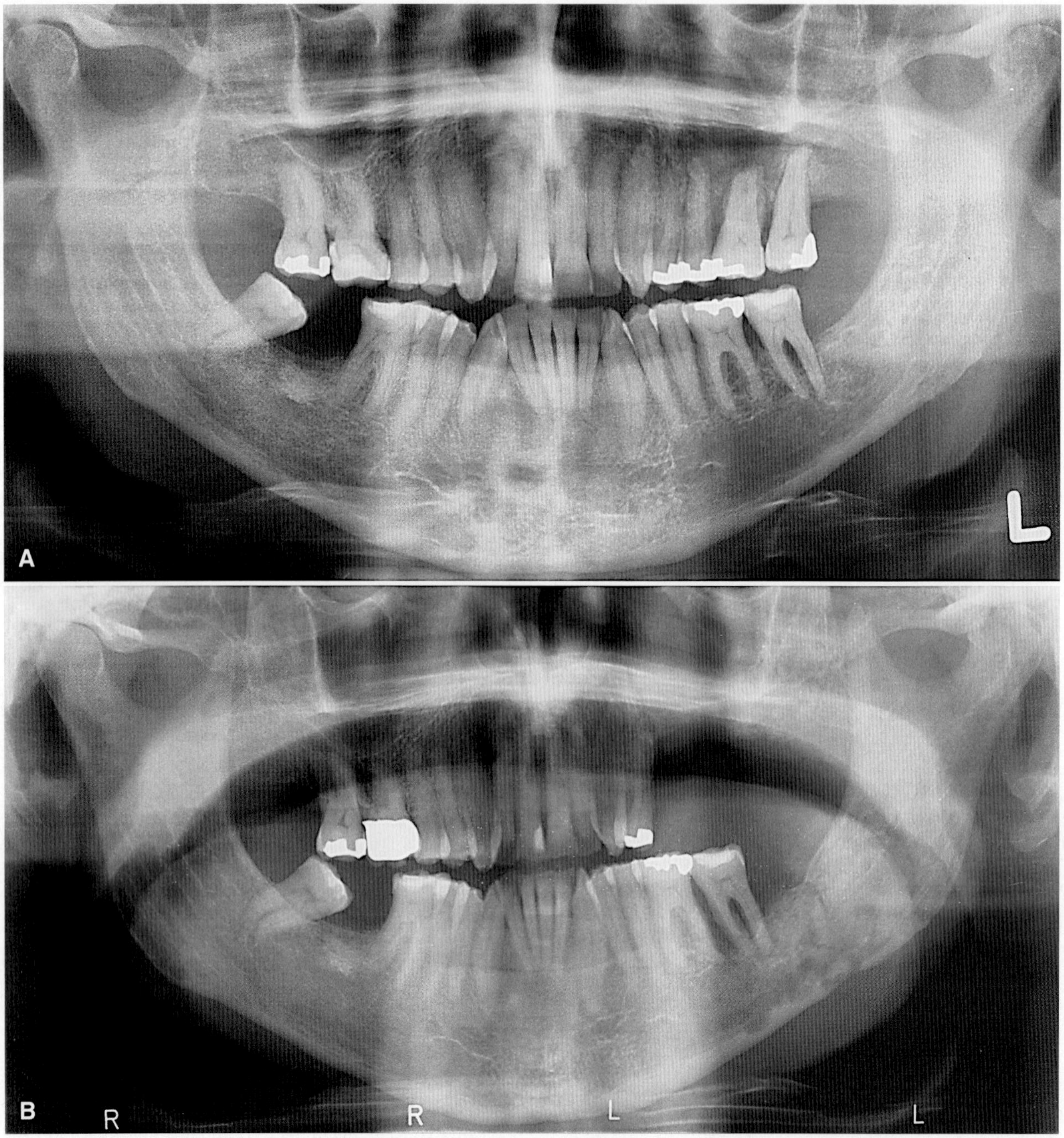

Fig. 2.13 (A) Panoramic radiograph made soon after completion of radiation therapy. Note the presence of mild periodontal bone loss. (B) Panoramic radiograph of the same patient taken 3 years later shows extensive bone destruction in the left posterior mandible body-angle region, extending to the inferior mandibular cortex.

Preradiotherapy dental care is important to prevent pulp infections from spreading into irradiated tissues causing ORN. Carious teeth must be restored before radiation therapy. Preventive measures of good oral hygiene and daily topical fluoride application must be emphasized. Teeth with extensive caries or with poor periodontal support may be extracted, allowing 2–3 weeks for the extraction wounds to heal before beginning radiation therapy.

Posttherapy management is equally important. Periodic oral examinations and radiographs will allow early detection of caries and periapical inflammation. The radiation dose from such diagnostic exposures is negligible compared to the amount received during therapy and should not deter making radiographs when indicated. Extractions in an area of irradiated bone must be performed with minimal surgical trauma. Dentures may need to be adjusted to minimize the risk of denture sores.

Musculature

Radiation may cause inflammation and fibrosis, resulting in contracture and trismus in the muscles of mastication. The masseter or pterygoid muscles are most frequently involved. Restriction in mouth opening usually starts approximately 2 months after radiotherapy is completed and progresses thereafter. Exercises for mouth opening are helpful to minimize trismus.

BIBLIOGRAPHY

Hall EJ, Giaccia AJ. *Radiobiology for the Radiologist*. 8th ed. Lippincott Williams & Wilkins; 2018.

National Research Council. *Health Risks From Exposure to Low Levels of Ionizing Radiation: BEIR VII Phase*. The National Academies Press; 2006. https://nap.nationalacademies.org/catalog/11340/health-risks-from-exposure-to-low-levels-of-ionizing-radiation. Accessed August 15, 2023.

Radiation-Induced Cancer

Brenner DJ. What we know and what we don't know about cancer risks associated with radiation doses from radiological imaging. *Br J Radiol*. 2014; 87(1035):20130629.

Boice JD. The linear nonthreshold (LNT) model as used in radiation protection: an NCRP update. *Int J Radiat Biol*. 2017;93(10):1079-1092.

Calabrese EJ. The linear no-threshold (LNT) dose response model: a comprehensive assessment of its historical and scientific foundations. *Chem Biol Interact*. 2019;301:6-25.

Iglesias ML, Schmidt A, Ghuzlan AA, et al. Radiation exposure and thyroid cancer: a review. *Arch Endocrinol Metab*. 2017;61(2):180-187.

National Council on Radiation Protection and Measurements. *Implications of Recent Epidemiologic Studies for the Linear Nonthreshold Model and Radiation Protection*. National Council on Radiation Protection and Measurements; 2018.

Preston DL, Shimizu Y, Pierce DA, et al. Studies of mortality of atomic bomb survivors. Report 13: solid cancer and noncancer disease mortality: 1950–1997. *Radiat Res*. 2003;160:381-407.

Ron E, Lubin JH, Shore RE, et al. Thyroid cancer after exposure to external radiation: a pooled analysis of seven studies. 1995. *Radiat Res*. 2012; 178(2):AV43-AV60.

Veiga LH, Lubin JH, Anderson H, et al. A pooled analysis of thyroid cancer incidence following radiotherapy for childhood cancer. *Radiat Res*. 2012;178(4):365-376.

Veiga LH, Holmberg E, Anderson H, et al. Thyroid cancer after childhood exposure to external radiation: an updated pooled analysis of 12 studies. *Radiat Res*. 2016;185(5):473-484.

Heritable Effects

United Nations Scientific Committee on the Effects of Atomic Radiation. Hereditary effects of radiation. 2001. http://www.unscear.org/unscear/en/publications/2001.html. Accessed August 15, 2023.

Cell Killing

Eriksson D, Stigbrand T. Radiation-induced cell death mechanisms. *Tumour Biol*. 2010;31(4):363-372.

Hall EJ. The bystander effect. *Health Phys*. 2003;85(1):31-35.

Tissue Reactions: Embryo and Fetus

American College of Radiology. ACR–SPR Practice parameter for imaging pregnant or potentially pregnant patients with ionizing radiation. 2023. https://www.acr.org/-/media/ACR/Files/Practice-Parameters/pregnant-pts.pdf. Accessed August 15, 2023.

Kelaranta A, Ekholm M, Toroi P, et al. Radiation exposure to foetus and breasts from dental X-ray examinations: effect of lead shields. *Dentomaxillofac Radiol*. 2016;45(1):20150095.

Wagner LK, Lester RG, Saldana LR. *Exposure of the Pregnant Patient to Diagnostic Radiations. A Guide to Medical Management*. Medical Physics Publishing; 1997.

Cataracts

Dauer LT, Ainsbury EA, Dynlacht J, et al. Guidance on radiation dose limits for the lens of the eye: overview of the recommendations in NCRP Commentary No. 26. *Int J Radiat Biol*. 2017;93(10):1-9.

Neriishi K, Nakashima E, Akahoshi M, et al. Radiation dose and cataract surgery incidence in atomic bomb survivors, 1986–2005. *Radiology*. 2012; 265:167-174.

Radiotherapy Involving the Oral Cavity

Chan KC, Perschbacher SE, Lam EW, et al. Mandibular changes on panoramic imaging after head and neck radiotherapy. *Oral Surg Oral Med Oral Pathol Oral Radiol*. 2016;121(6):666-672.

Chung EM, Sung EC. Dental management of chemoradiation patients. *J Calif Dent Assoc*. 2006;34:735-742.

Dahllof G. Craniofacial growth in children treated for malignant diseases. *Acta Odontol Scand*. 1998;56:378.

Delanian S, Lefaix JL. The radiation-induced fibroatrophic process: therapeutic perspective via the antioxidant pathway. *Radiother Oncol*. 2004;73(2):119-131.

Jacobson AS, Buchbinder D, Hu K, et al. Paradigm shifts in the management of osteoradionecrosis of the mandible. *Oral Oncol*. 2010;46:795-801.

Kielbassa AM, Hinkelbein W, Hellwig E, et al. Radiation-related damage to dentition. *Lancet Oncol*. 2006;7:326-335.

Mallya SM, Tetradis S. Imaging of radiation- and medication-related osteonecrosis. *Radiol Clin North Am*. 2018;56:77-89.

Marx RE. Osteoradionecrosis: a new concept of its pathophysiology. *J Oral Maxillofac Surg*. 1983;41(5):283-288.

Schwartz HC, Kagan AR. Osteoradionecrosis of the mandible: scientific basis for clinical staging. *Am J Clin Oncol*. 2002;25(2):168-171.

3

Safety and Protection

Avni Bhula and Sanjay M. Mallya

Every year, more than 1 billion dental radiographic examinations are done worldwide, accounting for approximately 26% of all healthcare radiographic imaging procedures. The high frequency of these procedures emphasizes the need for dentists and allied dental personnel to be prepared to intelligently address radiation-related questions from patients. This includes the benefits and possible hazards involved with the use of x-rays and the steps taken to reduce these hazards. This chapter provides foundational content to understand the magnitude of radiation exposure from diagnostic imaging, the estimated radiation-associated risks, and the means to minimize exposure from radiographic examinations.

SOURCES OF RADIATION EXPOSURE

The general population is exposed to radiation primarily from natural background and medical sources (Table 3.1). These exposure sources provide a useful contextual framework to understand the magnitude of diagnostic radiation exposure.

Background Radiation

All life on Earth has evolved in a continuous exposure to natural background radiation (Fig. 3.1; see Table 3.1). There is considerable variation in background radiation exposure depending on geographic location—the global average is 2.4 mSv/year (Fig. 3.1A), with a range of 1–13 mSv. Background radiation from various sources yields an average annual effective dose of approximately 3.1 mSv in the United States (Fig. 3.1B). Daily background radiation dose provides a useful and easily comprehended benchmark to communicate the magnitude of radiation dose received by patients from diagnostic imaging.

Radon and Its Progeny

Radon-222 is a radioactive element produced as an intermediate step in the decay of uranium-238, one of the most significant naturally occurring radioactive elements in the Earth's crust. Radon, a gas, is released from the ground and enters homes and buildings. Radon-222 and its decay product polonium-218 emit α particles. Radon is the principal contributor to background radiation exposure and accounts for approximately 52%–74% of background radiation exposure. Radon and its decay products may become attached to dust particles that can be inhaled and deposited on the bronchial epithelium in the respiratory tract. Radon is the second most frequent cause of lung cancer and is estimated to cause 3%–14% of all lung cancers worldwide.

Cosmic Radiation

Cosmic rays, or space radiation, comprise protons, helium nuclei, and nuclei of heavier elements, as well as other particles generated by the interactions of primary space radiation with the Earth's atmosphere. Exposure from cosmic radiation is primarily a function of altitude, almost doubling with each 2000-m increase in elevation because less atmosphere is present to attenuate the radiation. At sea level, the exposure from cosmic radiation is approximately 0.33 mSv/year; at an elevation of 1600 m (approximately 1 mile, the elevation of Denver, Colorado), it is approximately 0.50 mSv/year. Air travel exposes passengers and crew to cosmic radiation. The magnitude of exposure varies with flight altitude and duration. Cosmic radiation contributes approximately 11%–16% of background exposure.

Internal Radionuclides

Another source of background radiation is radionuclides that are ingested. The greatest internal exposure comes from foods containing uranium and thorium and their decay products, primarily potassium-40 but also rubidium-87, carbon-14, tritium, and others. The total exposure from ingestion contributes approximately 9%–12% of background exposure.

Terrestrial Radiation

Terrestrial radiation exposure is derived from radioactive nuclides in the soil, primarily potassium-40 and the radioactive decay products of uranium-238 and thorium-232. Most of the γ-radiation from these sources comes from the top 20 cm of soil. Indoor exposure from radionuclides is close to the exposure occurring outdoors because the shielding provided by structural materials balances the exposure from radioactive nuclides contained within these shielding materials. Terrestrial exposure contributes approximately 7%–20% of background exposure.

Medical Exposure

Diagnostic imaging is the largest contributor to exposure from human-made sources of radiation (Fig. 3.2). Worldwide, approximately 4.2 billion x-ray and nuclear medicine examinations are performed annually. The use of medical and dental imaging per capita is higher in the United States relative to the global population. The average annual exposure to US population from diagnostic radiation is approximately 2.2 mSv, almost fourfold higher than the global average of 0.56 mSv.

The global growth of the medical imaging market has caused interesting trends in imaging practices. Worldwide, the estimated number of computed tomography (CT) examinations doubled from 2006 to 2016. CT accounts for 56%–61% of the dose from diagnostic imaging (Fig. 3.2). In the United States, approximately 9.2% of CT examinations encompass the head and neck region. Use of conventional radiography, excluding dental imaging, has decreased. Dental radiographs are among the most frequently performed radiographic procedures and account for 26% of the examinations globally and approximately

46% of examinations done in the United States. Notably, despite their high frequency of use, dental x-ray examinations contribute to less than 2% of the total exposure from medical imaging.

Encouragingly, recent estimates of the average effective dose to the US population from diagnostic radiation have decreased to 2.2 mSv, compared to the prior 2006 estimate of 3.1 mSv. This dose reduction reflects technological innovations and better practices to select patients for imaging and optimized radiation doses. It reinforces the principles conveyed in this chapter that simple practices contribute substantially to patient dose reduction.

TABLE 3.1 Average Annual Effective Dose of Ionizing Radiation

	DOSE (mSv)	
Source	**Global**	**United States**
Natural Background[a]		
Radon	1.3	2.3
Cosmic radiation	0.4	0.3
Internal radionuclides	0.3	0.3
Terrestrial	0.5	0.2
Subtotal background	***2.4***	***3.1***
Medical[b]		
Computed tomography	0.35	1.37
Interventional fluoroscopy	0.05	0.25
Conventional radiography	0.13	0.22
Dental	0.003	0.04
Nuclear medicine	0.03	0.41
Subtotal medical (rounded)	***0.56***	***2.2***
Consumer products and other[a]	0.01	0.1
Grand total	***3.1***	***5.4***

[a]Data for global population from United Nations Scientific Committee on the Effects of Atomic Radiation. *Sources and Effects of Ionizing Radiation: United Nations Scientific Committee on the Effects of Atomic Radiation: UNSCEAR 2008 Report to the General Assembly, with Scientific Annexes.* United Nations; 2010. Data for US population from National Council on Radiation Protection and Measurements. *Ionizing Radiation Exposure of the Population of the United States, NCRP Report 160.* National Council on Radiation Protection and Measurements; 2009.
[b]Data on patient doses from healthcare imaging from Mahadevappa M. et al. Patient Exposure from Radiologic and Nuclear Medicine Procedures in the United States and Worldwide: 2009–2018. Radiology. 307:e221263. 2023.

Consumer Products

Consumer products contain some of the most interesting and unsuspected sources of radiation. This group includes, in order of importance, radiation exposure from cigarette smoking, building materials, air travel, mining and agriculture, and combustion of fossil fuels. With increasing air travel, cosmic radiation becomes a more significant contributor to exposure. Typically, an airline flight of 5 hours at a cruising altitude of 12 km results in an exposure of approximately 20–50 μSv. Other minor sources of exposure from consumer products include ceramics, including dental porcelain and smoke alarms. In total, consumer products contribute approximately 2%–6% of the total average annual exposure.

Other Sources

Other sources of exposure affect caregivers or others in contact with patients receiving nuclear medicine treatments; people who work in nuclear power generation; individuals involved in areas of industrial, medical, educational, or research activities; workers in medical and dental x-ray facilities; workers in airport baggage inspection systems; and commercial flight personnel. All these sources of radiation combined contribute only approximately 0.1% of the total average annual exposure.

DENTOMAXILLOFACIAL RADIOLOGY: RISK AND DOSES

The basic principle of diagnostic imaging is that the benefit to the patient far outweighs the radiation-associated risks. To satisfy this principle, doses from dentomaxillofacial radiographic examination must be:

- Optimized to produce a diagnostically acceptable image
- Less than the threshold needed to cause any tissue reactions
- Minimized to keep the risk of stochastic effects within an acceptable range

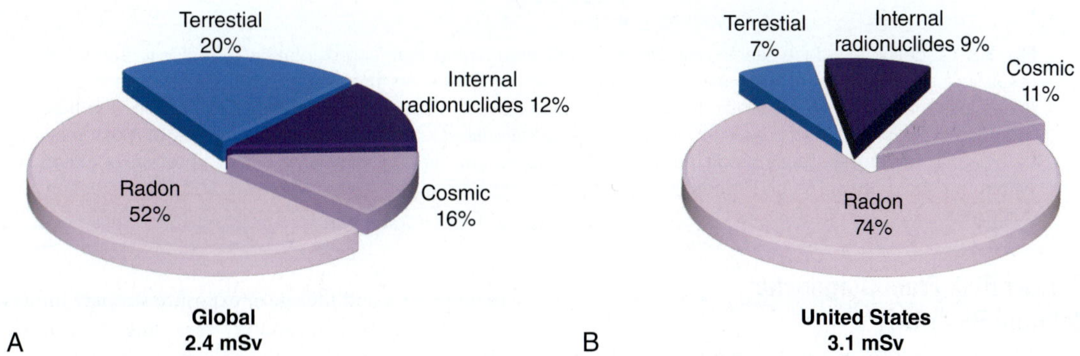

Fig. 3.1 Natural background radiation exposure of (A) global and (B) US populations. Average annual individual effective doses are 2.4 mSv globally and 3.1 mSv in the United States. Most exposure comes from radon, but there are significant contributions from cosmic radiation, ingested radionuclides, and terrestrial sources, including external radionuclides in the soil and building materials. (Data for global population from United Nations Scientific Committee on the Effects of Atomic Radiation. *Sources and Effects of Ionizing Radiation: United Nations Scientific Committee on the Effects of Atomic Radiation: UNSCEAR 2008 report to the General Assembly, with Scientific Annexes.* United Nations; 2010. Data for US population from National Council on Radiation Protection and Measurements. *Ionizing Radiation Exposure of the Population of the United States, NCRP Report 160.* National Council on Radiation Protection and Measurements; 2009.)

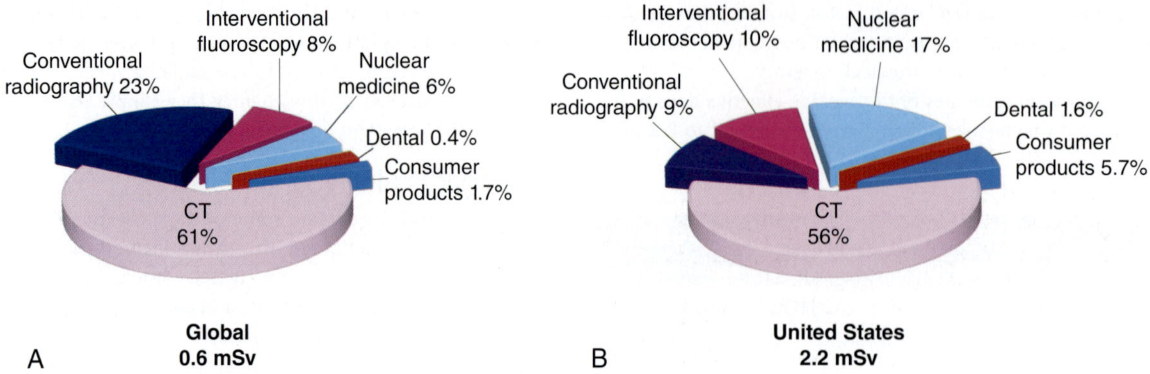

Fig. 3.2 Sources of ionizing radiation from diagnostic imaging and consumer products. (A) Global population and (B) US population. The average radiation dose to global and US populations from human-made sources of ionizing radiation are 0.6 and 2.2 mSv, respectively. The marked difference is a result of the relatively high number of imaging procedures done in the United States. Globally, most medical x-ray exposures come from computed tomography *(CT)*. Conventional and interventional radiography, fluoroscopy, and nuclear medicine are also significant contributors to dose. Exposures from dental examinations and from occupational, fallout, and nuclear power sources are small. Although individuals with exposures from natural background are fairly evenly distributed in the population, most medically exposed individuals are relatively old and sick. Data from Mahadevappa et al. Patient exposure from radiologic and nuclear medicine procedures in the United States and Worldwide: 2009–2018. Radiology. 307:e221263. 2023.

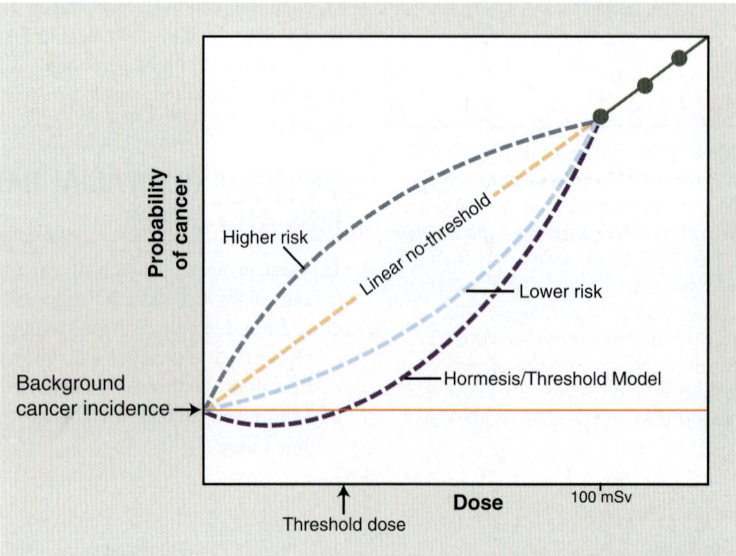

Fig. 3.3 Modeling low-dose cancer risk. Doses of radiation higher than approximately 100 mSv *(green dots)* result in a dose-dependent increase in the cancer rate. The linear no-threshold model (LNT) posits that at doses less than 100 mSv, there is a linear relationship between dose and risk *(orange dashed line)* and that there is no threshold dose below which there is no additional risk. Alternate models propose that risk may be higher or lower than those predicted by the LNT model and that low doses may have a protective effect with a threshold dose. The LNT model is currently accepted as the approach to develop radiation protection guidelines.

Estimating Cancer Risk From Diagnostic Dentomaxillofacial Radiology

The principal risk of dentomaxillofacial radiography is the unlikely chance of radiation-induced cancer. Cancer is the second leading cause of death and accounts for 16% of deaths worldwide. There were more than 19 million new cancer cases in 2020 globally. There is convincing evidence from studies of humans and research animals that links radiation exposure to development of solid neoplasms and leukemias (see Chapter 2). In general, experimental evidence shows that cancer risk increases linearly with protracted radiation exposures greater than 100 mSv. Certain tissues are more sensitive to radiation-induced carcinogenesis and the age at exposure strongly influences risk. However, there is great uncertainty regarding the extrapolation of these risks with exposures less than 100 mSv, the dose range of most diagnostic radiographic procedures. Estimating risks at low doses is practically meaningful—it provides the clinician with information to assess the balance of radiation-associated risk versus diagnostic benefit.

Current radiation protection policies and practices are based on the linear no-threshold (LNT) hypothesis, which predicts that there is a linear relationship between dose and the risk of inducing a new cancer, even at very low doses (Fig. 3.3). This hypothesis considers that there is no threshold or "safe dose" below which there is no added cancer risk. Proponents of this hypothesis argue that cancers are clonal in nature, arising from a single mutated cell. X-ray ionization events are sparse and physically separated (see Fig. 2.3A), the probability of causing double-strand breaks and clustered lesions—the likely precursors of cancer-causing mutations—is low but still exists (see Fig. 2.3B), and thus the basis for the absence of a threshold dose. *When applied to model cancer risk from diagnostic radiation, the LNT hypothesis favors a conservative approach to population radiation protection.*

The LNT model is not a demonstrated scientific fact, and its assumptions for low-dose effects have been contested. For example, there is evidence of cellular adaptive responses—stress responses induced by low-dose radiation that augment a cell's response to subsequent higher doses. These studies have prompted suggestions that low-dose radiation may have a protective effect (referred to as *hormesis*), that the risks are lower than those predicted by the LNT model, and that there is a threshold dose that must be exceeded to induce cancer. On the other hand, studies of cultured cells have suggested the presence of *bystander effects,* in which biologic effects occur in cells that are not directly irradiated. Such off-target effects could potentially yield a supralinear response, and the risk may potentially be higher than predicted by the LNT model. *Opponents of the LNT model argue that applying an overly conservative approach results in an inappropriate fear, which may compromise the full diagnostic benefits of imaging and increase costs for implementation of radiation protection programs.*

Despite its uncertainties in the low-dose range, policymakers need guidance to set dose limits for individuals exposed in the low-dose range, including from diagnostic imaging procedures and from occupational exposure. In the absence of data that conclusively support alternate models, most radiation protection organizations adopt the conservative estimates of the LNT model to guide radiation safety and protection policies. *The radiation safety practices described in this text have considered recommendations that are based on the LNT hypothesis.*

Patient Doses From Diagnostic Dentomaxillofacial Radiology

Radiation doses to the patient from radiographic imaging are usually reported as effective dose, a measure of the stochastic risks. Table 3.2 and Fig. 3.4 show typical effective doses from common dentomaxillofacial and medical radiographic examinations and the equivalent exposure in terms of days of natural background radiation. These effective doses consider the absorbed doses to various organs from a specific radiographic procedure and the relative sensitivity of the exposed organ to stochastic effects of radiation. Typically, the doses are measured using an anthropomorphic phantom or may be modeled by computational simulation. However, effective dose does not consider age, sex, and individual susceptibility factors and thus is not intended to represent an individual's radiation dose from that procedure. Nevertheless, effective dose is a convenient measure to compare the relative risks from different radiographic examinations and to convey the relative magnitude of the risk to patients. To assist healthcare providers and patients in categorizing the magnitude of radiation-associated risks, the American College of Radiology developed a categorization of relative radiation levels (Table 3.3). These levels categorize exposure based on a range of effective doses and also consider that cancer risks associated with pediatric radiation exposures are higher than for adults.

TABLE 3.2 Typical Effective Dose From Radiographic Examinations

Examination	Median Effective Dose	Equivalent Background Exposure[a]
Intraoral[b]		
Rectangular collimation		
Posterior bitewings: PSP or F-speed film	5 μSv	0.6 day
Full-mouth: PSP or F-speed film	40 μSv	5 days
Full-mouth: CCD sensor (estimated)	20 μSv	2.5 days
Round collimation		
Full-mouth: D-speed film	400 μSv	48 days
Full-mouth: PSP or F-speed film	200 μSv	24 days
Full-mouth: CCD sensor (estimated)	100 μSv	12 days
Extraoral		
Panoramic[b]	20 μSv	2.5 days
Cephalometric[b]	5 μSv	0.6 day
Chest[c]	100 μSv	12 days
Cone beam CT[b]		
Limited field of view (<6 cm)	50 μSv	6 days
Maxillofacial field of view (one or both jaws)	100 μSv	12 days
Craniofacial field of view (both jaws with cranium)	120 μSv	15 days
Multidetector CT		
Maxillofacial[b]	650 μSv	2 months
Head[c]	2 mSv	8 months
Chest[c]	7 mSv	2 years
Abdomen and pelvis, with and without contrast[c]	20 mSv	7 years

[a]Approximate equivalent background exposure is calculated based on an estimated background radiation dose of 3.1 mSv/year. Exposures more than the equivalent of 3 days are rounded off to the nearest day, month, or year.
[b]Median dose from dentomaxillofacial radiography with typical exposure protocols is calculated from data collated from multiple published studies. Doses in the range of 10–1000 μSv are rounded off to the nearest multiple of 10.
[c]RadiologyInfo, American College of Radiology and Radiologic Society of North America, https://www.radiologyinfo.org/en/info/safety-xray
CCD, Charge-coupled device; *CT*, computed tomography; *PSP*, photostimulable phosphor.

Communicating Radiation Risks to Patients

Although most patients readily accept dental radiographs as part of their diagnosis, some may have anxiety about radiation exposure for themselves or members of their families, particularly their children. With all the discussion of radiation risks in the general media and the availability of information via the internet, it is completely reasonable that an individual may be concerned. It is important to speak clearly and confidently with your patients to address these concerns, even if they seem misplaced or irrational.

- Importantly, allow the patient to fully express their thoughts. Do not interrupt the patient's comments or belittle the patient's concerns. Acknowledge their concerns and indicate that you understand their apprehension.
- Inform the patient why you need radiographs as part of their personal diagnosis—such as the detection of interproximal caries, the extent of bone loss from periodontal disease suggested by probing, periapical infections suggested by pain, or any anticipated findings specific to the patient's condition that are important and can be attained only by radiologic investigation. Assure new patients that you will contact their previous dentist to obtain previous radiographs that may assist you in their diagnosis without unnecessarily re-exposing the patient.

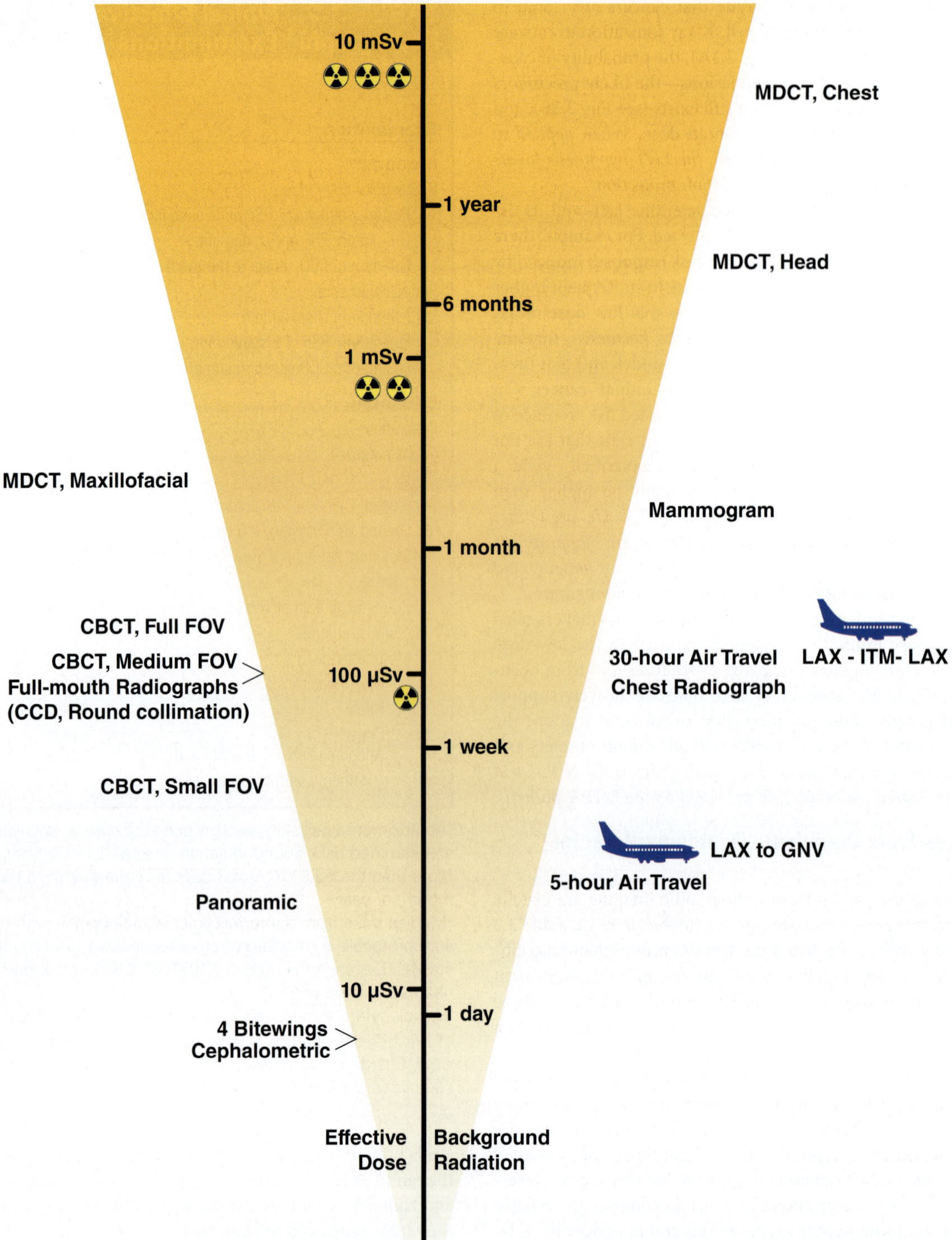

Fig. 3.4 Radiation doses from common dental and medical radiographic examinations. The *central axis* (log scale) shows the effective dose and the equivalent period of background radiation exposure. The radiation symbols adjacent to the dose identify the relative radiation level categories (see Table 3.3). *CBCT,* Cone beam computed tomography; *FOV,* field of view; *MDCT,* multidetector computed tomography.

TABLE 3.3 Relative Radiation Level Designations, American College of Radiology

Relative Radiation Level	Adult Effective Dose Range	Pediatric Effective Dose Range
☢	<100 μSv	<30 μSv
☢☢	100 μSv to 1 mSv	30–300 μSv
☢☢☢	1–10 mSv	300 μSv to 3 mSv
☢☢☢☢	10–30 mSv	3–10 mSv
☢☢☢☢☢	30–100 mSv	10–30 mSv

From ACR Appropriateness Criteria, Radiation Dose Assessment. https://www.acr.org/-/media/ACR/Files/Appropriateness-Criteria/RadiationDoseAssessmentIntro.pdf

- Emphasize that you will make only the exposures you specifically need for the patient's benefit guided by their symptoms and your clinical evaluation and not by a predetermined protocol (see Chapter 15).
- Educate and reassure the patient that you make consistent efforts to minimize their radiation dose by describing the many measures you take to reduce patient exposure. These may include using digital sensors or fast-speed film, rectangular collimation, and appropriate selection criteria.
- Convey the relative magnitude of the dose that the patient is likely to receive. Table 3.2 provides information on typical effective doses from dentomaxillofacial radiography. However, these doses are not easily comprehended by patients. Rather, convey the relative magnitude of the dose in terms of equivalent days, months, or years of natural background radiation (see Fig. 3.4). To help the patient place the risk in perspective, compare the magnitude of these risks with other sources of radiation exposure, such as an airline flight or other common imaging procedures. Note that dentomaxillofacial radiography delivers negligible to minimal doses, relative to other medical imaging procedures.

The provider-patient discussion should aim to address the patient's concerns and increase their confidence in the evidence-based care provided. Provided with the above information and assurances, most patients will appreciate your attention to their concerns and accept radiographic evaluation.

IMPLEMENTING RADIATION PROTECTION

Regulatory Agencies and Bodies

The International Commission on Radiological Protection (ICRP) is an independent, international organization that develops and disseminates recommendations and guidance on protection against ionizing radiation. Its recommendations are adopted or modified to establish radiation regulatory requirements in several countries worldwide. In the United States, the National Council on Radiation Protection and Measurements (NCRP), chartered by the US Congress, formulates guidance and recommendations on radiation protection and radiation measurements. The NCRP-recommended dose limits are incorporated into federal regulations (Title 10 of the Code of Federal Regulations, Part 20, Standards for protection against radiation). The current occupational exposure limits have been established to ensure that no individuals will have deterministic effects and that the probability for stochastic effects is as low as reasonably and economically feasible. Globally, it is important for dental personnel to be familiar with regulations and recommendations from their local and national radiation protection agencies.

Guiding Principles

There are three guiding principles in radiation protection:

1. Justification
2. Optimization
3. Dose limitation

The principle of **justification** means the dentist should identify situations where the benefit to a patient from the diagnostic exposure likely exceeds the risk of harm. In practice, this principle influences which patients are selected for radiographic examinations and what examinations are chosen. These matters are considered in Chapter 15.

The principle of **optimization** holds that dentists should use every reasonable means to reduce unnecessary exposure to their patients, their staff, and themselves. This philosophy of radiation protection is often referred to as the principle of ALARA (*a*s *l*ow *a*s *r*easonably *a*chievable). ALARA holds that exposures to ionizing radiation should be kept as low as reasonably achievable, with economic and social factors being taken into account. The means to accomplish this end are considered by dentists every day in their practices and are discussed later in this chapter (Box 3.1).

The principle of **dose limitation** provides dose limits for occupational and public exposures to ensure that no individuals are exposed to unacceptably high doses. This principle applies to dentists and their staff who are exposed occupationally but not to patients because there are no dose limits for individuals exposed for diagnostic purposes. Many of the steps described in the following sections that optimize exposures of the patient also reduce exposure to dentists and their staff.

BOX 3.1 Means for Reducing X-Ray Exposure

Use Good Clinical Judgment and Apply Evidence-Based Imaging Guidelines

- Make radiographs when they are likely to contribute to diagnosis and treatment planning
- Use selection criteria to assist in determining type and frequency of radiographic examinations

Use Best Practices in Radiographic Imaging

- Optimize your exposure settings to the patient's size and anatomic area to be imaged
- Intraoral radiography
  - Use E/F-speed film or digital sensors
  - Use holders to support film or digital sensors
  - Use rectangular collimation
  - Make exposures with 60–70 kVp
- Panoramic radiography
  - Use rare-earth screens for film imaging or use digital systems
- Cephalometric radiography
  - Use rare-earth screens for film imaging or use digital systems
- Cone beam computed tomography
  - Restrict the field of view to cover the region of interest only.
- Film-based imaging
  - Use time-temperature processing rather than "sight" processing, or use an automatic processor

Use Best Practices in Personnel Protection

- Stand behind a protective barrier or at least 6 feet (2 m) away from the patient and away from the x-ray machine when making an exposure
- For handheld devices, ensure the protective backscatter shield is in place and correctly positioned

The dentist in each facility is responsible for the design and conduct of the radiation protection program. In this section, methods of exposure and dose reduction are described that can be used in dental radiography. All methods that reduce exposure to patients also reduce exposure to the dental staff and usually improve the quality of the radiographs made.

Patient Protection

Patient Selection Criteria

Before conducting any type of radiographic examination, clinicians should complete a comprehensive clinical examination and patient assessment, with consideration of the patient's oral and medical histories, including previous radiographs, as well as the patient's specific oral disease risk[1].

The most effective approach to reduce unnecessary exposure is to reduce unnecessary radiographic examinations. Radiographs should be made only when they are likely to provide additional information that is likely to contribute to the diagnosis and treatment plan. The ADA has published radiographic selection criteria—clinical or historical findings that identify patients for whom a high probability exists that a radiographic examination would provide information affecting their treatment or prognosis. These criteria satisfy the principle of justification and are considered in Chapter 15.

When a decision is made to obtain a radiograph, the dentist should obtain the lowest dose image that would provide the necessary diagnostic information. Table 3.2 shows that there is a wide range of patient exposures from various dental examinations.

Conducting the Examination

When the dentist has determined that a radiographic examination is justified (using patient selection criteria), the specific radiographic protocol or the principle of optimization greatly influences patient exposure to radiation. Considerations for designing an optimal radiographic study include choice of imaging modality and equipment, choice of exposure settings, operation of equipment, and processing and interpreting the radiographic image.

Film and Digital Imaging

Digital rather than film-based imaging should be used because digital imaging allows for lower patient radiation exposure. If conventional film is used, only E-speed or F-speed film shall be used because they require substantially lower patient radiation exposure compared to D-speed film. D-speed film shall be eliminated from clinical use[1].

Intraoral dental x-ray film is available in two speed groups: D and E/F (see Chapter 4). Clinically, film of speed group E/F is approximately twice as fast (sensitive) as film of group D and thus requires only half the exposure (see Fig. 4.56). Fast films are effective for exposure reduction. Multiple studies have found that E/F-speed film provides the same useful density range, latitude, contrast, and image quality as D-speed films without sacrificing diagnostic information such that NCRP 177 (2019) recommended that image receptors of speeds slower than ANSI Speed Group E/F (i.e., speed group D) shall no longer be used for intraoral radiography. Current digital sensors (see Chapter 4) offer equal or greater dose savings than E/F-speed film and comparable diagnostic utility.

Intensifying Screens and Film

If film is used for panoramic or cephalometric imaging, rare-earth screens and high-speed film of 400 are recommended.

Contemporary intensifying screens used in extraoral radiography use the rare-earth elements gadolinium and lanthanum (see Chapter 4). Compared to the older calcium tungstate screens, rare-earth screens are more efficient in converting x-ray photons to light and decrease patient exposure by 50% in panoramic and cephalometric radiography.

Film-based panoramic and cephalometric imaging is being replaced with imaging using storage phosphors or charge-coupled device (CCD) sensors. However, unlike with intraoral radiography, dose reduction with these digital technologies is minimal.

Source-to-Skin Distance

Use of long source-to-skin distances of 40 cm, rather than short distances of 20 cm, decreases exposure by 10%–25% (ADA, 2006). The intraoral x-ray system shall be configured so that the distance from the x-ray tube focal spot to the skin entrance surface (source-to-skin distance) is not less than 20 cm[1].

Three standard focal source-to-skin distances have evolved over the years for use in intraoral radiography—20 cm (8 inches), 30 cm (12 inches), and 40 cm (16 inches). With a longer source-to-skin distance, the x-ray beam is less divergent, reducing the exposed tissue volume (Fig. 3.5). The use of a longer source-to-object distance also decreases image magnification (see Fig. 5.3).

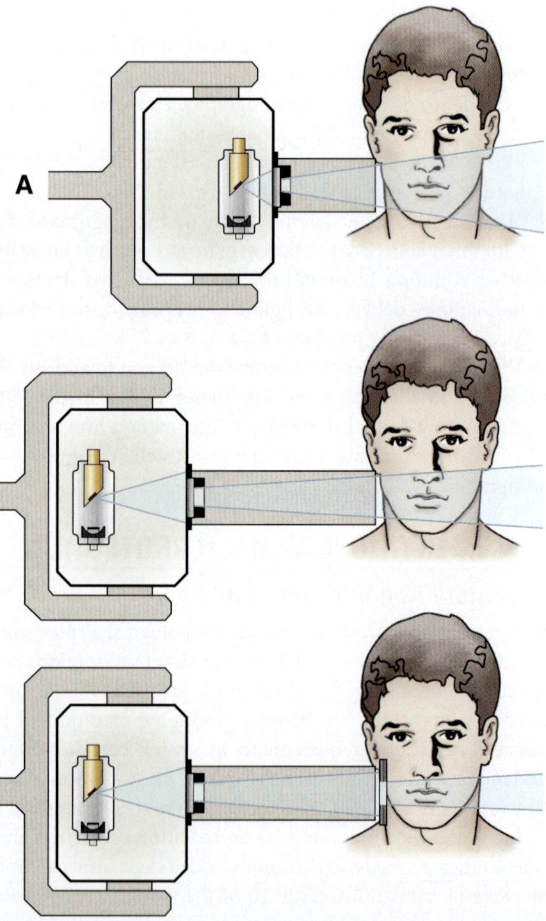

Fig. 3.5 Effect of source-to-skin distance and collimation on the volume of tissue irradiated. A larger volume of irradiated tissue results with the use of a short source-to-skin distance (A) compared to the use of a longer source-to-skin distance (B), which produces a less divergent beam. Using a rectangular collimator between the round position-indicating device and the patient (C) results in a smaller, less divergent beam and a smaller volume of tissue irradiated than in A or B.

Rectangular Collimation

Since a rectangular collimator decreases the radiation dose by up to fivefold as compared to a circular one, radiographic equipment should provide rectangular collimation for exposure of periapical and bitewing radiographs and occlusal radiographs when using a No. 2 receptor in children (ADA, 2012; NCRP, 2019). Use rectangular collimation whenever possible for intraoral imaging[1].

In the United States, the Code of Federal Regulations (21 CFR 1020) and most state regulations require that the x-ray beam used in intraoral radiography be collimated so that the field of radiation at the patient's skin surface is no more than 7 cm (2.75 inches) in diameter. The area of this circular field size is almost three times larger than the area of No. 2 intraoral film (3.2 cm × 4.1 cm) or digital sensor. Consequently, further limiting the size of the x-ray beam to the size of the image receptor significantly reduces unnecessary patient exposure. If the tissue volume exposed is decreased, the amount of scattered radiation is decreased, image fogging is decreased, and the resultant image has improved diagnostic quality. Rectangular collimation reduces the area of the patient's skin surface exposed by 60% over that of a round collimated (7-cm diameter) beam (Fig. 3.6A).

There are several means to limit the size of the x-ray beam. A simple approach is to use a rectangular collimator assembled onto the receptor holder (see Fig. 3.6B). This device can be used without modifying the round aiming cylinder of the x-ray tube. Some rectangular collimation devices are designed to attach to the aiming cylinder of the radiographic unit.

Filtration

The x-ray beam emitted from the radiographic tube consists of a spectrum of x-ray photons. Low-energy photons, which have little penetrating power, are absorbed mainly by the patient and do not contribute to the information on the image. The purpose of filtration is to preferentially remove these low-energy x-ray photons from the x-ray beam (see Chapter 1, Fig. 1.18). Filtration results in decreased patient exposure with no loss of radiographic information.

When an x-ray beam is filtered with 3 mm of aluminum, the surface exposure is reduced to approximately 20% of the exposure with no filtration. Federal regulations in the United States require the total filtration in the path of a dental x-ray beam to be equal to the equivalent of 1.5 mm of aluminum for a machine operating at 50–70 kVp and 2.5 mm of aluminum for machines operating at higher voltages.

Gonad Shielding

The ADA, American Academy of Oral and Maxillofacial Radiology, and the American Association of Physicists in Medicine recommend that patient gonadal and fetal shielding during diagnostic intraoral, panoramic, cephalometric, and cone beam computed tomography (CBCT) be discontinued.

Gonadal shielding is a long-standing practice during radiographic imaging in general and is currently mandated by law in many US states. In the early 1950s, lead aprons were recommended to limit exposure of the gonads to reduce the risk of radiation-induced heritable effects. Since then our understanding of radiation-induced heritable effects in humans has evolved. Studies of progeny of the atomic bomb survivors show no evidence of any disease associated with maternal or paternal radiation exposure, and it is well accepted that there is no evidence of radiation-induced heritable effects in humans. In the absence of any risk, there is no rationale to shield the gonads from radiation during diagnostic radiography.

Many states in the United States currently mandate the use of protective aprons and thyroid shielding. Compliance with state and local authority regulations is recommended until the regulations have been updated.

Thyroid Collars

The ADA and American Academy of Oral and Maxillofacial Radiology consider that risks from thyroid cancer are negligible with contemporaneous dentomaxillofacial imaging and recommend that thyroid shielding be discontinued during intraoral, panoramic, cephalometric, and CBCT imaging.

The thyroid gland is susceptible to radiation exposure during dental radiographic exams, given its anatomic position. Thyroid shielding seeks to reduce the risk of radiation-induced thyroid cancer—a risk corroborated by classic and contemporary evidence. Radiation exposure is a strong risk factor of benign and malignant tumors of the

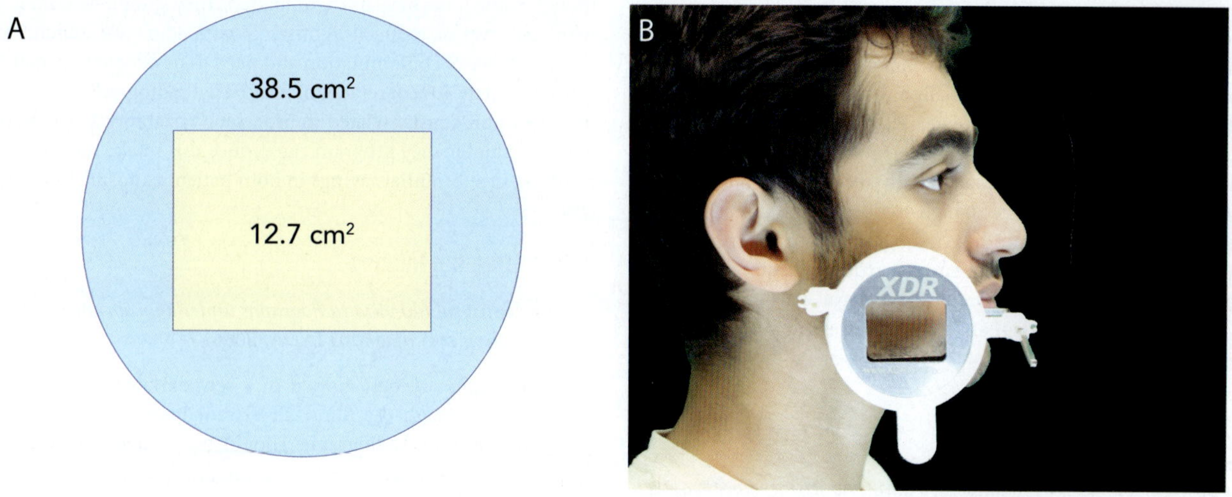

Fig. 3.6 Rectangular collimation. (A) Graphical representation of the surface areas of round collimation (7-cm diameter) and rectangular collimation (size 2 receptor). The rectangular collimated area is approximately 66% less than the round collimation field. (B) The XDR collimator, a metallic shield placed in the path of the beam limits the size of the exposure field to an area just larger than the film or sensor.

thyroid gland, particularly in the pediatric population. Multiple studies, including studies performed after the explosion of the Chernobyl reactor, have shown that the thyroid gland in children is highly sensitive to radiation-induced cancer. In consideration of dental imaging, the thyroid gland is exposed via the primary beam and internal scatter radiation. Shielding does not protect against internal scatter radiation, and it was found that compliance with other guiding principles of radiation safety in particular, rectangular collimation decreases thyroid dose from the primary beam by 50%. Thus if correct emphasis is placed on collimation, selection criteria, appropriate receptors, and other principles of radiation safety, then the overall exposure from dental imaging has negligible effects on thyroid carcinogenesis. In fact, thyroid shields may cause artifacts that degrade image quality and require retakes.

Film and Sensor Holders

Receptor holders that align the receptor precisely with the collimated beam are recommended for periapical and bitewing radiographs (ADA, 2006; NCRP, 2019).

Film or digital receptor holders should be used when intraoral radiographs are made because they improve the alignment of the film, or digital sensor, with teeth and the x-ray machine. The use of film and sensor holders allows the operator to control the position and alignment of the film or sensor with respect to the teeth and jaws. Their use results in a significant reduction in unacceptable images and thus avoidable retakes. This is especially important when used with the paralleling technique (see Chapter 6). In these cases, it is often desirable to position the receptor away from the teeth so as to get the best image and reduce patient discomfort. This requires the use of a film or sensor holder. Most of these devices have an external guide that shows the operator where to align the aiming cylinder. As a result, the x-ray beam is properly directed toward the receptors; this greatly reduces the chance of the beam partially missing the image receptor (a "cone-cut") and reduces image distortion (see Chapter 6). As discussed earlier, many film holder assemblies include a collimator to restrict the beam to the size of the image receptor.

Kilovoltage

Intraoral x-ray units should be operated at a minimum of 60 kV and not exceed 80 kV[1].

Kilovoltage (kVp) influences image contrast and patient dose. At lower kVp, the patient radiation dose is increased, but the image contrast is increased, which could potentially enhance diagnosis. At higher kVp, the patient radiation dose is decreased, but the image contrast is also decreased. Most intraoral x-ray units operate at 60–70 kVp, which provides adequate diagnostic quality with reduced radiation dose. Constant-potential (fully rectified), high-frequency, and direct current (DC) dental x-ray units can produce radiographs with lower kVp and at reduced levels of radiation. The surface exposure required to produce a comparable radiographic density using a constant-potential unit is approximately 25% less than that of a conventional self-rectified unit operating at the same kVp. Currently, several manufacturers produce DC units.

Milliampere-Seconds

The operator should set the amperage and time settings for exposure of dental radiographs of optimal quality (ADA, 2006).

Of the three settings on an x-ray machine (tube voltage, milliamperage, and exposure time), exposure time is the most crucial factor in influencing diagnostic quality. In terms of exposure, optimal image quality means that the radiograph is of diagnostic density, neither overexposed (too dark) nor underexposed (too light). Both overexposed and underexposed radiographs result in repeat exposures, leading to needless additional patient exposure. Image density is controlled by the quantity of x-rays produced, which is best controlled by the combination of milliamperage and exposure time, termed milliampere-seconds (see Chapter 1). Typically, a radiograph of correct density demonstrates very faint soft tissue outlines, and a gray scale that adequately distinguishes enamel, dentin, cortical bone, and trabecular bone. If the x-ray machine has a variable milliampere control, it should be set at the highest mA setting. Proper exposure times should be determined empirically when using optimal film processing conditions (see Chapter 4) or manufacturer's recommendations for digital sensors. A chart showing optimal exposure times for each region of the arch in children and adults should be mounted by each x-ray machine. As film-processing conditions are standardized and the mA and kVp settings are fixed, the only decision the dentist or the assistant needs to make is to select the proper exposure time for the age of the patient (less for young patients) and the region of the mouth being imaged (less in the anterior region).

Film Processing

All film should be processed following the film and processor manufacturer recommendations. Poor processing technique, including sight-developing, most often results in underdeveloped films, forcing the x-ray operator to increase the dose to compensate, resulting in patient and personnel being exposed to unnecessary radiation (ADA, 2012).

A major cause of unnecessary patient exposure is the practice of overexposing films and compensating by underdevelopment. This procedure results in both unnecessary exposure of the patient and films that are of inferior diagnostic quality because of incomplete development. Time-temperature processing is the best way to ensure optimal film quality (see Chapter 4). To help ensure optimal image quality, the dental assistant should follow the film manufacturer's recommendation for processing solutions.

The use of automatic film processing machines has become widespread, with more than 90% of dentists using such processors. Although some units have daylight loaders, they should be used in rooms with low-level or reduced lighting. Such loaders are difficult to keep clean and free of contamination and need to be adequately maintained. Approximately 30% of retakes of film-based radiographs are because of incorrect film density related to processor variability. Using a comprehensive maintenance program can reduce this retake rate significantly, resulting in substantial savings in both patient exposure and operating costs.

Interpreting the Images

The dentist should view radiographs under appropriate conditions for analysis and diagnosis (ADA, 2006).

Radiographs are best viewed in a semidarkened room with light transmitted through the films; all extraneous light should be eliminated. In addition, radiographs should be studied with the aid of a magnifying glass to detect even the smallest change in image density. Similarly, digital images are best interpreted on a computer screen in a darkened environment. Software features such as density, contrast enhancement, and magnification are useful for viewing all features of the radiographic image.

Personnel Protection

The dental practice shall develop and implement a radiation safety program that provides all staff with instructions and guidance for maintaining a safe x-ray imaging program. The program should be consistent with nationally established recommendations for the radiation protection of both patients and staff and adhere to all applicable state and local requirements, be developed and implemented under the guidance of a qualified expert, and should be regularly reviewed and updated to be current with applicable established guidance and regulations[1].

Dentists and their staff who operate radiographic equipment are occupationally exposed to radiation. This includes potential exposure from the primary beam and scattered radiation. Personnel must follow appropriate procedures to reduce the chance of occupational exposure.

Barriers

When barrier protection or shielding is not available for intraoral imaging, the operator shall stand at least 2 m from the tube head and out of the primary beam path[1].

Dentists should consult with a qualified expert to design and construct dental offices and clinics to meet the radiation shielding requirements specified by their state and national regulations. Primary barriers such as walls or mobile lead barriers provide the most effective method to protect the operator from primary and scattered radiation. The exposure switch should be located behind this barrier. The barrier should have a leaded window and allow the operator to maintain visual and verbal contact with the patient during the exposure.

If the office design does not permit the operator to leave the room or use an appropriate barrier, then strict adherence to the position-and-distance rule is required. The operator should stand at least 6 feet (2 m) from the patient, at an angle of 90–135 degrees to the central ray of the x-ray beam (Fig. 3.7). When applied, this rule not only takes advantage of the inverse square law to reduce x-ray exposure to the operator but also takes advantage of the fact that in this position the patient's head absorbs most scatter radiation. All practitioners should check their state's regulations for use of ionizing radiation regarding operator position during x-ray exposures. The operator should never hold films or sensors in place. Film or sensor-holding instruments should be used (see earlier section on rectangular collimation). If correct film placement and retention are still not possible, a parent or other individual responsible for the patient should be asked to hold the sensor in place rather than the dental radiographic personnel. Under no circumstances should this person be one of the office staff. The operator or the patient should not hold the radiographic tube housing during the exposure, except for specifically designed handheld intraoral radiographic units. Suspension arms should be adequately maintained to prevent housing movement and drift.

In addition to shielding the operator, radiation regulations also specify requirements for shielding of the walls to minimize radiation dose to non–occupationally exposed individuals (e.g., the office receptionist in the adjacent office). The NCRP recommendation states that walls must be of sufficient density or thickness so that the exposure to these non–occupationally exposed individuals is less than 0.02 mGy/week (1 mGy/year). In most instances, it is not necessary to line the walls with lead to meet this requirement. Walls constructed of gypsum wallboard (drywall or sheetrock), brick, or concrete are adequate for the average dental office.

Handheld Radiographic Devices

Handheld x-ray devices for intraoral imaging must be FDA cleared, used according to manufacturer's instructions, and restricted to use only by authorized operators with appropriate training in device use[1].

The use of handheld portable x-ray units for intraoral radiography requires special consideration. These battery-operated devices are designed to be held by the operator during use. The inherent design of the device offers primary protective shielding; however, to minimize exposure to the operator, secondary protective shielding is offered in the form of a backscatter shield. This is incorporated into the device at the end of the collimator ring and provides an operator protective zone, where scattered radiation is negligible. Importantly, the operator protective zone is directly associated with the positioning of the device and backscatter shield. For optimal operator protection, the device must be held in a horizontal position, oriented perpendicular to the operator, and with the backscatter shield placed close to the patient and parallel to the operator (Fig. 3.8A and B).

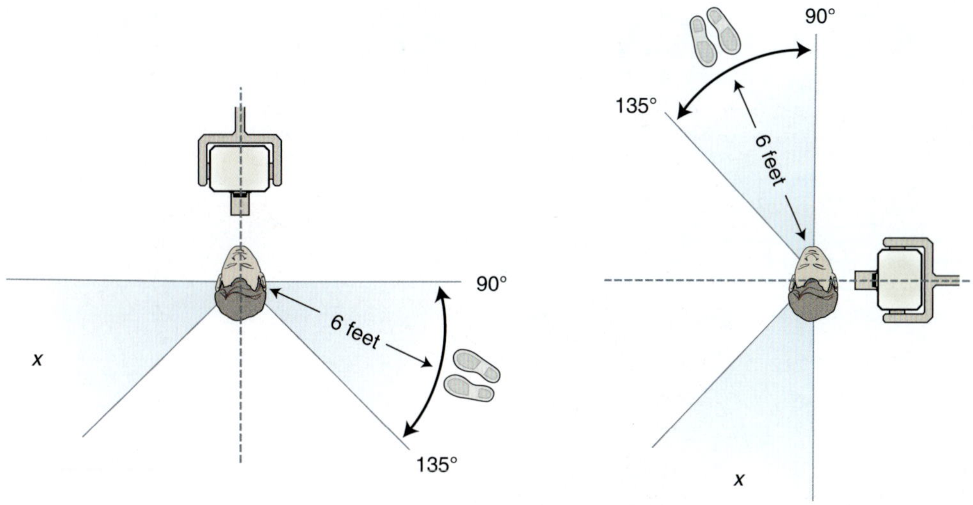

Fig. 3.7 Position-and-distance rule. The operator may be exposed from leakage radiation from the x-ray tube head, scattered radiation from the patient, and primary photons passing through the patient. If no barrier is available, the operator should stand at least 6 feet from the patient, at an angle of 90–135 degrees, to the central ray of the x-ray beam when the exposure is made because this region receives the least overall exposure.

Angling of the device changes the zone of protection and can expose the operator to scatter radiation. The protective zone also decreases when the shield is not positioned at the outer edge of the cone. In these situations, it may be necessary for the patient to angle their head instead and to use device positioning kits that do not require the shield to be slid back. In the United States, handheld devices have been approved for use by the Food and Drug Administration. Some states have additional regulatory requirements related to dose monitoring or personnel protective equipment that must be worn by the operators of these devices.

Personnel Monitoring Devices

The ADA and NCRP recommend that personal dose monitoring should be considered for radiation workers who are likely to receive an annual effective dose greater than 1 mSv. Personal dosimeters shall be provided for pregnant occupationally exposed personnel, and occupational exposure should be limited to 0.5 mSv/month once pregnancy is declared (NCRP 177, 2019)[1].

Personnel-monitoring devices provide a means to measure the operator's occupational radiation dose and are used to ensure that staff

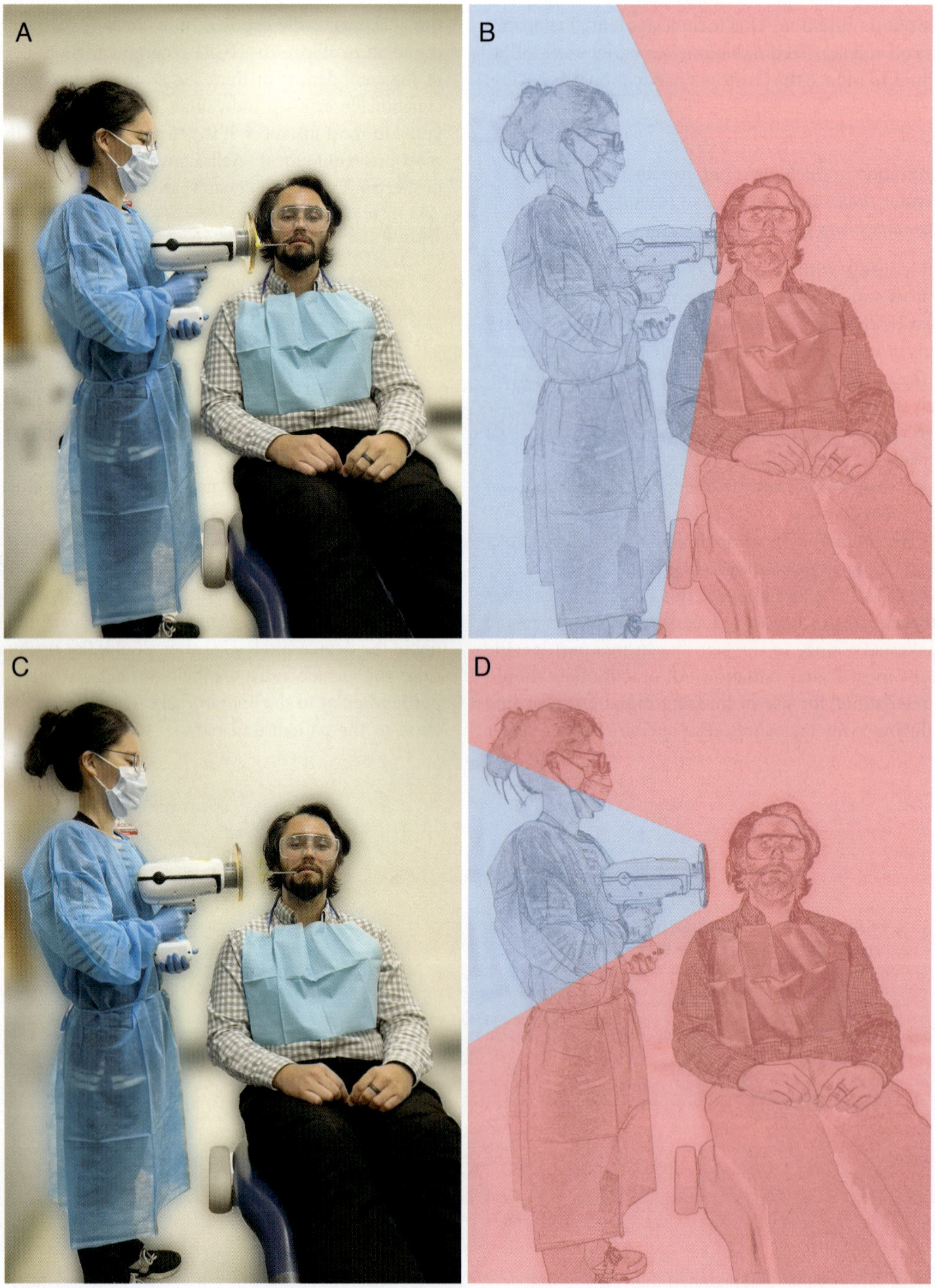

Fig. 3.8 Safe operation of handheld dental x-ray devices. The regions shaded in blue represent the area where scatter radiation is blocked by the shield. (A and B) Proper operation. The device is held horizontal with the collimator ring placed close to the patient's skin surface. (C and D) Improper handling. The device is held back away from the patient.

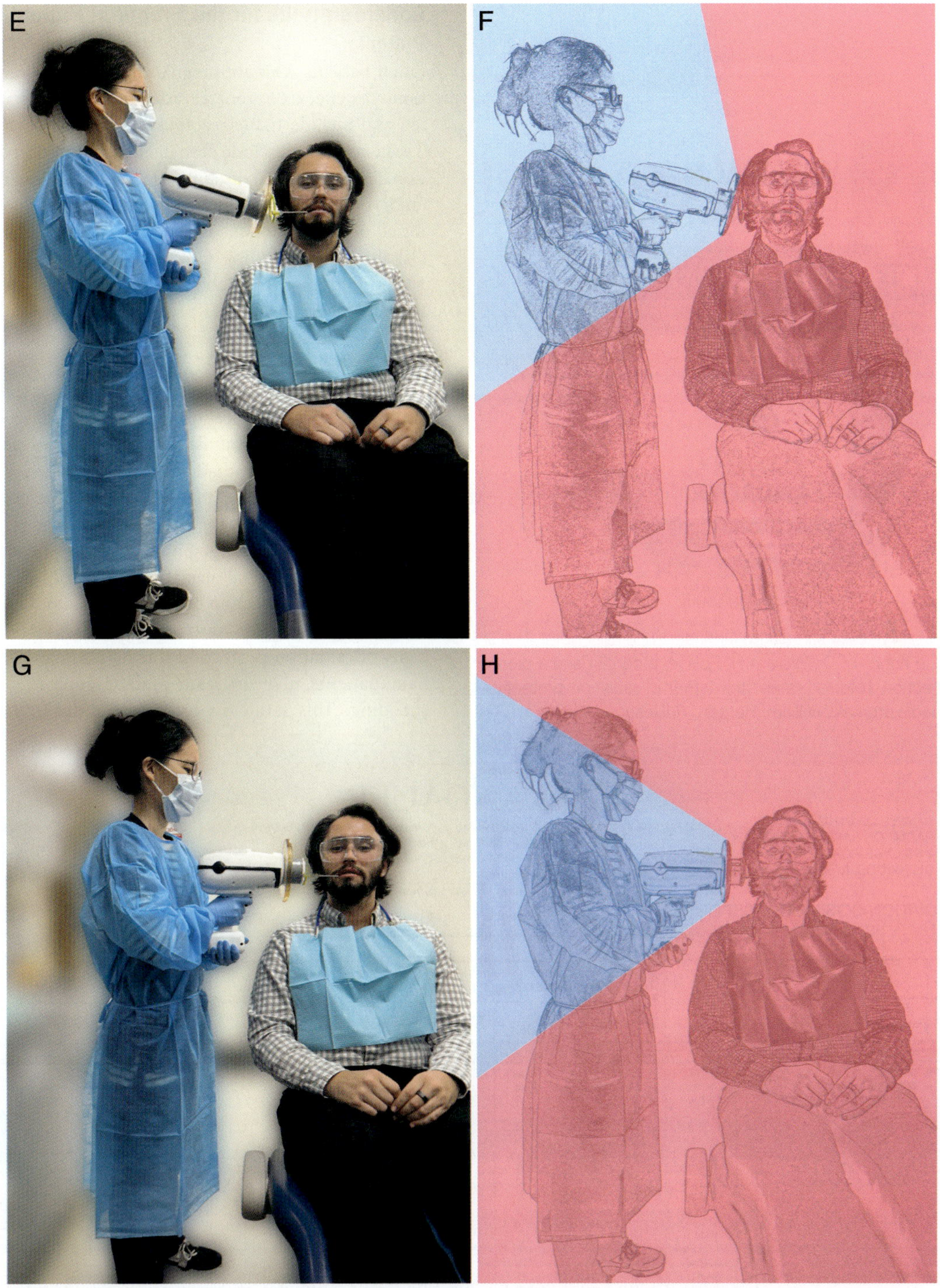

Fig. 3.8, cont'd (E and F) Improper handling. The device is held at an angle and the shield is not vertical. (G and H) Improper handling. The protective shield is slid back from the edge of the collimator ring.

consistently follow office radiation safety rules such as those described previously. Assuming optimal radiation safety procedures are used, most dental workers are not exposed to the occupation limits. However, the requirement to use personnel dosimeters is specified by state and national regulations. In the United States, the code of federal regulations requires that personnel likely to receive more than 10% of the annual dose limit be monitored.

Several companies in the United States offer dosimetry-monitoring services. The monitoring devices are worn clipped to clothing on the front of the chest. A widely used technology for personnel monitoring is the optically stimulated luminescent dosimeter (OSLD). The device consists of a strip of crystalline aluminum oxide (Al_2O_3:C) that luminesces in proportion to the amount of radiation exposure (Fig. 3.9). The device is sent to a service, typically at monthly intervals, where the accumulated dose is measured and reported back to the dental clinic (Fig. 3.10). Another technology for personnel monitoring is based on direct ion storage. The device incorporates the dosimeter with a USB interface allowing the end user to directly perform the dose reading via the internet. In contrast to previously used pocket ionization chambers, this device provides the advantage of immediate readings without loss of data after reading. Both OSLD and direct ion storage devices are sensitive to a dose as low as 10 μSv of x-rays.

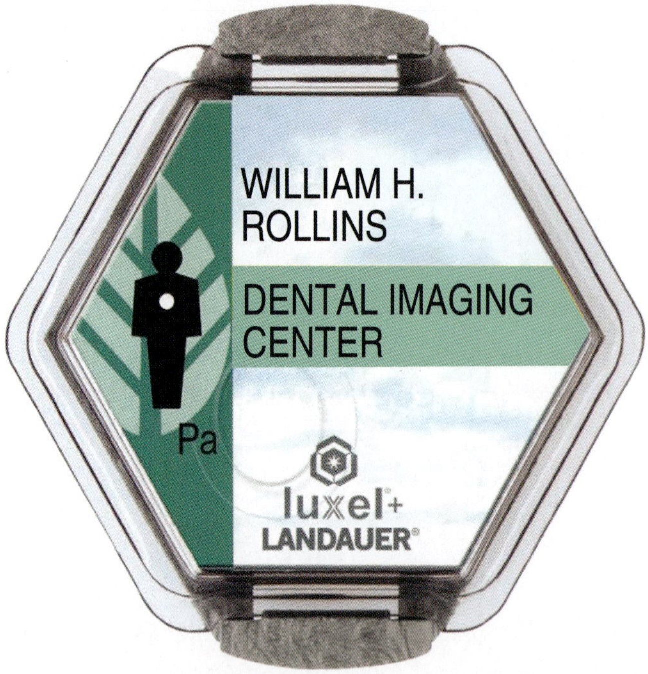

Fig. 3.9 A personal optically stimulated luminescence dosimeter. The image is modified in honor of Dr. William H. Rollins, a dentist and a pioneer in radiation protection, referred to as "the father of radiation protection." (https://en.wikipedia.org/wiki/William_Herbert_Rollins.)

Considerations for the Pregnant Patient/Personnel

Patients

Often patients who are pregnant may require radiographic examination. The effects of prenatal radiation exposure have been widely studied and include tissue reactions as well as radiation-induced cancer. Tissue reactions include prenatal death, microcephaly, growth retardation, and intellectual disability, depending on radiation exposure of the embryo/fetus during different periods of gestation. The threshold dose for all of these reactions is 100 mGy. Fetal dose from dentomaxillofacial imaging, including CBCT, is estimated at 0.01 mGy, which is 10,000-fold lower than the threshold dose. Radiation-induced cancer in utero, based on the LNT model, is not observed with doses less than 10 mGy. Thus diagnostic imaging of a pregnant patient poses no risk to the embryo/fetus.

Lead aprons do not protect the fetus from internal scatter radiation, and the relative radiation dose to the fetus during dentomaxillofacial imaging has been diminished to negligible levels. Importantly, the other measures of radiation protection such as selection criteria, appropriate receptors, and collimation must be strictly adhered to. Additionally, in alignment with the American College of Radiology's practice parameter of imaging pregnant patients, since the primary beam from dentomaxillofacial imaging does not directly expose the embryo/fetus, verification of pregnancy status is no longer required.

These changes are contradictory to previous well-accepted concepts of radiation protection during pregnancy. Undoubtedly, pregnant patients may question and be concerned about the lack of shielding. This is an opportunity for the oral healthcare team to

LANDAUER®

SAMPLE ORGANIZATION
RADIATION SAFETY OFFICER
2 SCIENCE ROAD
GLENWOOD, IL 60425

Landauer, Inc. 2 Science Road Glenwood, Illinois 60425-1586
Telephone: (708) 755-7000 Facsimile: (708) 755-7016
www.landauerinc.com

luxel®

RADIATION DOSIMETRY REPORT

ACCOUNT NO.	SERIES CODE	ANALYTICAL WORK ORDER	REPORT DATE	DOSIMETER RECEIVED	REPORT TIME IN WORK DAYS	PAGE NO.
103702	RAD	992150087	06/13/03	06/09/03	4	1

PARTICIPANT NUMBER	NAME / ID NUMBER, BIRTH DATE, SEX	DOSIMETER	USE	RADIATION QUALITY	DOSE EQUIVALENT (MREM) FOR PERIODS SHOWN BELOW			YEAR TO DATE DOSE EQUIVALENT (MREM)			LIFETIME DOSE EQUIVALENT (MREM)			RECORDS FOR YEAR	INCEPTION DATE (MM/YY)
					DEEP DDE	EYE LDE	SHALLOW SDE	DEEP DDE	EYE LDE	SHALLOW SDE	DEEP DDE	EYE LDE	SHALLOW SDE		
FOR MONITORING PERIOD:					05/01/03 - 05/31/03			2003							
0000H	CONTROL	J	CNTRL		M	M	M							5	07/97
	CONTROL	P	CNTRL		M	M	M								07/97
	CONTROL	U	CNTRL				M								07/97
00189	ADAMS, HEATHER 336235619 08/31/1968 F	P	WHBODY		M	M	M	9	10	12	29	31	42	5	07/01
00191	ADDISON, JOHN 471563287 10/04/1968 M	J	WHBODY	PN	90	90	90	100	100	100	200	200	200	5	07/01
				P	60	60	60	70	70	70	170	170	170		
				NF	30	30	30	30	30	30	30	30	30		
00202	HARRIS, KATHY 587582144 06/09/1960 F	P	WHBODY		M	M	M	M	M	M	M	M	M	5	02/02
		U	RFINGR				M			30			30		02/02
00005	MEYER, STEVE 982778955 07/15/1964 M	P	COLLAR	PL	119	119	113							5	08/97
		P	WAIST	P	10	11	11								08/97
			ASSIGN		19	119	113	33	185	174	1387	2308	2320		
			NOTE		ASSIGNED DOSE BASED ON EDE 1 CALCULATION										
		U	RFINGR				140			690			2180		08/97
00203	STEVENS, LEE 335478977 08/25/1951 M	P	WHBODY		ABSENT			M	M	M	M	M	M	4	07/02
		U	RFINGR		ABSENT					M			M		07/02
00204	WALKER, JANE 416995421 03/21/1947 F	P	WHBODY		3	3	3	12	11	11	22	21	21	5	11/02
00188	WEBSTER, ROBERT 355381469 05/15/1972 M	P	WHBODY		40	40	40	200	200	200	240	240	240	5	07/01
			NOTE		CALCULATED										

M: MINIMAL REPORTING SERVICE OF 1 MREM
ELECTRONIC MEDIA TO FOLLOW THIS REPORT

QUALITY CONTROL RELEASE: LMR   1 - PR 6774 - PT131 - N1   -21587

NVLAP®
NVLAP LAB CODE 100518-0**

Fig. 3.10 Sample radiation dosimetry report showing exposure received by various individuals during the month reported as well as the type of dosimeter, its location, and the dose distribution. The report also shows totals for the year-to-date and lifetime exposure. (Courtesy Landauer, Inc., Glenwood, IL.)

effectively communicate the absence of substantial risk and lack of benefit from such shielding. Emphasize that the diagnostic and treatment planning benefits are crucial to maintain oral health and that dental disease and its sequelae could have an adverse impact on the health of the unborn child. The provider-patient discussion should aim to address the patient's concerns and increase their confidence in the evidence-based care provided.

Personnel

The US Code of Federal Regulations requires that pregnant personnel be monitored if the dose to the embryo and fetus is likely to exceed 1 mSv during the entire period of pregnancy. Personnel monitoring is an effective approach to identify undesirable change in work habits and help to respond to office staff members who may be apprehensive about the risks from occupational radiation exposure (see Box 3.2).

Dose Limits

Recognizing the harmful effects of radiation and the potential risks involved with its use, several national, regional, and international organizations previously described established guidelines for limits on the amount of radiation received by occupationally exposed individuals and by the public (Table 3.4). These limits pertain to planned exposure situations, not to background radiation, and do not include radiation received for diagnostic or therapeutic purposes. Since their initial establishment in the 1930s, these dose limits have been revised downward several times, adapting to new knowledge on the harmful effects of radiation and the increased ability to use radiation more efficiently.

Occupational dose limits: Dentists and their staff who make diagnostic radiographs are considered as occupationally exposed individuals and thus should be familiar with regulatory dose limits in their region or country. The ICRP-established dose limit for occupationally exposed individuals is 20 mSv of whole-body radiation exposure. Although this level of exposure is considered to present only a minimal risk, every effort should be made to keep the radiation dose to all individuals as low as practical. The dental profession does well in limiting occupational exposure. The average dose for individuals occupationally exposed in the operation of dental x-ray equipment is 0.2 mSv—1% of the allowable dose limit. The section on protection of personnel describes approaches to minimize radiation dose to occupationally exposed staff.

Public dose limits: Support staff members (e.g., receptionists and auxiliary staff who do not perform radiography) and patients are subject to dose limits for members of the general public. The recommended limits for exposure to the public do not include natural background radiation and radiation received for individual medical and dental care. There are no limits on the exposure a patient can receive from diagnostic examinations, interventional procedures, or radiation therapy; this is because these exposures are made intentionally for the direct benefit of the recipient. Individual circumstances make the setting of limits inappropriate.

TABLE 3.4 Recommended Dose Limits for Human Exposure to Ionizing Radiation

	NCRP[a]	ICRP[b]
Occupational Exposure		
Annual effective dose	50 mSv/year	20 mSv, averaged over defined 5-year periods
Cumulative effective dose	10 mSv × age	100 mSv in 5 years *and* should not exceed 50 mSv[c] in any single year
Annual equivalent dose		
Lens of eye	Absorbed dose of 50 mGy	20 mSv, averaged over defined 5-year periods, *and* exposure in any single year should not exceed 50 mSv
Skin, hands, and feet	500 mSv	500 mSv
Pregnant workers	0.5 mSv/month to embryo/fetus	1 mSv to the embryo/fetus after declaration of pregnancy
Public Exposure[d]		
Annual effective dose	1 mSv (continuous or frequent exposure) 5 mSv (infrequent exposure)	1 mSv
Annual equivalent dose in:		
Lens of eye	15 mSv	15 mSv
Skin	50 mSv	50 mSv

[a]Recommendations from the National Council on Radiation Protection and Measurement. Report No. 116, Limitation of exposure to ionizing radiation, 1993. NCRP Commentary No. 26, Guidance on radiation dose limits for the lens of the eye, 2016.
[b]Recommendations of the International Commission on Radiological Protection. IRCP Publication 103. *Ann ICRP.* 2007;37:1-332. ICRP Statement on Tissue Reactions and Early and Late Effects of Radiation in Normal Tissues and Organs—Threshold Doses for Tissue Reactions in a Radiation Protection Context. ICRP Publication 118. *Ann ICRP.* 2012;41:1-322.
[c]The Atomic Energy Regulatory Board, Government of India, has set a lower dose limit of 30 mSv in any single year.
[d]Dose limits for public exposure do not include exposure from diagnostic or therapeutic radiation.
ICRP, The International Commission on Radiological Protection; *NCRP*, The National Council on Radiation Protection and Measurements.

BOX 3.2 Considerations for the Pregnant Patient/Personnel

Identify Risk

	Threshold Dose	Risk From Oral and Maxillofacial Imaging
Tissue Reaction	100 mGy	None, fetal dose is approximately 10,000-fold lower than threshold
Prenatal death		
Microcephaly		
Growth retardation		
Intellectual disability		
Stochastic Effect	In utero, not observed <10 mGy	Negligible, approximately 1 in 1.7 million
Radiation-induced cancer		

Recommendations for Pregnant Patients

- Lead aprons are no longer required due to negligible doses to the embryo/fetus during dentomaxillofacial radiology. The dosage that is received is from internal scatter radiation, and a lead apron does not offer protection against this.
- Verification of pregnancy status no longer required.
- All guiding principles of radiation protection and patient dose reduction measures must be strictly adhered to.

Recommendations in Pregnant Personnel

- US Code of Federal Regulations requires monitoring if the dose to the embryo/fetus is likely to be >1 mSv.

Increasing concern for minimizing patient exposure has led multiple institutions, including the NCRP, to issue diagnostic reference levels (DRLs) for medical and dental diagnostic imaging. **DRL** exposure values represent the acceptable upper limits for patient exposure (75th percentile of general practice), whereas **achievable doses** represent the median dose (50th percentile) in general practice. The NCRP recommends a DRL of 1.6 mGy entrance skin dose for intraoral periapical and bite-wing radiography. The NCRP further recommends an achievable dose of 1.2 mGy for intraoral radiography.

Quality Assurance

Staff of facilities using x-ray imaging equipment shall establish a quality assurance and quality control program, implemented and monitored by a qualified expert, and follow updated quality assurance and quality control guidance. A qualified expert should survey all conventional x-ray units at the time of installation and should survey the equipment at least every 4 years or in accordance with state and local law, whichever is more stringent[1].

Quality assurance is defined as a program for periodic assessment of the performance of all parts of the radiologic procedure. It is intended to ensure that a dental office consistently produces high-quality images with minimum exposure to patients and personnel (see Chapter 14). Studies have indicated that dentists may be needlessly exposing their patients to compensate for improper exposure techniques, film processing practices, and darkroom procedures. One study reported that only 33% of panoramic radiographs that accompanied biopsy specimens were of acceptable diagnostic quality. However, when demands were placed on dentists to improve their techniques, the number of unsatisfactory radiographs was significantly reduced. Two studies by a dental insurance carrier demonstrated that after claims were rejected for unsatisfactory radiographs and the dentist was made aware of the errors and ways in which they could be corrected, the number of satisfactory radiographs submitted doubled. This study suggests that when the dentist is presented with guidelines for quality assurance, along with proper motivation, patient exposure can be dramatically reduced. Commercial mail-in devices are available to dentists and radiation protection agencies to measure dental image quality and dose of their radiographs.

Some states require dental offices to establish written guidelines for quality assurance and to maintain written records of quality assurance tests. Regardless of requirements, each dental office should establish maintenance and monitoring procedures, as outlined in Chapter 14.

Continuing Education

Practitioners should remain informed about safety updates and the availability of new equipment, supplies, and techniques that could further improve the diagnostic quality of radiographs and decrease radiation exposure (ADA, 2006).

Individuals who administer ionizing radiation must be familiar with the magnitude of exposure encountered in medicine, dentistry, and everyday life; the possible risks associated with such exposure; and the methods used to affect exposure and dose reduction. Although this chapter presents some of this information, acquiring knowledge and developing and maintaining skills are lifelong processes.

REFERENCE

1. Benavides E, Krecioch JR, Connolly RT, et al. Optimizing radiation safety in dentistry: clinical recommendations and regulatory considerations. *J Am Dent Assoc.* 2024;155(4):280-293.e4. https://doi.org/10.1016/j.adaj.2023.12.002.

BIBLIOGRAPHY

Acharya S, Pai KM, Acharya S. Repeat film analysis and its implications for quality assurance in dental radiology: an institutional case study. *Contemp Clin Dent.* 2015;6:392-395.

American Dental Association Council on Scientific Affairs. The use of dental radiographs: update and recommendations. *J Am Dent Assoc.* 2006;137:1304–1312.

American Dental Association and the US Food and Drug Administration. *Dental Radiographic Examinations: Recommendations for Patient Selection and Limiting Radiation Exposure.* https://www.fda.gov/media/84818/download. Accessed 7 July, 2024.

Benavides E, Bhula A, Gohel A, et al. Patient shielding during dentomaxillofacial radiography: recommendations from the American Academy of Oral and Maxillofacial Radiology. *J Am Dent Assoc.* 2023;154:826-835.e2. https://doi.org/10.1016/j.adaj.2023.06.015.

Code of Federal Regulations, Title 10, Chapter I, Part 20. Standards for protection against radiation. https://www.ecfr.gov/cgi-bin.

Committee to Assess Health Risks from Exposure to Low Levels of Ionizing Radiations. In: *Health Risks from Exposure to Low Levels of Ionizing Radiation: BEIR VII.* National Academy Press; 2006.

Dental radiographs: benefits and safety. *J Am Dent Assoc.* 2011;142:1101.

Environmental Protection Agency. Calculate your radiation dose. http://www.epa.gov/radiation/calculate-your-radiation-dose.

Hall EJ. Is there a place for quantitative risk assessment? *J Radiol Prot.* 2009;29(2A):A171-A184.

Hall EJ, Giaccia AJ. *Radiobiology for the Radiologist.* 6th ed. Lippincott Williams & Wilkins; 2006.

Horner K, Rushton VE, Walker A, et al. European guidelines on radiation protection in dental radiology: the safe use of radiographs in dental practice. *Radiat Prot.* 2004;136:1-115.

Mossman KL. The LNT debate in radiation protection: science vs. policy. *Dose Response.* 2012;10(2):190-202.

National Council on Radiation Protection and Measurements. *Control of Radon in Houses, NCRP Report 103.* National Council on Radiation Protection and Measurements; 1989.

National Council on Radiation Protection and Measurements. *Quality Assurance for Diagnostic Imaging, NCRP Report 99.* National Council on Radiation Protection and Measurements; 1990.

National Council on Radiation Protection and Measurements. *Limitation of Exposure to Ionizing Radiation, NCRP Report 116.* National Council on Radiation Protection and Measurements; 1993.

National Council on Radiation Protection and Measurements. *Dental X-Ray Protection, NCRP Report 145.* National Council on Radiation Protection and Measurements; 2003.

National Council on Radiation Protection and Measurements. *Ionizing Radiation Exposure of the Population of the United States, NCRP Report 160.* National Council on Radiation Protection and Measurements; 2009.

National Council on Radiation Protection and Measurements. *Reference Levels and Achievable Doses in Medical and Dental Imaging: Recommendations for the United States, NCRP Report 172.* National Council on Radiation Protection and Measurements; 2012.

Nationwide Evaluation of X-Ray Trends (NEXT): Tabulation and Graphical Summary of the 1999 Dental Radiography Survey, CRCPD Publication E-03-6. Center for Devices and Radiological Health, U.S. Food and Drug Administration; 2003.

Preston RJ. Radiation biology: concepts for radiation protection. *Health Phys.* 2005;88:545-556.

SEDENTEXCT. Guidelines on CBCT for dental and maxillofacial radiology. http://www.sedentexct.eu/.

Sources and Effects of Ionizing Radiation, UNSCEAR 2008 Report: Volumes I and II. https://www.unscear.org/unscear/uploads/documents/unscear-reports/UNSCEAR_2008_Report_Vol.I-CORR.pdf.

The 2007 recommendations of the International Commission on Radiological Protection. ICRP Publication 103. *Ann ICRP.* 2007;37:1-332.

4

Image Receptors

André Mol and Sanjay M. Mallya

The imaging chain refers to the multiple components that collectively contribute to formation and display of a radiographic image. This includes the x-ray source, the image receptor and, in the case of digital images, the image display device. Image receptors detect radiation transmitted through the patient to record a radiographic image. Characteristics of an image receptor include:

- X-ray sensitivity: The detector should be sensitive to x-rays so that an image can be recorded with low patient radiation.
- X-ray attenuation: The detector should attenuate most of the radiation transmitted through the patient.
- Latitude: The detector should discriminate between attenuation of metal restorations, enamel, dentin, bone pulp and bone marrow spaces.
- Image resolution: The detector should provide the contrast and spatial resolution for the intended diagnostic task.
- Linear response: The relationship between radiation dose and image density should be linear.
- Infection control: When used for intraoral radiography, receptors are placed in the oral cavity. The general physical and material construct of the receptor should allow for infection control and appropriate disinfection and sterilization.
- Receptor handling: The receptor should be easy to handle with appropriate training.
- Cost-effectiveness: The receptor and associated computer systems should be economically viable.

For several decades, radiographic film was used as the image receptor and served as a permanent record of the image. Over the last two decades, digital imaging has gradually replaced film-based imaging, and it is estimated that more than 90% of dental offices in the United States use digital radiography, with similar trends across the world. Numerous forces have driven the shift from film to digital systems, including the decreased cost of the digital imaging systems. The detrimental effects of inadequate film processing on diagnostic quality and the difficulty of maintaining high-quality chemical processing are well documented. Digital imaging does not require chemical processing, thus eliminating hazardous wastes in the form of processing chemicals and lead foil from film. Images can be electronically transferred to other health care providers without any alteration of the original image quality. In addition, digital intraoral receptors require less radiation than film, thus reducing patient exposure. Finally, digital imaging allows enhancements, measurements, and corrections not available with film.

Digital systems do have a few disadvantages compared to film. The initial expense of setting up a digital imaging system is relatively high. Certain components, such as the electronic x-ray receptor used in some intraoral systems, are susceptible to rough handling and are costly to replace. Because digital systems use evolving technologies, there is a risk—perhaps even a likelihood—of systems becoming obsolete. The latter is true for most electronic devices, including computers.

Computers play a vital role in most dental practices, and that role is expanding as various functions—including appointment scheduling, procedure billing, and patient charting—are integrated into third-party applications for practice management and artificial intelligence-based radiographic analyses. This has made the adoption of digital imaging in dentistry easier, and for many dental practices, digital imaging is the preferred technology. This chapter describes digital and film-based image receptors, display options, and digital image processing.

ANALOG VERSUS DIGITAL

The term *digital* in digital imaging refers to the numeric format of the image content and its discreteness. Conventional film imaging can be considered an analog medium in which differences in the size and distribution of black metallic silver result in a continuous density spectrum. Digital images are numeric and discrete in two ways, in terms of (1) the spatial distribution of the picture elements (*pixels*) and (2) the different shades of gray of each of the pixels. A digital image consists of a large collection of individual pixels organized in a matrix of rows and columns (Fig. 4.1). Each pixel has a row and column coordinate that uniquely identify its location in the image matrix. The term *dexel* refers to the smallest element in the digital detector that records radiographic exposure. The formation of a digital image requires several steps. At each dexel of an electronic detector, the absorption of x-rays generates a small voltage. More x-rays generate a higher voltage and vice versa. At each dexel, the voltage can fluctuate between a minimum and maximum value and is therefore an analog signal (Fig. 4.2A). Signals from adjacent dexels can be combined, a process called binning, to create a larger dexel and thus a larger image pixel. Most manufacturers of digital dental receptors use image pixels to describe technical specifications of their products.

Production of a digital image requires a process called analog-to-digital conversion (ADC). ADC consists of two steps: (1) sampling and (2) quantization. Sampling means that a small range of voltage values are grouped together as a single value (see Fig. 4.2B). Narrow sampling better mimics the original signal but leads to larger memory requirements for the resulting digital image (see Fig. 4.2C). Once sampled, the signal is quantized, which means that every sampled signal is assigned

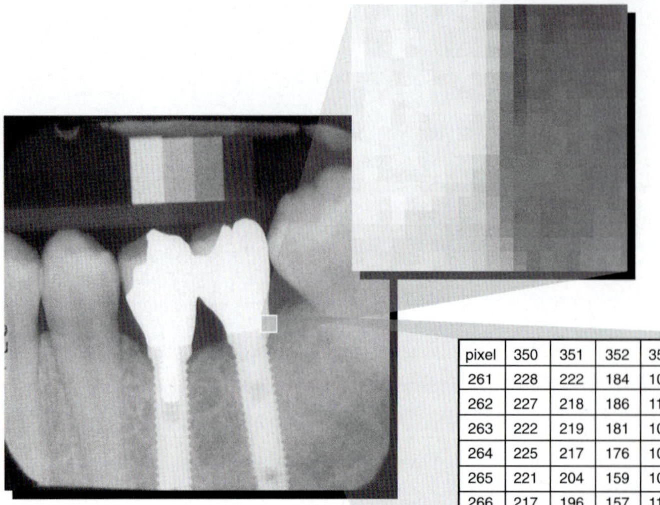

pixel	350	351	352	353	354	355	356	357
261	228	222	184	107	76	92	90	98
262	227	218	186	110	90	104	103	98
263	222	219	181	107	97	107	102	104
264	225	217	176	107	98	100	100	107
265	221	204	159	107	105	101	107	102
266	217	196	157	114	105	104	106	100
267	209	190	154	114	107	103	97	100
268	202	195	166	118	102	102	92	94
269	197	196	168	122	98	102	90	94
270	195	190	166	130	104	105	92	97
271	199	190	172	144	111	107	100	106
272	201	193	177	160	120	103	112	106
273	203	195	181	166	129	102	111	106
274	201	200	186	172	133	110	112	102

Fig. 4.1 A digital image is made up of a large number of discrete picture elements (pixels). The pixels are so small that the image appears smooth at normal magnification. The location of each pixel is uniquely identified by row and column coordinates within the image matrix. The value assigned to a pixel represents the intensity (gray level) of the image at that location.

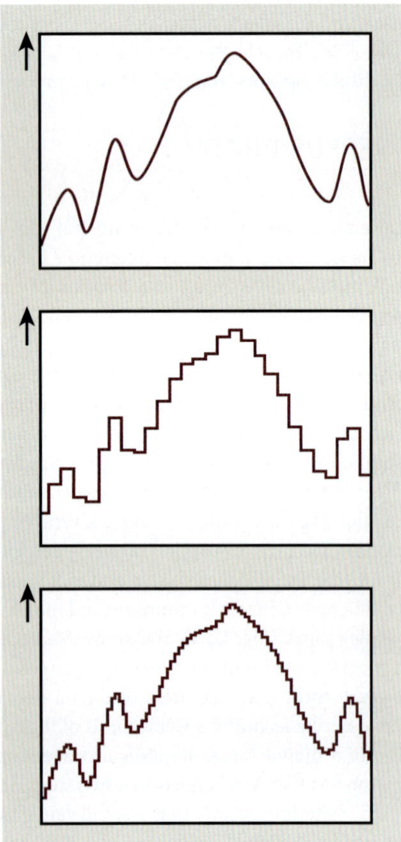

Fig. 4.2 (A) Illustration of an analog voltage signal generated by a detector. (B) Sampling of the analog signal discards part of the signal. (C) Sampling at a higher frequency preserves more of the original signal.

a value. These values are stored in the computer and represent the image. For the clinician to see the image, the computer organizes the pixels in their proper locations and displays a shade of gray that corresponds to the number that was assigned during the quantization step.

To understand the strengths and weaknesses of digital radiography, one must establish which elements of the radiographic imaging chain stay the same and which change. The imaging chain can be conceptualized as a series of interconnecting links beginning with the generation of x-rays. Exposure factors, patient factors, and the projection geometry determine how the x-ray beam is attenuated. A portion of the unattenuated x-ray beam is captured by the image receptor to form a latent image. This latent image is processed and converted into a real image, which is viewed and interpreted by the clinician. The use of digital detectors changes the way in which we acquire, store, retrieve, and display images. However, besides an adjustment of the exposure time, digital detectors do not fundamentally change the way in which x-rays are selectively attenuated by the tissues of the patient. The physics of the interaction of x-rays with matter and the effects of the projection geometry on the appearance of the radiographic image are unaltered and remain critically important for understanding image content and optimizing image quality. Elements in this part of the imaging chain that limit diagnostic performance affect both film-based radiography and digital radiography. Tables 4.1 and 4.2 compare the image receptor options available for projection radiography.

DIGITAL IMAGE RECEPTORS

Digital image receptors encompass numerous different technologies and come in many different sizes and shapes. Different and sometimes confusing names are in use to identify these receptors in medicine and dentistry. The most useful distinction is that between two main technologies:

- *Solid-state technology.* Although solid-state detectors can be subdivided further, these detectors have in common certain physical properties and the ability to generate a digital image in the computer

TABLE 4.1 Clinical Comparison of Intraoral Imaging Alternatives

Imaging Step	Film	CCD/CMOS	PSP
Receptor preparation	None	1. Place protective plastic sleeve over receptor envelope 2. Receptor must be connected to computer and patient-identifying information entered for acquisition/archiving software	1. "Erase" plates 2. Package plates in protective plastic
Receptor placement	1. Numerous generic film-holding devices are available 2. Film may be bent to accommodate anatomy	1. Specialized receptor holder specific for manufacturer's receptor may limit options 2. Receptor inflexibility and bulk limit placement options 3. Receptor cable must be carefully routed out of patient's mouth 4. Patient discomfort more likely than with film or PSP	1. Many receptor holders used for film may be adapted for PSP plates 2. Bending of receptor may irreversibly damage it
Exposure	1. Simple exposure	1. Computer must be activated before exposure	1. Simple exposure
Processing	1. Dark, light-safe environment in form of darkroom or daylight loader required 2. Processor chemistry must be prepared or replenished 3. Chemical temperature must be warmed, or processing time must be adjusted to accommodate temperature 4. Films must be removed from wrapper; lead foil must be separated for recycling	1. Image acquisition and display almost immediate	1. Dimly lit environment to prevent loss of image information 2. Processor must be programmed with patient information so that the images are stored properly. Alternatively, plates can be preprogrammed with patient information using RFID 3. Processor must be programmed with detector information so that the images are preprocessed 4. Protective wrapper must be removed from plates
Display preparation	1. Films may be placed in a variety of film mounts 2. Mounts must be labeled with patient-identifying information	1. Software may be configured to place image in appropriate position in digital mount when exposures are made in a predetermined sequence; otherwise images must be individually placed in the mount	1. Images must be individually placed in mount 2. Images may have to be digitally rotated to achieve proper orientation
Display	1. A room with subdued lighting and a masked viewbox are optimal 2. Any light source (including the operatory window or ceiling light) permits quick evaluation of the image	The same considerations apply to all digital receptor types: 1. A room with subdued lighting is optimal for interpretation activities 2. Computer with appropriate software and a display with adequate resolution are necessary; viewing is restricted to the location of the computer 3. Laptop computers increase flexibility of computer placement 4. Size of display restricts the numbers of images that may be viewed simultaneously; more time is required to open/close or expand/contract images when interpreting a series of images	
Image duplication	1. Quality of duplication is always inferior to original and is sometimes nondiagnostic	1. Electronic copies may be stored on various media without loss of image quality 2. Output on film or paper is inferior and is often nondiagnostic unless appropriate combinations of high-resolution printers and papers or film are used	

CCD, Charge-coupled device; *CMOS*, complementary metal oxide semiconductor; *PSP*, photostimulable phosphor; *RFID*, radio-frequency identification.

without any other external device. In medicine, the use of solid-state detectors is referred to as digital radiography. In dentistry, intraoral solid-state detectors are often called *sensors*.

- *Photostimulable phosphor (PSP) technology.* This technology consists of a phosphor-coated plate in which a latent image is formed after x-ray exposure. The latent image is converted to a digital image by a scanning device through stimulation by laser light. This technology is sometimes referred to as *storage phosphor* on the basis of the notion that the image information is temporarily stored within the phosphor. Other times, the term *image plates* is used to differentiate them from film and solid-state detectors. The use of PSP plates in medicine is referred to as *computed radiography*.

SOLID-STATE DETECTORS

Solid-state detectors collect the charge generated by x-rays in a solid semiconducting material (Fig. 4.3). The key clinical feature of these detectors is the rapid availability of the image after exposure. The matrix and its associated readout and amplifying electronics of intraoral detectors are enclosed within a plastic housing to protect

TABLE 4.2 Comparison of Physical Properties of Film, Charge-Coupled Devices, Complementary Metallic Oxide Semiconductors, and Photostimulable Phosphor Receptors

Feature	Technical Comment	Clinical Comment
Spatial resolution	Intraoral systems: Film > CCD = CMOS > PSP Panoramic systems: Film = CCD = PSP Cephalometric systems: Film > CCD = PSP	Limits of resolution for digital systems are readily appreciated when magnifying these images. With magnification, a "blocky" or "pixelated" appearance is evident. Resolution of panoramic systems is limited by mechanical motion to about 5 lp/mm
Exposure latitude	PSP ⪢ CCD ≥ CMOS > film	Because of the wide latitude of PSP and the automatic brightness and contrast "optimization" by image acquisition software, use of more x-ray exposure than is necessary is possible
Receptor dimensions	For equivalent imaged area, film = PSP < CCD = CMOS	"Active area" of CCD and CMOS receptors is smaller than surface area because of other electronic components within the plastic housing
Time for image acquisition	CCD = CMOS ⪡ PSP = film	Rapid image acquisition may be important for endodontic procedures or during implant placement
Image quality	Subjective quality is best with film when carefully exposed and well processed	Digital and film imaging are not significantly different when used for common diagnostic tasks
Image adjustment/ processing	Improves appearance of digital images	Takes time; may not improve diagnostic performance
Cost	Initial costs of digital systems are greater than those of film. Subsequent costs vary greatly depending on receptor wear and tear or abuse	Manufacturers' estimates of life expectancy of reusable receptors may be overly optimistic
Reliability	Mechanical problems affect digital PSP and film systems. Software reliability varies greatly among manufacturers. Changes in unrelated computer components and software can cause digital systems to malfunction	Digital systems fail when problems occur with receptors during image acquisition or with computers during image processing, archiving, and display
Image storage and retrieval	Data backup and security is critical for digital systems	Films can be misfiled and lost or be damaged by poor storage conditions. Digital data can be lost as a result of failures in power supplies or storage media and operator error
Transmitting images to others	Rapidly done with digital images	Facilitates communication between colleagues or with insurance companies

CCD, Charge-coupled device; *CMOS*, complementary metal oxide semiconductor; *lp*, line pairs; *PSP*, photostimulable phosphor.

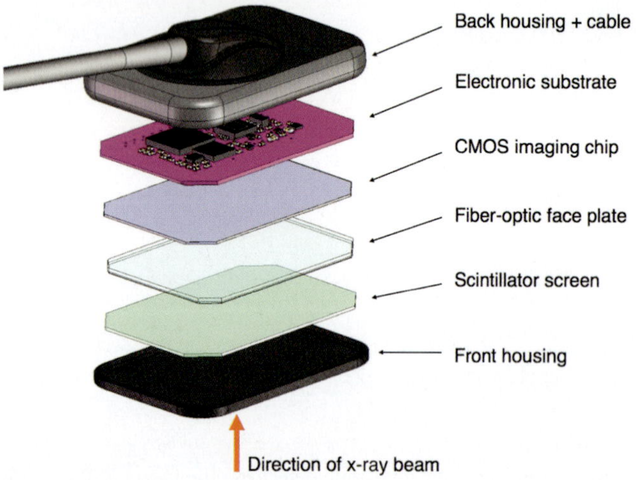

Fig. 4.3 Exploded view of complementary metal oxide semiconductor *(CMOS)* sensor. The front and back housings form a watertight and light-tight barrier to protect the sensor components. The scintillator screen fluoresces when exposed to x-rays and forms a visible light radiographic image. The fiberoptic faceplate couples the scintillator screen to the CMOS chip to reduce image noise. The CMOS imaging chip captures the light from the scintillator and creates a charge in each pixel proportional to the exposure. The sensor electronics read the charge in each pixel and transmit it to a computer. (Courtesy XDR Radiology, Los Angeles, CA, https://www.xdrradiology.com.)

them from the oral environment. These elements of the detector consume part of the real estate of the sensor so that the active area is smaller than its total surface area. Sensor bulk, although reduced by continued miniaturization of the electronic components, is a potential drawback of intraoral solid-state detectors. In addition, most detectors incorporate an electronic cable to transfer data to the computer. The presence of a cable makes positioning of the sensor more challenging and requires some adaptation. It also results in increased vulnerability of the device to fail due to wear of the cable connections from normal use. Manufacturers have addressed these issues in various ways. Some manufacturers have changed the location of the cable attachment to the corner of the sensor. Others offer sensors with magnetic connectors, induction connectors, or reinforced cables to reduce accidental damage to the device. Wireless radiofrequency transmission also has been introduced to eliminate the cable altogether. Wireless transmission frees the detector from a direct tether to the computer, but it necessitates some additional electronic components, thus increasing the overall bulk of the sensor.

Many manufacturers produce detectors with varying active sensor areas roughly corresponding to the different sizes of intraoral film. Detectors without flaws are relatively expensive to produce, and the expense of the detector increases with increasing matrix size (total number of pixels). Pixel size ranges from less than 20 μm to 70 μm. Three types of solid-state sensors are in common use.

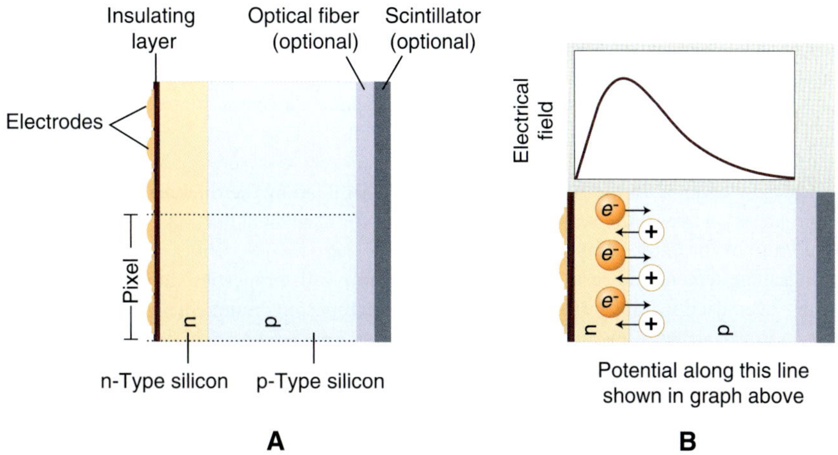

Fig. 4.4 (A) Basic structure of a charge-coupled device. The electrodes are insulated from an n-p silicon sandwich. The surface of the silicon typically incorporates a scintillating material to improve x-ray capture efficiency and fiberoptics to improve resolution. One pixel uses three electrodes. (B) Excess electrons from the n-type layer diffuse into the p-type layer, whereas excess holes in the p-type layer diffuse into the n-type layer. The resulting charge imbalance creates an electric field in the silicon with a maximum just inside the n-type layer.

Charge-Coupled Device

The charge-coupled device (CCD), introduced to dentistry in 1987, was the first digital image receptor to be adapted for intraoral imaging. The CCD uses a thin wafer of silicon as the basis for image recording. The silicon crystals are formed in a pixel matrix (Fig. 4.4). When exposed to radiation, the covalent bonds between silicon atoms are broken, producing electron-hole pairs (Fig. 4.5). The number of electron-hole pairs that are formed in an area is proportional to the amount of x-ray exposure that area receives. The electrons are attracted toward the most positive potential in the device, where they create "charge packets." Each packet corresponds to one pixel. The pattern of charge packets formed from the individual pixels in the matrix represents the latent image (Fig. 4.6). The image is read by transferring each row of pixel charges from one pixel to the next in "bucket brigade"

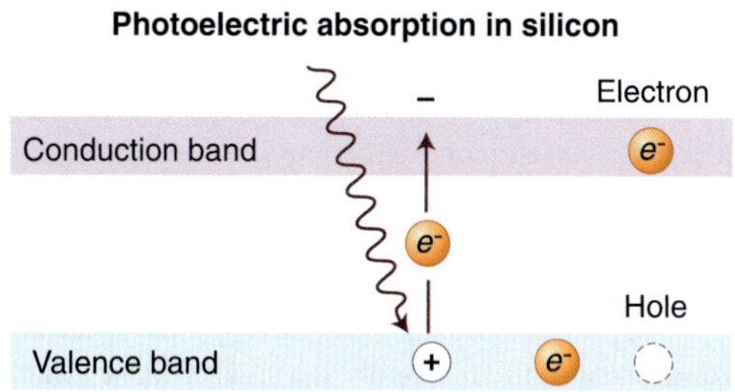

Fig. 4.5 X-ray or light photons impart energy to electrons in the valence band, releasing them into the conduction band. This generates an "electron hole" charge pair.

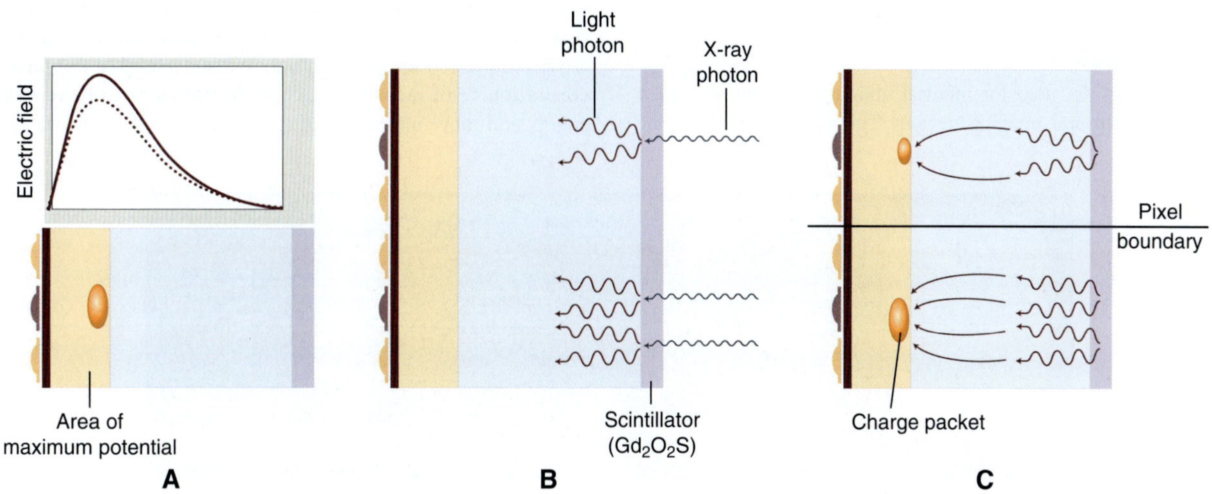

Fig. 4.6 (A) Before exposure, the central electrode of each pixel is turned on, creating an area of maximal potential or a potential well. (B) X-ray photons are absorbed in the scintillating material and converted to light photons. Light photons are absorbed in the silicon through photoelectric absorption. (C) Electrons released from the valence band collect selectively near the n-p layer interface in the area of maximum potential to form a charge packet. During charge-coupled device readout, the electrical potential of the pixel electrodes is sequentially modulated to shift the charge packet from pixel to pixel.

fashion. As a charge reaches the end of its row, it is transferred to a readout amplifier and transmitted as a voltage to the analog-to-digital converter located within or connected to the computer. Voltages from each pixel are sampled and assigned a numeric value representing a gray level (ADC). Because CCD detectors are more sensitive to light than to x-rays, most manufacturers use a layer of scintillating material coated directly on the CCD surface or coupled to the surface by a fiberoptic plate. This scintillating material increases the x-ray absorption efficiency of the detector. Gadolinium oxybromide compounds similar to those used in rare earth radiographic screens and cesium iodide are examples of scintillators that have been used for this purpose.

CCDs have also been made in linear arrays a few pixels wide and many pixels long for panoramic and cephalometric imaging. In the case of panoramic units, the CCD is fixed in position opposite to the x-ray source with the long axis of the array oriented parallel to the fan-shaped x-ray beam. Some manufacturers provide CCD sensors that may be retrofitted to older panoramic units. In contrast to film imaging, the mechanics for cephalometric imaging are different. Construction of a single CCD of a size that could simultaneously capture the area of a full skull would be prohibitively expensive. Combining a linear CCD array and a slit-shaped x-ray beam with a scanning motion permits scanning of the skull over several seconds. One disadvantage of this approach is the increased possibility of patient movement artifacts during the several seconds required to complete a scan.

Complementary Metal Oxide Semiconductors

Complementary metal oxide semiconductor (CMOS) technology is the basis for typical consumer-grade digital cameras. These detectors are also silicon-based semiconductors but are fundamentally different from CCDs in the way that pixel charges are read. Each pixel is isolated from its neighboring pixels and is directly connected to a transistor. Similar to the CCD, electron-hole pairs are generated within the pixel in proportion to the amount of x-ray energy that is absorbed. This charge is transferred to the transistor as a small voltage. The voltage in each transistor can be addressed separately, read by a frame grabber, and stored and displayed as a digital gray value. CMOS technology is widely used in the construction of computer central processing unit chips and digital camera detectors, and the technology is less expensive than that used in the manufacture of CCDs. Most manufacturers currently use this technology for intraoral imaging applications (Fig. 4.7).

Flat-Panel Detectors

Flat-panel detectors are used for medical imaging but have also been used in several extraoral imaging devices. The detectors can provide relatively large matrix areas with pixel sizes less than 100 μm; this allows direct digital imaging of larger areas of the body, including the head. Two approaches have been taken in selecting x-ray–sensitive materials for flat-panel detectors. Indirect detectors are sensitive to visible light, and an intensifying screen (gadolinium oxysulfide or cesium iodide) is used to convert x-ray energy to light. The performance of these devices is determined by the thickness of the intensifying screen. Thicker screens are more efficient but allow greater diffusion of light photons, leading to less sharp images. Direct detectors use a photoconductor material (selenium) with properties similar to silicon and a higher atomic number, which permits more efficient absorption of x-rays. Under the influence of an applied electrical field, the electrons that are freed during x-ray exposure of the selenium are conducted in a direct line to an underlying thin film transistor (TFT) detector element. Direct detectors using selenium ($Z = 34$) provide higher resolution but are less efficient compared to indirect detectors using intensifying screens with gadolinium ($Z = 64$) or cesium ($Z = 55$). The electrical energy generated in flat-panel detectors is proportional to the x-ray exposure and is stored at each pixel in a capacitor. The energy is released and read out by applying appropriate row and column voltages to a particular pixel's transistor. Flat-panel detectors are relatively expensive and currently limited to specialized imaging tasks, such as cone beam computed tomography.

Direct Photon Counting Detectors

These detectors directly convert x-ray photon energy into an electric charge without using a scintillator intermediate. This increases image spatial resolution. With these detectors, the energy of each photon is recorded individually, rather than integrated. In computed tomography devices, photon counting detectors can provide multienergy imaging.

PHOTOSTIMULABLE PHOSPHOR

PSP plates absorb and store energy from x-rays and release this energy as light (phosphorescence) when stimulated by another light of an appropriate wavelength. To the extent that the stimulating light and phosphorescent light wavelengths differ, the two may be distinguished, and the phosphorescence can be quantified as a measure of the amount of x-ray energy that the material has absorbed.

The PSP material used for radiographic imaging is "europium-doped" barium fluorohalide. Barium in combination with iodine, chlorine, or bromine forms a crystal lattice. The addition of europium (Eu^{2+}) creates imperfections in this lattice. When exposed to a sufficiently energetic source of radiation, valence electrons in europium can absorb energy and move into the conduction band. These electrons migrate to

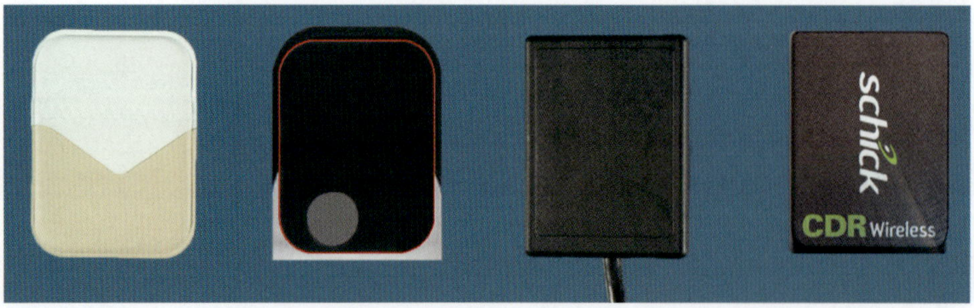

A B C D

Fig. 4.7 (A) Carestream (Kodak) No. 2 film. (B) Soredex OpTime No. 2 PSP plate (outlined in *red*) placed on a barrier envelope to demonstrate packaged size. (C) Gendex No. 2 charge-coupled device sensor. (D) Schick No. 2 complementary metal oxide semiconductor wireless sensor. (A, Courtesy Carestream Health, Inc., exclusive manufacturer of Kodak dental systems; B, Courtesy Soredex, Milwaukee, WI; C, Courtesy Gendex, Hatfield, PA; D, Courtesy Schick, Sirona Dental Inc., Charlotte, NC.)

nearby halogen vacancies (F-centers) in the fluorohalide lattice and may become trapped there in a metastable state. While in this state, the number of trapped electrons is proportional to x-ray exposure and represents a latent image. When stimulated by red light of around 600 nm, the barium fluorohalide releases trapped electrons to the conduction band. When an electron returns to the Eu^{3+} ion, energy is released as light in the green spectrum between 300 and 500 nm (Fig. 4.8). Fiberoptics conduct the light from the PSP plate to a photomultiplier tube. The photomultiplier tube converts this light into electrical energy. A red filter at the photomultiplier tube selectively removes the stimulating laser light, and the remaining green light is detected and converted to a varying voltage. The variations in voltage output from the photomultiplier tube correspond to variations in stimulated light intensity from the latent image. The voltage signal is quantified by an analog-to-digital converter and stored and displayed as a digital image. In practice, the barium fluorohalide material is combined with a polymer and spread in a thin layer on a base material to create a PSP plate. For intraoral radiography, a polyester base similar to radiographic film is used.

When they are manufactured in standard intraoral sizes, these plates provide handling characteristics similar to intraoral film. PSP plates are also made in sizes commonly used for panoramic and cephalometric imaging. Some PSP processors accommodate a full range of intraoral and extraoral plate sizes. Other processors are limited to intraoral or extraoral formats.

Before exposure, PSP plates must be erased to eliminate residual images from prior exposures. This erasure is accomplished by flooding the plate with a bright light. Current PSP systems integrate automatic plate erasing within the scanner. Plates can also be erased by placing them on a dental viewbox with the phosphor side of the plates facing the light for 1 or 2 minutes. More intense light sources can be used for shorter periods of time. Inadequate plate erasure results in double images and usually renders the image undiagnostic. Erased plates are placed in light-tight containers before exposure. In the case of intraoral plates, sealable polyvinyl envelopes that are impervious to oral fluids and light are used for packaging. For large-format plates, conventional cassettes without intensifying screens are used. After exposure, plates should be processed as soon as possible because trapped electrons spontaneously release over time. The rate of loss of electrons is greatest shortly after exposure. The rate varies depending on the composition of the storage phosphor and the environmental temperature. Some phosphors lose 23% of their trapped electrons after 30 minutes and 30% after 1 hour. Because loss of trapped electrons is uniform across the plate surface, early loss of charge does not typically result in clinically meaningful image deterioration. However, underexposed images may have noticeable image degradation in the form of increased image noise. Adequately exposed images may be stored for 12–24 hours and retain acceptable image quality. A more important source of latent image fading is exposure to ambient light during plate preparation for processing. A semidark environment is recommended for plate handling. The more intense the background light and the longer the exposure of the plate to this light, the greater the loss of trapped electrons and the more degraded the resultant image. Red safelights found in most darkrooms are not safe for exposed PSP plates, which are most sensitive to the red light spectrum.

Photostimulable Phosphor Scanners

A number of approaches have been adopted for "reading" the latent images on PSP plates. Soredex (Milwaukee, WI) in its Digora and OpTime systems and Air Techniques (Melville, NY) in its ScanX system use a rapidly rotating multifaceted mirror that reflects a beam of red laser light. As the mirror revolves, the laser light sweeps across the plate. The plate is advanced, and the adjacent line of phosphor is scanned. The direction of the laser scanning the plate is termed the *fast scan direction*. The direction of plate advancement is termed the *slow scan direction*.

These scanners, as well as the Carestream (Atlanta, GA) CS 7600 scanner and the Planmeca (Helsinki, Finland) ProScanner, also include

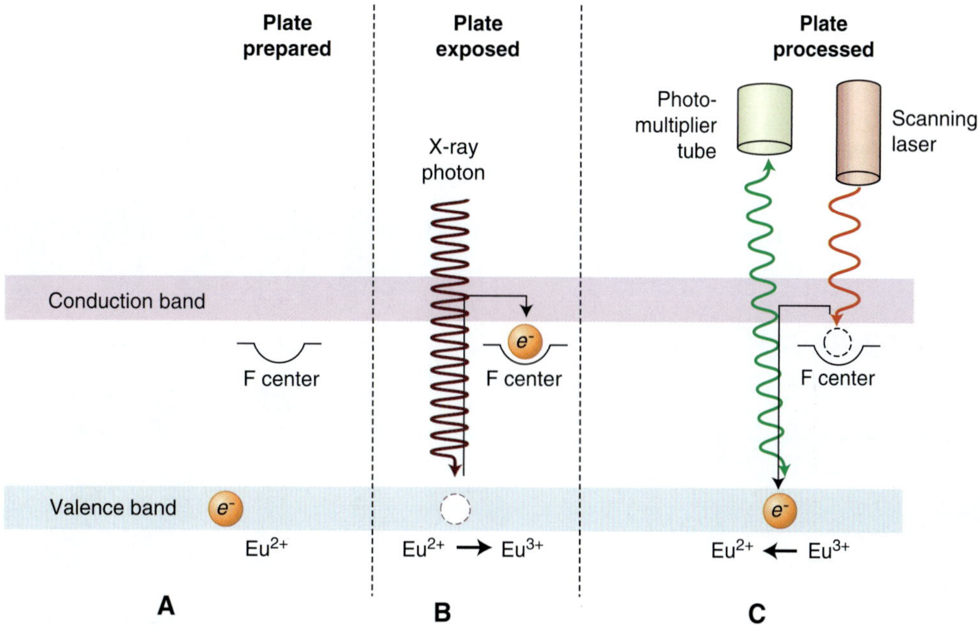

Fig. 4.8 Photostimulable phosphor (PSP) image formation. (A) Initially, the PSP plate is flooded with white light to return all electrons to the valence band. (B) Exposure to x-rays imparts energy to europium valence electrons, moving them into the conduction band. Some electrons become trapped at "F centers." (C) A red scanning laser imparts energy to electrons at the F centers, promoting them to the conduction band, from which many return to the valence band. With the electron's return to the valence band, energy is released in the form of light photons in the green spectrum. This light is detected by a photomultiplier tube or diode with a red filter to screen out the scanning laser light.

automatic plate clearance after scanning. Automatic plate clearance improves work flow and reduces potential plate damage from manual erasing. The mechanism used for plate intake in the Soredex OpTime scanner requires a metal disk on the back of the plate. This disk also serves as a marker to indicate when a plate was exposed backward. Carestream and Planmeca use radio-frequency identification (RFID) technology to link patient information to the plates. This prevents plates from being scanned into the wrong patient file. The RFID chip also serves to alert the operator when a plate is accidentally exposed backward.

Current PSP scanners all use individual plate loading. An alternative approach to plate reading involves a rapidly rotating drum that can hold multiple plates. Although some of these systems are likely still being used, they are no longer produced by the leading manufactures.

DIGITAL DETECTOR CHARACTERISTICS

Contrast Resolution

Contrast resolution is the ability to distinguish different densities in the radiographic image; this is a function of the interaction of the following factors:

- Attenuation characteristics of the tissues imaged.
- Capacity of the imaging system to distinguish differences in numbers of x-ray photons and translate them into gray values.
- Ability of the computer display to portray differences between gray levels.
- Ability of the observer to recognize those differences.

Current digital detectors capture data at 8, 10, 12, or 16 bits. The bit depth is a power of 2 (Fig. 4.9). This means that the detector can theoretically capture 256 (2^8) to 65,536 (2^{16}) different attenuation levels. In practice, the actual number of meaningful attenuation levels that can be captured is limited by inaccuracies in image acquisition—that is, noise. Regardless of the number of attenuation differences that a detector can capture, conventional computer monitors are capable of displaying a grayscale of only 8 bits. Because operating systems such as Windows reserve many gray levels for the display of system information, the actual number of gray levels that can be displayed on a monitor is 242. A more important limiting factor is the human visual system, which is capable of distinguishing only about 60 gray levels at any time under ideal viewing conditions. Considering the typical viewing environment in the dental operatory, the actual number of gray levels that can be distinguished decreases to less than 30. Human visual limitations are also present for film viewing; however, the luminance (brightness) of a typical radiograph viewbox is much greater than that of a typical computer display. Therefore, the ambient lighting of the room in which the image is viewed theoretically has a lower impact on film than on digital displays.

A B C D

Fig. 4.9 Contrast resolution. Examples of grayscale ramps representing distinct gray levels from black to white. Bit depth controls the number of possible gray levels in the image. The actual number of distinct gray levels that are displayed depends on the output device and image processing. The perceived number of gray levels is influenced by viewing conditions and the visual acuity of the observer. (A) 6 bits/pixel = 64 gray levels. (B) 5 bits/pixel = 32 gray levels. (C) 4 bits/pixel = 16 gray levels. (D) 3 bits/pixel = 8 gray levels.

Spatial Resolution

Spatial resolution is the capacity for distinguishing fine detail in an image. Resolution is often measured and reported in units of line pairs per millimeter. Test objects consisting of sets of very fine radiopaque lines separated from each other by spaces equal to the width of a line are constructed with a variety of line widths (Fig. 4.10). A line and its associated space are called a line pair (lp). At least two columns of pixels are required to resolve a line pair, one for the bright line and one for the dark space. Typical observers are able to distinguish about 6 lp/mm (line pairs per millimeter) without benefit of magnification. Intraoral film is capable of providing more than 20 lp/mm of resolution. Unless a film image is magnified, the observer will be unable to appreciate the extent of the detail in the image.

With solid-state digital imaging systems, the theoretic resolution limit is determined by the pixel size: the smaller the size of the pixel, the higher the maximally attainable resolution. A sensor with 20-μm pixels can obtain a maximum theoretical resolution of 25 lp/mm: One line pair requires two pixels, in this case 2 × 20 μm, which equals 40 μm. Thus, the maximal resolution would be 1 lp/40 μm, which is equal to 25 lp/mm (Box 4.1). Alternatively, resolution can be expressed in dots per inch (DPI) or points per inch (PPI). At best, there is one dot or point per pixel. Thus if the pixel size is 20 μm, there is one dot or point per 20 μm. This is equal to 1270 DPI or PPI because there are 25,400 μm in 1 inch (25,400/20 = 1270). However, in practice, actual detector resolution is lower than these theoretical limits for a variety of reasons, including (1) electronic noise; (2) diffusion of photons in the scintillator coating; and (3) potentially imperfect optical coupling between the scintillator, the fiberoptic screen (when present), and the photodetector. Currently, the highest-resolution intraoral solid-state detector for dentistry has a measured resolution of approximately 20 lp/mm; however,

A B C D

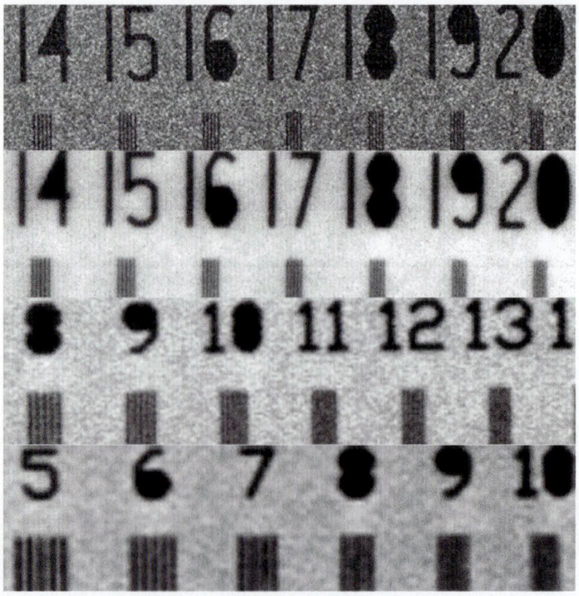

Fig. 4.10 Images of a line-pair resolution test phantom made with various receptors. (A) Kodak (Atlanta, GA) InSight film. (B) Trophy RVGui (Kodak) high-resolution charge-coupled device. (C) Gendex (Hatfield, PA). DenOptix photostimulable phosphor (PSP) scanned at 600 dots per inch (DPI). (D) Gendex DenOptix PSP scanned at 300 DPI.

BOX 4.1 Conversion Between Pixel Size and Theoretical Limit of Resolution

	THEORETICAL LIMIT OF RESOLUTION	
Pixel Size (μm)	Line Pairs Per Millimeter (lp/mm)	Dots or Points Per Inch (DPI or PPI)
20	25	1270
50	10	508
A	1000/(A × 2)	25,400/A
1000/(B × 2)	B	B × 2 × 25.4
25,400/C	C/(2 × 25.4)	C

this does not mean that this level of resolution is obtained clinically. Clinical spatial resolution depends not only on detector characteristics but also on the size of the focal spot, the source-to-object distance, and the object-to-image distance (see Chapter 5).

Resolution in PSP systems is influenced by the thickness of the phosphor material. Thicker phosphor layers cause more diffusion and yield a lower resolution. A thicker layer enhances x-ray absorption efficiency, resulting in a faster image receptor. Resolution is also inversely proportional to the diameter of the laser beam. Effective beam diameter is increased by vibration in the rotating mirror and drum scanner designs. Slow scan motion influences resolution by the increment of plate advancement. This increment may be adjusted to increase or reduce resolution in some systems. Current PSP systems are capable of providing more than 10 lp/mm of resolution.

Software displays of all digital images permit magnification of images. A periapical image filling the display of a computer monitor may be magnified by a factor of 10 times or more. At this level of magnification, the image takes on a building-block pattern or pixelated appearance, and the limits of resolution of the imaging system are evident.

Detector Latitude

The ability of an image receptor to capture a range of x-ray exposures is termed *latitude*. A desirable quality in intraoral image receptors is the ability to record a broad range of tissue attenuation differences—from gingiva to enamel. At the same time, subtle differences in attenuation within these tissues should be visually apparent. The useful range of densities in film radiography is two orders of magnitude, from 0.5 to 2.5. The dynamic range of film actually extends for more than four orders of magnitude, but densities of 3 and 4, which transmit only 1/1000 to 1/10,000 of the incident light, require intensified illumination or hot lighting to be distinguished from a density of 2.5. Such devices are not commonly used in general practice. The latitude of CCD and CMOS detectors is similar to the latitude of film and can be extended with digital enhancement of contrast and brightness. PSP receptors enjoy larger latitudes and have a linear response to five orders of magnitude of x-ray exposure (Fig. 4.11).

Detector Sensitivity

The sensitivity, or speed, of a detector is its ability to respond to small amounts of radiation. Intraoral film speed is classified according to speed group based on criteria developed by the International Organization for Standardization. Extraoral screen-film combinations use a classification system developed by Eastman Kodak. Currently, there are no classification standards for dental digital x-ray receptors. As a result, the reported sensitivity of systems by equipment manufacturers is difficult to compare, and the performance that can be achieved in routine practice may be exaggerated. The useful sensitivity of digital receptors is affected by numerous factors, including detector efficiency,

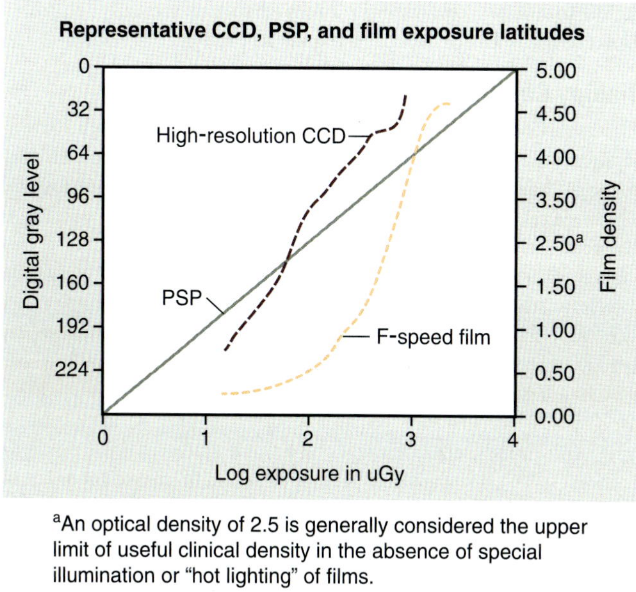

Fig. 4.11 Representative exposure latitudes of charge-coupled device, photostimulable phosphor *(PSP)*, and intraoral film sensors. The clinically useful optical density of film has an upper limit of 2.5. Use of a more intense viewbox or "hot lighting" can extend the upper end of the usable density range and expand useful film latitude. PSP plates are unique in responding linearly to exposure.

pixel size, and system noise. Current PSP systems for intraoral imaging allow dose reductions of about 50% compared to F-speed film with similar diagnostic performance. Subjectively, most observers prefer intraoral PSP images with a higher level of x-ray exposure. Paradoxically, patient doses may increase if the level of x-ray exposure is determined by image criteria that are based on the subjective perception of "attractiveness." Additionally, patient exposure may increase with CCD systems because of the ease of making repeat exposures. In general, solid-state detectors require less exposure than PSP systems or film. CCD and PSP systems for extraoral imaging require exposures similar to exposures needed for 200-speed screen-film systems.

DIGITAL IMAGE VIEWING

Electronic Displays

Contemporary desktop and laptop displays use liquid crystal display (LCD) and light-emitting diode (LED) technology. LCD uses TFT technology, similar to what is used in flat-panel detectors. The process involves sending signals to the transistor associated with each pixel, which causes the associated LCD to transmit light of an intensity proportional to the transistor voltage. Subpixels composed of red, green, and blue phosphors are subjected to varied voltages and in combination create a pixel output of a particular hue and intensity. In an LED display, each pixel is associated with a diodes that produces light. The viewing angle of LED displays is limited, and the observer must be positioned squarely in front of the display for optimum viewing quality. Current laptop displays are of sufficient quality to be used for typical dental diagnostic tasks. Desktop versions of TFT LCD displays have overcome problems of brightness and viewing angle but consume more power and thus are not suited for laptop configurations. Most modern flat-panel displays have sufficient brightness and contrast and have viewing angles of 160 degrees. Most flat-panel displays incorporate a digital video interface, which allows direct display of digital information without digital-to-analog conversion. These displays virtually eliminate signal loss and distortion from digital-to-analog conversion.

Display Considerations

The display of digital images on electronic devices is a straightforward engineering issue. Positioning an image in the context of other diagnostic and demographic information and in useful relationships with other images is a more complex challenge that may vary according to diagnostic task, practice pattern, and practitioner preference. These challenges are answered with varying degrees of success by image display software. The quality, capabilities, and ease of use of display software vary from vendor to vendor. Even with the same software, the display of images can vary dramatically depending on how the software handles resizing of windows or the size and resolutions of different displays. For instance, on some displays, it may be impossible to view a full-mouth series of images on a single screen at normal magnification (100%). Software may permit reduction in image size or scrolling around the window to compensate for smaller display areas. These approaches are not as fast or flexible as shifting a film mount around on a viewbox. The visibility of electronic displays is degraded by many of the same elements that degrade viewing of film images. Bright background illumination from windows or other sources of ambient light reduces visual contrast sensitivity. Light reflecting off a monitor surface may reduce the visibility of image contrast further. Images are best viewed in an environment in which lighting is subdued and indirect.

In using electronic displays for viewing digital images or other patient-related information, the design and layout of the practice must be such that access to protected health information (PHI) by other patients or unauthorized individuals is prevented. In the United States, this is necessary to comply with the Health Insurance Portability and Accountability Act (HIPAA). This can be challenging in practices that use an open bay layout.

HARD COPIES

The need to print digital images for sharing with other clinicians or with third parties is decreasing rapidly as digital technology has become mainstream. However, when digital image sharing is not feasible, digital image printing is an economical solution for making digital radiographs transferable. Any time a digital image is modified, including the process of printing it in hard copy, there must be sufficient assurance that the image retains relevant diagnostic information. The requirements for quality vary with the diagnostic task at hand. For instance, assessment of the impaction status of a third molar puts a lower demand on the image quality than caries detection. There is limited scientific evidence to support the diagnostic efficacy of printed images. The large number of variables that influence the quality of the printed image (e.g., printing technology, printer quality, printer settings, and type of media) makes the printing process a much more complicated process than it initially appears to be. When images must be printed, it is imperative to use a printing system that is designed for its intended use and to follow the manufacturer's recommendations. It is always preferable to transfer images digitally when possible. The main types of printing technologies available for image printing include laser, inkjet, and dye sublimation with the use of either film or paper.

Film Printers

Radiologists have traditionally relied on film images for common interpretive tasks. High-quality film printers that use laser or dye sublimation technologies are expensive, and low-cost alternatives have less diagnostic quality. Current film transparencies produced with inkjet technology appear to be suboptimal for tasks such as caries diagnosis.

Paper Printers

Although printing on film allows radiographs to be evaluated in a traditional manner with the transmitted light of a viewbox, paper-printed digital radiographs require reflective light from a normally lit room. Because most dental operatories are not well equipped to control the ambient light level for viewing film images on a viewbox, paper-printed digital radiographs offer a substantial advantage. By printing digital radiographs on paper, the dentist is able to use technologies developed for the digital photography domain.

Photographic printers vary widely in price and quality. Although more costly models usually provide higher resolution, printer resolution is only one of many factors determining the final quality of the printed image. Inkjet printers are the most dominant in the market and offer the most economical alternative. Dye sublimation printers provide excellent image quality but are generally more expensive.

For any printing technology, the printing resolution is usually defined as the number of DPI the printer can print. A printer with a higher DPI number is capable of laying the ink down more tightly than a printer with a lower DPI number. As a result, printers with a higher DPI number can print smaller objects and thus are said to have higher resolution. The resolution of the digital radiograph can never be increased by a printer that prints at a higher resolution than that of the image itself. Printing digital radiographs at a lower resolution may reduce the final resolution of the image unless the printed size of the image is increased. Spatial resolution is preserved as long as the image prints pixel for pixel.

The same cannot be said of contrast resolution, which is always reduced by the printing process. The reason for this reduction in contrast resolution is that the printer is not printing with shades of gray but instead is printing varying numbers of black dots. Typically, an 8 × 8 pixel page array is assigned to each image pixel (Fig. 4.12). The number of elements in the array that are filled with a black ink dot determines the relative gray level of the array. The 8 × 8 array provides for 0–64 ink dots or 65 gray values. With an 8 × 8 dot array, it may not be possible to print all pixels of an image on a single page. For instance, a PSP panoramic image with a physical size of 15 cm × 30 cm might be scanned at 150 DPI. For each pixel of this image to print within the same dimensions, a printer resolution of 1200 DPI (8 × 150) is required. If the maximal resolution of the printer is 1200 DPI, images with higher resolutions must be printed at a larger size to obtain full spatial resolution. Likewise, a bite-wing image scanned at 300 DPI must be printed at twice its physical size of 30 mm × 40 mm to

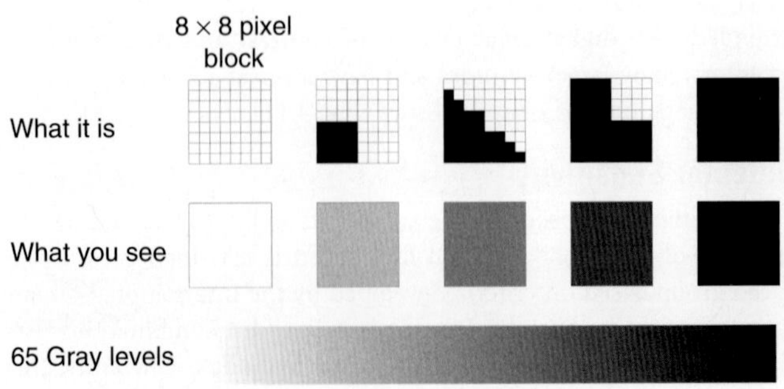

Fig. 4.12 Grayscale printing. Each image pixel is assigned to an 8 × 8 pixel array on the printed page. From 0 to 64, *black ink dots* can be used to fill each array, resulting in 65 potential gray levels. This means that an 8-bit (256 gray levels) image is reduced to 6 bits with a concomitant loss of contrast resolution during the printing process.

preserve the original resolution. Resizing of an image to fit on a printed page leads to interpolation of pixels and can result in a significant loss of resolution.

A final drawback of paper prints is the limited contrast ratio owing to the physics of the reflective process used for viewing images. The darkest inks absorb at most 96% of the incident visible light. If the paper were able to reflect 100% of the incident light, the maximum reflective contrast ratio achievable would be only 25:1.

IMAGE PROCESSING

Any operation that acts to improve, restore, analyze, or in some way change a digital image is a form of image processing. The use of digital imaging in dental radiography involves various image processing operations. Some of these operations are integrated in the image acquisition and image management software and are hidden from the user. Others are controlled by the user with the intention to improve the quality of the image or to analyze its contents. The fact that some of the image processing steps are hidden from the user may have consequences that have no analog in film. One such consequence is the difficulty in assessing underexposure or overexposure in digital radiographs. For film, this condition is readily apparent, but a suboptimally exposed digital image rarely appears too light or too dark because image processing usually includes automatic grayscale leveling. Other metrics, such as the data histogram or noise measurements, should be employed.

Image Restoration

When the raw image data enter the computer, they are usually not yet ready for storage or display. A number of preprocessing steps must be performed to correct the image for known defects and to adjust the image intensities so that they are suitable for viewing. For example, some of the pixels in a CCD sensor are always defective. The image is restored by substituting the gray values of the defective pixels with some weighted average of the gray values from the surrounding pixels. Depending on the quality of the sensor and the choices made by the manufacturer, various other operations may be applied to the image before it becomes visible on the display. These operations are executed very rapidly and are unnoticed by the user. Most preprocessing operations are set by the manufacturer and cannot be changed.

Image Enhancement

The term *image enhancement* implies that the adjusted image is an improved version of the original one. Most image enhancement operations are applied to make the image visually more appealing (subjective enhancement). This can be accomplished by increasing contrast, optimizing brightness, improving sharpness, and reducing noise. Subjective image enhancement does not improve the accuracy of image interpretation. Image enhancement operations are often task-specific: what benefits one diagnostic task may reduce the image quality for another task. For example, increasing contrast between enamel and dentin for caries detection may make it more difficult to identify the contour of the alveolar crest. Image enhancement operations are also dependent on viewer preference.

Brightness and Contrast

Digital radiographs do not always use the full range of available gray values effectively. They can be relatively dark or light, and they can show too much contrast in certain areas or not enough. Although the brightness and contrast can be judged visually, the image histogram is a convenient tool to determine which of the available gray values the image is using (Fig. 4.13). The minimum and maximum values and the shape of the histogram indicate the potential benefit of brightness- and contrast-enhancement operations.

Digital imaging software commonly includes a histogram tool and tools for the adjustment of brightness and contrast. Some tools also allow adjustment of the gamma value. Changing the gamma value of an image selectively enhances image contrast in either the brighter or the darker areas of the image. Adjustment of brightness, contrast, and gamma value changes the original intensity values of the image (input) to new values (output). The operator can choose to make these changes permanent or to restore the image to its original settings. Fig. 4.14 is a graphic representation of the relationship between input values (horizontal axis) and output values (vertical axis) with the corresponding images and their histograms. Digital imaging software usually also includes tools for histogram equalization and grayscale inversion. Histogram equalization is an enhancement operation that increases contrast between the image intensities abundantly present within the image while reducing contrast between image intensities that are used only sparsely. The actual effect of histogram equalization depends on the image content and may sometimes lead to unexpected degradation of image quality. Grayscale inversion changes a radiographic positive image into a radiographic negative image. Although this may affect the subjective perception of the image content, the altered appearance is foreign to interpretive practice and is little used.

The effect of contrast enhancement on the diagnostic value of digital radiographs is controversial. Some studies show substantial benefits

A

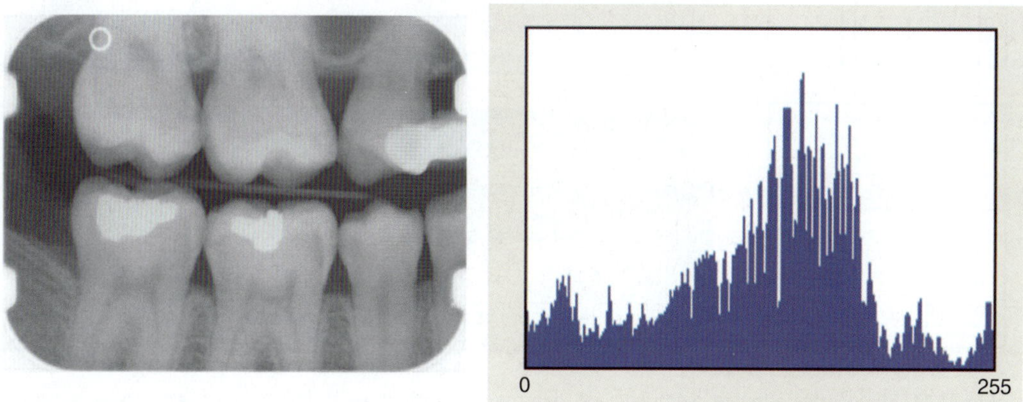

B

Fig. 4.13 Digital image (A) with image histogram (B). Horizontal axis represents image gray levels (8 bits = 256 levels); vertical axis represents number of pixels. Each *bar* indicates the number of pixels in the image with that particular gray level.

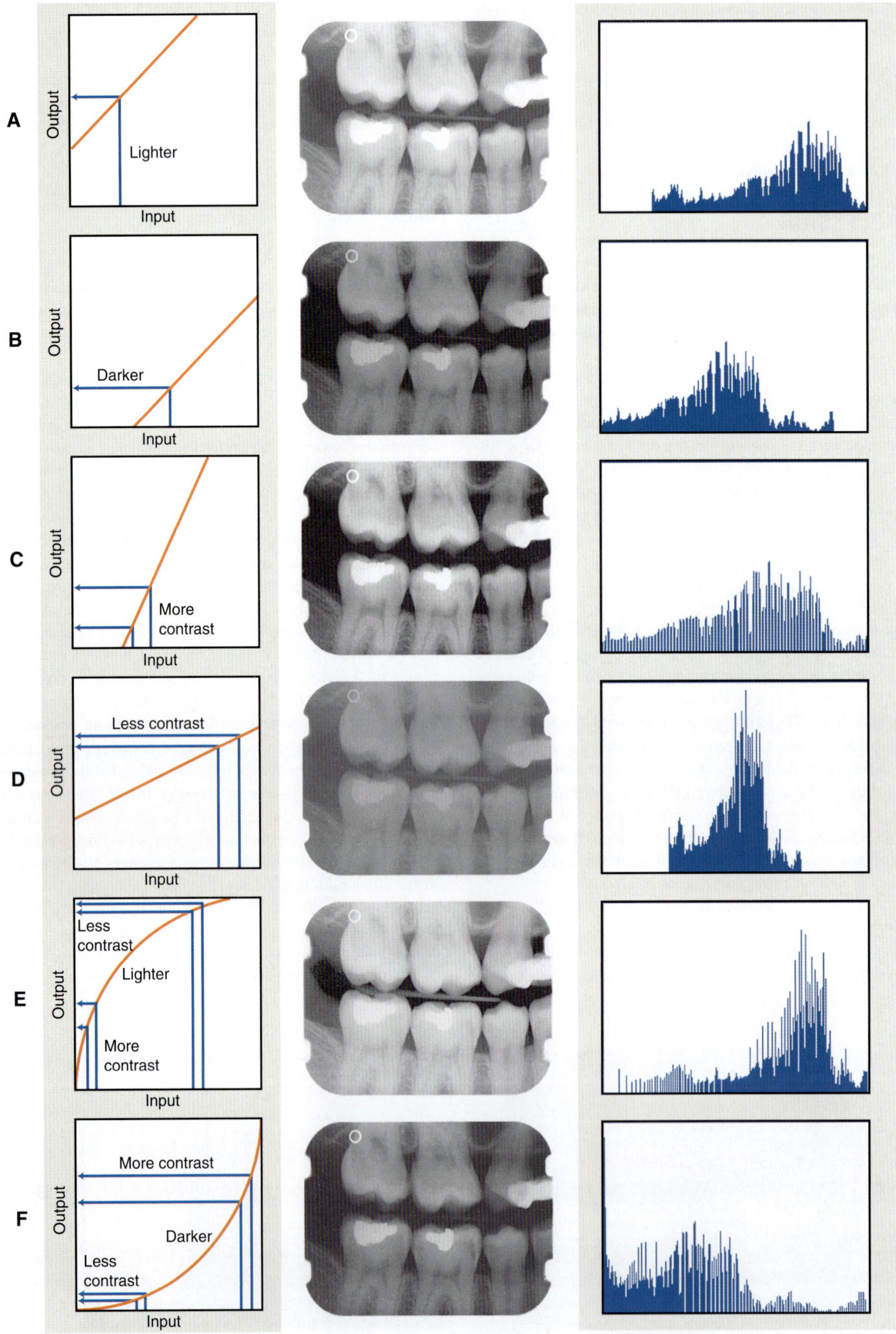

Fig. 4.14 Effect of brightness, contrast, and gamma adjustment as illustrated by image transformation graphs *(left column)*, digital images *(middle column)*, and image histograms *(right column)*. The image adjustments are relative to those of Fig. 4.13. (A) Increase in brightness. (B) Decrease in brightness. (C) Increase in contrast. (D) Decrease in contrast. (E) Increase in gamma. (F) Decrease in gamma.

of contrast enhancement operations, whereas others have found only limited value or no improvement at all. The effect of contrast enhancement cannot be predicted easily. The key to successful image enhancement is to enhance relevant radiographic signs selectively without simultaneously enhancing distracting features.

Sharpening and Smoothing

The purpose of sharpening and smoothing filters is to improve image quality by removing blur or noise. Noise represents random intensity variation and is often categorized as high-frequency noise (small-scale intensity variations) or low-frequency noise (gradual or large-scale intensity variations). Speckling is a special type of high-frequency noise that is characterized by isolated small regions surrounded by lighter or darker regions. Filters that smooth an image are sometimes called noise or despeckling filters because they are designed to remove high-frequency noise. Filters that sharpen an image either remove low-frequency noise or enhance boundaries between regions with different intensities (edge enhancement). For the purposeful application of filters, it is important to know what type of noise the filters reduce and how that affects radiographic features of interest. Without this knowledge, important radiographic features may degrade or disappear as noise is removed. Similarly, edge enhancement of radiographic features of interest may enhance noise or enhance local contrast to the extent that it simulates disease. Sharpening and smoothing filters may make the dental radiographic images subjectively more appealing; however, there is no scientific evidence suggesting an increase in diagnostic value. The indiscriminate use of filters made available in most imaging software packages should be avoided if there is no scientific support for their clinical usefulness.

Color

Most digital systems on the market provide opportunities for color conversion of grayscale images, also called pseudocolor. Humans can distinguish many more colors than shades of gray. Transforming the gray values of a digital image into various colors theoretically could enhance the detection of objects within the image; however, this works only if all the gray values representing an object are unique for that object. Because this is rarely the case, boundaries between objects may change, and new boundaries may be created. In most cases, these changes distract the observer from seeing the real content of the image and result in degraded image interpretation. Therefore, color conversion of radiographs is neither diagnostically nor educationally useful. Some useful applications of color do exist. When objects can be uniquely identified on the basis of a set of image features, color can be used to label or highlight these objects. The development of such criteria is a complex task, and only a few successful studies have been reported in the literature.

Digital Subtraction Radiography

When two images of the same object are registered and the image intensities of corresponding pixels are subtracted, a uniform difference image is produced. If there is a change in the radiographic attenuation between the baseline and follow-up examinations, this change shows up as a brighter area when the change represents gain and as a darker area when the change represents loss, such as loss of enamel and dentin owing to caries or loss of alveolar bone height with periodontitis. The strength of digital subtraction radiography (DSR) is that it cancels out the complex anatomic background against which this change occurs and reveals subtle changes. However, for DSR to be diagnostically useful, the baseline projection geometry and image intensities must be closely reproduced—a requirement that is difficult to achieve clinically.

IMAGE ANALYSIS

Image analysis operations are designed to extract diagnostically relevant information from the image. This information can range from simple linear measurements to fully automated diagnosis. The use of image analysis tools brings with it the responsibility to understand their limitations. The accuracy and precision of a measurement are limited by the extent to which the image is a truthful and reproducible representation of the patient and by the operator's ability to make an exact measurement.

Measurement

Digital imaging software provides numerous tools for image analysis. Digital rulers, densitometers, and various other tools are readily available. These tools are usually digital equivalents of existing tools used in endodontics, orthodontics, periodontology, implantology, and other areas of dentistry (Fig. 4.15). Digital imaging has also added new tools that were not available with film-based radiography. The size and image intensity of any area within a digital radiograph can be measured. Tools are also being developed for measuring the complexity of the trabecular bone pattern. Such measurements can be useful as screening tools for osteoporosis assessment and for detecting other diseases.

Diagnosis

One of the most challenging areas of research is the development of tools and procedures that automate the detection, classification, and quantification of radiographic signs of disease. The rationale for the use of such methods is early and accurate disease detection through use of reproducible and objective criteria. The development of automated image analysis operations is very complex and requires a thorough understanding of anatomy, pathology, and radiographic image formation. The three basic steps of image analysis are segmentation, feature extraction, and object classification. Of these, segmentation is the most critical step. The goal of segmentation is to simplify the image and reduce it to its basic components. This involves subdividing the image, thus separating objects from the background. Objects of interest are defined by the diagnostic task (e.g., a tooth, a

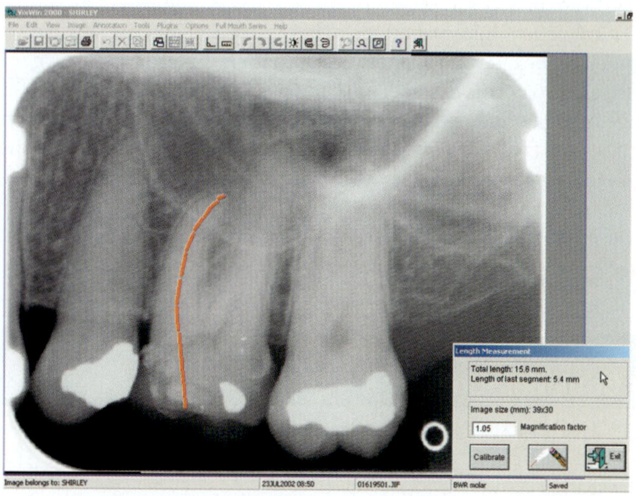

Fig. 4.15 Example of a measurement tool to determine the length of the crown and mesiobuccal root of the first molar. The measurement has been calibrated for a magnification factor of 1.05. The digital measurement tool is more versatile than the analog ruler; however, for both types of measurement tools, the apparent length remains dependent on the projection geometry.

carious lesion, a bone level, or an implant). When image segmentation results in the detection of an object, a variety of features can be measured that assist in determining what the object represents. Such features may include measures of size and shape, relative location, average density, homogeneity, and texture. A unique set of values for a certain combination of features can lead to classification of the object. Automated cephalometric landmark identification is an example of this technology. Other dental examples include caries detection, classification of periodontal disease, and detection and quantification of periapical bone lesions. The success of many of these applications is highly dependent on specific imaging parameters; very few provide reliable results when used clinically. This situation underscores the complexity of the radiographic image interpretation process.

IMAGE STORAGE

The use of digital imaging in dentistry requires an image archiving and management system very different from that used for film radiography. Storage of diagnostic images on magnetic or optical media raises new issues that must be considered, such as capacity, reliability, data integrity, and security. The file size of dental digital radiographs varies considerably, ranging from approximately 200 kilobytes for intraoral images to 6 megabytes for extraoral images. Storage and retrieval of these images in an average-sized dental practice is not a trivial issue. The development of new storage media and the continuing decrease in the price of a unit of storage has alleviated the capacity issue in dental radiography.

The simplicity with which digital images can be modified through image processing poses a potential risk with respect to ensuring the integrity of the diagnostic information. Once in a digital format, critical image data can be deleted or modified. It is important that the software prevents the user from permanently deleting or modifying original image data, whether intentionally or unintentionally. Not all software programs provide such a safeguard. As the use of digital imaging in dentistry continues to expand, the implementation of standards for preserving original image data becomes urgent. It is also imperative that images and other important patient-related information are duplicated to prevent permanent loss of data in case of a hardware or software malfunction. The use of computers for storing critical patient information mandates the design and use of a backup protocol. Box 4.2 shows some issues that must be considered when a backup protocol is designed. Backup media suitable for external storage of digital radiographs include external hard drives, digital tapes, CDs, and DVDs. The use of cloud-based software is rapidly gaining popularity because it offers a seamless solution for primary and secondary storage with the ability to access the data from any location. These solutions need to be HIPAA compliant and require reliable, secure, and sufficiently fast network connections.

BOX 4.2 Digital Image Backup Considerations

- Type of backup media
- Time and method of backup
- Backup interval
- Storage location of backup media
- Recovery time
- Recovery reliability
- Security
- Future compatibility of backup technology

Image Compression

The purpose of image compression is to reduce the size of digital image files for archiving or transmission. In particular, storing extraoral images in a busy clinic may pose a challenge to storage capacity and speed of image access. The purpose of file compression is to reduce the file size significantly while preserving critical image information.

Compression methods are generally classified as lossless or lossy. Lossless methods do not discard any image data, and an exact copy of the image is reproduced after decompression. Most compression techniques take advantage of redundancies in the image, which can be expressed in simpler terms. The maximum compression rate for lossless compression is usually less than 3:1. Lossy compression methods achieve higher levels of compression by discarding image data; empiric evidence suggests that this does not affect the diagnostic quality of an image. Compression rates of 12:1 and 14:1 were shown to have no appreciable effect on caries diagnosis. For determining endodontic file length, a rate of 25:1 was diagnostically equivalent to the uncompressed image. A compression rate of 28:1 was acceptable for the subjective evaluation of image quality and the detection of artificial lesions in panoramic radiographs.

Version 3.1 of the Digital Imaging and Communications in Medicine (DICOM) standard adopted Joint Photographic Experts Group (JPEG) as the compression method, which provides a range of compression levels. Other types of image compression methods, such as wavelet compression, are being investigated for their use in medical imaging. Although low and medium levels of lossy compression appear to have little effect on the diagnostic value of dental images, lossy compression should be used with caution and only after its effect for specific diagnostic tasks has been evaluated. With the continuing increase in the capacity of storage media and the widespread use of high-speed data communication lines, lossy compression of dental radiographs is rapidly becoming obsolete. At the same time, new digital image receptors are generating images with more and more pixels and more bits per pixel, thus increasing storage needs. Image compression negates to some extent the gain from such high-end detectors. Diagnostic criteria should dictate the need for high-resolution detectors and use of image compression. Current evidence suggests that detector quality and moderate image compression have a limited impact on diagnostic outcomes.

SYSTEMS COMPATIBILITY

The development of digital imaging systems for dental radiography has largely been driven by industry. Manufacturers have adopted and developed technologies according to individual needs and philosophies. As a result, image formats among systems from different vendors are not standardized, and image archival, retrieval, and display systems are often incompatible. Despite the proprietary nature of imaging software, it is possible to transfer images from one vendor's system to the other. Most systems provide image export and import tools using a variety of generic image formats, such as JPEG and tagged image file format (TIFF). However, the process of transferring images through export-import procedures is cumbersome. It requires many steps, and the operator needs to ensure that the right images are imported into the proper patient folder. Also, it cannot be assumed that the display and calibration of imported and native images will be the same.

Exporting and importing is not the method of choice when digital imaging is going to be used on a large scale. It has long been recognized that the adoption of a standard for transferring images and associated information between digital imaging devices in medicine and dentistry is necessary. The American College of Radiology and the

National Electrical Manufacturers Association formed a joint committee to develop a standard for digital imaging systems. Numerous professional organizations have contributed to this complex development process, which has resulted in the current DICOM standard. Various dental organizations, including the American Dental Association, are playing an active role in defining aspects of the DICOM standard related to dentistry. The DICOM standard is not a static set of rules dictating to manufacturers how to build imaging devices. Rather, it is an evolving document addressing the interoperability of medical and dental imaging and information systems. Manufacturers of digital imaging systems for dental radiography are responding to the call to adopt the DICOM standard. Currently most systems conform to the DICOM standard, although some may not conform to every aspect of the standard. The successful adoption of digital imaging in dentistry requires interoperability of all devices. It is likely that manufacturers do not want to be left behind and that the market will weed out the systems that are noncompliant. Dentists using different vendors with DICOM-compliant imaging devices are able to exchange images seamlessly. The exchange of any data that are considered PHI must be done in a secure HIPAA-compliant manner.

CLINICAL CONSIDERATIONS

Some fundamental differences from film in the clinical handling of digital receptors should be noted (Tables 4.1 and 4.2). Because digital receptors are intended to be reusable, they must be handled with greater care than their film counterparts. In certain situations, film may be intentionally damaged through bending to accommodate patient anatomy. This situation never occurs with digital receptors, as bending sensors would damage them. Instead, allowances must be made for sensor rigidity, such as placement of the sensor toward the midline to allow for greater clearance or to modify beam angulation to account for the smaller imaging area of digital sensors. Examples of common image artifacts found on images made with solid state or PSP systems are presented in Box 4.3. PSP plates are susceptible to bending and scratching during handling—defects that induce permanent artifacts in the receptor. These artifacts obscure information of potential diagnostic importance and may necessitate disposal of the receptor and repeat imaging of the patient. Because of the inability of digital detectors to be bent to accommodate patient anatomy, new imaging strategies must be used for some patients. It may not be possible to capture the distal surface of the canine on premolar views consistently. An additional projection may be required to visualize this surface adequately.

A significant potential problem with PSP systems is the inability to distinguish images from plates that have been exposed backward. In contrast to film packets, which incorporate a lead foil with a characteristic embossed pattern that results in an underexposed image of the anatomy with the pattern artifact when exposed backward, PSP images have little x-ray attenuation from the polyester base. It is much too easy for inattentive radiographers to mount these digital images on the

BOX 4.3 Common Problems in Digital Image Receptor Exposure, Processing, and Handling

Enrique Platin

Noisy Images

Although the brightness of these images has been adjusted to display similar average gray values, notice the noisy appearance of the underexposed periapical radiograph (Fig. 4.16A, 0.032 s) compared to the properly exposed radiograph (see Fig. 4.16B, 0.32 s).

Two PSP bite-wing radiographs (Fig. 4.17). Image A was processed properly and image B was exposed to excessive ambient light prior to scanning, causing it to fade. Exposed PSP plates must be protected from ambient light prior to scanning to prevent trapped electrons being released from their metastable state.

Nonuniform Image Density

Partial exposure of PSP plates to excessive ambient light before scanning results in nonuniform image density (Fig. 4.18A). This happens when plates are overlapped while exposed to ambient light (see Fig. 4.18B).

Distorted Images

Bending of PSP plates during intraoral placement: moderate bending (Fig. 4.19A), retake of image *A* (see Fig. 4.19B), severe bending (see Fig. 4.19C), and retake of image *C* (see Fig. 4.19D).

Double Images

PSP double image on incisor periapical radiograph resulting from incomplete erasure of previous image of posterior periapical region (Fig. 4.20A) and retake of image (see Fig. 4.20B).

Another example of a double image resulting from incomplete erasure of a PSP receptor: posterior periapical radiograph with double image (Fig. 4.21A), and retake of image A (see Fig. 4.21B).

Damaged Image Receptors

Scratched phosphor surface mimicking root canal filling (Fig. 4.22A) and retake of image (see Fig. 4.22B).

Image artifacts resulting from excessive bending of the PSP plate (Fig. 4.23A). Excessive bending has resulted in permanent damage to the phosphor plate (see Fig. 4.23B).

PSP circular artifact as a result of plate damage (Fig. 4.24A). The plate shows localized swelling of the protective coating as a result of ethylene oxide gas used to disinfect the plates (see Fig. 4.24B). Most likely a pinhole was present in the protective coating allowing the gas to infiltrate and separate the protective coating from the phosphor layer.

PSP image artifact resulting from exposure of the plate to liquid disinfectant (Fig. 4.25A). The disinfectant caused damage to the protective coating and the phosphor layer (see Fig. 4.25B). Plates should be protected from harsh disinfectants.

Malfunctioning CCD sensor resulting from incorrect exposure or misinterpretation of the incoming data by the processing software (Fig. 4.26A and B). The sensor was not damaged.

Improper Use of Image Processing

Straight radiopaque line artifact on PSP image as a result of dust on the lens of the scanner's photomultiplier (Fig. 4.27). After removal of the scanner cover, the lens can be cleaned according to manufacturer's recommendations.

Improper use of image processing tools, such as filters, may result in false-positive findings. An edge enhancement filter was applied to the panoramic image, which produced radiolucencies at restoration edges simulating recurrent caries (Fig. 4.28A). These radiolucencies are not present in a follow-up intraoral image (see Fig. 4.28B).

Effect of Image Scanning Resolution

Settings for the resolution of PSP scanning may have a significant impact on image quality. Scanning at 150 DPI (Fig. 4.29A) produces an image that lacks detail and appears pixelated when magnified. Scanning at 300 DPI provides increased detail through higher resolution (see Fig. 4.29B). Box 4.1 shows how to convert from DPI (scanner) to lp/mm (image resolution).

Continued

BOX 4.3 Common Problems in Digital Image Receptor Exposure, Processing, and Handling—cont'd

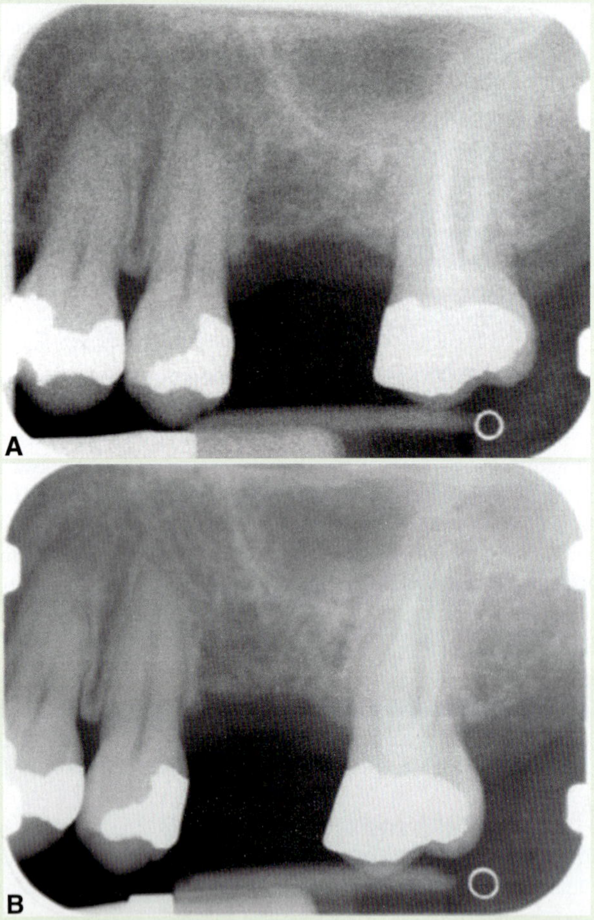

Fig. 4.16

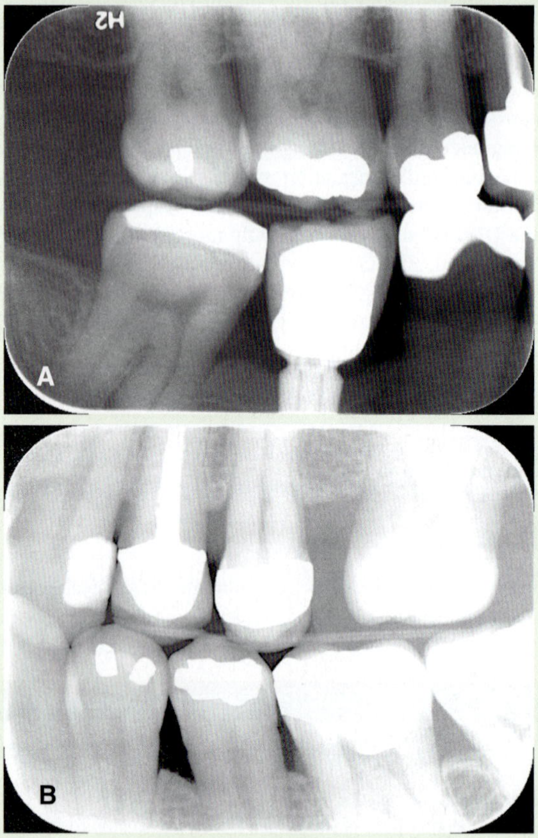

Fig. 4.17

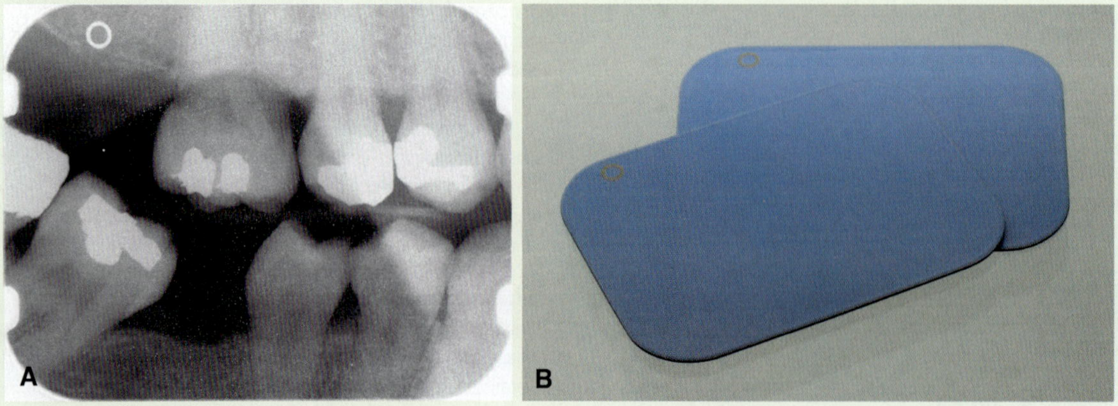

Fig. 4.18

BOX 4.3 **Common Problems in Digital Image Receptor Exposure, Processing, and Handling—cont'd**

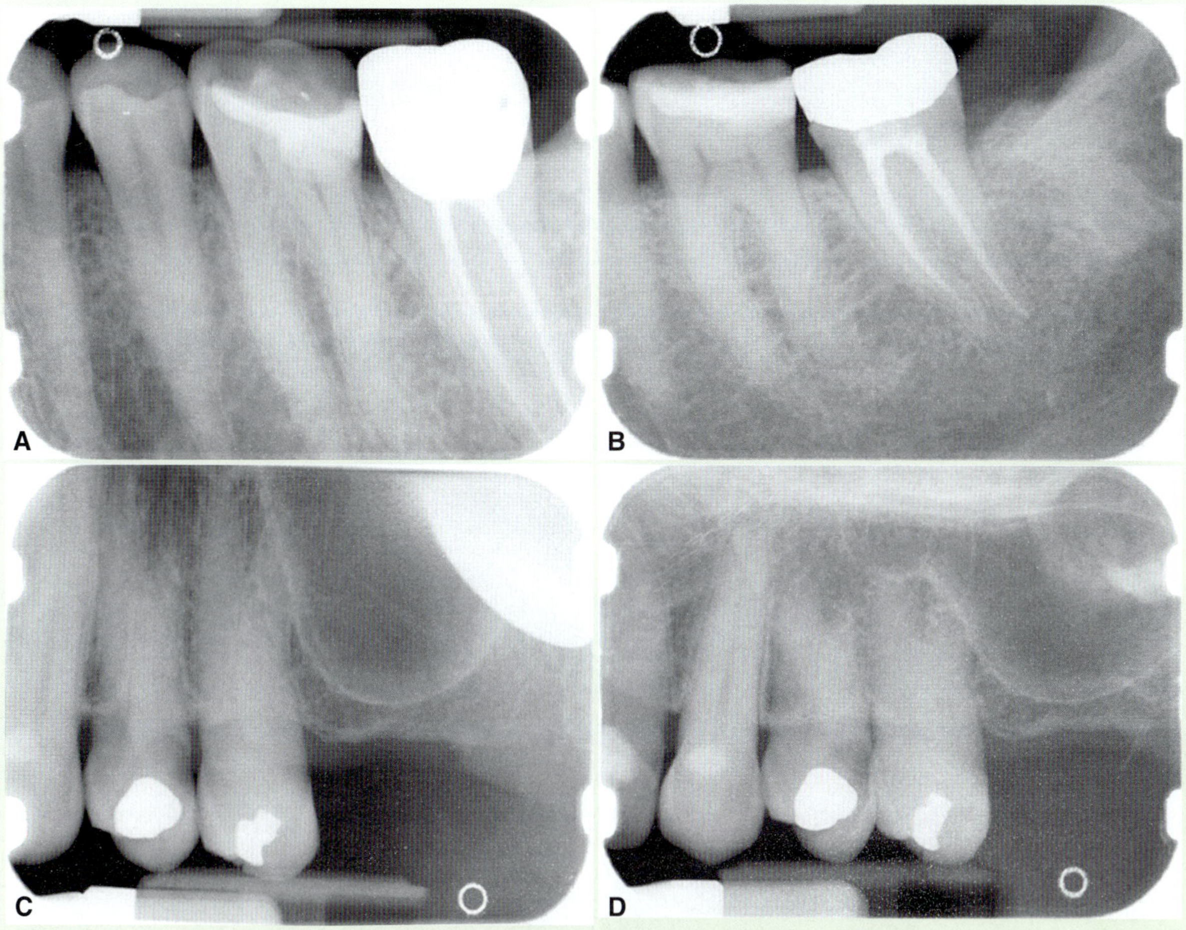

Fig. 4.19

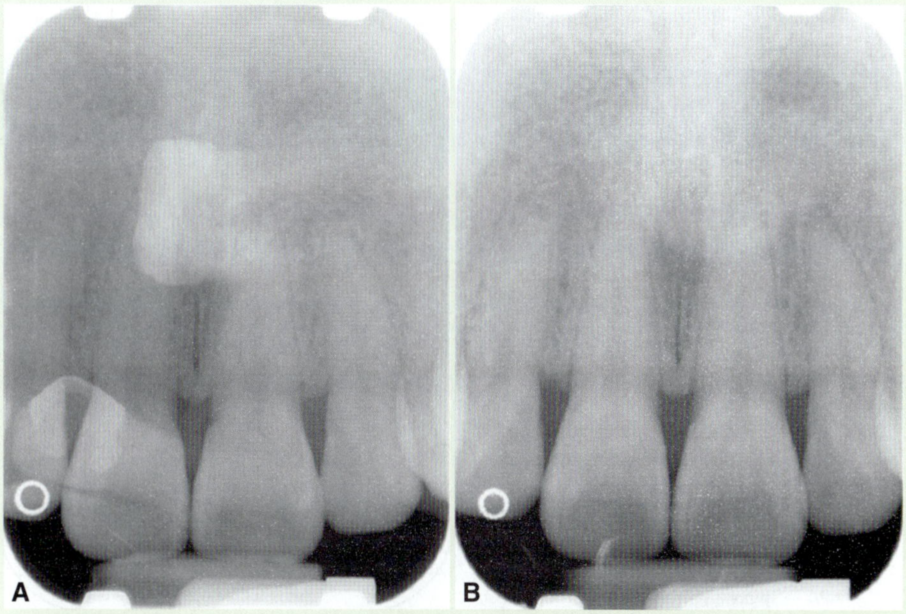

Fig. 4.20

Continued

BOX 4.3 Common Problems in Digital Image Receptor Exposure, Processing, and Handling—cont'd

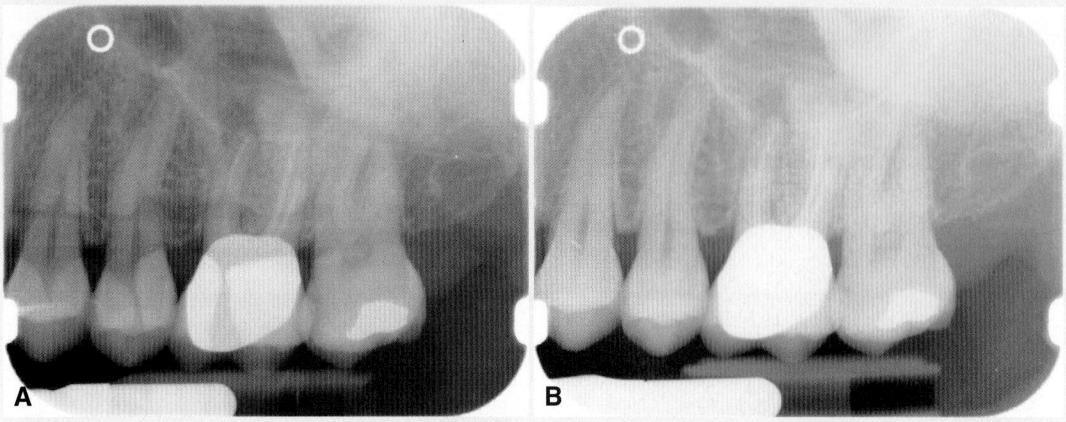

Fig. 4.21

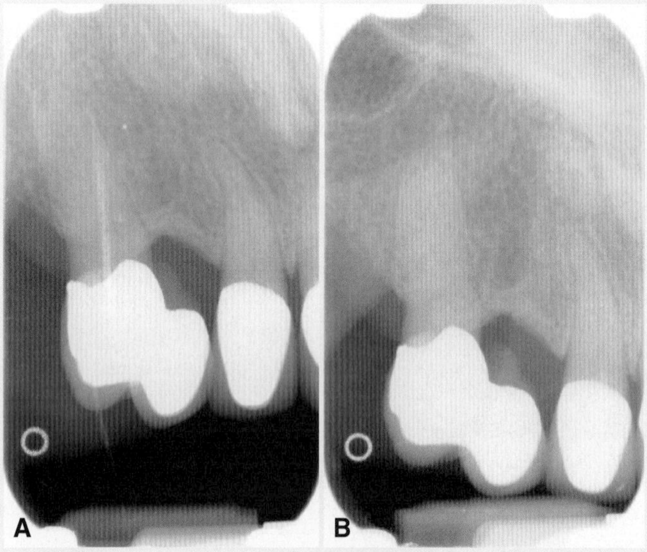

Fig. 4.22

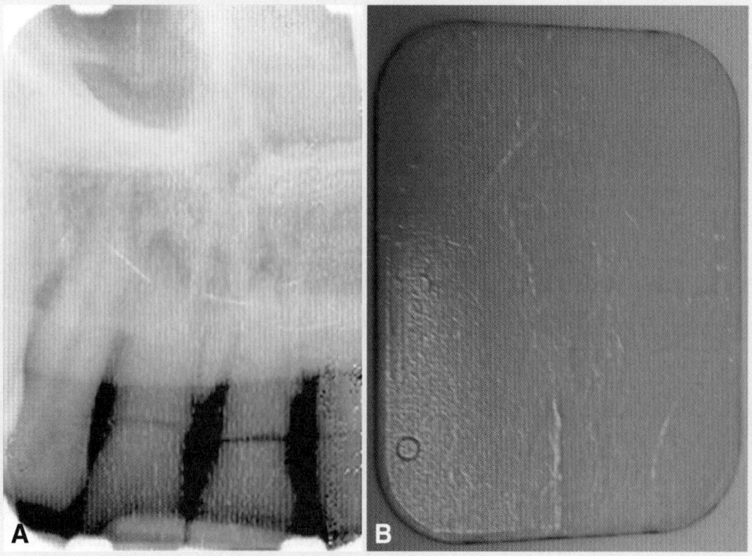

Fig. 4.23

BOX 4.3 Common Problems in Digital Image Receptor Exposure, Processing, and Handling—cont'd

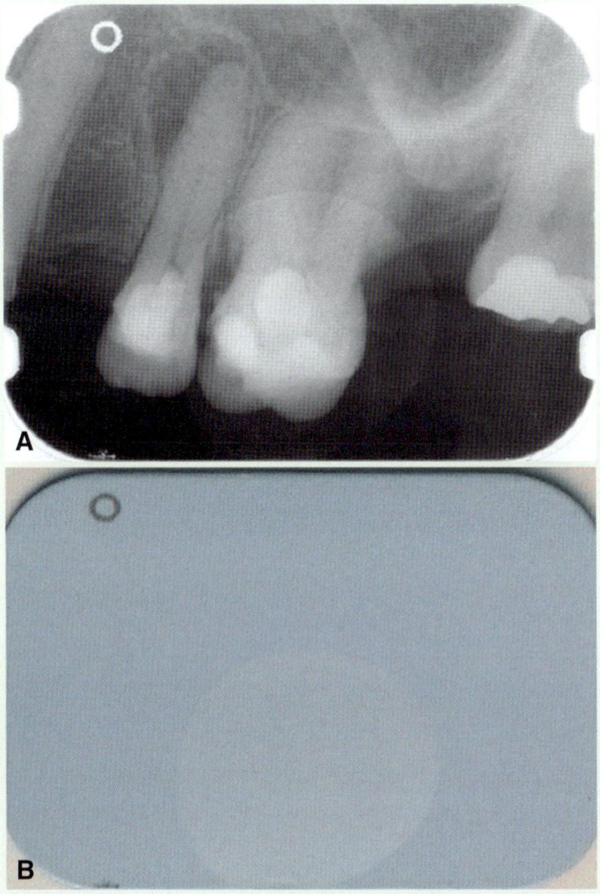

Fig. 4.24

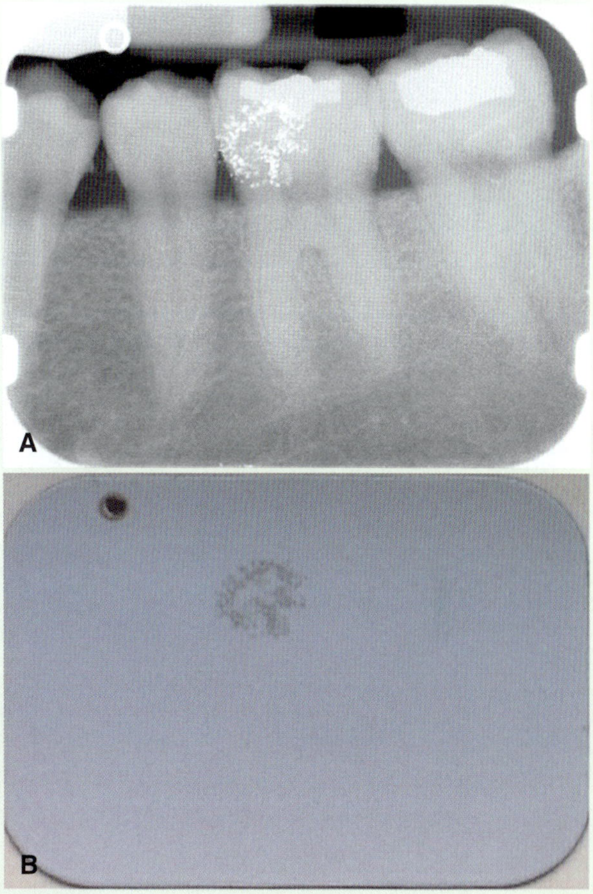

Fig. 4.25

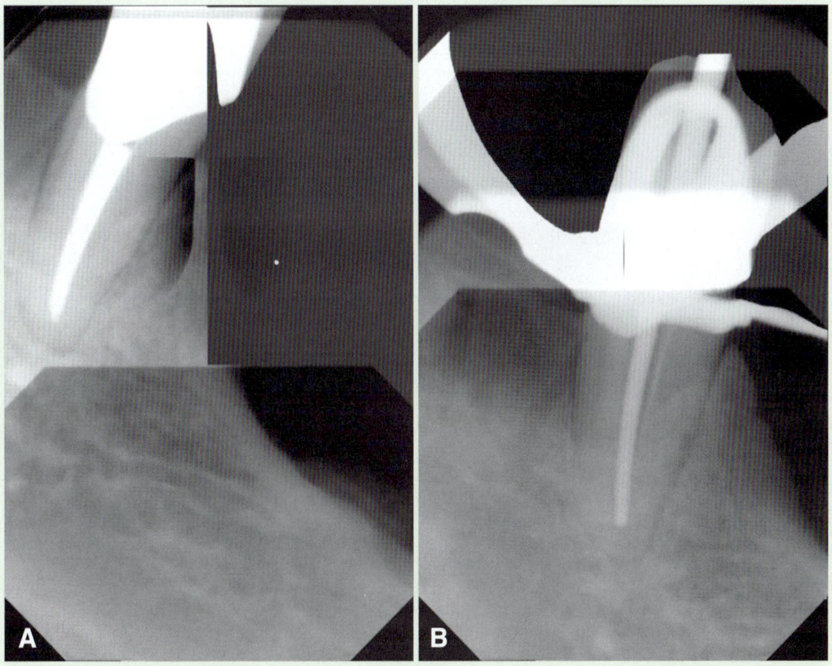

Fig. 4.26

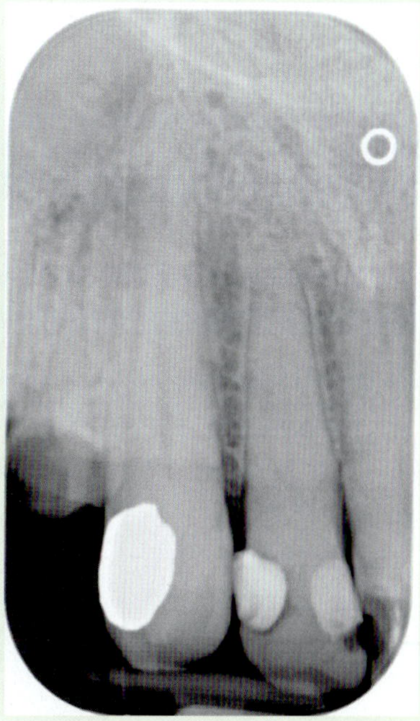

Fig. 4.27

Continued

BOX 4.3 Common Problems in Digital Image Receptor Exposure, Processing, and Handling—cont'd

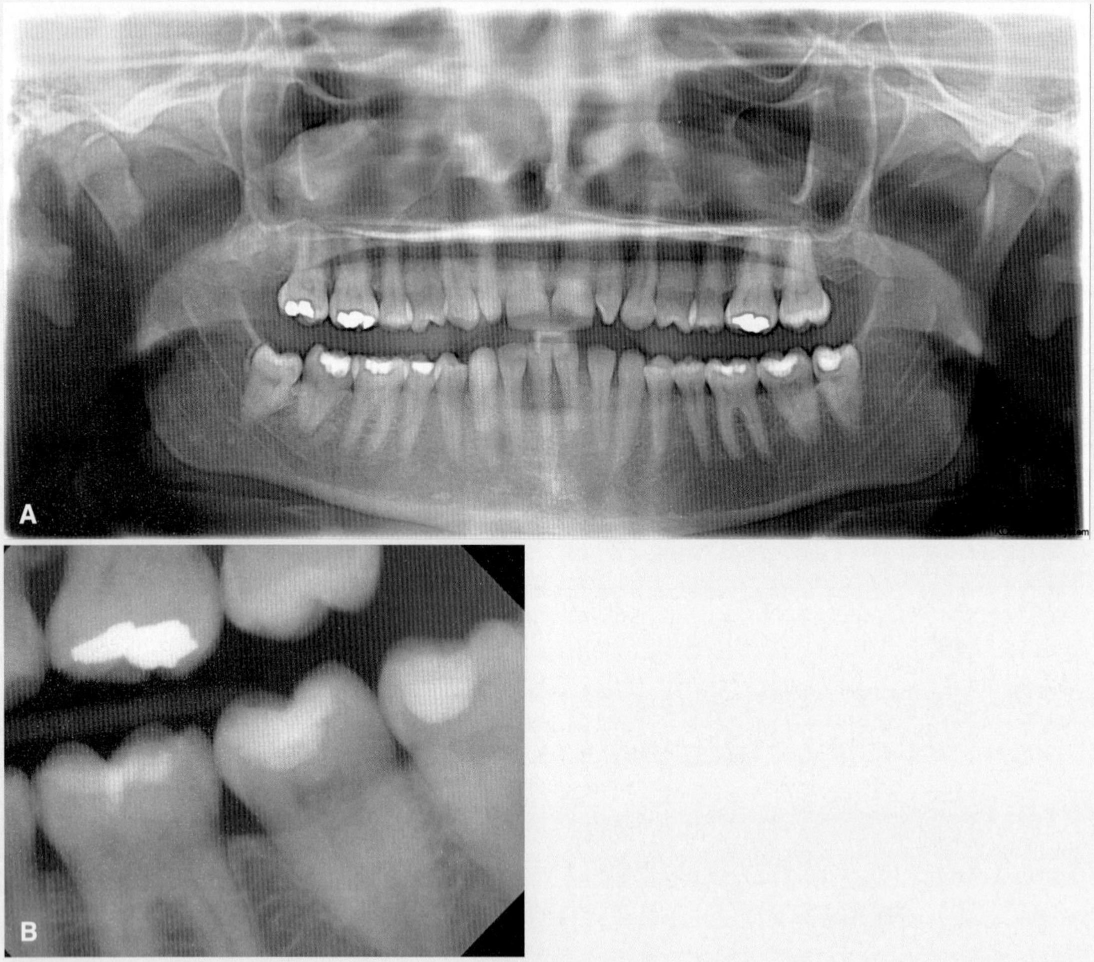

Fig. 4.28

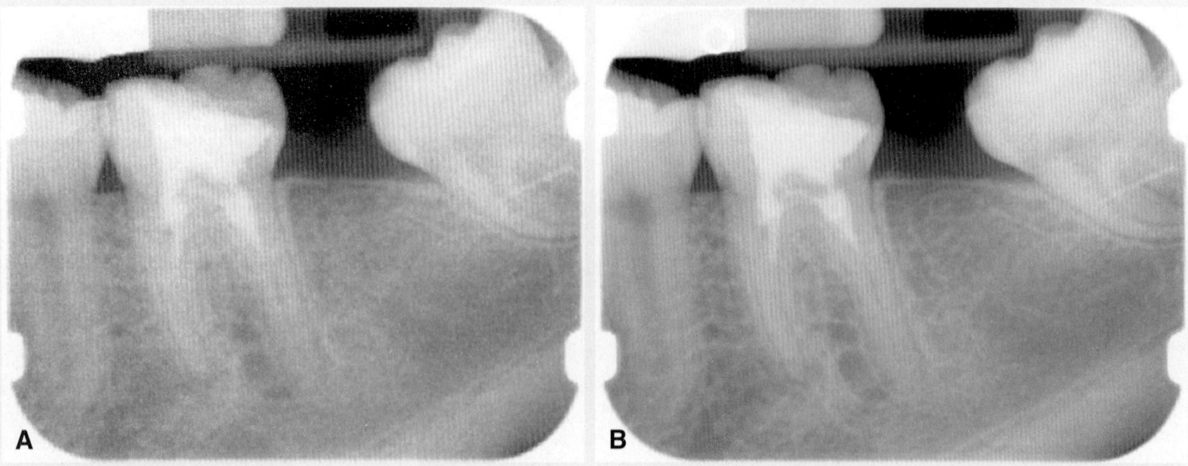

Fig. 4.29

CCD, Charge-coupled device; *PSP*, photostimulable phosphor.

contralateral position from their true side. One can imagine the liability that could occur from diagnosing and treating disease on the opposite side of the actual lesion. The Soredex OpTime system has addressed this issue by incorporating a round metal disk on the back of intraoral plates (see Fig. 4.7). This marker becomes visible on the image if the imaging plate is exposed backward. The appearance of the marker on the image does not fully obscure the anatomic information, and these images can be "mirrored" with imaging software tools without the need for repeated exposure. Carestream and Planmeca use RFID technology in their PSP plates, which also serves to identify plates that have been exposed backward.

Infection control is also an issue with digital receptors. Digital receptors cannot be sterilized by conventional means. They may be disinfected by wiping with disinfectants such as isopropyl alcohol or glutaraldehyde but should not be immersed in disinfecting solutions. The adage that "you can autoclave a digital receptor … once" stems from the fact that heat ruins electronic components in CCD and CMOS sensors and distorts the polyester base of PSP plates. Although each of the preceding concerns is of potential importance, the advantage of eliminating chemical processing in digital systems should not be overlooked. The time required to monitor and maintain a film processor properly is significant. Too often insufficient attention is paid to this critical aspect of film radiography. Digital systems may not save the time gained by eliminating film processing, but they do eliminate the loss in diagnostic quality that occurs when insufficient time and effort are spent on film processing quality assurance.

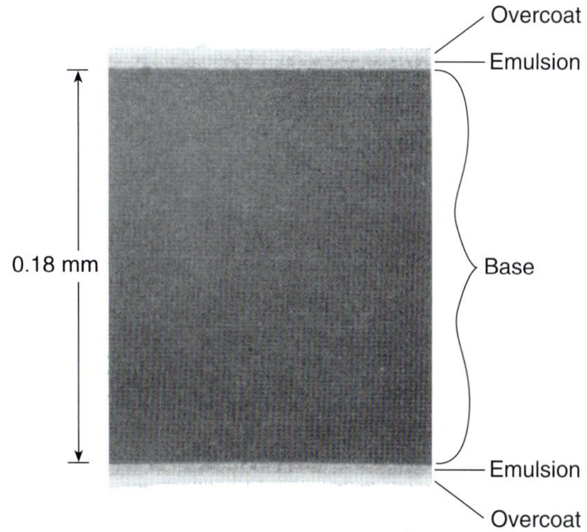

Fig. 4.30 Scanning electron micrograph of INSIGHT dental x-ray film (original magnification 300×). Note the overcoat, emulsion, and base on this double-emulsion film. (Courtesy Carestream Dental, a division of Carestream Health, Inc., Atlanta, Georgia.)

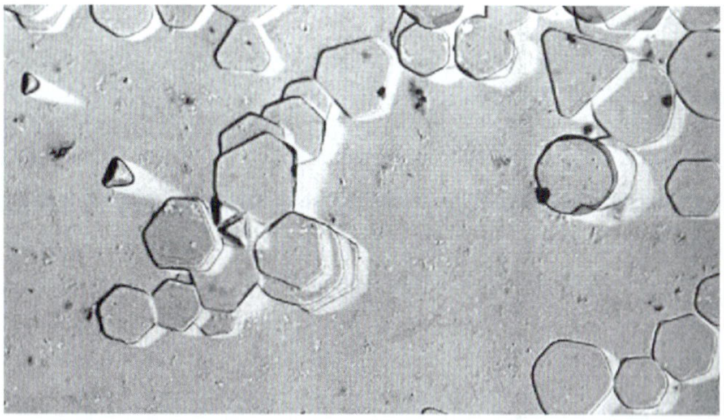

Fig. 4.31 Scanning electron micrograph of emulsion of INSIGHT film showing flat tabular silver bromide crystals, which capture incident photons. (Courtesy Carestream Dental, a division of Carestream Health, Inc., Atlanta, Georgia.)

FILM-BASED RADIOGRAPHIC IMAGING

Early radiation workers used photosensitive emulsions coated onto glass plates to record radiation. Subsequent to the discovery of x-rays, these emulsions were used to make radiographs. Radiographic film uses a silver halide emulsion on plastic to record and to display the image. Unlike digital receptors, radiographic film cannot be reused. Globally, film-based radiography is being replaced with digital imaging.

X-RAY FILM

Composition

X-ray film has two principal components: (1) emulsion and (2) base. The emulsion is sensitive to x-rays and visible light and records the radiographic image. The base is a plastic support onto which the emulsion is coated (Fig. 4.30).

Emulsion

The two principal components of emulsion are silver halide grains, which are sensitive to x-radiation and visible light, and a vehicle gelatinous matrix in which the crystals are suspended. The silver halide grains are composed primarily of crystals of silver bromide. The silver halide grains in INSIGHT film and Ultra-speed film (Carestream Dental, a division of Carestream Health, Inc., Atlanta, Georgia) are flat, tabular crystals with a mean diameter of approximately 1.8 μm (Fig. 4.31). The tabular grains are oriented parallel with the film surface to offer a large cross-sectional area to the x-ray beam. INSIGHT film has approximately twice the number of silver grains so that it requires only half the exposure of Ultra-speed film.

The silver halide grains are suspended in a surrounding vehicle that is applied to both sides of the supporting base. During film processing (described later in this chapter), the vehicle absorbs processing solutions, allowing the chemicals to reach and react with the silver halide grains. An additional layer of vehicle is added to the film emulsion as an overcoat (see Fig. 4.31). This barrier helps to protect the film from damage by scratching, contamination, or pressure from rollers when an automatic processor is used.

Film emulsions are sensitive to both x-ray photons and visible light. Film intended to be exposed by x-rays is called direct exposure film. All intraoral dental film is direct exposure film. Screen film is used with intensifying screens (described later in this chapter) that emit visible light. Screen film and intensifying screens are used for extraoral projections, such as panoramic and cephalometric radiographs.

Base

The function of the film base is to support the emulsion. The base for dental x-ray film is made of polyester polyethylene terephthalate, which provides the proper degree of flexibility to allow easy handling of the film. The film base must also withstand exposure to processing solutions without becoming distorted. The base is uniformly translucent and casts no pattern on the resultant radiograph.

Intraoral X-Ray Film

Intraoral dental x-ray film is made as a double-emulsion film (i.e., both sides of the base are coated with an emulsion). With a double layer of emulsion, less radiation is required to produce an image. Direct exposure film is used for intraoral examinations because it provides higher resolution images than screen-film combinations. Some diagnostic tasks, such as detection of incipient caries or early periapical disease, require this higher resolution.

One corner of each dental film has a small, raised dot that is used for film orientation (Fig. 4.32). The manufacturer orients the film in the packet so that the convex side of the dot is toward the front of the packet and faces the x-ray tube. The side of the film with the depression is thus oriented toward the patient's tongue. After the film has been exposed and processed, the dot is used to orient the patient's right- and left-side images properly. When mounting radiographs, each film is oriented with the convex side of the dot toward the viewer, and on the basis of the features of the teeth and anatomic landmarks in the adjacent bone, the films are arranged in their normal sequential relationship in the mount.

Intraoral x-ray film packets contain either one or two sheets of film (Fig. 4.33). When double film packs are used, the second film serves as a duplicate record that can be sent to insurance companies or to a colleague. The film is encased in a protective black paper wrapper and then in an outer moisture-resistant paper or plastic wrapping. The outer wrapping clearly indicates the location of the raised dot and identifies which side of the film should be directed toward the x-ray tube.

A thin lead foil backing with an embossed pattern is between the wrappers in the film packet. The foil is positioned in the film packet behind the film (see Fig. 4.33), away from the tube. This lead foil serves several purposes.

- It shields the film from backscatter (secondary) radiation, which fogs the film and reduces image contrast (image quality).
- It reduces patient exposure by absorbing some of the residual x-ray beam.
- Most importantly, if the film packet is placed backward in the patient's mouth so that the tube side of the film is facing away from the x-ray machine, the lead foil will be positioned between the subject and the film. In this circumstance, most of the radiation is absorbed by the lead foil, and the resulting radiograph is light and shows the embossed pattern in the lead foil (Fig. 4.34). This combination of a light film with the characteristic pattern indicates that the film packet was exposed backward in the patient's mouth and that the patient's right side–left side designation indicated by the film dot is reversed.

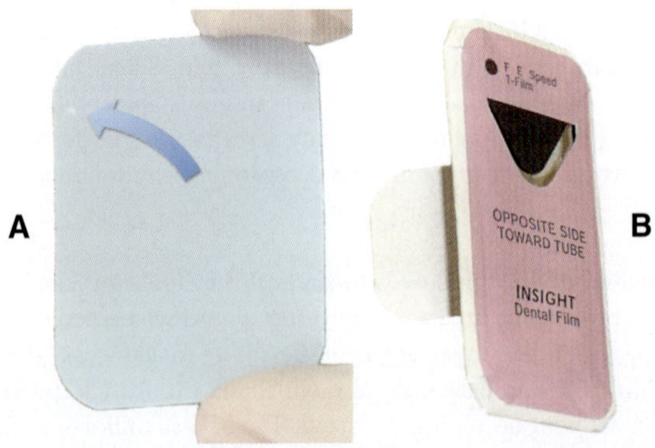

Fig. 4.32 (A) The raised film dot *(arrow)* indicates the tube side of the film and identifies the patient's right and left sides. (B) The location of this dot is clearly marked with a *black circle* on the outside of every film packet. (Courtesy of Carestream Dental, a division of Carestream Health, Inc., Atlanta, Georgia.)

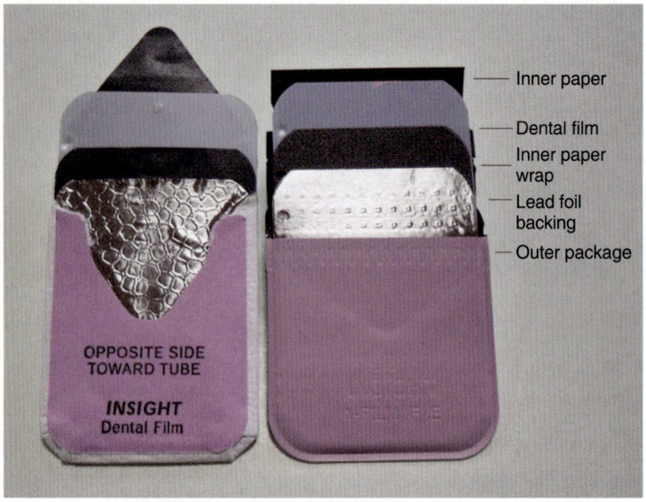

Fig. 4.33 Moisture-proof and lightproof packets, paper on the left and vinyl on right, contain an opening tab on the side opposite the tube. Inside is an interleaf paper wrapper that is folded around the film as well as a sheet of lead foil. Film is packaged with one or two sheets of film. The foil is positioned between the back side of the packet and the paper wrapper. In this position, it absorbs radiation that has passed through the film and prevents scatter radiation from blurring the image. If the film packet is inadvertently placed backward in the patient's mouth, the mottled image of the foil shows on the resultant image. (Courtesy of Carestream Dental, a division of Carestream Health, Inc., Atlanta, Georgia.)

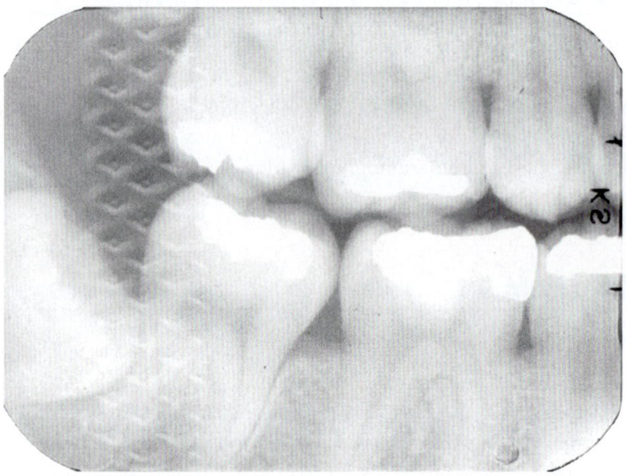

Fig. 4.34 Placing a film backward in the patient's mouth when the exposure was made results in a radiograph that is too light and shows the characteristic markings caused by exposure through the lead foil in the film packaging. In such an image, the left and right sides of the patient are reversed when using the dot as the orientation guide.

Periapical View

Periapical views record the crowns, roots, and surrounding bone. Film packs come in three sizes (Fig. 4.35):

- Size 0 for small children (22 mm × 35 mm).
- Size 1, which is relatively narrow and used for views of the anterior teeth (24 mm × 40 mm).
- Size 2, the standard film size used for adults (30.5 mm × 40.5 mm).

Bite-Wing View

Bite-wing (interproximal) views record the coronal portions of the maxillary and mandibular teeth in one image. They are used to detect interproximal caries and evaluate the height of alveolar bone. Size

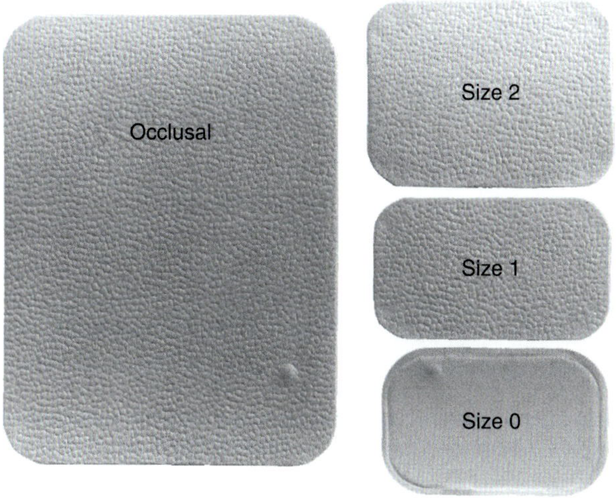

Fig. 4.35 Dental x-ray film is commonly supplied in various sizes. *Left*, Occlusal film. *Top right*, Size 2 for adult posterior film. *Middle right*, Size 1 for adult anterior film. *Bottom right*, Size 0 for child-size film (in vinyl wrapping).

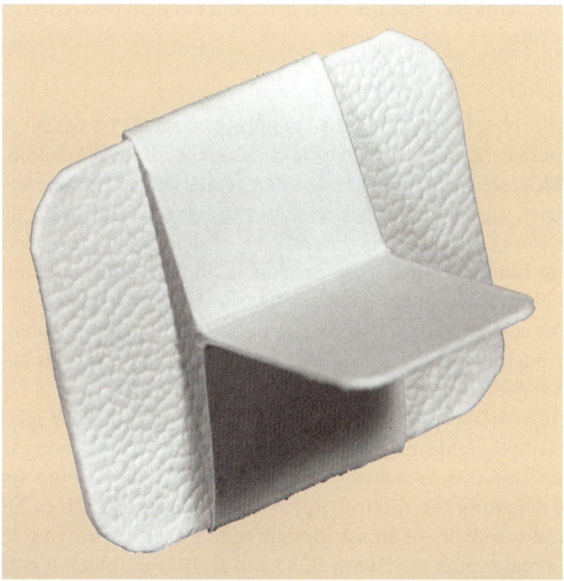

Fig. 4.36 Paper loop placed around a size 2 adult film to support the film when the patient bites on the tab for a bite-wing projection. This projection reveals the tooth crowns and alveolar crests.

2 film is normally used in adults; the smaller size 1 is preferred in children. In small children, size 0 may be used. A relatively long size 3 is also available.

Bite-wing films often have a paper tab projecting from the middle of the film on which the patient bites to support the film (Fig. 4.36). This tab is rarely visualized on the image and does not interfere with the diagnostic quality of the image. Film-holding instruments for bite-wing projections also are available.

Occlusal View

Occlusal film, size 4, is more than three times larger than size 2 film (see Fig. 4.36). It is used to show larger areas of the maxilla or mandible than may be seen on a periapical film. These films also are used to obtain right-angle views to the usual periapical view. The name derives from the fact that the film is held in position by having the patient bite lightly on it to support it between the occlusal surfaces of the teeth (see Chapter 6).

Screen Film

The extraoral projections used most frequently in dentistry are panoramic and cephalometric views. For these projections, screen film is used with intensifying screens (described later in this chapter) to reduce patient exposure (Fig. 4.37). Screen film is different from dental intraoral film. It is designed to be sensitive to visible light because it is placed between two intensifying screens when an exposure is made. The intensifying screens absorb x-rays and emit visible light, which exposes the film. Silver halide crystals are inherently sensitive to ultraviolet (UV) and blue light (300–500 nm) and thus are sensitive to screens that emit UV and blue light. When film is used with screens that emit green light, the silver halide crystals are coated with sensitizing dyes to increase absorption. It is important to use the appropriate screen-film combination recommended by the screen and film manufacturer so that the emission characteristics of the screen match the absorption characteristics of the film.

Contemporary screen films use tabular-shaped (flat) grains of silver halide (Fig. 4.38) to capture the image. The tabular grains are oriented with their relatively large, flat surfaces facing the radiation source, providing a larger cross section (target) and resulting in increased speed without loss of sharpness. To increase the sharpness of images, some manufacturers add an absorbing dye in the film emulsion. This dye reduces light from one screen crossing through the film to reach the emulsion on the opposite side. EVG film (enhanced visualization, green sensitive) from Carestream Dental is an example of this type of film.

INTENSIFYING SCREENS

Early in the history of radiography, scientists discovered that various inorganic salts or phosphors fluoresce (emit visible light) when

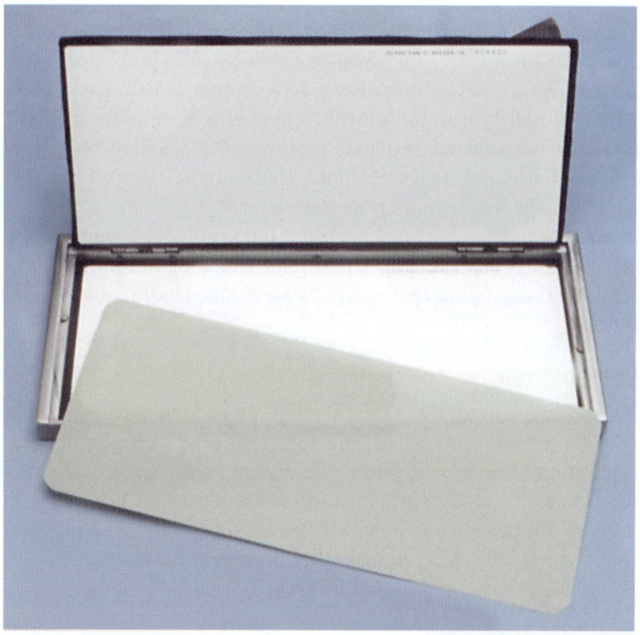

Fig. 4.37 Cassette for 8-inch × 10-inch film along with a sheet of screen film. When the cassette is closed, the film is supported in close contact between the two white intensifying screens seen on the inside of the cassette. These intensifying screens absorb most of the incident x-ray beam and then fluoresce and expose the film.

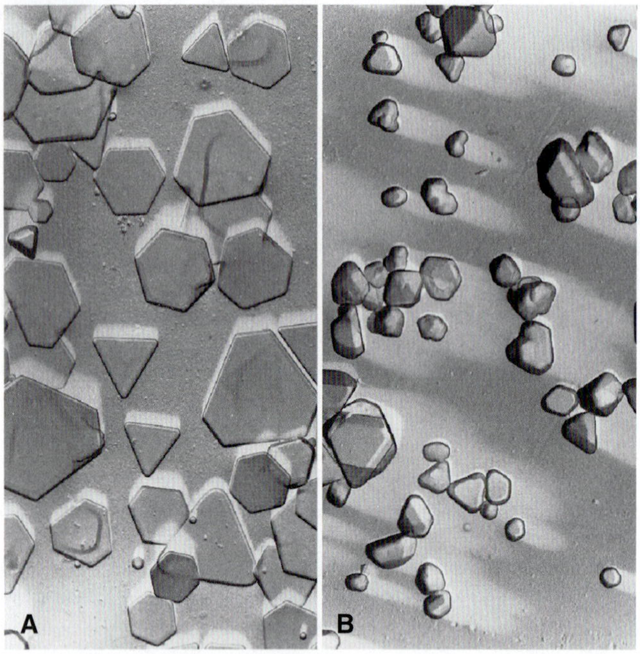

Fig. 4.38 Tablet grains of silver halide in an emulsion of T-MAT film (A) are larger and flatter than the smaller, thicker crystals in an emulsion of older conventional film (B). The flat surfaces of the tablet grains are oriented parallel with the film surface, facing the radiation source. (Courtesy of Carestream Dental, a division of Carestream Health, Inc.)

exposed to an x-ray beam. The intensity of this fluorescence is proportional to the x-ray energy absorbed. These phosphors are incorporated into intensifying screens for use with screen film. The sum of the effects of the x-rays and the visible light emitted by the screen phosphors exposes the film in an intensifying cassette (see Fig. 4.37).

Function

The presence of intensifying screens creates an image receptor system that is 10–60 times more sensitive to x-rays than is the film alone. Consequently, use of intensifying screens substantially reduces the dose of x-radiation to the patient. Intensifying screens are used with films for virtually all extraoral radiography, including panoramic, cephalometric, and skull projections. However, the use of an intensifying screen decreases image resolution.

Intensifying screens are not used intraorally with periapical or occlusal films because their use would reduce the resolution of the resulting image below that necessary for detailed evaluation of dental disease.

Composition

Intensifying screens are made of a base-supporting material, a phosphor layer, and a protective polymeric coat (Fig. 4.39). In all dental applications, intensifying screens are used in pairs, one on each side of the film, and they are positioned inside a cassette (see Fig. 4.37). The purpose of a cassette is to hold each intensifying screen in close contact with the x-ray film to maximize the sharpness of the image.

Base

The base material of most intensifying screens is some form of polyester plastic that is approximately 0.25 mm thick. The base provides mechanical support for the other layers. In some intensifying screens, the base also is reflective; thus it reflects light emitted from the phosphor layer back toward the x-ray film (see Fig. 4.39). This reflective

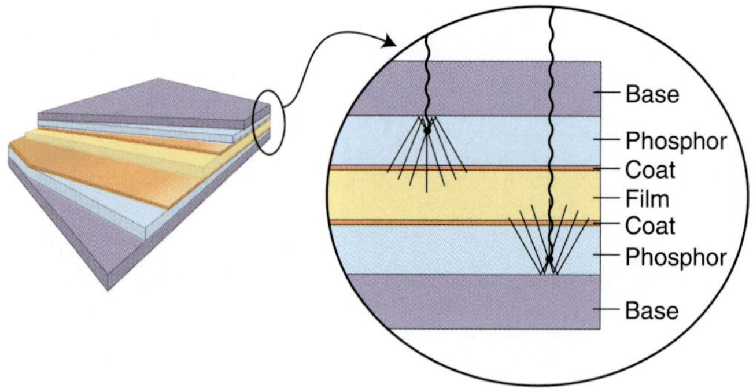

Fig. 4.39 Image on the *left* shows a schematic of two intensifying screens enclosing a film *(yellow)*. An intensifying screen is composed of a supporting base *(purple)*, a layer containing the phosphors *(light blue)*, and a protective coat *(orange)*. The detailed view on the *right* shows x-ray photons entering at the top, traveling through the base, and striking phosphors in the base. The phosphors emit visible light, exposing the film. Some visible light photons may reflect off the reflecting layer of the base.

base increases the light exposing the film but also results in some image "unsharpness" because of the divergence of light rays reflected back to the film.

Phosphor Layer

The phosphor layer is composed of phosphorescent crystals suspended in a polymeric binder. When the crystals absorb x-ray photons, they fluoresce (see Fig. 4.39). The phosphor crystals often contain rare earth elements, most commonly lanthanum and gadolinium. Their fluorescence can be increased by the addition of small amounts of elements, such as thulium, niobium, or terbium. Common phosphor combinations used in intensifying screens are shown in Table 4.3. Rare earth screens convert each absorbed x-ray photon into approximately 4000 lower-energy, visible-light (green or blue) photons. These visible photons expose the film.

Different phosphors fluoresce in different portions of the spectrum. For example, light emission from Lanex rare-earth intensifying screens ranges from 375 to 600 nm and peaks sharply at 545 nm (green). Fig. 4.40 shows the spectral emission of a rare-earth screen and the spectral sensitivity of an appropriate film. Other intensifying screens have a major peak at 350 nm (UV) and at 450 nm (blue). It is important to match green-emitting screens with green-sensitive films and blue-emitting screens with blue-sensitive films.

Intensifying screens are described in terms of their speed—their ability to convert x-ray photons to visible light photons. Fast screens have large phosphor crystals and efficiently convert x-ray photons to visible light but produce images with lower resolution. As the size of the crystals or the thickness of the screen decreases, the speed of the screen also declines, but image sharpness increases. Fast screens also have a thicker phosphor layer and a reflective layer, but these properties also decrease sharpness. In deciding on the combination to use, the practitioner must consider the resolution requirements of the task for which the image will be used. Screen-film combinations are rated for

TABLE 4.3 Rare-Earth Elements Used in Intensifying Screens

Emission	Phosphor
Green	Gadolinium oxysulfide, terbium activated
Blue and ultraviolet	Yttrium tantalite, niobium activated

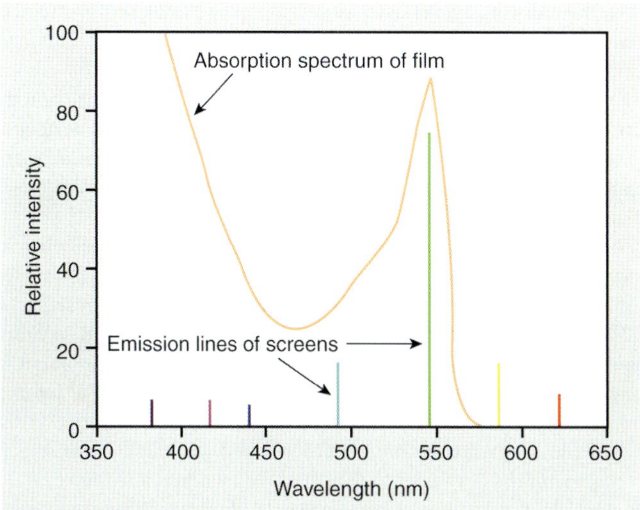

Fig. 4.40 Relative sensitivity of T-MAT film *(orange line)* and emission lines (shown in their visual colors) of Carestream Dental LANEX and EV screens (gadolinium oxysulfide, terbium activated). Intensifying screens emit light as a series of relatively narrow line emissions. The maximal emission of the screen at 545 nm *(green)* corresponds well to a high-sensitivity region of the film. (Data from Carestream Dental, a division of Carestream Health, Inc.)

speed, a measure of the amount of radiation required for a proper exposure. For dental extraoral diagnostic tasks, it is recommended to use screen-film combinations that have a speed of 400 or faster.

Protective Coat

A protective polymer coat ($\leq$15 μm thick) is placed over the phosphor layer to protect the phosphor and to provide a surface that can be cleaned. The intensifying screens should be routinely cleaned because any debris, spots, or scratches may cause light spots on the resultant radiograph.

FORMATION OF THE LATENT IMAGE

When a beam of photons exits the patient and exposes an x-ray film (either direct exposure film or screen film exposed by light photons), it chemically changes the photosensitive silver halide crystals in the film emulsion. These chemically altered silver bromide crystals constitute the latent (invisible) image on the film. Before exposure, film emulsion consists of photosensitive crystals containing primarily silver bromide (Fig. 4.41A). These silver halide crystals also contain a few free silver ions (interstitial silver ions) and trace amounts of sulfur compounds bound to the surface of the crystals. Along with physical irregularities in the crystal produced by iodide ions, sulfur compounds create sensitivity sites, sites in the crystals that are sensitive to radiation.

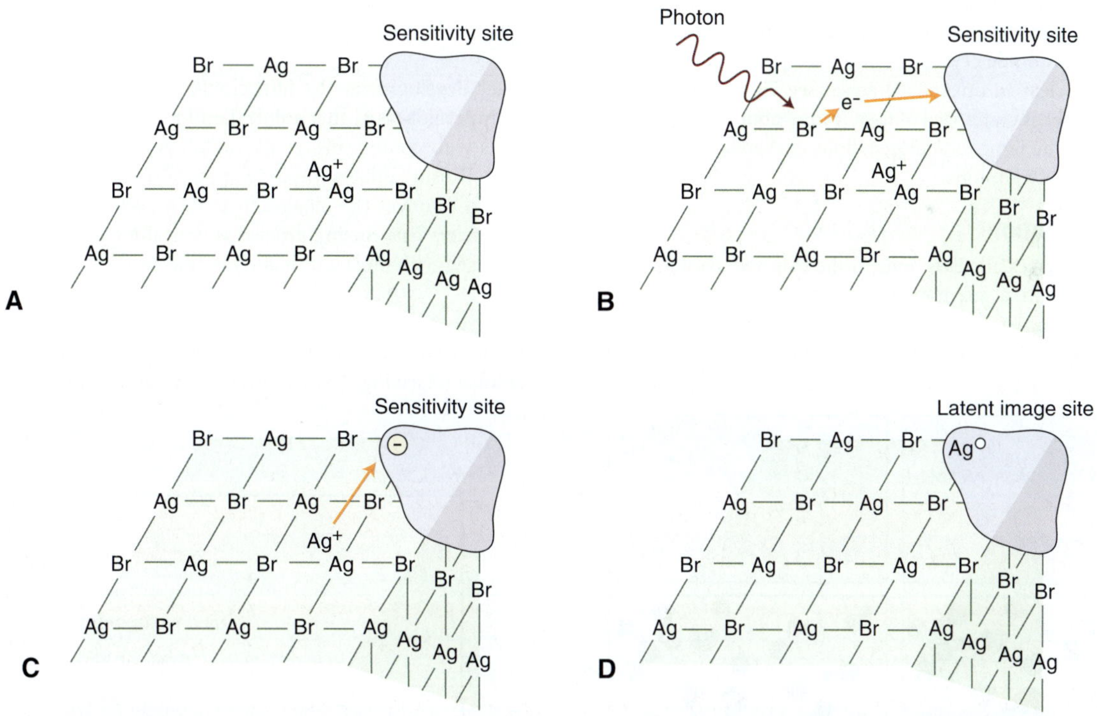

Fig. 4.41 (A) A silver bromide crystal in the emulsion of an x-ray film contains mostly silver and bromide ions in a crystal lattice. There are also free interstitial silver ions and areas of trace chemicals that form sensitivity sites. (B) Exposure of the crystal to photons in an x-ray beam results in the release of electrons, usually by interaction of the photon with a bromide ion. The recoil electrons have sufficient kinetic energy to move about in the crystal. When electrons reach a sensitivity site, they impart a negative charge to this region. (C) Free interstitial silver ions (with a positive charge) are attracted to the negatively charged sensitivity site. (D) When the silver ions reach the sensitivity site, they acquire an electron and become neutral silver atoms. These silver atoms now constitute a latent image site. The collection of latent image sites over the entire film constitutes the latent image. Developer causes the neutral silver atoms at the latent image sites to initiate the conversion of all the silver ions in the crystal into one large grain of metallic silver. The bromine dissolves in the developer.

Each crystal has many sensitivity sites. When the silver halide crystals are irradiated, x-ray photons release electrons from the bromide ions (see Fig. 4.41B). The free electrons move through the crystal until they reach a sensitivity site, where they become trapped and impart a negative charge to the site. The negatively charged sensitivity site attracts positively charged free interstitial silver ions (see Fig. 4.41C). When a silver ion reaches the negatively charged sensitivity site, it is reduced and forms a neutral atom of metallic silver (see Fig. 4.41D). The sites containing these neutral silver atoms are now called latent image sites. This process occurs numerous times within a crystal. The overall distribution of crystals with latent image sites in a film after exposure constitutes the latent image. Processing the exposed film in developer and fixer converts the latent image into the visible radiographic image.

PROCESSING SOLUTIONS

Film processing involves the following procedures:

1. Immerse exposed film in developer.
2. Rinse developer off film in water bath.
3. Immerse film in fixer.
4. Wash film in water bath to remove fixer.
5. Dry film and mount for viewing.

Following exposure, each grain of silver halide in film emulsion (Fig. 4.42A) contains neutral silver atoms at their latent image sites (see Fig. 4.42B). These latent image sites render the crystals sensitive to development and image formation. Developer converts silver bromide crystals with neutral silver atoms deposited at the latent image sites into black, solid silver metallic grains (see Fig. 4.42C). These solid silver grains block light from a viewbox. Fixer removes unexposed, undeveloped silver bromide crystals (crystals without latent image sites), leaving the film clear in unexposed areas (see Fig. 4.42D). Thus, the radiographic image is composed of light (radiopaque) areas, where few photons reached the film, and dark (radiolucent) areas of the film that were struck by many photons.

Developing Solution

The developer reduces all silver ions in the exposed crystals of silver halide (crystals with a latent image) to metallic silver grains (see Fig. 4.42). To produce a diagnostic image, this reduction process must be restricted to crystals containing latent image sites; to accomplish this, the reducing agents used as developers are catalyzed by the neutral silver atoms at the latent image sites (see Fig. 4.42B). Individual crystals are developed completely or not at all during the recommended developing times (see Fig. 4.42C). Variations in density on the processed radiographs are the result of different ratios of developed (exposed) and undeveloped (unexposed) crystals. Areas with many exposed crystals are darker because of their higher concentration of black metallic silver grains after development.

When an exposed film is developed, the developer initially has no visible effect (Fig. 4.43). After this initial phase, the density increases, rapidly at first and then more slowly. Eventually, all the exposed crystals develop (are converted to black metallic silver), and the developing agent starts to reduce the unexposed crystals. The development of unexposed crystals results in chemical fog on the film. The interval between maximal density and fogging explains why a properly exposed film does not become overdeveloped, although it may be in contact with the developer longer than the recommended interval.

The chemical components of the developing solution and their functions are described in Table 4.4.

Developer Replenisher

The developing solution of both manual and automatic developers should be replenished with fresh solution each morning to prolong the life of the used developer. The recommended amount to be added daily is 8 ounces of fresh developer (replenisher) per gallon of developing solution. This assumes the development of an average of 30 periapical or 5 panoramic films per day. Some of the used solution may need to be removed to make room for the replenisher.

Rinsing

After development, the film emulsion swells and becomes saturated with developer. At this point, the films are rinsed in water for 30 seconds with continuous, gentle agitation before they are placed in the fixer. Rinsing dilutes the developer, slowing the development process. It also removes the alkali activator, preventing neutralization of the acid fixer. This rinsing process is typical for manual processing but is not used with most automatic processors.

Fixing Solution

Fixing solution removes undeveloped silver halide crystals from the emulsion (see Fig. 4.42D). If these crystals are not removed, the image

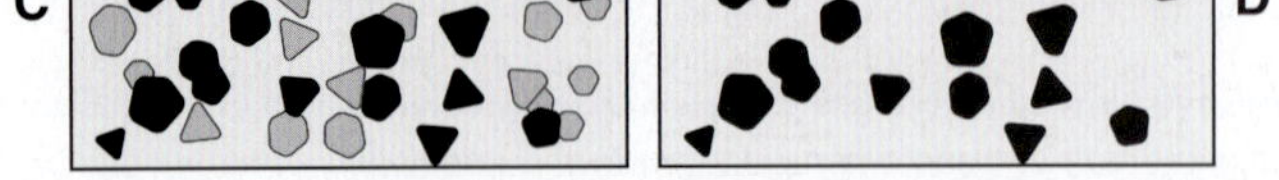

Fig. 4.42 Emulsion changes during film processing. (A) Before exposure, many silver bromide crystals *(gray)* are present in the emulsion. (B) After exposure, the exposed crystals containing neutral silver atoms at latent image sites (*orange dots* within some crystals) constitute the latent image. (C) The developer converts the exposed crystals containing neutral silver atoms at the latent image sites into solid grains of metallic silver *(black)*. (D) The fixer dissolves the unexposed, undeveloped silver bromide crystals, leaving only the solid silver grains that form the radiographic image.

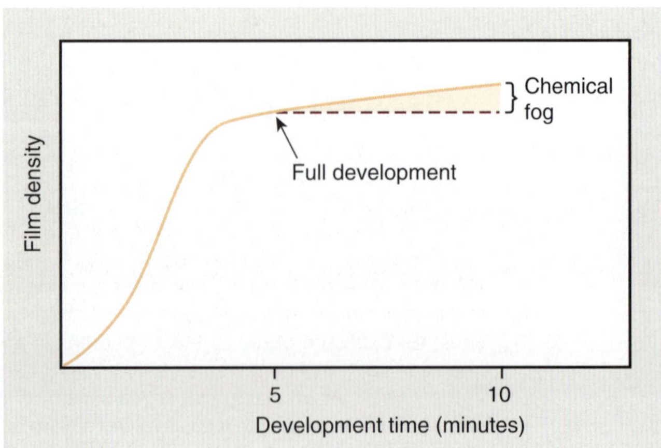

Fig. 4.43 Relationship between film density and development time. The density of film increases quickly initially in the developer. After full development, the density continues to increase slowly because of chemical fog.

TABLE 4.4 Components and Function of Radiographic Developer Solution

Component	Ingredient	Function
Developer	Phenidone	Serves as the first electron donor that converts silver ions to metallic silver at the latent image site. This electron transfer generates the oxidized form of phenidone
	Hydroquinone	Hydroquinone provides an electron to reduce the oxidized phenidone back to its original active state so that it can continue to reduce silver halide grains to metallic silver
Activator	Sodium hydroxide or potassium hydroxide	Maintains an alkaline pH (approximately 10) for activity of developer. Causes the gelatin to swell so that the developing agents can diffuse more rapidly into the emulsion to reach silver bromide crystals
Preservative	Sodium sulfite	Antioxidant that extends life of developing solution. Combines with oxidized developer to produce a compound that subsequently stains images brown if not washed out
Restrainer	Bromine-containing compounds	Restrains development of unexposed silver halide crystals. Acts as antifog agents and increases contrast

on the resultant radiograph is dark and nondiagnostic (Fig. 4.44). Fixer also hardens and shrinks the film emulsion.

The chemical components of the developing solution and their functions are described in Table 4.5. As with developer, fixer should be replenished daily at the rate of 8 ounces per gallon.

Washing

After fixing, the processed film is washed in water to remove all thiosulfate ions and silver thiosulfate complexes. Washing efficiency declines rapidly when the water temperature decreases to less than 60°F. Any silver compound or thiosulfate that remains because of improper washing discolors and causes stains, which are most apparent in the radiopaque (light) areas.

DARKROOM AND EQUIPMENT

A conventional darkroom with manual wet processing tanks should be convenient to the x-ray machines and dental operatories and should be at least 4 feet × 5 feet (1.2 m × 1.5 m).

DARKROOM

One of the most important requirements is that the darkroom be lightproof. If it is not, stray light can cause film fogging and loss of image contrast. To make the darkroom lightproof, a light-tight door or doorless maze (if space permits) is used. The door should have a lock to prevent accidental opening, which might allow an unexpected flood of light that can ruin opened films. The darkroom must also be well ventilated to provide a comfortable working environment and to exhaust moisture from drying films. In addition, a comfortable room temperature helps to maintain optimal conditions for developing, fixing, and washing solutions.

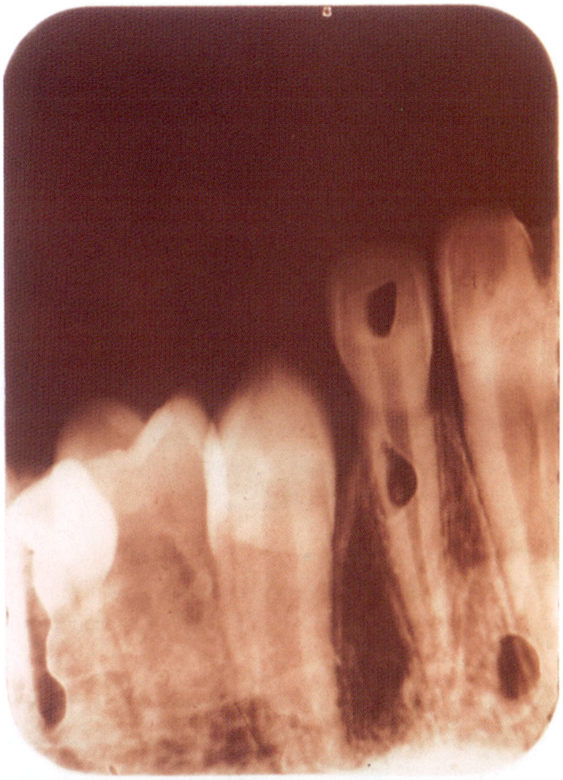

Fig. 4.44 Incomplete fixation results in images that are dark and discolored, making them nondiagnostic. This film was also poorly positioned in the patient's mouth, cutting off most apices of the teeth. Staining may also be caused by using depleted developer or fixer or using contaminated solutions.

TABLE 4.5 Components and Function of Radiographic Fixer Solution

Component	Ingredient	Function
Clearing agent	Ammonium thiosulfate	Dissolves the unexposed silver halide grains Excessive fixation (hours) results in a gradual loss of film density because the grains of silver slowly dissolve in the fixing solution
Acidifier	Acetic acid	Maintain an acidic pH (approximately 4–4.5) Promotes good diffusion of thiosulfate into the emulsion and of silver thiosulfate complex out of the emulsion Inactivates any residual developing agents
Preservative	Ammonium sulfite	Prevents oxidation of ammonium thiosulfate, which is unstable in the acidic environment
Hardener	Aluminum sulfate	Complexes with the gelatin during fixing to prevent damage to the gelatin overcoat during subsequent handling

Safelights

The processing room should have both white illumination and safelights. A safelight is low-intensity illumination of relatively long wavelength (red) that does not rapidly affect open film but permits one to see well enough to work in the area (Fig. 4.45). To minimize the fogging effect of prolonged exposure, the safelight should have a frosted 15-W bulb or a clear 7.5-W bulb and should be mounted at least 4 feet above the surface where opened films are handled.

X-ray films are very sensitive to the blue-green region of the spectrum and are less sensitive to red wavelengths. The red GBX-2 filter is recommended as a safelight in darkrooms where either intraoral or extraoral films are handled because this filter transmits light only at the red end of the spectrum (Fig. 4.46). Film handling under a safelight should be limited to approximately 5 minutes because film emulsion shows some sensitivity to light from a safelight with prolonged exposure. The older ML-2 filters (yellow light) are not appropriate for fast intraoral dental film or extraoral panoramic or cephalometric film.

Manual-Processing Tanks

Dental offices that use automatic film processors should maintain the capability to manually process film. The tank must have hot

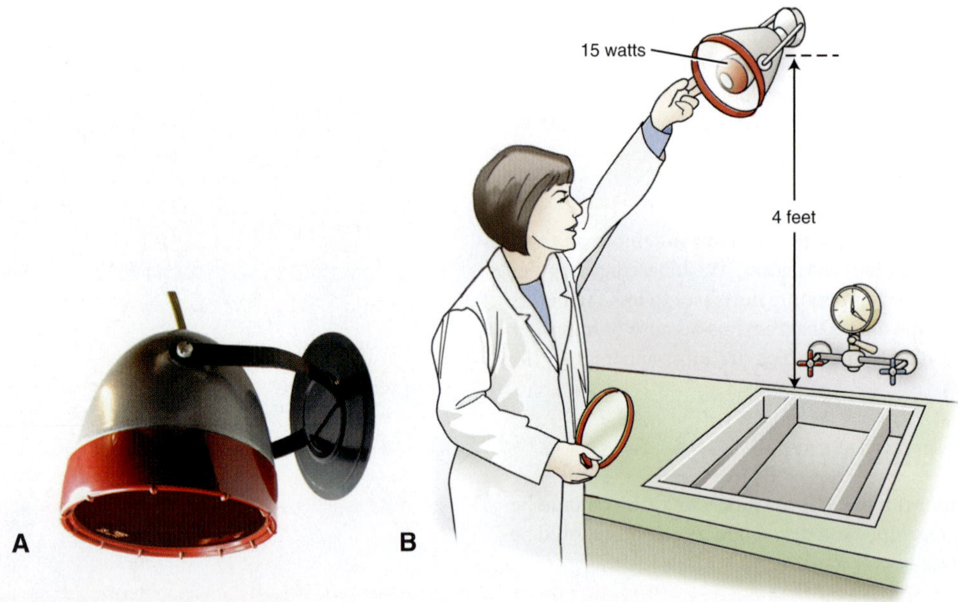

Fig. 4.45 (A) A safelight may be mounted on the wall or ceiling in the darkroom and should be at least 4 feet from the work surface. (B) The safelight uses a GBX-2 filter and 15-W bulb.

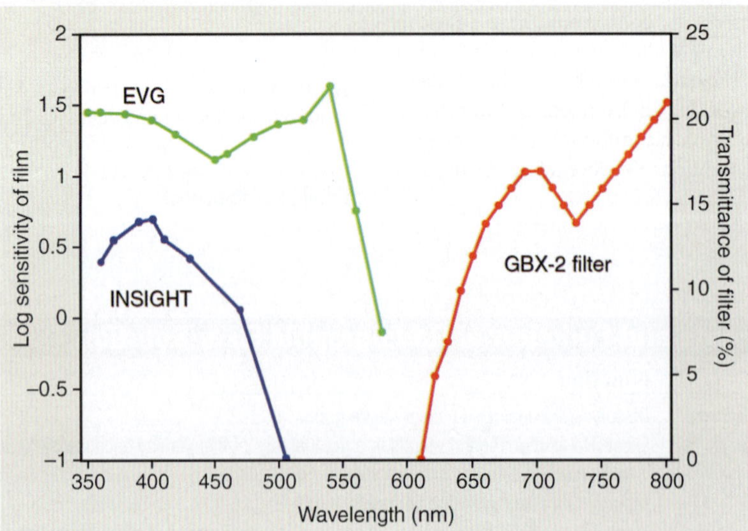

Fig. 4.46 Spectral sensitivities of EVG film *(green line)* and INSIGHT film *(blue line)* shown with the transmission characteristics of a GBX-2 filter *(red line)*. The films are more sensitive in the blue-green portion of the spectrum (shorter than 600 nm), whereas the GBX-2 filter transmits primarily at the red end of the spectrum (longer than 600 nm).

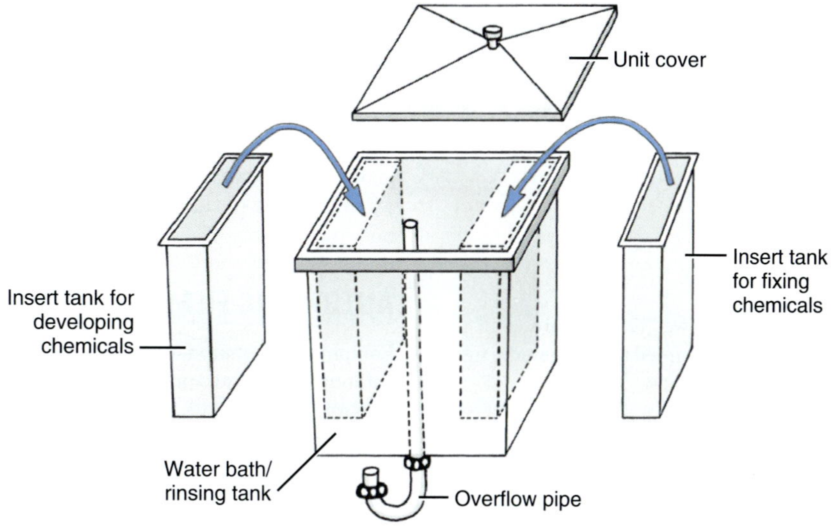

Fig. 4.47 Processing tank. The developing and fixing tanks are inserted into a bath of running water with an overflow drain. The water bath may be maintained at a stable and optimal temperature for film processing.

and cold running water and a means of maintaining the temperature between 60°F and 75°F. A practical size for a dental office is a master tank approximately 20 cm × 25 cm (8 inches × 10 inches) that can serve as a water jacket for two removable inserts that fit inside (Fig. 4.47). The insert tanks usually hold 3.8 L (1 gallon) of developer or fixer and are placed within the outer, larger master tank. The outer tank holds the water for maintaining the temperature of the developer and fixer in the insert tanks and for washing films. The developer customarily is placed in the insert tank on the left side of the master tank, and the fixer is placed in the insert tank on the right. All three tanks should be made of stainless steel, which does not react with the processing solutions and is easy to clean. The master tank should have a cover to reduce oxidation of the processing solutions, protect the developing film from accidental exposure to light, and minimize evaporation of the processing solutions.

Thermometer

The temperature of the developing, fixing, and washing solutions should be closely controlled. A thermometer can be left in the water circulating through the master tank to monitor the temperature and ensure that the water temperature regulator is working properly. The most desirable thermometers clip onto the side of the tank. Thermometers may contain alcohol or metal, but they should not contain mercury because they could break and contaminate the processor or solutions.

Timer

The x-ray film must be exposed to the processing chemicals for specific intervals. An interval timer is indispensable for controlling development and fixation times.

Drying Racks

Two or three drying racks can be mounted on a convenient wall for film hangers. Drip trays are placed underneath the racks to catch water that may run off the wet films. An electric fan can be used to circulate the air and speed the drying of films, but it should not be pointed directly at the films.

MANUAL-PROCESSING PROCEDURES

Manual processing of film requires the following nine steps:

1. *Replenish solutions.* The first step in manual tank processing is to replenish the developer and fixer. Check the solution levels to ensure that the developer and fixer cover the films on the top clips of the film hangers.
2. *Stir solutions.* Stir the developer and fixing solution to mix the chemicals and equalize the temperature throughout the tanks. To prevent cross-contamination, use a separate paddle for each solution. It is best to label one paddle for the developer and the other for the fixer.
3. *Mount films on hangers.* Using only safelight illumination in the darkroom, remove the exposed film from its lightproof packet or cassette. Hold the films by their edges only to avoid damage to the film surface. Clip the bare film onto a film hanger, one film to a clip (Fig. 4.48). Label the film racks with the patient' name and the exposure date.

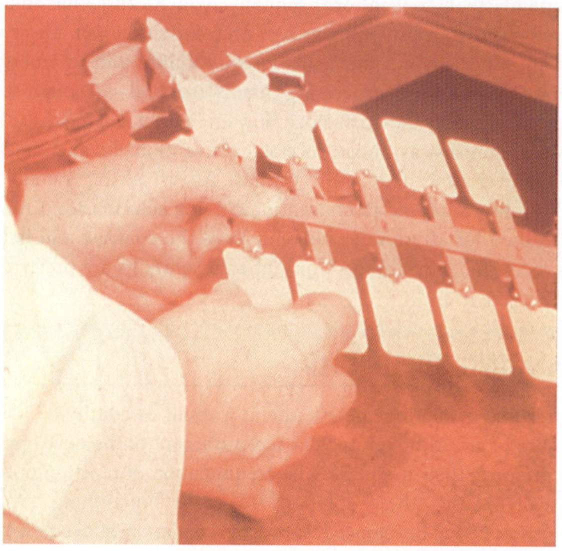

Fig. 4.48 Films are mounted securely on film clips. Film is always held by its edges to avoid fingerprints on the image. (Courtesy C. L. Crabtree, DDS, Bureau of Radiological Health, Rockville, MD.)

4. *Set timer.* Check the temperature of the developer, and set the interval timer to the time indicated by the manufacturer for the solution temperature, typically:

Temperature (°F)	Development Time (Minutes)
68	5
70	4½
72	4
76	3
80	2½

   Processing films at either higher or lower temperatures and for longer or shorter times than recommended by the manufacturer reduces the contrast of the processed film.
5. *Develop.* Start the timer mechanism, and immerse the hanger and films immediately in the developer. Agitate the hanger mildly for 5–10 seconds to remove air bubbles from the film. Do not agitate the film during development.
6. *Rinse.* After development, remove the film hanger from the developer, draining excess into the water bath, and place in the running water bath for 30 seconds. Agitate the films continuously in the rinse water to remove excess developer, thus slowing development and minimizing contamination of the fixer.
7. *Fix.* Place the hanger and film in the fixer solution for 2–4 minutes and agitate for 5 of every 30 seconds. Agitation eliminates bubbles and brings fresh fixer into contact with the emulsion. When the films are removed, drain the excess fixer into the wash bath.
8. *Wash.* After fixation of the films is complete, place the hanger in running water for at least 10 minutes to remove residual processing solutions. After the films have been washed, remove surface moisture by gently shaking excess water from the films and hanger.
9. *Dry.* Dry the films in circulating, moderately warm air. After drying, the films are ready to mount.

RAPID-PROCESSING CHEMICALS

Rapid-processing solutions typically develop films in 15 seconds and fix them in 15 seconds at room temperature. They have the same general formulation as conventional processing solutions but often contain a higher concentration of hydroquinone. They also have a more alkaline pH than conventional solutions, which causes the emulsion to swell more, thus providing greater access to developer. These solutions are especially advantageous in endodontics and in emergency situations, when short processing time is essential. Although the resultant images may be satisfactory, they often do not achieve the same degree of contrast as films processed conventionally, and they may discolor over time if not fully washed. After viewing, rapidly processed films are placed in conventional fixing solution for 4 minutes and washed for 10 minutes; this improves the contrast and helps to keep them stable in storage. Conventional solutions are preferred for most routine use.

CHANGING SOLUTIONS

All processing solutions deteriorate as a result of continued use and exposure to air. Although regular replenishment of the developer and fixer prolongs their useful life, the accumulation of reaction products eventually causes these solutions to cease functioning properly. Exhaustion of the developer results from oxidation of the developing agents, depletion of the hydroquinone, and buildup of bromide. With regular replenishment, solutions may last 3–4 weeks before they must be changed.

A simple procedure can help to determine when solutions should be changed. A double film packet is exposed on one projection for the first patient radiographed after new solutions have been prepared. One film is placed in the patient's chart, and the other is mounted on a corner of a viewbox in the darkroom. As successive films are processed, they are compared to this reference film. Loss of image contrast and density become evident as the solutions deteriorate, indicating when it is time to change them. The fixer is changed when the developer is changed.

AUTOMATIC FILM PROCESSING

Equipment that automates all processing steps is available (Fig. 4.49). Although automatic processing has numerous advantages, the most important is the time saved. Depending on the equipment and the temperature of operation, an automatic processor requires only 4–6 minutes to develop, fix, wash, and dry a film. Many dental automatic processors have a light-shielded (daylight loading) compartment in which the operator can unwrap films and feed them into the machine without working in a darkroom. However, special care must be taken to maintain infection control when using these daylight-loading compartments (see Chapter 14).

When extraoral films are processed, the light-shielded compartment is removed to provide room for feeding the larger film into the processor. Another attractive feature of the automatic system is that the density and contrast of the radiographs tend to be consistent. However, because of the higher temperature of the developer and the artifacts caused by rollers, the quality of films processed automatically often is not as high as the quality of films carefully developed manually. With automatically processed films, if more grain is evident in the final image, the correct choice of processing solutions may be able to help minimize the issue.

Whether automatic processing equipment is appropriate for a specific practice depends on the dentist and the nature and volume of the practice. The equipment is expensive and must be cleaned frequently, as described by the processor manufacturer. In addition, automated equipment may break down, and conventional darkroom equipment may still be needed as a backup system.

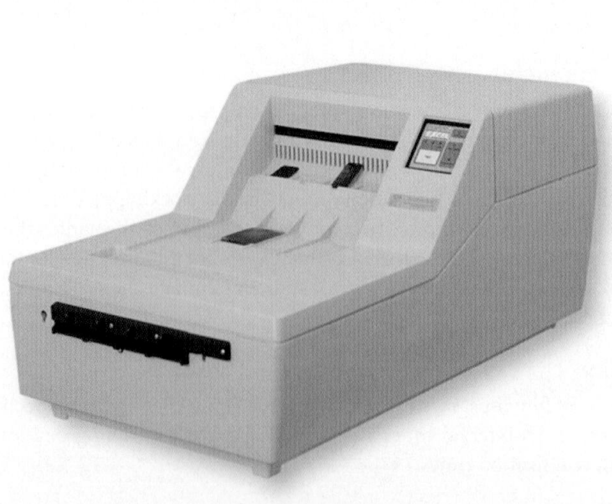

Fig. 4.49 Dent-X 810 AR film automatic film processor. The operator opens the film packet in a darkroom and inserts the film into the opening on the left end of the machine. The exposed film is carried on a roller apparatus through processing solutions, and the processed and dried film is returned through the upper right opening in 4.5 minutes. (Courtesy ImageWorks, Elmsford, NY.)

Mechanism

Automatic processors have an in-line arrangement consisting of a transport mechanism that picks up exposed, unwrapped film and passes it through the developing, fixing, washing, and drying sections (Fig. 4.50). The transport system most often used is a series of rollers driven by a motor that operates through gears, belts, or chains. The rollers often consist of independent assemblies of multiple rollers in a rack, with one rack for each step in the operation. Although these assemblies are designed and positioned so that the film crosses over from one roller to the next, the operator may remove them independently for cleaning and repairing.

The primary function of the rollers is to move the film through the developing solutions, but they also serve at least three other purposes. First, their motion helps to keep the solutions agitated, which contributes to the uniformity of processing. Second, in the developer, fixer, and water tanks, the rollers press on the film emulsion, forcing some solution out of the emulsion. The emulsions rapidly fill again with solution, thus promoting solution exchange. Finally, the top rollers at the crossover point between the developer and fixer tanks remove developing solution, minimizing carryover of developer into the fixer tank. This feature helps to maintain the uniformity of processing chemicals.

The chemical compositions of the developer and fixer are modified to operate at higher temperatures than the temperatures used for manual processing and to meet the more rapid development, fixing, washing, and drying requirements of automatic processing. The quality of the fixer is very important. High-quality fixers contain an additional hardener that helps the emulsion withstand the rigors of the transport system and improves transport. Poor-quality fixers containing no hardener produce more film artifacts, and film may slip and jam during transport.

Operation

Successful operation of an automatic processor requires standardized procedures and regular maintenance. The processor and surrounding area should always be kept clean so that no chemicals contaminate hands or films. The solution level and temperature should be checked each morning before films are processed. Hands should be dry when handling film, and films should be touched on their edges only. The better processors have automatic replenishment systems. A daily, weekly, and quarterly maintenance routine (see Chapter 14) should be followed, including cleaning the rollers and other working parts. It is vital to run a large roller transport cleanup film daily through the processor to clean the top and bottom rollers.

ESTABLISHING CORRECT EXPOSURE TIMES

When radiographs are first made with a new x-ray machine, it is important to examine the exposure guidelines that come with the machine. Typically, such guidelines provide a table listing the various anatomic regions (incisors, premolars, or molars), patient size (adult or child), and the length of the aiming cylinder. For each of these combinations, there is a suggested exposure time. It is also important to start out using fresh processing chemicals and optimal processing conditions as previously described. After the first images are made on patients, it may be necessary to adjust exposure time. If optimal film processing techniques are being followed and the images are consistently dark, exposure times should be decreased until optimal images are obtained. If images are consistently light, exposure times should be increased. When the optimal times have been determined, these values should be posted by the control panel.

MANAGEMENT OF RADIOGRAPHIC WASTES

To prevent environmental damage, many communities and states have passed laws governing the disposal of wastes. In the United States, such laws often derive from the federal Resource Conservation and Recovery Act of 1976. Although dental radiographic waste constitutes only a small potential hazard, it should be discarded properly. The primary ingredient of concern in processing solutions is the dissolved silver found in used fixer. Another material of concern is the lead foil found in film packets.

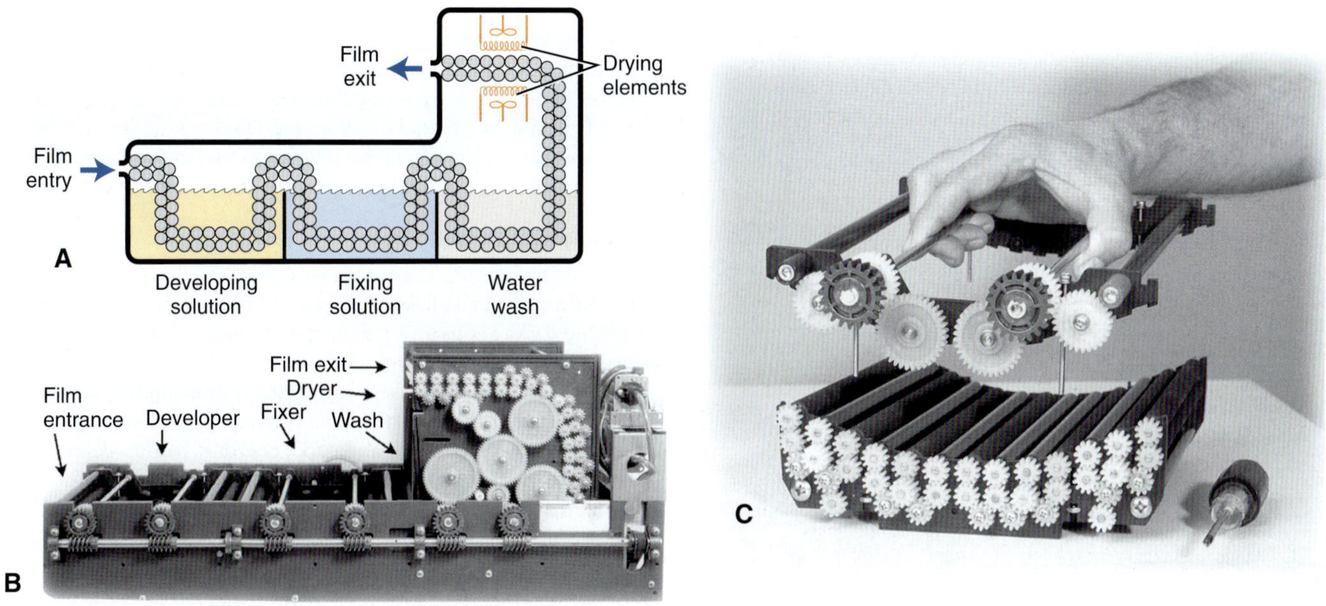

Fig. 4.50 (A) Automatic film processors typically consist of a roller assembly that transports the film through developing, fixing, washing, and drying stations. (B) Assembly of film transport mechanism. (C) One roller assembly. (B and C, Courtesy ImageWorks, Elmsford, NY.)

IMAGE CHARACTERISTICS

Processing an exposed x-ray film causes it to become dark in the exposed area. The degree and pattern of film darkening depend on numerous factors, including the energy and intensity of the x-ray beam, composition of the subject imaged, film emulsion used, and characteristics of film processing. This section describes the major imaging characteristics of x-ray film.

Radiographic Density

When a film is exposed by an x-ray beam (or by light, in the case of screen-film combinations) and then processed, the silver halide crystals in the emulsion that were struck by the photons are converted to grains of metallic silver. These silver grains block the transmission of light from a viewbox and give the film its dark appearance. The degree of darkening or opacity of an exposed film is referred to as optical density, defined as follows:

$$\text{Opticaldensity} = \log_{10} \frac{I_0}{I_t}$$

where I_0 is the intensity of incident light (e.g., from a viewbox) and I_t is the intensity of the light transmitted through the film. With an optical density of 0, 100% of the light is transmitted; with a density of 1, 10% of the light is transmitted; with a density of 2, 1% of the light is transmitted; and so on.

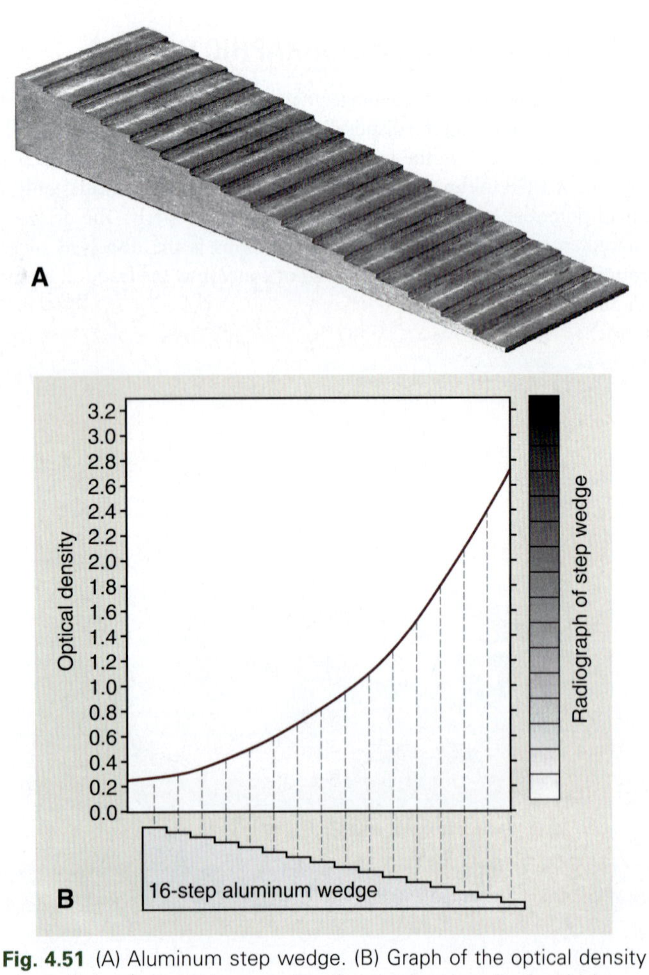

Fig. 4.51 (A) Aluminum step wedge. (B) Graph of the optical density of a radiograph made by exposing the step wedge. As the thickness of the aluminum decreases, more photons are passed through the wedge and are available to expose the film, and the image becomes progressively darker.

A plot of the relationship between film optical density and exposure is called a characteristic curve, or Hurter-Driffield curve (see Fig. 4.51). It usually is shown as the relationship between the optical density of the film and the logarithm of the corresponding exposure. As exposure of the film increases, its optical density increases. A film is of greatest diagnostic value when the structures of interest are imaged on the relatively straight portion of the graph, between 0.6 and 3.0 optical density units. The characteristic curves of films reveal much information about film contrast, speed, and latitude.

An unexposed film, when processed, shows some density. This appearance is caused by the inherent density of the base and added tint and the development of a few unexposed silver halide crystals. This minimal density is called base plus fog and typically is 0.2–0.3. Radiographic density is influenced by exposure and the thickness and density of the imaged structure.

Exposure

The overall film density depends on the number of photons absorbed by the film emulsion. Increasing the milliamperage (mA), peak kilovoltage (kVp), or exposure time increases the number of photons reaching the film and thus increases the density of the radiograph. Reducing the distance between the focal spot and film also increases film density.

Subject Thickness

The thicker the subject, the more the beam is attenuated, and the lighter the resultant image (Fig. 4.51). If exposure factors intended for adults are used on children or edentulous patients, the resultant films are dark because a smaller amount of absorbing tissue is in the path of the x-ray beam. The dentist should vary exposure time according to the patient's size to produce radiographs of optimal density.

Subject Density

Variations in the density of the subject exert a profound influence on the image. The greater the density of a structure within the subject, the greater the attenuation of the x-ray beam directed through that subject or area. In the oral cavity, the relative densities of various natural structures, in order of decreasing density, are enamel, dentin and cementum, bone, muscle, fat, and air. Metallic objects (e.g., restorations) are far denser than enamel and hence better photon absorbers. Because an x-ray beam is differentially attenuated by these absorbers, the resultant beam carries information that is recorded on the radiographic film as light and dark areas. Dense objects (which are strong absorbers) cause the radiographic image to be light and are said to be radiopaque. Objects with low densities are weak absorbers. They allow most photons to pass through, and they cast a dark area on the film that corresponds to the radiolucent object.

Radiographic Contrast

Radiographic contrast is a general term that describes the range of densities on a radiograph. It is defined as the difference in densities between light and dark regions on a radiograph. An image that shows both light areas and dark areas has high contrast; this also is referred to as a short grayscale of contrast because few shades of gray are present between the black-and-white images on the film. Alternatively, a radiographic image composed only of light gray and dark gray zones has low contrast, also referred to as having a long grayscale of contrast (Fig. 4.52). The radiographic contrast of an image is the result of the interplay of subject contrast, film contrast, scattered radiation, and beam energy.

Subject Contrast

Subject contrast is the range of characteristics of the subject that influences radiographic contrast. It is influenced largely by the subject's thickness, density, and atomic number. The subject contrast of a

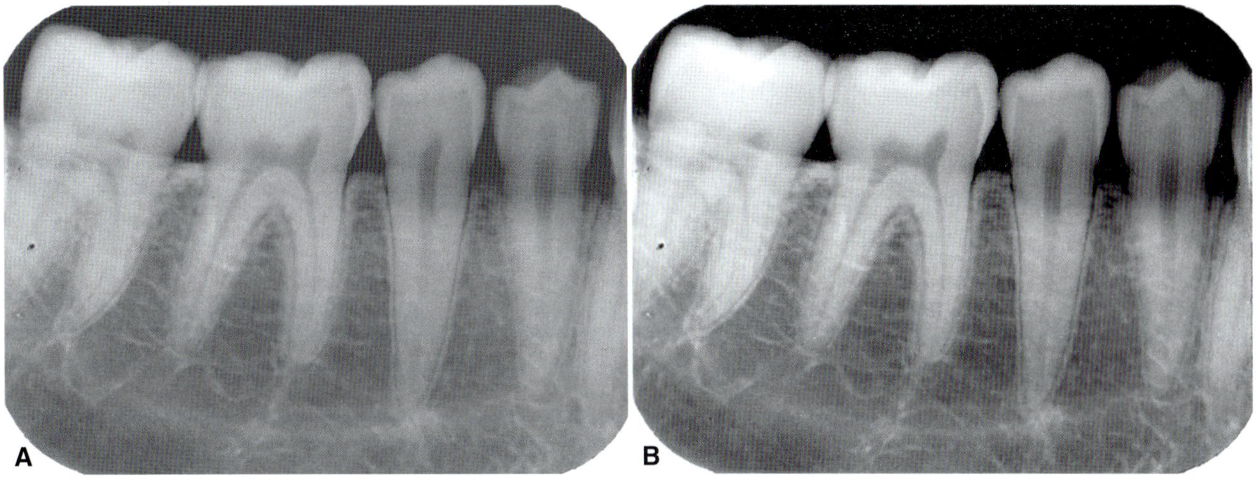

Fig. 4.52 Radiograph of a dried mandible revealing low contrast (A) and high contrast (B).

patient's head and neck exposed in a lateral cephalometric view is high. The dense regions of the bone and teeth absorb most of the incident radiation, whereas the soft tissue facial profile transmits most of the radiation.

Subject contrast also is influenced by beam energy and intensity. The energy of the x-ray beam, selected by the kVp, influences image contrast. Fig. 4.53 shows an aluminum step wedge exposed to x-ray beams of differing energies. Because increasing the kVp increases the overall density of the image, the exposure time has been adjusted so that the density of the middle step in each case is approximately the same. As the kVp of the x-ray beam increases, subject contrast decreases. Similarly, when relatively low kVp energies are used, subject contrast increases. A kVp in the range of 60–80 is optimal for dental imaging. At higher kVp, the exposure time is reduced, but the loss of contrast may be objectionable because subtle changes may be obscured. Changing the time or mA of the exposure (and holding the kVp constant) also influences subject contrast. If the film is excessively light or dark, contrast of anatomic structures is diminished.

Film Contrast

Film contrast describes the inherent capacity of radiographic films to display differences in subject contrast (i.e., variations in the intensity of the remnant beam). A high-contrast film reveals areas of small difference in subject contrast more clearly than a low-contrast film does. Film contrast usually is measured as the average slope of the diagnostically useful portion of the characteristic curve (Fig. 4.54): the greater the slope of the curve in this region, the greater the film contrast. In Fig. 4.54, film *A* has a higher contrast than film *B*. When the slope of the curve in the useful range is greater than 1, the film exaggerates subject contrast. This desirable feature, which is found in most diagnostic film, allows visualization of structures that differ only slightly in density. For example, the remnant beam in the region of a tooth pulp chamber is more intense (greater exposure) than the beam from the surrounding enamel crown. A high-contrast film shows a greater contrast (difference in optical density) between these structures than a low-contrast film. As can be seen in Fig. 4.55, film contrast also depends on the density range being examined. With dental direct exposure film, the slope of the curve continually increases with increasing exposure. As a result, properly exposed films have more contrast than underexposed (light) films. Films used with intensifying screens typically have a slope in the range of 2–3.

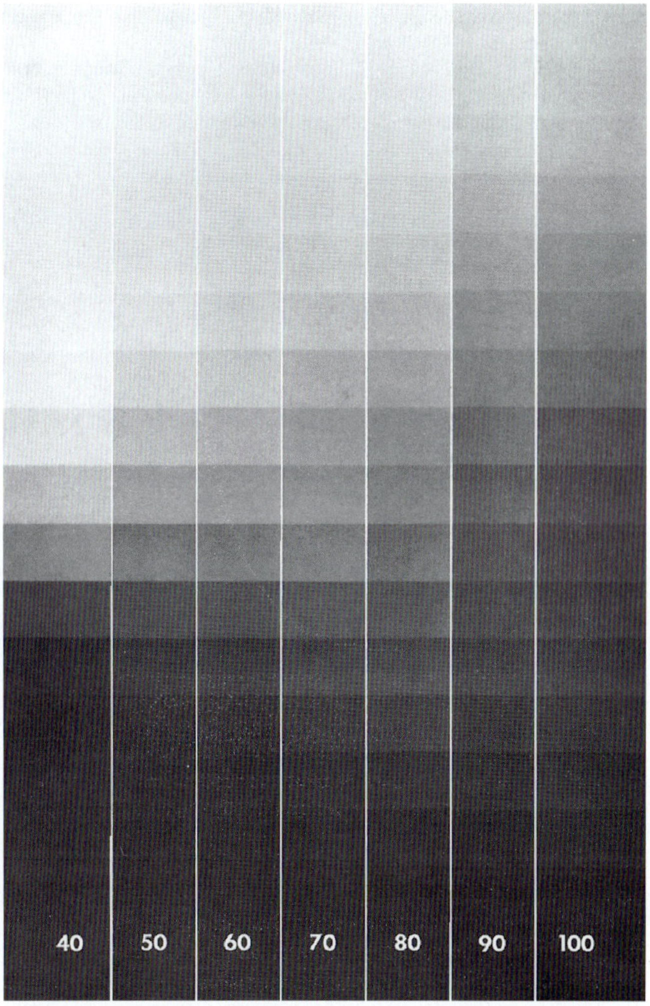

Fig. 4.53 Seven radiographs of a step wedge made at 40–100 peak kilovoltage (kVp) shown side by side. As the kVp increased, the milliamperage was reduced to maintain an approximately uniform middle-step density. Note the long grayscale (low contrast) image with high kVp and the short scale (high contrast) image when using low kVp. (Courtesy of Carestream Dental, a division of Carestream Health, Inc.)

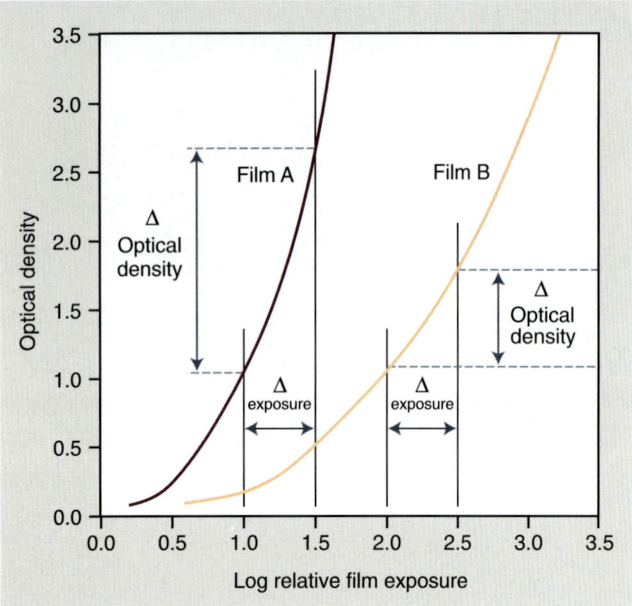

Fig. 4.54 Characteristic curves of two films demonstrating the greater inherent contrast of film *A* compared to film *B*. The slope of film *A* is greater than the slope of film *B*; film *A* shows a greater change in optical density than film *B* for a constant change in exposure. The fact that film *A* is faster than film *B* in this figure is unrelated to film contrast.

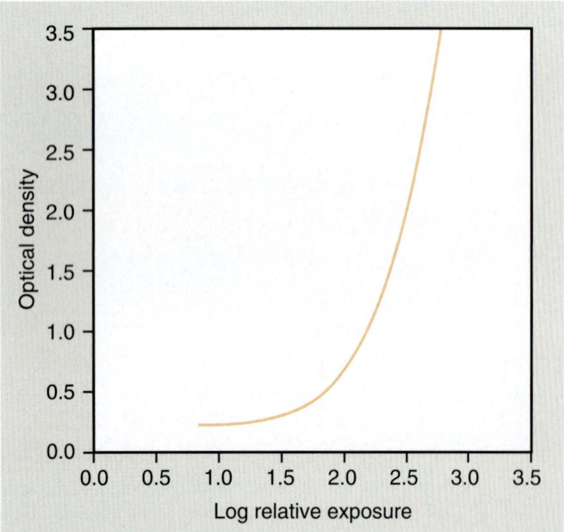

Fig. 4.55 Characteristic curve of direct exposure film. The contrast (slope of the curve) is greater in the high-density region than in the low-density region.

Film processing is another factor that influences film contrast. Film contrast is maximized by optimal film processing conditions. Incomplete or excessive development diminishes contrast of anatomic structures. In addition, storage at too high a temperature, exposure to excessively bright safelights, and light leaks in the darkroom degrade film contrast.

Fog on an x-ray film results in increased film density arising from causes other than exposure to the remnant beam and reduces film contrast. Common causes of film fog are improper safelighting, storage of film at too high a temperature, expired film, exhausted processing chemicals, and development of film at an excessive temperature or for a prolonged period. Film fog can be reduced by proper film processing and storage.

Scattered Radiation

Scattered radiation results from photons that have interacted with the subject by Compton or coherent interactions. These interactions cause the emission of photons that travel in directions other than that of the primary beam. This scattered radiation causes fogging of a radiograph—an overall darkening of the image—and results in loss of radiographic contrast. In most dental applications, the best means of reducing scattered radiation are to use a relatively low kVp and to collimate the beam to the size of the receptor to prevent scatter from an area outside the region of the image.

Radiographic Speed

Radiographic speed refers to the amount of radiation required to produce an image of a standard density. Film speed frequently is expressed as the reciprocal of the exposure (in roentgens) required to produce an optical density of 1 above base plus fog. A fast film requires a relatively low exposure to produce a density of 1, whereas a slower film requires a longer exposure for the processed film to have the same density. Film speed is controlled largely by the size of the silver halide grains and their silver content.

The speed of dental intraoral x-ray film is indicated by a letter designating a particular group (Table 4.6). Currently used intraoral x-ray films have a speed rating of D or E/F (i.e., it is right on the border between the E- and F-speed categories). Only films with a D or faster speed rating are appropriate for intraoral radiography. E/F-speed film is preferred because it requires approximately half the exposure time and thus half the radiation dose of D-speed film. In the United States, the most widely used films are Ultra-speed (D-speed) and INSIGHT (E/F speed). INSIGHT F-speed film is faster than Ultra-speed D-speed film because it has double the amount of tabular crystal grains. The characteristic curves in Fig. 4.56 show that INSIGHT film (curve on the left) is faster than Ultra-speed film (curve on the right) because less exposure is required to produce the same level of density, although the two films have similar contrast.

Film Latitude

Film latitude is a measure of the range of exposures that can be recorded as distinguishable densities on a film. A film optimized to display wide latitude records a wide range of subject contrasts. A film with a characteristic curve that has a long straight-line portion and a shallow slope has wide latitude (Fig. 4.57). As a consequence, wide variations in the

TABLE 4.6 Intraoral Film Speed Classification Per ISO 3665 and ISO 5799

Film Speed Group	Speed Range (Reciprocal Roentgens[a])
C	No longer listed because it is no longer offered
D	14–27.9
E	28–55.9
F	56–111.9

[a]Reciprocal roentgens are the reciprocal of the exposure in roentgens required to obtain a film with an optical density of 1.0 above base plus fog after processing. ISO 3665, Third edition, 2011-09-01.

Data from National Council on Radiation Protection and Measurements, Report No. 145, Appendix E, 2004. *ISO*, International Organization for Standardization.

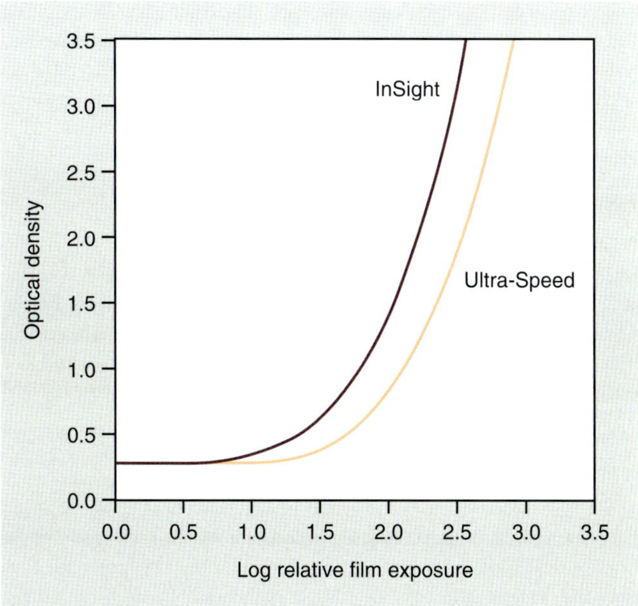

Fig. 4.56 Characteristic curves for INSIGHT and Ultra-speed film. INSIGHT film is faster and has essentially the same contrast (slope) as Ultra-speed film. INSIGHT film requires only half as much patient exposure and is the preferred film. (Courtesy of Carestream Dental, a division of Carestream Health, Inc.)

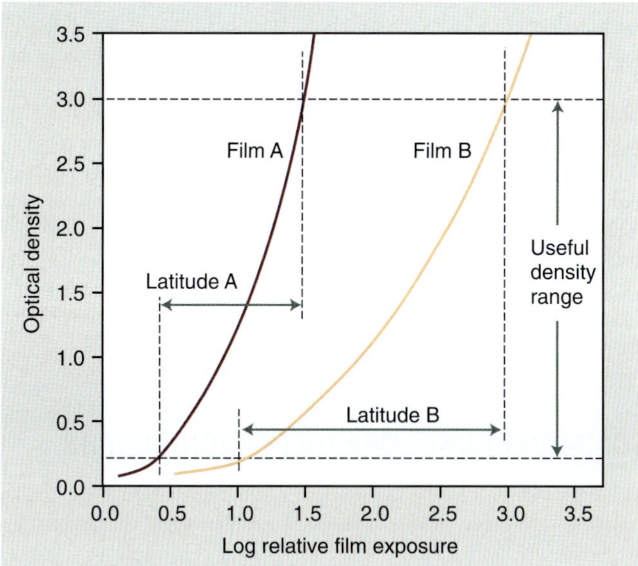

Fig. 4.57 Characteristic curves for two films demonstrating greater inherent latitude of film *B* compared to film *A*. The slope of film *B* is less steep than the slope of film *A*; film *B* records a greater range of exposures within the useful density range than film *A*.

amount of radiation exiting the subject can be recorded. Films with wide latitude have lower contrast than films with a narrow latitude. Wide-latitude films are useful when both the osseous structures of the skull and the soft tissues of the facial region must be recorded.

Radiographic Noise

Radiographic noise is the appearance of uneven density of a uniformly exposed radiographic film. It is seen on a small area of film as localized variations in density. The primary causes of noise are radiographic mottle and radiographic artifact. Radiographic mottle is uneven density resulting from the physical structure of the film or intensifying screens. Radiographic artifacts are defects caused by errors in film handling, such as fingerprints or bends in the film, or errors in film processing, such as splashing developer or fixer on a film or marks or scratches from rough handling.

On intraoral dental film, mottle may be seen as film graininess, which is caused by the visibility of silver grains in the film emulsion, especially when magnification is used to examine an image. Film graininess is most evident when high-temperature processing is used.

Radiographic mottle is also evident when the film is used with fast intensifying screens. Two important causes of the phenomenon are quantum mottle and screen structure mottle. Quantum mottle is caused by a fluctuation in the number of photons per unit of the beam cross-sectional area absorbed by the intensifying screen. Screen structure mottle is graininess caused by screen phosphors. Quantum mottle and screen structure mottle are each most evident when fast film-screen combinations are used.

Radiographic Sharpness and Resolution

Sharpness is the ability of a radiograph to precisely define an edge (e.g., the dentin-enamel junction, or a thin trabecular plate). Resolution, or resolving power, is the ability of a radiograph to record separate structures that are close together. It usually is measured by radiographing an object made up of a series of thin lead strips with alternating radiolucent spaces of the same thickness. The groups of lines and spaces are arranged in the test target in order of increasing numbers of lines and spaces per millimeter (Fig. 4.58). The resolving power is measured as the highest number of line pairs (a line pair being the image of an absorber and the adjacent lucent space) per millimeter that can be distinguished on the resultant radiograph when examined with low-power magnification. Typically, direct exposure

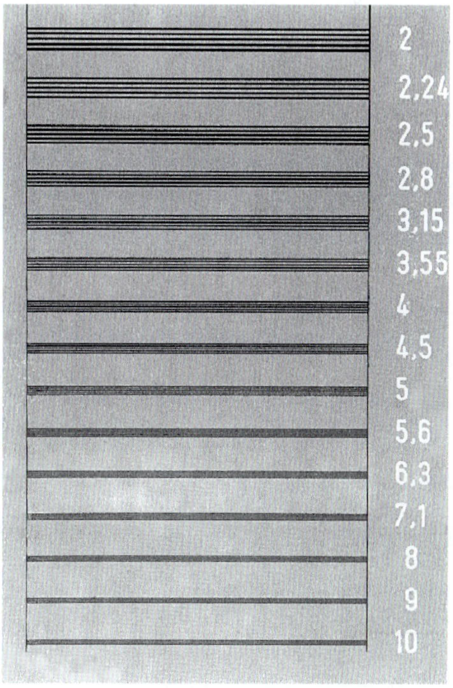

Fig. 4.58 Radiograph of a resolving power target consisting of groups of radiopaque lines and radiolucent spaces. Numbers at each group indicate the number of line pairs per millimeter represented by the group.

films used for intraoral radiography can delineate 20 lp/mm or more. Screen-film combinations for panoramic and cephalometric radiography resolve approximately 5 lp/mm.

Radiographic blur is the loss of sharpness. It can be caused by image receptor (film and screen) blurring, motion blurring, or geometric blurring.

Image Receptor Blurring

With intraoral dental x-ray film, the size and number of the silver grains in the film emulsion determines image sharpness: the finer the grain size, the finer the sharpness. In general, slow-speed films have fine grains, and faster films have larger grains.

Use of intensifying screens in extraoral radiography has an adverse effect on image sharpness. Some degree of sharpness is lost because visible light and UV radiation emitted by the screen spread out beyond the point of origin and expose a film area larger than the phosphor crystal (see Fig. 4.39). The spreading light causes a blurring of fine detail on the radiograph. Intensifying screens with large crystals are relatively fast, but image sharpness is diminished. Fast intensifying screens have a relatively thick phosphor layer, which contributes to dispersion of light and loss of image sharpness. Diffusion of light from a screen can be minimized and image sharpness maximized by ensuring as close a contact as possible between the intensifying screen and the film.

The presence of an image on each side of a double-emulsion film also causes a loss of image sharpness through parallax (Fig. 4.59). Parallax results from the apparent change in position or size of a subject when it is viewed from different perspectives. Because dental film has a double coating of emulsion and the x-ray beam is divergent, the images recorded on each emulsion vary slightly in size. When intensifying screens are used, parallax distortion contributes to image unsharpness because light from one screen may cross the film base and reach the emulsion on the opposite side. This problem can be solved by incorporating dyes into the base that absorb the light emitted by the screens.

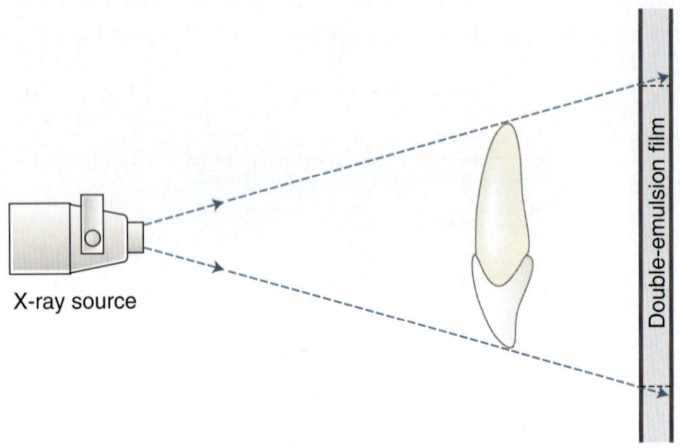

Fig. 4.59 Parallax unsharpness results when double-emulsion film is used because of the slightly greater magnification of the object on the side of the film away from the x-ray source. Parallax unsharpness is a minor problem in clinical practice.

Motion Blurring

Image sharpness also can be lost through movement of the film or subject during exposure. Movement of the x-ray source in effect enlarges the focal spot and diminishes image sharpness. Patient movement can be minimized by stabilizing the patient's head with the chair headrest during exposure. Use of a higher mA and correspondingly shorter exposure times also helps to resolve this problem.

Geometric Blurring

Several geometric factors influence image sharpness. Loss of image sharpness results in part because photons are not emitted from a point source (focal spot) on the target in the x-ray tube. The larger the focal spot, the greater the loss of image sharpness. In addition, image sharpness is improved by increasing the distance between the focal spot and the object and reducing the distance between the object and the image receptor. Various means of optimizing projection geometry are discussed in Chapter 5.

Image Quality

Image quality describes the subjective judgment by the clinician of the overall appearance of a radiograph. It combines the features of density, contrast, latitude, sharpness, resolution, and perhaps other parameters. Various mathematic approaches have been used to evaluate these parameters further, but a thorough discussion of them is beyond the scope of this text. The detective quantum efficiency is a basic measure of the efficiency of an imaging system. It encompasses image contrast, blur, speed, and noise. Often a system can be optimized for one of these parameters, but this usually is achieved at the expense of others. For instance, a fast system typically has a high level of noise. However, even with these and other sophisticated approaches, more information is needed for complete understanding of all the factors responsible for the subjective impression of image quality.

COMMON CAUSES OF FAULTY RADIOGRAPHS

Although film processing can produce radiographs of excellent quality, inattention to detail may lead to many problems and images that are diagnostically suboptimal. Poor radiographs contribute to a loss of diagnostic information and loss of professional and patient time. Box 4.4 presents a list of common causes of faulty radiographs. The steps necessary for correction are self-evident.

BOX 4.4 Common Problems in Film Exposure and Development

Light Radiographs (Fig. 4.60)

Processing Errors

Underdevelopment (temperature too low; time too short; thermometer inaccurate)
Depleted developer solution
Diluted or contaminated developer
Excessive fixation (hours)

Underexposure

Insufficient mA
Insufficient kVp
Insufficient exposure time
Film-source distance too long
Film packet reversed in mouth (see Fig. 4.34)

BOX 4.4 Common Problems in Film Exposure and Development—cont'd

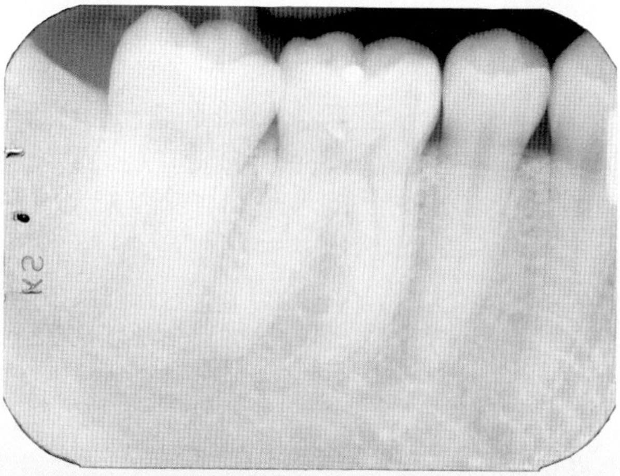

Fig. 4.60 Radiograph that is too light because of inadequate processing or insufficient exposure.

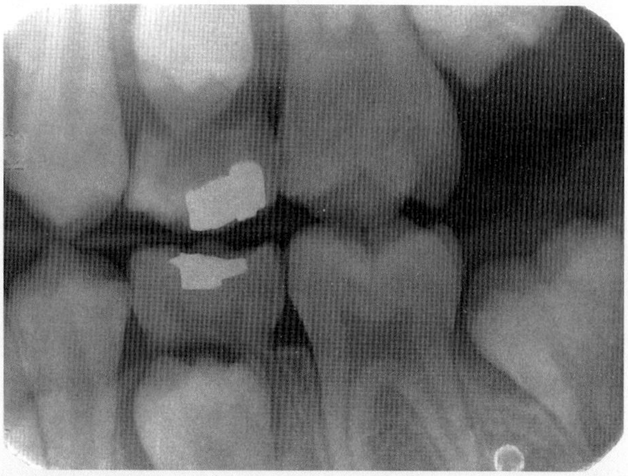

Fig. 4.62 Radiograph with insufficient contrast, showing gray enamel and gray pulp chambers.

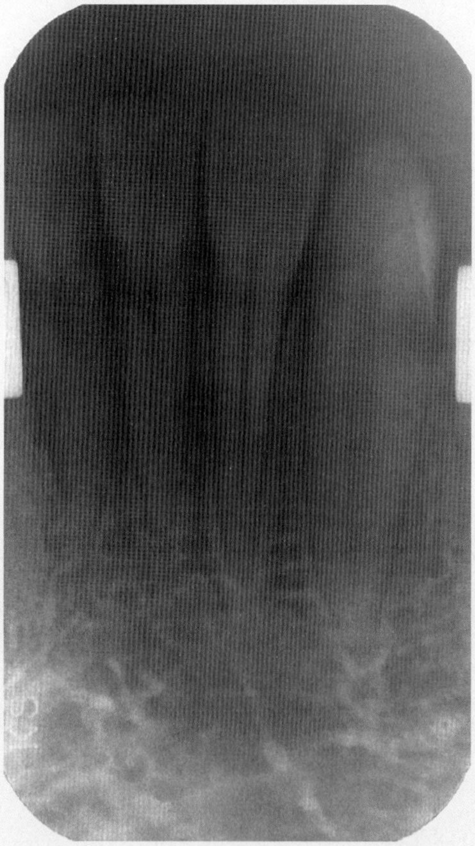

Fig. 4.61 Radiograph that is too dark because of overdevelopment or overexposure.

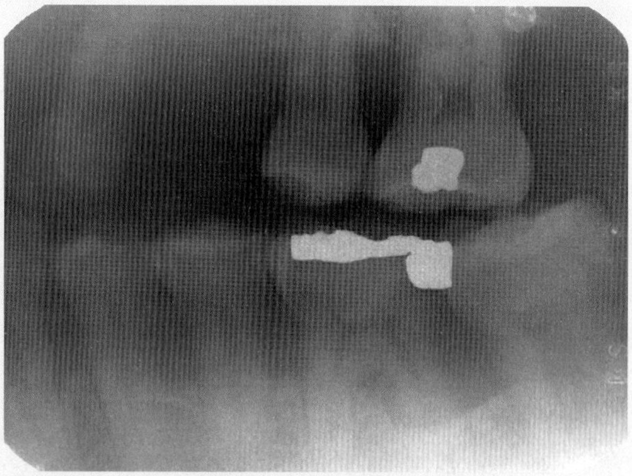

Fig. 4.63 Fogged radiograph marked by darkening and lack of image detail.

Dark Radiographs (Fig. 4.61)

Processing Errors

Overdevelopment (temperature too high; time too long)
Developer concentration too high
Inadequate time in fixer
Accidental exposure to light
Improper safelighting
Storage of films without shielding, at too high a temperature, or past expiration date

Overexposure

Excessive mA
Excessive kVp
Excessive exposure time
Film-source distance too short

Insufficient Contrast (Fig. 4.62)

Underdevelopment
Underexposure
Excessive kVp
Excessive film fog

Film Fog (Fig. 4.63)

Improper safelighting (improper filter; excessive bulb wattage; inadequate distance between safelight and work surface; prolonged exposure to safelight)
Light leaks (cracked safelight filter; light leaks from doors, vents, or other sources)
Overdevelopment
Contaminated solutions
Deteriorated film (stored at high temperature; stored at high humidity; exposed to radiation; past expiration date)

Dark Spots or Lines (Fig. 4.64)

Fingerprint contamination

Continued

BOX 4.4 Common Problems in Film Exposure and Development—cont'd

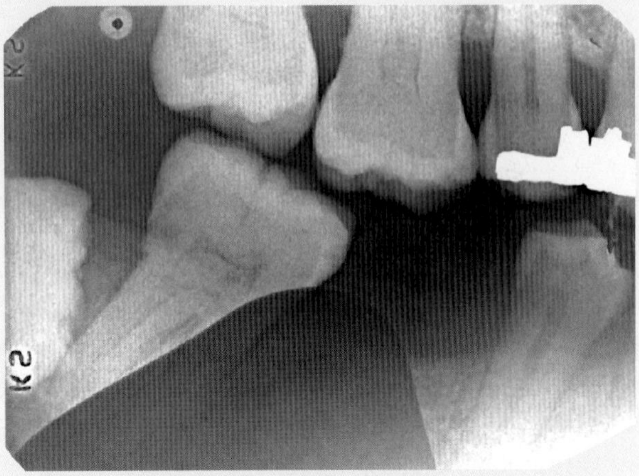

Fig. 4.64 Dark spot on an x-ray film caused by film contact with the tank wall during fixation. This contact prevented the fixer from dissolving the unexposed silver bromide crystals on the emulsion in contact with the tank wall.

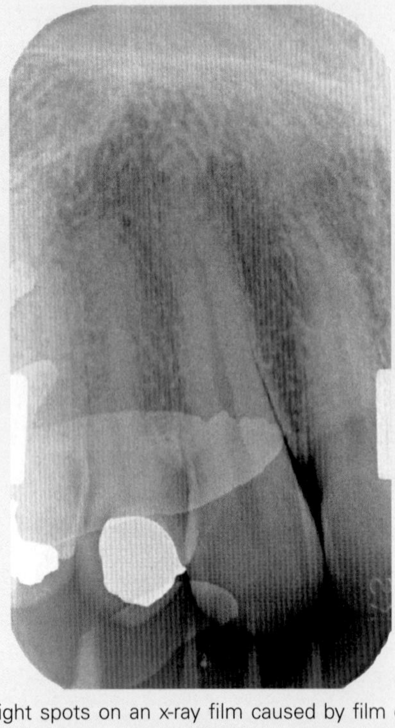

Fig. 4.65 Light spots on an x-ray film caused by film contact with drops of fixer before processing. The fixer removed the unexposed silver bromide grains on one emulsion but did not affect the opposite side, so there is still an image.

Protective wrapping paper sticking to film surface
Film in contact with tank or another film during fixation
Film contaminated with developer before processing
Excessive bending of film
Static discharge to film before processing
Excessive roller pressure during automatic processing
Dirty rollers in automatic processing

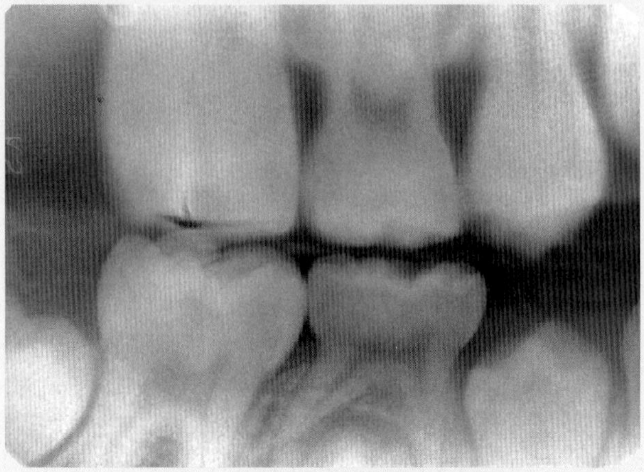

Fig. 4.66 Blurred radiograph caused by movement of the patient during exposure.

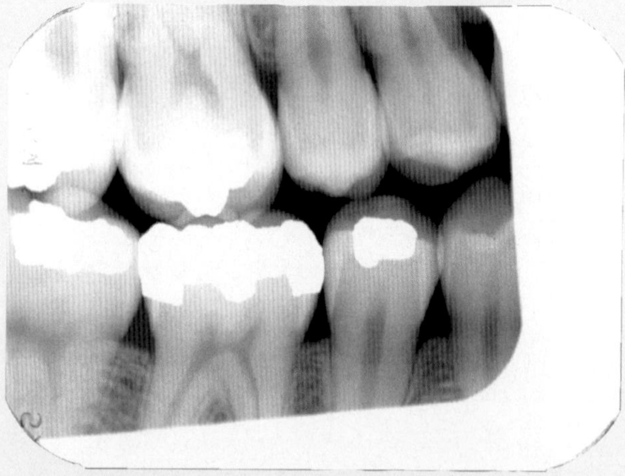

Fig. 4.67 Partial image caused by poor alignment of the tube head with the film rectangular collimator.

Light Spots (Fig. 4.65)
Film contaminated with fixer before processing
Film in contact with tank or another film during development

Yellow or Brown Stains (see Fig. 4.44)
Depleted developer
Depleted fixer
Insufficient washing
Contaminated solutions

Blurring (Fig. 4.66)
Movement of patient
Movement of film (film not stabilized)

Partial Images (Fig. 4.67)
Top of film not immersed in developing solution
Misalignment of x-ray tube head ("cone-cut")

Emulsion Peel
Abrasion of image during processing
Excessive time in wash water

kVp, Peak kilovoltage; *mA*, milliamperage.

MOUNTING RADIOGRAPHS

Film-based radiographs must be preserved and maintained in a satisfactory condition. Periapical, interproximal, and occlusal films are best handled and stored in a film mount (Fig. 4.68). The operator can handle them with greater ease, and there is less chance of damaging the emulsion. Mounts are made of plastic or cardboard and may have a clear plastic window that covers and protects the film. However, the window may have scratches or imperfections that interfere with radiographic interpretation. The operator can arrange several films from the same individual in a film mount in the proper anatomic relationship. This facilitates correlation of the clinical and radiographic examinations. Opaque mounts are best because they prevent stray light from the viewbox from reaching the viewer's eyes.

The preferred method of positioning periapical and occlusal films in the film mount is to arrange them so that the images of the teeth are in the anatomic position and have the same relationship to the viewer as when the viewer faces the patient. The radiographs of the teeth in the right quadrants should be placed in the left side of the mount, and the radiographs of the teeth of the left quadrants should be placed in the right side. This system, advocated by the American Dental Association, allows the examiner's gaze to shift from radiograph to tooth without crossing the midline. The alternative arrangement, with the images of the right quadrants on the right side of the mount and the images of the left quadrant on the left side, is not recommended.

DUPLICATING RADIOGRAPHS

Occasionally, film radiographs must be duplicated; this is best accomplished with duplicating film. The film to be duplicated is placed against the emulsion side of the duplicating film, and the two films are held in position by a glass-topped cassette or photographic printing frame. The films are exposed to light, which passes through the clear areas of the original radiograph and exposes the duplicating film. The duplicating film is processed in conventional x-ray processing solutions. In contrast to conventional x-ray film, duplicating film gives a positive image. Thus, areas exposed to light come out clear, as on the original radiograph. Duplication typically results in images with less resolution and more contrast than the original radiograph. The best images are obtained when a circular, UV light source is used. In contrast to the usual negative film, images on duplicating film that are too dark or too light are underexposed or overexposed, respectively.

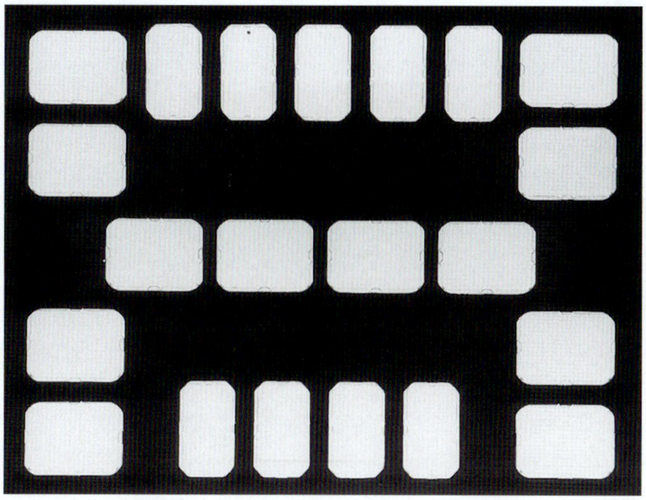

Fig. 4.68 Film mount for holding nine anterior periapical views, eight posterior periapical views, and four bite-wing views. An opaque film mount blocks extraneous light from a viewbox when examining the radiographs.

CONCLUSION

Although film remains an acceptable means to acquire and display dental radiographic image, the adoption of digital imaging is now widespread and will be the sole technology of the future. Comparison of imaging systems based on technical properties like resolution, contrast, and latitude is somewhat confounded by a lack of standardization in the assessment of these characteristics. From a diagnostic standpoint, most studies suggest that digital performance is not clinically different from film for typical diagnostic tasks, such as caries diagnosis. The "look and feel" of digital displays is distinctly different from film viewing, and some practitioners may find this difference disconcerting. A basic understanding of computers and a mastery of common computing skills are essential for viewing digital images. Beyond this, learning the peculiarities and vagaries of a particular acquisition and display software takes time and may not be intuitive. Multiple mouse clicks through multiple menus may be required to view a full-mouth series of images. This activity may modestly increase the time required to complete the interpretative process.

In selecting an imaging system, other issues should be considered. Digital images avoid environmental pollutants encountered with film processing, but what about the environmental impact associated with the disposal of broken or obsolete electronic equipment? The initial financial outlay for digital imaging hardware makes these systems more expensive than film. Manufacturers point out that the costs of film or digital systems should be amortized over the life of the equipment and consumables; however, the life expectancy of newer digital systems is speculative. Mishandling of digital system components can catastrophically shorten any projected life expectancy. Additionally, what price should we place on the ability to transmit images instantly and to integrate them into a fully electronic record? There are no universal answers to these questions. They must be asked and answered according to the needs and objectives of individual dental practices. As practice patterns and technology change with time, the answers will also change. Although the details of the image in our crystal ball have yet to resolve, the trends of increasing adoption of digital imaging and continuing technologic innovation make the future of digital imaging in dentistry certain.

BIBLIOGRAPHY

Digital Detectors and Displays

Abreu M Jr, Mol A, Ludlow JB. Performance of RVGui sensor and Kodak Ektaspeed Plus film for proximal caries detection. *Oral Surg Oral Med Oral Pathol Oral Radiol Endod.* 2001;91:381-385.

Butt A, Mahoney M, Savage NW. The impact of computer display performance on the quality of digital radiographs: a review. *Aust Dent J.* 2012; 57(suppl 1):16-23.

Couture RA, Hildebolt C. Quantitative dental radiography with a new photostimulable phosphor system. *Oral Surg Oral Med Oral Pathol Oral Radiol Endod.* 2000;89:498-508.

Hildebolt CF, Couture RA, Whiting BR. Dental photostimulable phosphor radiography. *Dent Clin North Am.* 2000;44:273-297.

Mol A, Yoon DC. Guide to digital radiographic imaging. *J Calif Dent Assoc.* 2015;43:503-511.

Sanderink GC, Miles DA. Intraoral detectors: CCD, CMOS, TFT, and other devices. *Dent Clin North Am.* 2000;44:249-255.

Vandenberghe B, Jacobs R, Bosmans H. Modern dental imaging: a review of the current technology and clinical applications in dental practice. *Eur Radiol.* 2010;20:2637-2655.

Van der Stelt PF. Principles of digital imaging. *Dent Clin North Am.* 2000;44:237-248.

Digital Image Processing

Analoui M. Radiographic image enhancement, I: spatial domain techniques. *Dentomaxillofac Radiol.* 2001;30:1-9.

Analoui M. Radiographic digital image enhancement, II: transform domain techniques. *Dentomaxillofac Radiol.* 2001;30:65-77.

Gonzalez R, Wood R. *Digital Image Processing.* 3rd ed. Prentice Hall; 2007.

Mol A. Image processing tools for dental applications. *Dent Clin North Am.* 2000;44:299-318.

Russ JC. *The Image Process Handbook.* 5th ed. CRC Press; 2006.

Film-Based Imaging

American Dental Association Council on Scientific Affairs. Dental radiographic examinations: recommendations for patient selection and limiting radiation exposure. Revised 2012. https://www.fda.gov/media/84818/download.

Baghele ON, Phadke S, Deshpande AA, et al. A simplified model for biomedical waste management in dental practices—a pilot project at Thane, India. *Eur J Gen Dent.* 2013;2:235-240. https://www.thieme-connect.de/products/ejournals/abstract/10.4103/2278-9626.115992.

Bushberg JT. *The Essential Physics of Medical Imaging.* 4th ed. Wolters Kluwer; 2021.

Bushong SC. *Radiologic Science for Technologists: Physics, Biology, and Protection.* 11th ed. Mosby; 2020.

Castro VM, Katz JO, Hardman PK, et al. In vitro comparison of conventional film and direct digital imaging in the detection of approximal caries. *Dentomaxillofac Radiol.* 2007;36:138-142.

de Carvalho FP, da Silveira MM, Frazao MA, et al. Effects of developer exhaustion on DFL Contrast FV-58 and Kodak Insight dental films. *Dentomaxillofac Radiol.* 2011;40:358-361.

Fitterman AS, Brayer FC, Cumbo PE. *Processing Chemistry for Medical Imaging, Technical and Scientific Monograph No. 5, N-327.* Eastman Kodak; 1995.

Ludlow JB, Platin E, Mol A. Characteristics of Kodak InSight, an F-speed intraoral film. *Oral Surg Oral Med Oral Pathol Oral Radiol Endod.* 2001;91:120-129.

Madalli VB, Annigeri RG, Basavaraddi SM. The evaluation of effect of developer age in the detection of approximal caries using three speed dental x-ray films: an in-vitro study. *J Clin Diagn Res.* 2014;8:236-239.

Mees DEK, James TH. *The Theory of the Photographic Process.* Macmillan; 1977.

Nair MK, Nair UP. An in-vitro evaluation of Kodak InSight and Ektaspeed Plus film with a CMOS detector for natural proximal caries: ROC analysis. *Caries Res.* 2001;35:354-359.

Pontual AA, de Melo DP, de Almeida SM, et al. Comparison of digital systems and conventional dental film for the detection of approximal enamel caries. *Dentomaxillofac Radiol.* 2010;39:431-436.

Syriopoulos K, Velders XL, Sanderink GC, et al. Sensitometric evaluation of four dental x-ray films using five processing solutions. *Dentomaxillofac Radiol.* 1999;28:73-79.

Thunthy KH, Ireland EJ. A comparison of the visibility of caries on Kodak F-speed (InSight) and D-speed (Ultra-Speed) films. *LDA J.* 2001;60:31-32.

US Food and Drug Administration. *Dental Radiography: Doses and Film Speed.* https://www.fda.gov/Radiation-EmittingProducts/RadiationSafety/NationwideEvaluationofX-RayTrendsNEXT/ucm116524.htm. Article IV.

Clinical Considerations

Wenzel A. A review of dentists' use of digital radiography and caries diagnosis with digital systems. *Dentomaxillofac Radiol.* 2006;35:307-314.

Wenzel A, Møystad A. Work flow with digital intraoral radiography: a systematic review. *Acta Odontol Scand.* 2010;68:106-114.

5

Projection Geometry

Anita Gohel and Sanjay M. Mallya

A conventional radiograph is made with a stationary x-ray source and displays a two-dimensional image of an anatomic region. Such images are often called *plain* or *projection* views (in contrast to ultrasound, computed tomography [CT], magnetic resonance imaging, or nuclear medicine). In plain views, the entire volume of tissue between the x-ray source and the image receptor (digital sensor or film) is projected onto a two-dimensional image. Intraoral radiographs (periapical, bite-wing, and occlusal radiographs; Chapter 6) and cephalometric and skull radiographs, Chapter 7) are examples of projection views commonly made in general and specialty dental practices.

Radiography provides an image of the internal anatomy that is not visible on clinical examination. To interpret a radiograph, the clinician must use their knowledge of normal anatomy to mentally reconstruct a three-dimensional image of the anatomic structures using information from one or more two-dimensional views. Using high-quality radiographs greatly facilitates this task. The term *image quality* refers to the reliability of the image to represent the true state of the anatomic region examined. Parameters that define radiographic image quality include image sharpness, spatial resolution, contrast resolution, magnification, and distortion. For optimal diagnosis, the radiographic imaging system should make an image that has minimal magnification and distortion, and with a contrast and spatial resolution that is adequate for the intended diagnostic task.

The five basic principles of projection geometry (Box 5.1) are based on the effects of focal spot size and relative positions of the object and image receptor (digital sensor or film) on image clarity, magnification, and distortion. Clinicians use these principles to maximize radiographic image quality and facilitate accurate radiographic diagnoses.

IMAGE SHARPNESS AND RESOLUTION

Several geometric considerations contribute to image sharpness and spatial resolution. *Sharpness* measures how well a boundary between two areas of differing radiodensity is revealed. Image *spatial resolution* measures how well a radiograph reveals small objects that are close together. Although sharpness and spatial resolution are two distinct parameters, they are interdependent, being influenced by the same geometric variables. For clinical diagnosis, it is desirable to optimize conditions that result in images with the optimal sharpness and resolution for the diagnostic task.

When x-rays are produced at the target in an x-ray tube, they originate from all points within the area of the focal spot. Because these rays originate from different points and travel in straight lines, their projections of an object do not superimpose at the same location on an image receptor. As a result, the image of the edge of an object is slightly blurred rather than sharp and distinct. Fig. 5.1 shows the path of photons that originate at the margins of the focal spot and provide an image of the edges of an object. The resulting blurred zone at the edge of the image causes a loss in image sharpness, and is referred to as *geometric unsharpness* or *penumbra*. The larger the focal spot area, the wider the zone of geometric unsharpness.

There are three means to maximize image sharpness (Box 5.2):

1. *Use as small an effective focal spot as practical.* The effective focal spot sizes in dental x-ray machines range from 0.4 to 0.7 mm. Using an x-ray unit with a smaller focal spot size adds to image sharpness. As described in Chapter 1, the size of the effective focal spot is a function of the angle of the target with respect to the long axis of the electron beam. A large angle distributes the electron beam over a larger surface and decreases the heat generated per unit of target area, thus prolonging tube life; however, this results in a larger radiation source and loss of image clarity (Fig. 5.2). A small angle has a greater wearing effect on the target but results in a smaller source and increased image sharpness.
2. *Increase the distance between the source and the object by using a long, open-ended cylinder.* Increasing the source-to-object distance reduces geometric unsharpness by reducing the divergence of the x-ray beam (Fig. 5.3). A longer source-to-object distance yields photons whose paths are almost parallel at the object and minimizes unsharpness. To facilitate making images with a longer source-to-object distance, many manufacturers locate the x-ray tube recessed within the x-ray tube housing. The benefits of using a source-to-object distance support the use of long, open-ended cylinders as aiming devices on dental x-ray machines. For intraoral x-ray units, the distance from the source to the edge of the aiming rim ranges from 8 to 16 inches.
3. *Minimize the distance between the object and the image receptor.* As the object-to-image receptor distance is reduced, the divergence of x-ray photons at the object is less, resulting in a decrease in the width of the unsharp zone (Fig. 5.4).

BOX 5.1 Basic Principles of Projection Geometry for Radiography

1. The focal spot should be as small as possible.
2. The source-receptor distance should be as long as possible.
3. The object-receptor distance should be as small as possible.
4. The receptor should be parallel to the long axis of the object.
5. The central beam should be perpendicular to the object and the receptor.

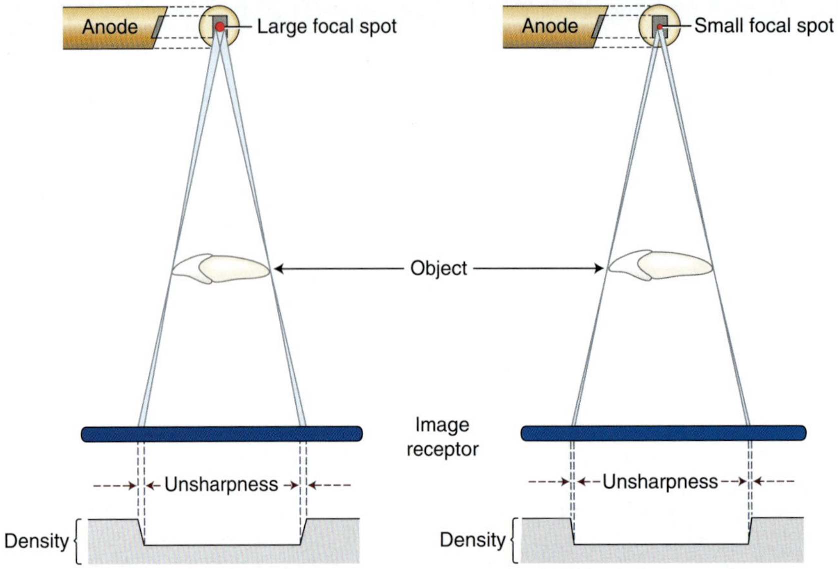

Fig. 5.1 Photons originating at different places on the focal spot *(red)* result in a zone of unsharpness on the radiograph. The density of the image changes from a high background value to a low value in the area of an edge of enamel, dentin, or bone. On the left, a large focal spot size results in a wide zone of unsharpness compared with a small focal spot size on the right, which results in a sharper image (narrow zone of unsharpness).

BOX 5.2 Factors Affecting Image Sharpness and Image Magnification

		Image Sharpness	Image Magnification
Focal spot	Small	Increases	–
	Large	Decreases	–
Source-receptor distance	Short	Decreases	Increases
	Long	Increases	Decreases
Object-receptor distance	Short	Increases	Decreases
	Long	Decreases	Increases

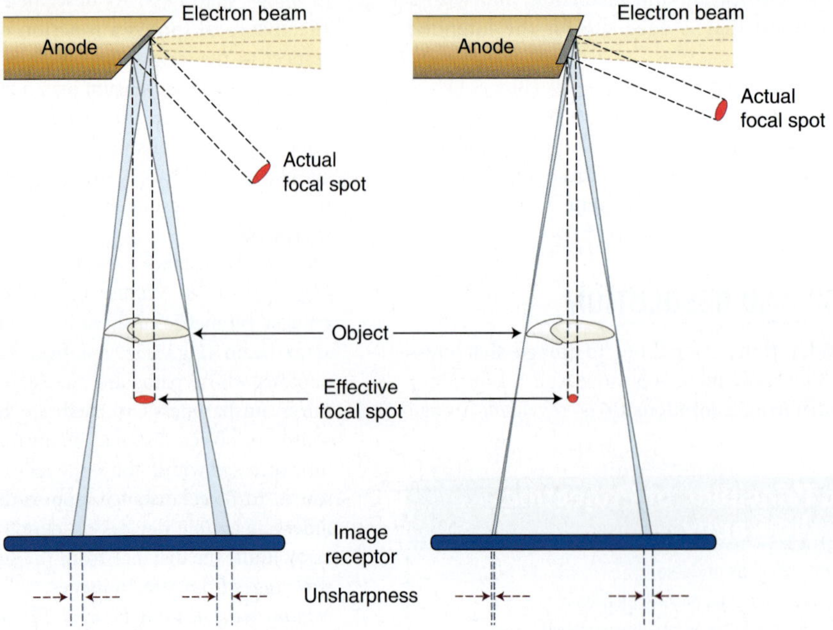

Fig. 5.2 As the angle of the target becomes closer to perpendicular to the long axis of the electron beam (as shown on the *right*), the actual focal spot becomes smaller, which decreases heat dissipation and tube life. The more perpendicular angle also decreases the effective focal spot size, increasing the sharpness of the resulting image.

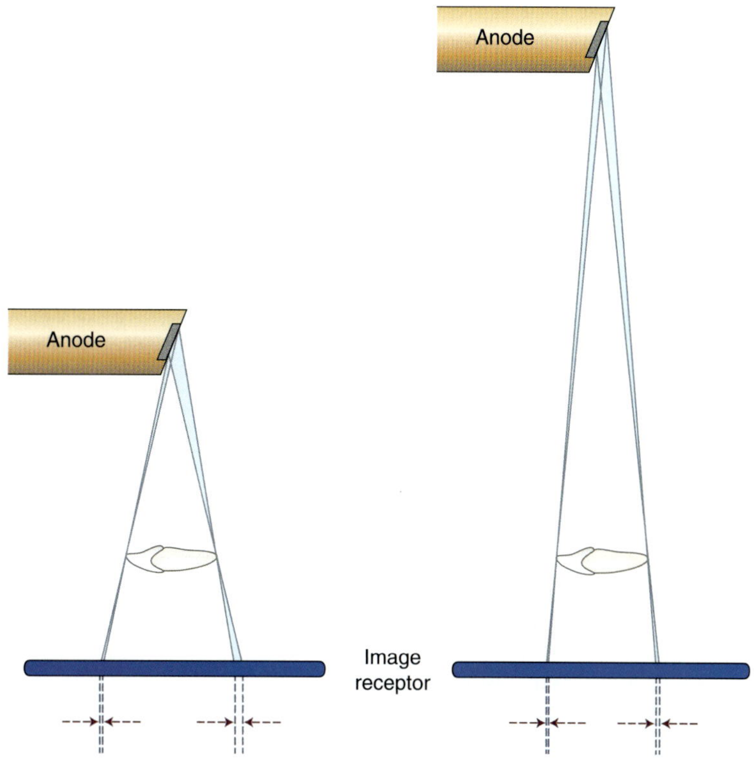

Fig. 5.3 Increasing the distance between the source and the object results in an image with increased sharpness and less magnification of the object, as seen on the *right*.

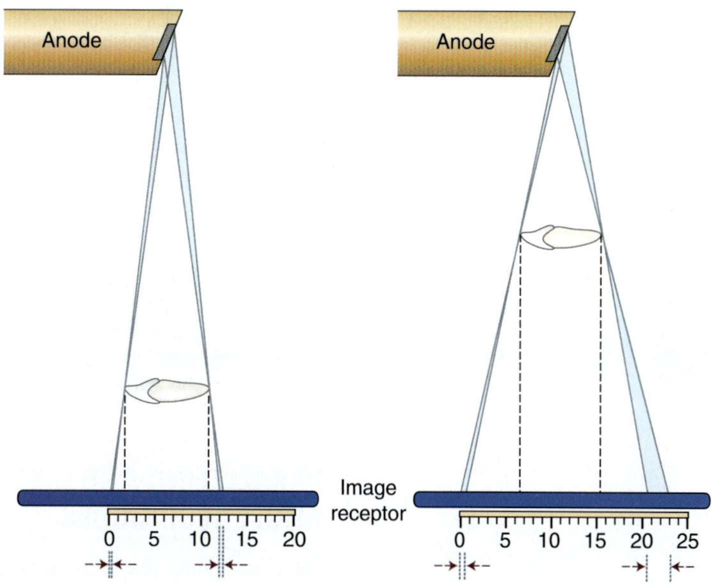

Fig. 5.4 Decreasing the distance between the object and the image receptor increases the sharpness and results in less magnification of the object, as seen on the *left*.

IMAGE SIZE DISTORTION

Image size distortion (magnification) is the increase in size of the image on the radiograph compared with the actual size of the object. The divergent paths of photons in an x-ray beam cause enlargement of the image on a radiograph. Image size distortion results from the relative distances of the source-to-object and object-to-image receptor (see Figs. 5.3 and 5.4). Increasing the source-to-object distance and decreasing the object-to-image receptor distance minimizes image magnification. The use of a long, open-ended cylinder as an aiming device on an x-ray machine thus reduces the magnification of images on a periapical view. As previously mentioned, this technique also improves image sharpness by increasing the distance between the focal spot and the object. The principle of maintaining a long source-to-object distance is applied during cephalometric radiography, where the distance between the source to midsagittal plane is 150 cm or higher to yield images with minimal magnification.

When imaging the facial bones, a posteroanterior projection is preferable to position the facial bones closer to the receptor and minimize their magnification.

IMAGE SHAPE DISTORTION

Image shape distortion is the result of unequal magnification of different parts of the same object. This situation arises when not all the parts of an object are at the same source-to-object distance. The physical shape of the object may often prevent its optimal orientation, resulting in some shape distortion. Such a phenomenon is seen by the differences in appearance of the image on a radiograph compared with the true shape. To minimize shape distortion, the practitioner should align the x-ray tube, object, and image receptor according to the following guidelines:

1. *Position the image receptor parallel to the long axis of the object.* Image shape distortion is minimized when the long axes of the image receptor and tooth are parallel. Fig. 5.5 shows that the central ray of the x-ray beam is perpendicular to the image receptor, but the object is not parallel to the image receptor. The resultant image is distorted because of the unequal distances of the various parts of the object from the image receptor. This type of shape distortion is called *foreshortening* because it causes the radiographic image to be shorter than the object. Fig. 5.6 shows the situation when the x-ray beam is oriented at right angles to the object but not to the image receptor; this results in *elongation*, with the object appearing longer on the image receptor than its actual length.
2. *Orient the central ray perpendicular to the object and image receptor.* Image shape distortion occurs if the object and image receptor are parallel, but the central ray is not directed at right angles to each. This distortion is most evident on maxillary molar views (Fig. 5.7), where the divergence of the buccal and palatal roots precludes placing all roots parallel to the receptor, and the palatal roots appear disproportionately longer than the buccal roots.

The practitioner can prevent shape distortion errors by aligning the object and image receptor parallel with each other and the central ray perpendicular to both.

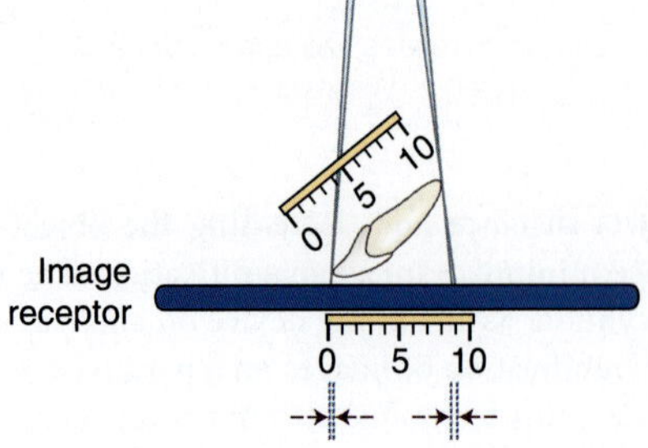

Fig. 5.5 Foreshortening of a radiographic image results when the central ray is perpendicular to the image receptor but the object is not parallel with the image receptor.

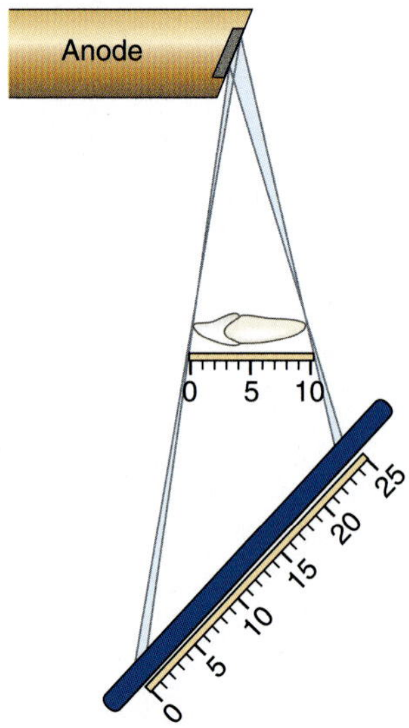

Fig. 5.6 Elongation of a radiographic image results when the central ray is perpendicular to the object but not to the image receptor.

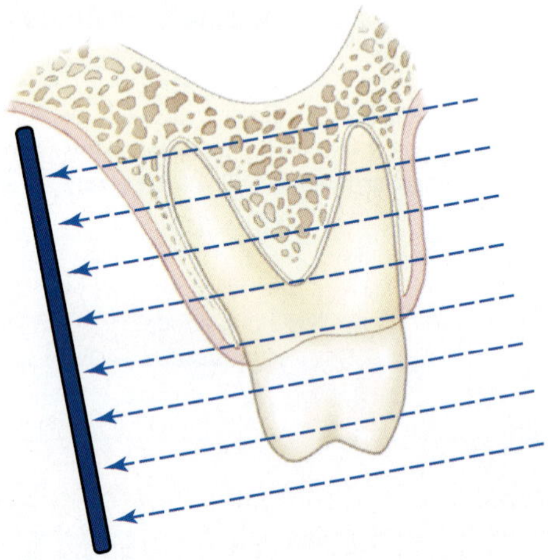

Fig. 5.7 The central ray should be perpendicular to the long axes of both the tooth and the image receptor. If the direction of the x-ray beam is not at right angles to the long axis of the tooth, the appearance of the tooth is distorted, typically by apparent elongation of the length of the palatal roots of upper molars and distortion of the relationship of the height of the alveolar crest relative to the cementoenamel junction.

PARALLELING AND BISECTING ANGLE TECHNIQUES

The clinical objective of intraoral periapical radiography is to produce images of the dentoalveolar structures with minimal size and shape distortion.

The *paralleling technique* is the preferred method for making intraoral radiographs. This technique seeks to minimize distortion by placing the image receptor parallel to the long axis of the tooth, and directs the central x-ray beam perpendicular to both the long axis of the tooth and the receptor (Fig. 5.8) and best incorporates the imaging principles described in the first three sections of this chapter (see Box 5.1).

To achieve this parallel orientation, the practitioner often must position the image receptor toward the middle of the oral cavity, away from the teeth. Although this allows the teeth and image receptor to be parallel, it increases the object-to-receptor distance, which will result

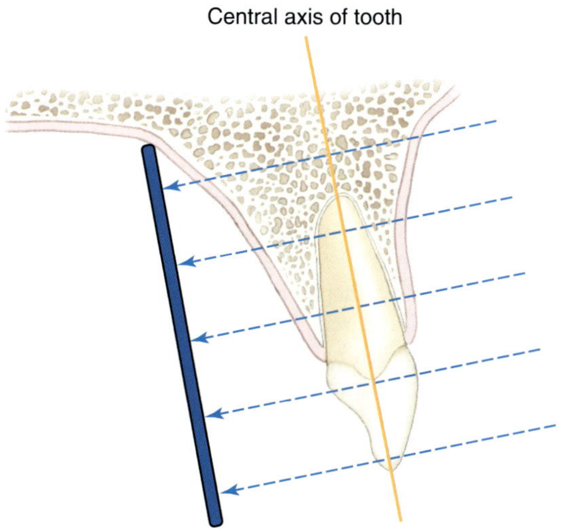

Fig. 5.8 In the paralleling technique, the central ray is directed at a right angle to the central axes of the object and the image receptor. This technique requires a device to support the film in position.

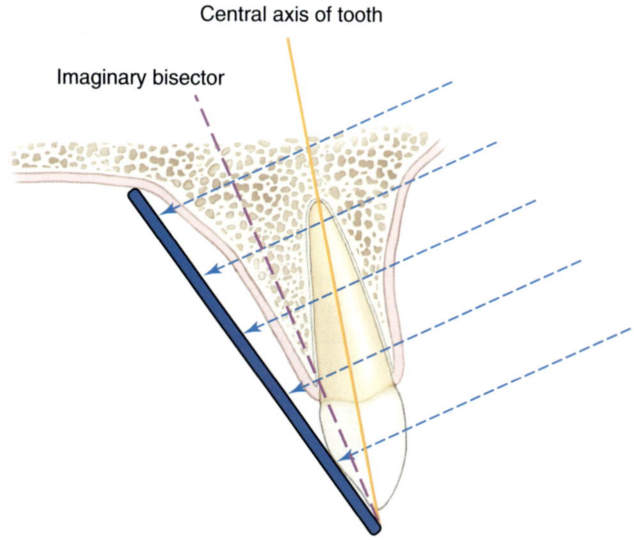

Fig. 5.10 In the bisecting angle technique, the central ray is directed at a right angle to the imaginary plane that bisects the angle formed by the image receptor and the central axis of the object. This method produces an image that is the same length as the object but results in some image distortion.

in some image magnification and geometric unsharpness. To overcome these limitations, the paralleling technique also uses a relatively long open-ended aiming cylinder ("cone") to increase the source-to-object distance. This "cone" directs only the most central and parallel rays of the beam to the image receptor and teeth and reduces image magnification while increasing image sharpness. For intraoral imaging, these extension cones are designed to yield source-object distances of 8, 12, or 16 inches. Fig. 5.9 shows the relationship between image magnification, the source-object distance, and the object-receptor distance. To facilitate the parallel position of the receptor, image-receptor holders are used to support the image receptor in the patient's mouth (see Chapter 6).

A second method to minimize image distortion and magnification in intraoral radiography is the *bisecting angle technique* (Fig. 5.10). In this method, the image receptor is placed as close to the teeth as possible without deforming it. However, when the image receptor is in this position, it is not parallel to the long axes of the teeth. This arrangement inherently causes distortion. Nevertheless, by directing the central ray perpendicular to an imaginary plane that bisects the angle between the teeth and the image receptor, the practitioner can make the length of the tooth's image on the image receptor correspond to the actual length of the tooth. This angle between a tooth and the image receptor is especially apparent when teeth are radiographed in the maxilla or anterior mandible. Although the projected length of a tooth is correct, these images display a distorted image of the position of alveolar crest with respect to the cementoenamel junction of a tooth. In recent years, the bisecting angle technique is used less frequently for general periapical radiography as use of the paralleling technique has increased.

OBJECT LOCALIZATION

Most often, conventional periapical and bite-wing radiographs are the first radiographic images made of the teeth and supporting bone. An inherent limitation of plain radiography is the two-dimensional nature of the image. Often, the dentist needs to derive three-dimensional information that describes the spatial relationship of the structures imaged. For example, the dentist may need to determine the location of an impacted tooth, or a foreign object within the jaw. Three

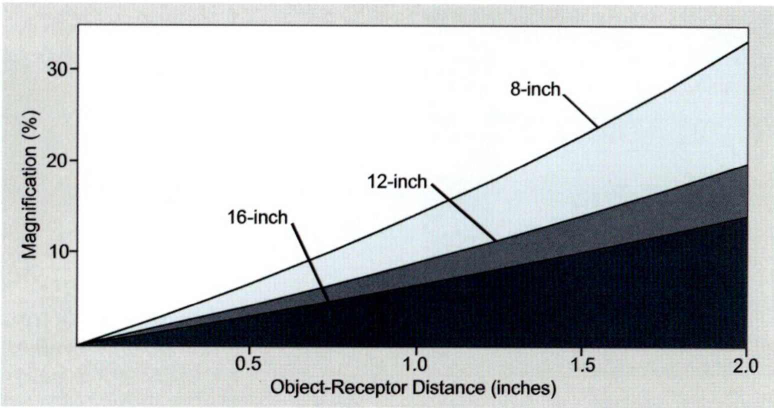

Fig. 5.9 Graph showing change in image magnification with change in the object-receptor distance, using source-object distances of 8, 12, and 16 inches. Magnification caused by an increased object-receptor can be minimized by increasing the source-object distance.

> **BOX 5.3 Approaches to Decipher Three-Dimensional Relationships by Radiography**
>
> - Examine two conventional images projected at right angles to each other.
> - Use the tube-shift technique employing conventional periapical views.
> - Image the anatomic region with a three-dimensional imaging modality.

approaches are frequently used to obtain such three-dimensional information (Box 5.3). The first two approaches combine information from two or more conventional projection radiographs to decipher the three-dimensional spatial location of an object, and are discussed in detail in this chapter. The third approach requires imaging the patient with a three-dimensional imaging modality such as cone beam computed tomography or multidetector computed tomography. Dentists must be familiar with the application of the first two approaches—these techniques are valuable because CT imaging may not be easily accessible or even necessary if the dentist already has multiple periapical views of the region of interest.

Examine two images projected at right angles to each other. In this approach, the clinician identifies the position of the object of interest relative to surrounding anatomic landmarks on both projections, and combines information from both projections to spatially locate the object. For radiography of the teeth and supporting structures, the two projections used are periapical and cross-sectional occlusal radiographs (see Chapter 6).

Fig. 5.11 demonstrates application of this method to spatially define the relationships of an impacted maxillary canine to the adjacent teeth. The periapical radiograph localizes the impacted canine in the mesiodistal and superoinferior dimensions, and the maxillary occlusal radiograph provides information in the mesiodistal and buccolingual dimensions. The combined information allows the clinician to locate the impacted tooth in all three dimensions, which is necessary for planning the surgical approach to expose the canine crown for subsequent orthodontic tooth movement.

This approach is best suited for the mandible, where making cross-sectional occlusal radiographs is easier. On a maxillary cross-sectional occlusal view, the superimposition of features in the anterior part of the skull frequently obscures the area of interest.

The principle of obtaining two projections at right angles can also be applied to cephalometric radiography—the combined analysis of lateral and posteroanterior projections provides information on skeletal relationships in all three planes.

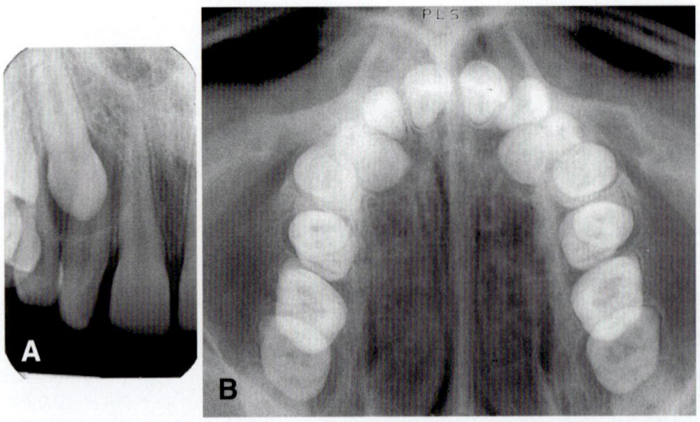

Fig. 5.11 (A) Periapical radiograph shows impacted canine lying apical to roots of lateral incisor and first premolar. (B) Maxillary cross-sectional occlusal view shows that the canine lies palatal to the roots of the lateral incisor and first premolar.

Use the tube-shift technique employing conventional periapical and/or bitewing views. A second approach to identify the spatial position of an object is the *tube-shift technique.* Other names for this procedure are the *buccal-object rule* and *Clark's rule* (Clark described this method in 1910). The rationale for this procedure derives from the manner in which the relative positions of radiographic images of two separate objects change when the projection angle at which the images were made is changed. The beam angulation changes opposite to the direction of tube movement.

Fig. 5.12 shows two radiographs of an object, located lingual to the premolar, exposed at different angles. Compare the positions of the object in question on each radiograph with a reference structure—for example, the apex of the second premolar. In the first radiograph, the object is superimposed over the apex of the second premolar. The x-ray tube head is then shifted and directed from a more mesial angulation. In the resultant radiograph, the image of the object in question has moved mesially with respect to the apex of the second premolar. *When an object lies lingual to the reference object, its image appears to move in the direction of the tube shift.*

Fig. 5.13 shows two radiographs of an object, now located buccal to the premolar. In the first projection, the object is superimposed over the apex of the second premolar. When the x-ray tube is moved mesially, the image of the object appears to move distal relative to the apex of the second premolar. *When the object lies buccal to the reference object, its image appears to move in the direction opposite to the tube shift.*

The application of this principle can be easily remembered by the acronym *SLOB*: same lingual, opposite buccal. Thus, if the object in question appears to move in the *same* direction with respect to the reference structures as does the x-ray tube, it is on the *lingual* aspect of the reference object; if it appears to move in the *opposite* direction as the x-ray tube, it is on the *buccal* aspect. If it does not move with respect to the reference object, it lies at the same depth (in the same vertical plane) as the reference object. The application of this method works equally well when the x-ray tube is moved vertically, instead of horizontally. In this case, the movement of the object's image in the

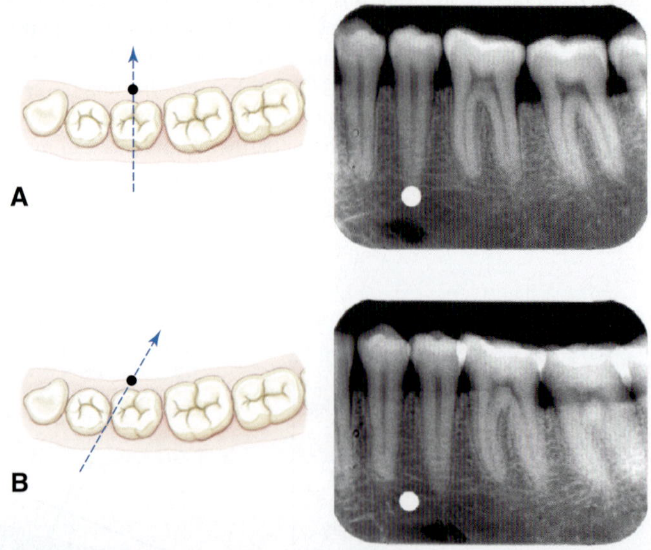

Fig. 5.12 The Position of an Object may be Determined with Respect to Reference Structures with Use of the Tube Shift Technique. (A) A radiopaque object on the lingual surface of the mandible *(black dot)* may appear apical to the second premolar. (B) When another radiograph is made of this region angulated from the mesial, the object appears to have moved mesially with respect to the second premolar apex ("same lingual" in the acronym SLOB).

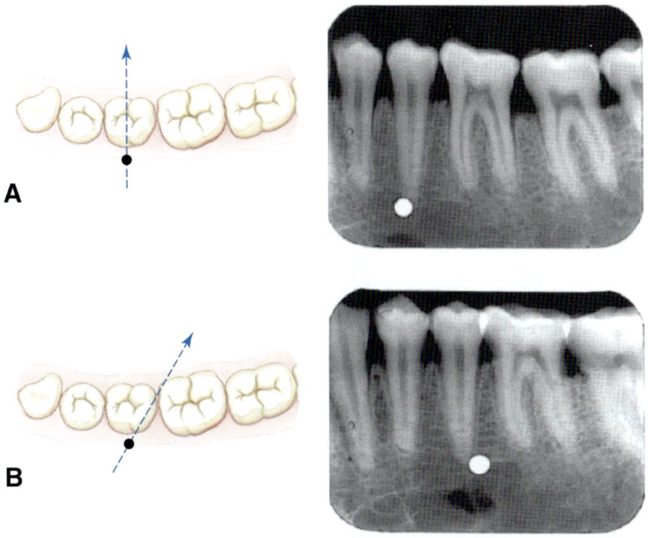

Fig. 5.13 The Position of an Object can be Determined with Respect to Reference Structures with Use of the Tube Shift Technique. (A) An object on the buccal surface of the mandible may appear apical to the second premolar. (B) When another radiograph is made of this region angulated from the mesial, the object appears to have moved distally with respect to the second premolar apex ("opposite buccal" in the acronym SLOB).

vertical plane (superior or inferior to the reference structure) is evaluated.

A conventional full-mouth radiographic series consists of images of an anatomic region taken at different angles. Dentists can use this principle to decipher the location of anatomic structures. For example, the mental foramen is often superimposed over the apex of the adjacent premolar, and may mimic a periapical radiolucency. However, the projection of the adjacent radiograph, taken at a different angle, will demonstrate movement of the radiolucency away from the apex, and allows it differentiation from a true periapical radiolucency. Likewise, the same principle can be applied to examine superimposition of the incisive foramen over the apex of a maxillary central incisor.

This technique assists in determining the position of impacted teeth, the presence of foreign objects, and identification of multiple pulp canals. Fig. 5.14 shows two periapical radiographs of the mandibular molar region taken at slightly different horizontal angulations. In the first projection (see Fig. 5.14A), the object of interest (impacted second premolar) is superimposed over the furcation and mesial root of the mandibular permanent first molar. The second projection (see Fig. 5.14B) represents movement of the x-ray tube toward the mesial, and the image of the impacted premolar is now superimposed over the distal root (image has moved distally, opposite to the direction of tube movement). Applying the *SLOB* rule indicates that the impacted premolar is located *buccal* to the roots of the mandibular first molar. Also note the distal movement of the image of the orthodontic bracket anchored on the buccal surface of the molar.

The dentist may have two radiographs of a region of the dentition that were made at different angles, but no record exists of the orientation of the x-ray machine. Comparison of the anatomy displayed on the images helps distinguish changes in horizontal or vertical angulation. The relative positions of osseous landmarks with respect to the teeth help identify changes in horizontal or vertical angulation. Fig. 5.15 shows the inferior border of the zygomatic process of the maxilla over the molars. This structure lies buccal to the teeth and appears to move mesially as the x-ray beam is oriented more from the distal. Similarly, as the angulation of the beam is increased vertically, the zygomatic process is projected occlusally over the teeth. Several buccal anatomic structures such as the zygomatic process of the maxilla, buccal cusps of multicusped teeth, buccal roots of maxillary multirooted posteriors, external oblique ridge will also appear to move in the opposite direction of the tube. These structures can be used as reference structures to determine tube movement or object localization.

EGGSHELL EFFECT

Plain radiographs—images that project a three-dimensional volume onto a two-dimensional receptor—may produce an eggshell effect of corticated structures (Fig. 5.16A). Fig. 5.16B shows a schematic view of an egg being exposed to an x-ray beam. The top photon has a tangential path through the apex of the egg and a much longer path through the shell of the egg than does the lower photon, which strikes the egg at right angles to the surface and travels through two thicknesses of the shell. As a result, photons traveling through the periphery of a curved surface are more attenuated than photons traveling at right angles to the surface. Fig. 5.16C shows an expansile lesion on the buccal surface of the mandible on an occlusal view. The periphery of the expanded cortex is more opaque than the region inside the expanded border. The cortical bone is not thicker on the cortex than over the rest of the lesion, but rather the x-ray beam is more attenuated in this region because of the longer path length of photons through the bony cortex on the periphery. This eggshell effect accounts for why normal structures such as the lamina dura, the border of the maxillary sinuses and nasal fossa, and abnormal structures, including the corticated walls of cysts and benign tumors, are

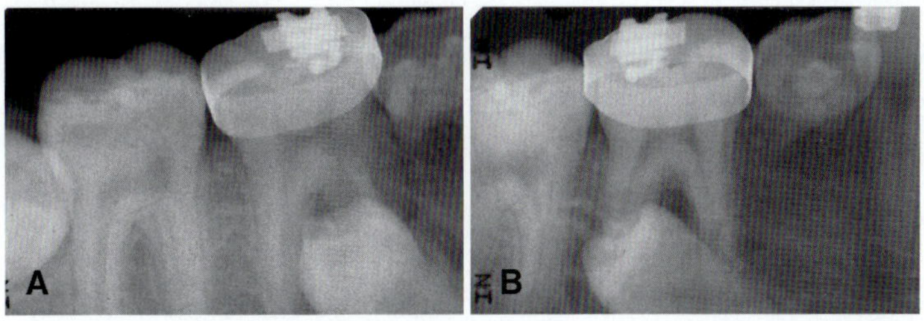

Fig. 5.14 Application of the Tube Shift Technique to Localize an Impacted Premolar. (A) Periapical radiograph of the mandibular molar region showing an impacted second premolar superimposed over the mesial root and furcation. (B) Another radiograph of this region angulated from the mesial; the impacted premolar appears to have moved distally with respect to the mandibular molar roots and indicates a relative buccal position. Note the apparent distal movement (opposite to tube movement) of the orthodontic bracket on the buccal surface of the tooth.

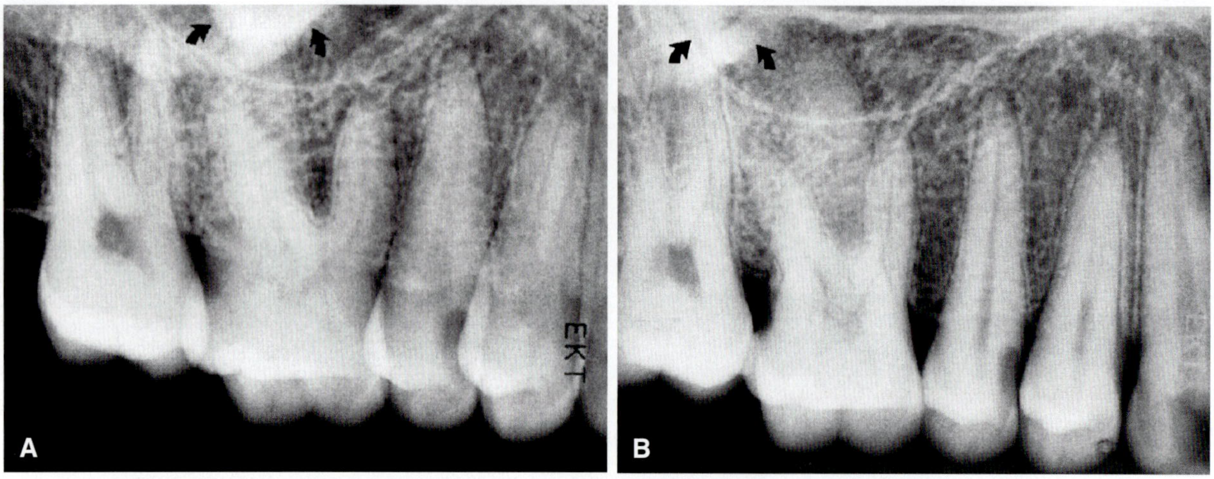

Fig. 5.15 The Position of the Maxillary Zygomatic Process in Relation to the Roots of the Molars can Help in Identifying the Orientation of Views. (A) The inferior border of the zygomatic process lies over the palatal root of the first molar. (B) The inferior border of the zygomatic process lies posterior to the palatal root of the first molar. This difference in position of the zygomatic process in relation to the palatal root indicates that when the image in *A* was made, the x-ray tube was positioned more posterior (distal) than when the image in *B* was made. The same conclusion can be reached independently by examining the roots and cusps of the first molar. The palatal root is superimposed over the distobuccal root in the image in *A*, but it lies between the two buccal roots in the image in *B*. The buccal cusps are mesial to the lingual cusps in A; they have moved distally and are aligned with the lingual cusps in image B.

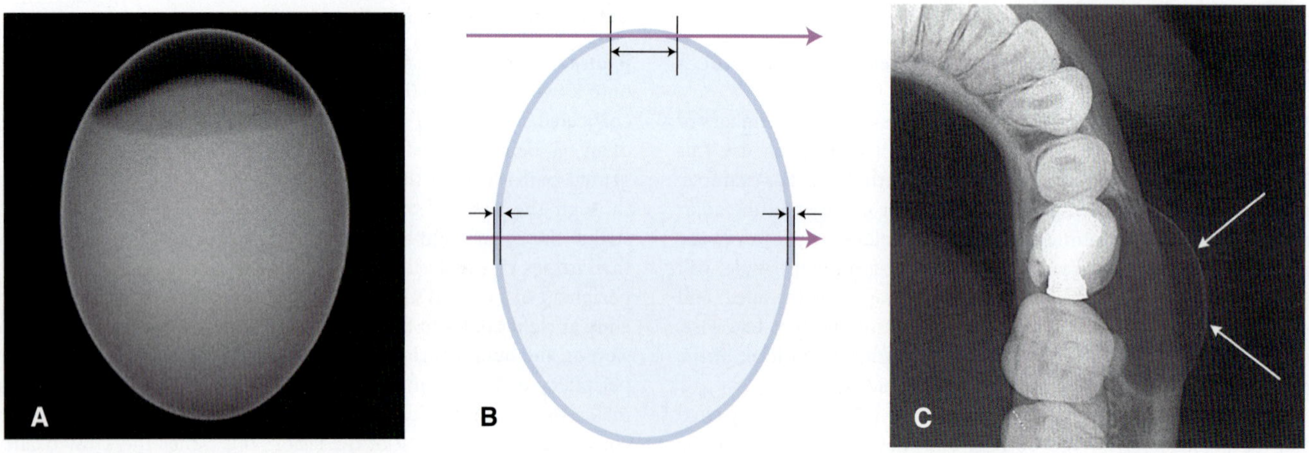

Fig. 5.16 Eggshell Effect. (A) Radiograph of a hard-boiled egg. Note how the rim of the eggshell is opaque even though it is uniform in thickness. (B) Schematic view of the egg being exposed to an x-ray beam. The top photon has a tangential path through the apex of the egg and a longer path through the shell of the egg than the lower photon. As a result, photons traveling through the periphery of a curved surface are more attenuated than the photons traveling at right angles to the surface. (C) An expansile lesion on the buccal surface of the mandible on a cross-sectional occlusal view. The expanded cortex is more opaque than the region inside the border as a result of the eggshell effect.

well demonstrated on plain radiographs. Soft tissue masses, such as the nose and tongue, do not show an eggshell effect because they are uniform rather than being composed of a dense layer surrounding a more lucent interior.

BIBLIOGRAPHY

Buccal-Object Rule

Clark CA. A method of ascertaining the relative position of unerupted teeth by means of film radiographs. *Proc R Soc Med Odontol Sect.* 1910;3:87-90.

Gutmann JL, Endo C. Clark's rule vis a vis the buccal object rule: its evolution and application in endodontics. *J Hist Dent.* 2011;59(1):12-15.

Jacobs SG. Radiographic localization of unerupted maxillary anterior teeth using the vertical tube shift technique: the history and application of the method with some case reports. *Am J Orthod Dentofacial Orthop.* 1999;116:415-423.

Jacobs SG. Radiographic localization of unerupted teeth: further findings about the vertical tube shift method and other localization techniques. *Am J Orthod Dentofacial Orthop.* 2000;118:439-447.

Katz JO, Langlais RP, Underhill TE, et al. Localization of paraoral soft tissue calcifications: the known object rule. *Oral Surg Oral Med Oral Pathol.* 1989;67:459-463.

Khabbaz MG, Serefoglou MH. The application of the buccal object rule for the determination of calcified root canals. *Int Endod J.* 1996;29:284-287.

Ludlow JB. The buccal object rule. *Dentomaxillofac Radiol.* 1999;28:258.

Richards AG. The buccal object rule. *Dent Radiogr Photogr.* 1980;53:37-56.

Paralleling Technique

Forsberg J. A comparison of the paralleling and bisecting-angle radiographic techniques in endodontics. *Int Endod J.* 1987;20:177-182.

Forsberg J. Radiographic reproduction of endodontic "working length" comparing the paralleling and the bisecting-angle techniques. *Oral Surg Oral Med Oral Pathol.* 1987;64:353-360.

Forsberg J, Halse A. Radiographic simulation of a periapical lesion comparing the paralleling and the bisecting-angle techniques. *Int Endod J.* 1994;27:133-138.

Rushton VE, Horner K. A comparative study of radiographic quality with five periapical techniques in general dental practice. *Dentomaxillofac Radiol.* 1994;23:37-45.

Rushton VE, Horner K. The acceptability of five periapical radiographic techniques to dentists and patients. *Br Dent J.* 1994;177:325-331.

Schulze RK, d'Hoedt B. A method to calculate angular disparities between object and receptor in "paralleling technique". *Dentomaxillofac Radiol.* 2002;31:32-38.

6

Intraoral Projections

Sanjay M. Mallya and Mansur Ahmad

Intraoral radiographic imaging examinations are the backbone of diagnostic imaging for the general dentist. Intraoral radiographs can be divided into three categories:

- Periapical projections, which show the entire length of the tooth and the surrounding peri-radicular bone
- Bitewing projections, which show only the crowns of teeth and the adjacent alveolar crests
- Occlusal projections, which show an area of teeth and bone larger than periapical images.

A full-mouth radiographic series consists of periapical and bitewing projections (Fig. 6.1; Box 6.1). These projections, when well exposed and properly processed (if film based), can provide valuable diagnostic information to complement the clinical examination. As with any clinical procedure, the operator must clearly understand the goals of diagnostic imaging and the criteria for evaluating the quality of performance.

Radiographic images should be made only when the historical or clinical findings identify a need for the additional diagnostic information that can be provided by a radiograph. The imaging modality selected and the frequency of such examinations will vary with the individual circumstances of each patient (see Chapter 15).

CRITERIA OF QUALITY

Every radiographic examination should produce images of optimal diagnostic quality, incorporating the following features:

- *Radiographs should record the complete areas of interest on the image.* Periapical radiographs must show the full length of the roots and at least 2 mm of periapical bone. If evidence of an abnormality is present, the area of the entire abnormality plus some surrounding normal bone must be shown by the radiographic examination. When this is not possible to achieve on a periapical radiograph, an appropriate radiographic examination must be designed to meet this diagnostic objective. The additional imaging may include occlusal and panoramic radiographs and cone beam computed tomography (CBCT), as indicated (see Chapters 8, 9, and 15). Bitewing examinations should demonstrate each posterior proximal surface at least once. Overlap of adjacent proximal tooth surfaces should be less than one-third of the enamel thickness.
- *Radiographs should have the least possible amount of distortion.* Most distortion is caused by improper angulation of the x-ray beam rather than by the curvature of the structures being examined or inappropriate positioning of the receptor. Close attention to proper positioning of the receptor and x-ray tube, as described in the principles of projection geometry (Chapter 5), results in diagnostically useful images.
- *Images should have optimal density and contrast to facilitate interpretation.* Radiographic exposure settings, including peak kilovoltage (kVp), the milliamperage (mA), and exposure time (s) are crucial parameters that influence density and contrast for both digital- and film-based radiography. When film-based imaging is used, faulty processing can adversely affect the quality of a properly exposed radiograph (see Chapter 4). Likewise, improper application of digital image enhancements such as contrast and sharpening may produce artifacts that compromise diagnostic interpretation (see Chapter 4).

When evaluating radiographic images, the practitioner must assess whether the initial diagnostic objectives of the examination are adequately met and whether there is a need to retake specific views. For example, a single projection in a full-mouth radiographic series may fail to open a contact or show a periapical region. However, retakes are not necessary if that missing information is available on another view.

PERIAPICAL RADIOGRAPHY

Periapical radiographs are commonly used in dentistry and show the entire length of the tooth and the surrounding bone. The diagnostic objectives of periapical radiographs are summarized in Box 6.2.

Two intraoral projection techniques are commonly used for periapical radiography: (1) the ***paralleling technique*** and (2) the ***bisecting angle*** technique. Both techniques can be applied to digital- and film-based imaging. The paralleling technique is preferred because it provides images with less distortion of the dentition. When anatomic configuration (e.g., palate and floor of the mouth) precludes strict adherence to the paralleling concept, slight modifications may have to be made. If the anatomic constraints are extreme, the principles of the bisecting angle technique may be used to accomplish the required receptor placement and determine the vertical angulation of the tube.

The term **image receptor** refers to any medium used to capture an image, including film, charge-coupled devices (CCDs), complementary metal oxide semiconductor (CMOS) sensors, or storage phosphor plates. The principles for making projection radiographs are the same for each of these receptor types; thus this chapter uses the general term **receptor** to refer any of the image receptors.

Paralleling Technique

The central principle of the paralleling technique (also called the **right-angle technique** or **long-cone technique**) is that the x-ray receptor is supported parallel to the long axis of the teeth and the central ray of the x-ray beam is directed at right angles to the teeth and receptor (Fig. 6.2). This orientation of the receptor, teeth, and central ray minimizes geometric distortion and presents the teeth and supporting bone in their true anatomic relationships.

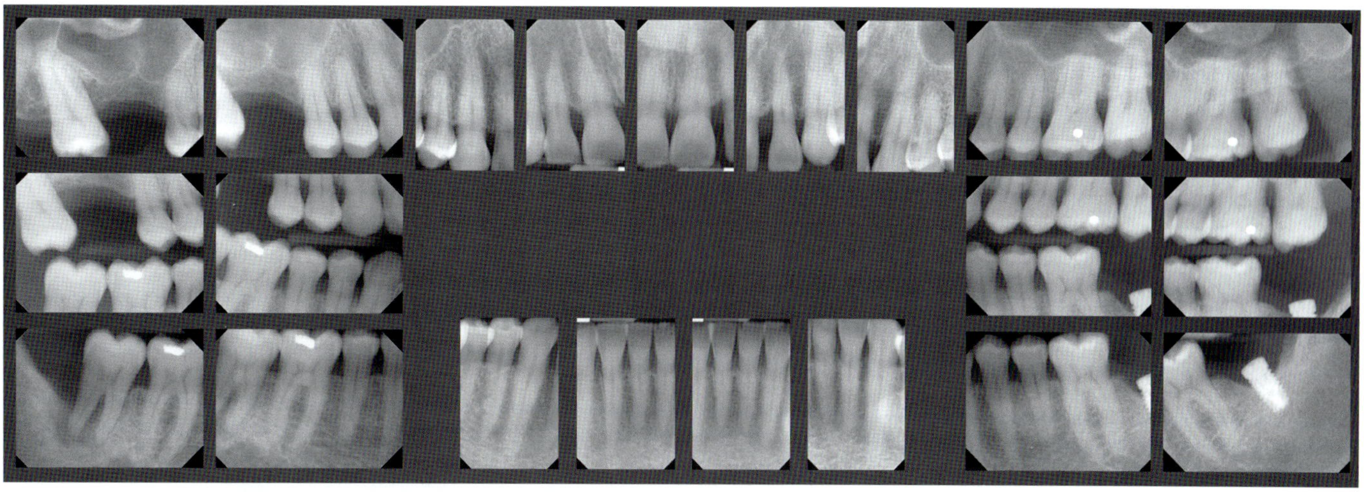

Fig. 6.1 Typical full-mouth set of radiographs consisting of 17 periapical views and 4 bitewing views.

BOX 6.1 Projections for a Typical Full-Mouth Radiographic Series

Anterior Periapical (Use No. 1 Receptor)

- Maxillary central incisors: one projection
- Maxillary lateral incisors: two projections
- Maxillary canines: two projections
- Mandibular central and lateral incisors: two projections
- Mandibular canines: two projections

Posterior Periapical (Use No. 2 Receptor)

- Maxillary premolars: two projections
- Maxillary molars: two projections
- Maxillary distomolar (as needed): two projections
- Mandibular premolars: two projections
- Mandibular molars: two projections
- Mandibular distomolar (as needed): two projections

Bitewing (Use No. 2 Receptor)

- Premolars: two projections
- Molars: two projections

BOX 6.2 Diagnostic Objectives of Periapical Radiography

- Assess extent of dental caries
- Detect presence and assess extent of periapical inflammation
- Evaluate consequences of traumatic injuries to the teeth and alveolar bone
- Assess periodontal bone loss
- Evaluate root morphology
- Assess implant osseointegration and peri-implant bone loss
- Evaluate unerupted and impacted teeth
- Evaluate external and internal root resorption
- Assess pulp morphology
- Determine length of endodontic instrumentation during treatment.

Due to anatomic constraints, this parallel orientation places the image receptor toward the middle of the oral cavity, away from the teeth. This increases the object-to-receptor distance and results in higher image magnification and poor geometric sharpness. To compensate for the resultant distortion and lack of sharpness, the paralleling technique is used with a relatively long source-to-object distance (see Fig. 6.3). The paralleling technique can be used effectively with film, CCD, or CMOS sensors or with storage phosphor plates.

Receptor-Holding Instruments

Receptor holders facilitate the positioning of the receptor in the patient's mouth. These holders stabilize the receptor to a bite block (Fig. 6.4). When the patient bites gently on this bite block, it places the receptor parallel to the tooth's long axis. Many of these receptor holders are specific for various brands of digital sensors, storage phosphor plates, or film. It is also important to use a receptor-holding instrument that has an external guiding ring. This guiding ring is used to align the x-ray collimator; it ensures that the beam is centered over receptor behind the teeth of interest and that the x-ray beam is perpendicular to the receptor and teeth (see Fig. 6.4). Rectangular collimators should be used to reduce patient radiation dose (see Chapter 3).

Receptor Placement

For optimal images, the receptor should be positioned parallel to the teeth and deep into the lingual vestibule or palatal vault; this is particularly important when rigid sensors are used because they are bulkier than film. For maxillary projections, the superior border of the receptor generally rests at the height of the palatal vault in the midline. Similarly, for mandibular projections, the receptor should be used to displace the tongue posteriorly or toward the midline to allow the inferior border of the receptor to rest on the floor of the mouth away from the mucosa on the lingual surface of the mandible.

Often anatomic variations do not allow the receptor to be placed deep enough to capture an image of the entire tooth length—for example, a shallow palate (Fig. 6.5), a shallow floor of the mouth, and tori. Another anatomic limitation is that all the roots of a multirooted tooth may not be placed parallel to the receptor, resulting in differential distortion of the roots (Fig. 6.6).

Angulation of the Tube Head

Orient the aiming cylinder of the x-ray machine in the vertical and horizontal planes to align with the aiming ring. The plane of the opening of the cylinder must be parallel to the plane of the aiming ring. The horizontal direction of the beam primarily influences the degree of overlapping of the images of the crowns at the interproximal spaces (Fig. 6.7).

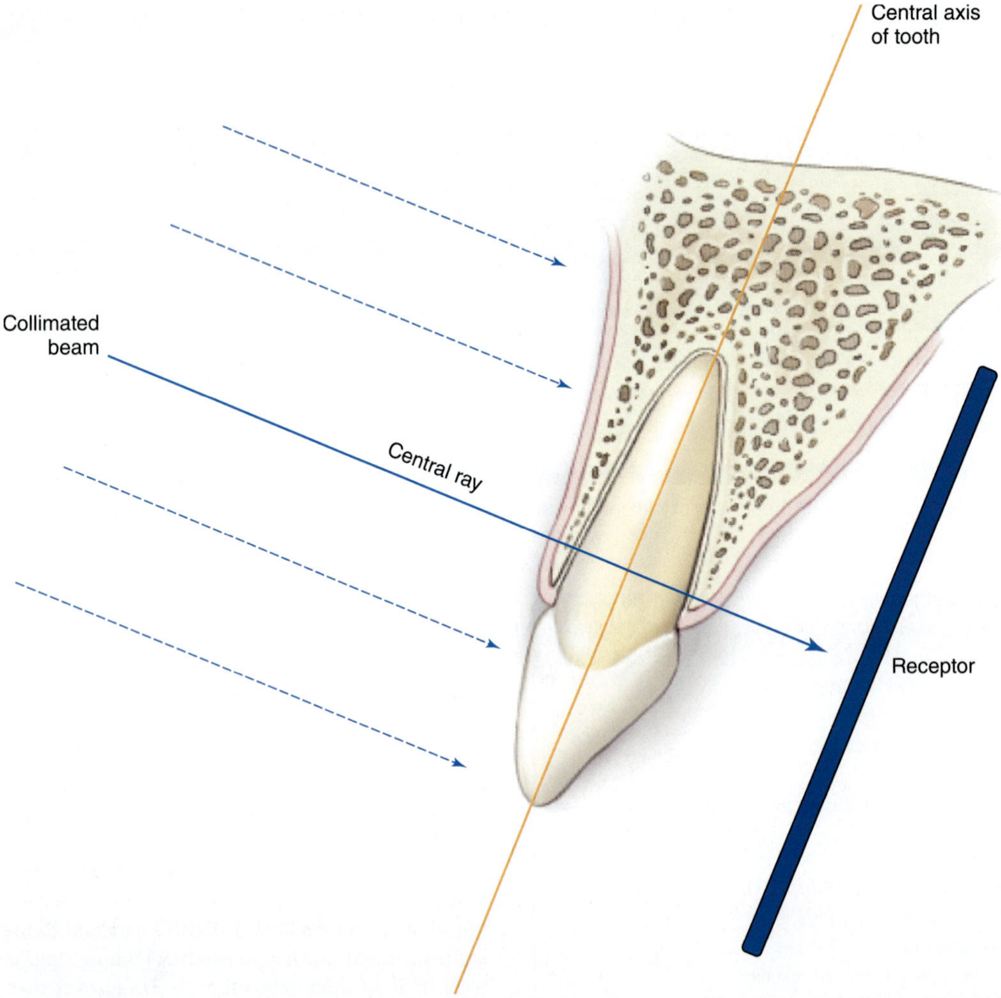

Fig. 6.2 Paralleling technique illustrates the parallelism between the long axis of the tooth and the receptor. The central ray is directed perpendicular to each. This technique minimizes image distortion but requires a receptor holder.

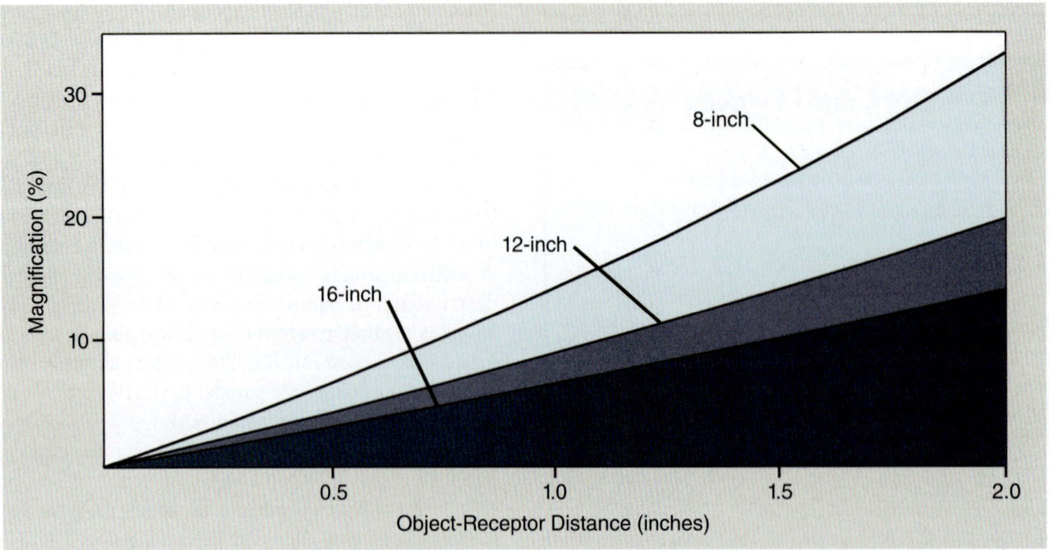

Fig. 6.3 Graph showing change in image magnification with change in the object-receptor distance, using source-object distances of 8, 12, and 16 inches. Magnification caused by an increased object-receptor can be minimized by increasing the source-object distance.

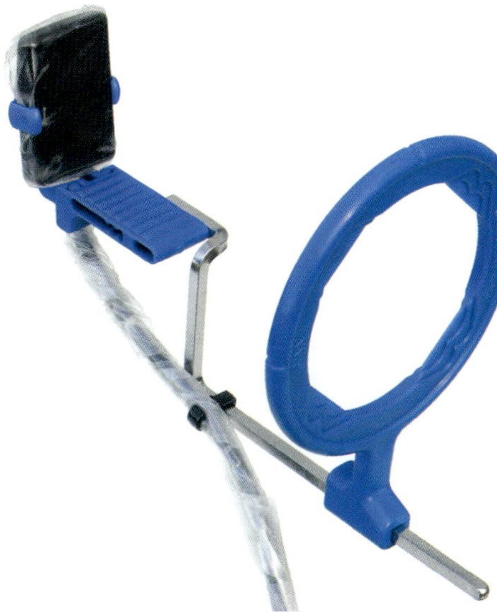

Fig. 6.4 Receptor-holding instruments. XCP instrument for anterior views shown with sensor and cord wrapped in disposable sensor cover for infection control and to protect the sensor from saliva. (Courtesy Dentsply Rinn, Elgin, IL.)

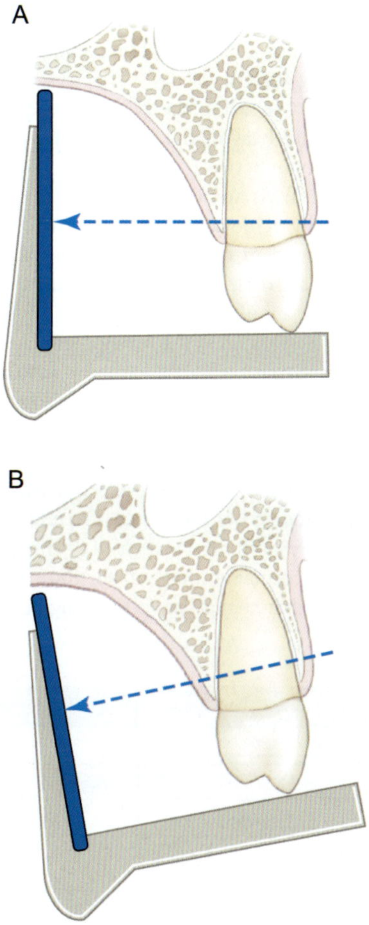

Fig. 6.5 Anatomic constraints in using the paralleling technique. (A) Optimal position of the receptor parallel to the long axis of the tooth. (B) A shallow palate limits placement of the receptor parallel to the tooth. Note that the x-ray beam is perpendicular to the receptor but not the tooth, resulting in distortion.

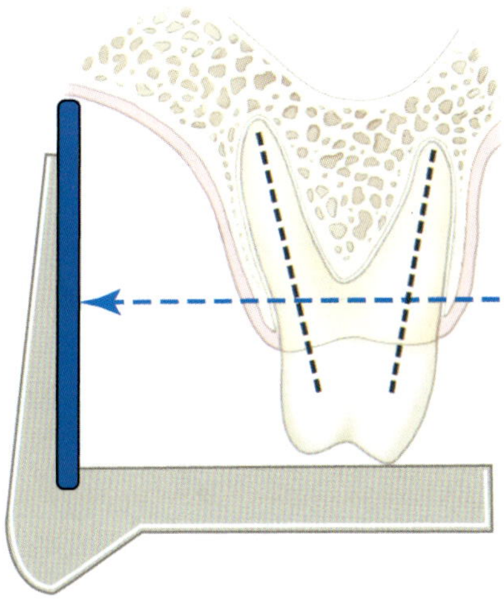

Fig. 6.6 The x-ray beam is parallel to the central axis of the tooth and the receptor. Note that the x-ray beam is at different angles to the buccal and palatal root of the molar, resulting in unequal distortion. Increasing the source-object distance by using a long cone will limit this distortion.

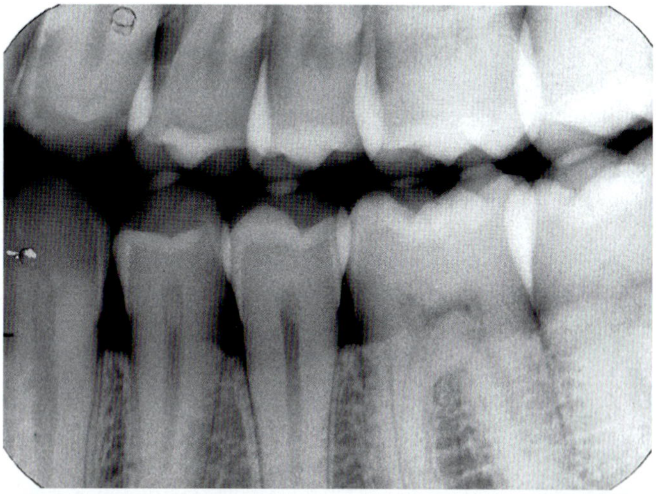

Fig. 6.7 Horizontal overlapping of crowns results from misdirection of the central ray in the horizontal plane.

Bisecting Angle Technique

In contemporary dental practice, the bisecting angle technique has been largely replaced by the paralleling technique. Nevertheless, the bisecting angle technique may be useful when the operator is unable to apply the paralleling technique because of large rigid sensors or the anatomy of the patient. The bisecting angle technique is based on a simple geometric theorem, Cieszynski's rule of isometry, which states that two triangles are equal when they share one complete side and have two equal angles. Dental radiography applies the theorem as follows. The receptor is positioned as close as possible to the lingual surface of the teeth, resting in the palate or in the floor of the mouth (Fig. 6.8). The plane of the receptor and the long axis of the teeth form an angle with its apex at the incisal edge or occlusal surface. Consider an imaginary line that bisects this angle and direct the central ray of the beam at right angles to this bisector. This creates two triangles with two equal angles and a common side (the imaginary bisector). The hypotenuses of the two triangles represent the actual tooth length and the image length; theoretically they are the same.

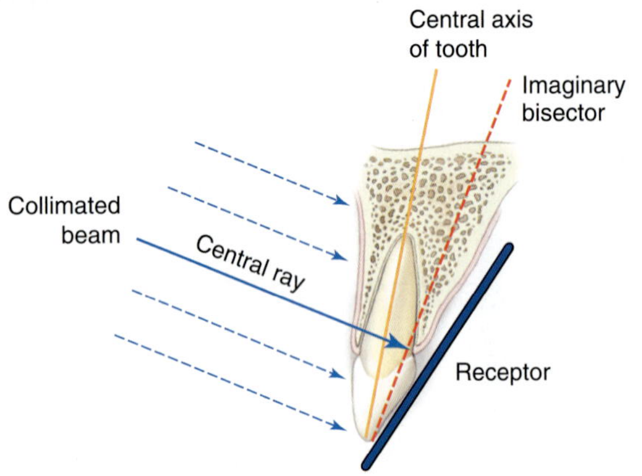

Fig. 6.8 Bisecting angle technique shows the central ray directed at a right angle to the plane that bisects the angle between the long axis of the tooth and the receptor.

To reproduce the length of each root of a multirooted tooth accurately, the central beam must be angled differently for each root. Another limitation of this technique is that the alveolar ridge often projects coronal to its true position and distorts the apparent height of the alveolar bone around the teeth.

Receptor-Holding Instruments

Several methods can be used to support receptors intraorally for bisecting angle projections. The preferred method is to use a receptor-holding bisecting angle instrument (BAI) with an external device to localize the x-ray beam and guide the appropriate vertical angle. BAI (Dentsply Rinn Corporation) uses an angled bite block and secures the receptor at an angle to the tooth. A metal arm attaches to the bite block and anchors an external aiming ring to ensure full coverage of the receptor by the primary x-ray beam. There are several other receptor holders and disposable bite blocks that can be used to support a receptor for this technique. It is undesirable to have the patient support the receptor from the lingual surface with his or her forefinger. Patients often use excessive force and may bend the film or storage phosphor plates, causing distortion of the image. Also, the receptor might slip, resulting in an improper image field. Finally, without an external guide to the position of the receptor, the x-ray beam may miss part of the receptor, resulting in a partial image (**cone cut**).

Positioning of the Patient

Maxillary projections. The patient should be seated upright in the dental chair with the sagittal plane vertical and the occlusal plane horizontal.

Mandibular projections. The patient should be seated upright in the dental chair with the sagittal plane vertical. The head is tilted back slightly to compensate for the changed occlusal plane when the mouth is opened.

Receptor Placement

Similar to the paralleling technique, the receptor is positioned lingual to the area of interest, with the apical end against the mucosa on the lingual or palatal surface. The occlusal or incisal edge is oriented against the teeth with an edge of the receptor extending approximately 1–2 mm beyond the teeth. If necessary for the patient's comfort, the anterior corner of a film can be softened by bending it before it is placed against the mucosa. Care must be taken not to bend the film excessively because this may result in considerable image distortion and in pressure defects in the emulsion that are apparent on the processed film. Such bending is less marked with storage phosphor plates, and the rigid structure of the CCD or CMOS sensors cannot be bent to adapt to the arch shape.

Angulation of the Tube Head

Horizontal angulation. When a receptor-holding device with a beam-localizing ring is used, it facilitates alignment with the x-ray beam, so that the central ray is directed through the interproximal contacts in the region being examined. If the receptor-holding device does not have a beam-localizing feature, the tube is angled in the horizontal plane to direct the central ray through the contacts. The edge of the x-ray beam collimator cone should be parallel to the buccal surfaces of the teeth being examined.

Vertical angulation. In using the bisecting angle technique, the goal is to aim the central ray of the x-ray beam perpendicular to a plane bisecting the angle between the receptor and the long axis of the tooth. However, if BAIs are not used, accurate orientation of the beam is not practically achievable for every single projection to be made. Instead, the clinician uses predetermined angles for specific anatomic regions (Table 6.1). Proper patient positioning is imperative when using these angulations—the patient must be positioned with the occlusal plane parallel to the horizontal plane. The predetermined angles are based on typical human jaw anatomy and are not customized to individual patients. Often the radiographer may need to adjust these angles to account for anatomic variations, such as proclination of the teeth.

Image distortion is likely and limits effective use of the bisecting angle technique. Furthermore, individual divergent roots of multirooted teeth will manifest different extents of distortion.

Diagnostically unacceptable image distortion may require retaking the radiograph with a change in vertical angulation. The pattern

TABLE 6.1 Angulation Guidelines for Bisecting Angle Projections

	REGION-SPECIFIC SETTINGS					
	North America		India[a]		Brazil[b]	
Projection	*Maxilla*	*Mandible*	*Maxilla*	*Mandible*	*Maxilla*	*Mandible*
Incisors	+40 degrees	−15 degrees	+45 degrees	−25 degrees	+45 to +55 degrees	−25 to −15 degrees
Canines	+45 degrees	−20 degrees	+45 degrees	−20 degrees	+40 to +50 degrees	−20 to −10 degrees
Premolars	+30 degrees	−10 degrees	+30 degrees	−15 degrees	+30 to +45 degrees	−10 to −5 degrees
Molars	+20 degrees	−5 degrees	+30 degrees	−10 to 0 degrees	+20 to +35 degrees	−5 to 0 degrees

[a]Data courtesy Dr. Freny Karjodkar, from *Essentials of Oral and Maxillofacial Radiology*, 2014, Jaypee Publishers.
[b]Data collated by Prof. Dr. Matheus Lima de Oliveira, UNICAMP—University of Campinas, Piracicaba Dental School.
The occlusal plane is oriented parallel with the floor. By convention, with a positive (+) angulation, the aiming cylinder points downward, and with a negative (−) angulation, it points upward.

of distortion should guide the radiographer to select an appropriate angle. Image foreshortening indicates that the vertical angulation is too high. In contrast, image elongation indicates insufficient vertical angulation.

General Steps for Making Intraoral Radiographs

The following steps describe the overall general procedure to obtain a full-mouth set of radiographs, made using the paralleling technique.

- *Prepare unit for exposure.* Place barriers for universal infection control (see Chapter 14) and have receptors and receptor-holding instruments ready at chairside.
- *Greet and seat the patient.* Position the patient upright in the chair with the back and head well supported, and briefly describe the procedures that are to be performed. Position the dental chair low for maxillary projections and elevated for mandibular projections. Ask the patient to remove eyeglasses and all removable dental appliances. Jewelry in the path of the x-ray beam, such as nose, lip, and tongue rings, should be removed.
- *Adjust the x-ray unit setting.* Set the x-ray machine for the proper kVp, mA, and exposure time. Generally only the exposure time is adjusted for the various anatomic locations.
- *Wash your hands thoroughly and wear appropriate personal protective equipment.* Wash your hands with soap and water, preferably in front of the patient or at least in an area where the patient can observe or be aware of this step. Put on disposable gloves and a disposable gown or coat.
- *Examine the oral cavity.* Before placing any receptors in the mouth, examine the teeth to estimate their axial inclination, which influences the placement of the receptor. Also note tori or other obstructions that may modify receptor placement. Ensure that all removable dental appliances and intraoral jewelry are removed.
- *Position the x-ray tube head.* Bring the x-ray tube head to the side to be examined so that it is easily accessible for final positioning after the receptor has been placed in the mouth.
- *Position the receptor.* Insert the receptor into the holding device and position the receptor and holding device in the region of the patient's mouth to be examined. Angle the receptor holder such that the film or sensor is parallel to the occlusal plane. Leading with the apical end of the receptor, rotate it into the oral cavity. This technique avoids the need for the patient to open wide. For maxillary views, place the receptor in the mouth as far from the teeth as possible, near the midline of the palate, where there is the maximal space available. The added space allows the receptor to be oriented parallel to the long axis of the teeth. With the receptor now in the mouth, place it gently on the palate or floor of the mouth. For all bitewing and mandibular periapical images, it is useful to shift the mandible to the side being imaged; this decreases patient discomfort because there is now more room for the sensor on the lingual side of the mandible. After the sensor is positioned, rotate the receptor-holding instrument until the bite block rests on the teeth to be radiographed and place a cotton roll between the bite block and the opposing teeth. The cotton roll helps stabilize the receptor-holding instrument and decreases patient discomfort. Holding the instrument and receptor in place, ask the patient to close the mouth gently. Solid-state receptors (CCD or CMOS sensors) have approximately of 2–4 mm of "dead space" between the edge of the plastic casing and the image capture chip, and the captured anatomic region is smaller than the external sensor size. The width of the dead space varies with manufacturer.
- *Position the x-ray tube.* Adjust the vertical and horizontal angulation of the tube head to correspond to the receptor-holding instrument. The end of the aiming ring of the x-ray tube head must be flush or parallel to the guide ring instrument. Alignment is satisfactory when the aiming cylinder covers the port and is within the limits of the face shield. Caution the patient not to move.
- *Make the exposure.* Make the exposure with the preset exposure time. If the receptor is a film or storage phosphor plate, remove the receptor from the patient's mouth after exposure, dry it with a paper towel, remove the infection control sleeve, and place the receptor in an appropriate receptacle outside the exposure area. If the receptor is a CCD or CMOS sensor, you may keep it in the patient's mouth and reposition it for the next view. Ensure patient comfort after each exposure.

Individual Periapical Projections

A typical full-mouth radiographic series consists of 21 images (see Box 6.1 and Fig. 6.1). To facilitate work flow, it is useful to establish a regular sequence of projections in making exposures. It is practical to start with the anterior views because they cause less discomfort for the patient. The following section describes procedural details to make periapical radiographs using the paralleling technique. It describes the field encompassed in the image, the placement of the receptor, the projection of the central ray, and the positioning of the aiming ring.

PARALLELING TECHNIQUE

Maxillary Central Incisor Projection (Fig. 6.9)

Image field: The field of view on these radiographs should include both central incisors and their periapical areas (see Fig. 6.9A and B).

Receptor placement: Place a No. 1 receptor at about the level of the second premolars or first molars to take advantage of the maximal palatal height so that the entire length of the teeth can be projected on it. Have the receptor resting on the palate with its midline centered with the midline of the arch (see Fig. 6.9C). Position the receptor's long axis parallel to the long axis of the maxillary central incisors (see Fig. 6.9D).

Projection of central ray: Direct the central ray through the contact point of the central incisors and perpendicular to the plane of the receptors and roots of the teeth (see Fig. 6.9C). Because the axial inclination of the maxillary incisors is about 15–20 degrees, the vertical angulation of the tube should be at the same positive angle (see Fig. 6.9E). The tube should have no horizontal angulation (see Fig. 6.9C).

Point of entry: Direct the point of entry of the central ray high on the lip, in the midline, just below the septum of the nostril (see Fig. 6.9E). If the palatal vault is unusually low or a palatal torus is present, it may be necessary to tilt the receptor holder positively and compromise a completely parallel relationship between the receptor and the teeth to ensure that the periapical region is included on the image.

PARALLELING TECHNIQUE

Maxillary Lateral Projection (Fig. 6.10)

Image field: This projection should show the lateral incisor and its periapical field centered on the radiograph (see Fig. 6.10A and B). Include the mesial interproximal area with the distal aspect of the central incisor on the radiograph so that no overlap is evident.

Receptor placement: Place a No. 1 receptor deep in the oral cavity parallel with the long axis and the mesiodistal plane of the maxillary lateral incisor (see Fig. 6.10C and D).

Projection of central ray: Direct the central ray through the middle of the lateral incisor (see Fig. 6.10C), with no overlapping of the margins of the crowns at the interproximal space on its mesial aspect. Do not attempt to open the distal contact with the canine (see Fig. 6.10B).

Point of entry: Orient the central ray to enter high on the lip about 1 cm from the midline (see Fig. 6.10E).

PARALLELING TECHNIQUE

Maxillary Canine Projection (Fig. 6.11)

Image field: This projection should demonstrate the entire canine, with its periapical area, in the midline of the radiograph (see Fig. 6.11A and B). Open the mesial contact area. Ignore the distal contact because it will be viewed on other projections.

Receptor placement: Place a No. 1 receptor against the palate, well away from the palatal surface of the teeth (see Fig. 6.11C). Orient the receptor packet with its anterior edge at about the middle of the lateral incisor and its long axis parallel with the long axis of the canine (see Fig. 6.11D).

Projection of central ray: Position the holding instrument so that it directs the beam through the mesial contact of the canine (see Fig. 6.11C). Do not attempt to open the distal contact.

Point of entry: Direct the central ray through the canine eminence. The point of entry is at about the intersection of the distal and inferior borders of the ala of the nose (see Fig. 6.11E).

PARALLELING TECHNIQUE

Maxillary Premolar Projection (Fig. 6.12)

Image field: The radiograph of this region should include the images of the distal half of the canine and the premolars, with room for at least the first molar (see Fig. 6.12A and B).

Receptor placement: Place a No. 2 receptor in the mouth with the long dimension parallel with the occlusal plane and near the palatal midline (see Fig. 6.12C). The receptor should extend far enough forward to cover the distal half of the canine. It should also include the premolars and the first molar and maybe the mesial portion of the second molar (see Fig. 6.12B). The plane of the receptor should be nearly vertical to correspond with the long axis of the premolar teeth (see Fig. 6.12C). Position the receptor-holding device so that the long axis of the receptor is parallel with the buccal plane of the premolars. This establishes the proper horizontal angulation (see Fig. 6.12C).

Projection of central ray: Direct the central ray perpendicular to the receptor (see Fig. 6.12D). The horizontal angulation of the holding instrument should be adjusted to permit the beam to pass through the interproximal area between the first and second premolars (see Fig. 6.12C).

Point of entry: Place the holding instrument so that the central ray passes through the center of the second premolar root. This point is usually below the pupil of the eye (see Fig. 6.12E).

PARALLELING TECHNIQUE

Maxillary Molar Projection (Fig. 6.13)

Image field: The radiograph of this region should show the images of the distal half of the second premolar, the three maxillary permanent molars, and some of the tuberosity (see Fig. 6.13A and B). Include the same area on the receptor even if some or all molars are missing. If the third molar is impacted in an area other than the region of the tuberosity, a distal oblique or extraoral projection (e.g., panoramic or oblique lateral jaw view) may be required.

Receptor placement: When placing the No. 2 receptor for this projection, position the long dimension of the receptor nearly horizontal to minimize brushing the palate and dorsum of the tongue. When the receptor is in the region to be examined, rotate it into position with a firm and definite motion. This maneuver is important in avoiding the gag reflex, and resolute action by the operator enhances the patient's confidence. Place the receptor far enough posterior to cover the first, second, and third molar areas and some of the tuberosity. The anterior border should just cover the distal aspect of the second premolar (see Fig. 6.12B). To cover the molars from crown to apices, place the receptor at the midline of the palate (see Fig. 6.13C). In this position, room should be available to orient the receptor parallel with the molar teeth. The mesial or distal rotation of the receptor-holding device should ensure that the long axis of the receptor is parallel with the mean buccal plane of the molars (to establish the proper horizontal angulation). A shallow palate may require slight tipping of the holding instrument to avoid bending the receptor.

Note: In some cases, the size of the mouth (length of the arch) will not allow positioning of the receptor-holding device as far posterior as recommended for the molar projection. However, by placing the receptor-holding device so that half the tube alignment ring or face shield is behind the outer canthus of the eye, the molars and part of the tuberosity usually can be included in the image of the molar projection.

Projection of central ray: Direct the central ray perpendicular to the receptor (see Fig. 6.13D). Adjust the horizontal angulation of the receptor-holding device to direct the beam at right angles to the buccal surfaces of the molar teeth (see Fig. 6.13C).

Point of entry: The point of entry of the central ray should be on the cheek below the outer canthus of the eye and the zygoma at the position of the maxillary second molar (see Fig. 6.13E).

PARALLELING TECHNIQUE

Mandibular Centrolateral Projection (Fig. 6.14)

Image field: Center the image of the mandibular central and lateral incisors and their periapical areas on the receptor (see Fig. 6.14A and B). Because the space in this area is frequently restricted, use two size 1 receptors for the incisors on each side to provide good coverage with minimal discomfort. In addition, the incisor contact areas are better viewed on two narrower anterior receptors because the angulation of the central ray can be adjusted for the contact area on each side (see Fig. 6.14C).

Receptor placement: Place the long dimension of the No. 1 receptor vertically behind the central and lateral incisors with the contact area centered and the lower border below the tongue. Position the receptor posteriorly as far as possible, usually between the premolars (see Fig. 6.14C). With the receptor resting gently on the floor of the mouth as the fulcrum, tip the instrument downward until the receptor-holder bite block is resting on the incisors. Instruct the patient to close the mouth slowly. As the patient is closing slowly and the floor of the mouth is relaxing, rotate the instrument with the teeth as the fulcrum to align the receptor to be more parallel with the teeth (see Fig. 6.14D).

Projection of central ray: Orient the central ray through the interproximal space between the central and lateral incisors (see Fig. 6.14C).

Point of entry: The central ray enters below the lower lip and about 1 cm lateral to the midline (see Fig. 6.14E).

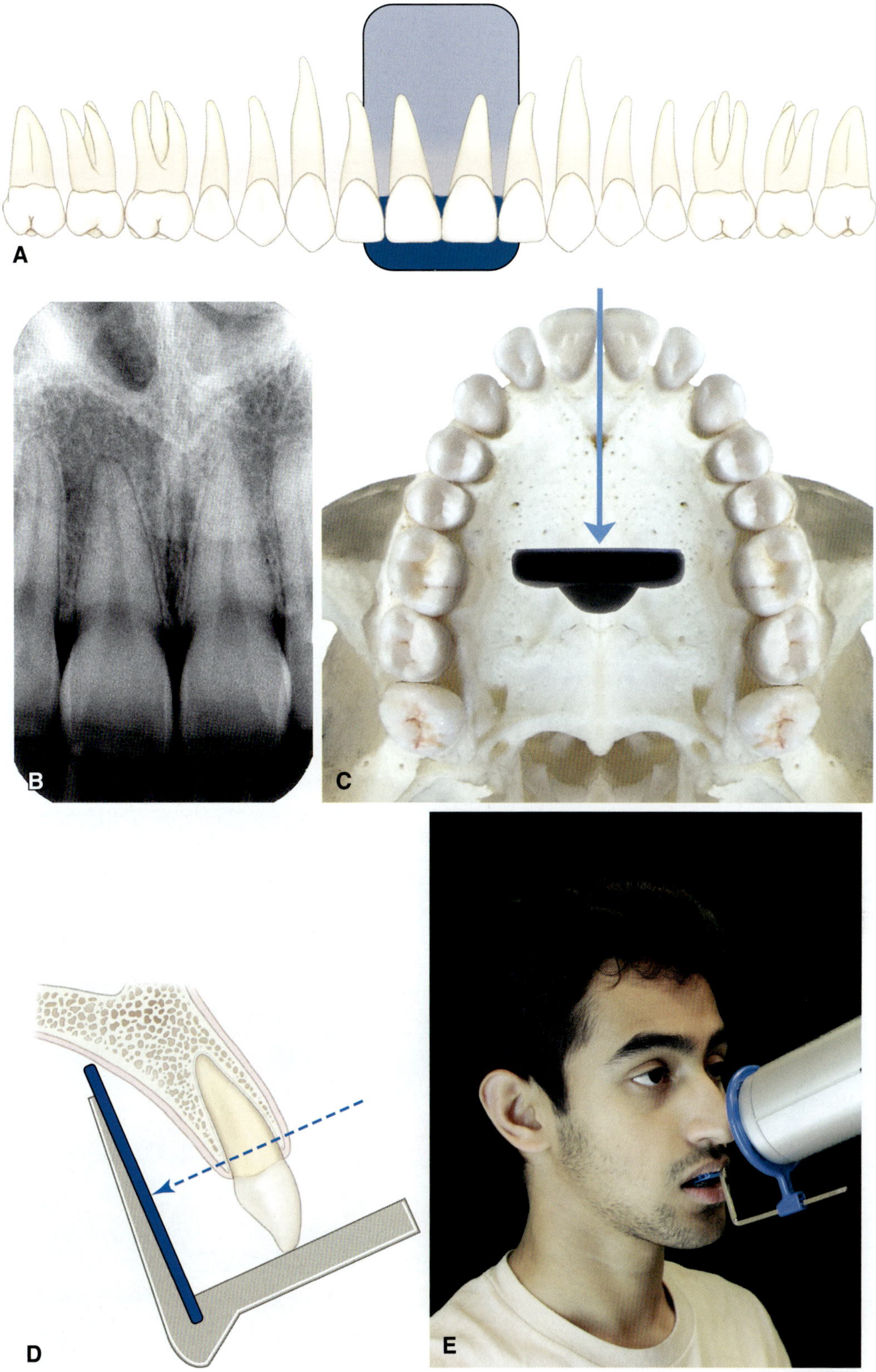

Fig. 6.9 Maxillary central incisor periapical projection. (A) The *shaded* area outlines the image field. (B) Periapical radiograph of the maxillary central incisor. (C) Position of the receptor in the oral cavity and direction of the x-ray beam (*blue arrow*). (D) Graphic representation of the image receptor and the x-ray beam relative to the long axis of the central incisor. (E) Position of the patient with the receptor holder in place and the aiming ring aligned for exposure.

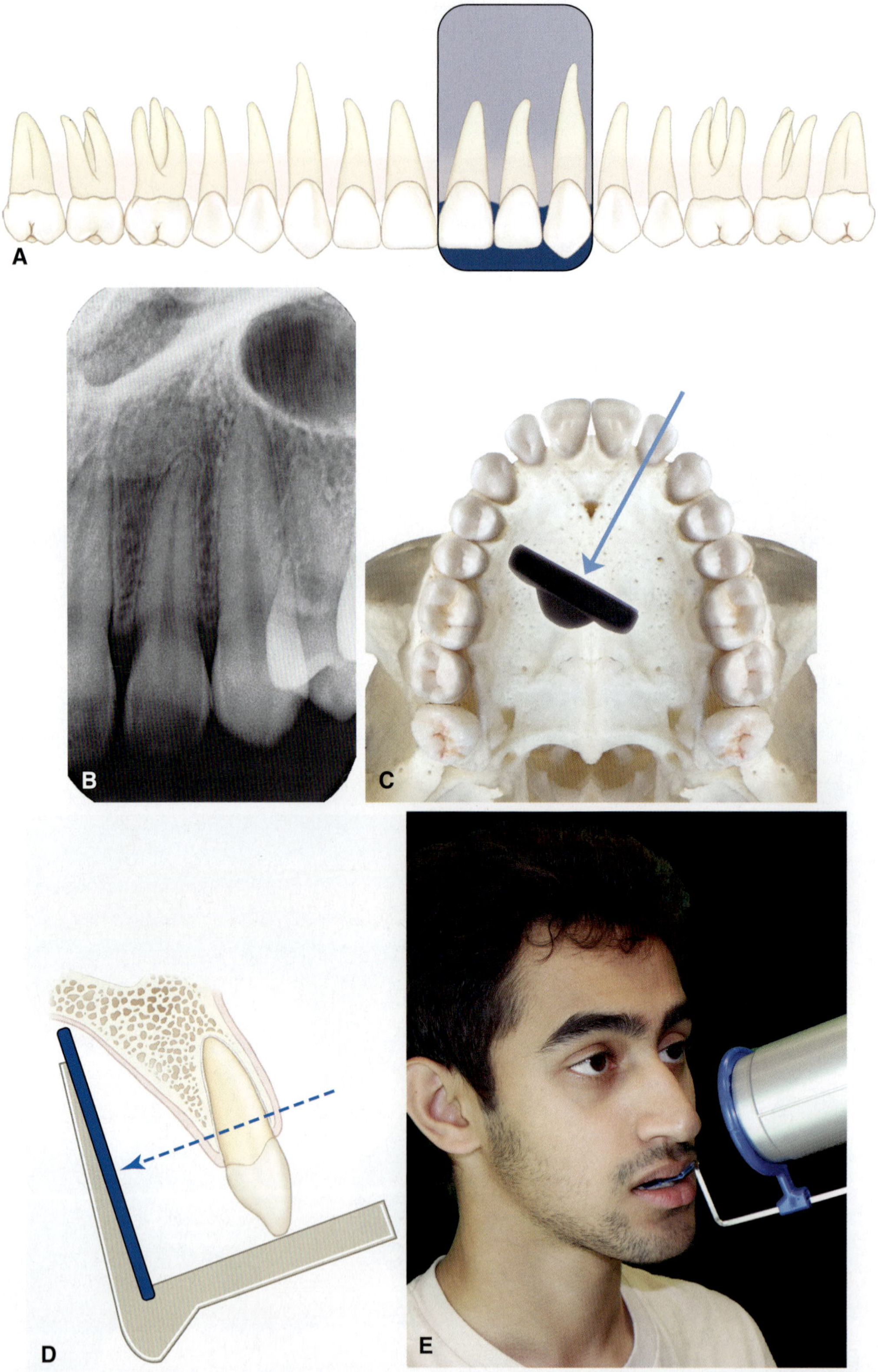

Fig. 6.10 Maxillary lateral incisor periapical projection. (A) The *shaded* area outlines the image field. (B) Periapical radiograph of the maxillary lateral incisor. (C) Position of the receptor in the oral cavity and direction of the x-ray beam (*blue arrow*). (D) Graphic representation of the image receptor and the x-ray beam relative to the long axis of the lateral incisor. (E) Position of the patient with the receptor holder in place and the aiming ring aligned for exposure.

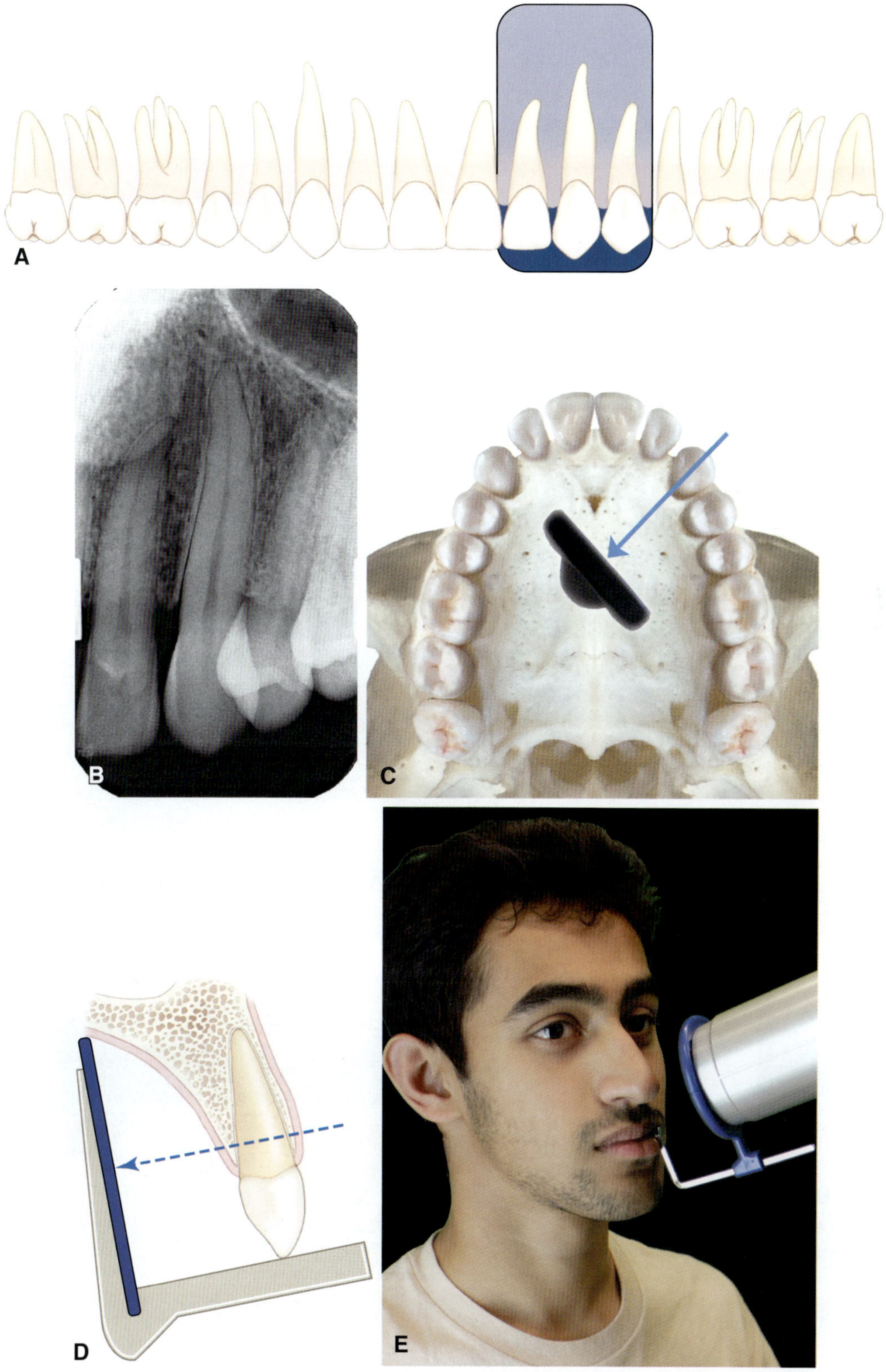

Fig. 6.11 Maxillary canine periapical projection. (A) The *shaded* area outlines the image field. (B) Periapical radiograph of the maxillary canine. (C) Position of the receptor in the oral cavity and direction of the x-ray beam (*blue arrow*). (D) Graphic representation of the image receptor and the x-ray beam relative to the long axis of the lateral incisor. (E) Position of the patient with the receptor holder in place and the aiming ring aligned for exposure.

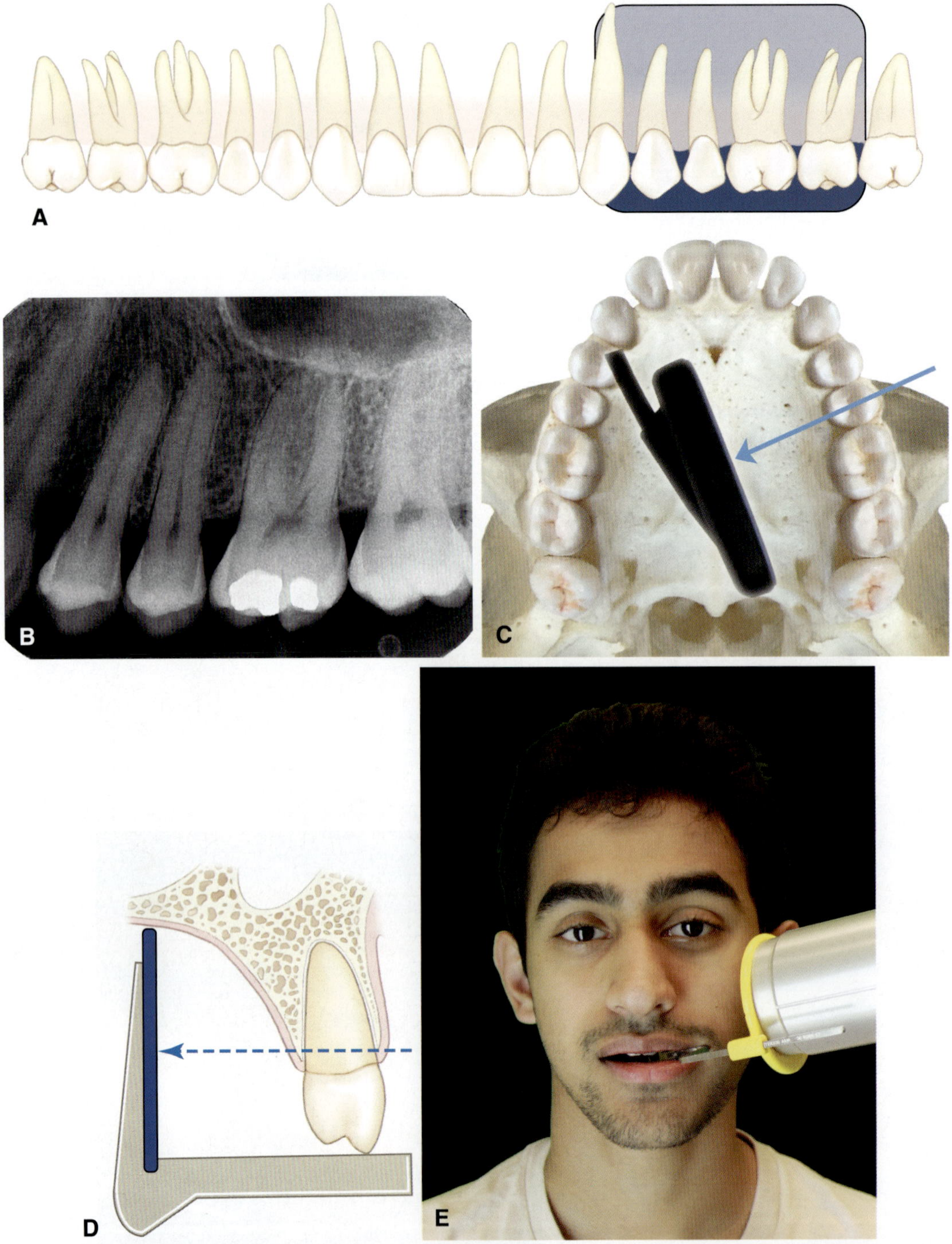

Fig. 6.12 Maxillary premolar periapical projection. (A) The *shaded* area outlines the image field. (B) Periapical radiograph of the maxillary premolar region. (C) Position of the receptor in the oral cavity and direction of the x-ray beam (*blue arrow*). (D) Graphic representation of the image receptor and the x-ray beam relative to the long axis of the premolar. (E) Position of the patient with the receptor holder in place and the aiming ring aligned for exposure.

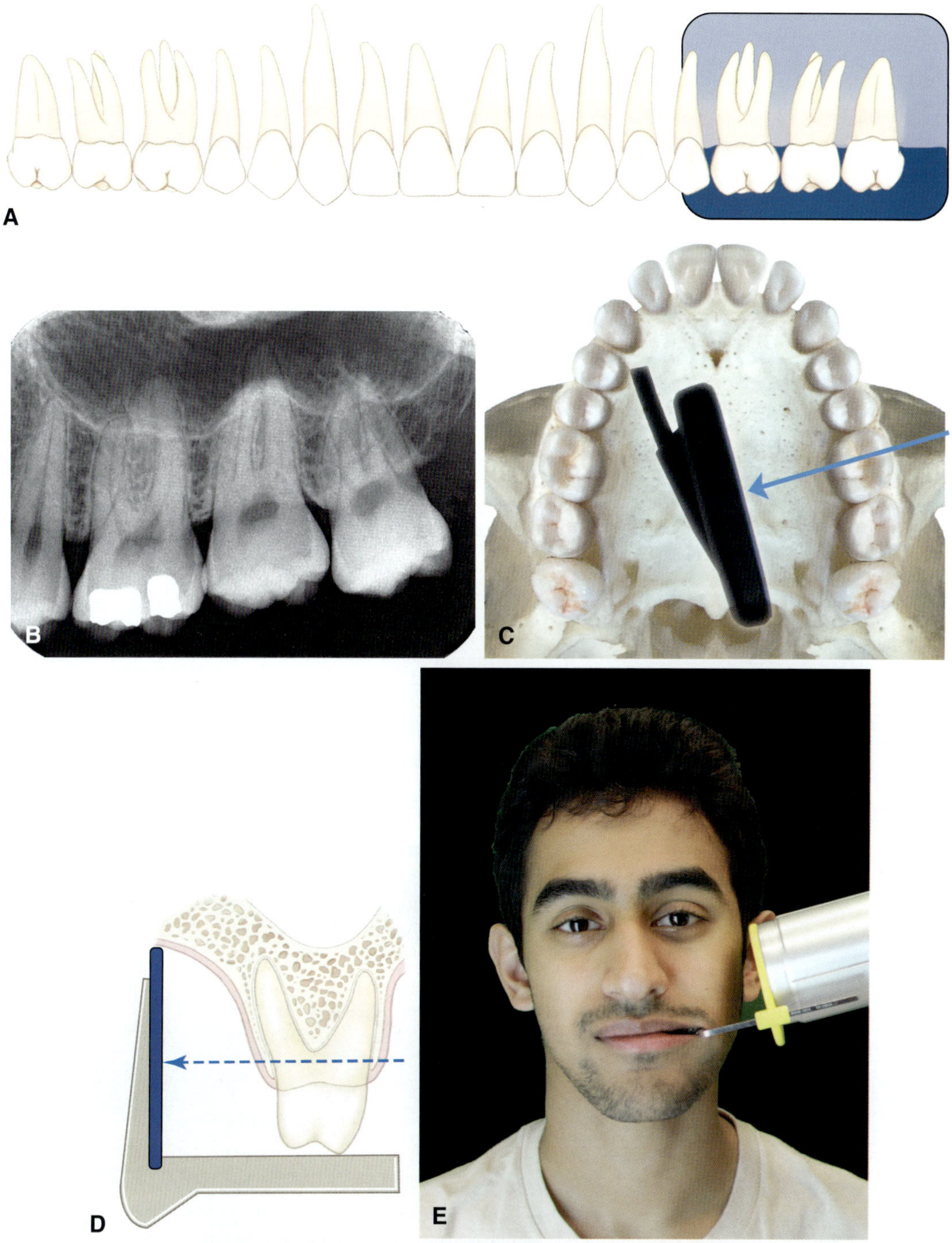

Fig. 6.13 Maxillary molar periapical projection. (A) The *shaded* area outlines the image field. (B) Periapical radiograph of the maxillary molar region. (C) Position of the receptor in the oral cavity and direction of the x-ray beam (*blue arrow*). (D) Graphic representation of the image receptor and the x-ray beam relative to the long axis of the molar. (E) Position of the patient with the receptor holder in place and the aiming ring aligned for exposure.

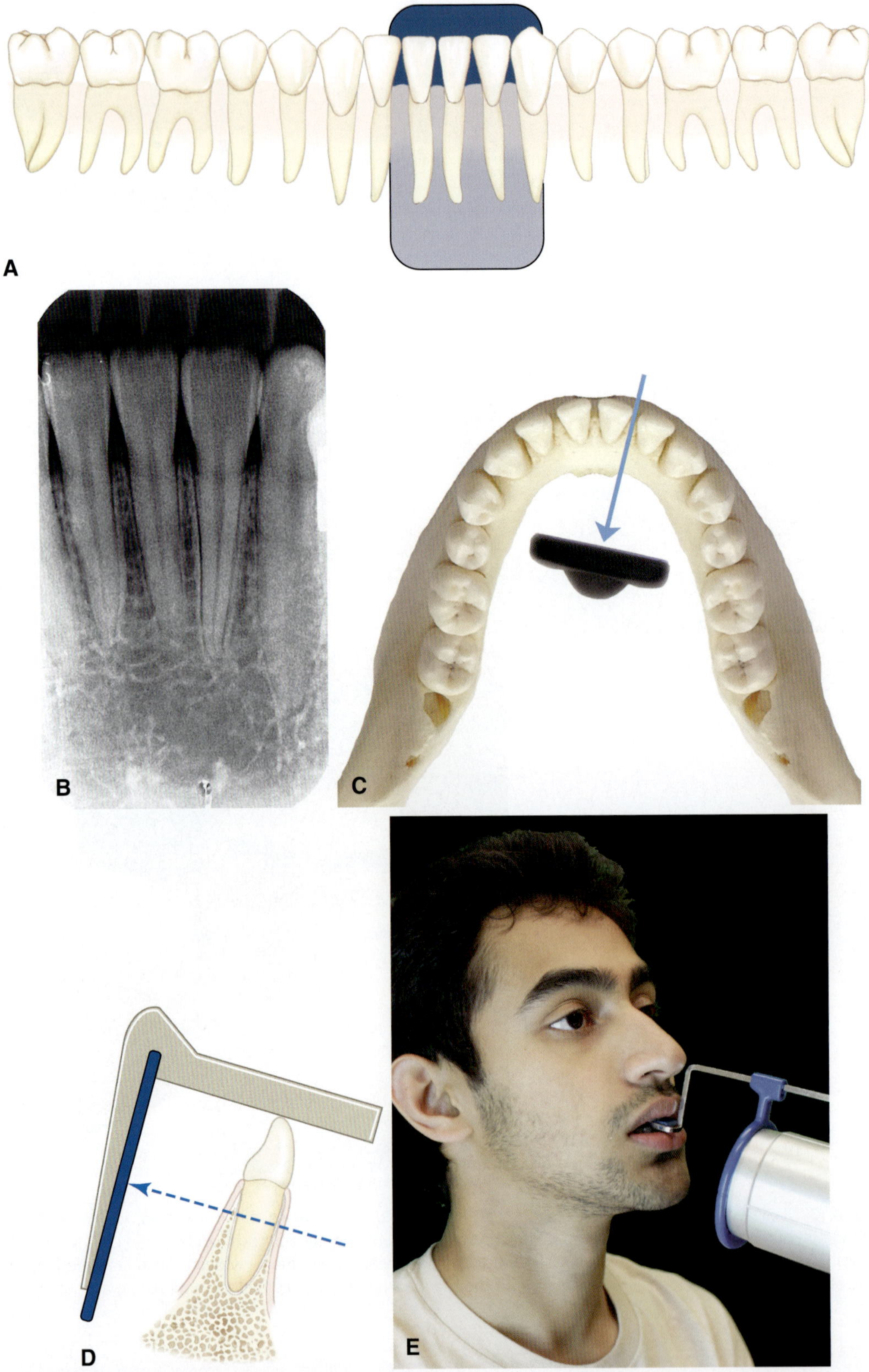

Fig. 6.14 Mandibular centrolateral incisor periapical projection. (A) The *shaded* area outlines the image field. (B) Periapical radiograph of the mandibular central and lateral incisors. (C) Position of the receptor in the oral cavity and direction of the x-ray beam (*blue arrow*). (D) Graphic representation of the image receptor and the x-ray beam relative to the long axis of the mandibular incisor. (E) Position of the patient with the receptor holder in place and the aiming ring aligned for exposure.

PARALLELING TECHNIQUE

Mandibular Canine Projection (Fig. 6.15)

Image field: This image should show the entire mandibular canine and its periapical area (see Fig. 6.15A and B). Open its mesial contact area. The distal contact is included on other projections.

Receptor placement: Place a No. 1 receptor packet in the mouth with its long dimension vertical and the canine in the midline of the receptor. Position it as far lingual as the tongue and contralateral alveolar process permit (see Fig. 6.15C), with its long axis parallel and in line with the canine (see Fig. 6.15D). The instrument must be tipped with the bite block on the canine before the patient is asked to close.

Projection of central ray: Direct the central ray through the mesial contact of the canine without regard to the distal contact (see Fig. 6.15C).

Point of entry: The point of entry is nearly perpendicular to the ala of the nose, over the position of the canine, and about 3 cm above the inferior border of the mandible (Fig. 6.15E).

PARALLELING TECHNIQUE

Mandibular Premolar Projection (Fig. 6.16)

Image field: The radiograph of this area should show the distal half of the canine, the two premolars, and the first molar (see Fig. 6.16A and B).

Receptor placement: Bring the No. 2 receptor into the mouth with its plane nearly horizontal. Rotate the lead edge to the floor of the mouth between the tongue and the teeth with the anterior border near the midline of the canine. Place the receptor away from the teeth to position it in the deeper portion of the mouth (see Fig. 6.16C). Placing the receptor toward the midline also provides more room for the anterior border of the receptor in the curvature of the jaw as it sweeps anteriorly. Prevent the anterior border from contacting the very sensitive attached gingiva on the lingual surface of the mandible.

Projection of central ray: Position the receptor-holding instrument to project the central ray through the second premolar molar area. The vertical angulation should be small, nearly parallel with the occlusal plane, to keep the receptor as nearly parallel with the long axis of the teeth as possible (see Fig. 6.16D). Adjust the horizontal angulation and the placement of the receptor-holding device to direct the beam through the premolar contact points (see Fig. 6.16C).

Point of entry: The point of entry of the central ray is below the pupil of the eye and about 3 cm above the inferior border of the mandible (see Fig. 6.16E).

PARALLELING TECHNIQUE

Mandibular Molar Projection (Fig. 6.17)

Image field: The radiograph of this region should include the distal half of the second premolar and the three mandibular permanent molars (see Fig. 6.17A and B). In the case of an impacted third molar or a pathologic condition distal to the third molar, a distal oblique molar projection or even additional extraoral projections (panoramic or lateral ramus) may be required to demonstrate the area adequately. If the molar area is edentulous, place the receptor far enough posterior to include the retromolar area in the examination.

Receptor placement: Place the No. 2 receptor in the mouth with its plane nearly horizontal. Rotate the inferior edge downward beneath the lateral border of the tongue, displacing it medially. The anterior edge of the receptor should be at about the middle of the second premolar (see Fig. 6.17C). In most cases, the tongue forces the receptor near the alveolar process and molars aligning it parallel with the long axis of the teeth and the line of occlusion.

Projection of central ray: Proper placement of the holding instrument directs the central ray through the second molar. Adjust the horizontal angulation to project the beam through the contact areas (see Fig. 6.17C). Because of the slight lingual inclination of the molars, the central ray may have some slight positive angulation (approximately 8 degrees; see Fig. 6.17E).

Point of entry: Direct the point of entry of the central ray below the outer canthus of the eye about 3 cm above the inferior border of the mandible (see Fig. 6.17E).

BITEWING RADIOGRAPHY

Bitewing (also called *interproximal*) radiographs include the crowns of the maxillary and mandibular teeth and the alveolar crest on the same receptor. The long axis of bitewing receptors usually is oriented horizontally but may be oriented vertically. The beam is directed through the interproximal spaces and parallel with the occlusal plane. The receptor is placed parallel to the buccal and lingual surfaces of the teeth being examined and is perpendicular to the x-ray beam.

The diagnostic objectives of bitewing radiographs are listed in Box 6.3.

Receptor-Holding Instruments

Receptor holders are used to position and stabilize the receptor adjacent to the teeth being examined. The bitewing instruments have a bite plate and an external guide ring to aid positioning the tube head (Fig. 6.18). The bite block facilitates positioning of the receptor parallel to the facial surfaces of the teeth being radiographed. Separate bite plates are used for film and storage phosphors, and solid-state digital sensors. The external guide ring helps to align the beam, reduce overlap between proximal surfaces, and reduces the possibility of partially exposing the receptor.

A receptor fitted with a bitewing tab or loop may be used instead of a holding device. These disposable tabs are made of stiff cardboard or plastic, and available for film, storage phosphor plates, and digital sensors (Fig. 6.19).

Positioning of the Patient

The patient should be seated upright in the dental chair with the sagittal plane vertical and the occlusal plane horizontal. When receptor holders with external guiding rings are used, the patient's head position is less important. However, when bitewing tabs are used, external guidance to position the x-ray cone is not available; thus standardization of the patient's head position is important.

Receptor Placement

Horizontal bitewing projections. Typically, bitewing radiographs are made with the receptor in a horizontal orientation. Separate views are made for the premolar and molar regions. The receptor is placed in the lingual vestibule adjacent to the teeth to be radiographed, and the receptor bite block or tab is rested onto the mandibular occlusal surface. The receptor is adjusted to be parallel to the buccal surfaces of the teeth being radiographed. The edge of the receptor holders or the tab can be used to assist in this parallel orientation. Once the receptor is positioned, the patient is asked to gently occlude onto the bite block. When using the cardboard bitewing tabs, it is important to direct the patient to close gently to ensure sufficient separation of the maxillary and mandibular teeth.

Two posterior bitewing views, a premolar and a molar, are recommended for each quadrant. However, for children 12 years of age or younger, one bitewing receptor (No. 2) usually suffices. The premolar projection should include the distal half of the canines and the crowns of the premolars. Because the mandibular canines usually are more mesial than the maxillary canines, the mandibular canine is used as the guide for placement of the premolar bitewing receptor. The molar bitewing receptor is placed 1 or 2 mm beyond the most distally erupted molar (maxillary or mandibular). The anterior edge of the receptor is used to guide the position to encompass the appropriate interproximal contacts. When using film or storage phosphor plates, the imaging area of the film or plate is approximately 2 mm from the edge of the packet. When using solid-state sensors, there is approximately 2 to 4 mm of dead space between the edge of the plastic casing and the image capture chip; this varies with manufacturer. One manufacturer, XDR Radiology, has a patented technology that provides less dead space toward mesial imaging end, and this facilitates imaging of the canine/premolar contact.

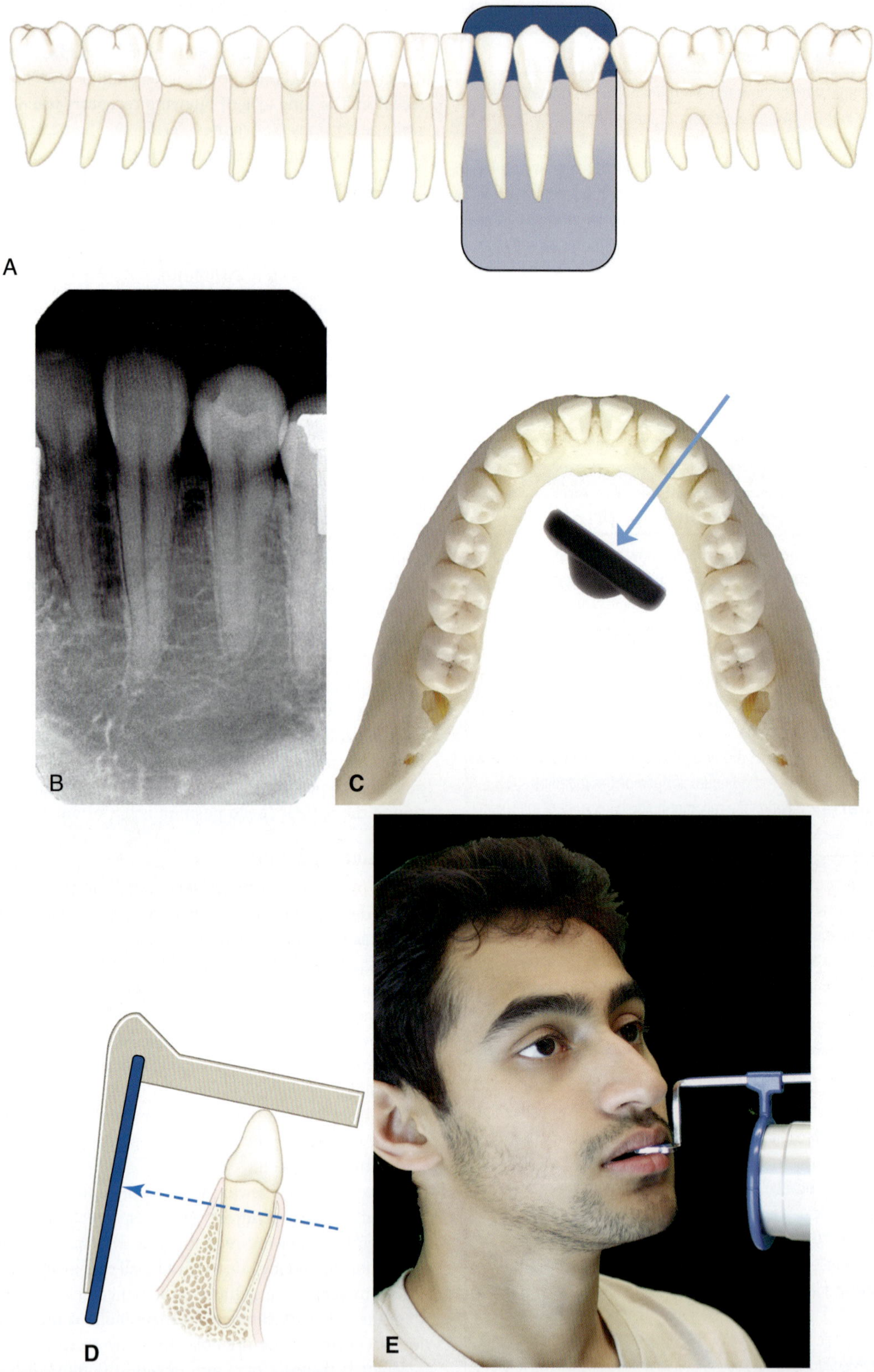

Fig. 6.15 Mandibular canine periapical projection. (A) The *shaded* area outlines the image field. (B) Periapical radiograph of the mandibular canine. (C) Position of the receptor in the oral cavity and direction of the x-ray beam (*blue arrow*). (D) Graphic representation of the image receptor and the x-ray beam relative to the long axis of the mandibular canine. (E) Position of the patient with the receptor holder in place and the aiming ring aligned for exposure.

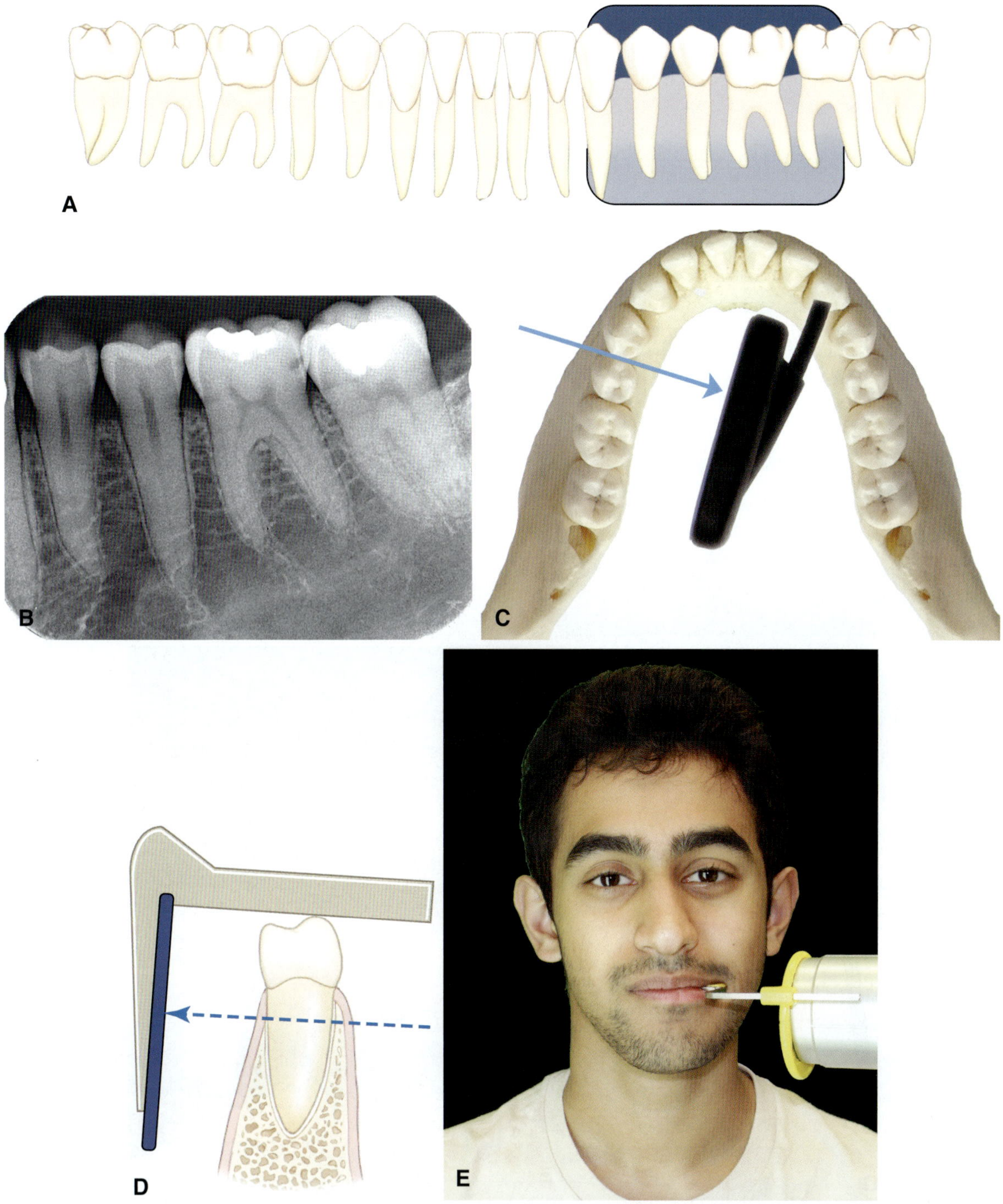

Fig. 6.16 Mandibular premolar periapical projection. (A) The *shaded* area outlines the image field. (B) Periapical radiograph of the mandibular premolar region. (C) Position of the receptor in the oral cavity and direction of the x-ray beam (*blue arrow*). (D) Graphic representation of the image receptor and the x-ray beam relative to the long axis of the mandibular premolar. (E) Position of the patient with the receptor holder in place and the aiming ring aligned for exposure.

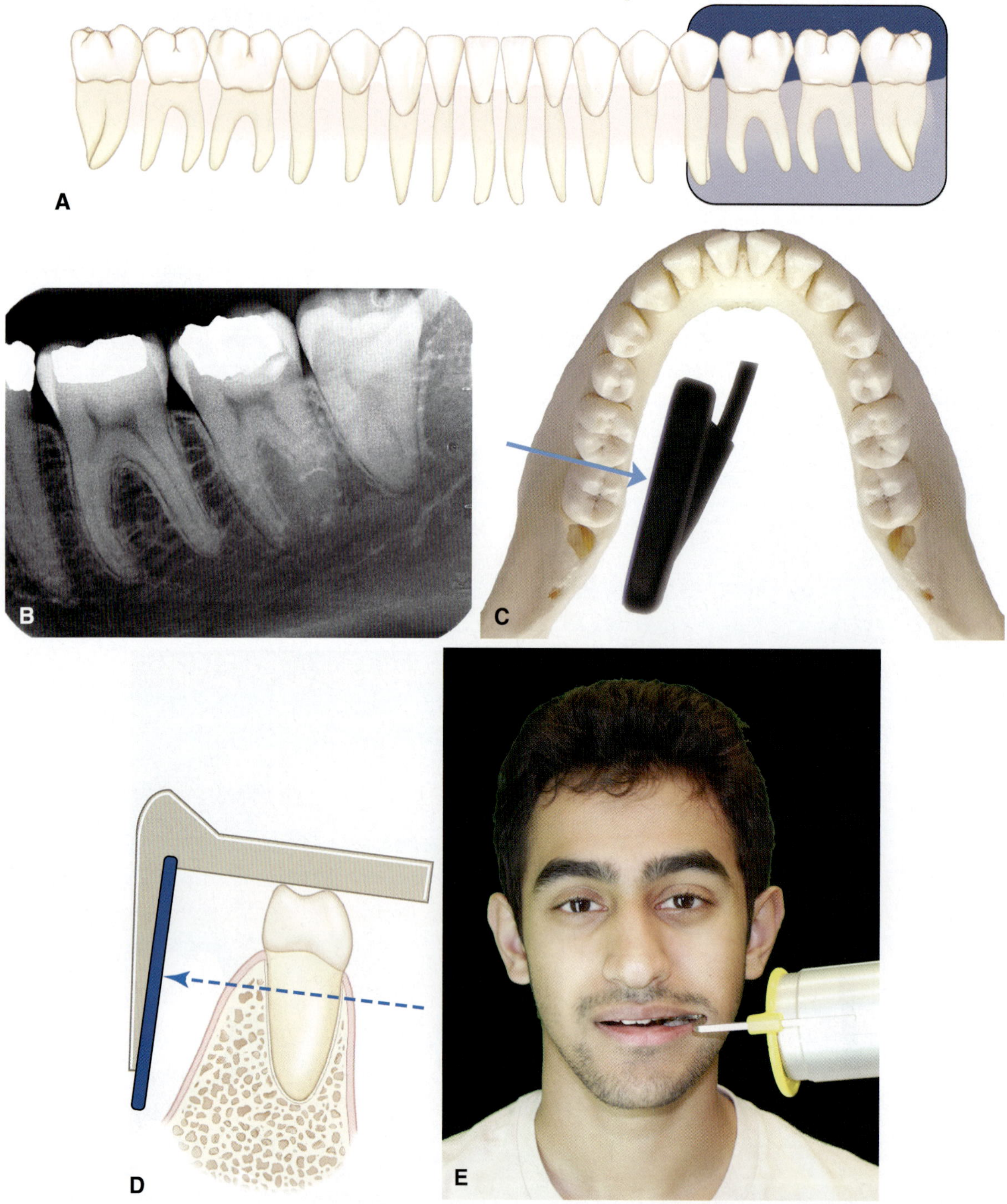

Fig. 6.17 Mandibular molar periapical projection. (A) The *shaded* area outlines the image field. (B) Periapical radiograph of the mandibular molar region. (C) Position of the receptor in the oral cavity and direction of the x-ray beam (*blue arrow*). (D) Graphic representation of the image receptor and the x-ray beam relative to the long axis of the mandibular molar. (E) Position of the patient with the receptor holder in place and the aiming ring aligned for exposure.

BOX 6.3 Diagnostic Objectives of Bitewing Radiography

- Detect early interproximal caries before it becomes clinically apparent
- Detect secondary caries below restorations
- Assess loss of the interdental and furcation bone

Vertical bitewing projections. Vertical bitewing projections are used when the patient has moderate to severe alveolar bone loss. Orienting the length of the receptor vertically increases the likelihood that the residual alveolar crests in the maxilla and the mandible will be recorded on the radiograph (Fig. 6.20). The principles for positioning the receptor and orienting the x-ray beam are otherwise the same as for horizontal bitewing projections. Bite blocks specifically designed for vertical orientation of the sensor are available.

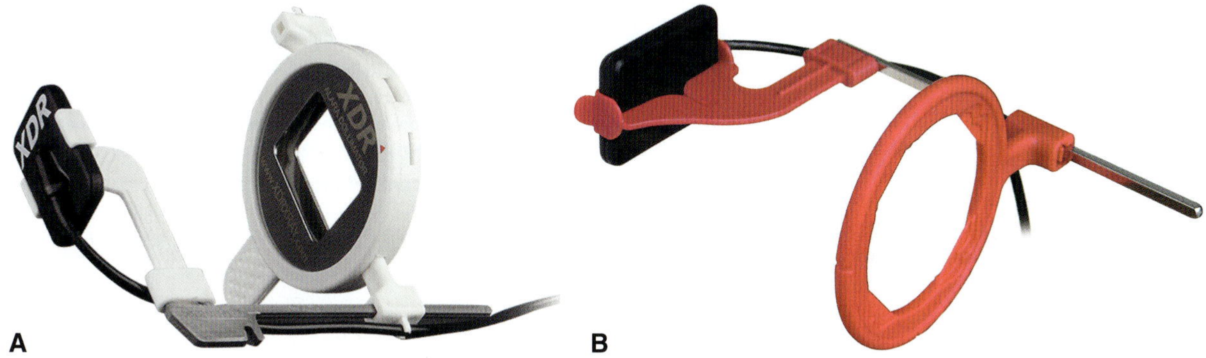

Fig. 6.18 Receptor-holding devices for bitewing radiography. (A) A wired sensor is held in position with a bite block. The aiming ring guides beam alignment and incorporates rectangular collimation to minimize patient radiation dose. (B) XCP Bitewing Holder, with external localizing ring to guide position of the aiming tube of the x-ray machine to ensure that the entire receptor is in the x-ray beam. Disposable barriers have been removed to show the detector and wire. (A, Courtesy XDR Radiology, Los Angeles, CA. B, Courtesy Dentsply Rinn, Elgin, IL.)

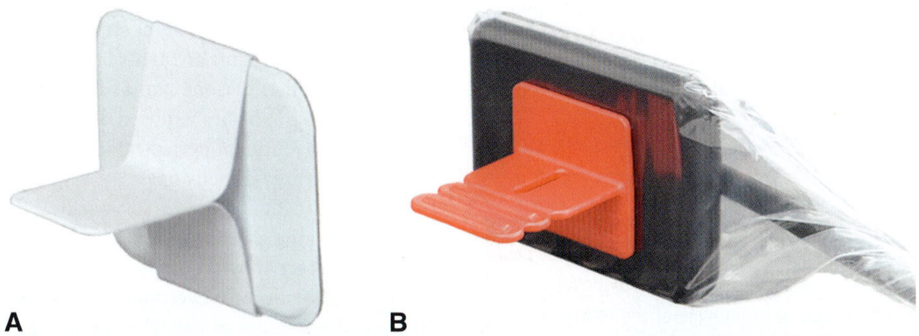

Fig. 6.19 Disposable bitewing tabs showing the tab that the patient bites on to support the receptor during exposure. (A) Cardboard loop for film and storage phosphor plates. (B) Plastic adhesive tab for use with solid-state sensors. Image shows use with the infection-control sleeve over the sensor and wire. (Courtesy Dentsply Rinn, Elgin, IL.)

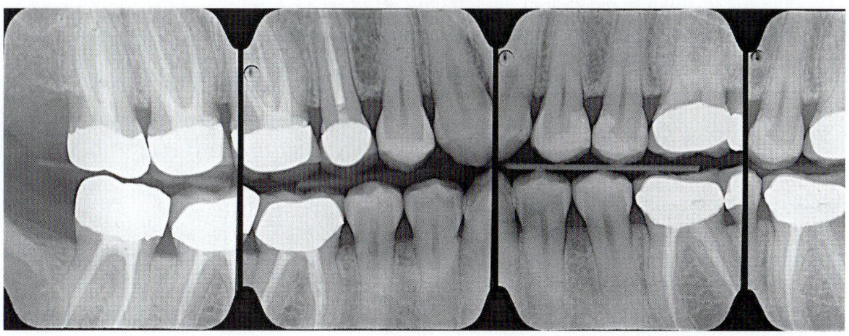

Fig. 6.20 Set of vertical bitewing views. Orienting the length of the receptor vertically increases the likelihood that the residual alveolar crests in the maxilla and the mandible will be recorded on the radiograph even in patients with extensive alveolar bone loss.

Angulation of the Tube Head

Horizontal angulation. To effectively image the interproximal tooth surface without superimposition, the x-ray beam is directed through the contacts. Some difference may exist in the curvature of the mandibular and maxillary arches. However, when the x-ray beam is accurately directed through the mandibular premolar contacts, overlapping is minimal or absent in the maxillary premolar segment. A few degrees of tolerance are available in the horizontal angulation before overlapping becomes critical. Typically less than one-third of the proximal enamel thickness should be overlapped. The contact between the maxillary first and second molars often is angled a few degrees more anteriorly than between the mandibular first and second molars.

When using receptor holders that have an external aiming ring, guide the horizontal position of the x-ray cone to the predetermined direction that passes the x-ray beam through the interproximal spaces. When using bitewing tabs, the horizontal orientation is less straightforward and the operator must ensure accurate horizontal orientation of the tube head to direct the beam through the interproximal spaces and encompass the entire surface of the receptor to prevent cone cuts.

Vertical angulation. The aiming cylinder is positioned about +10 degrees to project the beam parallel with the occlusal plane (occlusal dentinoenamel junction). This orientation minimizes overlapping of the opposing cusps onto the occlusal surface and thus improves the probability of detecting early occlusal lesions at the dentinoenamel junction.

Individual Bitewing Projections

Separate bitewing projections are made of the premolars and molars. The following section describes procedural details to make bitewing radiographs. It describes the field encompassed in the image, the placement of the receptor, the projection of the central ray, and the positioning of the aiming ring.

PREMOLAR BITEWING PROJECTION (FIG. 6.21)

Image field: This projection should cover the distal portion of the mandibular canine anteriorly and show equally the crowns of the maxillary and mandibular premolar teeth (see Fig. 6.21A and B).

Receptor placement: Place the receptor between the tongue and the teeth, far enough from the lingual surface of the teeth to prevent interference by the palate on closing. The receptor should be parallel to the long axes of the teeth (see Fig. 6.21C). The anterior border of the receptor should extend beyond the contact area between the mandibular canine and the first premolar (see Fig. 6.21D). Hold the receptor in place until the patient's mouth is completely closed. Holding the receptor while closing prevents it from being displaced distally.

Projection of central ray: Adjust the horizontal angulation of the cone to project the central ray to the center of the receptor through the premolar contact areas (see Fig. 6.21D). To compensate for the slight inclination of the receptor against the palatal mucosa, the vertical angulation should be about +5 degrees. (In the drawing, the mandibular teeth are shown in *dashed* lines.)

Point of entry: Identify the point of entry by retracting the cheek and determining that the central ray will enter the line of occlusion at the point of contact between the second premolar and the first molar (see Fig. 6.21E).

MOLAR BITEWING PROJECTION (FIG. 6.22)

Image field: This projection should show the distal surface of the most posterior erupted molar and equally the crowns of the maxillary and mandibular molars (see Fig. 6.22A and B). Because the maxillary and mandibular molar contact areas may not be open from the same horizontal angulation, they may not be visible on one image. In this case, it may be desirable to open the maxillary molar contacts because the mandibular molar contacts usually are open on the periapical receptors.

Receptor placement: Place the receptor between the tongue and teeth as far lingual as practical to avoid contacting the sensitive attached gingiva (see Fig. 6.22C). The distal margin of the receptor should extend 1–2 mm beyond the most posterior erupted molar (see Fig. 6.22D). When using the XCP, adjust the horizontal angulation by placing the guide bar parallel with the direction of the central ray to open the contact area between the first and second molars.

Projection of central ray: Project the central ray to the center of the receptor and through the contact of the first and second maxillary molars (see Fig. 6.22D). Angle the central ray slightly from the anterior because the molar contacts usually are not oriented at right angles to the buccal surfaces of these teeth. A vertical angulation of +10 degrees is recommended.

Point of entry: The central ray should enter the cheek below the lateral canthus of the eye at the level of the occlusal plane (see Fig. 6.22E).

OCCLUSAL RADIOGRAPHY

An occlusal radiograph displays a relatively large segment of a dental arch. It may include the palate or floor of the mouth and a reasonable extent of the contiguous lateral structures. Occlusal radiographs also are useful when patients are unable to open wide enough for periapical images or for other reasons cannot accept periapical receptors. Because occlusal radiographs are exposed at a steep angulation, they may be used with conventional periapical images to determine the location of objects in all three dimensions.

The diagnostic objectives of occlusal radiographs are listed in Box 6.4. With the growth of CBCT in dentistry, many of these diagnostic objectives are now accomplished with CBCT imaging rather than occlusal radiography. Nevertheless, occlusal radiographs continue to be used where access to CBCT imaging may be limited.

To make an occlusal radiograph, a large receptor (7.7 cm × 5.8 cm [3 inches × 2.3 inches]) is inserted between the occlusal surfaces of the teeth. Occlusal receptors are made of film or storage phosphor plates. CCD or CMOS sensors of this size are not manufactured. As its name implies, the receptor lies in the plane of occlusion. The "tube" side of this receptor is positioned toward the jaw to be examined, and the x-ray beam is directed through the jaw to the receptor. Because of its size, the receptor allows examination of relatively large portions of the jaw. Standardized projections are used, which stipulate a desired relationship between the central ray, receptor, and region being examined. However, the clinician should feel free to modify these relationships to meet a specific clinical requirement.

Individual Occlusal Projections

The following section describes procedural details to make specific occlusal radiographic projections. It describes the field encompassed in the image, the placement of the receptor, the projection of the central ray, and the positioning of the aiming ring.

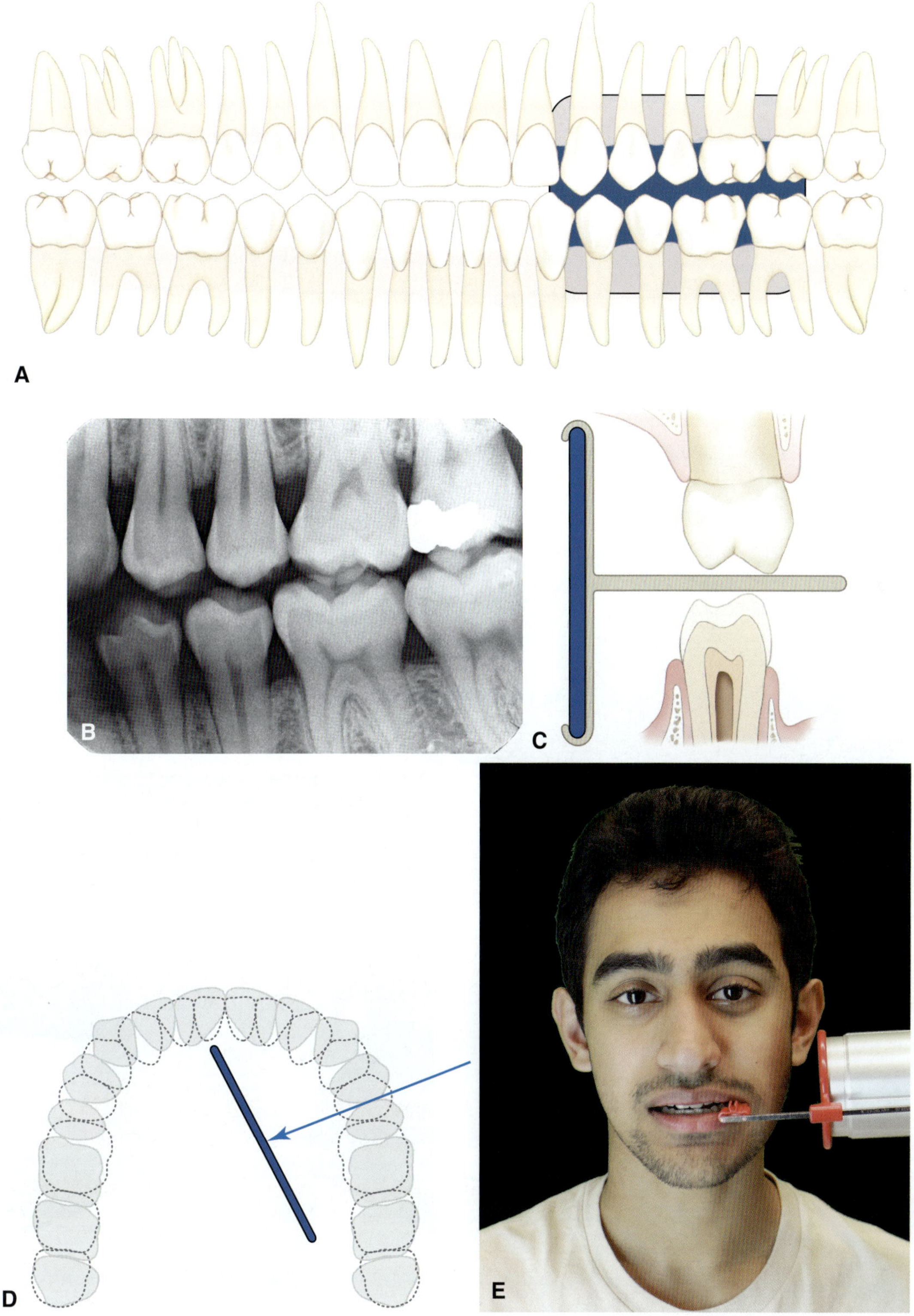

Fig. 6.21 Premolar bitewing projection. (A) The *shaded* area outlines the image field. (B) Bitewing radiograph of the premolar region. (C and D) Graphic representations of the image receptor and the x-ray beam relative to the crowns of the maxillary and mandibular premolar. (E) Position of the patient with the receptor holder in place and the aiming ring aligned for exposure.

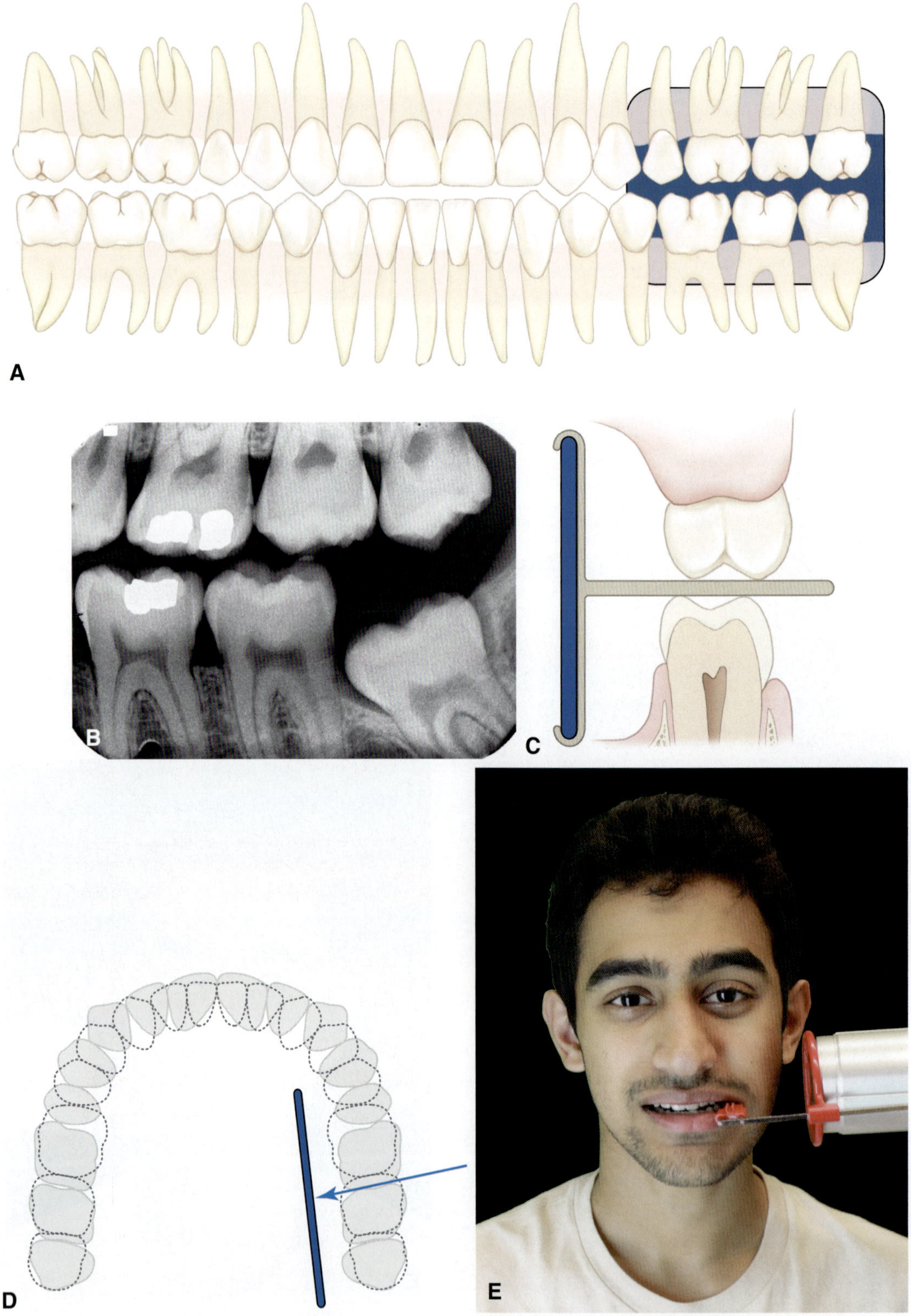

Fig. 6.22 Molar bitewing projection. (A) The *shaded* area outlines the image field. (B) Bitewing radiograph of the molar region. (C and D) Graphic representations of the image receptor and the x-ray beam relative to the crowns of the maxillary and mandibular molar. (E) Position of the patient with the receptor holder in place and the aiming ring aligned for exposure.

BOX 6.4 Diagnostic Objectives of Occlusal Radiography

- To locate supernumerary, unerupted, and impacted teeth
- To localize foreign bodies in the jaws and floor of the mouth
- To identify and determine the full extent of disease (e.g., cysts, osteomyelitis, malignancies) in the jaws, palate, and floor of the mouth
- To evaluate and monitor changes in the midpalatal suture during orthodontic palatal expansion. To detect and locate sialoliths in the ducts of sublingual and submandibular glands
- To evaluate the integrity of the anterior, medial, and lateral outlines of the maxillary sinus
- To aid in the examination of patients with trismus, who can open their mouths only a few millimeters; this condition precludes intraoral radiography, which may be impossible or at least extremely painful for the patient
- To obtain information about the location, nature, extent, and displacement of fractures of the mandible and maxilla

ANTERIOR MAXILLARY OCCLUSAL PROJECTION (FIG. 6.23)

Image field: The primary field of this projection includes the anterior maxilla and its dentition and the anterior floor of the nasal fossa and teeth from canine to canine (see Fig. 6.23A and B).

Receptor placement: Adjust the patient's head so that the sagittal plane is perpendicular and the occlusal plane horizontal to the floor (see Fig. 6.23C). Place the receptor in the mouth with the exposure side toward the maxilla, the posterior border touching the rami, and the long dimension of the receptor perpendicular to the sagittal plane. The patient stabilizes the receptor by gently closing the mouth.

Projection of central ray: Orient the central ray through the tip of the nose toward the middle of the receptor with approximately +45 degrees vertical angulation and 0 degree horizontal angulation (see Fig. 6.23C).

Point of entry: The central ray enters the patient's face approximately through the tip of the nose (see Fig. 6.23C).

TOPOGRAPHIC MAXILLARY OCCLUSAL PROJECTION (FIG. 6.24)

Image field: This projection shows the palate, zygomatic processes of the maxilla, anteroinferior aspects of each antrum, nasolacrimal canals, teeth from second molar to second molar, and nasal septum (see Fig. 6.24A and B).

Receptor placement: Seat the patient upright with the sagittal plane perpendicular to the floor and the occlusal plane horizontal. Place the receptor, with its long dimension perpendicular to the sagittal plane, crosswise in the mouth. Gently push the receptor in backward until it contacts the anterior border of the mandibular rami. The patient stabilizes the receptor by gently closing the mouth (see Fig. 6.24C).

Projection of central ray: Direct the central ray at a vertical angulation of +65 degrees and a horizontal angulation of 0 degree to the bridge of the nose just below the nasion, toward the middle of the receptor (see Fig. 6.24C).

Point of entry: Generally, the central ray enters the patient's face through the bridge of the nose (see Fig. 6.24C).

LATERAL MAXILLARY OCCLUSAL PROJECTION (FIG. 6.25)

Image field: This projection shows a quadrant of the alveolar ridge of the maxilla, inferolateral aspect of the antrum, tuberosity, and teeth from the lateral incisor to the contralateral third molar (see Fig. 6.25A and B). In addition, the zygomatic process of the maxilla superimposes over the roots of the molar teeth.

Receptor placement: Place the receptor with its long axis parallel to the sagittal plane and on the side of interest, with the tube side toward the side of the maxilla in question. Push the receptor posteriorly until it touches the ramus. Position the lateral border parallel with the buccal surfaces of the posterior teeth, extending laterally approximately 1 cm past the buccal cusps. Ask the patient to close gently to hold the receptor in position (see Fig. 6.25C).

Projection of central ray: Orient the central ray with a vertical angulation of +60 degrees, to a point 2 cm below the lateral canthus of the eye, directed toward the center of the receptor (see Fig. 6.25C).

Point of entry: The central ray enters at a point approximately 2 cm below the lateral canthus of the eye (see Fig. 6.25C).

ANTERIOR MANDIBULAR OCCLUSAL PROJECTION (FIG. 6.26)

Image field: This projection includes the anterior portion of the mandible, the dentition from canine to canine, and the inferior cortical border of the mandible (see Fig. 6.26A and B).

Receptor placement: Seat the patient tilted back so that the occlusal plane is 45 degrees above horizontal. Place the receptor in the mouth with the long axis perpendicular to the sagittal plane and push it posteriorly until it touches the rami. Center the receptor with the exposure side down and ask the patient to bite lightly to hold the receptor in position (see Fig. 6.26C).

Projection of central ray: Orient the central ray with −10 degrees angulation through the point of the chin toward the middle of the receptor; this gives the ray −55 degrees of angulation to the plane of the receptor (see Fig. 6.26C).

Point of entry: The point of entry of the central ray is in the midline and through the tip of the chin (see Fig. 6.26C).

TOPOGRAPHIC MANDIBULAR OCCLUSAL PROJECTION (FIG. 6.27)

Image field: This projection includes the soft tissue of the floor of the mouth and reveals the lingual and buccal plates of the mandible from second molar to second molar (see Fig. 6.27A and B). When this view is made to examine the floor of the mouth (e.g., for sialoliths), the exposure time should be reduced to half the time used to create an image of the mandible.

Receptor placement: Seat the patient in a semireclining position with the head tilted back so that the ala-tragus line is almost perpendicular to the floor. Place the receptor in the mouth with its long axis perpendicular to the sagittal plane and with the tube side toward the mandible. The anterior border of the receptor should be approximately 1 cm beyond the mandibular central incisors. Ask the patient to bite gently on the receptor to hold it in position (see Fig. 6.27C).

Projection of central ray: Direct the central ray at the midline through the floor of the mouth approximately 3 cm below the chin, at right angles to the center of the receptor (see Fig. 6.27C).

Point of entry: The point of entry of the central ray is in the midline through the floor of the mouth approximately 3 cm below the chin (see Fig. 6.27C).

LATERAL MANDIBULAR OCCLUSAL PROJECTION (FIG. 6.28)

Image field: This projection covers the soft tissue of half the floor of the mouth, the buccal and lingual cortical plates of half of the mandible, and the teeth from the lateral incisor to the contralateral third molar (see Fig. 6.28A and B). When this view is used to provide an image of the floor of the mouth, the exposure time should be reduced to half that used to provide an image of the mandible.

Receptor placement: Seat the patient in a semireclining position with the head tilted back so that the ala-tragus line is almost perpendicular to the floor (see Fig. 6.28C). Place the receptor in the mouth with its long axis initially parallel with the sagittal plane and with the exposure side down toward the mandible. Place the receptor as far posterior as possible, then shift the long axis buccally (right or left) so that the lateral border of the receptor is parallel with the buccal surfaces of the posterior teeth and extends laterally approximately 1 cm.

Projection of central ray: Direct the central ray perpendicular to the center of the receptor through a point beneath the chin, approximately 3 cm posterior to the point of the chin and 3 cm lateral to the midline (see Fig. 6.28C).

Point of entry: The point of entry of the central ray is beneath the chin, approximately 3 cm posterior to the chin and approximately 3 cm lateral to the midline (see Fig. 6.28C).

IMAGING OF CHILDREN

Radiation protection is especially important for children because of their greater sensitivity to irradiation. The best way to reduce unnecessary exposure is for the dentist to make the minimal number of radiographs required for the individual patient. These judgments are based on a careful clinical examination and consideration of the patient's age, medical history, growth considerations, and general oral health as well as whether caries is present and the time elapsed since previous examinations (see Chapter 15). Bitewing examinations for caries assessment are not required when the contacts are open and the proximal surfaces can be visually examined. The frequency should be determined partly by the patient's caries rate. A periapical survey is often recommended for children early in the mixed dentition stage. Special attention should be paid to procedures that reduce exposure (see Chapter 3), including use of fast receptor, proper processing, and beam-limiting devices.

Radiography in a child can be a challenging experience. Although the principles of periapical radiography for children are the same as for adults, in practice children present special considerations because of their small anatomic structures and possible behavioral problems. The smaller size of the arches and dentition requires the use of smaller periapical receptors. The relatively shallow palate and floor of the mouth may require further modification of receptor placement. Special radiographic examinations using an occlusal receptor for extraoral projections have been suggested.

Patient Management

Children are often apprehensive about the radiographic examination, much as they are about many other types of dental procedures. The radiographic examination usually is the first manipulative procedure performed on a young patient. If this examination is nonthreatening and comfortable, subsequent dental experiences are usually accepted with little or no apprehension. Such apprehension is best allayed by familiarizing the child with the procedure, which is done by explaining it in a manner that he or she can comprehend. It often is wise to

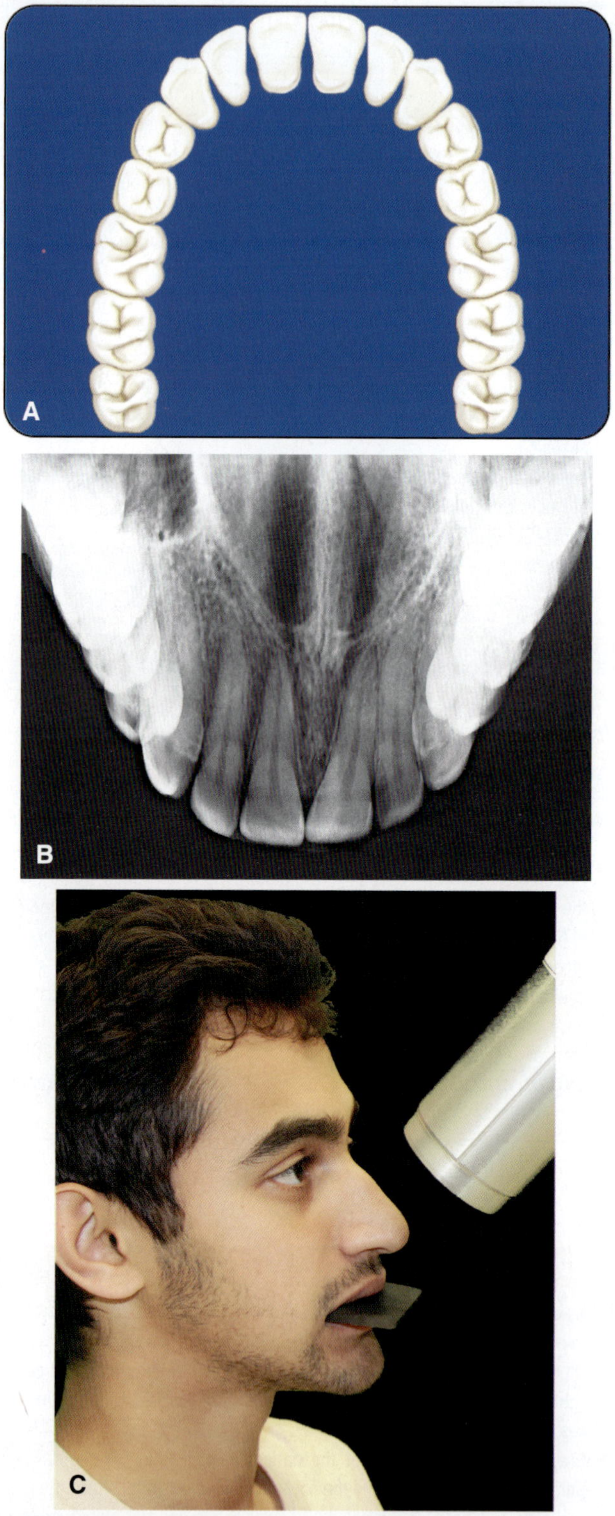

Fig. 6.23 Anterior maxillary occlusal projection. (A) The *shaded* area outlines the image field. (B) Anterior maxillary occlusal radiograph. (C) Position of the patient with the receptor in place and the aiming ring aligned for exposure.

describe the x-ray machine as a "camera used to take pictures of teeth." The child can become more comfortable with the receptor and x-ray machine by touching them before the examination. The operator should carry on a conversation with the child as a distraction and to gain their confidence. It may be advantageous for the child to watch an

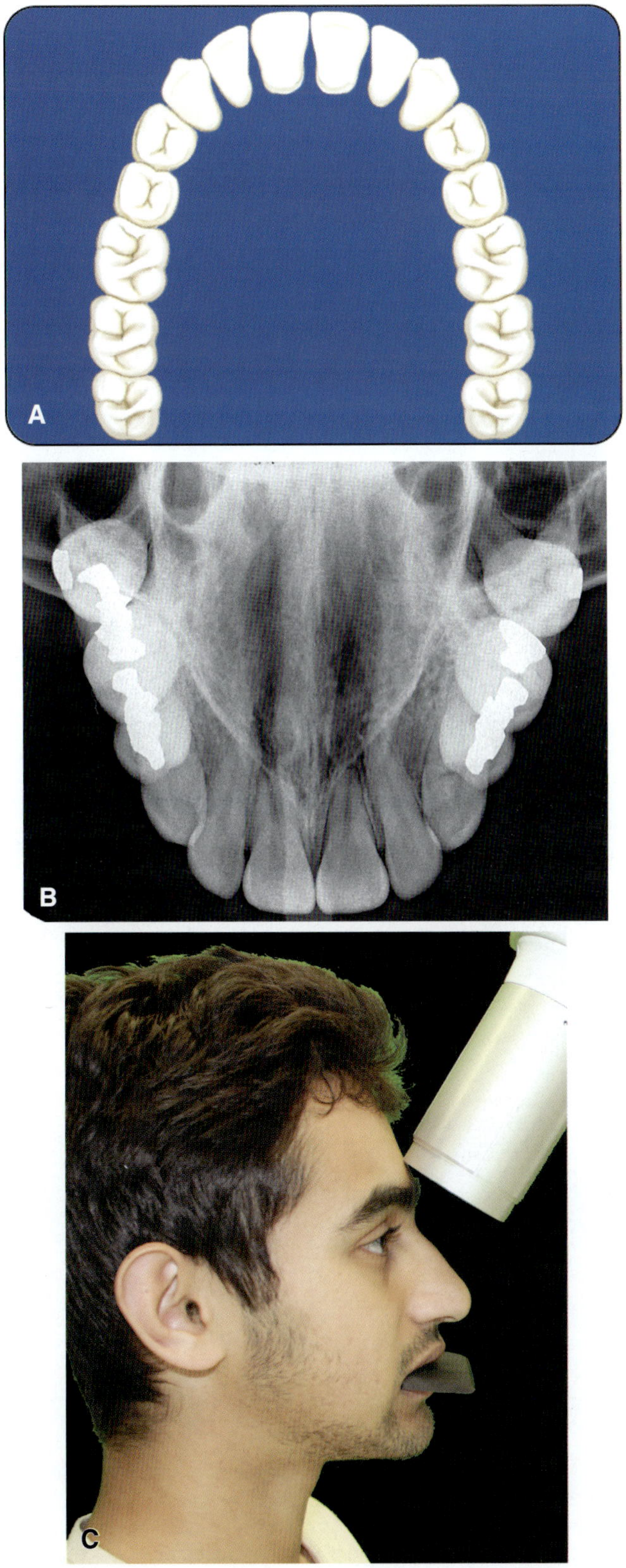

Fig. 6.24 Topographic maxillary occlusal projection. (A) The *shaded* area outlines the image field. (B) Topographic maxillary occlusal radiograph. (C) Position of the patient with the receptor in place and the aiming ring aligned for exposure.

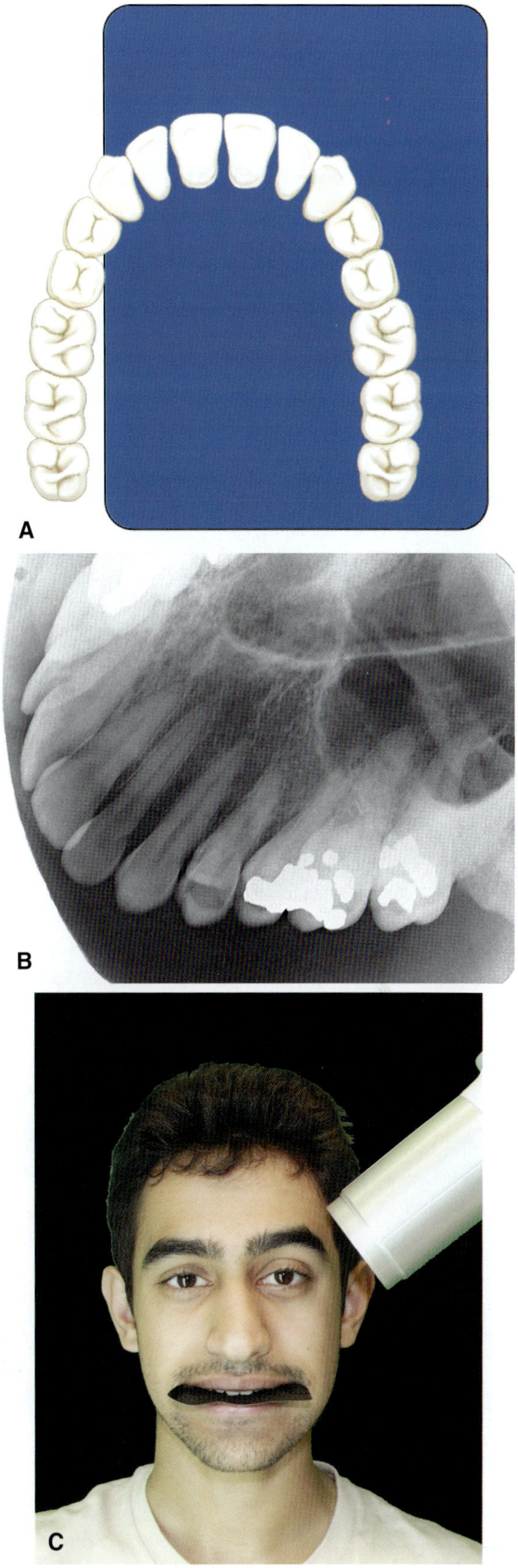

Fig. 6.25 Lateral maxillary occlusal projection. (A) The *shaded* area outlines the image field. (B) Lateral maxillary occlusal radiograph. (C) Position of the patient with the receptor in place and the aiming ring aligned for exposure.

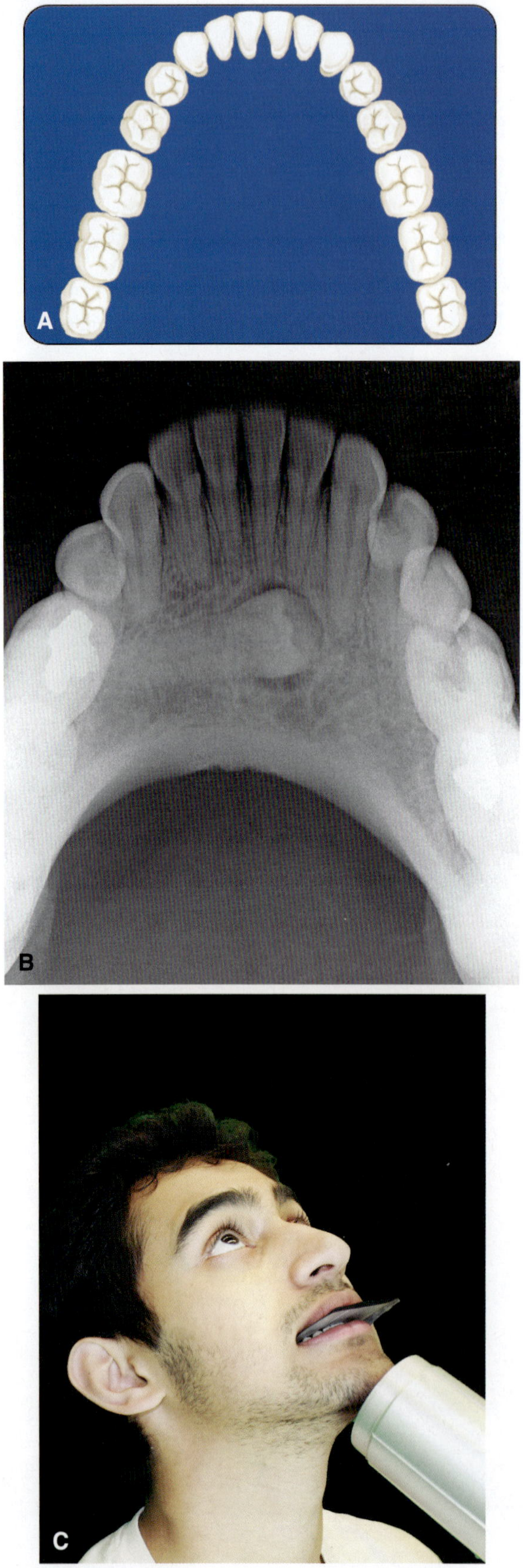

Fig. 6.26 Anterior mandibular occlusal projection. (A) The *shaded* area outlines the image field. (B) Anterior mandibular occlusal radiograph. (C) Position of the patient with the receptor in place and the aiming ring aligned for exposure.

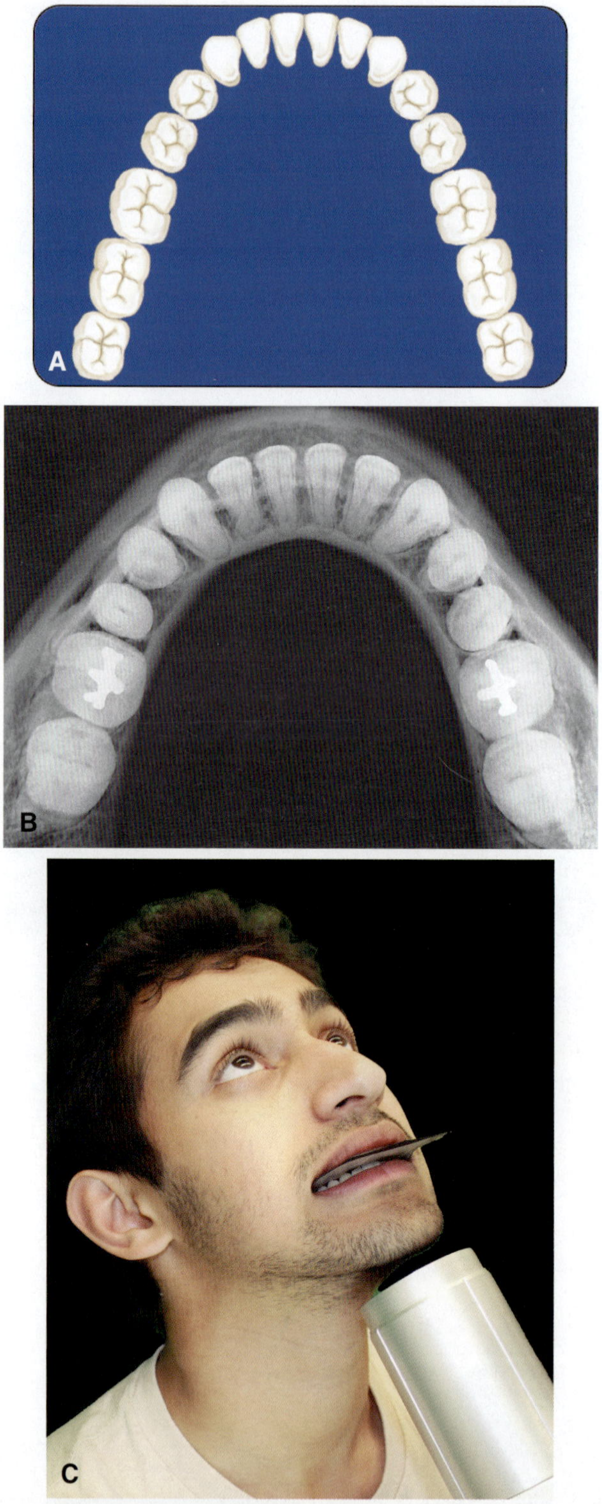

Fig. 6.27 Topographic mandibular occlusal projection. (A) The *shaded* area outlines the image field. (B) Topographic mandibular occlusal radiograph. (C) Position of the patient with the receptor in place and the aiming ring aligned for exposure.

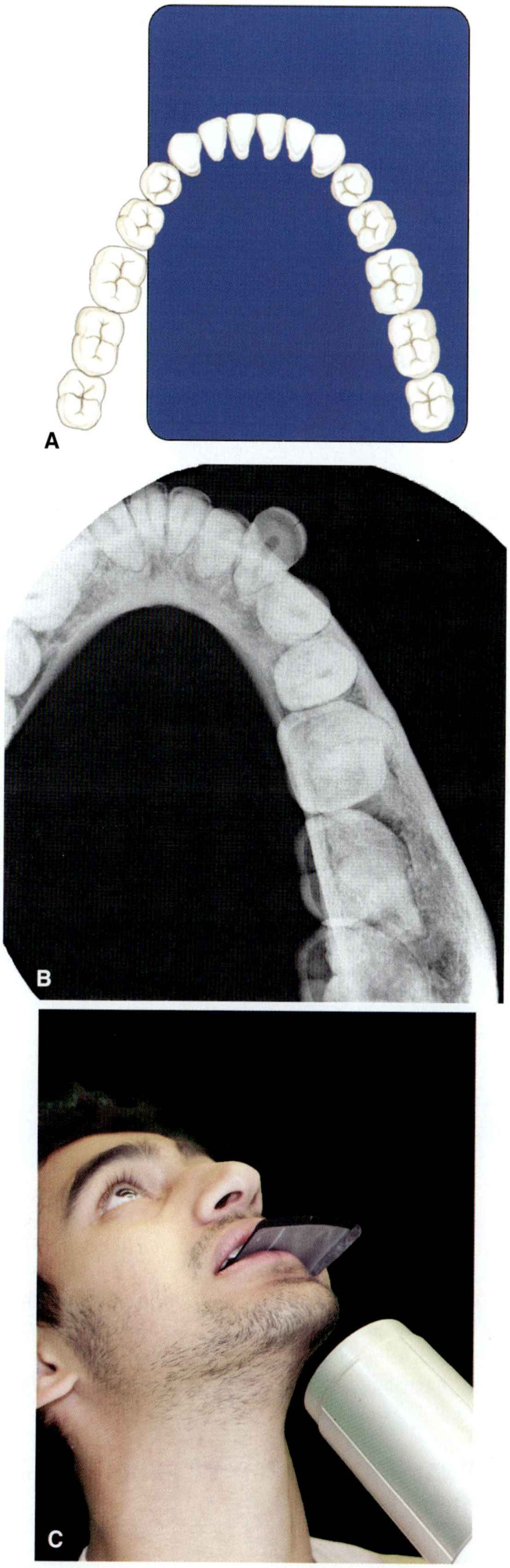

Fig. 6.28 Lateral mandibular occlusal projection. (A) The *shaded* area outlines the image field. (B) Lateral mandibular occlusal radiograph. (C) Position of the patient with the receptor in place and the aiming ring aligned for exposure.

older sibling being radiographed or to have the parent or dental assistant serve as a model. Children who feel a gagging sensation can be asked to breathe through the nose. Techniques to distract their attention, such as asking them to curl their toes or make a fist, can be effective. However, if the procedure is postponed until the next appointment, the gag reflex may not be encountered; often it may then be much easier for the patient to control. It is especially important to explain to the patient that the procedure will be much easier the next time—plant the positive thought.

Examination Coverage

When a complete radiographic survey is necessary, it should show the periapical region of all teeth, the proximal surfaces of all posterior teeth, and the crypts of the developing permanent teeth. The number of projections required depends on the child's size. Also, an exposure appropriate to the child's size should be used. For example, a 50% reduction in the milliamperes used for an average young adult gives the proper density for patients younger than 10 years. Exposure settings (mA or s) are reduced about 25% for children 10–15 years old.

Primary Dentition (3–6 Years)

A combination of projections can be used to provide adequate coverage for the pediatric dental patient. This examination may consist of two anterior occlusal receptors, two posterior bitewing receptors, and up to four posterior periapical receptors as indicated (Fig. 6.29). For the maxillary and interproximal projections, the child is seated upright with the sagittal plane perpendicular to and the occlusal plane parallel with the floor (horizontal plane). For mandibular projections other than the occlusal, the child is seated upright with the sagittal plane perpendicular. The tragus corner of the mouth line is oriented parallel to the floor. Some dentists find that a panoramic view, rather than the four periapicals, is more informative and results in less exposure to the child (see Chapter 3).

Maxillary anterior occlusal projection. A No. 2 receptor should be placed in the mouth with its long axis perpendicular to the sagittal plane and the exposure surface toward the maxillary teeth. The receptor is centered on the midline with the anterior border extending just beyond the incisal edges of the anterior teeth. The central ray is directed at a vertical angulation of +60 degrees through the tip of the nose toward the center of the receptor.

Mandibular anterior occlusal projection. The child should be seated with the head tipped back so that the occlusal plane is about 25 degrees above the plane of the floor. A No. 2 receptor is placed with the long axis perpendicular to the sagittal plane and the exposure surface toward the mandibular teeth. The central ray is oriented at −30 degrees vertical angulation and through the tip of the chin toward the receptor.

Bitewing projection. A No. 0 receptor is used with a paper loop receptor holder. The receptor is placed in the child's mouth as in the adult premolar bitewing projection. The image field should include the distal half of the canine and the deciduous molars. A positive vertical angulation of +5 to +10 degrees should be used. The horizontal angle is oriented to direct the beam through the interproximal spaces.

Deciduous maxillary molar periapical projection. A No. 0 receptor in a modified XCP or BAI (Dentsply Rinn, Elgin, IL) bite block is used, either with or without the aiming ring and indicator bar. The receptor is positioned in the midline of the palate with the anterior border extending to the maxillary primary canine. The image field of this projection should include the distal half of the primary canine and both primary molars.

Deciduous mandibular molar projection. A No. 0 receptor is positioned in a modified XCP or BAI bite block with or without the aiming ring and indicator bar between the posterior teeth and tongue. The exposed radiograph should show the distal half of the mandibular primary canine and the primary molar teeth.

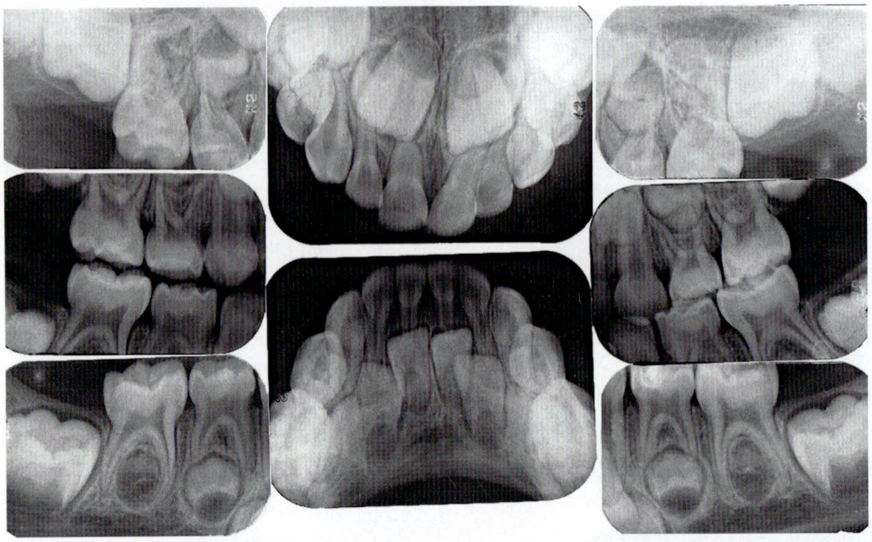

Fig. 6.29 Radiographic examination of primary dentition consists of two anterior occlusal views, four posterior periapical views, and two bitewing views. Often it is preferable to make a bitewing and panoramic examination followed by selected periapical views as indicated.

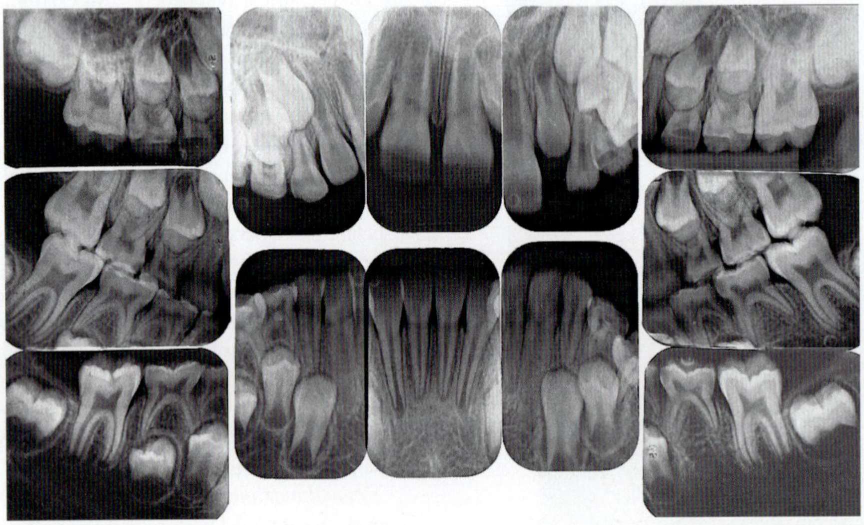

Fig. 6.30 Radiographic examination of mixed dentition consists of two incisor views, four canine views, four posterior views, and two bitewing views. Often it is preferable to make a bitewing and panoramic examination followed by selected periapical views as indicated.

Mixed Dentition (7–12 Years)

A complete examination of the mixed dentition, if indicated, consists of two incisor periapical views, four canine periapical views, four posterior periapical views, and two or four posterior bitewing views (Fig. 6.30). For the maxillary and interproximal projections, the child should be seated upright with the sagittal plane perpendicular and the occlusal plane parallel to the floor. For the mandibular projections, the child should be seated upright with the sagittal plane perpendicular and the ala-tragus line parallel to the floor. XCP instruments are used for larger children. Bisecting angle bite blocks may be more comfortable for smaller individuals.

Maxillary anterior periapical projection. A No. 1 receptor should be placed in the mouth behind the maxillary central and lateral incisors. The receptor should be centered on the embrasure between the central incisors.

Mandibular anterior periapical projection. A No. 1 receptor should be positioned behind the mandibular central and lateral incisors.

Canine periapical projection. A No. 1 receptor should be positioned behind each of the canines.

Deciduous and permanent molar periapical projection. A No. 1 or No. 2 receptor (if the child is large enough) should be positioned with the anterior edge behind the canine.

Posterior bitewing projection. Bitewing projections should be exposed in the premolar region with a No. 1 or No. 2 receptor as previously described, using either bitewing tabs or the Rinn bitewing instrument. Four bitewing projections should be exposed when the second permanent molars have erupted.

INTRAORAL RADIOGRAPHY WITH HANDHELD X-RAY DEVICES

The use of handheld radiographic devices for intraoral radiography has increased over the last decade. These devices offer advantages for mobile radiography, for example, in nursing homes, hospital inpatient units, or at disaster scenes, where the portable device can be taken directly to the patient. Combining such a portable x-ray generator with digital imaging provides rapid, self-contained, and mobile imaging capability.

Portable battery-powered x-ray generators are manufactured worldwide, and several devices have been approved by the US Food and Drug Administration (FDA) for intraoral radiography (see Fig. 6.31). Clinical use of these devices has shown that they can be held stable and produce clinically acceptable images. There are several considerations for incorporating handheld x-ray devices into the dental clinic's imaging armamentarium and workflow.

Device mobility: Handheld x-ray devices offer the advantage of mobility, and a single unit can serve several adjacent operatories, with the convenience of imaging the patient in the treatment chair. With added mobility, it is important to ensure that infection control protocols are followed rigorously. Mobile x-ray devices must be maintained securely to prevent its unauthorized use or theft.

Operating parameters: Most handheld devices operate with fixed kilovolt and milliampere setting. For example, the NOMAD Pro 2 operates at 60 kVp and 2.5 mA, lower than typical settings of wall-mounted intraoral radiographic machines. As battery charge decreases, the actual radiation output during operation also decreases, and potentially may yield underexposed, nondiagnostic images. A dental clinic that performs several imaging procedures during the day should consider additional batteries as a backup to prevent this undesirable outcome.

Manual handling: Proper handling of the device is key to safe operation of these devices (see Chapter 3). While handheld devices offer convenience, device handling may be cumbersome, especially when performing full-mouth examinations. These devices weigh approximately 2.7 kilograms (6 pounds), and prolonged handling may lead to operator fatigue. Devices that are improperly handled or dropped may be damaged.

Users must be familiar with national and local guidance for use of handheld x-ray devices. Several states in the United States have additional requirements related to training and radiation dose documentation when using handheld x-ray devices.

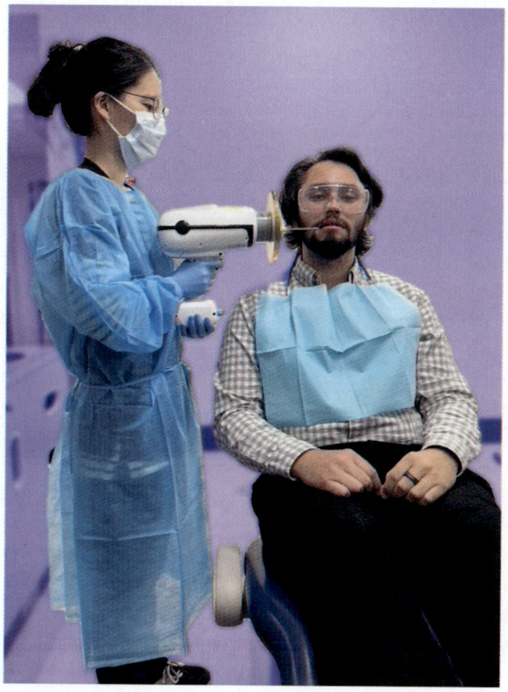

Fig. 6.31 Handheld x-ray machine for intraoral radiography. With appropriate handling, operator dose is minimized by a shield on the aiming cylinder to reduce backscatter. (Courtesy Dr. Somyung Ji and Dr. Conor Kemp, UCLA School of Dentistry, Los Angeles, CA.)

SPECIAL CONSIDERATIONS

The radiographic procedures described in this chapter may need to be modified for patients who have unusual difficulties or special needs. Specific modifications depend on the patient's physical and emotional characteristics. However, as with any dental procedure, the dental assistant begins the examination by showing appreciation of the patient's condition and compassionate recognition of problems that might occur. If the assistant is kind but firm, the patient's confidence increases, which helps the patient to relax and cooperate. Following are a few conditions and circumstances that may be encountered, with recommendations and suggestions that may help the clinician achieve an adequate radiographic examination.

Infection

Infection in the orofacial structures may result in edema and lead to trismus of some of the muscles of mastication. As a result, intraoral radiography may be painful to the patient and difficult for both the patient and the radiologist. Under such circumstances, panoramic or occlusal techniques may offer the only possibility of an examination. In the case of edema in an area to be examined, exposure time should be increased to compensate for the increased x-ray attenuation due to tissue swelling.

Trauma

A patient who has undergone trauma may have a dental or facial fracture. Dental fractures are depicted on periapical or occlusal radiographs. Special care must be taken in making these views because of the condition of the patient. Skeletal fractures are usually best seen with panoramic or other extraoral views or a computed tomography examination. In some cases, patients with fractures of the facial skeleton may be nonambulatory because of other injuries. Consequently an extraoral radiographic examination with the patient in the supine position may be necessary. However, the circumstances need not compromise the techniques, and satisfactory intraoral images can be produced if the proper relative positions of the tube, patient, and receptor are observed.

Patients With Mental Disabilities

Patients with mental disabilities may cause some difficulty that usually is the result of the patient's lack of coordination or inability to comprehend what is expected. When the radiographic examination is performed speedily, unpredictable moves by the patient can be minimized. In some cases sedation may be required.

Patients With Physical Disabilities

Patients with physical disabilities (e.g., loss of vision, loss of hearing, loss of the use of any or all extremities, congenital defects such as cleft palate) may require special handling during a radiographic examination. These patients are usually cooperative and eager to assist. They may be accustomed to so much discomfort and inconvenience that their tolerance level is high, and they are not challenged by the relatively slight irritation represented by the x-ray procedures. Generally intraoral and extraoral radiographic examinations may be performed for these patients if a good rapport between the patient and radiology technician is established and maintained. Members of the patient's family are often helpful in assisting the patient into and out of the examination chair and in receptor positioning and holding inasmuch as they are usually familiar with the patient's condition and accustomed to coping with it.

Gag Reflex

Occasionally patients who need a radiographic examination manifest a gag reflex at the slightest provocation. These patients are usually very apprehensive and frightened by unknown procedures; others simply seem to have very sensitive tissue that precipitates a gag reflex when stimulated. This sensitivity is manifested when the receptor is placed in the oral cavity. To overcome this disability, the radiologist should try to relax and reassure the patient. The radiologist can describe and explain the procedures. Often gagging can be controlled if the operator bolsters the patient's confidence by demonstrating technical competence and showing authority tempered with compassion. The gag reflex is often worse when a patient is tired; therefore it is advisable to perform the examination in the morning, when the individual is well rested, especially in the case of children.

Stimulating the posterior dorsum of the tongue or the soft palate usually initiates the gag reflex. Consequently, during the placement of the receptor, the tongue should be very relaxed and positioned well to the floor of the mouth; this can be accomplished by asking the patient to swallow deeply just before opening the mouth for placement of the receptor. (The dentist should never mention the tongue or ask patients to relax the tongue; this usually makes them more conscious of it and precipitates involuntary movements.) The receptor is carried into the mouth parallel to the occlusal plane. When the desired area is reached, the receptor is rotated with a decisive motion, bringing it into contact with the palate or the floor of the mouth. Sliding it along the palate or tongue is likely to stimulate the gag reflex. Also, the dentist must keep in mind that the longer the receptor stays in the mouth, the greater the possibility that the patient will start to gag. The patient should be advised to breathe rapidly through the nose because mouth breathing usually aggravates this condition.

Any little exercise that can be devised which does not interfere with the x-ray examination but shifts the patient's attention from the receptor and the mouth is likely to relieve the gag reaction. Asking patients to hold their breath or to keep a foot or arm suspended during receptor placement and exposure can often create such a distraction. In extreme cases, topical anesthetic agents in mouthwashes or spray can be administered to produce temporary numbness of the tongue and palate to reduce gagging. However, in our experience, this procedure gives limited results. The most effective approach is to reduce apprehension, minimize tissue irritation, and encourage rapid breathing through the nose. If all measures fail, an extraoral examination may be the only means, short of administering general anesthesia, to examine the patient radiographically.

Imaging for Endodontics

Radiographs are essential for endodontic diagnosis and treatment planning. Additionally, intraoperative radiographs may be taken during the endodontic procedure to assist in confirming the working length of the endodontic instrumentation or to identify additional canals. The presence of a rubber dam, rubber dam clamp, and root canal instruments may complicate an intraoral periapical examination by impairing proper receptor positioning and aiming cylinder angulation. Despite these obstacles, certain requirements must be observed:

1. The tooth being treated must be centered in the image.
2. The receptor must be positioned as far from the tooth and apex as the region permits to ensure that the apex of the tooth and some periapical bone are apparent on the radiograph.

For maxillary projections, the patient is seated so that the sagittal plane is perpendicular and the occlusal plane is parallel to the floor. For mandibular projections, the patient is seated upright with the sagittal plane perpendicular and the tragus-to-corner of the mouth line parallel to the floor. Specially designed receptor holders for endodontic images are available (Fig. 6.32). These instruments fit over files, clamps, and the rubber dam without touching the subject tooth. The aiming cylinder is aligned to direct the central ray perpendicular to the receptor.

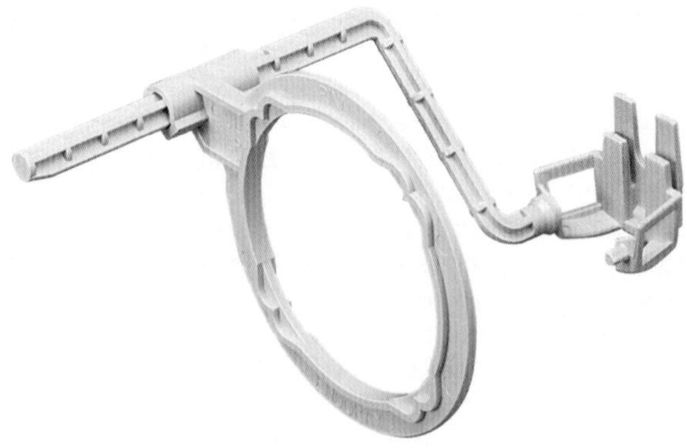

Fig. 6.32 EndoRay receptor holder used for endodontic images. This device provides room for files to be in place while making the image (Courtesy Dentsply Rinn, Elgin, IL.)

Often a single radiograph of a multirooted tooth made at the normal vertical and horizontal projection does not display all the roots. In these cases, when it is necessary to separate the roots on multirooted teeth, a second projection may be made. The horizontal angulation is altered 20 degrees mesially for maxillary premolars, 20 degrees mesially or distally for maxillary molars, or 20 degrees distally for an oblique projection of mandibular molar roots.

If a sinus tract is encountered, its course is tracked by threading a gutta-percha cone through the tract before the radiograph is made. It also is possible to localize and determine the depth of periodontal defects with this gutta-percha tracking technique.

A final radiograph of the treated tooth is made to demonstrate the quality of the root canal filling and the condition of the periapical tissues after removal of the clamp and rubber dam. This radiograph serves as a baseline for comparison with subsequent radiographic examinations to monitor outcomes of endodontic treatment.

Pregnancy

Although a fetus is sensitive to ionizing radiation, the amount of exposure received by an embryo or fetus during dental radiography is extremely low. There have been no reports of damage to a fetus from dental radiography. Nevertheless, prudence suggests that such radiographic examinations be kept to a minimum consistent with the mother's dental needs. As with any patient, radiographic examination is limited during pregnancy to cases with a specific diagnostic indication. With optimal radiation safety techniques patient radiation doses are minimal (see Chapter 3), and an intraoral or extraoral examination can be performed whenever a reasonable diagnostic requirement exists.

Edentulous Patients

Radiographic examination of edentulous patients is important, whether the area of interest is one tooth or an entire arch. These areas may contain roots, residual infection, impacted teeth, cysts, or other pathologic entities that may adversely affect the usefulness of prosthetic appliances or the patient's health. After a determination has been made that these entities are not present, repeated examinations to detect them are not warranted in the absence of signs or symptoms.

If available, a panoramic examination of the edentulous jaws is most convenient. If abnormalities of the alveolar ridges are identified, the higher resolution of the periapical receptor is used to make intraoral projections to supplement the panoramic examination.

In a completely or partly edentulous patient, a receptor-holding device is used for intraoral radiography of the alveolar ridges. Placement of the receptor-holding instrument may be complicated by its tipping into the voids normally occupied by the crowns of the missing teeth. To manage this difficulty, cotton rolls are placed between the ridge and the receptor holder, supporting the holder in a horizontal position. An orthodontic elastic band to hold cotton rolls to the bite block on the receptor holder often is useful when several such projections must be exposed. With elastics, it is simple to maneuver the cotton rolls into the areas that require support. The patient may steady the receptor-holding instrument with a hand or an opposing denture.

If panoramic equipment is unavailable, an examination consisting of 14 intraoral views provides an excellent survey. The exposure required for an edentulous ridge is approximately 25% less than that for a dentulous ridge. This examination consists of seven projections in each jaw (adult No. 2 receptor) as follows:

Central incisors (midline): one projection
Lateral canine: two projections
Premolar: two projections
Molar: two projections

Intraoral Radiography: Common Errors

Figures 6.33 to 6.37 demonstrate common errors due to receptor misplacment and incorrect x-ray beam angulation.

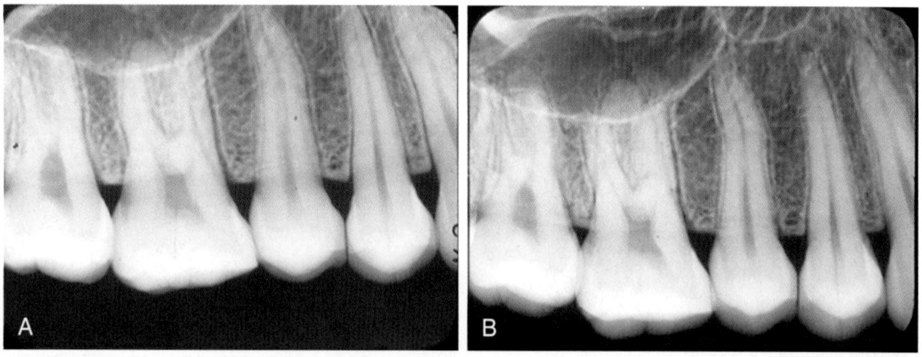

Fig. 6.33 Receptor placement error. (A) Receptor is placed too far toward the occlusal plane. Note that premolar apices and periapical bone are not seen. (B) Correct placement of receptor. The occlusal table and periapical regions are encompassed.

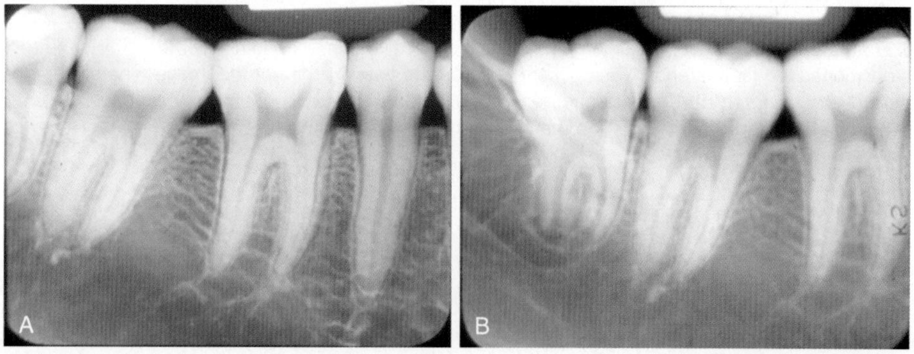

Fig. 6.34 Receptor placement error. (A) Receptor is placed too far anterior for the molar projection. Note that the third molar is only partly encompassed. (B) Correct placement of receptor. The radiograph now includes the entire third molar and surrounding bone.

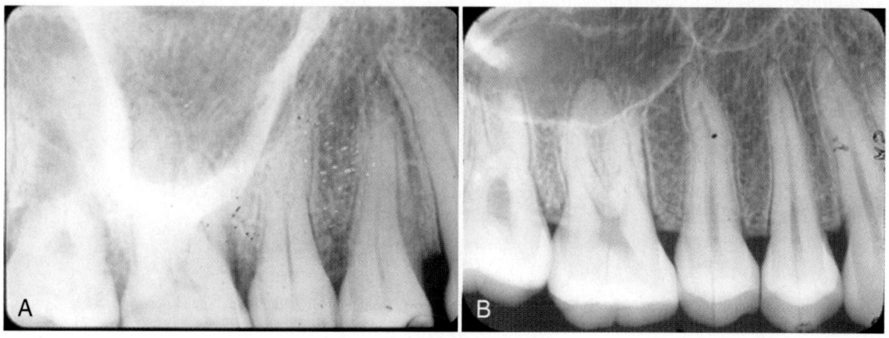

Fig. 6.35 Vertical beam angulation error. (A) Excessive vertical angulation. Note that the zygomatic process of the maxilla is supperimposed over the molar apices and the occulsal table is not projected on the image. (B) Correct vertical beam angulation. The occlusal table is included and the molar periapical regions are better viewed without supierimposition.

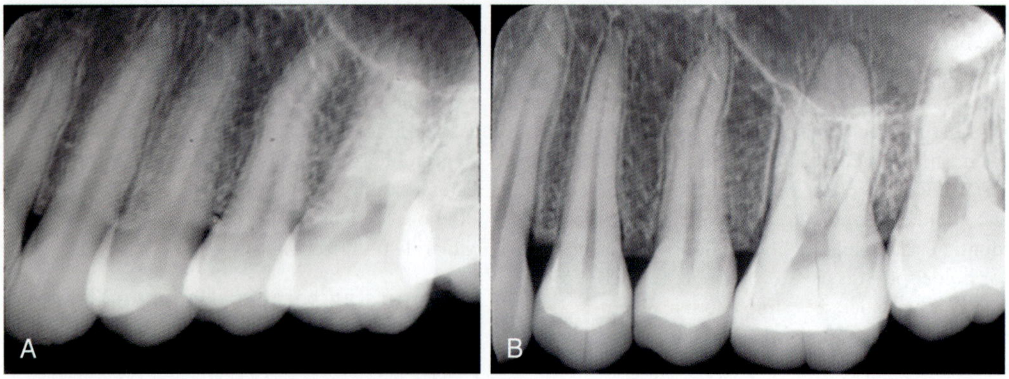

Fig. 6.36 Horizontal beam angulation error. (A) Incorrect horizontal angulation. Note supperimposition of the enamel on the proximal surfaces of premolar and molar teeth. (B) Correct horizontal beam angulation. The x-ray beam is directed through the interproximal contacts. The separation of proximal surfaces allows assessment for caries and interproximal bone loss.

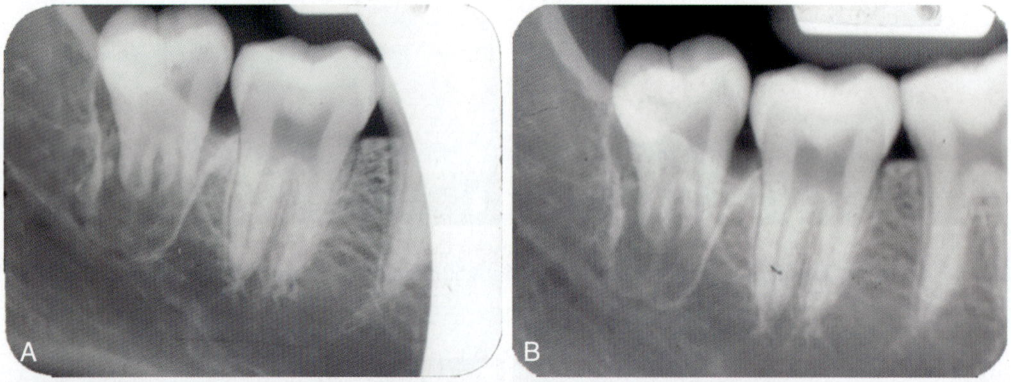

Fig. 6.37 Improper beam-receptor alignment. (A) The x-ray collimator cone is not centered over the receptor and is positioned too far posterior. Note a "cone cut" on the anterior third of the image where there was no exposure of the receptor. (B) Correct beam-receptor alignment. The x-ray beam now exposes the entire receptor surface to record the image of the mandibular molar and retromolar regions.

BIBLIOGRAPHY

Adriaens PA, De Boever J, Vande Velde F. Comparison of intra-oral long-cone paralleling radiographic surveys and orthopantomographs with special reference to the bone height. *J Oral Rehabil.* 1982;9:355-365.

Biggerstaff RH, Phillips JR. A quantitative comparison of paralleling long-cone and bisection-of-angle periapical radiography. *Oral Surg Oral Med Oral Pathol.* 1976;62:673-677.

Forsberg J, Halse A. Periapical radiolucencies as evaluated by bisecting-angle and paralleling radiographic techniques. *Int Endod J.* 1997;30(2):115-123. doi:10.1046/j.1365-2591.1997.00059.x.

Kazzi D, Horner K, Qualtrough AC, Martinez-Beneyto Y, Rushton VE. A comparative study of three periapical radiographic techniques for endodontic working length estimation. *Int Endod J.* 2007;40(7):526-531. doi:10.1111/j.1365-2591.2007.01251.x.

Scandrett FR, Tebo HG, Miller JT, et al. Radiographic examination of the edentulous patient, 1: review of the literature and preliminary report comparing three methods. *Oral Surg Oral Med Oral Pathol.* 1973;35:266-274.

Schulze RK, d'Hoedt B. A method to calculate angular disparities between object and receptor in "paralleling technique". *Dentomaxillofac Radiol.* 2002;31:32-38.

Cephalometric and Skull Imaging

Sanjay M. Mallya

This chapter discusses cephalometric and various planar radiographs to evaluate the skull, midface, and jaw bones. Cephalometric projections are used in dentistry, predominantly for orthodontic diagnosis and treatment planning. The use of other planar radiographs of the craniofacial skeleton has decreased over the years. Considering the complex anatomy of the skull and midface, computed tomography (CT) has replaced these projections as the preferred modality to evaluate trauma, pathoses, and sinonasal disease. Nevertheless, such projection radiographs often constitute part of the patient's historical health record and continue to be used in communities where CT imaging is not readily available. Thus, the oral and maxillofacial radiologist must be competent in evaluation of these imaging studies.

CEPHALOMETRIC RADIOGRAPHY

Cephalometric radiographs are made with a standard projection geometry and known magnification, and allow for reproducible imaging of the craniofacial region. This radiographic technique, designed independently by B. Holly Broadbent and Herbert Hofrath in 1931, was developed to apply anthropometric techniques to evaluate patient growth and orthodontic treatment-associated changes. The development of this technique was driven by the need to make skull radiographs with minimal magnification and with high reproducibility to enable temporal comparisons.

The Cephalostat

All cephalometric radiographs are made with a cephalostat (Fig. 7.1A), a device that maintains a constant relationship between the skull, the receptor, and the x-ray beam. The cephalostat is equipped with two ear rods to stabilize the patient's head in the desired position. For lateral cephalometric radiographs, a nasion stabilizer is used to restrict craniocaudal head movement (Fig. 7.1A). Radiopaque markers or a measurement scale is incorporated within the nasion stabilizer to allow determination of magnification directly on the radiograph. Manufacturers attach cephalostats onto panoramic and cone beam computed tomography (CBCT) machines—these multipurpose devices use a single x-ray source to serve panoramic, CBCT, and cephalometric imaging needs (Fig. 7.1B).

Cephalometric Projection Geometry

Cephalometric projections use a long source-to-object distance of 150 cm or higher to minimize image magnification (Fig. 7.2) The object-to-receptor distance is typically 15–20 cm and must be maintained constant for all sequential radiographs of the same patient. For contemporary digital units, these distances are fixed and cannot be changed by the user (Table 7.1). The source-to-object and object-to-receptor distances used in the cephalometric machine vary with manufacturer and determine the image magnification, which can be calculated from the projection geometry specifications provided by the manufacturer. Typically, this ranges from 10% to 15% in the center of the craniostat (Table 7.1). For lateral cephalometric radiographs, this magnification can be applied to midline anatomy (Fig. 7.2A). Structures located closer to the receptor are magnified less, whereas structures located closer to the source are magnified more. Applying this same principle to view craniofacial anatomy in the coronal plane, cephalometric views are made with a posteroanterior (PA) beam direction. This places the facial anatomy closest to the receptor decreasing magnification of the structures of interest (Fig. 7.2B).

Cephalometric radiographs may be made using film, photostimulable phosphor (PSP) plates, or solid-state detectors. When using film or PSP plates, the x-ray beam is collimated to the size of the receptor and a projection image is acquired with a short exposure. When using direct digital acquisition, two approaches are used. One approach uses a large area detector made of scintillator material, typically cesium iodide or gadolinium oxysulfide, as the primary interaction with the x-ray photons. These compounds absorb x-rays and produce visible light that is transmitted via fiber optic cables to tiled complementary metal-oxide semiconductor (CMOS) detectors. With this technique, termed "one-shot" by vendors, the exposure time is approximately 1 second, minimizing the likelihood of patient motion during imaging. A second approach uses a narrow, vertical array of CMOS detectors, usually 4–7 mm wide. The x-ray beam is collimated at the source and with secondary collimators to restrict the beam to the dimensions of the detector array. During exposure, coordinated linear movement of the x-ray beam, collimators, and detector array acquire sequential vertical images that are digitally assembled into the final image. The total exposure time varies from approximately 4 seconds to as much as 20 seconds depending on the specific device and image resolution mode. Although a longer image capture time may increase the possibility of patient motion, this has not been a practical limitation to this technique.

The principles of cephalometric analyses are the same, irrespective of the mode of acquisition. Skeletal, dental, and soft tissue anatomic landmarks delineate the lines, planes, angles, and distances used to generate measurements and to classify patients' craniofacial morphology. At the beginning of treatment, these measurements are compared with an established standard or norm; during treatment, the measurements are compared with measurements from previous cephalometric radiographs of the same patient to monitor growth and treatment-induced changes.

Lateral Cephalometric Projection

The lateral cephalometric projection is the most commonly used craniofacial projection radiograph in dentistry. It is used predominantly

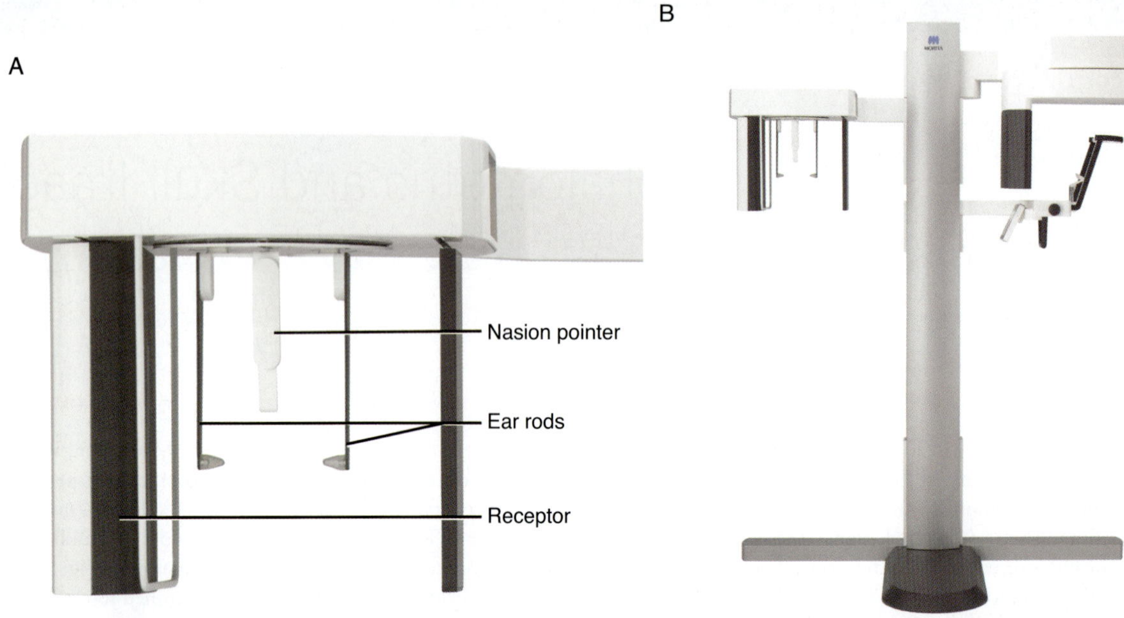

Fig. 7.1 (A) Cephalostat. The ear rods and nasion pointer help stabilize the patient's head in a standard position and are shown in the configuration for making lateral cephalometric radiographs. The assembly can be rotated at its base to turn the ear rods 90 degrees and position the patient for a posteroanterior projection. (B) Veraview X800, a multipurpose imaging device combining cephalometric, panoramic, and cone beam computed tomography imaging. (Images courtesy of J. Morita Corporation, Kyoto, Japan).

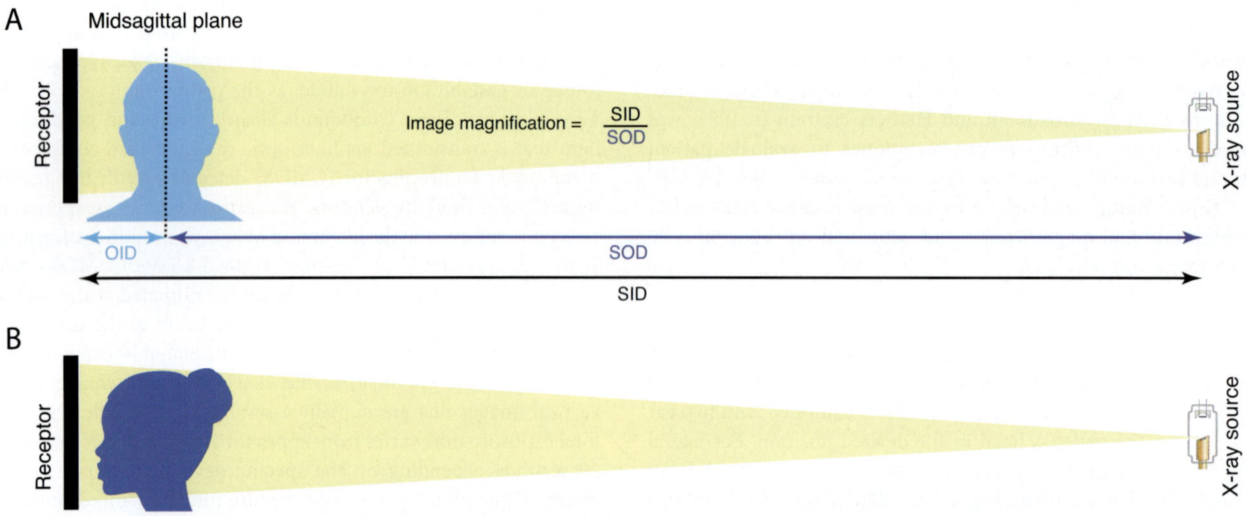

Fig. 7.2 Projection geometry for cephalometric radiography. (A) Position for lateral cephalometric radiograph. To limit magnification, the source to midsagittal plane is long and the distance between the midsagittal plane and receptor is short. Image magnification in the midsagittal plane can be calculated as *Image magnification* = *Source-to-image distance* (SID) ÷ *Source-to-object distance* (SOD). (B) Position for posteroanterior cephalometric radiograph. The structures of interest in the facial skeleton are positioned closer to the receptor to minimize magnification.

for growth assessment, and for orthodontic and orthognathic diagnosis and treatment planning.

Indications

- Evaluate the anteroposterior (AP) and vertical relationships between the dentition, maxilla, mandible, and cranial base to identify skeletal discrepancies.
- Assess skeletal and soft-tissue relationships.
- Evaluate the AP dimensions of the nasopharyngeal and oropharyngeal airways.
- Assess skeletal growth stage via cervical spine maturation.
- Monitor growth-associated skeletal and soft-tissue profile changes.
- Monitor treatment progress.
- Monitor treatment outcomes.

TABLE 7.1 Cephalometric Projection Geometry and Image Magnification in Select Cephalometric X-Ray Units

Manufacturer	Model(s)	SID[a](cm)	SOD[b] (cm)	Image magnification[c]
Gendex	GXDP-700	174.5	152	14.8%
Instrumentarium	OP10	174.5	152.4	14.5%
J. Morita	Veraviewepocs 2D Veraview X800 Veraviewepocs 3D R100	165	150	10%
Midmark	Extraoral imaging system (EOIS)	165	150*	10%
Planmeca	ProCeph	170	154.5*	10%
Sirona	Orthophos SL	171.4	155.8	10%
Vatech	PHT-30CSS	174.5	152.4	14.5%

[a]SID, Source-to-image receptor distance.
[b]SOD, Source-to-object (midsagittal plane) distance.
[c]Image magnification in midsagittal plane on lateral cephalometric projection = SID ÷ SOD.
*Value calculated from manufacturer specifications.

Image Receptor and Patient Placement (Fig. 7.3A and B)

The patient is positioned in the cephalostat with the ear rod tips securely within the external auditory canal. The midsagittal plane is oriented vertical and the Frankfort plane horizontal. The patient is asked to occlude in a normal intercuspation position. The image receptor is positioned parallel to the midsagittal plane. Cephalometric machines may have the source located on the patient's right or left side. By convention, cephalometric machines marketed in the United States are assembled with the x-ray source located to the left of the patient.

When using film, PSP plates and nonscanning digital cephalometric imaging, a wedge filter is positioned at the x-ray source to decrease radiation intensity in the anterior aspect and depict the soft tissue facial profile. For scanning digital cephalometric techniques, the scanning speed is increased when imaging the anterior region, decreasing x-ray intensity per unit area for better soft-tissue attenuation.

Position of the Central X-Ray Beam (Fig. 7.3A)

The central beam is perpendicular to the patient's midsagittal plane and to the plane of the image receptor and is centered over the external auditory meatus.

Resultant Image (Fig. 7.4)

Exact superimposition of right and left sides is impossible because the structures on the side near to the image receptor are magnified less than the same structures on the side of the x-ray source. Bilateral structures close to the midsagittal plane demonstrate less discrepancy in size compared with bilateral structures farther away from the midsagittal plane. Structures close to the midsagittal plane (e.g., the clinoid processes and inferior turbinates) should be nearly superimposed.

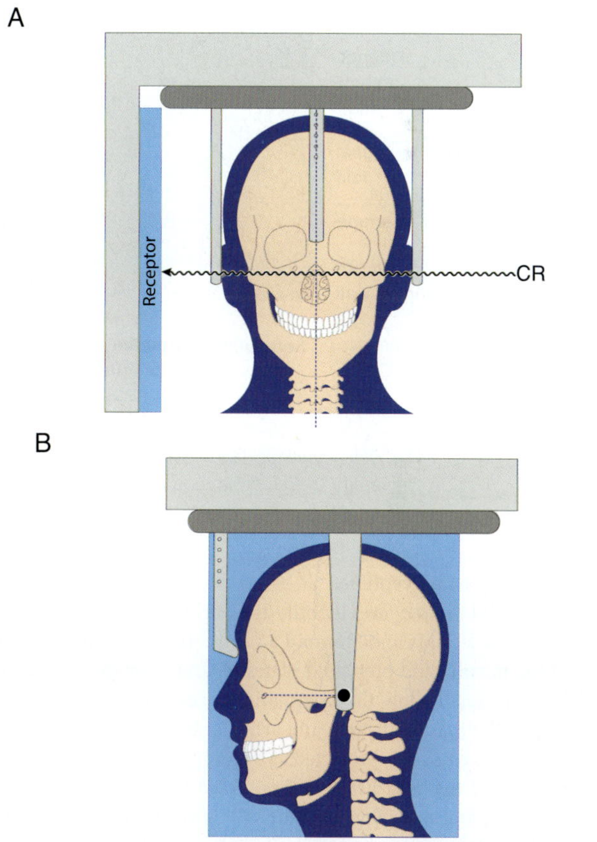

Fig. 7.3 Patient position for lateral cephalometric radiography. (A) Coronal view. The midsagittal plane is parallel to the plane of the receptor. Teeth are in intercuspation. The entry and direction of the central ray (CR) is shown. (B) Sagittal view. The Frankfort plane is horizontal and the nasion pointer contacts the soft tissue of the bridge of the nose.

Radiologic Evaluation

The primary purpose of making a lateral cephalometric radiographic is to infer relationships between the skull, jaws, and teeth via specific cephalometric analyses. However, before performing these analyses, the lateral cephalometric radiograph must be systematically evaluated to identify relevant anatomic variants and potential incidental pathoses. The evaluation must systematically encompass all of the anatomic regions listed below.

- *Calvarium.* Trace the contour of the calvarium and identify the diploic space—the medullary cavity between the inner and outer cortices of the skull. Trace the sutures, where visible. Vessel grooves may appear as tortuous radiolucent channels. Identify any intracranial calcifications.
- *Skull base.* Identify the mastoid air cells. The external auditory meatuses are superimposed and appear as oval radiolucencies, superior to the mastoid cells. Trace the cortical contour of the clivus, clinoid processes, sella turcica, and roof of the orbit.
- *Paranasal sinuses.* The sinus cavities should appear radiolucent with cortical borders, although the borders of the bilateral sinuses are superimposed. Trace the outlines of the sphenoid, ethmoid, frontal,

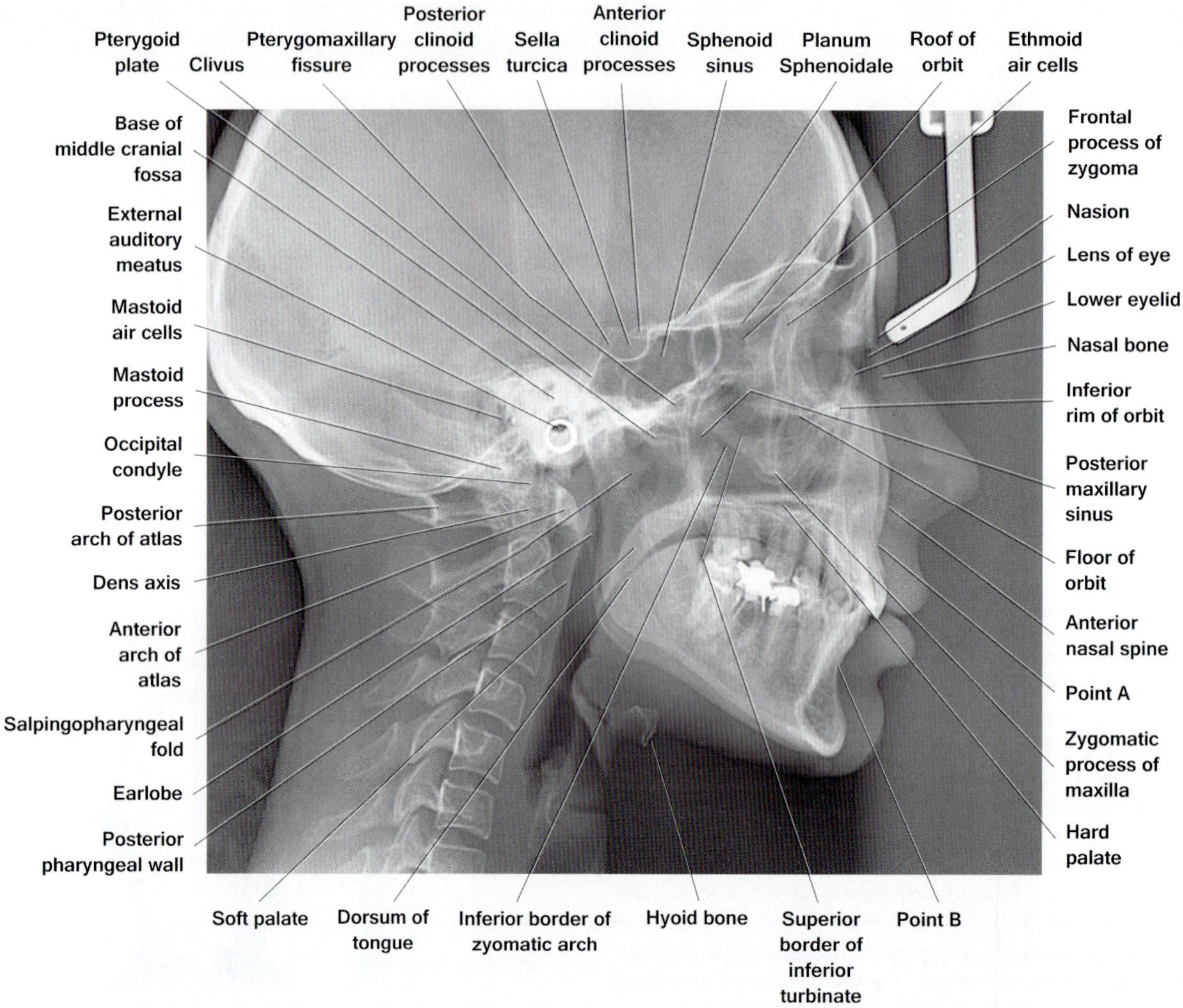

Fig. 7.4 Anatomic landmarks identified in the lateral cephalometric projection. (Courtesy Ms. Lucy Gao, University of California, Los Angeles.)

and maxillary sinuses. Due to superimposition, the ethmoid air cells are least perceptible.

- *Upper and middle face.* Identify the orbits, superimposed over the maxillary sinuses and ethmoid air cells. Trace the posterior border of the maxilla and pterygoid plates separated by the pterygomaxillary fissures. Follow the zygomatic process of the maxilla posteriorly to the zygomatic arch and articular eminence. The hard palate (floor of the nose) is projected as a radiopaque line over the inferior portion of the maxillary sinuses. Trace the line anteriorly to the anterior nasal spine. Evaluate the soft tissue profile of the upper and middle face.
- *Lower face.* Follow the outline of the mandible from the condylar and coronoid processes to the rami; to the mandibular angles and bodies; and finally, to the mandibular symphysis. Evaluate the soft-tissue profile of the lower face and determine lip competence.
- *Craniovertebral junction and cervical spine.* Evaluate the craniovertebral junction. Identify the odontoid process and the anterior arch of the atlas. The intervening space should be less than 3 mm in adults and less than 5 mm in children. The intervertebral spaces should be of uniform thickness. Assess alignment of the vertebral bodies.
- *Airway.* Identify the nasal turbinates. Outline the nasopharynx, soft palate, and dorsum of tongue. These are perceptible as sharp air-tissue contrasts and outline the nasopharyngeal and oropharyngeal airway spaces. Assess the anteroposterior dimension of the airway space. Identify the hyoid bone.
- *Alveolar bone and teeth.* Note the labial inclination of the incisors and the boundaries of the alveolar bone in the maxilla and mandible. Although superimposed, apical periodontitis and periodontal bone loss are often visible, although these lesions are better evaluated with intraoral and panoramic imaging.

Posteroanterior Cephalometric Projection

The PA cephalometric projection is made at a right angle to the lateral cephalometric projection. The combined information from lateral and PA cephalometric radiographs allow assessment of the craniofacial skeleton in all three dimensions.

Indications

- Evaluate craniofacial asymmetry.
- Assess maxillomandibular relationship in the mediolateral and vertical dimensions.
- Monitor treatment progress.
- Monitor treatment outcomes.

Image Receptor and Patient Placement (Fig. 7.5)

The patient is positioned in the cephalostat with the ear rods securely within the external auditory canal and facing the image receptor.

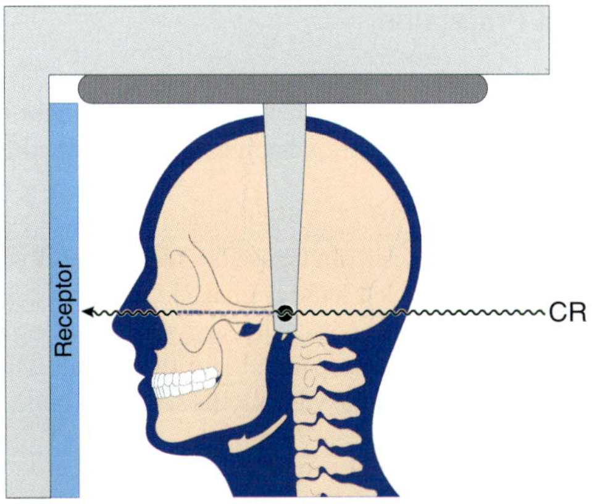

Fig. 7.5 Sagittal view of patient position for posteroanterior cephalometric radiography. The Frankfort plane is horizontal and the midsagittal plane is vertical. Teeth are in intercuspation. The entry and direction of the central ray (CR) is shown.

Placing the facial structures closer to the receptor minimizes their magnification. The patient's midsagittal plane is oriented vertical and perpendicular to the image receptor. The Frankfort plane is aligned horizontal and perpendicular to the image receptor.

Position of the Central X-Ray Beam (Fig. 7.5)

The central beam is perpendicular to the image receptor, directed from posterior to anterior (hence the name PA), through the midsagittal plane, and centered through the level of the external auditory meatus.

Resultant Image (Fig. 7.6)

In this PA view, the anterior structures of interest—the midfacial skeleton and mandible—are positioned closer to the receptor and are magnified less relative to more posterior structures. The midsagittal plane is projected vertical and divides the right and left halves of the craniofacial skeleton to facilitate detection of asymmetry. When the Frankfort plane is aligned horizontal, the superior border of the petrous ridge should be projected over the lower third of the orbit.

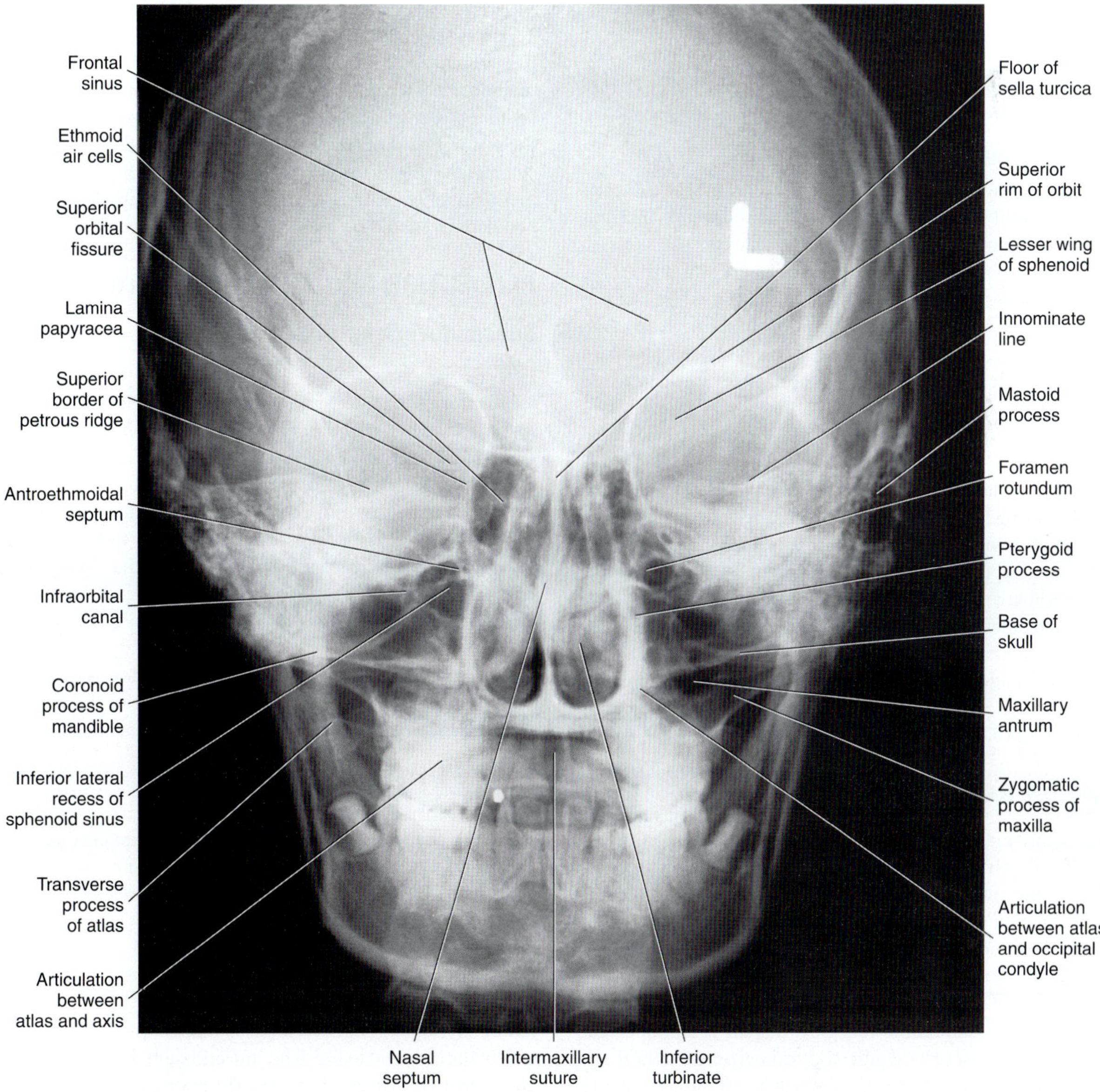

Fig. 7.6 Anatomic landmarks identified in the posteroanterior cephalometric projection.

Radiologic Evaluation

Similar to lateral cephalometric radiographs, PA cephalometric images must be systematically evaluated to identify relevant anatomic variants and potential incidental pathoses. The evaluation must encompass all of the anatomic regions listed below.

- *Calvarium.* Trace the contour of the calvarium. Trace the sutures, where visible. Vessel grooves may appear as tortuous radiolucent channels. Identify any intracranial calcifications.
- *Skull base.* Identify the mastoid air cells. Trace the cortical contour of the sphenoid bone and roof of the orbit.
- *Paranasal sinuses.* The sinus cavities should appear radiolucent with cortical borders. The sphenoid sinus is obscured by superimposition. Identify the ethmoid, frontal, and maxillary sinuses.
- *Upper and middle face.* Assess symmetry of the orbits, zygomatic processes, and nasal cavity.
- *Lower face.* Follow the outline of the mandible from the condyle on one side across the mandibular midline to the condyle of the opposite side. Assess symmetry and its relationship to the maxillary midline.
- *Alveolar bone and teeth.* The anterior dentition is superimposed over the cervical spine. The posterior dentition, in particular the mandibular third molars, are better visible. Pathoses associated with third molars, such as dentigerous cysts are common, and thus, partly developed and unerupted teeth must be evaluated in detail.

Cephalometric Analyses

Cephalometric radiographs allow the clinician to assess the relationships of the skull base, jaws, and teeth, and their contributions to the patient's malocclusion. Cephalometric analyses use skeletal, dental, and soft-tissue anatomic landmarks (Fig. 7.7 and Box 7.1) to delineate lines, planes, angles, and distances that form the basis to classify craniofacial morphology. At the beginning of treatment, these measurements are compared with an established standard or norm; during treatment, the measurements are compared with measurements from previous cephalometric radiographs of the same patient to monitor growth and treatment-associated changes.

Cephalometric analyses were initially performed by manually marking and drawing landmarks onto a sheet of acetate tracing paper placed over an illuminated cephalometric radiograph on a view box. Computer-assisted applications for cephalometric analyses provide automated landmark identification and decrease personnel time needed for cephalometric tracing. Augmented intelligence-based programs for fully automated cephalometric analyses are also available. These systems can identify landmarks and perform cephalometric tracing and analyses of two-dimensional cephalometric radiographs within few minutes (Figs. 7.7 and 7.8).

HAND-WRIST RADIOGRAPHY

Skeletal age or bone age is a measure of biologic maturation in the growing child, and is frequently performed to evaluate growth in pediatric patients with endocrine disturbances. This is usually accomplished by evaluation of skeletal maturity indicators on hand-wrist radiographs and is a more reliable marker for maturation than chronologic age, height, dental development and eruption, and pubertal markers. During adolescence, there is a spurt in facial growth. Prediction of the timing and duration of this growth spurt is an important consideration in planning orthodontic and orthognathic surgical approaches. Although not necessary routinely, hand-wrist projections are occasionally used to predict timing of growth for individual patients undergoing orthodontic treatment.

Hand-Wrist Projection

Indications

Assess skeletal maturation to predict intensity and duration of facial growth for planning orthodontic treatment and orthognathic surgery.

Image Receptor and Patient Placement

A cephalometric x-ray device can be used to make a hand-wrist radiograph. By convention, the left hand is imaged. The hand is positioned flat on the receptor, with the digits, palm, and wrist touching the receptor. The individual digits are separated and the thumb is positioned away from the palm to facilitate viewing the sesamoid bone.

Position of the Central X-Ray Beam

The central beam is perpendicular to the image receptor, directed from dorsal to palmar surface, and centered on the third metacarpal.

Resultant Image (Fig. 7.9)

The image should encompass all phalanges and metacarpals, the carpal bones and the distal ulna and radius.

Radiologic Evaluation

To assess skeletal age, the patient's radiograph is compared with established standards. The Greulich–Pyle Atlas and Tanner Whitehouse method are two commonly used standards. For practical application in orthodontic treatment planning, the assessment may simply focus on the maturation events relative to the timing of the growth spurt and its completion (Fig. 7.10). Importantly, these methods were developed in predominantly White populations, and its application to different populations should be used with caution.

PROJECTION SKULL RADIOGRAPHY

Submentovertex (Base) Projection

Indications

Submentovertex (SMV) radiographs display the base of the skull, the zygomatic arches, and the sphenoid sinuses and are indicated to:

- Demonstrate osseous changes from skull base tumors.
- Fractures of the zygomatic arches.
- Evaluate integrity and aeration of the sphenoid sinuses.

In contemporary practice, these imaging indications are largely achieved by CT decreasing the application of the SMV projection (see Chapter 9).

Image Receptor and Patient Placement (Fig. 7.11)

The patient is positioned with the neck extended as far back as possible. The image receptor is positioned parallel to the Frankfort plane and perpendicular to the midsagittal and coronal planes.

Position of the Central X-Ray Beam (Fig. 7.11)

The central beam is perpendicular to the image receptor, directed from below the mandible toward the vertex of the skull (hence the name SMV) and centered about 2 cm anterior to a line connecting the right and left condyles. The source-to-receptor distance is 100 cm.

Resultant Image (Fig. 7.12)

The midsagittal plane is projected vertical, represented by an imaginary line extending from the interproximal space between the maxillary central incisors through the nasal septum to the middle of the anterior arch of the atlas and to the dens. The midsagittal plane should divide the image into two symmetric halves. The buccal and lingual cortical plates of the mandible should be projected as uniform opaque lines and the middle cranial base is projected posterior to the hard palate.

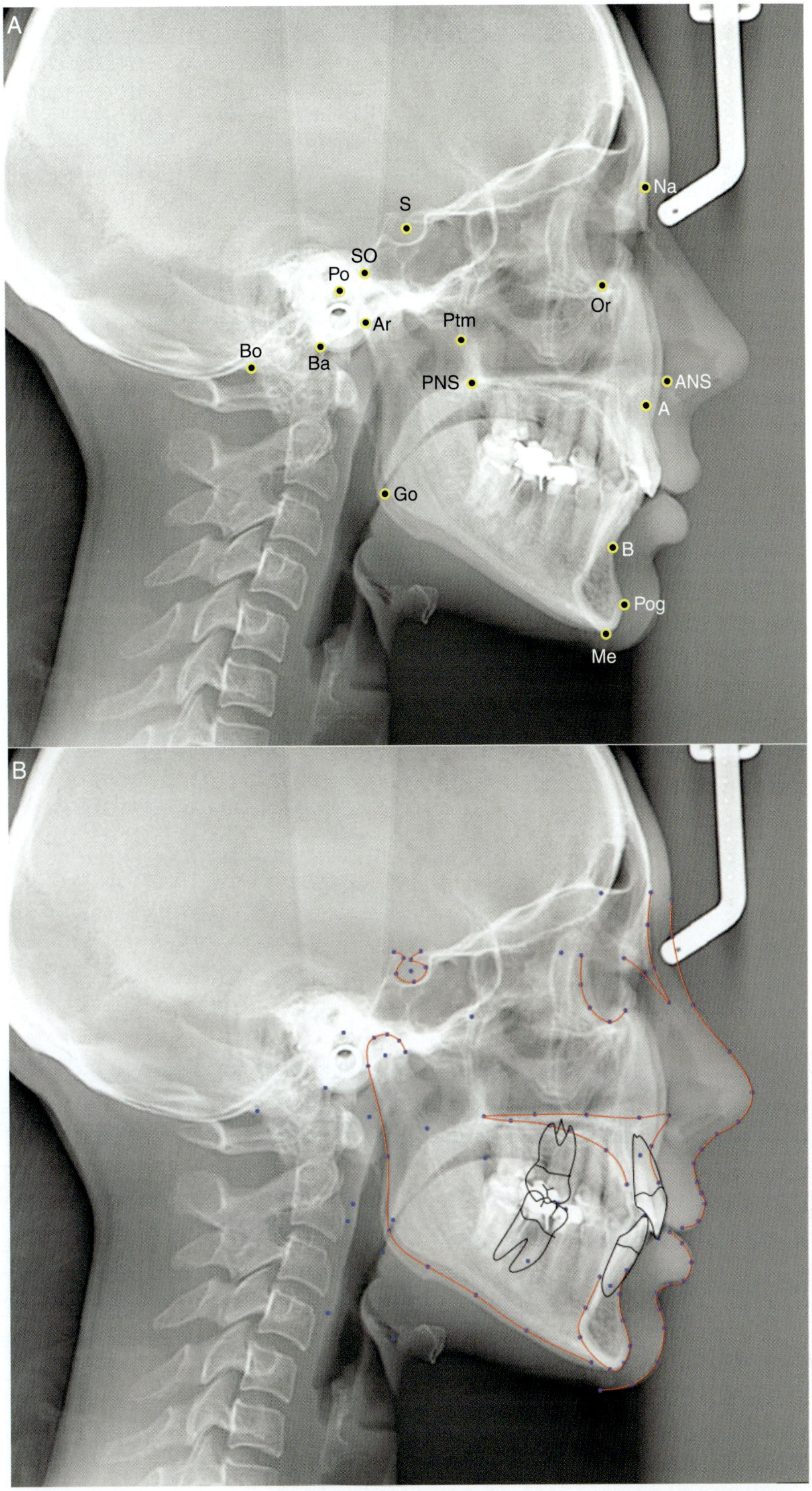

Fig. 7.7 (A) Basic landmarks identified on a lateral cephalometric radiograph. See Box 7.1 for definitions of the landmarks. (B) Computer-assisted automated tracing of a lateral cephalometric radiograph. The system automatically identifies landmarks and traces the contours of the soft tissues and relevant bones and allows for manual adjustment. The radiograph used in this figure is the same as Fig. 7.4.

BOX 7.1 Definition of Cephalometric Landmarks

Bo: Bolton point, the highest point in the upward curvature of the retrocondylar fossa of the occipital bone

Ba: Basion, the lowest point on the anterior margin of the foramen magnum

Ar: Articulare, point of intersection between the shadow of the zygomatic arch and the posterior border of the mandibular ramus

Po: Porion, the midpoint of the upper contour of the external auditory canal

SO: Spheno-occipital synchondrosis

S: Sella, the midpoint of the cavity of sella turcica

Ptm: Point at the base of the pterygomaxillary fissure where the anterior and posterior walls meet

Or: Orbitale, the lowest point on the inferior margin of the orbit

N: Nasion, the most anterior point of the nasofrontal suture

ANS: Anterior nasal spine, the most anterior point of the premaxilla

PNS: Posterior nasal spine, the most posterior point on the horizontal plate of the palatine bone

Point A: Innermost point on the contour of the premaxilla between anterior nasal spine and the maxillary incisor

Point B: Innermost point on the contour of the mandible between the mandibular incisor and the mandibular symphysis

Pog: Pogonion, the most anterior point on the contour of the mandibular symphysis

Me: Menton, the most inferior point on the mandibular symphysis

Go: Gonion, the midpoint of the contour connecting the ramus and body of the mandible

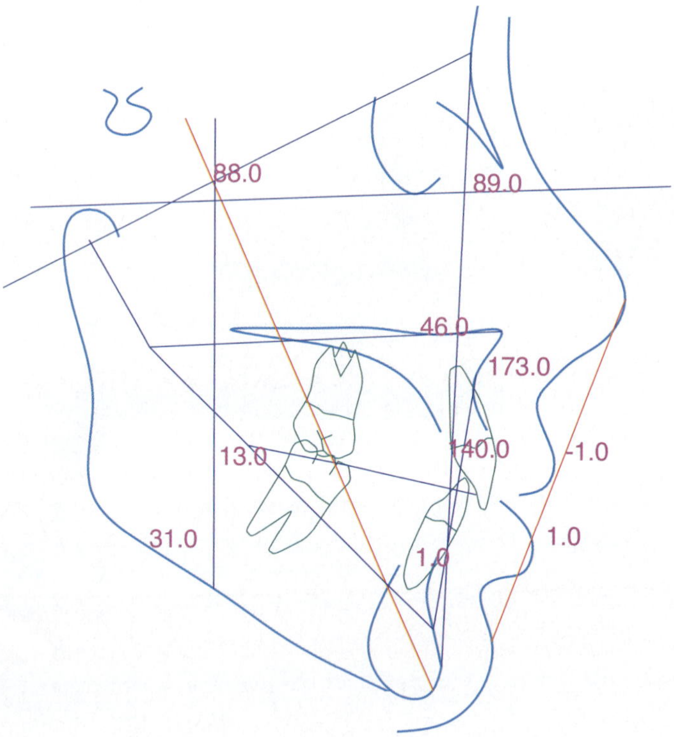

Descriptor	Meas.	Type	Mean	Sd	Patient	Graph	Comment
MAX. POSITION							
MAX DEPTH	FH to N-A	Deg	95.0	5.0	88.88	-(*I)+	Maxilla distal to Base
MAX HEIGHT	N-PTV to A pt	Deg	54.0	5.0	61.64	-(I*)+	Large Max height
SN TO PALATAL PLANE		Deg	3.0	5.0	10.49	-(I*)+	
MAND. POSITION							
FACIAL DEPTH	FH to N-Pog	Deg	90.0	4.0	85.37	-(*I)+	Retrognathic Mandible
FACIAL AXIS	Na-Ba to PTV-Gn pt	Deg	90.0	4.0	88.33	-(*)+	
FACIAL TAPER	Na-Gn-Go	Deg	67.0	4.0	64.51	-(*)+	
MAND. PLANE	FH-GoGn	Deg	28.0	3.0	30.81	-(*)+	
CORPUS LENGTH	Xi to Pm	mm	70.0	5.0	71.97	-(*)+	
MAND. ARC	DC-Xi to Xi-Pm	Deg	27.0	5.0	15.83	-(* I)+	Closed Arc
MAX.TO MAND RELATIONSHIP							
A pt. CONVEXITY	A to N-Pog	mm	3.0	2.0	3.5	-(*)+	
LOW.FACE.HEIGHT	ANS-Xi-Pog	Deg	47.0	5.0	46.46	-(*)+	
DENTURE RELATIONSHIP							
MAX.1 to APo		mm	6.0	3.0	4.68	-(*)+	
MAX.6 to PTV		mm	12.0		12.85	-( )+	
MAND. 1 to APo		mm	1.0	2.0	0.25	-(*)+	
HINGE AXIS ANGLE	DC - Go - LI	Deg	90.0	3.0	88.05	-(*)+	
MAX.1 to MAND.1		Deg	131.0	5.0	140.1	-(I*)+	Incisors too vertical
OVERJET		mm	2.5	2.0	3.74	-(*)+	
OVERBITE		mm	2.5	2.0	5.95	-(I*)+	
ESTHETICS							
UPPER LIP to E-LINE		mm	-4.0	2.0	-1.5	-(I*)+	Upper lip protruded
LOWER LIP to E-LINE		mm	-2.0	2.0	0.81	-(I*)+	Lower lip protruded

Fig. 7.8 Sample cephalometric analysis. Cephalometric tracings and Rickett's analysis were done using CephX, an artificial intelligence-based program. The radiograph in Fig. 7.4 was used for this analysis.

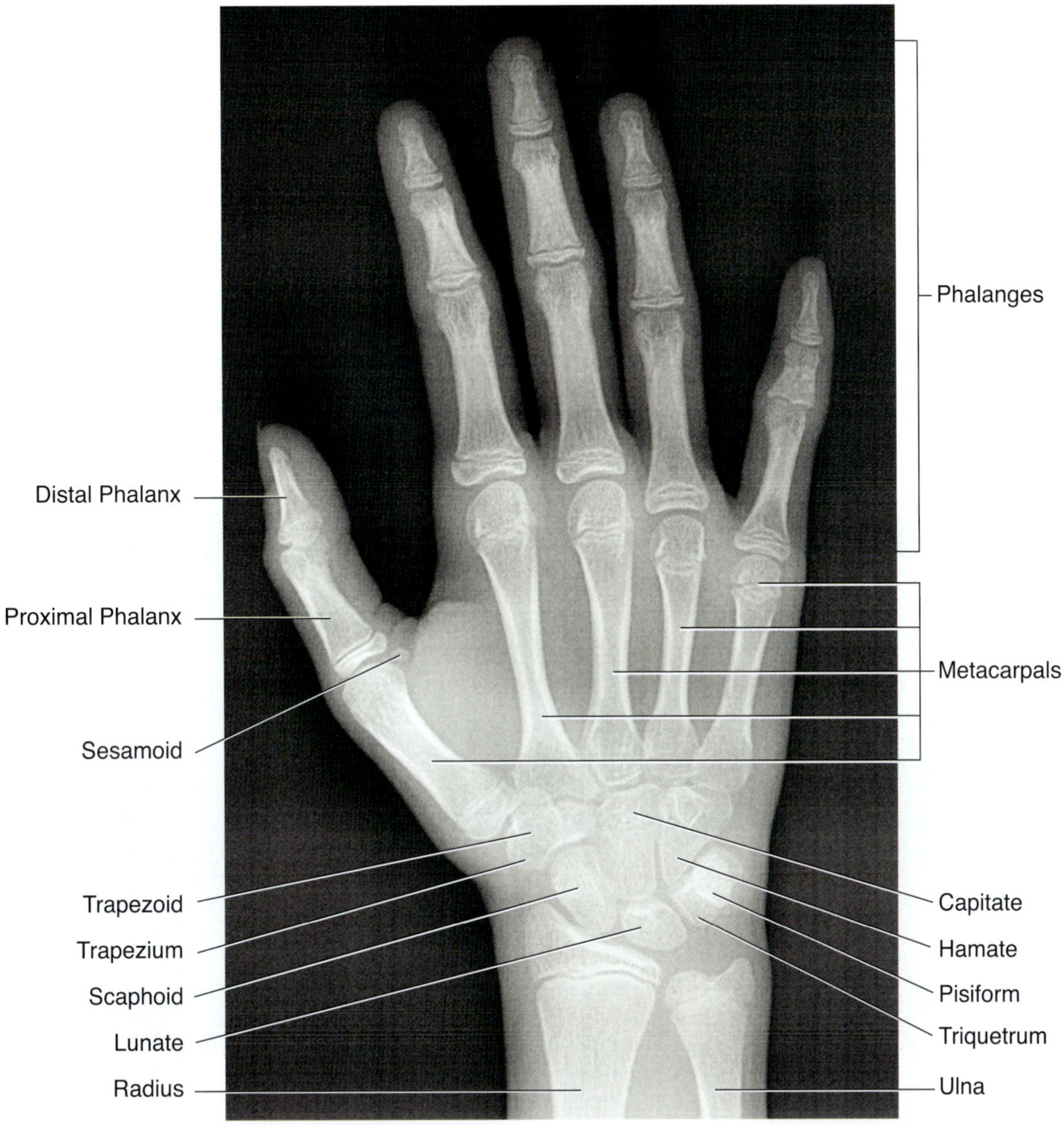

Fig. 7.9 Bones of the hand and wrist. Analysis of skeletal maturity indicators (see Fig. 7.10) indicates that the patient is at the peak of the growth phase.

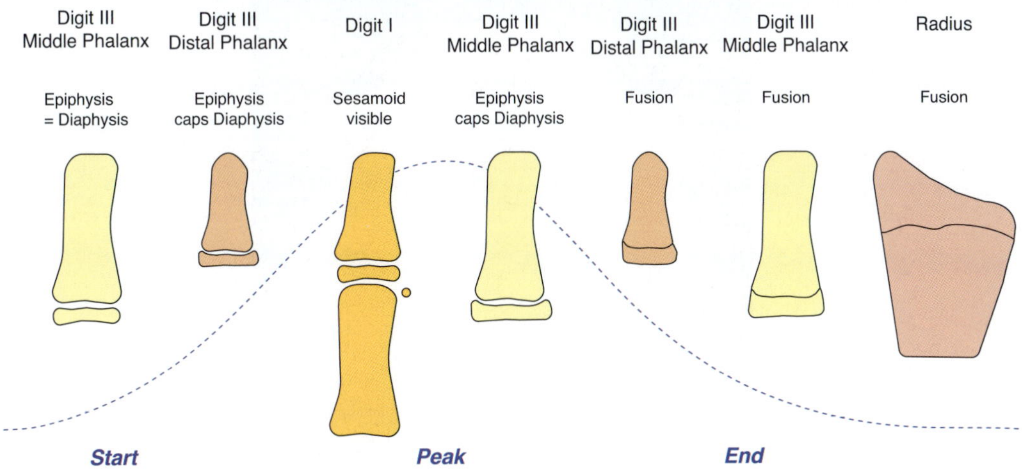

Fig. 7.10 Simple approach to assess skeletal growth analysis based on maturation events in select phalanges and the radius. The sequence of events is graphically represented superimposed over the growth spurt period. Analysis of these maturity indicators on the hand-wrist radiograph in Fig. 7.9 indicates that the patient is at the peak of the growth phase. (Based on Fishman LS. Radiographic evaluation of skeletal maturation: a clinically oriented method based on hand-wrist films. *Angle Orthod.* 1982;52(2):88-112.)

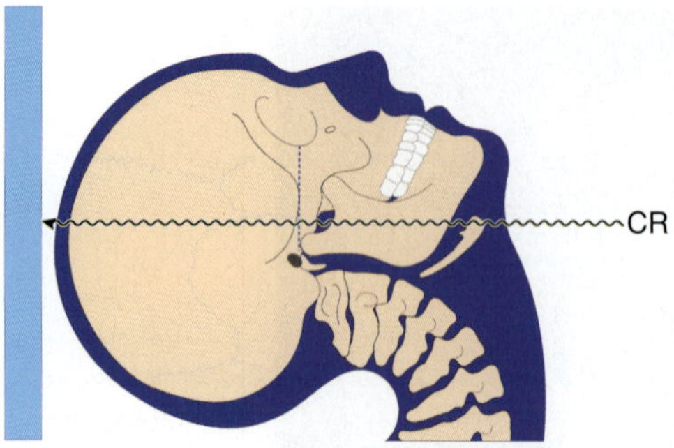

Fig. 7.11 Patient position for submentovertex projection. The patient's head is extended backward until the canthomeatal line is parallel to the receptor and the midsagittal plane is vertical. The entry and direction of the central ray (CR) is shown.

When made to evaluate the zygomatic arches, the x-ray beam intensity is markedly decreased to allow depiction of the zygomatic arches that are projected on either side of the maxilla, termed "jug handle" view. The decreased x-ray intensity underexposes the cranial base and these structures appear radiopaque.

Interpretation

When exposed for the skull base, identify the petrous ridges of the temporal bone and the mastoid air cells. The foramen ovale, foramen spinosum, and carotid canal can be viewed, bilaterally. Assess symmetry. The sphenoid sinus and ethmoid air cells are also visible. When exposed for the zygomatic arches, the skull base is opaque and the zygomatic arches on either side are seen contrasted against the radiolucent infratemporal fossa. The two arches appear as handles, and thus the colloquial term "jug handle" view for this projection.

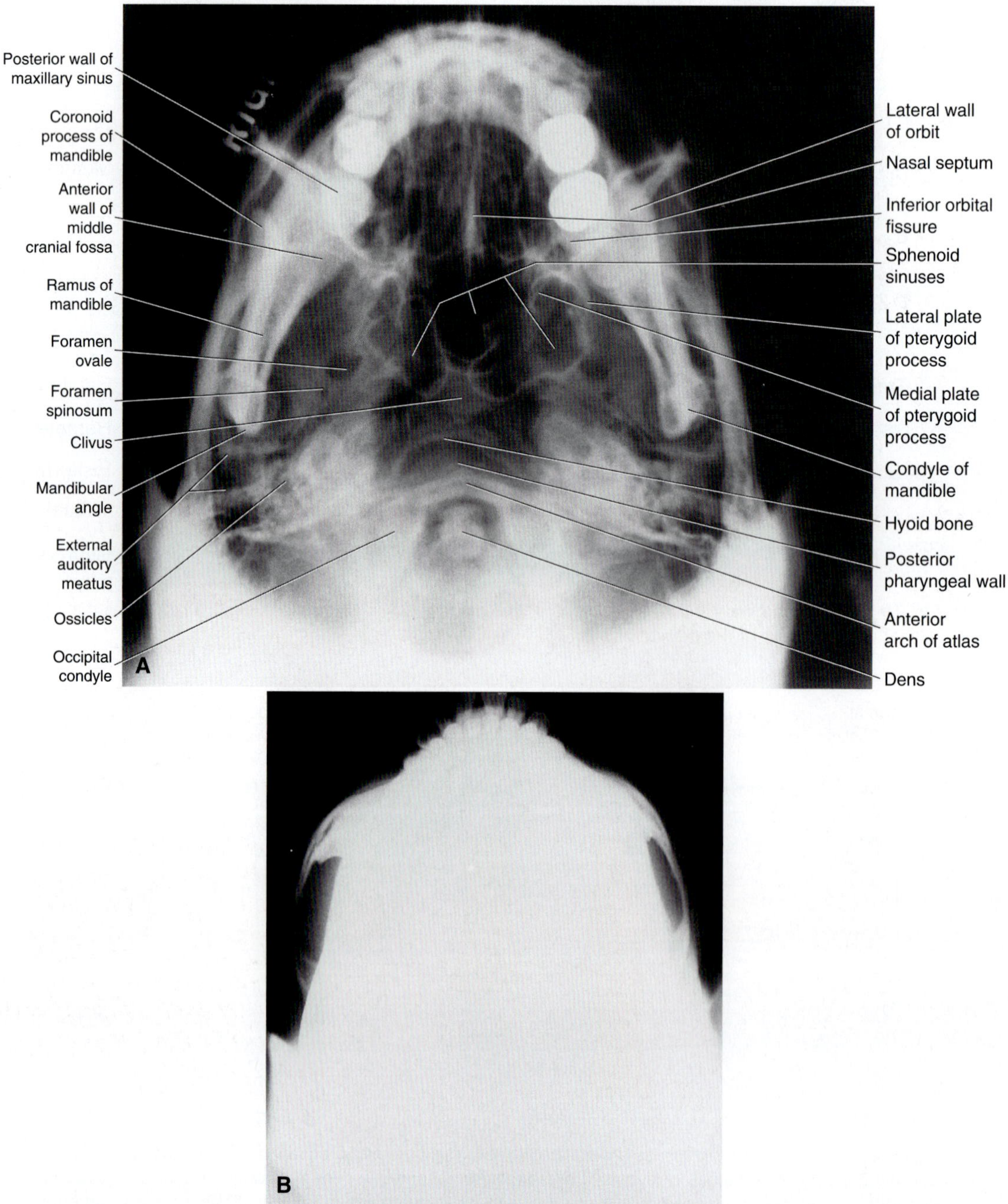

Fig. 7.12 (A) Anatomic landmarks identified in the submentovertex projection. (B) Underexposed submentovertex view reveals the zygomatic arches.

Waters Projection

Indications

The Waters projection, also referred to as the occipitomental projection, displays the paranasal sinuses, predominantly the maxillary sinus and to a lesser extent the frontal sinus and ethmoid air cells. It also demonstrates the midfacial bones and orbits (Fig. 7.9). A Waters projection is indicated to:

- Evaluate paranasal sinuses, in particular, the maxillary, ethmoid, and frontal sinuses.
- Evaluate midfacial fractures, in particular tripod and Le Fort fractures.

In contemporary practice, these diagnostic objectives are better accomplished by CT (see Chapter 9). Thus, the American College of Radiology Appropriateness Criteria considers that the Waters projection is usually not appropriate for the evaluation of trauma, orbits, and sinonasal disease.

Image Receptor and Patient Placement (Fig. 7.13)

The image receptor is placed in front of the patient and perpendicular to the midsagittal plane. The patient's head is tilted upward so that the canthomeatal line forms a 37-degree angle with the image receptor. This can be accomplished with the chin touching the receptor and the tip of the nose approximately 1–1.5 cm away from the receptor. If the patient's mouth is open, the sphenoid sinus is seen superimposed over the palate.

Position of the Central X-Ray Beam (Fig. 7.13)

The central beam is perpendicular to the image receptor and directed from the occipital bone toward the mental region of the mandible (hence the term occipitomental) and centered over the maxillary sinuses. The source-to-receptor distance is 100 cm.

Resultant Image (Fig. 7.14)

The Waters view is an inclined PA projection. Anterior structures are projected with less magnification and are projected higher relative to more posterior structures. The midsagittal plane (represented by an imaginary line extending from the interproximal space of the maxillary central incisors through the nasal septum and the middle of the bridge of the nose) should divide the skull image into two symmetric halves. The petrous ridge of the temporal bone should be projected below the floor of the maxillary sinus. The orbital floor and the orbital rim are depicted as two sharp radiopaque lines, with the orbital rim projected higher.

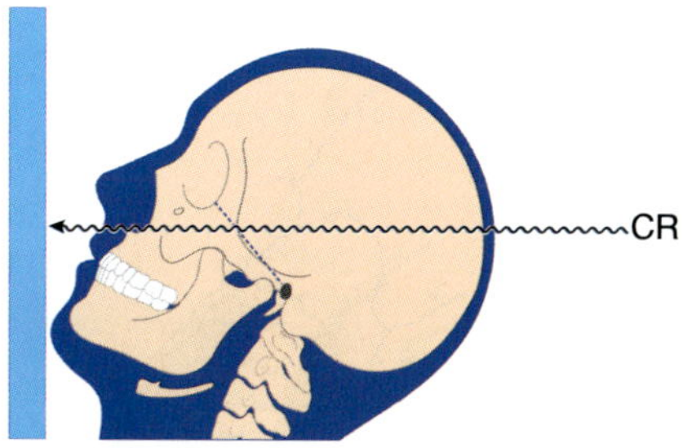

Fig. 7.13 Patient position for Waters projection. The patient's head is extended upward with the canthomeatal line forming an angle of 37 degrees with the receptor and the midsagittal plane is vertical. The entry and direction of the central ray (CR) is shown.

Reverse Towne Projection (Open Mouth)

Indications

The reverse Towne projection is used to evaluate patients with suspected fractures of the condyle and condylar neck. In contemporary practice, radiologic evaluation of maxillofacial trauma is best achieved by CT (see Chapter 9), decreasing the application of the reverse Towne projection.

Image Receptor and Patient Placement (Fig. 7.15)

The image receptor is placed in front of the patient, perpendicular to the midsagittal plane. The patient's head is tilted downward so

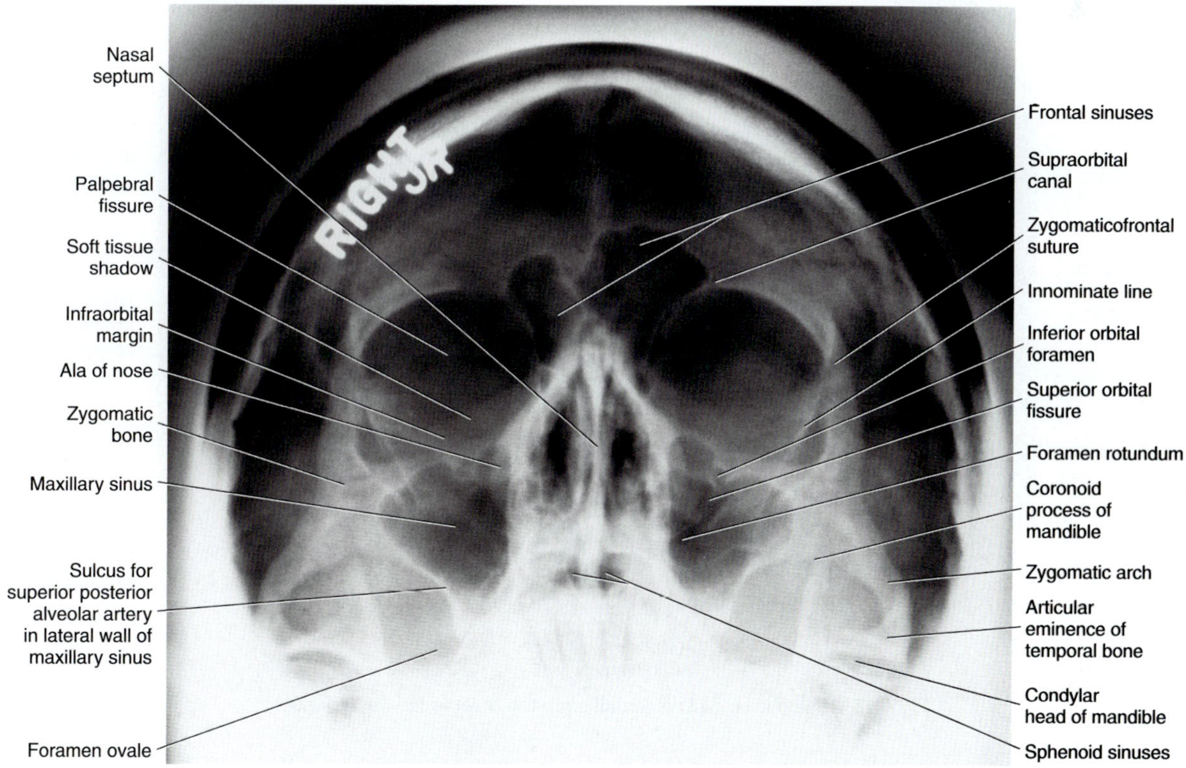

Fig. 7.14 Anatomic landmarks identified in the Waters view.

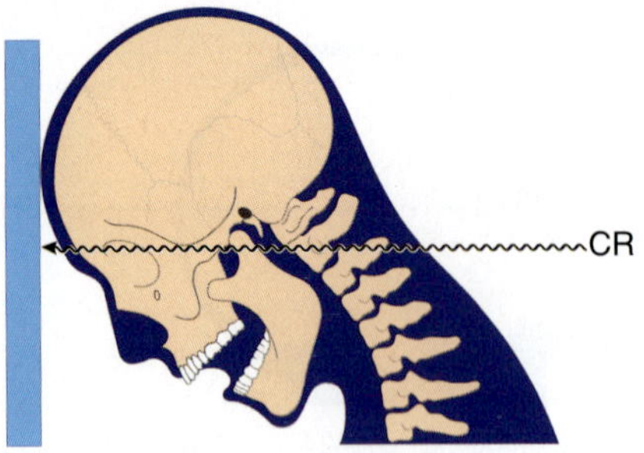

Fig. 7.15 Patient position for reverse Towne's projection. The patient's head is tipped downward with the canthomeatal line forming an angle of 30 degrees with the receptor. The midsagittal plane is vertical and the mouth is open. The entry and direction of the central ray (CR) is shown.

that the canthomeatal line forms a 30-degree angle with the image receptor. To improve the visibility of the condyles, the patient's mouth is opened so that the condylar heads are located inferior to the articular eminence. When requesting this image to evaluate the condyles, it is necessary to specify "open-mouth reverse Towne" to distinguish it from the standard Towne view of the occiput.

Position of Central X-Ray Beam (Fig. 7.15)

The central beam is perpendicular to the image receptor and through the patient's midsagittal plane; it is centered at the level of the condyles. The source-to-receptor distance is 100 cm.

Resultant Image (Fig. 7.16)

The midsagittal plane (represented by an imaginary line extending from the middle of the foramen magnum and the posterior arch

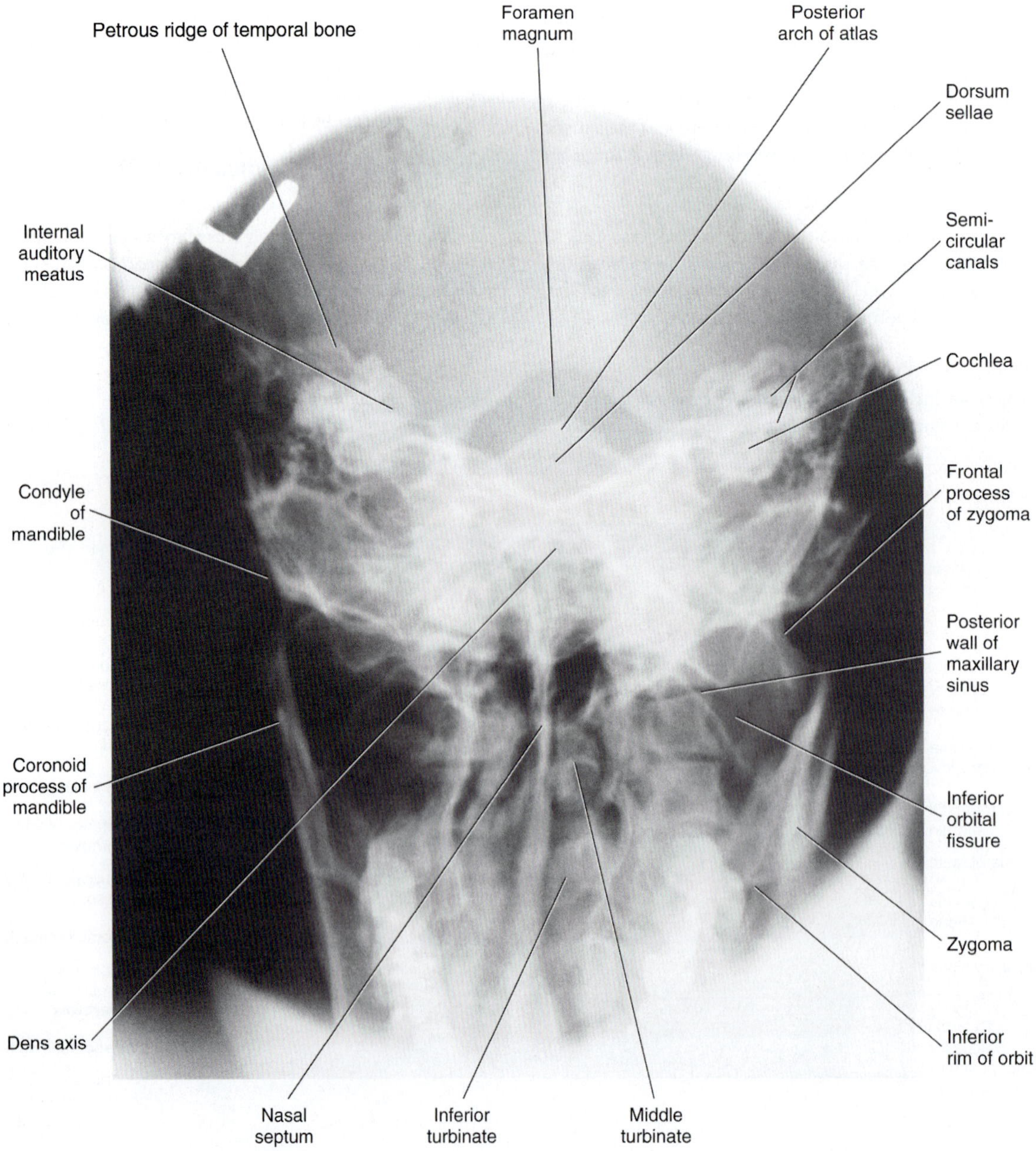

Fig. 7.16 Anatomic landmarks identified in the reverse Towne projection.

of the atlas through the middle of the bridge of the nose and the nasal septum) should divide the skull image in two symmetric halves. The petrous ridge of the temporal bone should be superimposed at the inferior part of the occipital bone, and the condylar heads should be projected inferior to the articular eminence. The condylar necks will appear elongated. This projection depicts fractures of the condylar head and neck and provides information of the mediolateral displacement of the fractured fragment.

BIBLIOGRAPHY

American College of Radiology. Appropriateness Criteria. https://acsearch.acr.org/list.

Broadbent BH. A new x-ray technique and its application to orthodontia. *Angle Orthod.* 1931;1:45-66.

Fishman LS. Radiographic evaluation of skeletal maturation: a clinically oriented method based on hand-wrist films. *Angle Orthod.* 1982;52(2):88-112.

Greulich WW, Pyle SI. *Radiographic Atlas of Skeletal Development of the Hand and Wrist.* 2nd ed. Stanford University Press; 1959.

Hofrath H. Die Bedeutung der Röntgenfern-und Abstandsaufnahme für die Diagnostik der Kieferanomalien. *Fortschritte der Orthodontik in Theorie und Praxis.* 1931;1:232-258.

Jacobson A, Jacobson RL. Radiographic Cephalometry: From Basics to 3D Imaging. Quintessence Publishing; 2007.

Kantor ML, Norton LA. Normal radiographic anatomy and common anomalies seen in cephalometric films. *Am J Orthod Dentofacial Orthop.* 1987;91:414-426.

Keats TE, Anderson MW. *Atlas of Normal Roentgen Variants That May Simulate Disease.* 9th ed. Mosby; 2012.

Miyashita K. *Contemporary Cephalometric Radiography.* Quintessence Publishing Co; 1996.

Proffit WR, Fields HW, Larson B, Sarver DM. *Contemporary Orthodontics.* 6th ed. Elsevier; 2018.

Rollins JH, Long BW, Curtis T. *Merrill's Atlas of Radiographic Positions and Radiologic Procedures.* Vol. 2. 15th ed. Mosby; 2023.

8

Panoramic Imaging

Aruna Ramesh and Sanjay M. Mallya

To access the videos in this chapter, please visit ebooks.health.elsevier.com.

Panoramic radiography (also called *pantomography*) is a body section imaging technique that results in a wide, curved image layer, depicting the maxillary and mandibular dental arches and their supporting structures (Fig. 8.1). This is achieved by using a single rotation of the x-ray source and image receptor around the patient's head (Fig. 8.2). Panoramic images are most useful for diagnostic challenges requiring broad coverage of the jaws (Box 8.1). Common clinical applications include evaluation of trauma including jaw fractures, location of third molars, extensive dental or osseous disease, known or suspected large lesions, tooth development and eruption (especially in the mixed dentition), impacted or unerupted teeth and root remnants (in edentulous patients), temporomandibular joint (TMJ) pain, and developmental anomalies. Panoramic imaging is often used in initial patient evaluation that can provide the required insight or assist in determining the need for other projections. Panoramic images are also useful for patients who do not tolerate intraoral procedures well.

The main disadvantage of panoramic radiography is the lack of fine anatomic detail available on intraoral periapical radiographs. Thus it is not as useful as periapical radiography for detecting small carious lesions, fine structure of the marginal periodontium, or early periapical disease. The availability of a panoramic radiograph for an adult patient often does not preclude the need for intraoral films for the diagnoses of most commonly encountered dental diseases. When a full-mouth series of radiographs is available for a patient requiring only general dental care, typically little or no additional useful information is gained from a simultaneous panoramic examination. A panoramic combined with bitewings or with a combination of bitewings and selected periapical radiographs could provide diagnostic information similar to a full-mouth series. Other problems associated with panoramic radiography include unequal magnification and geometric distortion across the image. Occasionally, the presence of overlapping structures, such as the cervical spine, can hide odontogenic lesions, particularly in the incisor regions. Clinically important objects may be situated outside the focal trough and may appear distorted or not be seen at all.

PRINCIPLES OF PANORAMIC IMAGE FORMATION

The principles of panoramic radiography were first described by Paatero and Numata independently in 1948 and 1933, respectively. Fig. 8.2 shows a schematic view of the relationships between the x-ray source, the patient, the secondary collimator, and the image receptor during panoramic image formation. The following illustrations explain the formation of the *focal trough* in a panoramic machine. Imagine an assembly containing a disk with upright physical objects (represented by letters) and an image receptor (Fig. 8.3). The receptor travels upward through the beam at the same speed as objects *A–C* rotate through the beam. A lead collimator in the shape of a slit located at the x-ray source limits the x-rays to a narrow vertical beam. Another collimator between the objects and the image receptor reduces scattered radiation from the objects to the image receptor. Consider first radiopaque objects *A–C*. As the disk rotates, their radiographic images are recorded sharply on the receptor that also moves through the beam at the same direction and speed. The spatial relationship of the shadows of these objects correctly represents the relationship of the actual objects. Because the source-receptor distance is constant and the object-receptor distance is the same for each object, all objects are magnified equally. Now consider objects *D–F*. They are located on the opposite side of the disk, between the x-ray source and the center of rotation of the disk. These objects move in the opposite direction of the receptor, so their shadows are reversed on the receptor. Because these objects are much closer to the x-ray source, their images are greatly magnified.

Fig. 8.4 shows that the same relationship between the rotating receptor and objects can be achieved if the disk is held stationary but the x-ray source and the receptor are rotated around the center of rotation in the disk. The x-ray beam still passes through the center of the disk and sequentially through objects *A–C*. Similarly, the receptor is still moved through the beam and at the same rate as the beam passes through *A–C*. In this situation, as before, objects *A–C* move through the x-ray beam in the same direction and at the same rate as the receptor. Objects *D–F* continue to be blurred, just as before.

Fig. 8.5 shows that a patient may replace the disk and objects *A–F* represent teeth and surrounding bone. The illustration demonstrates the positions of the x-ray source and the receptor early in an exposure cycle. The center of rotation is located off to the side of the arch, away from the objects being imaged. The rate of movement of the receptor is regulated to be the same as that of the x-ray beam sweeping through the dentoalveolar structures on the side of the patient nearest the receptor. Structures on the opposite side of the patient (near the x-ray tube) are distorted and appear out of focus because the x-ray beam sweeps through them in the direction opposite that in which the image receptor is moving. In addition, structures near the x-ray source are so magnified (and their borders so blurred) that they are not seen as discrete images on the resultant image. These structures appear only as diffuse phantom or ghost images. Because of both of these circumstances, only structures near the receptor are usefully captured on the resultant image.

Contemporary panoramic machines use a continuously moving center of rotation rather than multiple fixed locations (Fig. 8.6). This feature optimizes the shape of the focal trough to clearly image the teeth and supporting bone. This center of rotation is initially near the lingual surface of the right body of the mandible when the left TMJ region is being imaged. The rotational center moves anteriorly along an arc that ends just lingual to the symphysis of the mandible when the midline is imaged. The arc is reversed as the opposite side of the jaws is imaged.

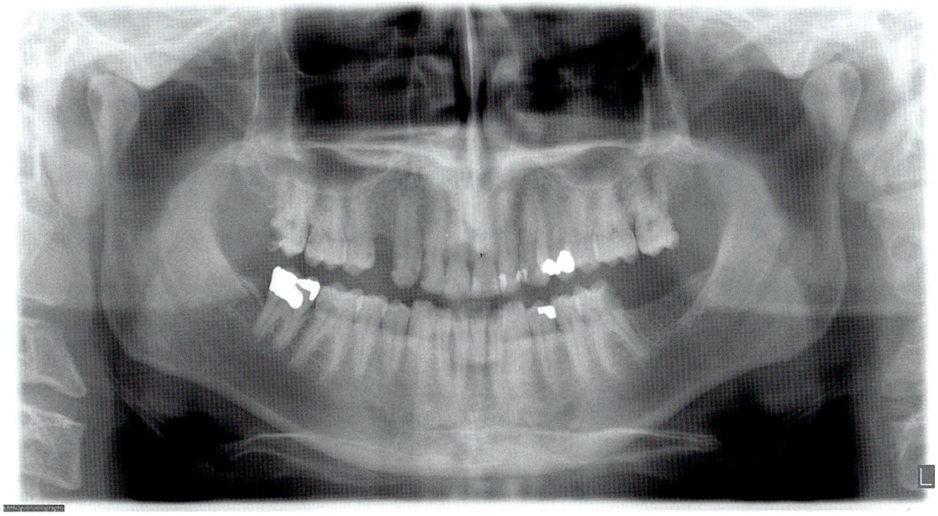

Fig. 8.1 Panoramic image demonstrating broad coverage of hard and soft tissues of adult orofacial region including maxilla, mandible, dentition, and adjacent structures. Panoramic images are made with a much lower dose than a full-mouth set and have broader coverage; however, they have lower spatial resolution.

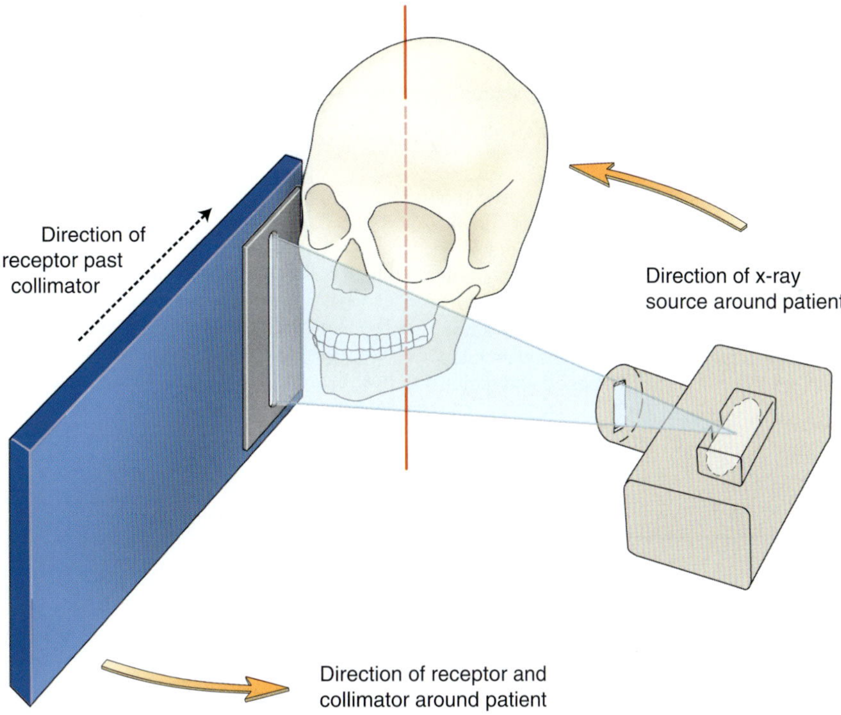

Fig. 8.2 Schematic view of relationships between the x-ray source, the patient, the secondary collimator, and image receptor. As the x-ray tube head moves around one side of the patient, the receptor assembly moves toward the opposite side. The image receptor slides past the collimator, sequentially producing a latent image. With a charge-coupled device (CCD) image receptor, there is a vertical CCD linear array behind the collimator that continuously reads out the exposure to produce an image.

This basic principle of image formation remains the same, regardless of the type of detector used to record the image. In the case where the receptor is a charge-coupled device (CCD) array, the film is replaced by a two-dimensional CCD array. Each column of the array is read out to construct the image. The key is to read out the columns at the same rate as an imaginary moving film would move past the array. The CCD array is read out continuously as the x-ray source and receptor travel around the patient. The resulting geometric projection characteristics are the same as in film or photostimulable phosphor (PSP) plate imaging.

Focal Trough (Image Layer)

The focal trough or image layer is a wide, three-dimensional curved zone, where the structures positioned within this zone are reasonably

BOX 8.1 Panoramic Imaging

Indications
- Overall evaluation of dentition
- Examine for intraosseous pathology, such as cysts, tumors, or infections
- Gross evaluation of temporomandibular joints
- Evaluation of position of impacted teeth
- Evaluation of eruption of permanent dentition
- Dentomaxillofacial trauma
- Developmental disturbances of maxillofacial skeleton

Advantages Compared to a Full-Mouth Examination
- Broad coverage of facial bones and teeth
- Low radiation dose
- Ease of panoramic radiographic technique
- Can be used in patients with trismus or in patients who cannot tolerate intraoral radiography
- Quick and convenient radiographic technique
- Useful visual aid in patient education and case presentation

Disadvantages
- Lower-resolution images that do not provide the fine details provided by intraoral radiographs
- Magnification across image is unequal, making linear measurements unreliable
- Image is superimposition of real, double, and ghost images and requires careful visualization to decipher anatomic and pathologic details
- Requires accurate patient positioning to avoid positioning errors and artifacts
- Difficult to image both jaws when patient has severe maxillomandibular discrepancy

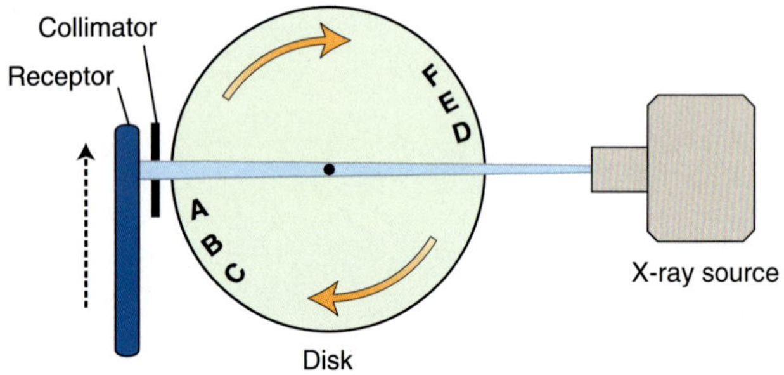

Fig. 8.3 Producing a panoramic image: In this conceptual view, the x-ray source and collimator are held stationary. The receptor moves through the beam, and the rotating disk also carries objects *A–F* through the beam. Objects *A–C* move through the beam at the same rate and direction as the image receptor and are imaged well. Objects *D–F* move through the beam at the same rate as the receptor but in the opposite direction, and so their images are blurred. The principles of panoramic image formation are the same for film-based and digital systems.

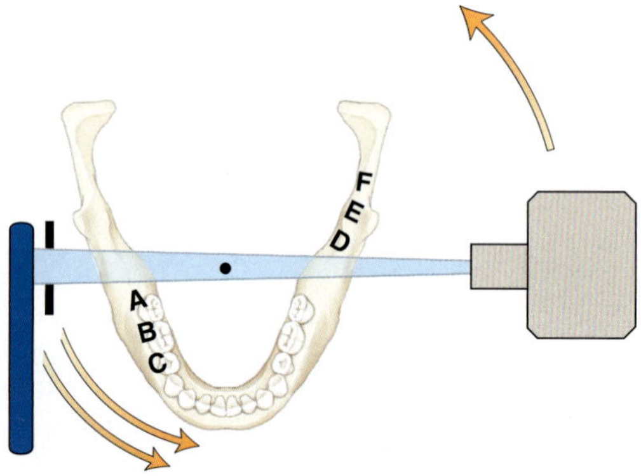

Fig. 8.5 Producing a panoramic image: The imaging geometry is the same as Figs. 8.3 and 8.4, but the disk and objects are replaced with a patient. The rate the receptor moves through the beam is the same as the rate the beam passes through objects *A–C*; thus only the dentition in the mandible near the receptor (objects *A–C*) is imaged well. Structures on the opposite side of the mandible (objects *D–F*) are blurred beyond recognition.

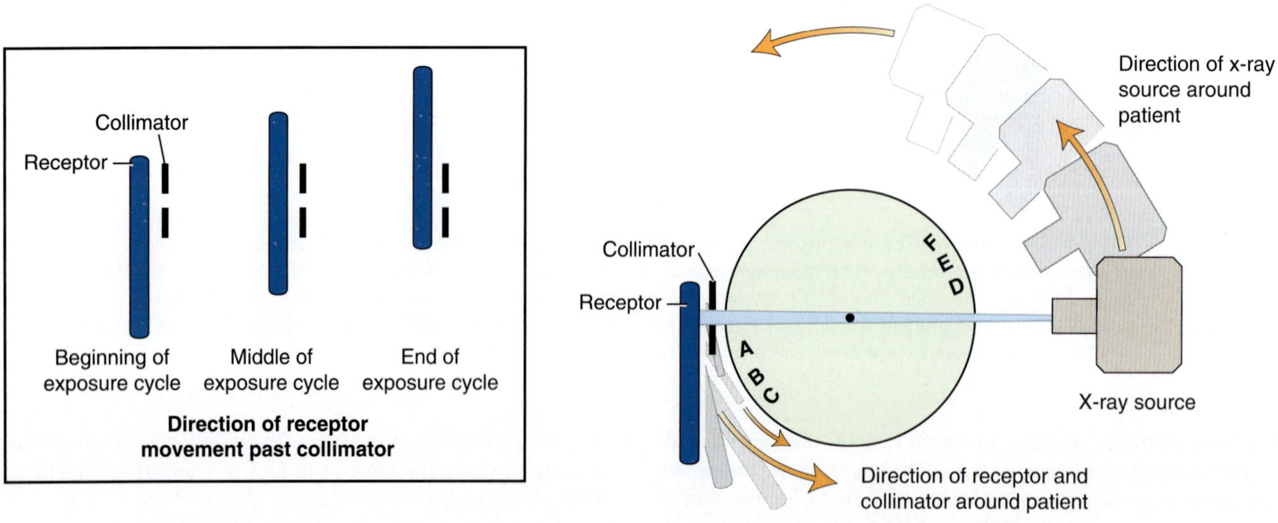

Fig. 8.4 Producing a panoramic image: The disk is held stationary while the x-ray source, receptor, and collimator rotate around the center of the disk. Nonetheless, the x-ray beam still passes through the objects to the image receptor in the same direction as in Fig. 8.3, and the same imaging results are obtained. The *inset* emphasizes how the receptor moves past the collimator during their motion around the disk.

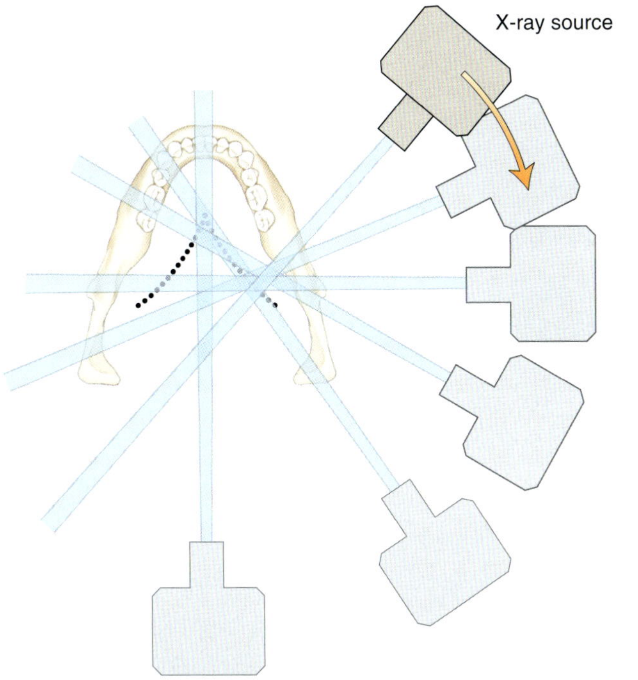

Fig. 8.6 Producing a panoramic image: In contrast to the preceding three schematic drawings shown in Figs. 8.3–8.5, the center of rotation of the x-ray source moves continuously as the tube and receptor rotate around the patient. Initially, the x-ray beam rotates on the end of the dotted arc on the tube side of the patient. As the x-ray source moves behind the patient, the center of rotation moves forward along the arc *(dotted line)*. The drawing shows the directions of the x-ray beam at various intervals for the first half of the exposure cycle. The x-ray source then continues to move around the patient to image the opposite side.

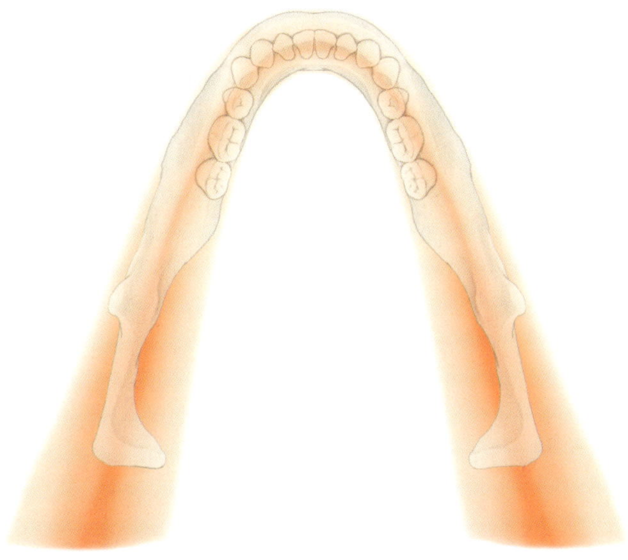

Fig. 8.7 Focal trough: The moving source and receptor generate a zone of sharpness, known as the focal trough or image layer. The closer an anatomic structure is positioned to the center of the trough, the more clearly it is imaged on the resulting radiograph. Panoramic machines typically provide laser lights to allow the operator to position the patient's dentition optimally in the focal trough.

well defined on the panoramic image (Fig. 8.7). The anatomic structures seen on a panoramic image are primarily those positioned within the focal trough during imaging. Structures positioned in the center of the focal trough are the clearest and those that are progressively farther from the center of the focal trough become progressively less clear. Objects outside the focal trough are blurred, magnified, or reduced in size and are sometimes distorted to the extent of not being recognizable. The shape of the focal trough varies with the brand of equipment used, as well as with the imaging protocol selected within each unit. The shape and width of the focal trough is determined by the path and velocity of the receptor and x-ray tube head, alignment of the x-ray beam, and collimator width. The location of the focal trough can change with extensive machine use, so recalibration may be necessary if consistently suboptimal images are being produced.

In some panoramic machines, the shape and size of the focal trough can be adjusted to conform better to the patients' maxillomandibular anatomy, allowing for better imaging of children, patients with atypical jaw morphology, or specific anatomic sites of interest such as the TMJ or the maxillary sinuses. This modification is achieved by decreasing the rotational arc of the x-ray source-receptor movement to reduce the focal trough size to better adapt to pediatric jaws. The decreased rotational arc also results in reduced patient radiation exposure. In some panoramic units, the projection angle of the x-ray beam is modified to yield images with decreased overlap of adjacent teeth and with minimal superimposition of structures from the opposite side of the jaw.

Real, Double, and Ghost Images

Because of the rotational nature of the x-ray source and receptor, the x-ray beam intercepts some anatomic structures twice during the single exposure cycle. Depending on their location, objects may cast three different types of images:

- *Real images:* Objects that lie between the center of rotation and the receptor form a real image. Within this zone, objects that lie within the focal trough cast relatively sharp images, whereas images of objects located outside the focal trough are blurred. Fig. 8.8A and C show the positions of the x-ray source during imaging of the left and right sides of the mandibular ramus, respectively. In Fig. 8.8A, the left ramus lies between the center of rotation and the receptor and casts a real image. Because it is within the focal trough, its image is sharp. Also demonstrated in Fig. 8.8A is the formation of the real images of the hyoid bone and cervical spine. However, because these structures are away from the center of the focal trough and closer to the x-ray source, their images are blurred and magnified. Fig. 8.8D shows in blue the anatomic region that makes real images.
- *Double images:* Objects that lie posterior to the center of rotation and that are intercepted twice by the x-ray beam form double images (green region in Fig. 8.8E). This region includes the hyoid bone, epiglottis, and cervical spine, all of which cast images on both the right and left side of the image.
- *Ghost images*: Some objects are located between the x-ray source and the center of rotation. These objects cast ghost images. On the panoramic image, ghost images appear on the opposite side of its true anatomic location and at a higher level because of the upward inclination of the x-ray beam. As the object is located outside of the focal plane and close to the x-ray source, the ghost image is blurred and significantly magnified. Several anatomic structures cast ghost images (orange region in Fig. 8.8F). For example, in Fig. 8.8A, the right mandibular ramus lies between the x-ray source and the center of rotation and its ghost image is superimposed over the left side of the image. Similarly, the ghost image of the left ramus is superimposed over the right side of the image (see Fig. 8.8C). The hyoid bone and cervical spine also form ghost images when the anterior regions of the jaws are imaged (see Fig. 8.8B). In addition, metallic accessories, such as earrings, necklaces, and hairpins, form ghost images, which appear as

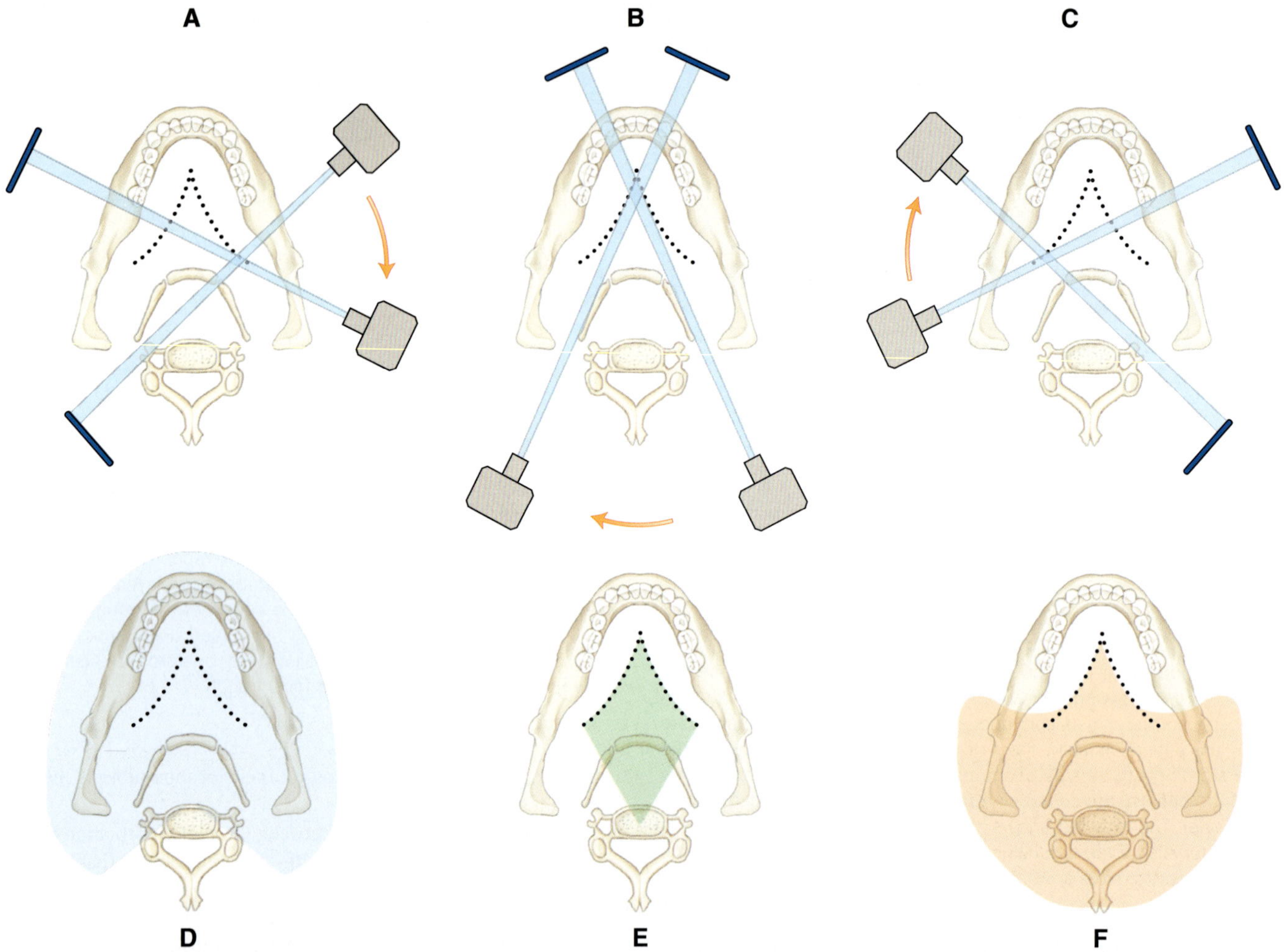

Fig. 8.8 Formation of real, double, and ghost images. (A–C) The exposure begins with the x-ray tube head on the patient's right side and continues with the tube head moving behind the patient and ending on the left side. The *dotted line* represents the path of the moving center of rotation during the exposure cycle. (D) Structures between the moving center of rotation and the receptor form real images *(blue zone)*. (E) Structures lying between the moving centers of rotation and the receptor that are imaged twice *(green zone)* cast double images. (F) Structures located between the x-ray source and moving center of rotation *(orange zone)* cast ghost images.

blurred radiopaque images that can obscure anatomic details, mask pathologic changes, or mimic pathologic changes. The ghost images of the hard palate and mandibular body and angle are clearly visualized in a panoramic image (Fig. 8.9). Some anatomic zones form both real double and ghost images. These zones are the regions of overlap between the orange and green regions in Fig. 8.8E and F.

Image Distortion

The panoramic image necessarily produces distortion of the size and shape of the object, making it unreliable for linear or angular measurements. The image distortion is influenced by several factors, including x-ray beam angulation, x-ray source-to-object distance, path of rotational center, and position of the object within the focal trough. These parameters vary among panoramic units and among different regions of the jaws for the same unit. They are also strongly dependent on patient anatomy and positioning of the patient in the unit. These variables make it impossible to apply preset magnification factors that can be used to make reliable measurements on panoramic radiographs.

Horizontal magnification is determined by the position of the object within the focal trough. The magnitude of the horizontal distortion depends on the distance of the object from the center of the focal trough and thus is strongly influenced by patient positioning. Fig. 8.10 illustrates the influence of anterior patient positioning on image size and shape. Fig. 8.10A and B show a mandible supporting a brass ring properly aligned in the center of the focal trough. A notched positioning device (bite-block) denotes the center of the anterior aspect of the focal trough. Note the even magnification of the ring and the images of the anterior teeth in proper proportion. Fig. 8.10C–E show the same mandible positioned 5 mm posterior to the center of the focal trough and a panoramic radiograph of a patient with the same error. This position causes distortion of the ring in the horizontal dimension, with the ring appearing broader with a commensurate increase in width of the images of the teeth. Fig. 8.10F–H show the same mandible positioned 5 mm anterior to the center of the focal trough and a panoramic radiograph of a patient with the same error. The horizontal distortion results in the ring appearing narrow with a commensurate decrease in width of the projected teeth. On these images, the vertical dimension, in contrast to the horizontal dimension, is little altered. These distortions result from the horizontal movements of the receptor and x-ray source. Thus, as a general rule, when the structure

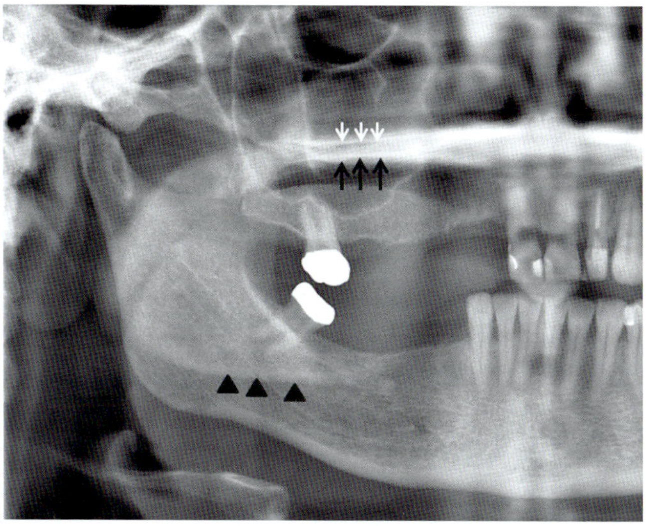

Fig. 8.9 Panoramic radiograph cropped to show the right posterior midfacial region. The hard palate appears as two radiopaque lines. The lower line *(black arrows)* represents the junction between the hard palate and lateral nasal wall on the receptor side of the patient. The upper line *(white arrows)* represents the junction between the nasal wall and hard palate on the tube side or ghost image of the opposite side. The *black arrowheads* indicate the ghost image of the opposite mandible.

of interest, in this case the mandible, is displaced to the lingual side of its optimal position in the focal trough, toward the x-ray source, the beam passes more slowly through it than the speed at which the receptor moves. Consequently, the images of the structures in this region are elongated horizontally on the image, and they appear wider. Alternatively, when the mandible is displaced toward the buccal aspect of the focal trough, the beam passes at a rate faster than normal through the structures. In the example shown, because the receptor is moving at the proper rate, the representations of the anterior teeth are compressed horizontally on the image, and they appear thinner.

The same principle applies to the patient's midsagittal plane being rotated in the focal trough. (Fig. 8.11A). The posterior structures on the side to which the patient's head is rotated are magnified in the horizontal dimension because the posterior structures are positioned away from the image receptor, whereas posterior structures on the opposite side are positioned closer to the image receptor and are reduced in horizontal dimension. The resulting image has horizontally (mesiodistally) large molar teeth and mandibular ramus and severe premolar overlap on one side and horizontally (mesiodistally) smaller molar teeth and mandibular ramus on the other side (this positioning artifact is demonstrated in Fig. 8.11B). This imaging appearance must not be confused with a congenital or developmental facial asymmetry.

The magnitude of horizontal distortion varies between the anterior and posterior regions of the jaws. In the anterior region, horizontal magnification increases markedly as the object moves away from the center of the focal trough. The degree of this magnification in the

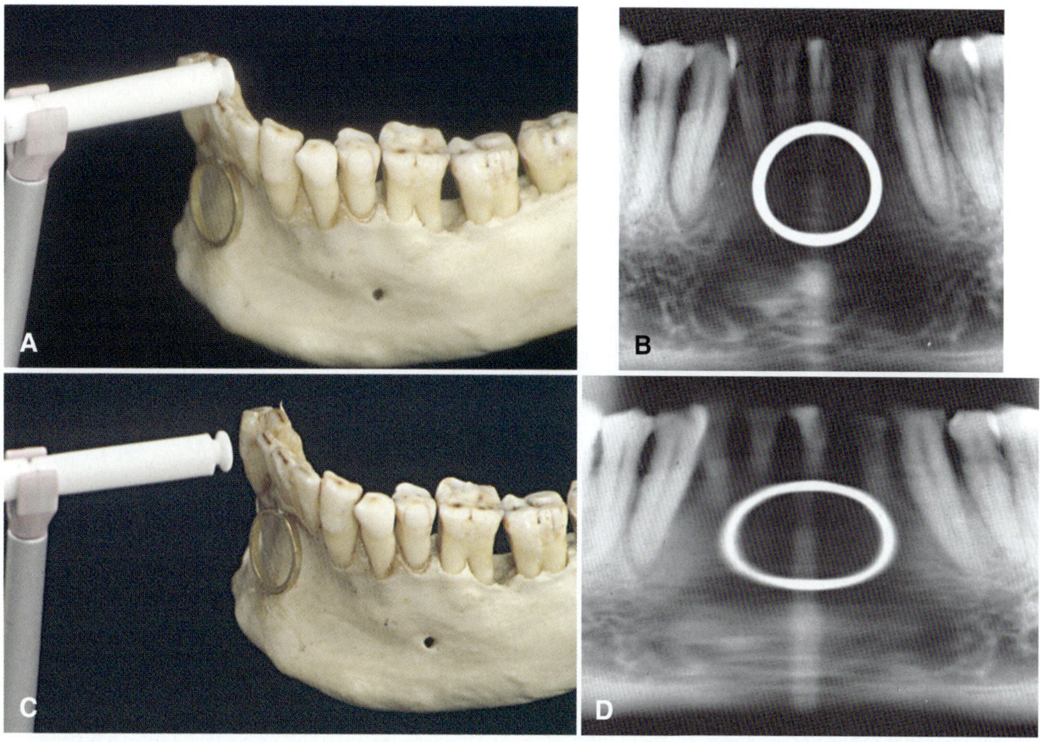

Fig. 8.10 Influence of an object's position on its radiographic size. (A) A mandible is supporting a metal ring positioned at the center of the focal trough. The mandible is positioned at the center of the focal trough by placing the incisal edges of the central incisors in a notch at the end of a bite rod-positioning device. (B) Resultant cropped panoramic radiograph shows minimal distortion of the metal ring. (C) The mandible and ring are positioned 5 mm posterior to the focal trough. (D) Resultant cropped panoramic radiograph demonstrates horizontal magnification of both the ring and the mandibular teeth.

Continued

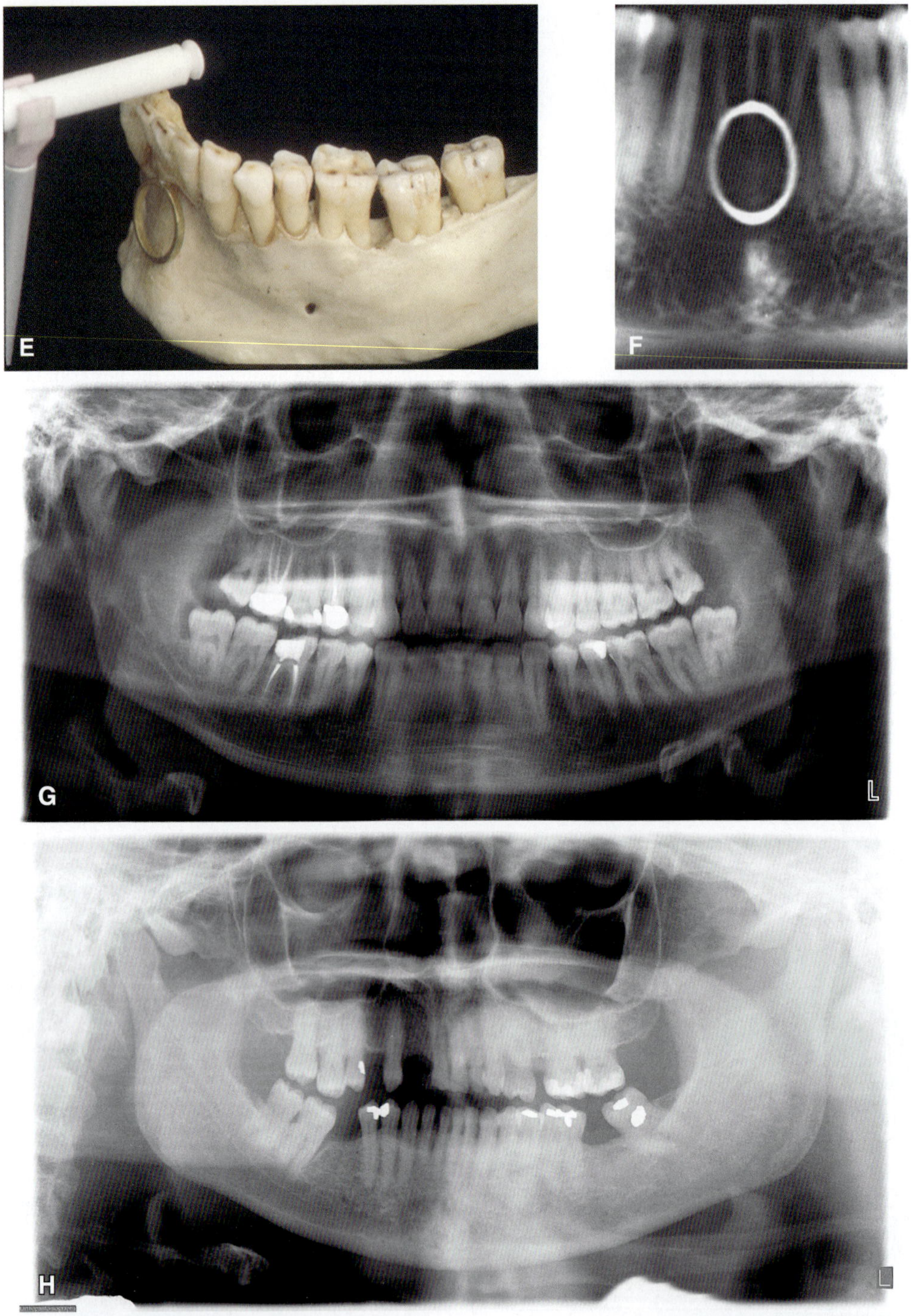

Fig. 8.10, cont'd (E) The mandible and ring are positioned 5 mm anterior to the notch in the bite block. (F) Resultant cropped panoramic radiograph demonstrates the horizontal minification of both the ring and the mandibular teeth. (G) Panoramic radiograph of a patient showing horizontal magnification of the anterior teeth due to patient positioning error as shown in *C*. (H) Panoramic radiograph of a patient showing decrease in horizontal dimension of the anterior teeth due to patient positioning error as shown in *E*. There is also a rotation to the left present in *H*.

posterior regions is less than that in the anterior region. Two identical objects located in the anterior and posterior regions may have different horizontal magnifications. Thus overall horizontal measurements made on panoramic radiographs are unreliable. Special attention must be paid to these considerations when following the progress of a bony lesion, especially in the anterior region. As a result of improper patient positioning, pathoses may appear relatively larger or smaller on successive images. The importance of careful alignment and positioning of the patient's dental arches within the focal trough is apparent.

Vertical magnification is determined by distance between the x-ray source and the object, similar to conventional radiography. In some panoramic units, this distance is maintained constant throughout the exposure cycle, resulting in a relatively constant vertical magnification in different areas of the image.

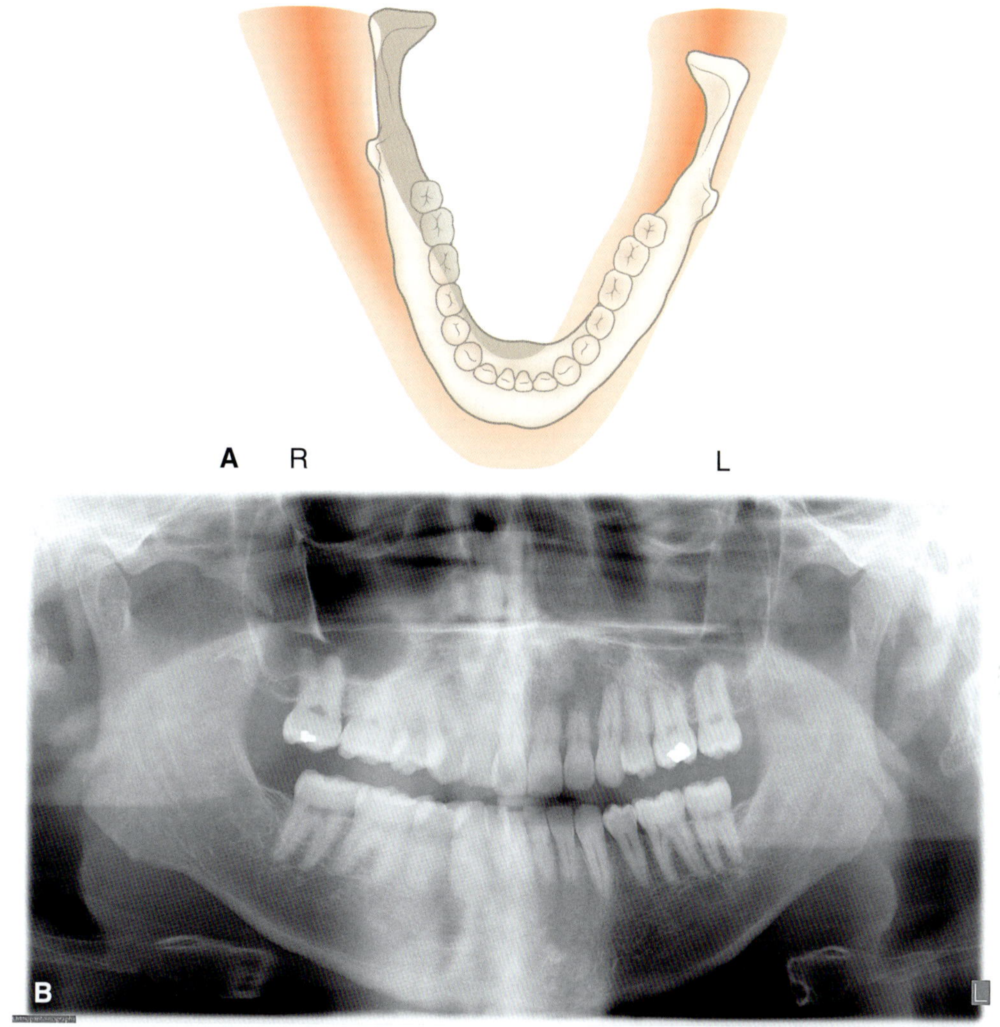

Fig. 8.11 (A) Schematic presentation of rotation of the patient's head to the right without a midline shift. Note that the right jaws are lingual to the focal trough and the left jaws are buccal to the focal trough. (B) Resultant panoramic radiograph shows horizontal magnification of the anterior and right posterior dentition. The horizontal dimension of the left posterior teeth is reduced.

The orientation of the panoramic x-ray beam has a slight caudocranial inclination. As a result of this beam angulation, structures that are positioned closer to the source are projected higher up on the image, relative to structures that are positioned farther away from the source of radiation. Thus the spatial relationships between the objects in the vertical dimension may not accurately represent true anatomic relationships, rendering assessment of vertical relationships in panoramic radiograph unreliable. Fig. 8.12 depicts a mandibular molar and three different positions of the mandibular canal, from lingual to buccal. All three positions are in the same horizontal plane (see Fig. 8.12A). However, owing to the angulation of the x-ray beam, the image of the lingually positioned canal (orange) is projected closer to the apex of the molar, whereas the image of the buccally positioned canal (green) is projected farther away from the root apex. Thus the distance between the root apex and the mandibular canal can be misrepresented on a panoramic radiograph.

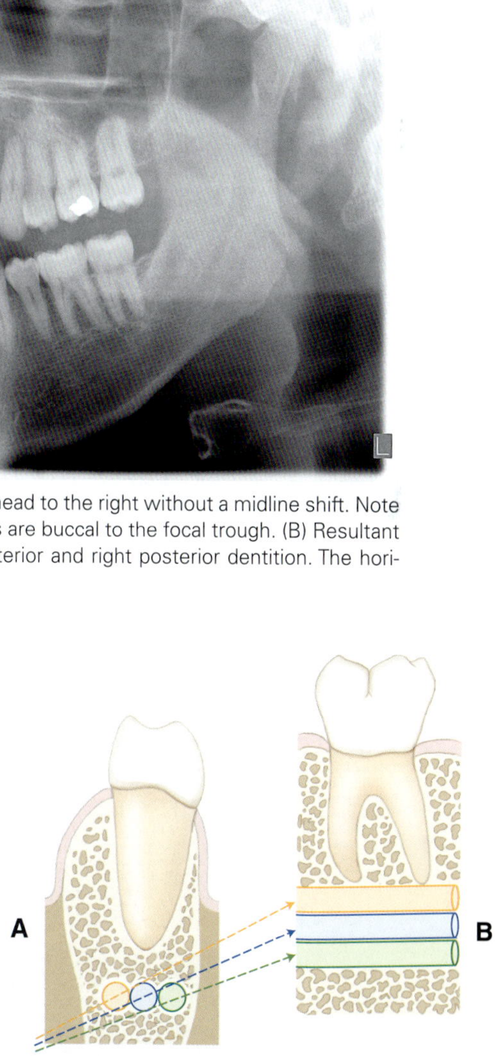

Fig. 8.12 Influence of projection geometry on spatial relationships in the vertical dimension. (A) Diagrammatic representation of a coronal cross section through the mandible. Three potential locations of the mandibular canal are shown. The locations lie in the same horizontal plane but differ in their buccolingual position. The x-ray beam *(dotted lines)* is angulated relative to the horizontal plane. (B) Apparent locations of the mandibular canals in the resultant image. When lingually positioned *(orange)*, the canal is projected more superiorly than when the canal is located buccally *(green)*.

PANORAMIC MACHINES

A number of manufacturers produce high-quality film-based and digital panoramic machines. Most of these units have the versatility to allow for adjustment of focal trough shape based on patient size (adult vs child) for panoramic image and produce tomographic cross-sectional images of selected areas of the facial skeleton. One such unit is presented in Fig. 8.13A. As mentioned previously, in addition to producing standard panoramic images of the jaws, some of these units have the capability of adjusting to patients of various sizes and making frontal and lateral images of TMJs, tomographic views through the sinuses, and cross-sectional views of the maxilla and mandible. These views are acquired by having special x-ray source and receptor movements programmed into the machine. "Extraoral bitewing" views are also offered by a few of the panoramic units that are designed to decrease overlap between the proximal surfaces of posterior teeth (see Fig. 8.13). Each machine also has the capability for adding on a cephalometric attachment to allow exposure of standardized skull views. Some machines have the capability of automated exposure control; this is accomplished by measuring the amount of radiation passing through the patient's mandible during the initial part of the exposure and adjusting the imaging factors (kilovoltage peak, milliamperage, and speed of imaging movements) to obtain an optimally exposed image. Finally, all of these machines are available in CCD-digital configurations, and some have cone beam imaging capability (see Chapter 9).

Patient Positioning and Head Alignment

Proper patient preparation and positioning within the focal trough are essential to obtaining diagnostic panoramic radiographs. Dental appliances, earrings, necklaces, hairpins, and any other metallic objects in the head and neck region should be removed. It may also be wise to demonstrate the machine to the patient by cycling it while explaining the need to remain still during the procedure. This is particularly important for children, who may be anxious. Children should be instructed to look forward and not to follow the tube head with their eyes.

The anteroposterior head position is achieved typically by having patients place the incisal edges of their maxillary and mandibular incisors into a notched positioning device (bite stick). The patient's midsagittal plane must be centered within the focal trough without any lateral shift in the mandible when making this protrusive movement. Most panoramic units have laser beams to facilitate alignment of the

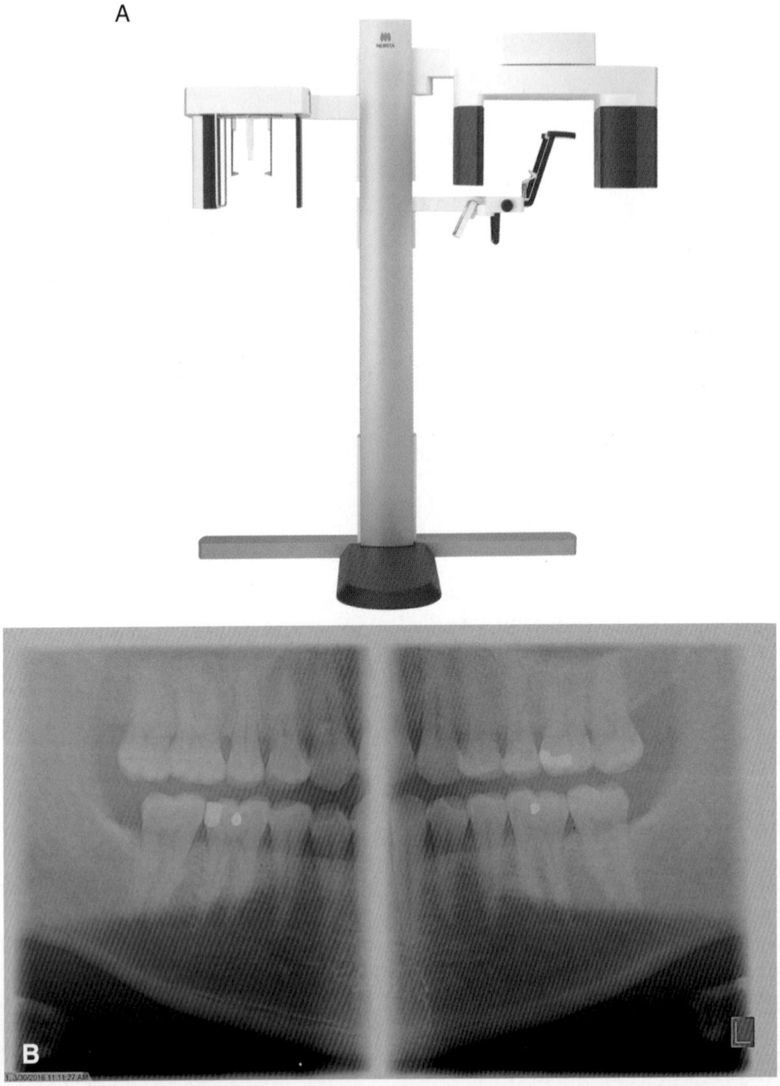

Fig. 8.13 (A) Veraview X800, a multipurpose imaging device combining cephalometric, panoramic, and cone beam computed tomography imaging. (B) "Extraoral bitewings" with open interproximal contacts in the posterior teeth as well as the periapical areas. (A, Courtesy J. Morita Corporation, Kyoto, Japan; B, Courtesy Planmeca ProMax 3D, Planmeca Inc., Wood Dale, IL.)

patient's midsagittal plane, Frankfort plane, and anteroposterior position within the focal trough.

Placement of the patient either too far anterior or too far posterior relative to the focal trough results in significant dimensional aberrations in the images. Too far posterior positioning results in magnified mesiodistal dimensions *("fat" teeth)* through the anterior sextants (see Fig. 8.10D). Too far anterior positioning results in reduced mesiodistal dimensions *("thin" teeth)* through the anterior sextants (see Fig. 8.10F). Failure to position the midsagittal plane in the rotational midline of the machine results in a radiograph showing right and left sides that are unequally magnified in the horizontal dimension (see Fig. 8.11). Poor midline positioning is a common error, causing horizontal distortion in the posterior regions, excessive tooth overlap in the premolar regions, and, occasionally, nondiagnostic, clinically unacceptable images. A simple method for evaluating the degree of horizontal distortion of the image is to compare the apparent mesiodistal width of the mandibular first molars bilaterally. The smaller side is too close to the receptor, and the larger side is too close to the center of rotation or rotational center.

The patient's chin and occlusal plane must be properly positioned to avoid distortion. The occlusal plane is aligned so that it is slightly lower anteriorly. A general guide for chin positioning is to position the patient so that a line from the tragus of the ear to the outer canthus of the eye is parallel with the floor. If the chin is tipped too high, the occlusal plane on the radiograph appears flat or inverted, and the resultant image of the mandible is distorted (Fig. 8.14A). In addition, the radiopaque shadow of the hard palate is superimposed on the roots of the maxillary teeth. If the chin is tipped too low, the occlusal plane shows an exaggerated smile line, the teeth become severely overlapped, the symphyseal region of the mandible may be cut off the film, and both mandibular condyles may be projected off the superior edge of the film (see Fig. 8.14B).

Patients are positioned with their backs and spines as erect as possible and their necks extended. Props such as a cushion for back support, foot support, or to straighten the spine minimize the artifact produced by vertebral shadow. Proper neck extension is best accomplished by using a gentle upward force on the mastoid eminences when positioning the head with a slight lower inclination of the chin. Allowing patients to slump their heads and necks forward causes a large opaque artifact in the midline created by the superimposition of the cervical vertebrae. This shadow obscures the entire symphyseal region of the mandible and may require that the radiograph be retaken (Fig. 8.15A). Finally, after patients are positioned in the machine, they should be instructed to swallow and hold the tongue flat against the

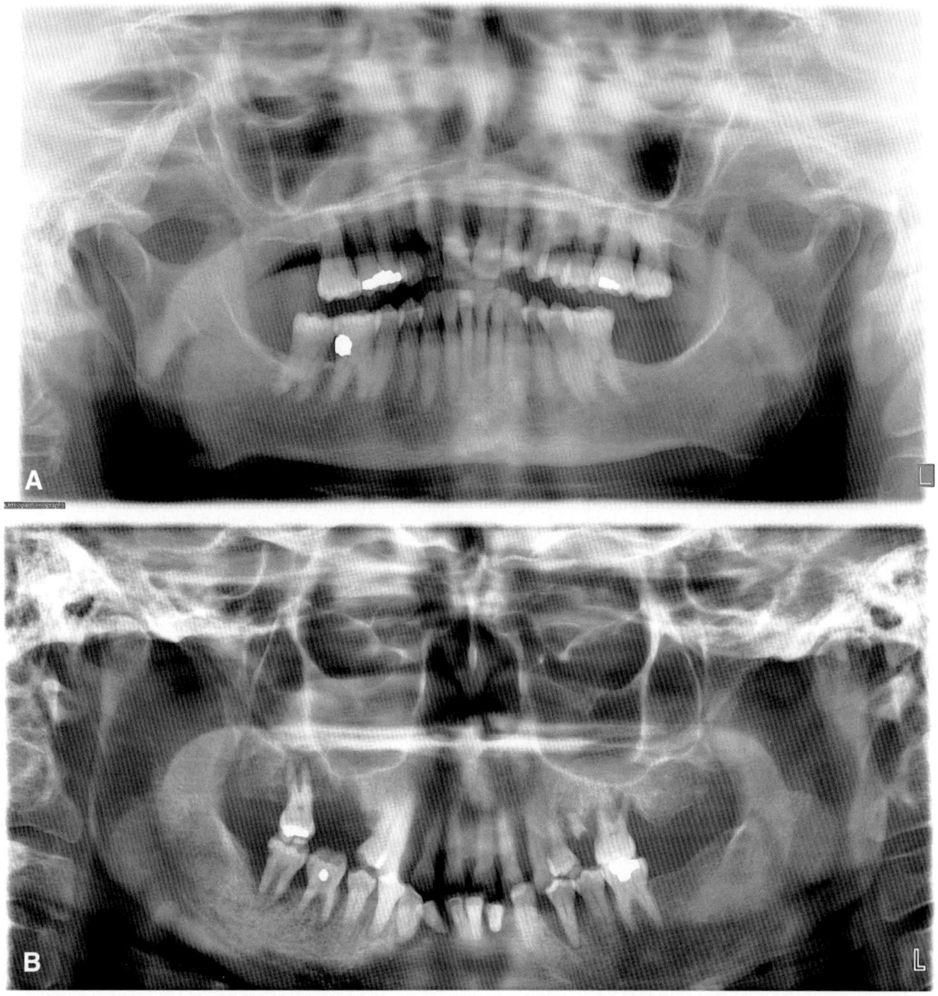

Fig. 8.14 Panoramic radiographs demonstrating poor patient head alignment. (A) The chin and occlusal plane are rotated upward, resulting in overlapping images of the teeth and an opaque shadow (the hard palate) obscuring the roots of the maxillary teeth. (B) The chin and occlusal plane are rotated downward, cutting off the symphyseal region on the radiograph and distorting the anterior teeth.

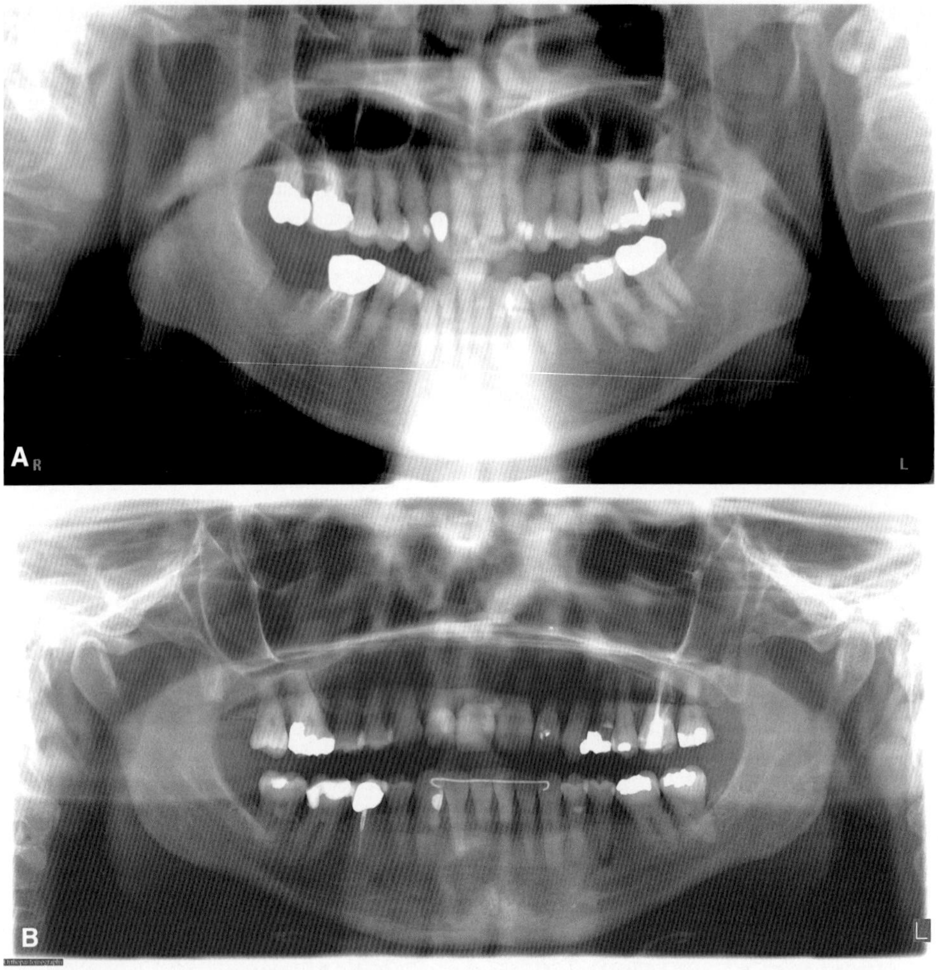

Fig. 8.15 (A) Panoramic radiograph demonstrating improper neck positioning. Note the large radiopaque region in the middle because the patient has the neck angled forward. This ghost image of the cervical spine could have been eliminated by having the patient sit straight and align or stretch the neck. (B) Panoramic radiograph showing improper tongue positioning, where the dorsum of the tongue was not positioned flat against the hard palate, resulting in the airspace below the hard palate hindering visualization of the apices of the maxillary teeth.

roof of the mouth. This raises the dorsum of the tongue to the hard palate, eliminating the airspace and providing optimal visualization of the apices of the maxillary teeth. Fig. 8.15B presents improper tongue positioning with an airspace below the hard palate, hindering visibility of the maxillary teeth apices.

Image Receptors

The use of digital image receptors in panoramic imaging has become very common. Both PSP and solid-state detectors (CCD or complementary metal oxide semiconductor device) are used in panoramic imaging (see Chapter 4). In indirect digital acquisition with the film-sized PSP plate, the image is processed by reading the latent image off of the PSP plate, yielding a digital image. Alternatively, direct digital acquisition panoramic machines use an array of solid-state detectors that transmit an electronic signal to the controlling computer, which is transmitted to the display screen, as it is being acquired. Digital modalities allow postacquisition processing to enhance the image characteristics, including contrast and density adjustments, white/black inversion, magnification, edge enhancement, and color rendering. Most units are capable of exporting the digital image in DICOM (Digital Imaging and Communications in Medicine) format or in a variety of standard image formats, such as Tagged Image File Format or Joint Photography Experts Group, allowing easy exchange of radiographic images. DICOM is a standard that specifies handling, storage, printing, and transmission of medical images. The American Dental Association endorses the use of DICOM as the standard for exchange of all dental digital images and recommends that all new digital x-ray units be DICOM compliant.

Intensifying screens (see Chapter 4) are used in film-based panoramic radiography because they significantly reduce the amount of radiation required for properly exposing a radiograph. Fast films combined with high-speed (rare earth) screens are indicated for most examinations. In most cases, the manufacturer provides panoramic machines with intensifying screens. The type of screen (manufacturer and model) is printed in black letters on each screen and clearly projected onto the radiograph. With rare earth screens and fast films, the patient's skin exposure from panoramic radiography is approximately equivalent to four bitewing views using F-speed film.

All panoramic radiographs must have a mechanism to indicate the patient's name, date of birth, the right and left side of the patient, date of examination, and the name of the dentist, without obscuring anatomic structures. No parts of the image should be trimmed to make the film fit the patient's chart.

Panoramic Film Darkroom Techniques

Special darkroom procedures are needed when panoramic film is being processed. These films are far more light sensitive than intraoral films, especially after they have been exposed. A reduction in darkroom lighting from that used for conventional intraoral film is necessary. A Kodak GBX-2 (Carestream Dental LLC, Atlanta, GA) filter can be installed with a 15-watt bulb at least 4 feet from the working surface. Panoramic film should be developed either manually or in automatic film processors according to the manufacturers' recommendations in order to obtain optimal images.

INTERPRETING PANORAMIC IMAGES

The need for appropriate ambient lighting and a quiet viewing room applies equally to viewing digital images on a computer display and traditional film radiographs on a view box. Image interpretation starts with a systematic analysis of the image and a thorough understanding of the appearances of the normal anatomic structures and their variants on the image. Panoramic images are quite different from intraoral images and demand a disciplined and focused approach to their interpretation. Recognizing normal anatomic structures on panoramic radiographs is challenging because of the complex anatomy of the midface, the superimposition of various hard and soft structures, and the changing projection orientation with real, double, and ghost images. The many potential artifacts associated with machine and patient movement and patient positioning must be identified and understood.

Routine imaging in dentistry is predominantly limited to two-dimensional representation of three-dimensional structures. On a posteroanterior skull film, orbital rims, nasal conchae, teeth, cervical vertebrae, and petrous ridges are all in sharp focus on the image, although they may be 8 inches apart from each other. Despite this presenting less interpretation challenge in a panoramic view, which is a curved image "slice" of the maxillomandibular complex, there is still the thickness to the tomogram that must be considered. The clinician must relate the structures on the image to their relative positions in the midfacial skeleton. An example of this three-dimensionality is the relative positioning of the external oblique and mylohyoid ridges in the mandible: On the panoramic image, they generally both appear sharp, whereas physically, the external oblique ridge is on the mandibular buccal surface and the mylohyoid ridge is on the mandibular lingual surface, separated by several millimeters. When panoramic images are viewed, it is important for the clinician to remember this principle and to attempt mental visualization of the structures three-dimensionally.

It is helpful to view the image as if looking at the patient, with the structures on the patient's right side positioned on the viewer's left (Fig. 8.16), similar to the orientation of periapical and bitewing images, making the interpretation more comfortable. It is important to recognize the planes of the patient that are represented in different parts of the panoramic image. The panoramic image represents the curved jaw that is unfolded onto a flat plane. In the posterior regions, the panoramic image depicts a sagittal (lateral) view of the jaws, whereas in the anterior sextant, it represents a coronal (anteroposterior) view.

Dentition

One of the strengths of the panoramic image is the demonstration of the complete dentition. Although there is a rare situation where positioning of the patient or an ectopic tooth places the tooth out of the focal trough, all the teeth are generally seen on the image. Thus the interpretation must always include identification of all erupted and developing teeth (Fig. 8.17). The teeth should be examined for abnormalities of number, position, and anatomy. Existing dentistry, including endodontic obturations, crowns, and other fixed restorations, should be noted. Excessively wide or narrow anterior teeth suggest malposition of the patient in the focal trough. Similarly, teeth that are wider on one side than the other suggest that the patient's sagittal plane was rotated. Gross caries and periapical and periodontal disease may be evident. However, the resolution of a panoramic radiograph is lower than that of intraoral radiographs, and additional intraoral radiographs may be needed to detect subtle disease. The proximal surfaces of the premolar teeth often overlap, which interferes with caries interpretation.

It is particularly important to examine impacted third molars closely. The orientation of the molars; the numbers and configurations of the roots; the relationships of the tooth components to critical anatomic structures, such as the mandibular canal, floor and posterior wall of the maxillary sinus, maxillary tuberosity, and adjacent teeth; and the presence of abnormalities in the pericoronal or periradicular bone must be carefully studied. However, given the two-dimensional nature of the panoramic image, such findings may need additional imaging with cone beam computed tomography (CBCT) to define precisely the spatial relationships of the roots of the impacted molars to the vital structures.

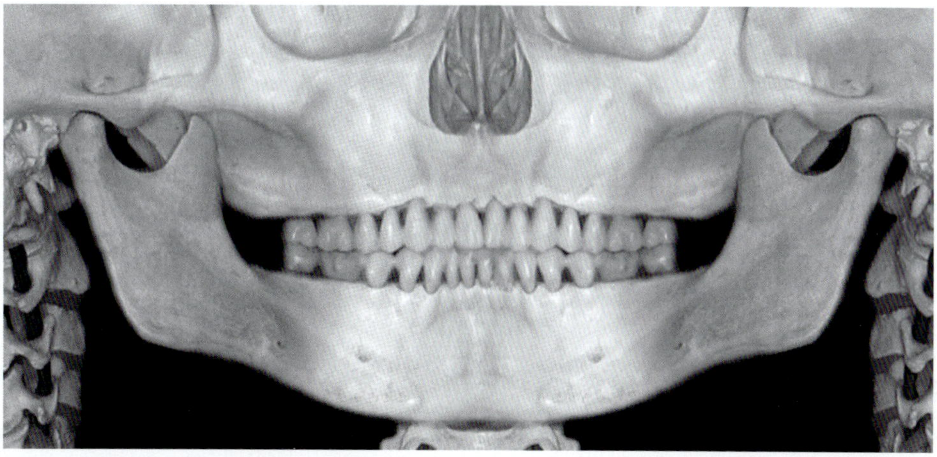

Fig. 8.16 The bones of the mandible, midface, cervical spine, and skull base as they appear on a panoramic image. The image is composed of left and right lateral views of the facial bones posterior to the canines and a coronal view anterior to the premolars.

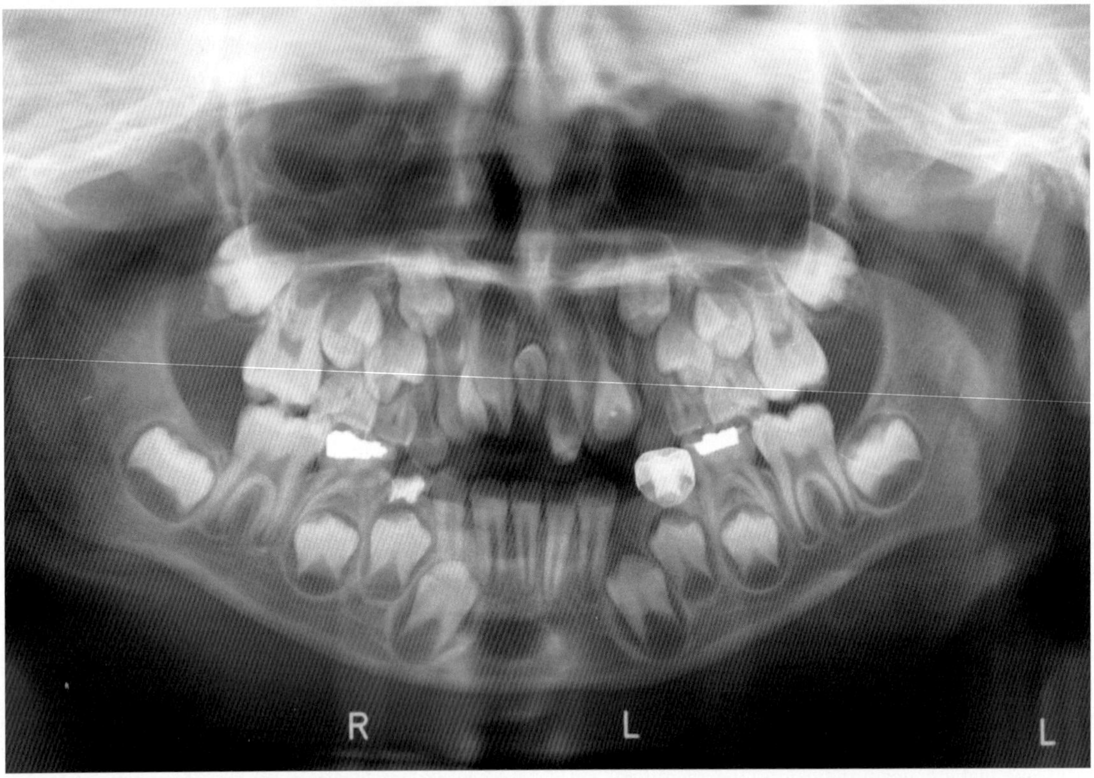

Fig. 8.17 Panoramic image showing late mixed dentition of an 8-year-old patient. The panoramic image can be useful in identifying the presence or absence of the permanent dentition, as well as assessing their developmental status. Note impacted and inverted mesiodens in the maxillary midline and malalignment of incisors.

Midfacial Region

The midface is a complex mixture of bones, air cavities, and soft tissues, all of which appear on panoramic images (Fig. 8.18). Individual bones that may appear on the panoramic image of the midface include temporal, zygoma, mandible, frontal, maxilla, sphenoid, ethmoid, vomer, nasal, nasal conchae, and palate; thus it is a misnomer to refer to the midfacial region on the panoramic image as "the maxilla." Maintaining the discipline and focus of a systematic examination of all aspects of the midfacial images is difficult and critical in the overall examination of the panoramic image.

This region can be compartmentalized into major sites for examination (see Fig. 8.18) as follows:

- Cortical boundary of the maxilla, including the posterior border and the alveolar ridge.
- Pterygomaxillary fissure.
- Maxillary sinuses.
- Zygomatic complex, including inferior and lateral orbital rims, zygomatic process of maxilla, and anterior portion of zygomatic arch.
- Nasal cavity and conchae.
- TMJs (also viewed in the mandible but visualizing important structures multiple times is always a good idea in image interpretation).
- Maxillary dentition and supporting alveolus.

Examining the cortical outline of the maxilla is a good way to center the examination of the midface. The posterior border of the maxilla extends from the superior portion of the pterygomaxillary fissure down to the tuberosity region and around to the other side. The posterior border of the pterygomaxillary fissure is the pterygoid spine of the sphenoid bone (the anterior border of the pterygoid plates). Occasionally, the sphenoid sinus may extend into this structure. The pterygomaxillary fissure itself has an inverted teardrop appearance; it is very important to identify this area on both sides of the image because maxillary sinus mucoceles and carcinomas characteristically destroy the posterior maxillary border, which is manifested as loss of the anterior border of the pterygomaxillary fissure. To clarify the three-dimensional anatomy of the pterygomaxillary fissure, Fig. 8.19 shows this structure in a dried skull, in an axial CT image, and in the panoramic image.

The maxillary sinuses are usually well visualized on panoramic images. The clinician should identify each of the borders (posterior, anterior, floor, roof) and note whether they are entirely outlined with cortical bone, approximately symmetric, and comparable in radiographic density. The borders should be present and intact. The medial border of the maxillary sinus is the lateral border of the nasal cavity; however, this interface is not demonstrated on the panoramic image. The superior border, or roof, of the maxillary sinus is the floor of the orbit; this interface is demonstrated on the panoramic image in its most anterior aspect. Although it is useful to compare right and left maxillary sinuses when looking for abnormalities, it is important to remember that bilateral asymmetry in size, shape, and presence or number of septae within the maxillary sinuses is a common anatomic variation. The posterior aspect of the sinus is more opaque because of superimposition of the zygoma. Each sinus should be examined for evidence of a mucous retention cyst, mucoperiosteal thickening, and other abnormalities.

The zygomatic complex, or "buttress" of the midface, is a very complex anatomic area, with contributions from the frontal, zygomatic, and maxillary bones. It includes the lateral and inferior orbital rims, the zygomatic process of the maxilla, and the zygomatic arch. The zygomatic process of the maxilla arises over the maxillary first and second molars. The maxillary sinus can pneumatize the zygomatic process of the maxilla up to the zygomaticomaxillary suture. This can result in the appearance of an elliptical, corticated radiolucency in the maxillary sinus, possibly superimposed over the roots of a molar tooth,

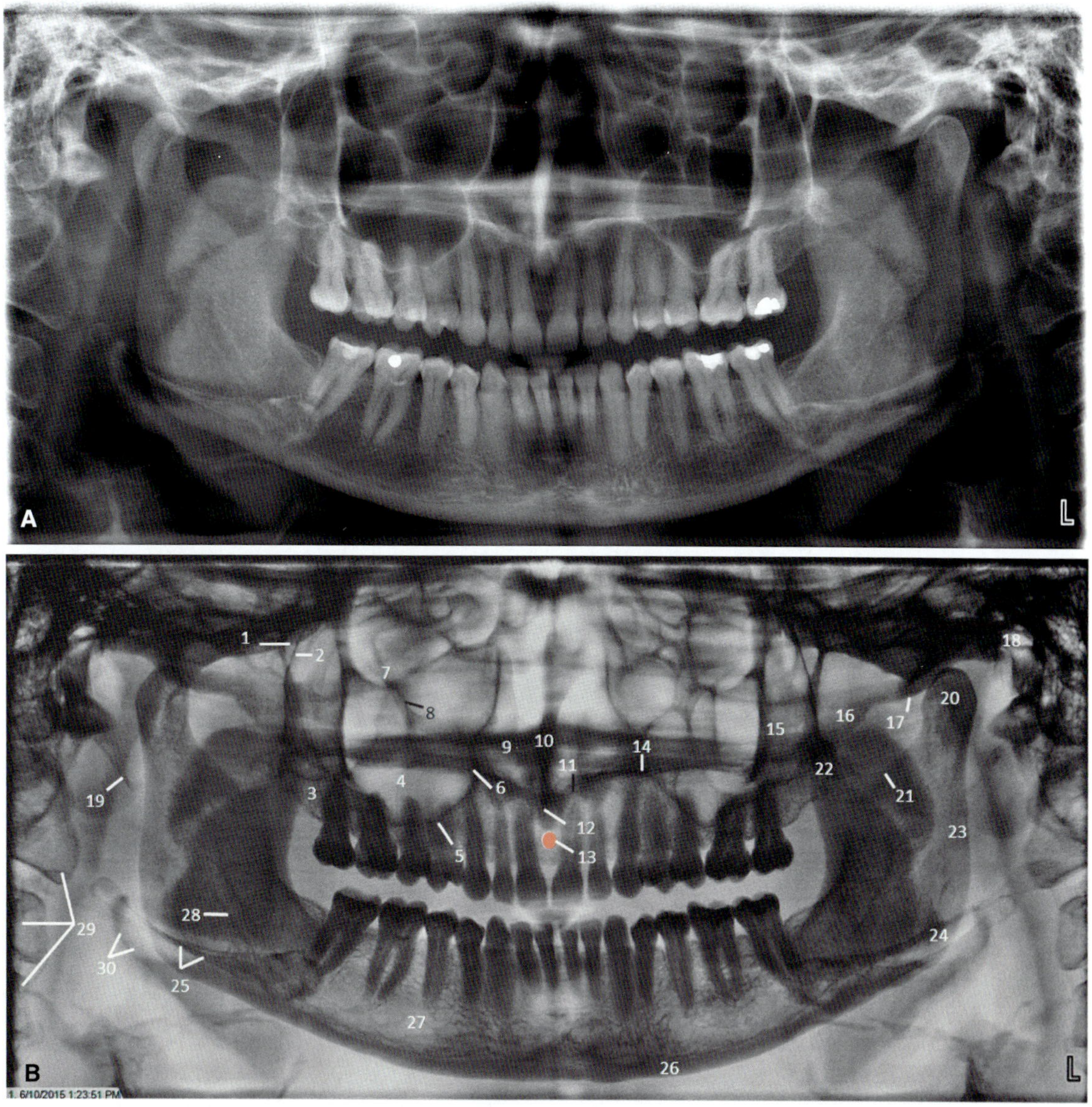

1. Pterygomaxillary fissure
2. Posterior border of maxilla
3. Maxillary tuberosity
4. Maxillary sinus
5. Floor of the maxillary sinus
6. Medial border of the maxillary sinus/ lateral border of the nasal cavity
7. Floor of the orbit
8. Infraorbital canal
9. Nasal cavity
10. Nasal septum
11. Floor of the nasal cavity
12. Anterior nasal spine
13. Incisive foramen
14. Hard palate/floor of the nasal cavity
15. Zygomatic process of maxilla
16. Zygomatic arch
17. Articular eminence
18. External auditory meatus
19. Styloid process
20. Mandibular condyle
21. Sigmoid notch
22. Coronoid process
23. Posterior border of the ramus
24. Angle of the mandible
25. Hyoid bone
26. Inferior border of the mandible
27. Mental foramen
28. Mandibular canal
29. Cervical vertebrae
30. Epiglottis

Fig. 8.18 (A) Properly acquired and displayed panoramic image of an adult patient. The patient's left side is indicated on the image, and the image is oriented as if the clinician were facing the patient. This is the same orientation used with a full-mouth series. (B) Inverted image of the same panoramic radiograph identifying midfacial and mandibular anatomic structures.

on a panoramic image. The inferior border of the zygomatic arch extends posteriorly from the inferior portion of the zygomatic process of the maxilla and continues posteriorly to the articular tubercle and glenoid fossa of the temporal bone. The superior border of the zygomatic arch, which curves anterosuperiorly to form the lateral aspect of the lateral orbital rim, should also be noted. The zygomaticotemporal suture lies in the middle of the zygomatic arch and may simulate a fracture if visualized on the image. In addition, the mastoid air cells occasionally pneumatize the temporal bone all the way to the zygomaticotemporal suture, giving the glenoid fossa of the TMJ the appearance of having a multilocular, or "soap-bubbly," radiolucency, which is a variant of normal.

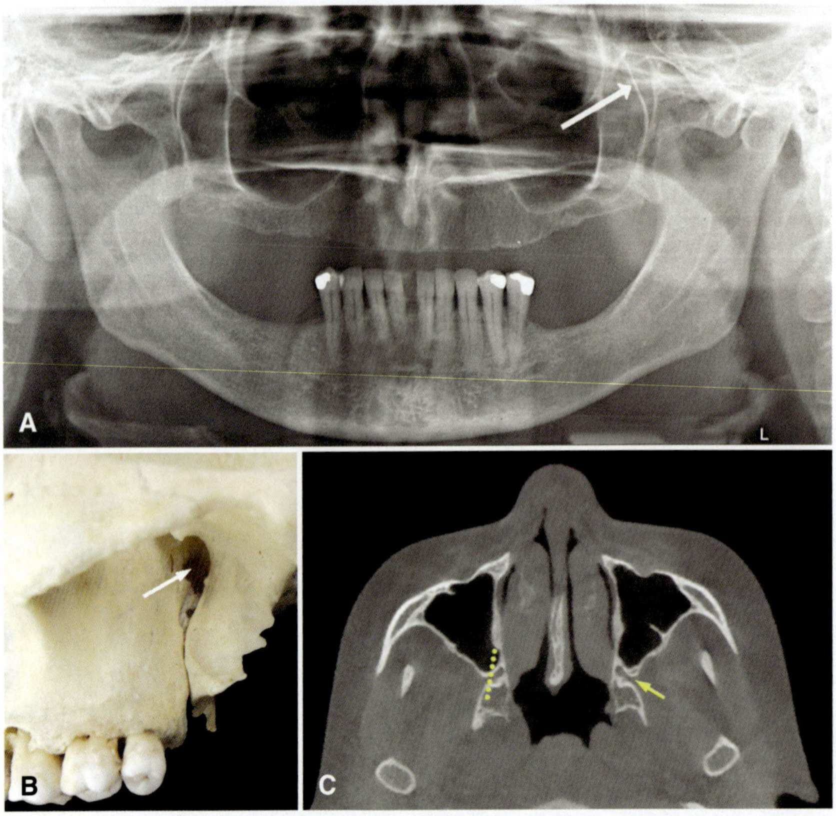

Fig. 8.19 Pterygomaxillary fissure, a space between the posterior surface of the maxilla and the anterior border of the pterygoid plates. (A) Inverted teardrop shape of the fissure on a panoramic image *(arrow)*. (B) The fissure on a dried skull *(arrow)*. (C) The approximate image section *(dotted line)* of the panoramic focal trough through the pterygomaxillary fissure *(arrow)* on an axial computed tomographic section.

The nasal fossa may show the nasal septum and inferior concha, including both the bone and its mucosal covering. In the anterior region, the lateral border and anterior rim of the nasal cavity are seen as a radiopaque line. The anterior nasal spine and the incisive foramen also may be seen. The floor of the nasal cavity or hard palate is seen as a horizontal radiopacity, superimposed over the maxillary sinus in the posterior regions; this is often seen as two radiopaque lines (see Fig. 8.9). The lower line is sharp and represents the junction between the lateral wall of the nasal cavity and hard palate on the tube side. The upper line is more diffuse and represents the junction on the opposite side. The conchae, composed of an internal bone, the turbinate, and covering cartilage and mucosa, are seen in a coronal manner in the anterior portion of the image and in a sagittal manner in the posterior portions of the panoramic image. They can appear as very large, homogeneous, soft tissue densities superimposed over the maxillary sinuses and occasionally the anterior nasopharynx.

Mandible

Assessment of the mandible (see Fig. 8.18) can be compartmentalized into the major anatomic areas of this curved bone, as follows:

- Condylar process and TMJ
- Coronoid process
- Ramus
- Body and angle
- Anterior sextant
- Mandibular dentition and supporting alveolus

The clinician should be able to follow a cortical border around the entire bone, with the exception of the dentate areas. This border should be smooth, without interruptions, and should have symmetric thicknesses in comparable anatomic areas (e.g., angles, inferior borders of bodies, posterior borders of rami). The trabeculation of the mandible tends to be more plentiful in the anterior regions, whereas the marrow compartment increases toward the angle and into the ramus; however, these trabecular patterns and densities should be relatively symmetric. This is especially true in children, who have very sparse trabeculation throughout the deciduous and mixed dentition stages.

The mandibular condyle is generally positioned slightly anteroinferior to its normal closed position because the patient has to open and protrude the mandible slightly to engage the positioning device in most panoramic machines. The TMJ can be assessed for gross anatomic changes of the condylar head and glenoid fossa; the soft tissues, such as the articular disk and posterior ligamentous attachment, cannot be evaluated. The glenoid fossa is part of the temporal bone, and it can be pneumatized by the mastoid air cells. This can result in the appearance of a multilocular radiolucency in the articular eminence and the roof of the glenoid fossa, which is a variant of normal. More definitive osseous assessment of the TMJ is accomplished by using CBCT imaging and multidetector computed tomography scan. Magnetic resonance imaging is the examination of choice for evaluation of the disk and pericondylar soft tissues.

Shadows of other structures that can be superimposed over the mandibular ramal area include the following:

- Oropharyngeal and nasopharyngeal airway shadows, the former specifically when the patient is unable to expel the air and place the tongue in the palate during the exposure.
- Posterior wall of the nasopharynx.
- Cervical vertebrae, especially in patients with pronounced anterior lordosis, typically seen in severely osteoporotic individuals.
- Earlobe.
- Nasal cartilage.

- Soft palate and uvula.
- Dorsum of the tongue.
- Ghost shadows of the opposite side of the mandible.
- Real and ghost shadows of metallic jewelry or other ear, nose, tongue decorations.

From the angle of the mandible, viewing should be continued anteriorly toward the symphyseal region. A fracture often manifests as a discontinuity ("step deformity") in the inferior border; a sharp change in the level of the occlusal plane indicates that the fracture passes through the tooth-bearing area, whereas a cant in the entire occlusal table without a step deformity in the occlusal plane indicates that the fracture is posterior to the tooth-bearing area. The width of the cortical bone at the inferior border of the mandible should be at least 3 mm in adults and of uniform density. There may be localized or generalized bone thinning indicating an expansile lesion such as a cyst or systemic diseases such as hyperparathyroidism and osteoporosis, respectively. The outlines of both sides of the mandible should be compared for symmetry. Asymmetry of size may result from improper patient positioning or conditions such as hemifacial hyperplasia or hypoplasia. The hyoid bone may be projected below or onto the inferior border of the mandible.

Trabeculation is most evident within the alveolar process. The mandibular canals and mental foramina are usually clearly visualized in the ramus and body regions of the mandible. Typically, the canals exhibit uniform width or gentle tapering from the mandibular foramina to the mental foramina. They may be less well demarcated in the first molar and premolar regions. When only one border of the canal is seen, it is typically the inferior border. The canals usually rise to meet the mental foramina, often looping several millimeters anterior to the mental foramina; this is termed the "anterior loop" of the mandibular canal, and its position and extent are considerations when planning dental implants in the mandibular canine regions. An expansion of the canal suggests neurovascular pathology; however, slight widening at the entry point of the canal into the body of the mandible from the ramus is a variation of normal. The mandible should be examined for radiolucencies or opacities. The midline is more opaque because of the mental protuberance, increased trabecular numbers, and attenuation of the beam as it passes through the cervical spine. Many modern panoramic machines automatically increase the exposure factors as they pass across the cervical spine region in an attempt to minimize this opacity; nevertheless, some opacity is generally seen in the anterior regions of the image. There are often depressions on the lingual surfaces of the mandible, which are occupied by the submandibular and sublingual glands. These depressions are termed the lingual salivary gland depressions, or fossae, and are often more radiolucent compared to adjacent areas. This anatomic feature is shown on a panoramic image, dry skull, coronal CT section, and periapical image in Fig. 8.20A–D.

Soft Tissues

Numerous opaque soft tissue structures may be identified on panoramic radiographs, including the tongue arching across the image under the hard palate (approximately extending from the right to the left mandibular angle), lip markings (in the middle of the image), the soft palate extending posteriorly from the hard palate over each ramus, the posterior wall of the oral and nasal pharynx, the nasal septum, the earlobes, the nose, and the nasolabial folds (Fig. 8.21A and B). Radiolucent airway shadows superimpose on normal anatomic structures and may be delineated by the borders of adjacent soft tissues. They include the nasal fossa, nasopharynx, oral cavity, and oropharynx. The epiglottis and thyroid cartilage are often seen in panoramic images (Fig. 8.22).

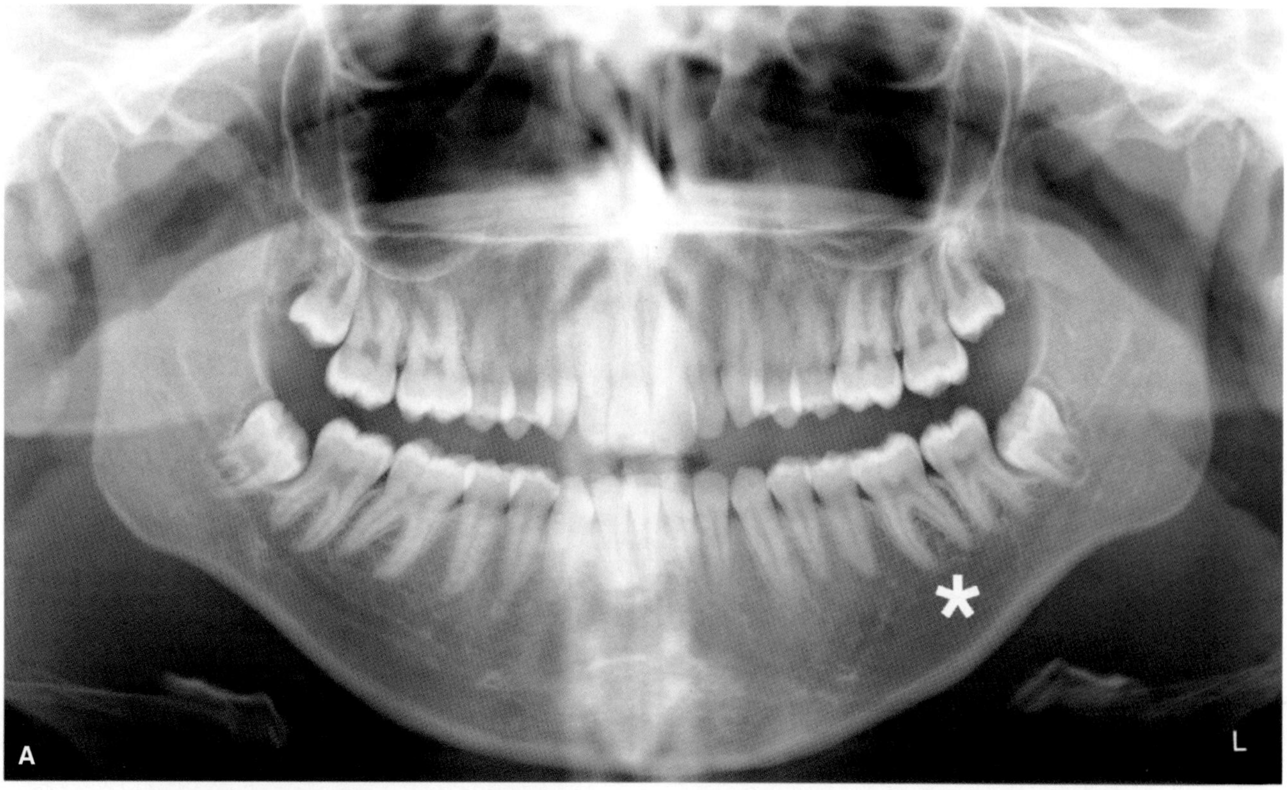

Fig. 8.20 The submandibular fossa (lingual salivary gland depression) is a concavity often found on the posterior lingual surface of the mandible. This triangularly shaped area is bounded by the mylohyoid ridge superiorly and the inferior border of the mandibular body and lies in the region of the roots of the molars and premolars. The *asterisk* indicates the area of the submandibular fossa on the various images. (A) Panoramic image.

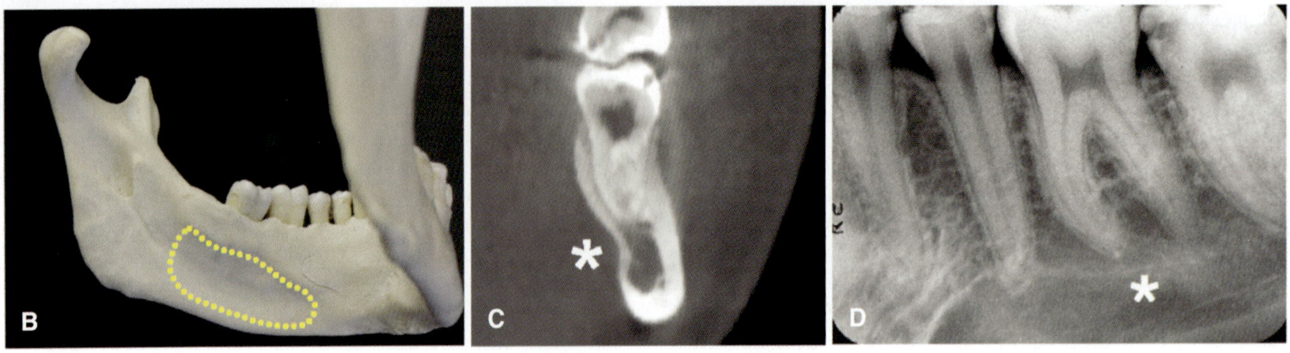

Fig. 8.20, cont'd (B) Photograph of the lingual side of a dried mandible. (C) Coronal computed tomographic scan through the molar region of the mandible. (D) Mandibular molar periapical image.

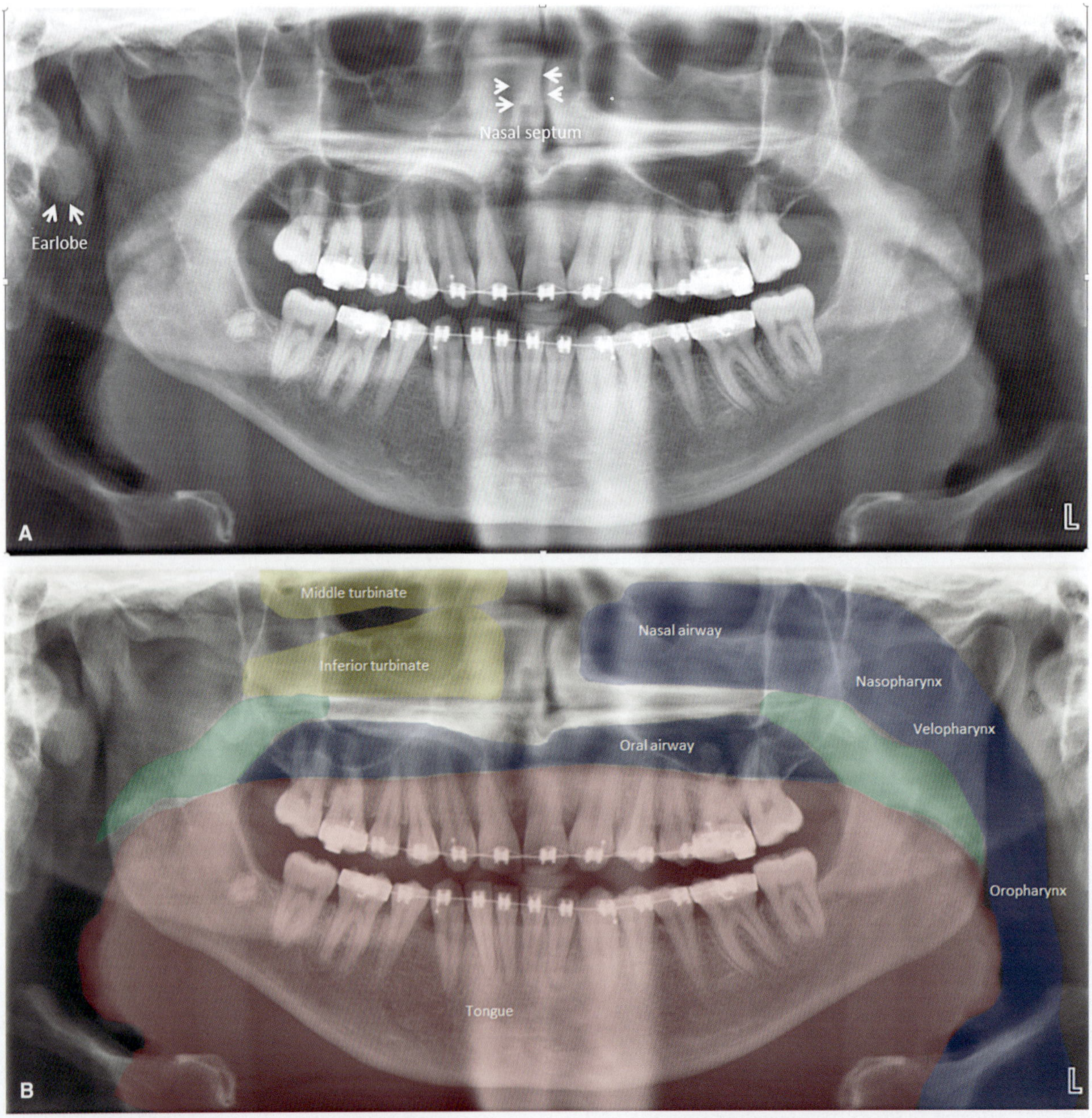

Fig. 8.21 Soft tissue images on a panoramic radiograph. (A) Properly acquired panoramic radiograph showing radiographically evident orofacial soft tissues. (B) The same panoramic image with an overlay indicating the components of the airway. The nasal airway surrounds the turbinates. The nasopharynx is posterior to the turbinates and above the level of the hard palate. The velopharynx is posterior to the soft palate. The oropharynx is below the uvula.

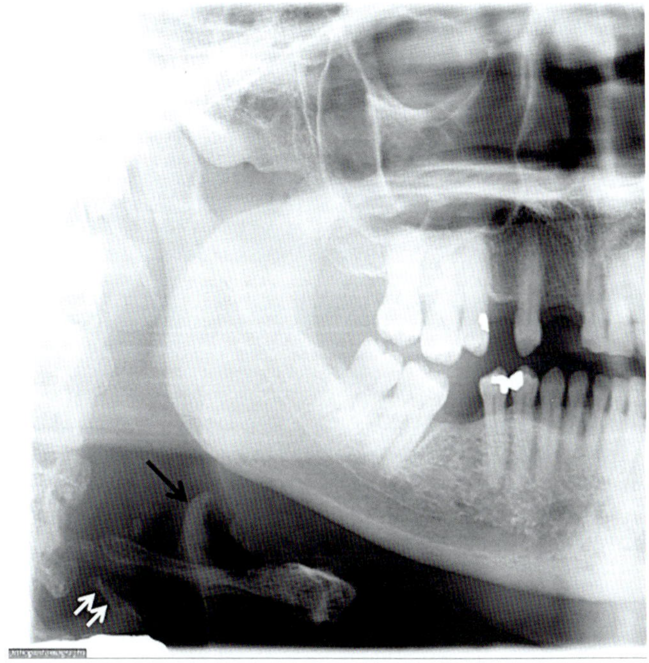

Fig. 8.22 Normal structures occasionally seen in the neck region on panoramic images. The superior aspect of the thyroid cartilage *(white arrows)* can be mistaken for a vascular calcification. The epiglottis *(black arrow)* lies posterior to the dorsum of the tongue.

BIBLIOGRAPHY

American Dental Association Council on Scientific Affairs. The use of dental radiographs: update and recommendations. *J Am Dent Assoc.* 2006;137(9): 1304-1312.

Chomenko AG. *Atlas for Maxillofacial Pantomographic Interpretation.* Quintessence; 1985.

Langland OE, Langlais RP, McDavid WD, et al. *Panoramic Radiology.* 2nd ed. Lea & Febiger; 1988.

McDavid WD, Dove SB, Welander U, et al. Dimensional reproduction in direct digital rotational panoramic radiography. *Oral Surg Oral Med Oral Pathol.* 1993;75:523-527.

McDavid WD, Langlais RP, Welander U, et al. Real, double and ghost images in rotational panoramic radiography. *Dentomaxillofac Radiol.* 1983;12:122-128.

Numata H. Consideration of the parabolic radiography of the dental arch. *J Shimazu Stud.* 1933;10:13.

Paatero YV. A new tomographic method for radiographing curved outer surfaces. *Acta Radiol.* 1949;32:177.

Paatero YV. The use of a mobile source of light in radiography. *Acta Radiol.* 1948;29:221.

Terry GL, Noujeim M, Langlais RP, et al. A clinical comparison of extraoral panoramic and intraoral radiographic modalities for detecting proximal caries and visualizing open posterior interproximal contacts. *Dentomaxillofac Radiol.* 2016;45(4):20150158.

9

Computed Tomography

William C. Scarfe and Sanjay M. Mallya

In 1972, Godfrey Hounsfield, an engineer, announced the invention of a revolutionary medical diagnostic radiographic imaging device to produce sequential narrow cross-sectional images of the head. The images were produced perpendicular to the cranio-caudal axis of the head, so the term computed axial tomography, or "CAT scan" was adopted. This was the first practical electronic medical application of the principles of tomography—derived from the Greek words "*tomos*" (slice) and "*graphe*" (drawing). Hounsfield shared the 1979 Nobel Prize in Physiology or Medicine with Allan Cormack, on whose work on image reconstruction mathematics two decades earlier laid the basis for computed tomography (CT). CT provides high-contrast images eliminating the superimposition of adjacent anatomic structures inherent in conventional plain projection radiography and the blur of film-based tomography. Cone beam computed tomography (CBCT) presents as a separate evolutionary arm to CT for the electronic production of cross-sectional images. Similarities exist between technologies, however, differences in the image acquisition beam shape, as well as the x-ray generator and detecting system used make CBCT systems stand independently as a simple and inexpensive approach to the concept of electronic sectional imaging focusing mostly on the maxillofacial region. This chapter discusses general principles of CT technology and CT image reconstruction. It discusses similarities and differences between current multidetector CT (MDCT) and CBCT regarding beam geometry, image acquisition, image detection, image reconstruction, and radiation dose with specific reference to maxillofacial applications.

GENERAL PRINCIPLES OF COMPUTED TOMOGRAPHY

Acquiring the Data

There are many commonalities in data acquisition with both MDCT and CBCT technologies:

- An x-ray source and an electronic detector revolve around the patient through a rotational arc (Figs. 9.1 and 9.2).
- The x-ray source is collimated to a varying degree to project onto the detector.
- The detector records photon attenuation by measuring the number of photons that exit the patient, registering this information at several hundred angles through the rotational arc.
- Each detector that records photon attenuation comprises multiple dexels (detector elements) as fundamental electronic units.
- Data recorded by the detector at each angle represents a composite of the absorption characteristics of all anatomic structures in the path of the x-ray beam.
- Reconstruction of the transmitted x-ray attenuation data in adjacent slices or local regions (in the case of MDCT) or the entire area (in the case of CBCT) by specific software algorithms produces a three-dimensional (3D) volumetric dataset represented by cuboidal voxels (volume elements), each with a location and attenuation value.
- When the volumetric dataset is represented visually on a computer monitor, the image comprises a square matrix of pixels (picture elements). Each pixel represents the location of the voxel and the degree of attenuation in that cuboidal region is displayed as a gray scale image intensity.

There are important differences in data acquisition between MDCT and CBCT technologies including device configuration, x-ray source, detector type and properties, image acquisition parameters such as field of view (FOV) and exposure settings, reconstruction algorithms and the use of contrast agents. These features have consequences in the characteristics of the images produced and patient dose provided by each modality and are described in subsequent sections of this chapter.

Data Manipulation and Image Reconstruction

After the attenuation data is acquired, it is mathematically adjusted to prepare it for image reconstruction. The first step is to apply a Radon transformation (named after the mathematician Johann Radon). Data recorded by the detector represent photon absorption along an x-ray beam projection path. Radon transformation calculates the line integrals of x-ray intensities at different paths to the detector at each projection angle. The output is a sinogram—a two-dimensional (2D) plot of the x-ray source rotation angle on the *x*-axis and the position along the detector array on the *y*-axis. Additional filters are applied to the sinogram to reduce artifacts and enhance spatial and contrast resolution. The filtered sinogram is transformed using the Fourier transformation. This operation breaks the signals within the sinogram into its fundamental frequencies, which allows better control of image contrast and resolution. The filtered sinogram is then "backprojected," where each line integral in the sinogram is projected back into the image matrix to an individual pixel, and a numerical value is contributed to that image pixel for each projected angle. As the backprojection continues, the contributions from each angle are summed and the cumulative summation from all angles provides a numerical value to each pixel through the image matrix. The data may be normalized to account for variations in the number of contributing projections to each pixel. Filtered backprojection (FBP) is computationally effective and provides rapid reconstruction of CT images.

There are some variations in the reconstruction algorithms used in MDCT and CBCT to account for differences in x-ray beam projection geometry. MDCT uses a fan beam geometry with multiple rows of detectors that sequentially acquire image data as they rotate around the patient (Fig. 9.1). Data from individual detector rows are acquired in parallel, and this requires high computing power. During the filtering step, specific reconstruction filters can be applied to modulate contrast and spatial resolution to accentuate features in bone or in soft tissues. Reconstruction algorithms for MDCT involve FBP and are designed to

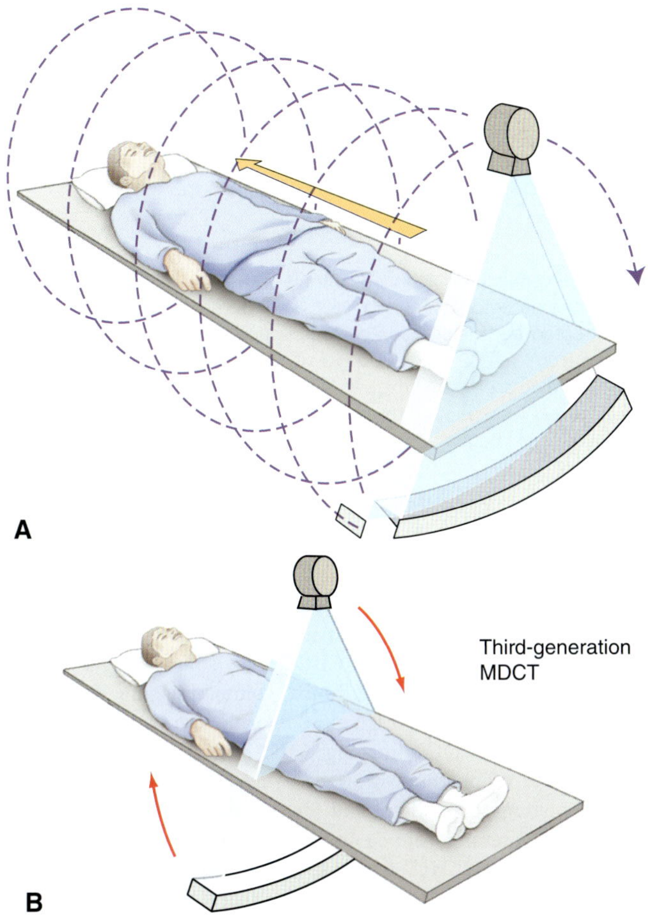

Fig. 9.1 (A) Helical computed tomography imaging. In helical scanners, the patient is moved continuously through the gantry, and the x-ray source moves continuously around the patient in a circle. The net effect is of helical scanning is volumetric imaging that is reconstructed into slices. (B) Multidetector computed tomography *(MDCT)* scanners. These scanners use a detector array, typically 64–640 rows in contemporary MDCT devices. In these scanners, all parts of the detector array arc are equidistant from the x-ray source.

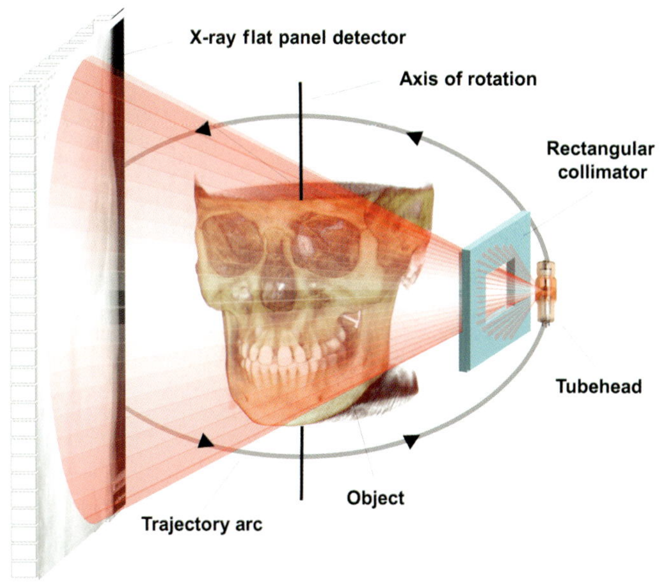

Fig. 9.2 Cone beam imaging geometry. A divergent x-ray beam created at the tube head is collimated in a rectangle into a three-dimensional pyramid. The x-ray projection is directed through the patient onto a solid-state flat panel detector. After a single two-dimensional projection is acquired by the detector, the x-ray source and detector rotate a small distance around the axis of rotation on a trajectory arc. At this second angular position, another basis projection image or frame is captured. This sequence continues around the object for the entire 360 degrees (full trajectory) or along a reduced or partial trajectory capturing hundreds of individual images.

account for the helical acquisition, fan beam geometry, and to provide speed of reconstruction.

CBCT systems use a wider cone beam geometry (Fig. 9.2) with a 2D detector and the entire image volume is acquired in a single rotation. Reconstruction algorithms account for the cone beam geometry. In addition to FBP, other methods include *Feldkamp-Davis-Kress* (FDK) algorithm. Iterative reconstruction methods use multiple iterations to minimize discrepancy between the acquired sinogram and the forward projection of the current image. Such methods may reduce noise and artifacts and optimize dose. The reconstruction process described is often referred to as the primary reconstruction. Subsequent processing of the image volume, for example, to generate orthogonal planes or curved "panoramic" images, is referred to as secondary reconstruction.

Properties of the Volumetric Dataset and DICOM Format

MDCT and CBCT data are 3D volumetric datasets represented by voxels, with each voxel representing the location and x-ray attenuation properties of the corresponding tissue location (Fig. 9.3). MDCT and CBCT data produce datasets with isometric voxels so individual voxels are cubical with equal dimensions in all three planes. With isotropic voxels, secondary reconstructions of the 3D volumetric data can be performed in virtually any plane without distortion. The pixel matrix for conventional MDCT (spatial resolution of 0.5 mm) is usually 512×512, however, with a high-resolution CT (HRCT) (spatial resolution of 0.23–0.35 mm), and now ultra high-resolution CT (U-HRCT) (spatial resolution as low as 0.15 mm) image grids are possible of 1024×1024 (HRCT) or even 2048×2048 (U-HRCT). Unlike conventional intraoral, panoramic, and cephalometric imaging, the reconstructed CT image has minimal geometric distortion and hence linear and angular measurements made on CT images are accurate and reliable. This is a major advantage of CT imaging.

CT data from individual devices can be exported in DICOM (digital imaging and communications in medicine) format. DICOM is a standard that specifies handling, storing, transmitting, and displaying medical images. In addition to the image itself, DICOM files include metadata to provide essential information about the image and the patient. Image data include device identifying information, exposure factors, slice thickness, and modality, among other information. Patient information includes demographics (name, age, sex) and may include other protected health information and personally identifying information. DICOM enables seamless interoperability and exchange of diagnostic imaging examinations and associated information. This interoperability is particularly important when using third-party software applications to view the CT dataset, perform in silico treatment simulations, and to generate files for printing of surgical guides (see Chapters 31 and 32).

Computed Tomography Numbers and Hounsfield Units

Each voxel of the CT volumetric dataset provides a gray scale intensity value that directly corresponds to the calculated linear attenuation

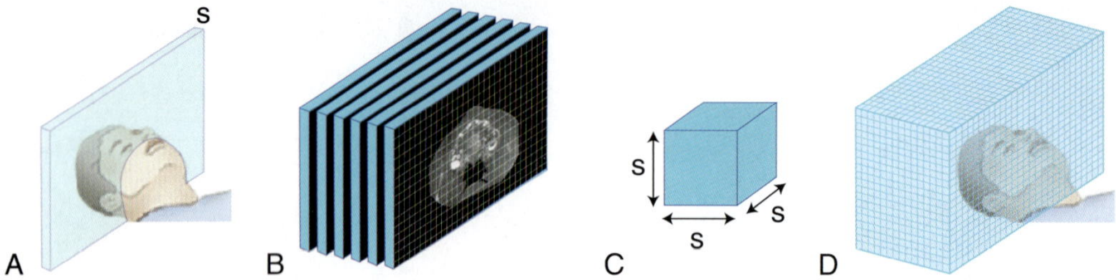

Fig. 9.3 (A) A single slice represents data reconstructed from multiple projections acquired during a 360-degree rotation around the patient. Slice thickness *(s)* is dependent on the detector row width (MDCT) or detector nominal dexel size (CBCT). (B) The sectional CT image is constructed from absorption characteristics of the subject and displayed as differences in optical density, ranging from −1000 to +3000 HU. (C) The image consists of a matrix of individual pixels representing the face of a volume called a voxel. In MDCT and CBCT, the voxels are isotropic (*cubical*). (D) Arrangement of individual voxels represents a three-dimensional image volume. This allows the formation of multiplanar and three-dimensional images.

coefficient of that tissue voxel. For MDCT, monitor pixels are assigned CT numbers expressed on a scale of arbitrary units—Hounsfield units (HU), in honor of Godfrey Hounsfield. On the HU scale, water is assigned a CT number of zero, and air is assigned a CT number of −1000. The upper end of the HU scale is not fixed and is determined by image bit depth. CT examinations with 12-bit images yield an HU scale with air at −1024 and an upper limit of 3071. With 16-bit images, the upper range is increased to 64,511. The mathematical derivation of CT numbers and HU of common tissues and materials with standard CT protocols are shown in Table 9.1.

The HU is not an SI unit and is dimensionless. Except for water and air, which have fixed values on the scale, the CT number for a given material varies with the physical tissue properties (effective atomic number and physical density; see Chapter 1) and with beam energy. In terms of image display, higher HU values appear as lighter shades of gray, whereas lower HU values correspond with darker shades. High attenuation material such as cortical bone and metal yield high CT numbers. When the beam energy (kVp) is increased, the CT numbers will decrease, in particular for high effective atomic number tissues such as enamel, dentin, and bone.

Pixel gray scale intensity values determined from CBCT images are less reliable indicators of tissue attenuation. This reflects the lower radiation dose output of CBCT x-ray sources, higher scatter radiation striking the detector, limited volume imaging, and the inherent limitations of reconstruction algorithms to correct for these variables. Unlike MDCT imaging, CBCT imaging focuses on hard tissue details. Attenuation within these high atomic number tissues is markedly energy dependent, and measurements of these tissues to infer tissue mineral density is unreliable. Many vendors provide the options to measure "HU" within a CBCT image, and users should recognize the limitations of using these quantitative values for clinical decision making.

TABLE 9.1 Range of Hounsfield Units (HU)[a] for Air, Water, and Various Tissues

Tissue	Hounsfield Units (CT Numbers)
Enamel	+1500 to +3000
Bone	+1000 to +3000 (cortical), +150 to +600 (cancellous)
Muscle	+20 to +140
Clotted blood	+13 to +30 (fluid), +50 to +75 (hemorrhage), +4 to +90 (hematoma)
Brain	+25 (white matter), +40 (gray matter)
Pus	0 to +45
CSF	+15
Water	0
Fat	−50 to −200
Lung	−600 to −800
Air	−1000

$$HU = 1000 \times \frac{\mu - \mu_{water}}{\mu_{water}}$$

where μ is the linear attenuation coefficient.

[a]The HU scale represents a 12-bit image. HU values for different tissues vary widely in the literature, so values are only approximate.
CSF, cerebrospinal fluid; *CT,* Computed tomography.

MULTIDETECTOR COMPUTED TOMOGRAPHY

Improvements in CT data acquisition has continued evolving over the past 5 decades, with advances in primary motion and geometric configuration between x-ray source and detector directed at faster image acquisition and better spatial and contrast resolution.

The prevailing tube head motion mode is *helical* or *spiral scanning,* also known as *volume acquisition*. These scanners require "slip-ring" technology which allows the continuous acquisition of projection data through a 3D volume of tissue by continuous rotation of the x-ray tube and detectors and simultaneous translation of the patient through the gantry opening. While the x-ray tube rotates in a circular arc, relative to the moving patient, it appears that it follows a spiral or helical trajectory (Fig. 9.1A). The tightness or spread of the spiral between the contiguous revolutions of the x-ray source and therefore voxel dimensions in the Z direction is determined by the speed of the table movement per 360-degree revolution, known as *table feed.*

The geometric configuration of most CT scanners is now MDCT or multislice CT (MSCT). These scanners have a wider x-ray beam projected onto multiple rows of detectors incorporated into the array along the long axis of the human body or the *z*-axis. The rows of detectors are frequently referred to as channels and range from 64 to 640 detector rows depending on the manufacturer and model. MDCT systems are now divided into four categories: 16-channel, 20- to 40-channel, 64- to 80-channel, and premium. This considers the number of rows but also criteria such as coverage, advanced applications, and acquisition capabilities. The detector configuration allows capture of multiple slices during each gantry rotation (see

Fig. 9.1B) and provides two main benefits. The first is faster scan times, ranging from a few seconds to a few minutes. This limits motion artifact from breathing, peristalsis, or heart contractions; this is important for patients who cannot hold their breath for long periods and for pediatric and trauma patients. The second is improved spatial resolution to submillimeter dimensions as low as 0.125 to 0.25 mm. Volumetric acquisition with isotropic imaging allows reformatting in planes different from the axial acquisition, without compromising image quality.

Device Configuration

MDCT devices are designed with a gantry and a patient table. The gantry is the main physical structure and resembles a large ring that houses the x-ray tube and detector and associated electrical and electronic components. The patient lies on a movable table that slides through the gantry during the scan. The gantry design acquires axial slices along the *z*-axis (craniocaudal axis) and can be angled to acquire direct coronal scans. However, when the scans are acquired with isotropic voxels and volumetric image acquisition, they can be reconstructed in any plane without distortion.

X-Ray Source

MDCT scanners operate at high tube voltage and tube current, and thus require special x-ray tubes to meet the high demands on heat production and cooling. MDCT units use x-ray tubes with rotating anodes (see Fig. 1.9), with a high heat capacity, up to 8 million heat units (compare with intraoral dental x-ray tubes of 20,000 heat units). They typically operate at 120 kVp (range 80–140 kVp) and at high tube currents (mA) (range 200–800 mA). The high x-ray output minimizes exposure time and improves image quality by increasing the signal-to-noise ratio. The high kVp also provides a wide dynamic range by reducing bone absorption compared with soft tissue and extends tube life by reducing tube loading. The tubes use three-phase or high-frequency generators and operate in continuous or pulsed exposure modes. To minimize patient exposure, the beam is collimated to a thin fan beam before it enters the patient. Some of the x-ray photons interact with the patient and are scattered. To improve image quality, the residual beam is again collimated to remove the scattered photons before it reaches the detector array.

Detectors

In MDCT, the attenuated x-ray beam exiting the patient is captured by an array of detectors. Structurally each detector has three layers: a scintillator, a solid-state photodiode, and a substrate to provide mechanical and electrical infrastructure. The detectors absorb x-ray photons and produce visible light (scintillator), which is then converted into an electronic signal (photodiode) that forms the data to be analyzed. Scintillators usually have a high-atomic number, such as gadolinium oxysulfide (Gd_2S_2O). Scintillation detectors have a high x-ray detection efficiency and absorb almost 90% of the incident photons. This increased efficiency allows for short scan times and increases image signal-to-noise ratio. Detectors may have a predetector collimator (antiscatter grid) to limit the amount of scattered radiation that strikes the scintillator. This decreases noise and improves image contrast. Photon counting (PhC) detectors is a new technology that replaces the scintillator and the photodiode with a direct conversion material. Incoming x-ray photons are directly converted to electrical signals, allowing the detector to capture not only the number of striking photons, but also their energy. PhC detectors operate at lower doses, as counting is less disturbed by electronic noise and produce images with improved contrast-to-noise ratio (CNR) by different energy weighting of the detected photons.

Image Acquisition Parameters

Field of View

The collimated x-ray beam or scan FOV must encompass the anatomic region of interest (ROI) to be imaged. The physical extent of a cylindrical FOV is defined by a ventrodorsal (diameter) and craniocaudal (vertical) dimensions. The typical diameter of the FOV for MDCT is 25 cm. For maxillofacial and mandibular MDCT protocols, the vertical FOV ranges from 7 to 25 cm, to include the entire maxillofacial skeleton from the cranial base to below the inferior border of the mandibular. Prior to the scan, a scout projection or localizer view is performed. Localizer scans can be lateral or anterior-posterior (AP) and appear similar to lateral or AP head projections. This scout projection allows customized adjustment of the FOV to minimize radiation exposure to the patient. Following acquisition, the entire FOV, or a part thereof, can be reconstructed into an image data set. Some automatic exposure control (AEC) techniques (see later) use information from this scout view to estimate tube current based on patient size and anatomy.

Exposure Settings (kVp and mA)

Most adult CT examinations are performed at a tube voltage of 120 kVp. Several pediatric MDCT protocols use a lower kVp (80–120 kVp). Lowering the kVp will decrease the radiation dose to the patient but will increase image noise and increase contrast. A more common method to minimize radiation dose is to decrease the milliampere setting (mA). Notably, some units offer AEC rather than using fixed mA settings, where the mA is automatically adjusted depending on patient size and body part being examined.

Detector Configurations and Slice Thickness

In MDCT, multiple slices are acquired in one gantry rotation, and the minimum slice thickness is dependent on the detector row width. Following acquisition, data from contiguous detector rows can be combined *(binning)* to reconstruct slices of different thicknesses. For example, if a 320-slice CT scanner has detector elements that are 0.5-mm wide, the beam width would be 160 mm (320×0.5 mm). The acquired volume can be reconstructed into 320×0.5 mm slices, 160×1 mm slices, or 80×2 mm slices. The diagnostic task determines the reconstructed slice thickness. For maxillofacial examinations, bone evaluation is typically accomplished with 0.5-mm thick slices, whereas 1-mm thick sections are adequate for soft-tissue examination.

The detector *pitch* is the table distance traveled in one 360-degree gantry rotation divided by beam collimation width and influences scan speed, overlapping of sections, and the radiation dose.

$$\text{Pitch} = \frac{\text{Distance moved by table per 360 degree rotation}}{\text{Beam width}}$$

When the pitch is one, x-ray beams are contiguous for adjacent rotations and there is no overlap between slices. At a pitch less than one, x-ray beams overlap, yielding images with higher resolution. However, the length of tissue imaged per gantry rotation is less, resulting in longer scan times to image the same anatomic region. Importantly, the radiation dose to the patient is increased. When the pitch is greater than one, the x-ray beams are not contiguous and helical acquisitions are separated. This allows for faster scan times for the same scan length and reduced radiation dose. However, the missing data between the helical rotations reduce image resolution in the *z*-axis.

MDCT Reconstruction Kernels

Various image processing algorithms, also referred to as *filters* or *kernels,* can be applied to highlight specific characteristics in the MDCT image.

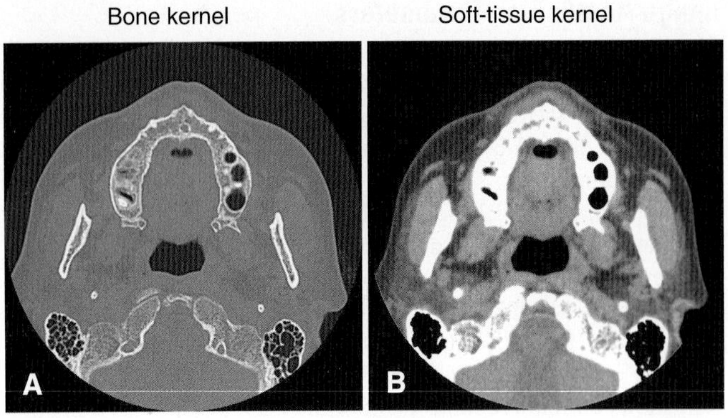

Fig. 9.4 (A) Axial MDCT images through the maxillary dentoalveolar arch, reconstructed with a bone kernel. Note details of bone trabeculation. (B) Axial slice from the same plane reconstructed with a soft-tissue kernel. Note enhanced contrast between muscles and subcutaneous fat.

These filters manipulate the contrast and spatial resolution to provide a reconstructed image that best serves a specific diagnostic purpose. These filters are denoted by their intended enhancement effect—*very smooth, smooth, medium, sharp,* and *ultra sharp*. Fig. 9.4 shows examples of a MDCT examination reconstructed with a bone *kernel* and a soft-tissue *kernel*. Application of the bone kernel will reconstruct an image with sharper detail to emphasize various features of bone, although with some increase in image noise. On the other hand, evaluation of soft-tissue areas requires delineation of minor differences in attenuation, and so soft-tissue kernels are applied that provide images with less noise and enhanced contrast resolution. The kernels are applied to the original sinogram data, before backprojection and separate reconstructions are generated for each kernel and each reconstruction should be evaluated separately. It is common for MDCT protocols to include several different reconstructions from a single scan. For example, an MDCT scan of the face, orbits, and sinus will acquire data using thin detector widths (typically 0.625 mm) at a pitch of 0.8 (overlapping data) and reconstruct the dataset to provide five sets of images:

- Axial sections, 3-mm thick, spaced 3 mm apart, reconstructed with smooth filters.
- Axial sections, 3-mm thick, spaced 3 mm apart, reconstructed with very sharp filters.
- Coronal sections, 3-mm thick, spaced 3 mm apart, reconstructed with very sharp filters.
- Axial sections, 0.75-mm thick, spaced 0.7 mm apart, reconstructed with very sharp filters.
- Coronal sections, 0.75-mm thick, spaced 0.7 mm apart, reconstructed with very sharp filters.

All reconstructions are applied to the original raw dataset, so while applying additional reconstructions increases the time to create the image series, it has no impact on patient radiation dose.

Contrast Agents

Contrast agents are injectable fluids used to improve radiographic visualization of specific soft tissue structures, the interface between anatomic structures or demonstrate relative vascularity. They are used almost exclusively in MDCT. Iodine-based intravenous (IV) contrast media are either ionic and nonionic and can be further classified as high or low osmolality, based on the concentration. The most common contrast agents are nonionic with low osmolality. The iodine in the contrast medium has a high atomic number ($Z = 53$) and efficiently attenuates x-rays by photoelectric absorption and appears bright (Fig. 9.5). Malignant maxillofacial tumors are often more vascularized than surrounding normal tissues; thus, the presence of the iodine perfusing through the vessels of these tissues increases their radiographic density and makes their margins more detectable. Contrast medium also helps to visualize enlarged lymph nodes containing metastatic carcinoma. The rate of acute adverse allergic-like (e.g., anaphylaxis and death) or physiologic reactions for low osmolarity is extremely low (approximately 0.6%) and the same for both ionic and nonionic agents, however, nonionic agents have a lower rate of minor reactions. The incidence of delayed adverse reactions (up to 1 week) ranges from 0.5% to 14%. Contrast-induced (within 6 hours) and contrast-associated (within 48 hours) acute kidney injury due to the nephrotoxicity of the contrast media may occur, particularly in elderly patients with preexisting severe renal insufficiency.

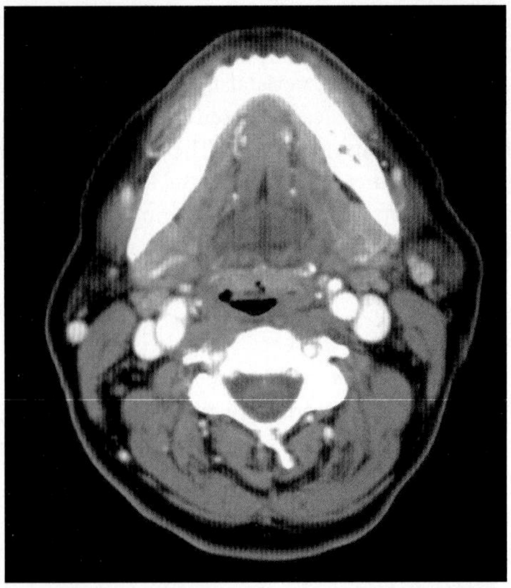

Fig. 9.5 Contrast agents. Iodine may be administered intravenously to enhance blood vessels and structures with a rich vascular supply, including the periphery of some tumors. Axial soft-tissue window computed tomography image at the level of the mandible after administration of iodine. Note prominent great vessels (white) lying just anterior and lateral to the cervical vertebrae and muscles of the floor of the mouth and neck.

CONE BEAM COMPUTED TOMOGRAPHY

CBCT imaging was originally developed for angiography in the early 1980s and subsequently used in other medical fields (e.g., radiotherapy, mammography). The first dental and maxillofacial units became commercially available in Europe in the late 1990s and subsequently in the early 2000s in the United States. There are almost 50 manufacturers of dental CBCT devices, with more than 200 models commercially available. With the reduced cost and small footprint of CBCT units, this modality continues to become increasingly available as an in-office imaging procedure and expanded the scope of its clinical application in dentistry. Technological changes have improved image quality and decreased radiation dose. Unlike intraoral, panoramic, and cephalometric radiography, CBCT acquires data volumetrically providing 3D radiographic imaging for the assessment of the dental and maxillofacial complex facilitating dental diagnosis. With expanding availability of third-party application software capable of importing data in DICOM file format, the role of maxillofacial CBCT has expanded to image guidance of operative and surgical procedures and, more recently, additive manufacturing (AM) of bio models and surgical guides.

CBCT imaging is performed using a rotating platform to which an x-ray source and detector are separated by a fixed distance. A divergent pyramidal- or cone-shaped source of ionizing radiation (similar in shape to the divergent beam of traditional 2D transmission imaging) is directed through the middle of the ROI and the transmitted, attenuated radiation is projected onto an area x-ray detector on the opposite side. The x-ray source and detector rotate around a rotation fulcrum, fixed within the center of the ROI. Unlike MDCT, the patient to be imaged does not move. This fulcrum acts as the center of the final acquired volume imaged. During the rotation, multiple sequential planar projection images covered by the detector, or the FOV are acquired in an arc of 180 degrees or greater. These single projection transmission images constitute the raw primary data and are individually referred to as basis, frame, or raw images. Basis images appear like cephalometric radiographic images, only each is slightly offset from the next. There are usually several hundred basis images with the complete series known as the projection data. The number of projections and the angular spacing between the projections are important determinants of image quality. Increasing the number of basis projections increases the image quality, but also increases patient radiation dose. This principle is used in many CBCT devices to provide low-dose imaging protocols by decreasing the number of projection angles. The basis images are integrated by software to construct an image volume and are very similar for CBCT and MDCT technologies. Only one rotational sequence of the gantry of 180 degrees or greater is necessary for CBCT to acquire enough data for volumetric image construction because the entire FOV is irradiated simultaneously.

Device Configuration

CBCT device configurations vary with manufacturer make and model. CBCT devices can be configured to be dedicated CT units or as hybrid multimodality systems that combine digital panoramic and/or cephalometric radiography with a small to medium FOV CBCT system (see Fig. 10.3). In most CBCT units, the x-ray source and the detector are mounted on a C-arm that rotates around a fixed axis centered within the anatomic ROI. The trajectory arc or rotational angle is ideally 360 degrees but can vary from 180 to 270 degrees. Because CBCT exposure incorporates the entire ROI, only one rotational scan of the gantry is necessary to acquire enough data for volumetric image construction. Some units with limited detector sizes may use two (vertical) or more (horizontal) consecutive scans to provide volumetric data which is then merged (registered and stitched together) into a larger FOV. In these instances, the patient rotation may be up to 720 degrees or more. Scan times average approximately 18 seconds (range 5–55 seconds), depending on CBCT model and the protocol selected. Scan time corresponds to the time between the first and last basis image acquisition and varies from exposure time, which is the period during the scan when the patient is exposed to radiation. Most CBCT units (80%) scan the patient while standing, 17% are performed with the patient sitting, and few (3%) scan the patient while supine (see Fig. 9.6). Supine units are physically larger, have a greater physical footprint, and may not be accessible for patients with some physical disabilities. Standing units may not be able to be adjusted to a height low enough to accommodate wheelchair-bound patients. Although seated units are the most comfortable, they may not allow scanning of physically disabled or wheelchair-bound patients. With all systems, immobilization of the patient's head is more important than patient positioning because any head movement degrades the final image. Immobilization of the head is achieved by using some combination of a chin cup, bite fork, or other head-restraint mechanism.

X-Ray Source

The x-ray generators used in CBCT machines are far simpler than those used in MDCT. Most units have adjustable kVp (range 80–120 kVp) and mA (range 1–32 mA) options with most of the units operating toward the lower end of these ranges which do not differ substantially from operating parameters in panoramic radiographic machines. Focal spot size for CBCT (nominal range 0.15–0.7 mm) is usually smaller than MDCT (nominal range 0.5–0.8 mm), however, unlike MDCT, the anode is stationary in most CBCT systems. During the scan rotation in CBCT imaging, each projection image set is made by sequential single-image capture of the remnant attenuated x-ray beam by the area detector. X-ray generation may be continuous but is most often pulsed to coincide with the detector activation and sampling. This is preferable in that it means that actual exposure time can be substantially less than scanning time, significantly reducing patient radiation dose.

Detectors

All current CBCT units use 2D array flat panel detectors (FPDs) to record projection images. FPDs employ an "indirect" detector based on a large-area solid-state detector panel coupled to an x-ray scintillator layer (see Chapter 4). The most common flat panel configuration consists of a cesium iodide scintillator applied to a thin film transistor made of amorphous silicon. X-rays are detected indirectly by means of a scintillator converting them to visible light that is registered in the photo diode array. The photodiodes produce an electrical charge proportional to the incident x-ray energy. The FPD area array of *dexels* record various levels of radiation attenuation and after preprocessing is represented on the image display matrix as shades of gray or intensity levels. The range of shades of gray captured is known as the bit depth and for CBCT FPDs ranges between 8 (256 shades) and 16 bits (65,536 shades) with 14 bits (16,384 shades) being the most common.

For each basis image, the detector records incident x-ray photons, collects a charge, and sends a signal to the computer. As rotation is usually performed within times equivalent or less compared to panoramic radiography (from 5 seconds to approximately 20 seconds), this means that each basis image is acquired and sent within milliseconds, and this occurs many hundreds of times within a single exposure rotation. The speed with which a detector performs this acquisition is called the *frame-rate*.

Cone Beam Computed Tomographic Image Acquisition Parameters

Field of View

The shape and size of the FOV or scan volume primarily depend on the detector size and shape, the beam projection geometry, and the ability to collimate the beam. The shape of almost all scan volumes is cylindrical. One manufacturer produces a convex triangular (rouleaux) scan volume for medium-sized FOVs which more closely matches the shape of the dental arches and compared to a cylindrical scan volume reduces radiation exposure. Mechanical collimation of the height and width of the primary x-ray beam limits radiation exposure to the ROI. It is desirable to limit the field size to the smallest volume that includes the ROI. This field size should be selected for each patient based on individual needs. This procedure reduces unnecessary exposure to the patient and produces optimal images by minimizing scattered radiation, which degrades image quality. CBCT units are classified according to the maximum FOV incorporated from the scan or scans (Fig. 9.7).

Manufacturers use three approaches to extend the size of the FOV to include a large ROI that is larger than the detector. The first method

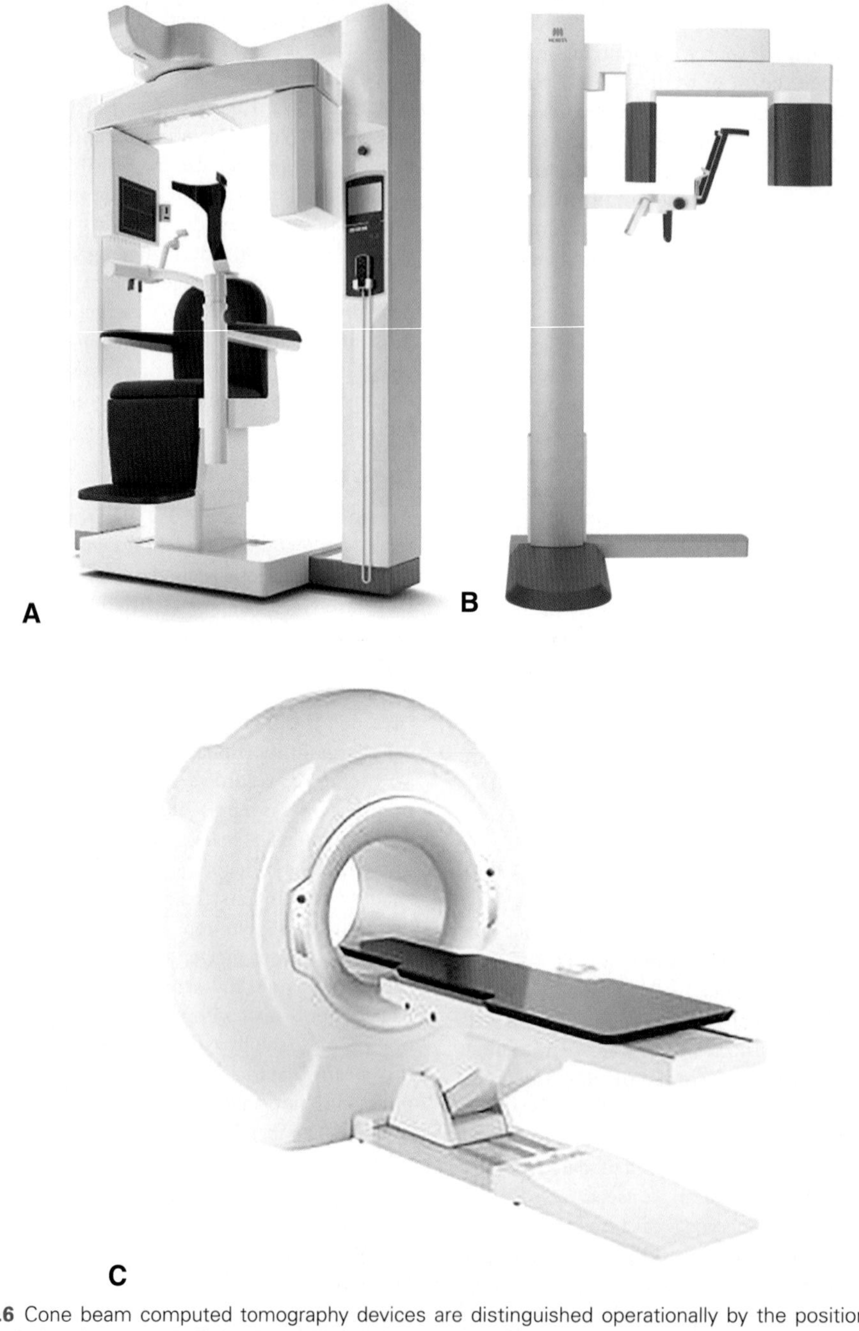

Fig. 9.6 Cone beam computed tomography devices are distinguished operationally by the position of the patient during the scan. (A) Sitting (e.g., 3D Accuitomo 170, J. Morita Corp., Kyoto, Japan). (B) Standing (e.g., X800 CBCT and panoramic device, J. Morita Corp., Kyoto, Japan). (C) Supine (e.g., Newtom 5G XL, Newtom | Cefla, Imola, Italy). Devices shown on panel (A) and panel (C) are dedicated CBCT devices. (3D Accuitomo and X800 images courtesy and copyright of J. Morita Corp., Kyoto, Japan; Newtom 5G XL image courtesy and copyright of Newtom | Cefla, Imola, Italy.)

involves combining or *stitching* two or more adjacent scans. In this approach, overlapping regions of adjacent scan volumes are registered using concordant reference landmarks and fused together (stitched) to create a larger scan volume. This involves an initial scan, physical translation of the gantry either vertically or horizontally while the patient is still restrained in the head holder, and immediate acquisition of a second scan to extend either the height or width of the FOV, respectively (Fig. 9.8). The disadvantage of stitching overlapped regions is that such overlapped regions are imaged twice, resulting in double the radiation dose in these areas. Approximately one-quarter of all CBCT units use this technique. A second method to increase the height or width of the FOV using a small area detector is to laterally offset the position of the detector, collimate the beam asymmetrically, and scan only half the patient's ROI in each of the two lateral offset scans (Fig. 9.9). In these scan volumes, there is variation in image quality (i.e., noise, contrast resolution, and artefact production) between the

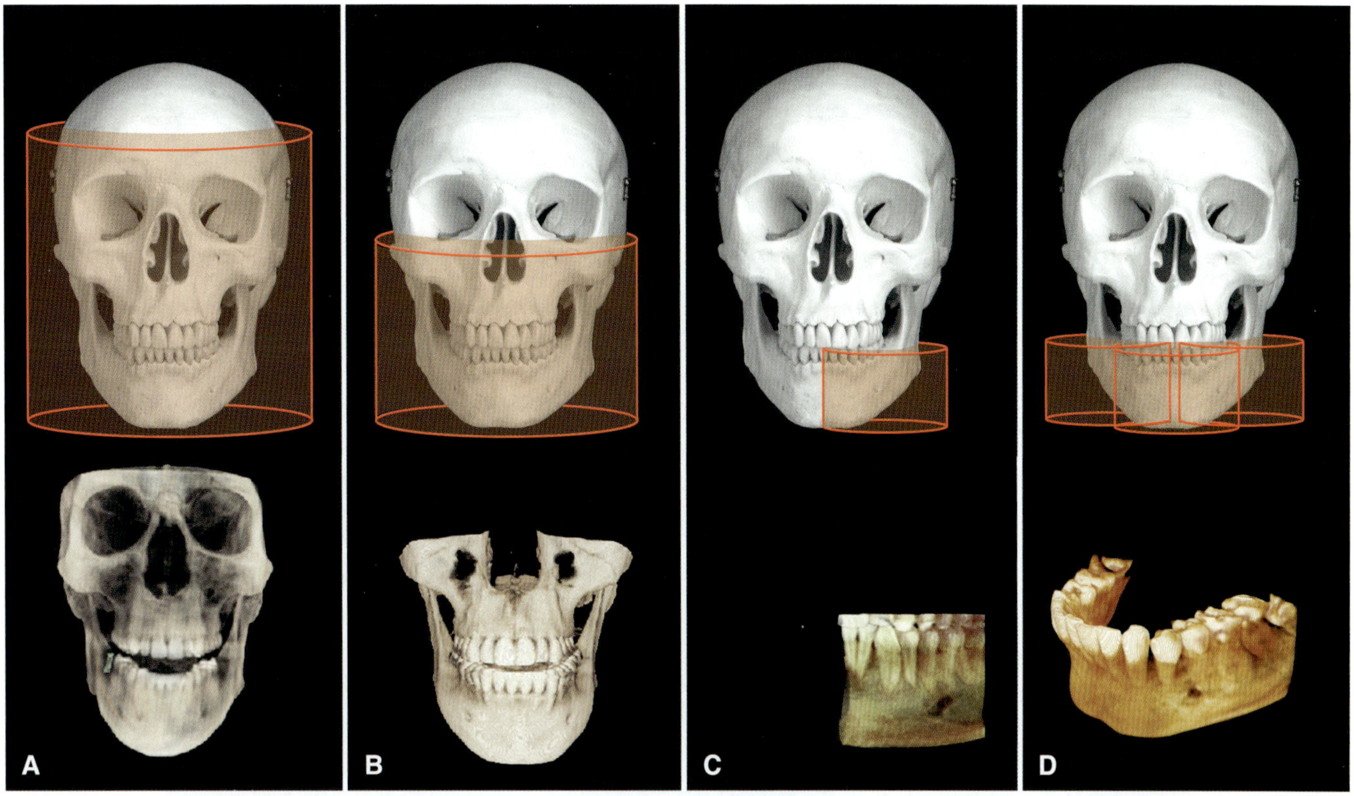

Fig. 9.7 Classification of cone beam computed tomography units according to the field of view (FOV). (A) Craniofacial FOV scans provide images of the entire craniofacial skeleton, enabling cephalometric analysis. (B) Maxillofacial FOV scans image the maxilla or mandible or both. (C) Limited FOV scans provide high-resolution images of limited regions. (D) Stitched scans from multiple limited FOV scans provide larger regions of interest to be imaged from superimposition of multiple scans. (Skull image courtesy and copyright of Primal Pictures, Ltd., London, UK: http://www.primalpictures.com.)

central and peripheral regions and therefore positioning of an object toward the center of the FOV becomes more critical.

Collimation of the CBCT primary x-ray beam by adjustment of the FOV enables limitation of the x-radiation to the ROI and can reduce patient radiation dose considerably. Adjustment in the FOV usually can be accomplished mechanically or, in some instances, electronically. Currently, most CBCT units use adjustable metallic shields acting as primary collimation at the radiation source to adjust the dimensions of the x-ray beam to the ROI. Electronic collimation involves cropping of data recorded on the detector that are peripheral to the area of interest. Electronic collimation is undesirable because it results in greater exposure of the patient to radiation than is necessary for the imaging task.

Reduction of the FOV to the ROI improves image quality because reduced scattered radiation is recorded (see Fig. 9.12). In addition, smaller FOVs have less beam divergence at the edge of the FOV, which results in improved peripheral image quality. More importantly, a reduction in FOV is usually associated with patient dose reductions ranging from 25% to 66% depending on machine, type of collimation (vertical or horizontal), amount of mechanical collimation, and location (maxilla vs. mandible; anterior vs. posterior).

Exposure Settings (kVp, mA)

Several parameters determine the energy and quantity of the x-ray beam and influence the quality of the projection image. These factors are both equipment dependent (e.g., focal spot size, source-object distance, object-detector distance, beam filtration, and beam frequency) and operator-dependent (e.g., exposure factors, such as tube current (mA), tube voltage (kVp), and exposure time (s). Most CBCT units operate at or below 90 kVp, whereas a few can operate at higher kVp, up to 120 kV. In general, low kVp units operate at a higher mA. Some CBCT manufacturers provide units with fixed, nonadjustable exposure settings, whereas others incorporate "preset" exposure settings for different-sized individuals or specific scanning protocols and allow operator "manual" adjustment of kVp or mA or both (Fig. 9.10). Operators who use CBCT units with operator-adjustable exposure settings must understand that these parameters affect both image quality (Fig. 9.11) and patient radiation dose and that careful selection is required to fulfill the ALARA (*As Low As Reasonably Achievable*) principle.

The ALARA principle of dose optimization necessitates that CBCT exposure factors should be adjusted to produce a diagnostically acceptable image based on patient size and specific diagnostic task. This adjustment can be primarily achieved by appropriate selection of mA, kVp, or both. In some cases, exposure time also can be adjusted to change scan time. Faster scans produce volumetric data sets from fewer basis images (see later section on scan modes). The variation in exposure parameters together with the presence of pulsed x-ray beam and size of the FOV are the primary determinants of patient exposure. Although commonplace in MDCT, AEC in maxillofacial CBCT units is currently extremely limited. AEC is a technique that modulates mA specifically for each patient according to the radiation intensity recorded by the detector by using a short preexamination (scout)

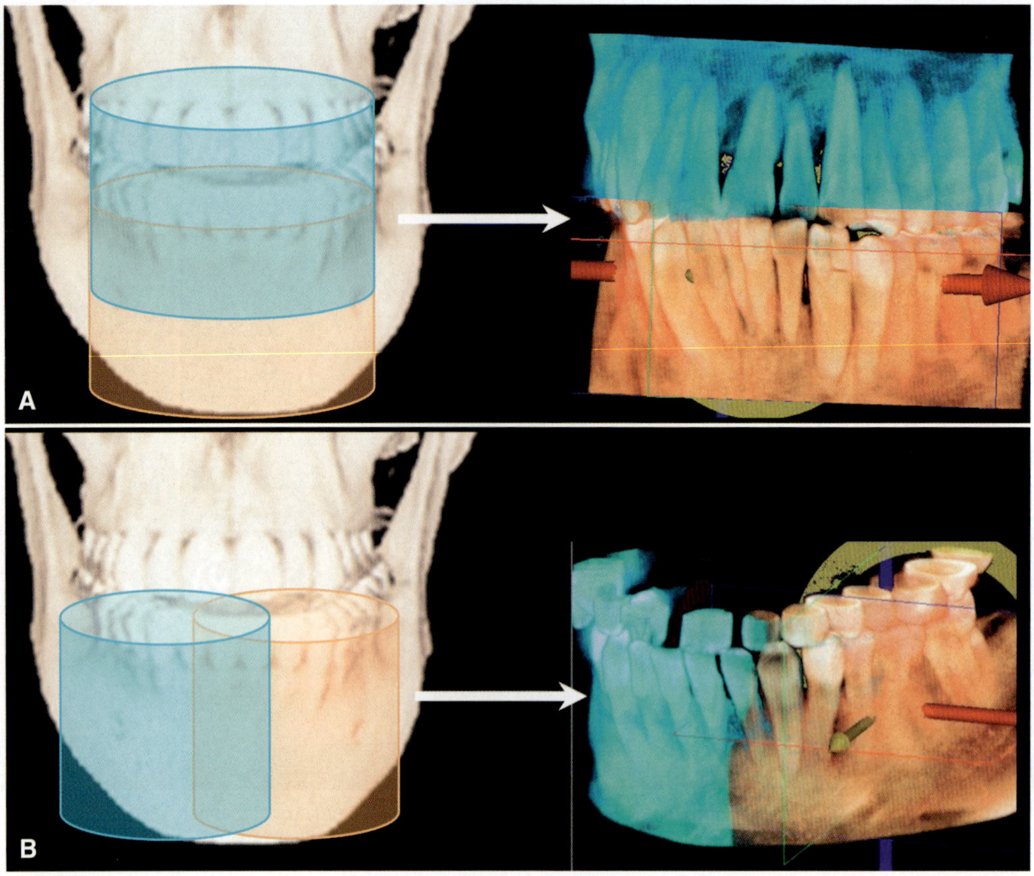

Fig. 9.8 Increasing field of view (FOV) by "stitching" volumetric datasets. Larger ROI can be acquired by small FOV cone beam computed tomography units by "stitching" adjacent limited area volumetric datasets. This process requires acquisition of separate scans *(left)*, registration of each volume by superimposition of fiducial landmarks, and fusion to provide a larger FOV *(right)*. Units may use this technique to increase either the vertical (A) or the horizontal (B) FOV. Shown here are adjacent *(orange and blue)* volumetric datasets (KODAK CS 9000 Carestream Dental, Atlanta, GA) stitched manually using proprietary software. (Invivo dental software, Osteoid, Santa Clara, CA.)

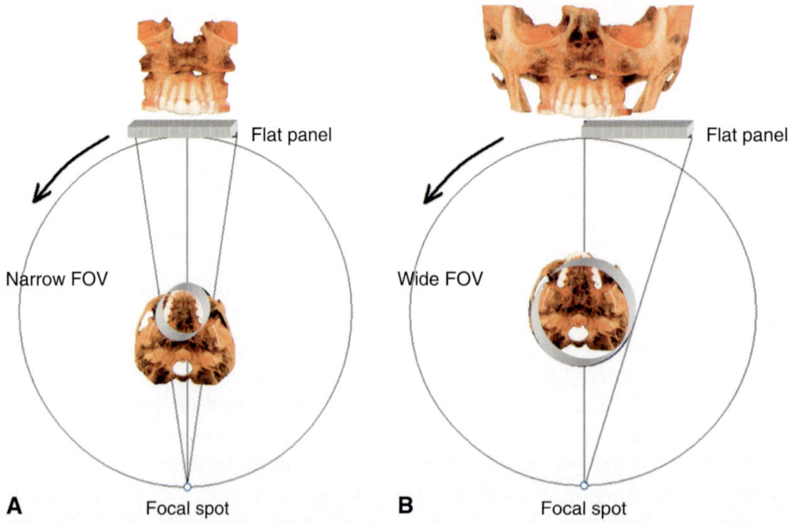

Fig. 9.9 Schematic of asymmetric cone beam computed tomography geometric configuration to increase field of view (FOV). (A) Conventional geometric arrangement whereby the central ray of the x-ray beam from the focal source is directed through the middle of the object to the center of the detector. The resultant image is limited to the region of the detector (dentition in this case). (B) Alternative method increasing image size involves shifting the location of the detector and collimating the x-ray beam laterally to extend the FOV to include a greater volume of the object. In this instance, the detector is shifted to the opposite side of the midline halfway through the exposure. The resulting image doubles the horizontal ROI. (Courtesy DEXIS Alpharetta, GA, previously SOREDEX, Tuusula, Finland.)

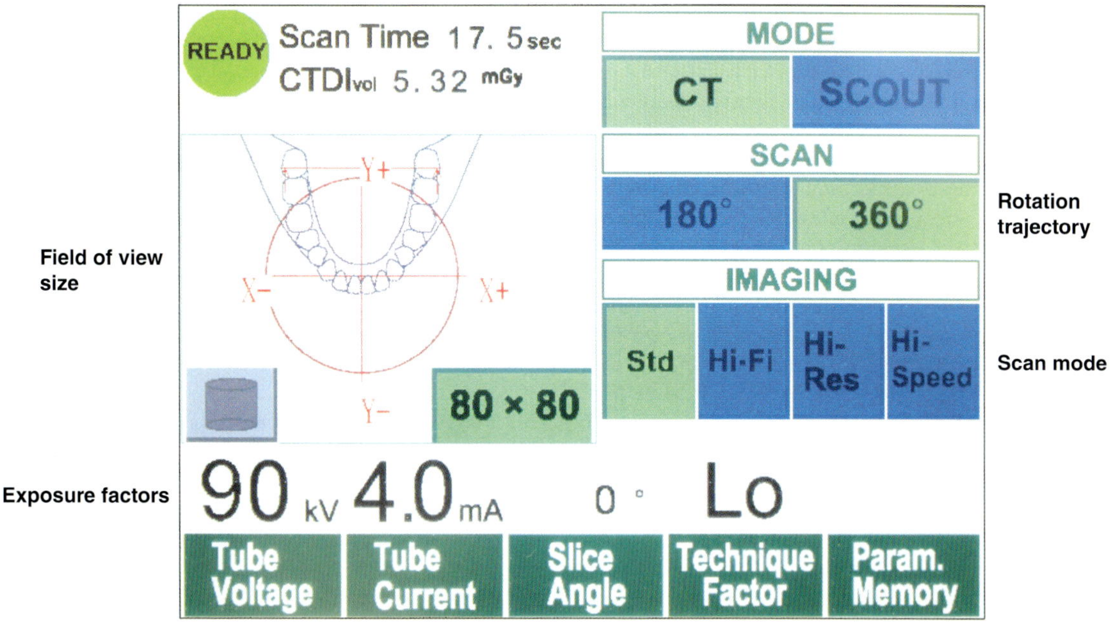

Fig. 9.10 Control panel for a cone beam computed tomography device (Accuitomo 170, J. Morita Corp., Kyoto, Japan). Icons in *light green* show the selected settings for a medium field of view (80 mm × 80 mm) with a rotation trajectory of 360 degrees, and a standard nominal resolution. The selected exposure factors (90 kV, 4 mA) can be adjusted to optimize for patient size. The scan time and the radiation dose (computed tomography dose index, CTDI) for these settings are displayed in the *top left* corner.

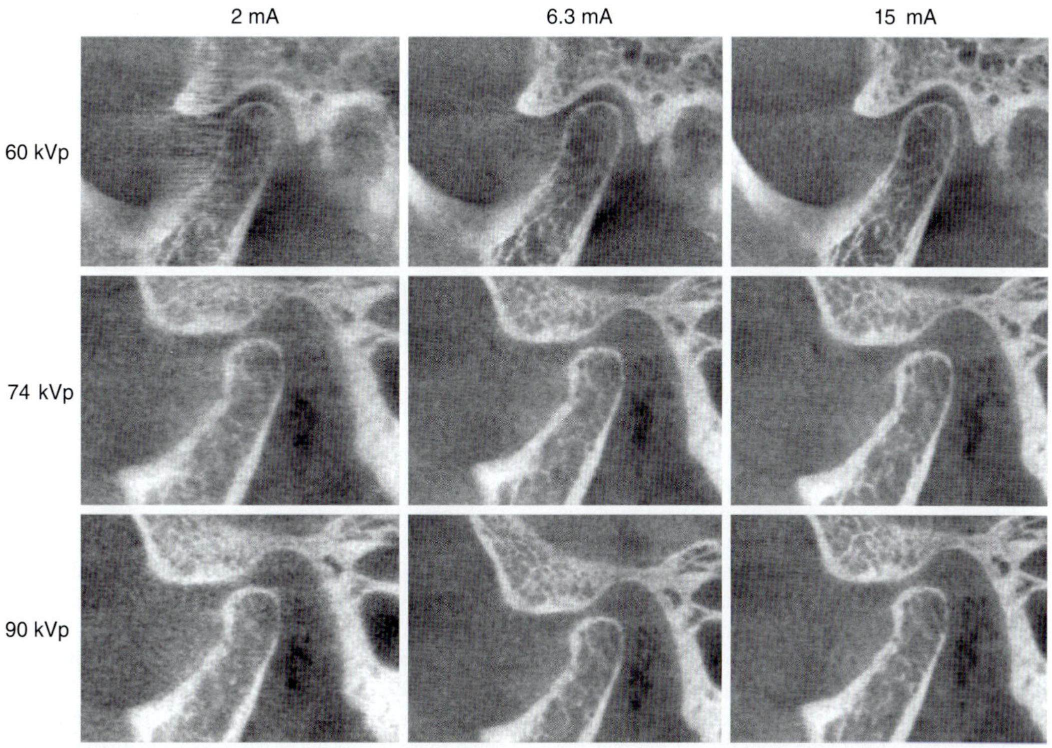

Fig. 9.11 Effect of exposure parameters on image quality. Representative 0.076 mm parasagittal slices of the left temporomandibular joint demonstrate the effect of changing mA (columns) and kVp (rows) on image quality for high-density (cortical bone) and low-density (cancellous bone) structures. Although all images are adequate for visualization of gross morphologic changes at all values, there is increased graininess (noise) of the images occurring at low kVp and mA, making discernment of the fine trabecular pattern or surface irregularities of cortical plates more difficult. Little improvement in subjective image quality is achieved at settings greater than 74 kVp and 6.3 mA despite appreciable associated increases in dose.

exposure or using an exposure modulation during the rotation. Implementation of AEC in maxillofacial is extremely limited, however, widespread adoption would avoid the need for manual adaptation of exposure parameters based on patient size and minimize patient radiation exposure.

In clinical practice, mA changes are preferable to kVp changes when exposure reduction is necessary to compensate for differences in patient size. This is because the increase in noise for a given dose reduction is smaller for mA than kVp. mA adjustments affect effective dose proportionately. Higher kVp may be considered in patients with high-density objects, such as teeth with root canal fillings or dental implants, to reduce beam-hardening artifacts from these materials. Adjustment of kVp has an even greater effect on dose than does mA, with each increase in 10 kVp approximately doubling the dose if all other parameters remain the same. Exposure parameters should be appropriate for both the given patient size and the diagnostic task that motivated image selection.

Detector Dexel Size and Voxel Size

The detector nominal *dexel* size influences the final spatial resolution of a CBCT image. A CBCT volumetric dataset is composed of a 3D matrix of discrete spatial units, called a *voxel*, each possessing a location (a spatial coordinate) and an intensity value (associated with the radiographic density at that coordinate). When represented as a 2D image area matrix on a display monitor, each *voxel* is represented as a *pixel*. All CBCT units provide voxel resolutions that are isotropic—equal in all three dimensions. The principal determinants of nominal voxel size in a CBCT image are the dimensions of the matrix and size of each dexel on the detector. Detectors with smaller dexels capture fewer x-ray photons per voxel and result in more image noise. Consequently, CBCT imaging using higher resolutions may be designed to use higher dosages to achieve a reasonable signal-to-noise ratio for improved diagnostic image quality. In addition, CBCT units may offer a selection of voxel sizes. For these choices, the image detector collects information over a series of dexels in the horizontal and vertical directions and averages the data. This collation or binning results in a substantial reduction in data processing, reducing secondary reconstruction times. Therefore, voxel size should be specified as either acquisition or reconstruction. Although increased image resolution in some CBCT units does not affect changes in exposure parameters, some manufacturers incorporate reduced dose exposure protocols for low-resolution settings.

Scan Modes

The number of basis images that constitute the projection data from the scan is determined by the detector frame rate (number of images acquired per second), the extent of the rotational arc (180–360 degrees), and the rotational speed. The number of basis images of a projection dataset may be fixed or variable. Longer scan times provide for higher frame rates which have both desirable and undesirable effects. Higher frame rates increase the signal-to-noise ratio, producing images with less noise and reducing metallic artifacts (Fig. 9.12). However, a higher frame rate results in a greater patient radiation dose. Since more data are obtained, primary reconstruction time is increased. In contrast, some "quick scan" or "fast scan" protocols use markedly lower frame rates with considerable reduction in patient radiation dose. However, the image resolution from these scans may not be adequate for all diagnostic tasks.

CBCT units may have fixed or variable rotation angles. Most CBCT units have fixed scan angles. These units may be a full rotation (360 degrees) or partial trajectory arcs (range 200–270 degrees). CBCT imaging with a full scan arc acquires adequate projection data to provide high-fidelity reconstruction. CBCT units based on panoramic platforms may provide fixed partial trajectory arcs. While scan time and patient radiation dose is reduced in these units, images produced by this method may have greater noise and reconstruction interpolation artifacts. Units providing variable rotation angles usually provide two options: a complete or a partial scan arc. Reconstructed images from incomplete, limited, or truncated scanning trajectories of less than 360 degrees may have limited-angle artifacts because of missing information. These include greater peripheral unidirectional streaking artifacts and more pronounced midplane cupping and photon starvation artifacts. Missing data can be compensated for with many approaches, including use of statistical knowledge of the patient's anatomy and use of numerous algorithm projection completion techniques.

It is desirable to reduce CBCT scan times to as short as possible to reduce motion artifact resulting from patient movement. Patient movement can be substantial and may be a limiting factor in image resolution. Decreased scanning times may be achieved by increasing the detector frame rate, reducing the number of projections, or reducing the scan arc. The first method provides images of the highest quality, whereas the latter methods increase image noise.

CBCT Reconstruction Kernels

In most CBCT units, the acquired dataset is reconstructed with a default primary reconstruction algorithm that cannot be controlled by the user. Recently, some CBCT models have introduced iterative or deep learning–based reconstruction methods. These techniques, which involve multiple applications of image reconstruction algorithms ("iterations"), produce images with reduced noise and both metal and motion-related artifacts. Some CBCT devices allow the selection of secondary reconstruction algorithms to enhance detail or contrast. Some vendors provide the option to apply metal artifact reduction (MAR) to reduce artifacts from highly attenuating materials such as dental implants and gutta percha and motion artifact correction (MAC) algorithms to mitigate against image artifacts due to head motion during the scan. Motional artifact reduction convolutional neural network based on deep learning shows promise and potential application in improving CBCT image quality.

CLINICAL APPLICATIONS OF COMPUTED TOMOGRAPHY

CT is indicated in diagnosis and management of several diseases and conditions (Table 9.2). MDCT and CBCT are both CT technologies that provide high resolution imaging of the maxillofacial hard tissues. MDCT has higher contrast resolution, enabling soft-tissue evaluation to assess pathoses that cannot be adequately evaluated by CBCT. The use of IV contrast media is limited to MDCT and improves the sensitivity of detection of numerous soft tissue conditions due to enhancement, including inflammation, malignancy, and lymph node involvement. The choice of MDCT versus CBCT is based primarily on the diagnostic objective. Many of these objectives can be accomplished by both MDCT and CBCT, however, modality choice should be based on the need for superior contrast resolution (MDCT) or spatial resolution (for CBCT). For most intraosseous pathologies in the bone, CBCT is adequate. MDCT provides better evaluation of soft tissues. Thus, when there is evident or suspected soft-tissue involvement, MDCT is the preferred CT modality. Table 9.3 compares the spatial resolution, contrast resolution, and radiation dose of MDCT and CBCT. Compared with CBCT, MDCT has a higher radiation dose, and lesser spatial resolution.

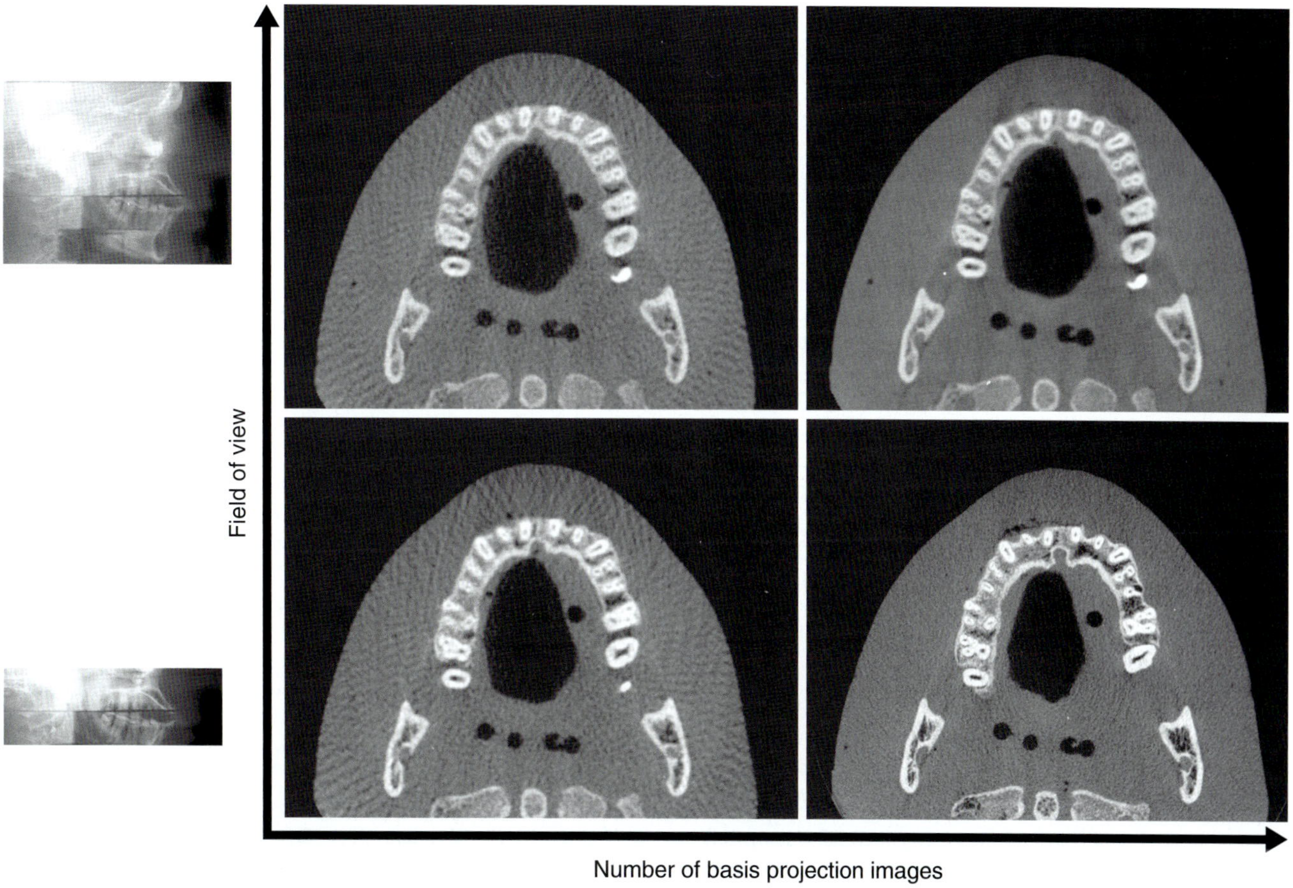

Fig. 9.12 Pictorial plot of the effect of number of basis projection images and size of field of view (FOV) on image quality. Increasing the number of projections in one 360-degree scan (*x*-axis) provides more data and reduces image noise; however, it increases patient dose proportionately. Reducing the number of projections creates undersampling and produces line patterns, which are more prominent at the periphery of the scan (moiré effects). Minimizing the FOV (*y*-axis) reduces patient exposure and resultant scatter radiation and results in images with increased contrast and decreased noise.

TABLE 9.2 Relative Clinical Indications for Computed Tomography Imaging

	MDCT	CBCT[a]		
		Limited FOV	Dentoalveolar FOV	Craniofacial FOV
Implant dentistry	++	+++	+++	++
Teeth and periodontal structures: Endodontics	−	+++	++	−
Teeth and periodontal structures: Periodontics	−	+++	++	−
Impacted teeth	+	+++	+++	+
Trauma: Dental	−	+++	++	−
Trauma: Dentoalveolar	+	+++	+++	+
Trauma: Maxillofacial	+++	−	++	+++
Pathoses: Intraosseous	++	++	+++	++
Pathoses: Soft tissue	+++	−	−	−
Craniofacial assessment	++	−	+	+++
TMJ evaluation (Condyle, eminence and fossa)	++	+++[b]	+++[c]	+++[d]
Paranasal sinuses	+++	−	+	++

[a]Use the smallest FOV that will encompass the anatomy of interest.
[b]Separate acquisitions for the right and left sides.
[c]FOV encompasses both TMJs, and may partially include the dental arches.
[d]Preferred when skeletal discrepancy or asymmetry present.
−, Not indicated in most situations and has an unfavorable risk-benefit ratio; +, may be not indicated in many circumstances and has an equivocal or slightly favorable risk-benefit ratio; ++, is indicated in many situations at a favorable risk-benefit ratio; +++, is indicated in most situations and provides optimal diagnostic information at a favorable risk-benefit ratio.

TABLE 9.3 Comparison of Multidetector Computed Tomography and Cone Beam Computed Tomography Parameters

Parameter	Multidetector Computed Tomography	Cone Beam Computed Tomography
Device footprint	Large	Small
Acquisition time	Less than 1 second	Typically 15–20 seconds
Craniomaxillofacial CT, standard protocol		
Spatial resolution	Inadequate for dental and periodontal assessment	Higher resolution of dental and periodontal structures
Image noise	Lower	High
Soft tissue contrast resolution	Excellent	Poor
Radiation dose	Standard protocol: 0.65 mSv Low-dose protocol: 0.18 mSv	Limited FOV: 0.05 mSv Maxillofacial FOV: 0.1 mSv Craniofacial FOV: 0.12–0.15 mSv

MDCT AND CBCT: COMPARISON OF STRENGTHS AND LIMITATIONS

While the data produced by CT technology is now essentially volumetric, there are numerous similarities and differences between MDCT and CBCT that provide advantages and disadvantages for each technology. These features translate to differences in size and cost of equipment, utility, image quality, and patient radiation dose.

Acquisition

MDCT and CBCT can be compared in all four steps of the image acquisition process:

- X-ray generation and projection geometry: MDCT systems rely on high power x-ray generators with beam energies of 120–140 kVp to acquire large volumes of data at high speeds and are operated at maximum power for a limited time only, approximately 30–60 seconds. Innovations in x-ray tube design, like the rotating envelope vacuum vessel (e.g., Straton tube), "flying focal spot," variable focal spot sizes, and improved heat dissipation have enabled longer exposures. CBCT x-ray generators are far simpler, in many instances the same as in panoramic units, with stationary focal spots operating at lower kVp and marked reduced mA. The primary rotational motion of the x-ray source and detector in MDCT is a complex spiral or helical motion and always scans the patient in the supine position. MDCT units consequently have a larger physical footprint and are 10–20 times more expensive than CBCT units. Both features make CBCT better suited for in-office imaging in dental practices and imaging centers. However, MDCT images are produced with better contrast, reduced noise, and fewer artifacts but at a higher dose.
- X-ray detection: The arrangement and structure of detectors in MDCT units is more complicated than CBCT with greater collimation and geometric correspondence between the x-ray beam and the detector. The efficiency and sensitivity of MDCT detectors is also higher, contributing to optimal soft tissue contrast imaging. FPD detectors used in CBCT unfortunately have limitations in their performance including linearity of response to the radiation spectrum, lack of uniformity of response throughout the area of the detector, and bad pixels. Consequently, high-resolution CBCT imaging often uses greater exposures to achieve a reasonable signal-to-noise ratio for diagnostic image quality. The effects of these factors on image quality are most noticeable at lower and higher exposures.
- Image reconstruction: While both CT technologies use FBP reconstruction operations, the process differs somewhat in spiral CT scanners. An additional preprocessing step (z-interpolation) is required to correct the inconsistencies present in the data set due to the continuous spiral motion and to create planar images from the spiral data at any random plane along the imaging volume. While postprocessing operations such as contrast, brightness, and edge enhancement can be applied to CBCT data after reconstruction to improve visualization, various reconstruction kernels can be applied to MDCT data to modify the frequency contents of projection data prior to FBP during image reconstruction for specific anatomic applications, influencing both resolution and contrast. This requires substantial workstation computing power rather than PC-based computers commonly used for CBCT.
- Display: Both MDCT and CBCT images are viewed on computer monitors using software programs in a default display and viewed interactively. The data are in DICOM file standard format which not only contains the image files but metadata. One element of the metadata is the calibration instructions for monitors to provide consistent display of images referred to as gray scale display function (GSDF). This is especially important for MDCT images which have high contrast resolution. Computer monitors for the display of medical images can be classified into primary and secondary display systems. Primary display systems (medical grade, DICOM conformant) are used for interpretation of MDCT medical images and must meet strict performance criteria according to ACR (American College of Radiology) standards. While under consideration, no such standards currently exist for CBCT display in dentistry. Most CBCT systems incorporate secondary display systems (consumer grade).

Acquisition Time

MDCT acquisition times are rapid with scanning of the maxillofacial region in less than 1 second. This rapid scanning time, along with the configuration of a patient bed, makes MDCT more suited to image patients with trauma (see Chapter 25) or nonambulatory patients. The typical scan time for CBCT units is typically 15–20 seconds. Some "fast scan" protocols have a scan time of 5 seconds, but image quality is markedly reduced and may not be adequate for specific diagnostic tasks. For some "high-resolution" CBCT protocols, the scan time may be as high as 40 seconds, increasing the possibility of image motion artifact due to patient movement during the scan.

Spatial Resolution

The spatial resolution of a CT image is primarily related to, but not exclusively determined by, the physical attributes of the detector *dexel* including the nominal dimensions and fill factor—the fraction of a dexel's area that is capable of recording light. Other factors affecting the maximum achievable resolution include the beam projection geometry, x-ray scatter, detector and patient motion, focal spot size, image acquisition settings (e.g., number of basis images, full arc vs. partial arc), and reconstruction algorithms. Both MDCT and CBCT are capable of providing submillimeter spatial resolution. With MDCT units, nominal detector width approaches 0.5 mm. With CBCT units, the nominal voxel resolution is typically 0.4 mm for larger fields of view. Some machines are capable of high-resolution imaging (nominal 0.076–0.125 mm voxel resolution) and may be required for tasks requiring discernment of fine detail anatomic structures (e.g., periodontal ligament space, root canal morphology) and disease processes (e.g., root resorption, ankylosis, or fracture).

Both MDCT and CBCT units in general provide voxel resolutions that are isotropic—equal in all three dimensions. The principal determinants of nominal voxel size in a CBCT image are the detector matrix dimensions and size of each dexel. Detectors with smaller dexels capture fewer x-ray photons per voxel and result in more image noise. Consequently, CBCT imaging using higher resolutions may require higher dosages to improve signal-to-noise ratio for adequate diagnostic image quality. In addition, CBCT units may offer a selection of voxel sizes. For these choices, the detector collects information over a series of dexels and converts one to one as voxels (acquisition resolution) and subsequently pixels. During reconstruction, the dimensional and image intensity values of corresponding adjacent pixels in the horizontal and vertical directions in the image matrix may be averaged (reconstructed or displayed resolution). This collation or *pixel binning* results in a substantial reduction in data processing, reducing secondary reconstruction times. Therefore, voxel size should be specified as either acquisition or reconstruction. Although increased image resolution in some CBCT units does not affect changes in exposure parameters, some manufacturers incorporate reduced dose exposure protocols for low-resolution settings.

Both the focal spot size and the geometric configuration of the x-ray source are important factors in determining the degree of geometric unsharpness, a limiting factor in spatial resolution. The cost of x-ray tubes—and therefore of the CT unit—increases substantially with small focal spot size tubes.

Reducing the object-to-detector distance and increasing source-to-object distance also minimizes geometric unsharpness. In maxillofacial CBCT imaging, the detector position is limited because it must be located far enough from the patient's head so that it freely rotates unobstructed by the patient's shoulders. Limitations also exist in extending the source-to-object distance because this increases the size of the CBCT unit. However, reducing source-to-object distance produces a magnified projected image on the detector, potentially increasing spatial resolution.

Patient motion during exposure decreases image resolution. Gantry rotation in MDCT is rapid, and the entire maxillofacial region can be acquired in less than 1 second. With CBCT, gantry rotation is much slower, typically 20–30 seconds.

The image reconstruction algorithm applied can enhance or degrade spatial resolution. The proprietary nature of image reconstruction algorithms contributes to differences in image quality from the different CBCT manufacturers.

Image Noise

Random variations of gray level intensity within the image are referred to as image noise, and are influenced by x-ray scatter, exposure factors (kVp, mA), slice thickness, detector factors (nominal detector width or pixel size), and electronic disturbances. Some noise can be reduced by *adaptive filtering* applied during reconstruction.

The signal-to-noise ratio is higher for MDCT than for CBCT. This reflects the robust signal produced in MDCT when using radiation outputs with higher beam energies. The cone beam projection acquisition geometry irradiates a larger tissue volume yielding more scatter radiation from Compton interactions. Much of this scattered radiation is produced omnidirectionally and recorded by detector pixels. Consequently, the number of photons detected at each pixel does not reflect the true attenuation of an object along a specific path of the x-ray beam, contributing to image noise and degradation. The amount of scattered radiation is generally proportional to the total mass of tissue contained within the primary x-ray beam; this increases with increasing object thickness and field size. The contribution of this scattered radiation to production of the CBCT image may be greater than that of the primary beam. In clinical applications, the scatter-to-primary ratios are about 0.01 for single-ray CT imaging, 0.05–0.15 for fan beam and spiral CT imaging, and may be 0.4–2 in CBCT imaging. For these reasons, it is always desirable to use the smallest FOV possible when making a CBCT image.

Additional sources of image noise in CT are statistical variations in the homogeneity of the incident x-ray beam (quantum mottle) and added noise of the detector system (electronic). The inhomogeneity of x-ray photons depends on the number of the primary and scattered x-rays absorbed, the primary and scattered x-ray spectra incident on the detector, and the number of basis projections. Electronic noise is due to the inherent degradations of the detector system related to the x-ray absorption efficiency of energy at the detector.

In addition, with CBCT, because of the increased divergence of the x-ray beam over the area detector, there is a pronounced heel effect. This effect produces a large variation or nonuniformity of the incident x-ray beam on the patient and resultant nonuniformity in absorption with greater signal-to-noise ratio (noise) on the cathode side of the image relative to the anode side.

Soft Tissue Contrast

Contrast resolution is the ability to determine subtle differences in radiodensity in an image. Variations in image intensity are a result of differential attenuation of x-rays by tissues that differ in density, atomic number, or thickness. MDCT produces images with high contrast resolution. Separate reconstructions (kernels) are applied to emphasize bone and soft tissue and allow evaluation of a wide range of contrasts, ranging from fat, muscle, and trabecular and cortical bone. MDCT is the preferred modality to image soft tissue pathoses and fascial space infections.

Two physical factors limit the contrast resolution of CBCT: The inherent geometric configuration and the use of 2D detector panels with no collimation. The geometric configuration of CBCT provides both a relatively short source-to-object and object-to-detector distance and, coupled with the divergence of the x-ray projection beam, results in a high amount of scatter radiation. Detection of scattered x-ray photons in areas not corresponding to x-ray photons attenuated by anatomy contribute to overall reduced image quality by adding background signals resulting in reduced subject contrast. CBCT units have noticeably less soft tissue contrast than MDCT units and are inadequate for critical evaluation of soft tissue pathoses. In addition, the inherent efficiency of CBCT detectors is lower than for MDCT detectors as well as the stability and linearity. Saturation (nonlinear pixel effects above a certain exposure), dark current (charge that accumulates over time with or without exposure), and bad pixels (pixels that do not react to exposure) contribute to nonlinearity of the response of the detectors in CBCT to x-radiation. In addition, the sensitivity of different regions of the panel to radiation (pixel-to-pixel gain variation) may not be uniform over the entire region.

Patient Radiation Dose

In general, patient radiation dose from MDCT is higher than that from CBCT. Doses from CBCT vary depending on the type and model of

CBCT equipment and parameters used in clinical practice, such as FOV, exposure (kVp and mA), and acquisition (e.g., rotational arc, number of basis images) settings. Median adult effective dose from CBCT for limited FOV (height <5 cm) is 29 μSv (range 5.5–197 μSv), for maxillofacial FOV (height 5.1–10 cm) is 65 μSv (range 3.9–716 μSv), and for craniofacial FOV (height >10 cm) is 118 μSv (range 8.8–1073 μSv). Doses from maxillofacial MDCT without contrast range from 650 μSv to 1 mSv. Typical doses from standard exposure protocols from CBCT and MDCT imaging are listed in Chapter 3 (Table 3.2 and Fig. 3.4). Patient radiation dose from CBCT imaging is less. Thus, when the diagnostic objective can be accomplished with CBCT, it should be the preferred modality.

IMAGE ARTIFACTS

Artifacts are systemic discrepancies between the CT numbers in reconstructed voxels and the true attenuation coefficients of the anatomic structures that they represent. It is a distortion or error in the image that is unrelated to the subject being studied. The clinical importance of identifying artifacts is that they may be misinterpreted as disease. Artifacts occur in both MDCT and CBCT images. Many artifacts occur due to inherent limitations of CT technology and reconstruction and are similar to both MDCT and CBCT. However, CBCT images inherently have more artifacts than MDCT images because of the lower energy spectra used; cone beam geometry; and the introduction of additional considerations such as aliasing artifacts caused by the cone beam divergence, scatter, and a generally higher noise level. Artifacts can be classified according to where they occur in the imaging chain and can appear as streaks, shadings, rings/bands, and miscellaneous (e.g., cupping, densitometric inaccuracy).

Inherent Artifacts

Artifacts can arise from limitations in the physical processes involved in the acquisition of CBCT data. The beam projection geometry of CBCT, reduced trajectory rotational arcs, and image reconstruction methods produce the following three types of artifacts:

- Scatter
- Partial volume averaging
- Cone beam effect

Scatter results from x-ray photons that are diffracted from their original path after interaction with matter. Because CBCT uses area detectors, they capture scattered photons that contribute to overall image degradation or "quantum noise" compared with MDCT imaging (Fig. 9.13). Scatter causes streak artifacts similar to artifacts of beam hardening.

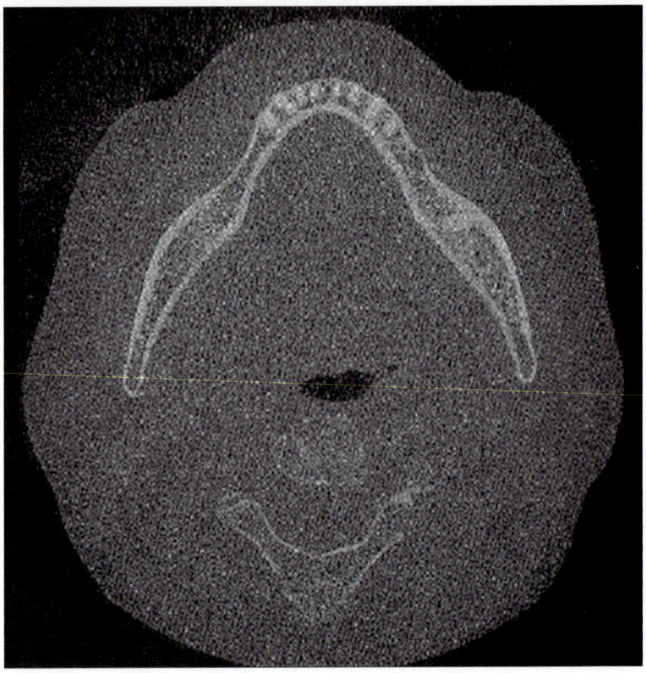

Fig. 9.13 Quantum noise cone beam computed tomography (CBCT) artifacts. Axial high-resolution CBCT image at default resolution (0.125 mm nominal voxel size) shows marked graininess or quantum noise caused by contamination of detector signal by scatter radiation.

Partial volume averaging is a feature of both MDCT and CBCT imaging. It occurs when the selected voxel size of the scan is larger than the size of the object being imaged. For instance, a voxel 1 mm on one side may contain both bone and adjacent soft tissue. In this case, the displayed pixel is not representative of either bone or soft tissue but rather becomes an average of the brightness values of the different tissues. Boundaries in the resultant image may have a "step" appearance or homogeneity of pixel intensity levels. Partial volume averaging artifacts occur in regions where surfaces are rapidly changing in the Z direction, for example, in the temporal bone. Selection of the smallest acquisition voxel can reduce the presence of these effects. Practically, this artifact may appear as partial disruption of a thin layer of cortical bone, for example, the bony walls of the ethmoid air cells or the temporal bone.

The cone beam effect is a potential source of artifacts, especially in the peripheral portions of the scan volume. Because of the divergence of the x-ray beam as it rotates around the patient in a horizontal plane, structures at the top or bottom of the image field are exposed only when the x-ray source is on the opposite side of the patient (Fig. 9.14). The result is image distortion, streaking artifacts, and greater peripheral noise. This effect is minimized by incorporation by manufacturers of various forms of CT reconstruction. Clinically, the effect can be reduced by positioning the ROI in the horizontal plane of the x-ray beam.

Procedure-Related Artifacts

Undersampling of the object can occur when too few basis projections are provided for image reconstruction or when rotational trajectory arcs are incomplete. A reduced data sample leads to misregistration, sharp edges, and noisier images as a result of aliasing, which appear as fine striations in the image (Fig. 9.15). Because increasing scan time (the number of basis projections) or reducing scan arc rotation results in proportional increase or decrease to patient exposure, respectively, the importance of this artifact should be considered in relation to the diagnostic information.

Typically, scanner-related artifacts appear as circular or ring streaks in the axial plane centered about the location of the axis of rotation resulting from imperfections in scanner detection or poor calibration (Fig. 9.16). Either of these problems results in a consistently repetitive reading at each angular position of the detector, resulting in a circular artifact.

Misalignment of the x-ray source to the detector creates a double contour artifact, similar to that created by patient motion. Repeated use of CBCT equipment over time may result in slight configuration changes, and components may need to be periodically geometrically realigned. Chapter 14 describes the periodic quality assurance procedures for CBCT devices.

Introduced Artifacts

As an x-ray beam passes through an object, lower energy photons are absorbed in preference to higher energy photons. This phenomenon,

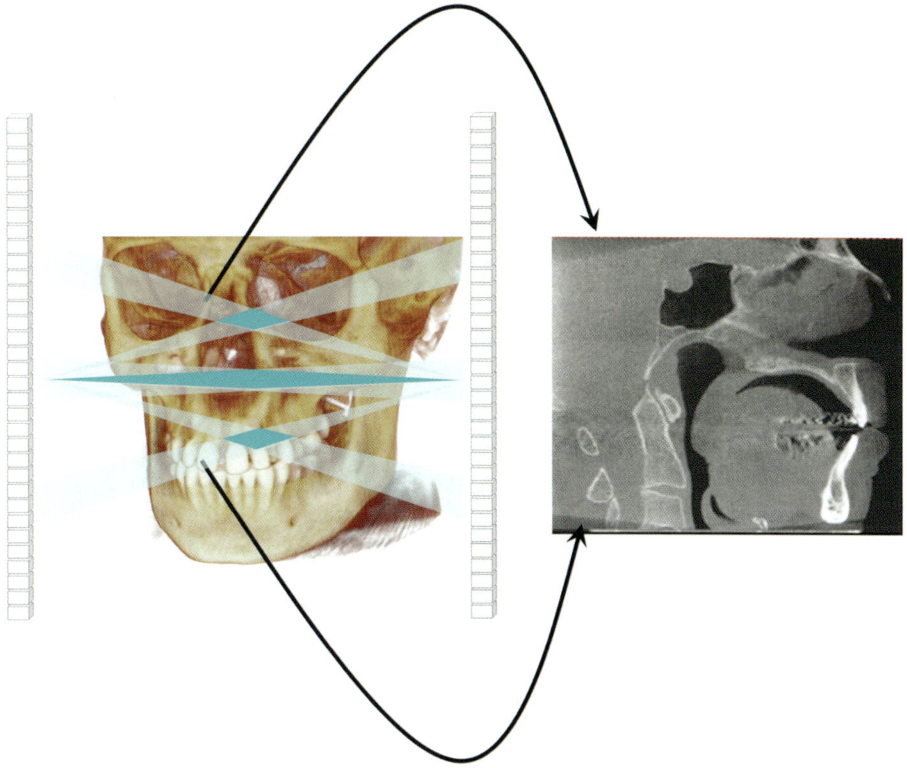

Fig. 9.14 Schematic of cone beam artifact. Exaggerated projection of three representative x-ray beams (one perpendicular, one angled inferiorly, and one angled superiorly) from the focal spot point of origin is shown at two positions of the x-ray tube rotation, 180 degrees apart. The optimal amount of data collected by the detector for reconstruction corresponds to the *solid blue* volume between the overlapping projections. Centrally, the amount of data acquired is maximal, whereas peripherally *(transparent blue)*, the amount of data collected is appreciably less. The midsagittal section image demonstrates the visual effects of data interpolation by the reconstruction algorithm owing to inadequate data obtained at the peripheral superior and inferior extensions of the volumetric dataset producing a peripheral "V" artifact of increased noise, distortion, and reduced contrast.

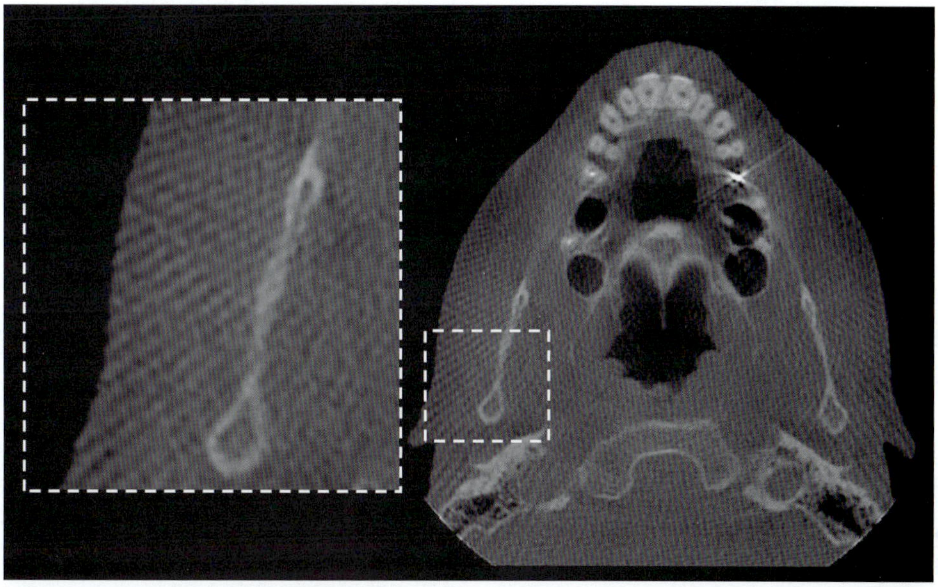

Fig. 9.15 Moiré artifact. Too few basis projections (undersampling) or an incomplete scanning trajectory can result in misregistration of data by the reconstruction software, known as aliasing. On the axial image, particularly at the periphery *(inset)*, fine alternating hyperdense and hypodense stripes appear to be radiating from the edge of the volumetric data, resulting in a characteristic "Moiré" pattern, a type of aliasing artifact.

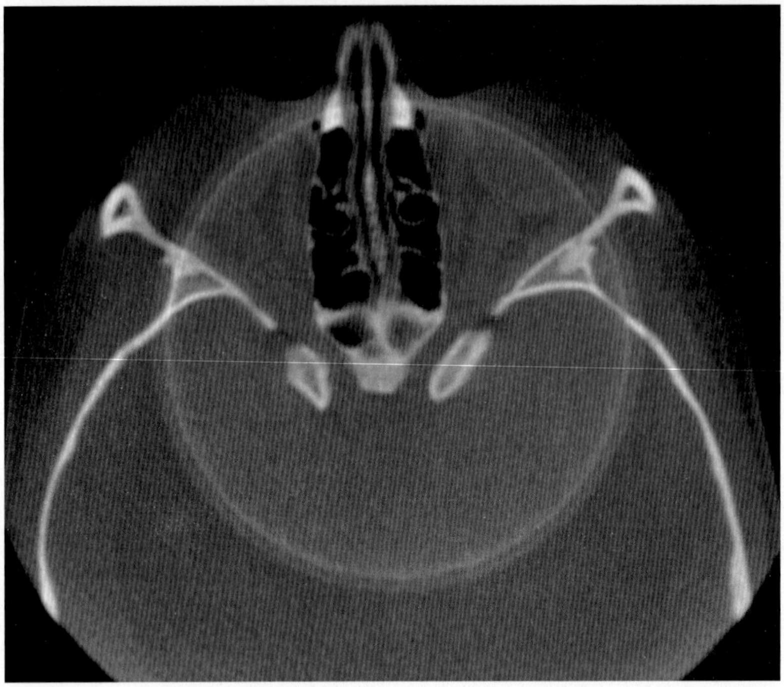

Fig. 9.16 Circular or ring artifacts. Visual appearance of scanner-related artifacts as circular rings on an axial image suggests imperfections in scanner detection due to poor calibration.

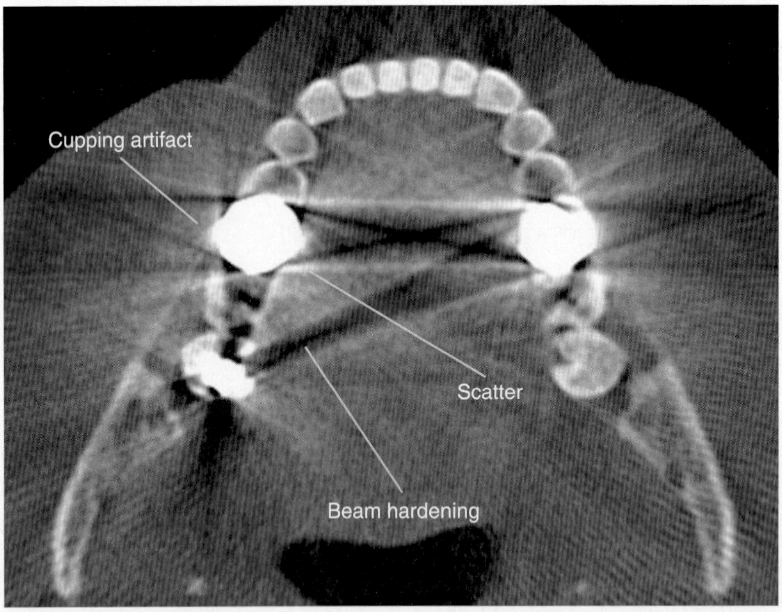

Fig. 9.17 Introduced artifacts. Axial view demonstrating beam hardening *(dark bands)*, scatter *(white streaks)*, and cupping (image distortion) artifacts.

called beam hardening, results in two types of artifacts: (1) distortion of metallic structures as a result of differential absorption, known as a cupping artifact, and (2) streaks and dark bands, which, when present between two dense objects, create extinction, photon starvation, or missing value artifacts (Fig. 9.17). In clinical practice, it is advised to reduce the field size, modify patient position, or separate the dental arches to avoid scanning regions susceptible to beam hardening (e.g., metallic restorations, dental implants). It is also important to remove metallic objects such as jewelry before scanning to reduce peripheral beam hardening effects superimposed on the ROI. When performing limited FOV CBCT, restorations or metallic prostheses and surgical hardware outside the ROI cause beam hardening peripheral to the image volume and can degrade image quality.

Patient Motion Artifacts

One of the most frequent artifacts in CBCT imaging results from patient motion. Patient motion can cause misregistration of data, which appear as double contours in the reconstructed image (Fig. 9.18).

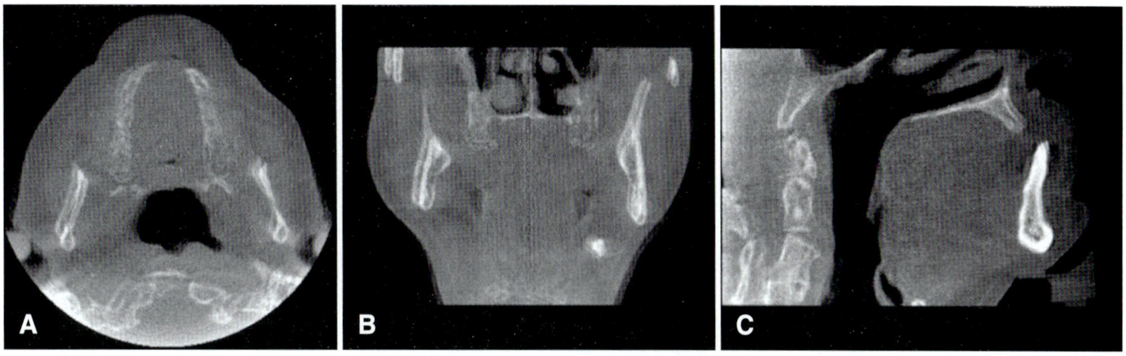

Fig. 9.18 Motion artifacts. Patient motion during the scanning exposure can result in misregistration artifacts, which appear as double contours in the reconstructed image as demonstrated in the axial (A), coronal (B), and sagittal (C) planes.

The smaller the voxel size (i.e., the higher the spatial resolution), the smaller the movement necessary to cause misalignment of structures. This problem can be minimized by restraining the head and using as short a scan time as possible.

POSTPROCESSING OF COMPUTED TOMOGRAPHIC DATA SETS

This section provides guidance on the use of dental software to display, investigate, and interpret volumetric data for task-specific clinical applications. CT imaging provides a volumetric data set that can be reformatted to present digital images in any plane. Both MDCT and CBCT provide isotropic voxel imaging, which allows the volumetric reconstruction without distortion. Most MDCT examinations will be performed in a hospital or imaging center and the dental team should request the volumetric dataset in DICOM format. The reconstruction protocols should be set to create overlapping or contiguous slices to provide a volumetric dataset with isotropic voxels. For hard-tissue diagnostic evaluation and treatment discussed here, use MDCT datasets with the thin slice width (0.5–0.75mm) and reconstructed with filters that enhance bone (bone kernels). The dental team should coordinate with hospital radiologic technologists to ensure that the exported dataset meets the needs for diagnostic evaluation, treatment planning and, when appropriate, 3D printing of bio models, surgical guides, or templates.

Most CBCT examinations will be conducted as in-office procedures. All CBCT devices are configured to provide isotropic, volumetric imaging. CBCT users should be familiar with the parameters that determine image quality so that the dataset generated is adequate for the diagnostic task and any additional applications such as 3D printing or CAD/CAM-designed surgical guides. CBCT users should be familiar with software-assisted dynamic image review, and reformatting according to task-specific protocols. Several software applications provide the ability to expand the use of this volumetric dataset to facilitate digital treatment planning, image guidance of operative and surgical procedures, and AM (see Chapter 32).

Stages in Volumetric Data Display

Most software programs display the CBCT volumetric dataset as secondary 2D contiguous reconstructed images in three orthogonal planes (axial, sagittal, and coronal) at a default thickness (Fig. 9.19). Typically, the default display view presents the three planes in three individual panels or *panes* (to keep the analogy with windows) in an interactive format with localizers within each orthogonal panel to spatially identify an anatomic location in all three panes. Often there is a fourth panel showing a 3D rendering with the three localizers. CBCT data should be considered as a volume that must be analyzed in its entirety, and from which selected images are extracted according to the task (i.e., task specific) to demonstrate specific findings. Technically, four stages provide an efficient and consistent systematic methodologic approach to optimize CBCT image display before image interpretation:

1. Reorient data
2. Correct data
3. Explore data
4. Format data

Reorient Data

One of the advantages of CBCT acquisition is that the resultant volumetric dataset can be reoriented in relation to three orthogonal planes using imaging software. As CBCT volumetric datasets are isotropic, imaging software may align the orthogonal planes with respect to anatomic features or according to a reference plane according to a specific diagnostic task (Fig. 9.20). The entire volume can be reoriented such that the patient's anatomic features are aligned to fixed orthogonal coordinates or alternately the orthogonal planes are adjusted in relation to the volumetric dataset. This stage is particularly important for aligning subsequent cross-sectional, transaxial images perpendicular to the structure of interest, such as to visualize single tooth pathoses, to measure the maximal height and width of the residual alveolar ridge in an edentulous segment for implant site assessment (Fig. 9.21), to compare temporomandibular joint (TMJ) condylar morphology, or to perform a craniofacial analysis.

Optimize Displayed Images

The overall density and contrast of orthogonal images varies between CBCT units and within the same unit depending on the patient size, degree of edentulism, and scan parameters selected. Therefore, to optimize image presentation and facilitate diagnosis, it is often necessary to adjust contrast (window width) and brightness (window level) parameters to favor bony structures. Although CBCT proprietary software may provide for window width and level presets, it is advisable that these parameters be adjusted for each scan. After these parameters are set, further enhancements can be performed by the application of sharpening, filtering, edge enhancement, noise reduction algorithms, and increasing slice thickness. The use of these functions must be weighed against the visual effects of increased noise in the image (Fig. 9.22) and other introduced artifacts such as overshoot (Uberschwinger). After these adjustments, secondary algorithms (e.g., annotation, measurement, magnification) can be applied with confidence.

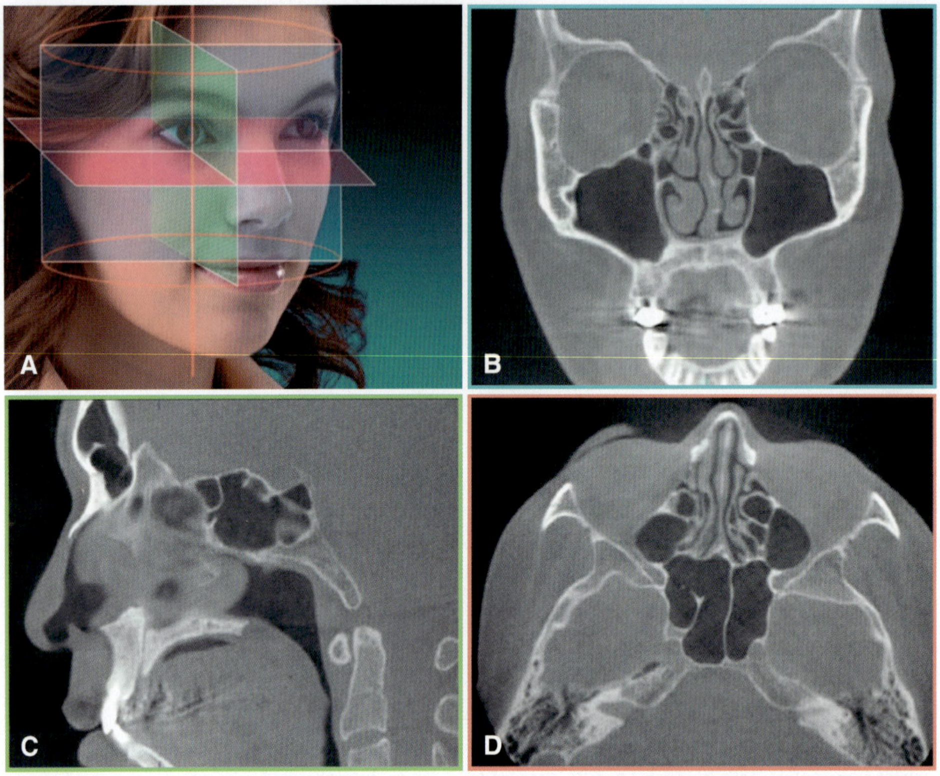

Fig. 9.19 Standard display modes of cone beam computed tomographic volumetric data. (A) Cylindrical three-dimensional volumetric dataset superimposed on a head showing the three orthogonal planes in relation to the reconstructed volumetric dataset: coronal *(teal)*, sagittal *(green)*, and axial *(pink)*. (B–D) Corresponding representative coronal *(teal)* (B), sagittal *(green)* (C), and axial *(pink)* (D) images. Each orthogonal plane has multiple contiguous thin-slice sections, which are interrelational. (Image of head and superimposed volumetric data set and orthogonal orientation courtesy J. Morita Corp., Kyoto, Japan.)

Explore the Data

Because there are numerous contiguous orthogonal images in each plane, it is impractical to display all slices on one display format. Therefore, each series must be reviewed dynamically by scrolling through the consecutive orthogonal image "stack." This is referred to as navigating through the volume in a "cine" or "paging" mode. It is recommended that scrolling be performed craniocaudally (i.e., from head to toe) and then in reverse, slowing down in areas of greater complexity (e.g., TMJ articulations and skull base). This scrolling process should be performed at least in two planes (e.g., coronal and axial). Viewing orthogonal projections at this stage is recommended as an overall survey for disease and to establish the presence of any asymmetry.

Format Data

All CBCT software, be it either proprietary acquisition and display original equipment manufacturer (OEM) or commercial third-party display programs, are capable of many formatting options, each directed toward visualizing specific components of the volumetric dataset. Acquisition or scan protocols incorporate FOV limitations and allow choice of specific exposure parameters. After acquisition, an image display protocol should be applied selectively on the volume to highlight anatomic features or functional characteristics for each specific diagnostic task. Overall, selection should be based on applying thin sections to show detail and thicker sections to demonstrate relationships. There are two basic format options (Fig. 9.23):

- Multiplanar reformation
- Volumetric rendering

Multiplanar reformation. Because of the isotropic nature of acquisition, the volumetric dataset can be sectioned nonorthogonally to provide 2D planar images referred to as multiplanar reformation (MPR). MPR modes include linear oblique and curved planar in relation to the axial image and may result in serial transaxial reformations. Several maxillofacial anatomic structures do not correspond to the standard orthogonal planes, in which case, oblique reformatting can be useful (Fig. 9.24). Linear oblique images are most often used to transect the mandibular condyle. Curved planar images are generated by manually drawing a planning line or spline by selecting multiple nodes along the centerline corresponding to the jaw arch on an appropriate axial image; this creates a "simulated" or reformatted dental panoramic image. Panoramic MPR-reformatted images are useful for jaw evaluation. Such reformatted images must be thick enough to include the entire mandible to avoid missing disease. Serial sequential images perpendicular to an arbitrary linear oblique or curved planar MPR provide a dynamic representation of the anatomic structure, minimizing parallax error. These images are referred to as transaxial, tangential, or, most commonly, cross-sectional images. Cross-sectional images have two characteristics, a slice thickness and distance between adjacent cross-sectional images (interslice interval). Cross-sectional images are optimal for examining teeth and alveolar bone.

Volume rendering

Volume rendering allows visualization of volumetric data by selective display of voxels within a dataset as a 2D projection. Two specific techniques are commonly used: indirect volume rendering (IVR) and direct volume rendering (DVR).

Text continued on page 178

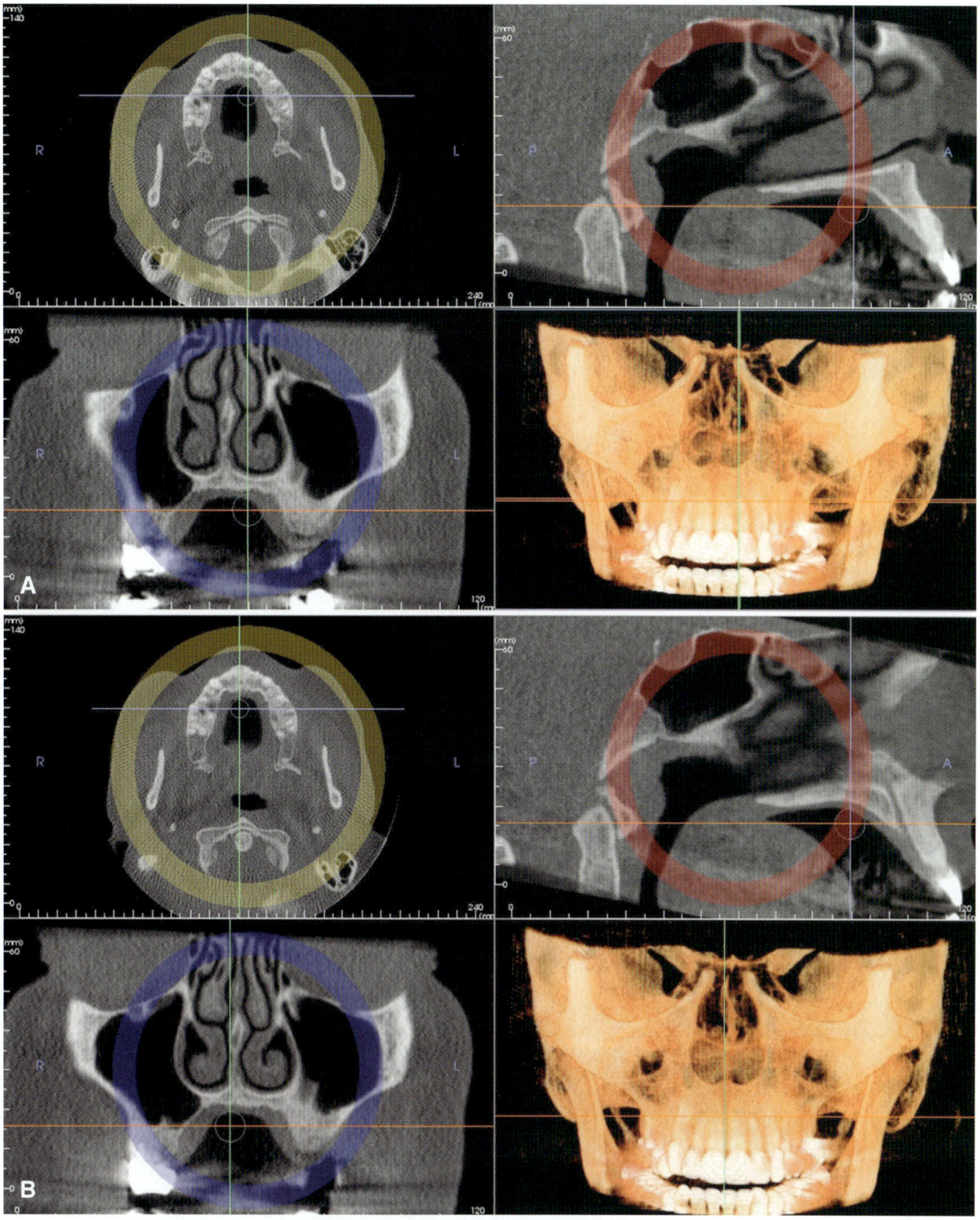

Fig. 9.20 Cone beam computed tomographic volumetric data reorientation. Axial, sagittal, and coronal orthogonal sectional images and three-dimensional volumetric rendering before (A) and after (B) reorientation of the CBCT dataset to fixed orthogonal coordinates. The circular rotational tool superimposed on the respective images is selected with the cursor and adjusted to align images according to specific reference lines. In this case, axial and sagittal orthogonal images were realigned such that the maxillary jaw was symmetrically repositioned, and the palatal plane was parallel to the floor. (Images created with Invivo dental software, Osteoid, Santa Clara, CA.)

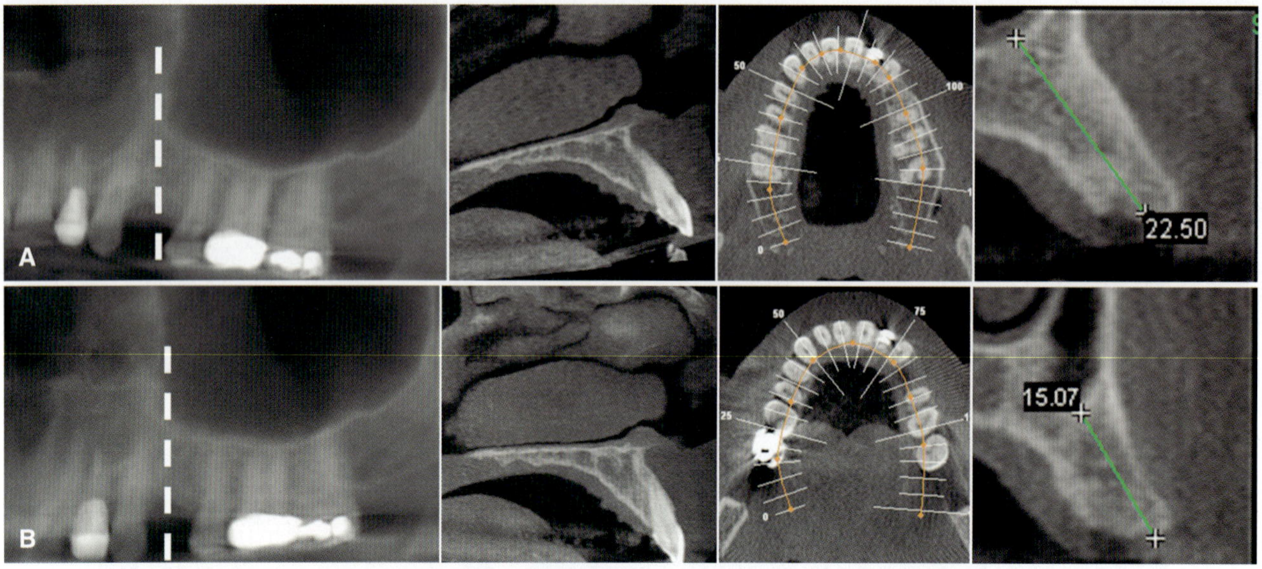

Fig. 9.21 Reorientation of sagittal plane to internal reference (occlusal plane). *(Left to right)* Reformatted panoramic, midsagittal, axial, and cross-sectional images of the same dataset at (A) original orientation and (B) after down-tilt of the volumetric data set in the sagittal plane such that the residual alveolar ridge is parallel to the occlusal plane. The lower set of images shows the appropriate relationship of the maxillary sinus to the alveolar ridge and a substantial difference in measured height of the alveolar bone.

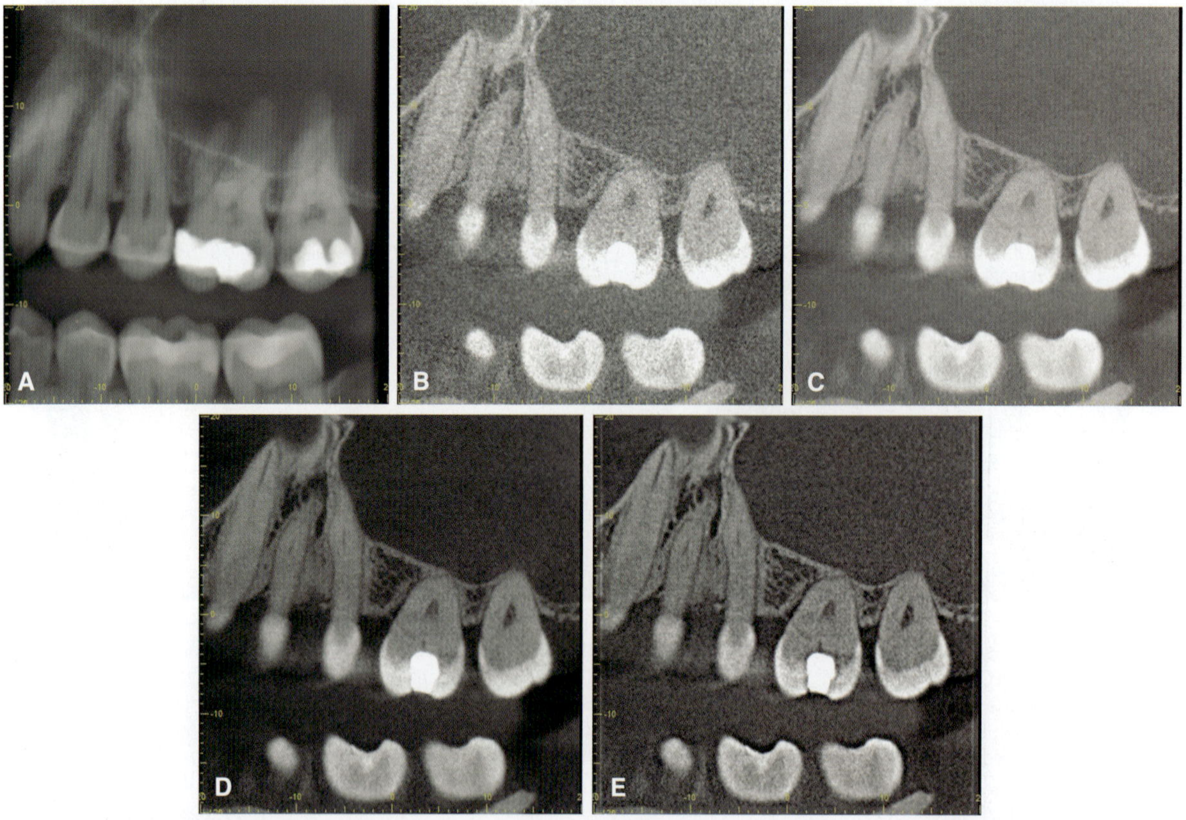

Fig. 9.22 Effect of image enhancement on cone beam computed tomographic images. The visual effect of four sequential adjustments on a multiplanar reformation cross-sectional image. (A) Default ray sum image of the left maxillary first molar tooth referred for clinical suspicion of fracture. (B) Parasagittal CBCT image at default resolution (0.08 nominal resolution) through the mesio-distal axis of the crown. (C) Same image as (B) but with slice thickness increased to 0.5 mm. Note vertical low-density line immediately below occlusal restoration and faint vertical oblique line extending to the mesial aspect of the alveolar crest. (D) Same image as (B) after adjustment of window level and width to correspond to histogram intensity distribution—previous features more clearly demonstrated. (E) Same image as (B) after addition of mild sharpen algorithm—vertical and mesial oblique fracture is now clearly evident. However, note the low density halo around the high density occlusal amalgam due to "Uberschwinger" artifact. (Images acquired using X800 and created with iDixel software, J. Morita Corp., Kyoto, Japan.)

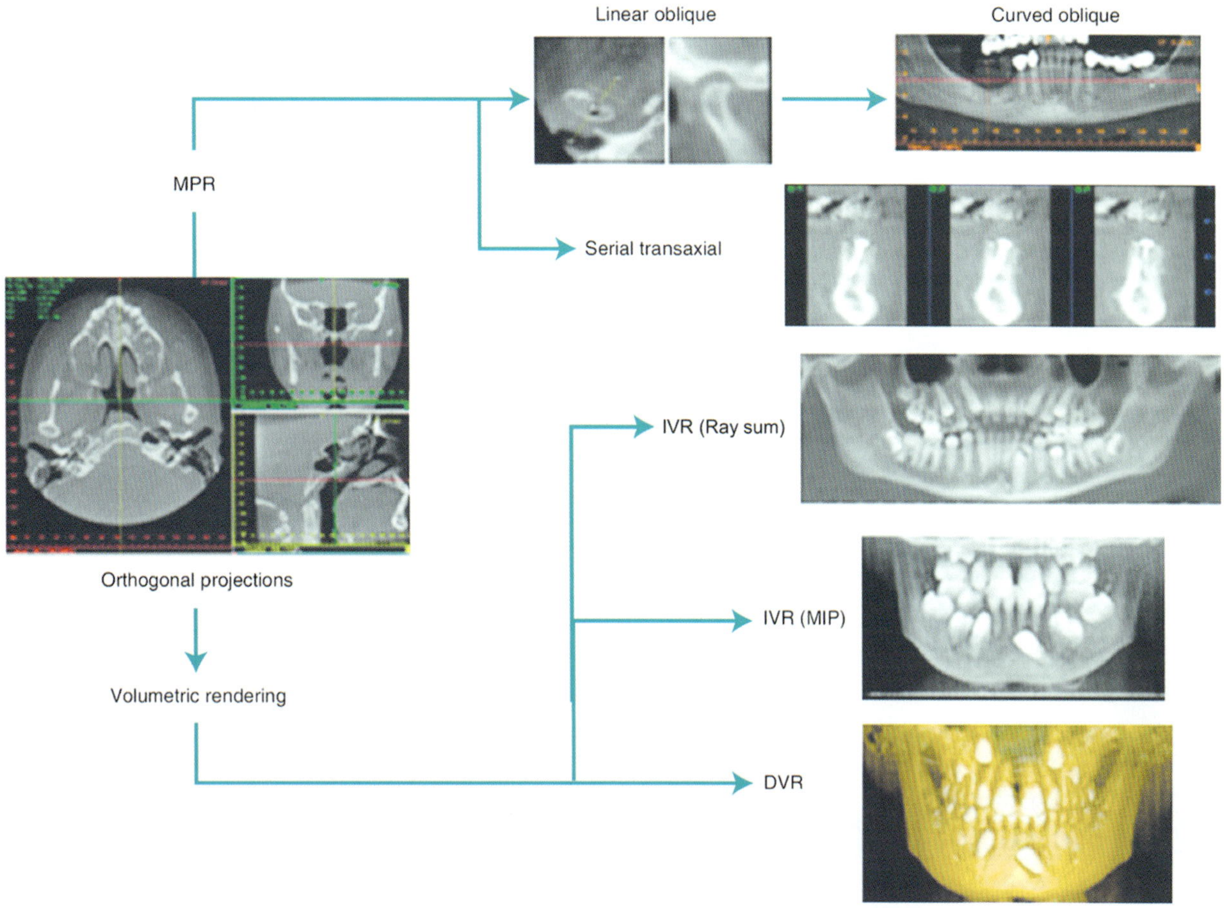

Fig. 9.23 Display mode options of cone beam computed tomographic volumetric data. Display modes can be divided into two categories: multiplanar reformation *(MPR)* consisting of linear, curved oblique, and serial transaxial images; and volumetric images including ray sum, comprising images of increased section thickness, indirect volume rendering *(IVR)*, the most common of which being maximum intensity projection *(MIP)*, and direct volume rendering *(DVR)*.

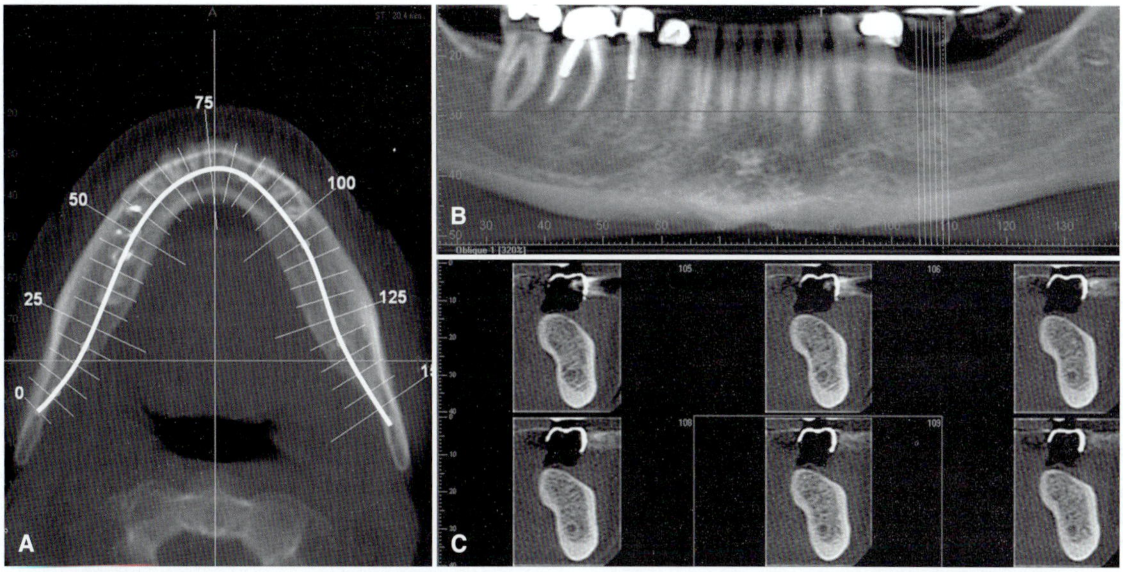

Fig. 9.24 Multiplanar reformation (MPR). (A) A thick axial image simulating an occlusal image with an MPR oblique curved line *(white solid line)*, (B) resultant "panoramic" image, and (C) serial cross-sectional 1-mm-thick images of a potential implant site in the lower left mandible. The axial and panoramic images are used as reference images to show the location of the cross-sectional images. The cross-sectional images demonstrate the volume of alveolar bone available, morphology of the bone including degree of lingual undercut and location of the inferior alveolar canal.

IVR is a complex process requiring selection of the intensity or density of the grayscale level of the voxels to be displayed within an entire dataset (called "segmentation"). This process is technically demanding and computationally difficult, requiring specific software; however, it provides a volumetric surface reconstruction with depth (Fig. 9.25). Two types of views are possible: views that are solid (surface rendering) and views that are transparent (volumetric rendering). This volumetric procedure is optimal for visualization and analysis of craniofacial conditions and determination of relationships of various anatomic features, such as the inferior alveolar canal (IAC) to the mandibular third molar.

DVR is a much simpler process that involves selecting an arbitrary threshold of voxel intensities, below or above which all gray values are removed. Numerous techniques are available; however, the most used are ray sum and maximum intensity projection (MIP).

The slice thickness of orthogonal or MPR images can be "thickened" by increasing the number of adjacent voxels included in the display (Fig. 9.26). This creates an image slab that represents

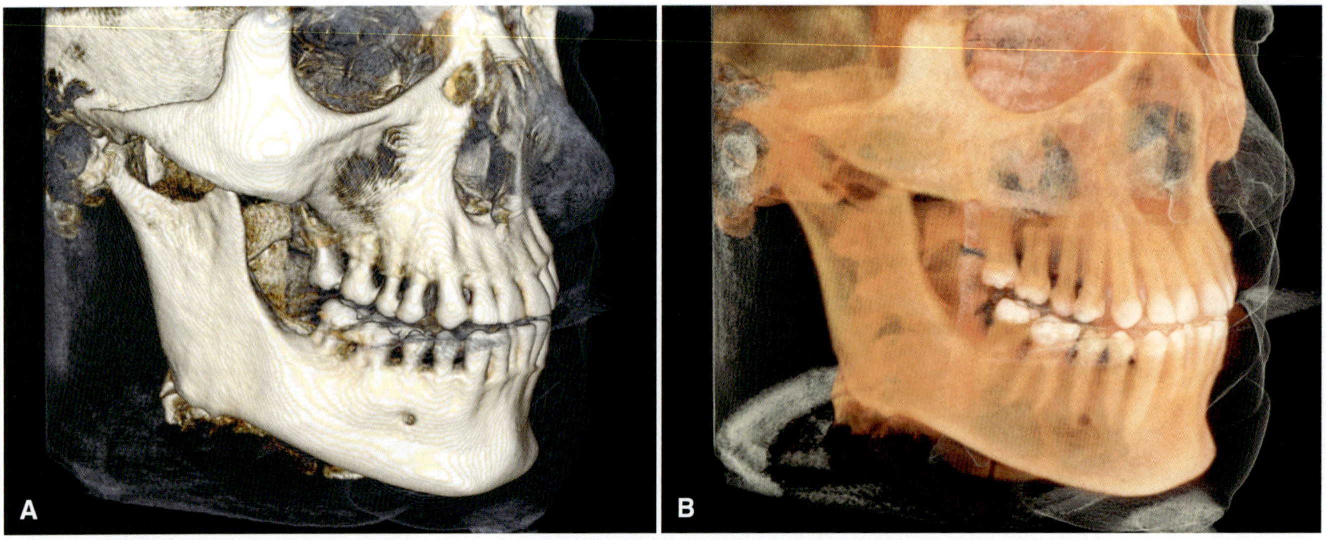

Fig. 9.25 Three-dimensional volumetric surface rendering. Manual segmentation is often accomplished by an adjustable scale determining the upper and lower limit and range of gray intensity values to include in the segmentation. The visual result of changes in this scale is displayed in "real time" so that the effects of incremental changes can be visualized. The segmentation may be optimized to reveal the objects of interest, including bone as a solid surface or (A) shaded surface display and bone and the dentition under the bone as a (B) transparency using volumetric imaging. (Segmentation performed with Invivo dental software, Osteoid, Santa Clara, CA.)

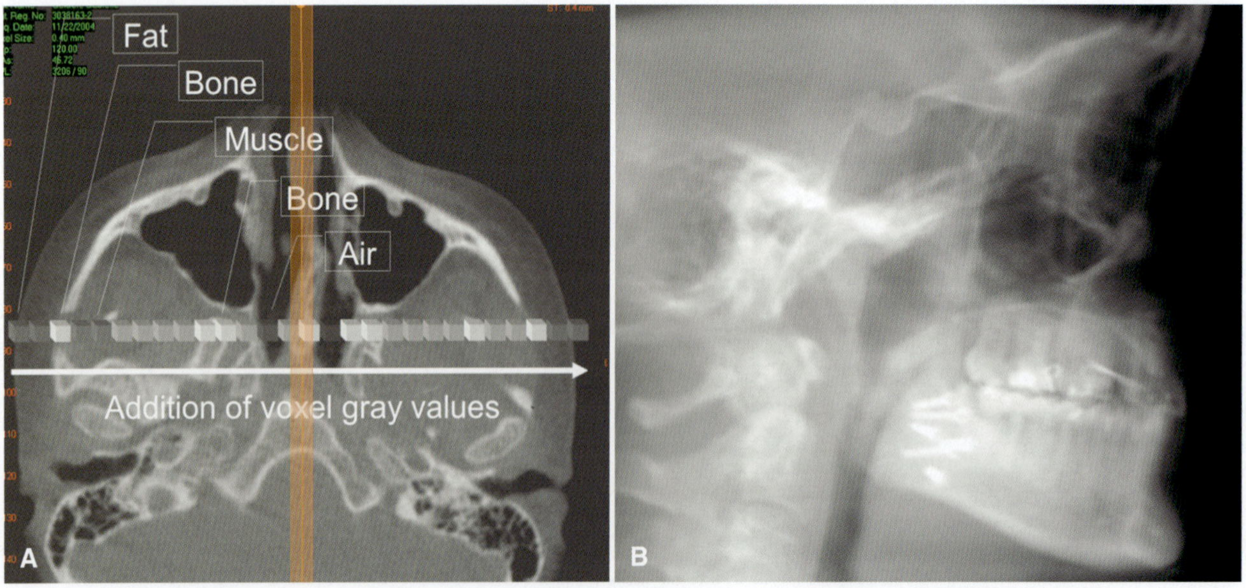

Fig. 9.26 Creation of ray sum images. (A) An axial projection is used as the reference image. A sectional slice is identified that in this case corresponds to the midsagittal plane, and the thickness of this slice is increased to include both left and right sides of the volumetric data set equally. As the thickness of the "slab" increases, adjacent voxels representing elements such as air, bone, and soft tissues are added. (B) The resultant image generated from a full-thickness ray sum provides a simulated lateral cephalometric image.

a specific volume of the patient, referred to as a ray sum. The thickness of the slab is usually determined by the thickness of the structure to be imaged. Full-thickness ray sum images in the sagittal and coronal planes can be used to generate simulated skull projections, such as lateral and posteroanterior cephalometric images (Fig. 9.27), respectively. In contrast to conventional radiographs, these ray sum images are without magnification and parallax distortion. However, this technique uses the entire volumetric dataset, and interpretation is negatively affected by "anatomic noise"—the superimposition of multiple structures—also present in conventional projection radiography.

MIP visualizations are achieved by evaluating each voxel value along an imaginary projection ray from the observer's eyes within a particular volume of interest and representing only the highest value as the display value. Voxel intensities that are below an arbitrary threshold are eliminated (Fig. 9.28). MIP images have great utility for demonstration of the location of impacted teeth, for TMJ evaluation, for identification of fractures, for craniofacial analysis, for surgical follow-up, for assessment of cervical spine anomalies, and for demonstration of soft tissue dystrophic calcifications.

INTERPRETIVE REPORT

Cone beam imaging comprises the technical component of patient exposure. It is the professional responsibility of a practitioner who operates a CBCT unit, or who requests a CBCT study, to interpret the entire image dataset. Documentation of the CBCT acquisition and interpretation by the inclusion of an interpretive report is an essential element of CBCT imaging and should form part of a patient's record. Patient diagnosis may often be complex, and management may involve numerous practitioners. An interpretation report serves as the optimal method of communication of interpretation findings for CBCT. Often this report includes selected images that best document significant findings.

It is imperative that all image data be systematically reviewed for disease. Competency in interpretation of both anatomic and pathologic findings on CBCT images varies depending principally on practitioner

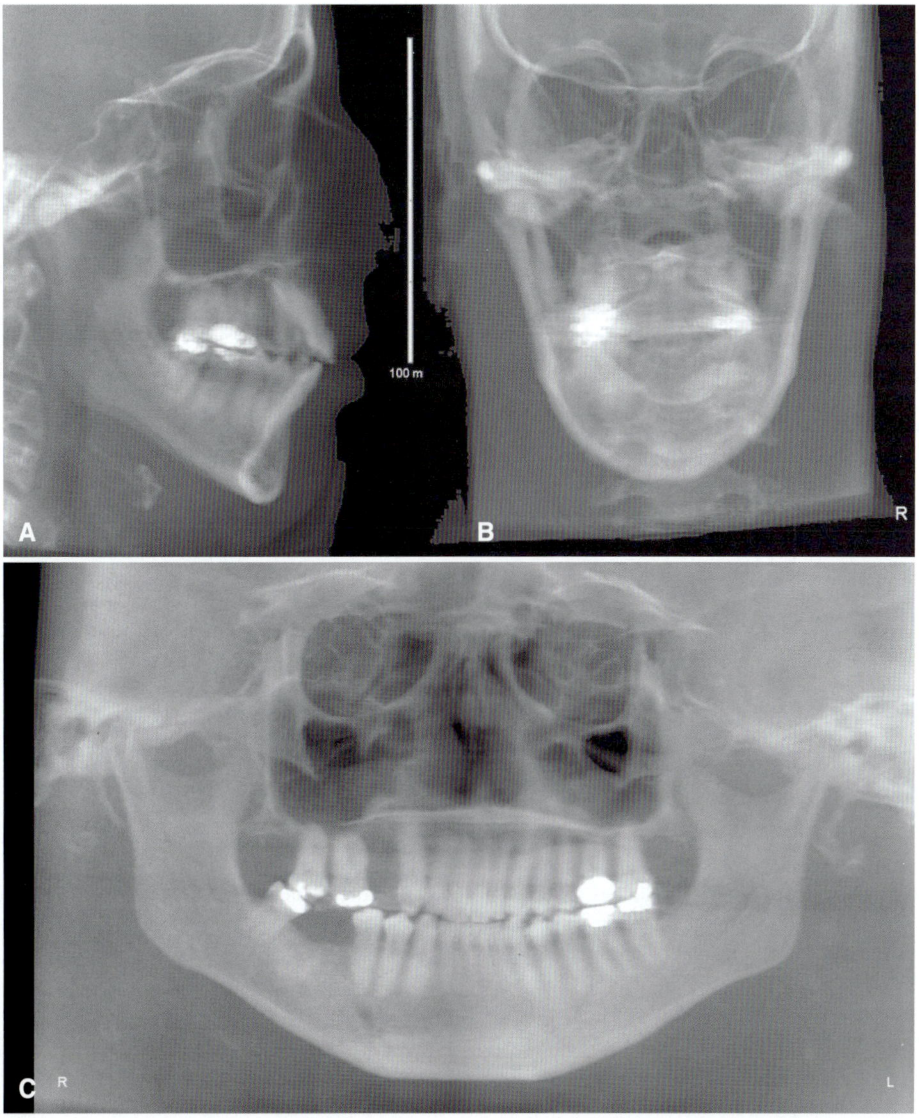

Fig. 9.27 Two-dimensional projections generated with cone beam dataset. This patient had an asymmetry of one side of the face. Ray sum reformation of the cone beam computed tomographic data was performed to provide multiple conventional images, such as the lateral cephalometric (A), frontal cephalometric or posteroanterior (B), and panoramic (C) projections. (Images generated with Dolphin 3D Imaging Software, Chatsworth, CA.)

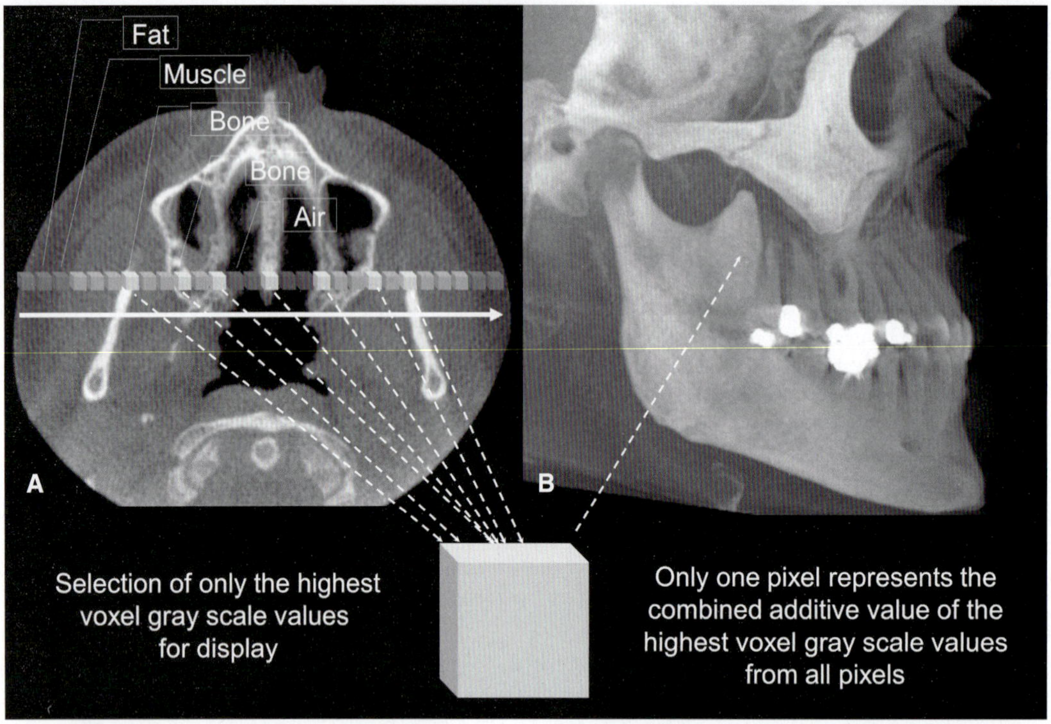

Fig. 9.28 Maximum intensity projection (MIP). This method produces a "pseudo" three-dimensional image by evaluating each voxel value along an imaginary projection ray from the observer's eyes within the dataset and then representing only the highest gray intensity as the display value. In this example, an axial projection (A) is used as the reference image. A projection ray is identified throughout the entire volumetric data set along which individual voxels are identified, each with varying grayscale intensity corresponding to various tissue densities, such as fat, muscle, air, and bone. The MIP algorithm selects only the values along the projection ray that have the highest values (usually corresponding to bone or metal) and represents this as only one pixel on the resultant image (B).

experience and the FOV of the scan. Qualified specialist oral and maxillofacial radiologists should be consulted when practitioners are not familiar with the image findings, or if they are unwilling to accept the responsibility to review the entire CBCT volume. The essential elements of a radiology report are described in Chapter 16 (see section on Writing a Diagnostic Imaging Report).

TASK-SPECIFIC APPLICATIONS

CBCT technology has been applied to diagnosis in all areas of dentistry. CBCT imaging is not a replacement for panoramic or conventional projection radiographic applications but rather is best used as a complementary modality for specific applications.

Diagnosis and Preoperative Assessment

Implant Site Assessment

The American Academy of Oral and Maxillofacial Radiology (AAOMR) recommends that "CBCT should be considered as the imaging modality of choice for preoperative cross-sectional imaging of potential implant sites" (see Chapter 15). Perhaps the greatest impact of CBCT has been on the planning of dental implant placements (see Chapters 31 and 32). CBCT provides cross-sectional images demonstrating alveolar bone height, width, and angulation and accurately depicts vital structures, such as the inferior alveolar dental nerve canal in the mandible or the sinus in the maxilla. The most useful series of images for implant site assessment include the axial, reformatted panoramic, and cross-sectional images at the specific location (Fig. 9.29). In many instances, a radiographic template with hyperdense markers is worn by the patient during the scan (Fig. 9.30). This stent provides a reference of the location of the proposed implants or teeth. Chapters 31 and 32 discuss in silico implant-treatment planning and fabrication of surgical guides to link the computer-based plan to the surgical implant placement. CBCT is now becoming the digital scaffold for the combination of all digital inputs including facial and intraoral optical surface scans.

Endodontics

The American Association of Endodontists and the AAOMR have published guidelines on the use of CBCT imaging for endodontic applications. Note that endodontic applications require high resolution and thus, limited FOV protocols are used. CBCT imaging in endodontics is indicated in the following clinical situations (Fig. 9.31, see Fig. 25.11):

- Patients who present with contradictory or nonspecific clinical signs and symptoms associated with untreated or previously endodontically treated teeth.
- For the initial treatment of teeth with the potential for extra canals and suspected complex morphology, such as mandibular anterior teeth, and maxillary and mandibular premolars and molars, and dental anomalies.
- For intra-appointment identification and localization of calcified canals.
- If clinical examination and 2D intraoral radiography are inconclusive in the detection of vertical root fracture.
- When evaluating the nonhealing of previous endodontic treatment to help determine the need for further treatment, such as nonsurgical, surgical, or extraction.
- For nonsurgical retreatment to assess endodontic treatment complications, such as overextended root canal obturation material, separated endodontic instruments, and localization of perforations.

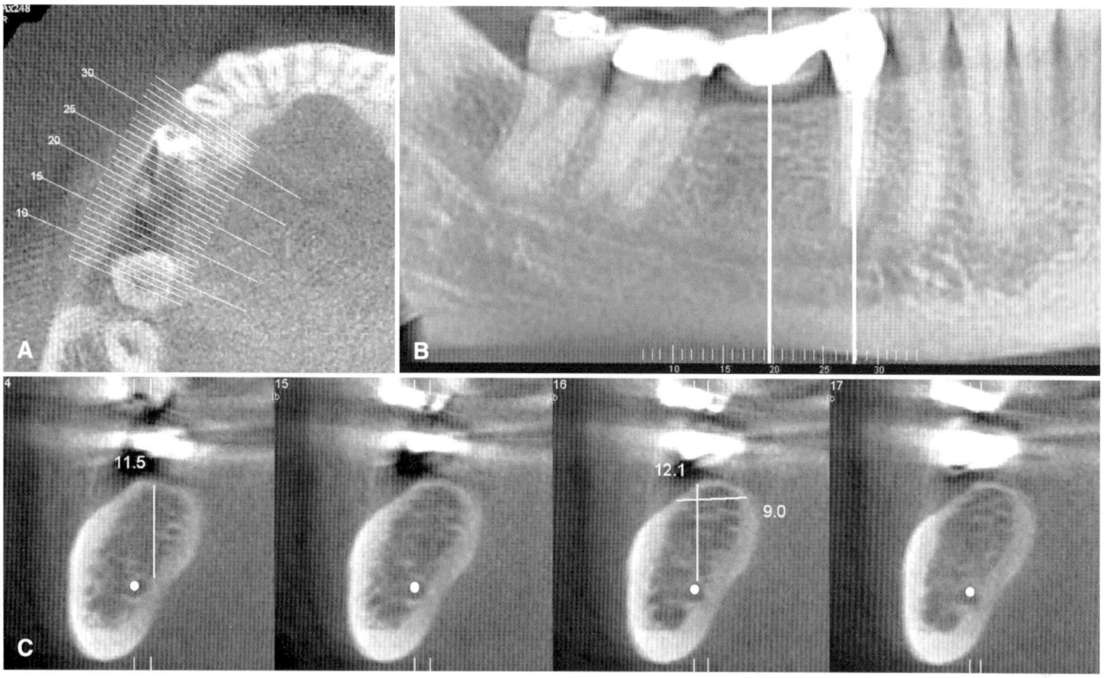

Fig. 9.29 Cone beam computed tomographic imaging for implant site assessment. A curved planar multiplanar reformation (MPR) is accomplished by aligning the long axis of the imaging plane with the dental arch (A), providing a regional panorama-like thin-slice image (B). In addition, serial thin slice transaxial images are often generated perpendicular to the curved planar MPR (C), which are useful in the assessment of specific morphologic features, such as the location of the inferior alveolar canal (shown with a *white dot*) for implant site assessment and for allowing measurement of the available alveolar bone height and width *(solid line)*. (Images created with NNT software, Newtom | Cefla, Imola, Italy.)

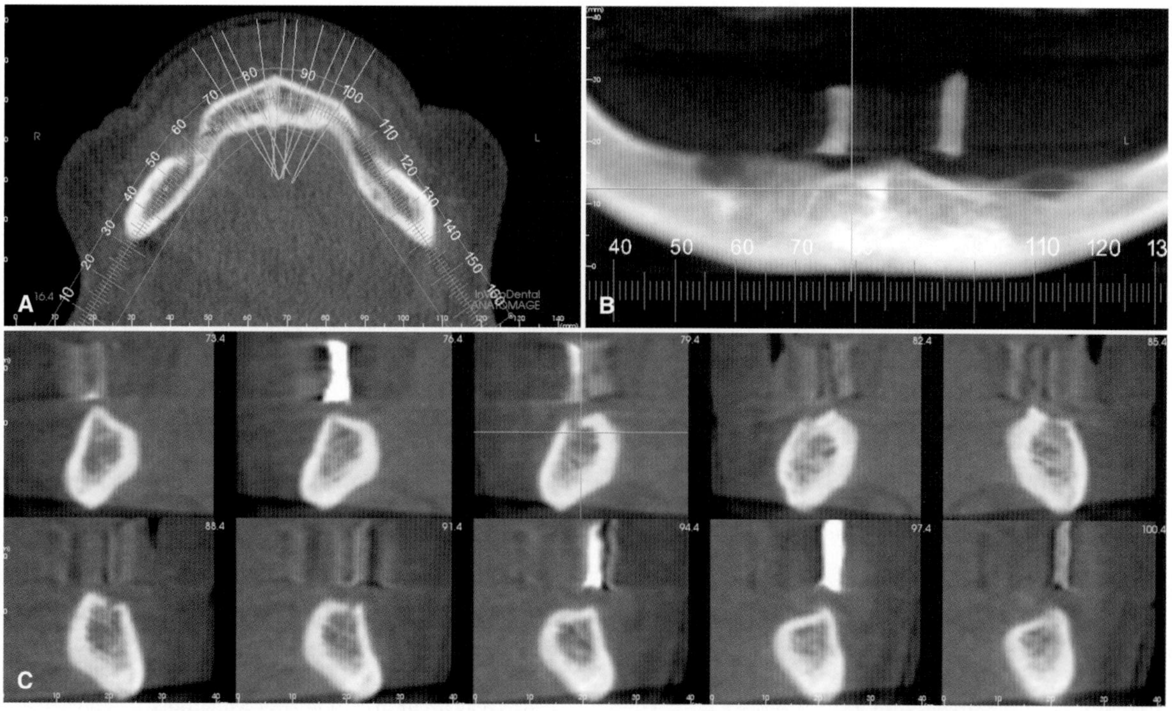

Fig. 9.30 Use of a radiographic template. Plastic intraoral appliances provide fiducial radiopaque landmarks that can be used to correlate proposed clinical location and angulation of implants with the available alveolar bone. The axial (A) and panoramic (B) projections provide an overview of location, whereas serial cross-sectional images (C) indicate alveolar bone height. In this example of an edentulous mandible, the radiograph has two markers at proposed implant sites; the 1-mm- thick transplanar images at 3-mm intervals of the mandibular anterior region (C) indicate that although the right trajectory is optimal (*upper left* cross-sectional image), the proposed placement trajectory of the right implant *(lower left)* is too far buccal to engage the available bone. (Images generated on Invivo dental software, Osteoid, Santa Clara, CA.)

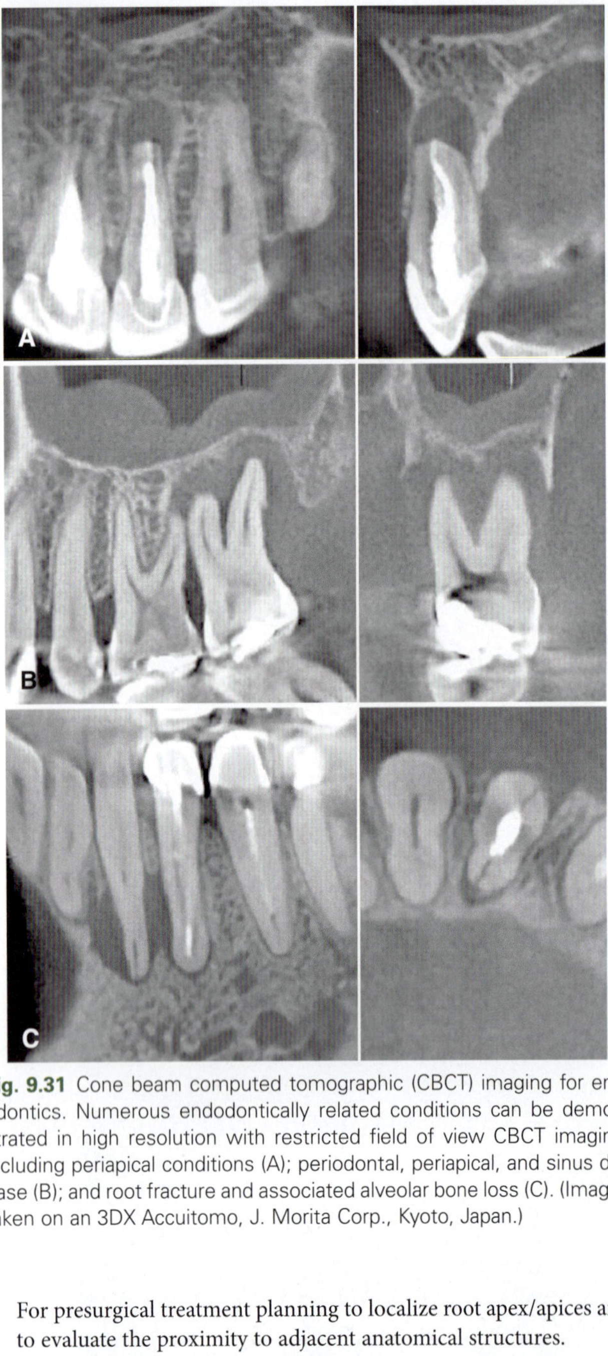

Fig. 9.31 Cone beam computed tomographic (CBCT) imaging for endodontics. Numerous endodontically related conditions can be demonstrated in high resolution with restricted field of view CBCT imaging, including periapical conditions (A); periodontal, periapical, and sinus disease (B); and root fracture and associated alveolar bone loss (C). (Images taken on an 3DX Accuitomo, J. Morita Corp., Kyoto, Japan.)

- For presurgical treatment planning to localize root apex/apices and to evaluate the proximity to adjacent anatomical structures.
- For the surgical placement of implants.
- For diagnosis and management of limited dentoalveolar trauma, root fractures, luxation, and/or displacement of teeth, and localized alveolar fractures, in the absence of other maxillofacial or soft tissue injury that may require other advanced imaging modalities.
- For the localization and differentiation of external and internal resorptive defects and the determination of appropriate treatment and prognosis.

Orthodontics and Three-Dimensional Cephalometry

CBCT imaging is used in the diagnosis, assessment, and analysis of maxillofacial orthodontic and orthopedic anomalies. The most common conditions in which CBCT is useful are the identification of dental structural anomalies, such as root resorption and display of the position of impacted and supernumerary teeth and their relationships to adjacent roots or other anatomic structures. CBCT imaging facilitates surgical exposure and planning of subsequent movement. Other applications include the assessment of palatal morphologic features and dimensions, tooth inclination and torque, characterization of alveolar bone for orthodontic mini-implant placement, and determining available alveolar bone width for buccolingual movement of teeth. CBCT imaging also provides adequate visualization of the TMJ, pharyngeal airway space, and soft tissue relationships.

CBCT imaging provides two unique contributions to orthodontic practice:

- Numerous projection images currently used in orthodontic diagnosis, cephalometric analysis, and treatment planning can be simulated from a single CBCT scan. This capability provides for greater clinical efficacy.
- CBCT data can be reconstructed to provide unique, previously unavailable images. Specific software provides 3D visualization and analysis of the maxillofacial skeleton and soft tissue boundaries, such as the airway and facial outline. The numerous potential benefits to 3D cephalometry include demonstrating and characterizing asymmetry and anteroposterior, vertical, and transverse dentoskeletal discrepancies, incorporating the soft tissue integument, and the potential for assessment of growth and development.

Oral and Maxillofacial Surgery

Assessment of third molars. The relationship of the IAC to the roots of mandibular third molar teeth is important when considering extractions and attempting to minimize the likelihood of nerve damage that may lead to permanent loss of sensation to one side to the lower lip. Accurate assessment of the position of the IAC in relation to the impacted third molar may reduce injuries to this nerve. Panoramic imaging may be adequate when intervening bone is present between the roots of the third molar and the IAC, but when radiographically superimposed, it is advisable to use a 3D imaging approach. Volumetric rendering with IAC annotation or "tracing" in combination with cross-sectional imaging provides useful visualization of the relationships of anatomic structures in these circumstances (Fig. 9.32).

Temporomandibular Joint. The AAOMR recommends that "CT imaging, preferably CBCT, should be used to evaluate osseous changes in patients with suspected TMJ arthritis." CT is the gold standard for identifying arthritis of the TMJ. Imaging can depict the features of degenerative joint disease (Fig. 9.33) and other arthritides, such as rheumatoid arthritis, and developmental anomalies of the condyle, and ankylosis. Appropriate imaging protocols should include reformatted panoramic and axial reference images; corrected parasagittal and paracoronal cross-sectional slices; and for cases in which asymmetry is suspected or surgery is contemplated, volumetric reconstructions.

Maxillofacial pathoses. CT imaging provides value to assess a variety of conditions and diseases that affect the face, mouth, and jaws. MDCT is the preferred modality for soft tissue pathoses, for example, dental infections with cellulitis and space infection. For intraosseous pathoses, the contrast resolution of CBCT is adequate. Most notably dental conditions such as impacted canines and supernumerary teeth, fractured or split teeth, periapical lesions, and periodontal disease are better imaged with CBCT than with MDCT. Benign calcifications (e.g., tonsilloliths, lymph nodes, salivary gland stones) can also be identified by location and differentiated from potentially significant calcifications, such as may occur in carotid artery atheroma. Although CBCT imaging does not provide suitable soft tissue contrast to distinguish the contents of paranasal soft tissue attenuations, the morphologic characteristics and extent of these lesions are particularly well seen (e.g., mucous extravasation cyst). CBCT imaging is useful for assessment of trauma (Fig. 9.34, see Chapter 25) and for evaluating bone infections (see Chapter 20), and benign odontogenic and nonodontogenic cysts and tumors (Fig. 9.35, see Chapters 21 and 22).

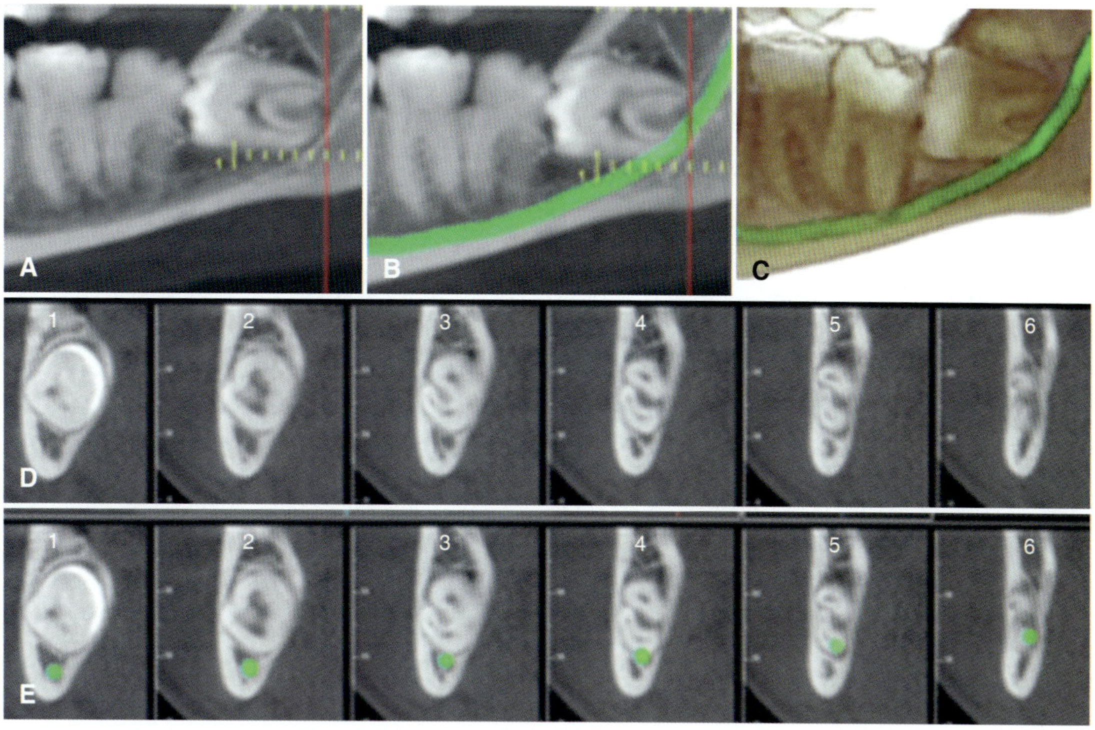

Fig. 9.32 Cone beam imaging for third molar assessment. Third-party software used to demonstrate the location of the inferior alveolar canal (IAC) *(green)*. Nonannotated (A) and annotated (B) panoramic multiplanar reformation reformatted, volumetric transparency reconstruction (C) images with corresponding nonannotated (D) and annotated field of view (E) cross-sectional images at 1-mm intervals. Cross-sectional slices with the IAC traced *(green)*. All images demonstrate the proximity and course of the IAC in relation to the root of the left mandibular, horizontally bony impacted third molar. (Images created with Dolphin 3D Imaging Software, Chatsworth, CA.)

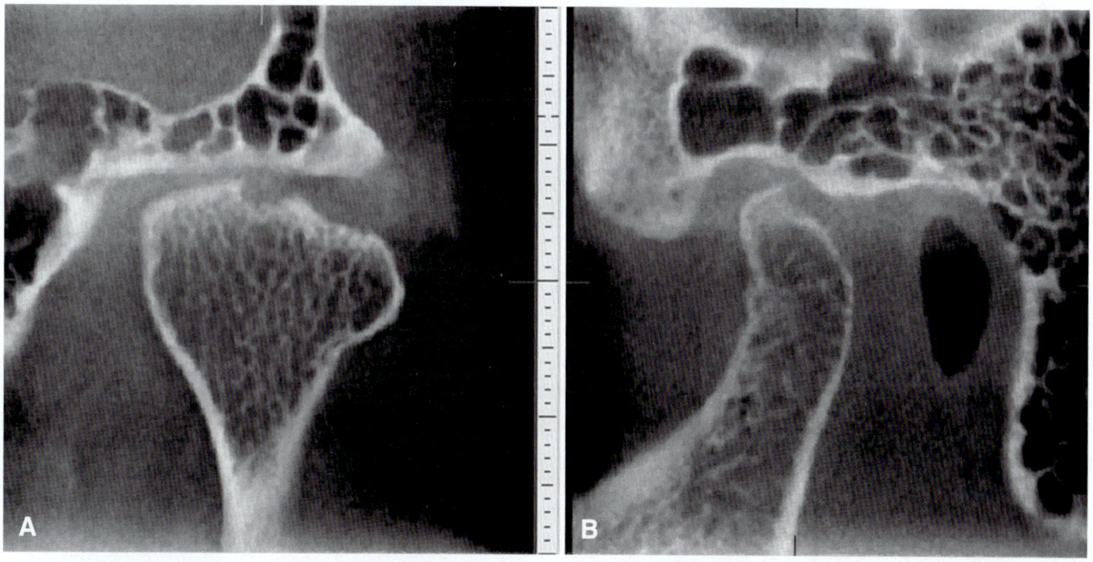

Fig. 9.33 Cone beam computed tomographic imaging of the temporomandibular joint (TMJ). Corrected coronal (A) and sagittal (B) images of a right TMJ with erosive defects on the superior cortical surface of the condyle associated with mild degenerative joint disease. (Images created with 3DX Accuitomo, J. Morita Corp., Kyoto, Japan.)

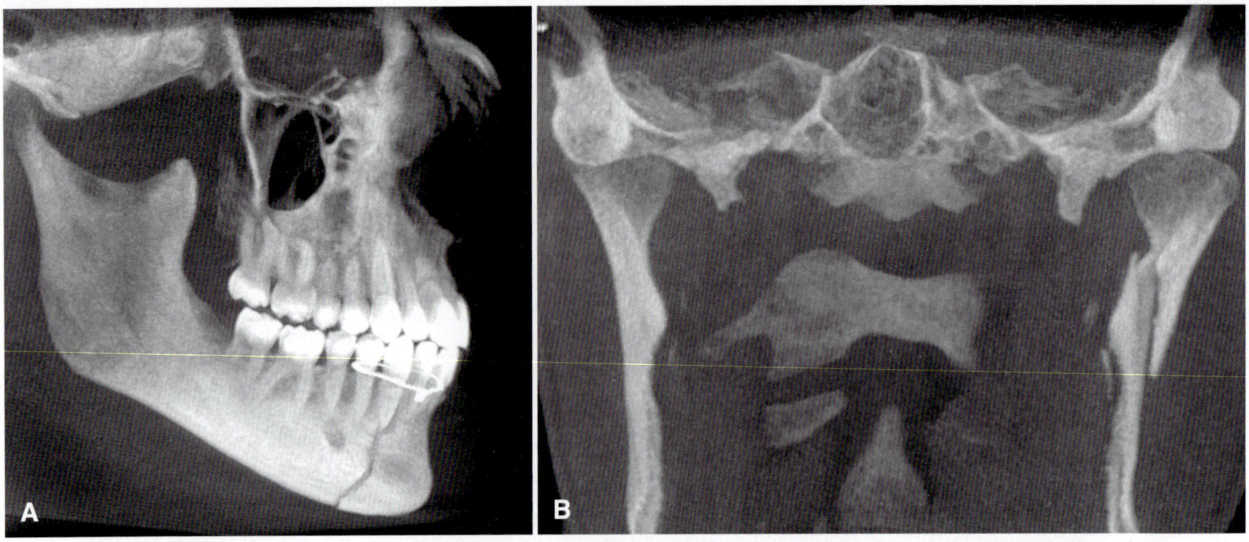

Fig. 9.34 Cone beam computed tomographic imaging of mandibular fractures. Use of maximum intensity projection (MIP) in the assessment of complex mandibular fractures. (A) Oblique thin slab multiplanar reformation image with MIP application demonstrates a simple, slightly displaced fracture of the right parasymphyseal region. (B) Coronal thin-slab MIP image demonstrates a comminuted displaced left subcondylar neck fracture. (Images created with i-CAT [Version; Next Generation 17-19] Imaging Science International, Hatfield, PA; created using XoranCAT software, Xoran Technologies, Inc., Ann Arbor, MI.)

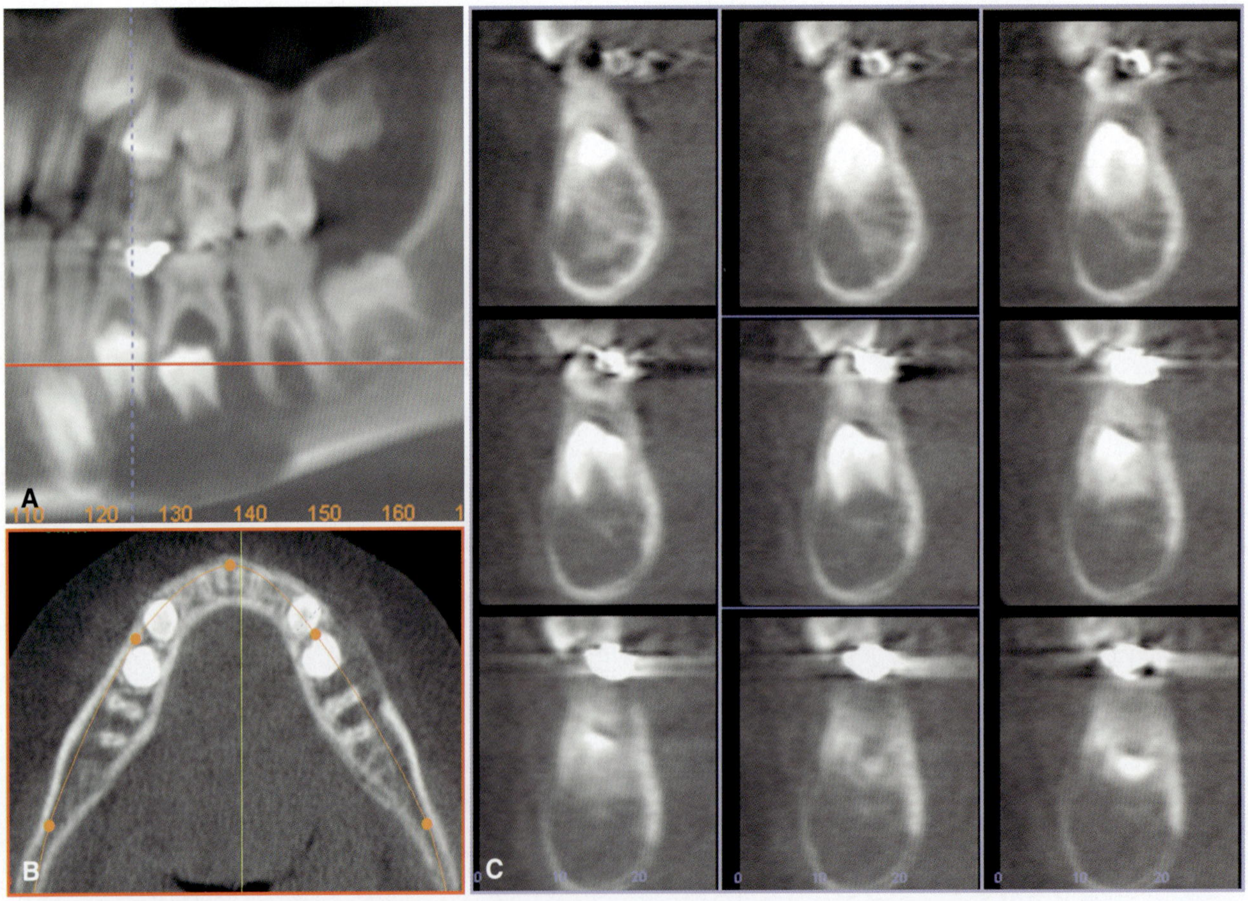

Fig. 9.35 Cone beam computed tomographic imaging of maxillofacial pathoses. (A) Cropped reformatted ray sum panoramic view. (B) Axial slice at level of *red horizontal line* on panoramic view and outline for midportion of cross-sectional images. (C) Serial 1-mm-thick cross-sectional slices (of a unilocular well-defined, noncorticated hypodensity) in the left premolar mandibular body of a patient in the mixed dentition phase.

BIBLIOGRAPHY

Multidetector Computed Tomography

American College of Radiology. *ACR-ASNR-SPR Practice Parameter for the Performance of Computed Tomography (CT) of the Extracranial Head and Neck*. 2021. https://www.acr.org/-/media/ACR/Files/Practice-Parameters/CT-Head-Neck.pdf. Accessed March 28, 2024.

Bushberg JT, Seibert JA, Leidholdt EM Jr, et al. *The Essential Physics of Medical Imaging*. 4th ed. Lippincott Williams & Wilkins; 2020.

Mahesh M. *MDCT Physics: The Basics - Technology, Image Quality and Radiation Dose*. Lippincott Williams & Wilkins; 2009.

Mahesh M. Search for isotropic resolution in CT from conventional through multiple-row detector. *Radiographics*. 2002;22(4):949-962.

American College of Radiology. *ACR manual on contrast media*. 2023. https://www.acr.org/-/media/ACR/Files/Clinical-Resources/Contrast_Media.pdf?1711275559636. Accessed March 27, 2024.

Cone Beam Computed Tomography

Scarfe WC, Angelopoulos C, eds. *Maxillofacial Cone Beam Computed Tomography: Principles, Techniques and Clinical Applications*. 1st ed. Springer International Publishing; 2018.

Gaêta-Araujo H, Alzoubi T, Vasconcelos KF, et al. Cone beam computed tomography in dentomaxillofacial radiology: a two-decade overview. *Dentomaxillofac Radiol*. 2020;49:20200145.

Gaêta-Araujo H, Leite AF, Vasconcelos KF, Jacobs R. Two decades of research on CBCT imaging in DMFR – an appraisal of scientific evidence. *Dentomaxillofac Radiol*. 2021;50:20200367.

Kaasalainen T, Ekholm M, Siiskonen T, Kortesniemi M. Dental cone beam CT: an updated review. *Phys Med*. 2021;88:193-217.

American Dental Association Council on Scientific Affairs. The use of cone-beam computed tomography in dentistry: an advisory statement from the American Dental Association Council on Scientific Affairs. *J Am Dent Assoc*. 2012;143(8):899-902.

Al-Okshi A, Horner K, Rohlin M. A meta-review of effective doses in dental and maxillofacial cone beam CT using the ROBIS tool. *Br J Radiol*. 2021;94(1123):20210042.

Radiologic Reports

American College of Radiology. ACR practice parameter for communication of diagnostic imaging findings. In: *Practice guidelines and technical standards*. American College of Radiology; 2014. https://www.acr.org/-/media/ACR/Files/Practice-Parameters/CommunicationDiag.pdf. Accessed January 31, 2024.

Carter L, Farman AG, Geist J, et al. American Academy of Oral and Maxillofacial Radiology executive opinion statement on performing and interpreting diagnostic cone beam computed tomography. *Oral Surg Oral Med Oral Pathol Oral Radiol Endod*. 2008;106:561-562.

European Society of Radiology (ESR). Good practice for radiological reporting. Guidelines from the European Society of Radiology. *Insights Imaging*. 2011;2:93-96.

Clinical Applications

Bornstein MM, Scarfe WC, Vaughn VM, et al. Cone beam computed tomography in implant dentistry: a systematic review focusing on guidelines, indications, and radiation dose risks. *Int J Oral Maxillofac Implants*. 2014;29(suppl):55-77.

Scarfe WC, Azevedo B, Toghyani S, et al. Cone Beam Computed Tomographic imaging in orthodontics. *Aust Dent J*. 2017;62(suppl 1):33-50.

Scarfe WC, Farman AG, Sukovic P. Clinical applications of cone-beam computed tomography in dental practice. *J Can Dent Assoc*. 2006;72:75-80.

Scarfe WC, Levin MD, Gane D, et al. Use of cone beam computed tomography in endodontics. *Int J Dent*. 2009;2009:634567.

Guidelines for Computed Tomography Imaging

American College of Radiology. *ACR–ASNR–SPR practice parameter for the performance of computed tomography (CT) of the extracranial head and neck*. 2021. https://www.acr.org/-/media/ACR/Files/Practice-Parameters/CT-Head-Neck.pdf. Accessed March 28, 2024.

American College of Radiology. *ACR–AAPM–SIIM Technical standard for Electronic Practice of Medical Imaging*. 2022. https://www.acr.org/-/media/ACR/Files/Practice-Parameters/Elec-Practice-MedImag.pdf. Accessed March 28, 2024.

American Academy of Oral and Maxillofacial Radiology. Clinical recommendations regarding use of cone beam computed tomography in orthodontics. Position statement by the American Academy of Oral and Maxillofacial Radiology. *Oral Surg Oral Med Oral Pathol Oral Radiol*. 2013;116:238-257.

Special Committee to Revise the Joint American Association of Endodontists/American Academy of Oral and Maxillofacial Radiology Position Statement on use of CBCT in Endodontics. AAE and AAOMR Joint Position Statement: use of cone-beam computed tomography in endodontics – 2015 update. *Oral Surg Oral Med Oral Pathol Oral Radiol*. 2015;120:508-512.

Swennen GR, Schutyser F. Three-dimensional cephalometry: spiral multislice vs cone-beam computed tomography. *Am J Orthod Dentofacial Orthop*. 2006;130:410-416.

The American Dental Association Council on Scientific Affairs. The use of cone-beam computed tomography in dentistry: an advisory statement from the American Dental Association Council on Scientific Affairs. *J Am Dent Assoc*. 2012;143:899-902.

Mallya SM, Ahmad M, Cohen JR, Kaspo G, Ramesh A. Recommendations for imaging of the temporomandibular joint. Position statement from the American Academy of Oral and Maxillofacial Radiology and the American Academy of Orofacial Pain. *Oral Surg Oral Med Oral Pathol Oral Radiol*. 2022;134:639-648.

Tyndall DA, Price JB, Tetradis S, et al. Position statement of the American Academy of Oral and Maxillofacial Radiology on selection criteria for the use of radiology in dental implantology with emphasis on cone beam computed tomography. *Oral Surg Oral Med Oral Pathol Oral Radiol*. 2012;113:817-826.

10

Magnetic Resonance Imaging

Shumei Murakami and Sanjay M. Mallya

1. INTRODUCTION

Magnetic resonance imaging (MRI) is a tomographic imaging technique that uses the principle of nuclear magnetic resonance (NMR).

A. History of Nuclear Magnetic Resonance

A charged particle in motion produces a magnetic field. When an atomic nucleus with a nonzero nuclear spin is placed in a magnetic field, it begins to precess. The frequency of precession is proportional to the magnetic flux density. When irradiated with a radio wave with the same frequency as the precession frequency, the atomic nucleus absorbs the energy of the radio wave. This phenomenon is called nuclear magnetic resonance (NMR). In 1946, Felix Bloch and Edward Mills Purcell applied the NMR principle to liquids and solids, a major development for which they were awarded the Nobel Prize in Physics in 1952.

When irradiation of the nucleus with the radio wave is stopped, the atomic nucleus returns to its original state through a process called relaxation. In 1971, Raymond Damadian's experiments in laboratory mice showed that the relaxation of tumors was different from that of normal tissue.

B. History of Magnetic Resonance Imaging

Based on Damadian's research, tomographic imaging was widely studied to identify a tumor's location and extent. In 1973, Paul Lauterbur proposed a technique to record NMR signals from different locations using "gradient magnetic fields." Sir Peter Mansfield invented the technique of slice selection the following year, and Richard Ernst invented a method to mathematically reconstruct images using a two-dimensional Fourier transform. Other than Damadian, these three scientists were awarded the Nobel Prize for their discoveries.

C. Clinical Magnetic Resonance Imaging

The target nuclei for clinical MRI are hydrogen nuclei (protons). Nuclei with odd numbers of protons or neutrons can be used for clinical MRI. However, hydrogen is the most suitable, considering its high sensitivity and natural abundance (Table 10.1). Importantly, hydrogen is present in large amounts in the human body in water and fat, thus providing rich sources for NMR signals. In addition to hydrogen, nuclei of phosphorus, sodium, and xenon have been targeted for MRI.

MRI is noninvasive as it does not involve exposure to ionizing radiation. It provides excellent soft tissue contrast and provides contrasts between tissues that cannot be differentiated on computed tomography (CT) or conventional radiography. Practical limitations of MRI include long scan times and artifacts from dental restorative materials and prostheses.

TABLE 10.1 Magnetic Properties of Abundant Biological Nuclei

Isotope	Abundance (%)	Gyromagnetic Ratio (MHz/T)
^{1}H	99	42.6
^{12}C	98	0[a]
^{16}O	99	0[a]
^{19}F	100	40.0
^{23}Na	100	11.3
^{31}P	100	17.2

[a]Isotopes with a gyromagnetic ratio of zero do not produce a magnetic resonance signal.

2. NUCLEAR MAGNETIC RESONANCE

An atomic nucleus with an odd number of protons or neutrons can be considered a magnet because it is charged and spinning. When placed in a magnetic field, the spin axes of atomic nuclei move in a precessional motion, analogous to the motion of a toy spinning top. The frequency of precession is proportional to the magnetic flux density (approximately the same as that of the magnetic field strength). When the precessing nucleus is irradiated with a radio wave of the same frequency as its precession frequency, the nucleus will absorb energy. When the frequencies differ even slightly, the atomic nucleus does not absorb any energy. This highly specific energy reception is called NMR.

A. Protons in Magnetic Field

For clinical MRI, the patient is placed in a strong magnetic field. Magnetic flux density ranges from 0.1 to 7 T (Tesla), with 1.5 and 3 T most commonly used in clinical imaging.

Hydrogen nuclei comprise a single unpaired proton, so they act as magnetic vectors. A tiny electric current is generated when a proton spins, so the spinning proton acts as a tiny magnet. Typically, these magnetic vectors are randomly oriented in space (Fig. 10.1). The protons can exist in one of two energy states: a low energy state (spin-up, a magnetic moment that follows the direction of the external magnetic field) and a high energy state (spin-down, a magnetic moment that opposes the direction of the external magnetic field).

At equilibrium, more protons have a magnetic moment in the direction of the external magnetic field because protons prefer to be in a lower energy state. In this situation, the net *longitudinal magnetization*, the sum of all magnetic moments from all protons, is in the direction of the magnetic field (Fig. 10.2). As the magnetic field's

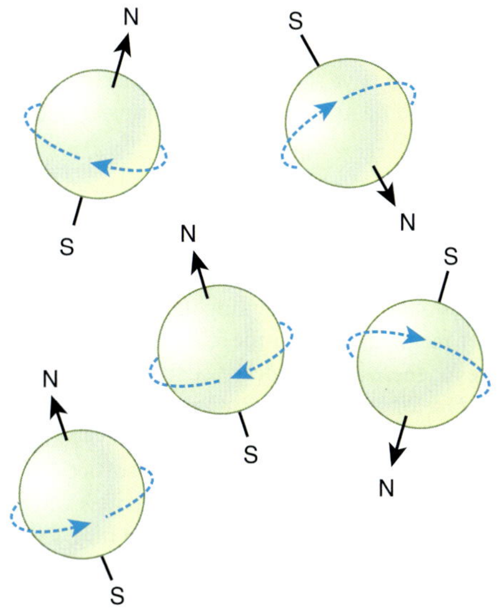

Fig. 10.1 Since protons are spinning, they can be thought of as tiny magnets. They are vectors because they have directions and magnitudes. Since the directions of the magnet's nuclear spins are random, the sum of the vectors is zero.

strength increases, the magnitude of longitudinal magnetization increases.

B. Precession

In addition to aligning in or against the direction of the external magnetic field, the magnetic moment of the protons also precesses around the external magnetic field. This motion resembles a spinning top, which rotates around an upright position as it slows down (Fig. 10.3).

Likewise, the external magnetic field's presence causes the spinning proton's axis to precess around the axis of the static magnetic field. The frequency of precession is called the *Larmor frequency* or resonance frequency and is defined by the Larmor equation. Practical applications of the Larmor equation to clinical MRI are discussed in Box 10.1.

C. Resonance

When protons are irradiated with radio waves of the same frequency as the proton's Larmor frequency, the protons absorb the radio wave energy. As a result, some protons in the lower energy state transition to higher energy states (Fig. 10.4). Furthermore, the phases of precession of individual protons are aligned. This phenomenon is called NMR.

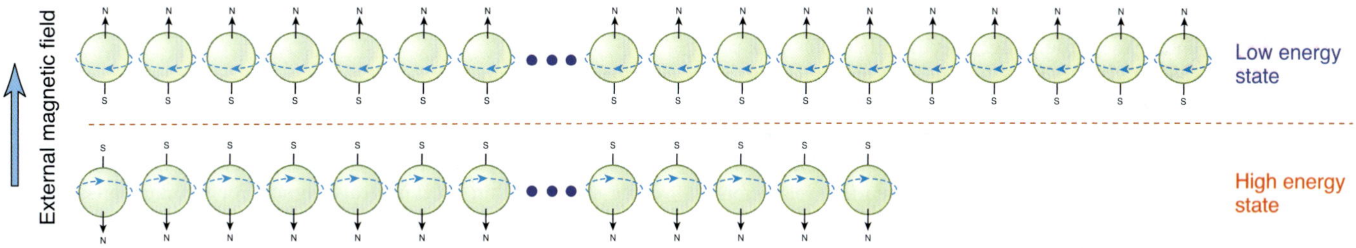

Fig. 10.2 In a magnetic field, the direction of the proton's magnetization vector is parallel to the external magnetic field. The number of magnetization vectors in the direction of the external magnetic field (spin-up) is slightly more than those in the opposite direction (spin-down). This is because protons tend to exist in a lower energy state.

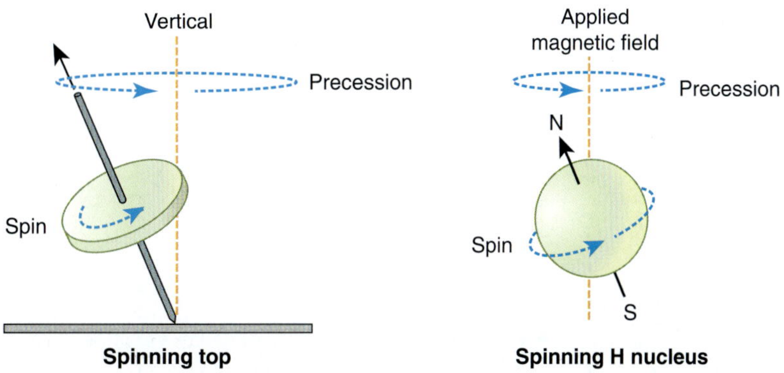

Fig. 10.3 Precession. Much as a top rotates around a vertical axis when spinning, the spin axis of a spinning hydrogen nucleus rotates around the direction of the external magnetic field. This movement is called precession, and the rate or frequency of precession is called the precessional, resonance, or Larmor frequency. The Larmor frequency depends on the strength of the external magnetic field and is specific for the nuclear species (see Box 10.1).

BOX 10.1 Practical Applications of the Larmor Equation in Clinical Magnetic Resonance Imaging

- Hydrogen nuclei are abundant and have a high gyromagnetic ratio, and thus, a high Larmor frequency, which permits efficient signal production to make a magnetic resonance image.
- The gyromagnetic ratio of each nucleus is unique (see Table 10.1). Thus, for a given magnetic field strength, the Larmor frequencies of different nuclei are also unique, and this allows for the selective excitation of hydrogen nuclei during clinical imaging.
- The Larmor frequency of a nuclear species is directly proportional to the strength of the external magnetic field. In magnetic resonance imaging, a local magnetic gradient is applied across an anatomic site. This spatially separates the tissue's protons into "slices" of varying Larmor frequencies—the basis for spatially encoding magnetic resonance signals into image slices.

$$\omega = \gamma \times \boldsymbol{B}_0$$

where $\boldsymbol{\omega}$ is the Larmor frequency, $\boldsymbol{\gamma}$ is the gyromagnetic ratio, and $\boldsymbol{B}_0$ is the strength of the external magnetic field.

The rotational frequency of proton precession is about 128 MHz at 3 T, which is similar to the frequency of a radio, so the electromagnetic waves sent to perturb precessing protons are called *radio frequency (RF)* pulses.

D. Relaxation

Resonant protons that receive energy and precess in phase (coherent) will return to their original state when the RF pulse is stopped. As the protons transfer energy to surrounding molecules, their phases of precession tend to separate out and the longitudinal magnetization increases. These processes are called *relaxation*, and there are two modes of relaxation—*T1 relaxation* and *T2 relaxation*. Each mode of relaxation is independent. T2 relaxation always occurs with T1 relaxation. However, T2 relaxation can also occur independent of T1 relaxation.

i. T1 Relaxation

When the irradiation with an RF pulse is stopped, the longitudinal magnetization of the protons is restored due to relaxation. This is achieved by transferring thermal energy from the resonant protons (spins) to the surrounding molecules (lattice). This is an exponential process. The time required for the longitudinal magnetization to return to 63% ($1 - 1/e$) of its original value is defined as the *T1 relaxation time* or *spin-lattice relaxation time* (Fig. 10.5).

The T1 relaxation time varies between tissues and reflects the ability of the proton to transfer excess energy to surrounding molecules (Table 10.2). Tissues with high water content tend to have longer T1 times because the high intrinsic energy of water inhibits the transfer of energy to the lattice. In contrast, tissues with high fat content, such as bone marrow, tend to have short T1 times, reflecting the low intrinsic energy of fat and the relatively easy energy transfer to the lattice.

ii. T2 Relaxation

When the RF pulse stops, the aligned in-phase precession of the protons starts to fall apart. The magnetic moments of adjacent protons begin to interfere with each other, causing the nuclear magnetic moments to precess out of phase, resulting in a loss of *transverse magnetization*, the net magnetization in the XY plane. The time required for the transverse magnetization to decrease to 37% ($1/e$) is defined as the *T2 relaxation time* or *spin-spin relaxation time* (Fig. 10.6).

As the transverse magnetization rapidly decays to zero, the amplitude and duration of the detected signal also decay. T2 relaxation occurs more quickly than T1 relaxation, so a tissue's T1 relaxation time is typically 5 times longer than its T2 relaxation time. Like T1 time, T2 time is also characteristic of the examined tissue. In fats, the molecules are tightly packed, resulting in stronger dephasing interactions between adjacent protons. Therefore, tissues with higher fat content have shorter T2 relaxation times. In contrast, tissues with more fluid have longer T2 relaxation times because the water molecule array is more widely spaced, resulting in less dephasing interactions.

E. How to Receive an MR Signal

The precession of the transverse magnetization M_{XY} induces a current in the receiver coil (Fig. 10.7)—Faraday's law of electromagnetic induction. The magnitude of this current is proportional to the overall density of protons within the tissue. The measured current serves as the signal needed to generate an MR image.

3. CLINICAL MRI

An MR image is a distribution of signal magnitudes in three-dimensional positions (X-, Y-, and Z-coordinates). Consider a patient lying supine within a cylindrical magnet. For standard imaging, the direction of the X-axis is left to right, the Y-axis is anterior to posterior, and the craniocaudal direction is the Z-axis (Fig. 10.8A). This chapter uses these three standard coordinates.

A. Creating Tomographic Sections

Consider a patient is placed in a magnetic field strength of 1.5 T—every proton in the patient will experience an external magnetic field strength of 1.5 T (Fig. 10.8B). At this time, all mobile protons will precess at a frequency of 64 MHz. If you apply a 64-MHz radio wave to the patient, you will receive signals from all mobile protons in the patient's body.

To create tomographic slices, a magnetic field gradient is applied in the Z-axis direction. The gradient is relatively small and in the

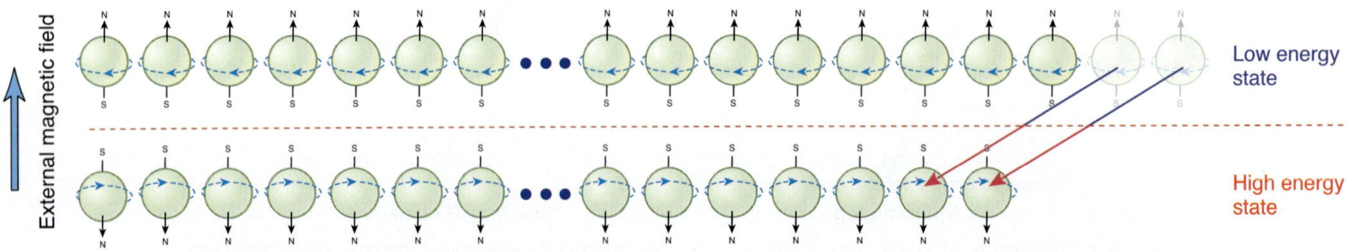

Fig. 10.4 Nuclear Magnetic Resonance. Protons placed in a strong magnetic field precess in response to the strength of the magnetic field. When a radio wave with frequency equal to the proton's precession frequency is applied, protons at a lower energy level transition to a higher energy level. This phenomenon of energy absorption and change in state of net magnetization is termed nuclear magnetic resonance.

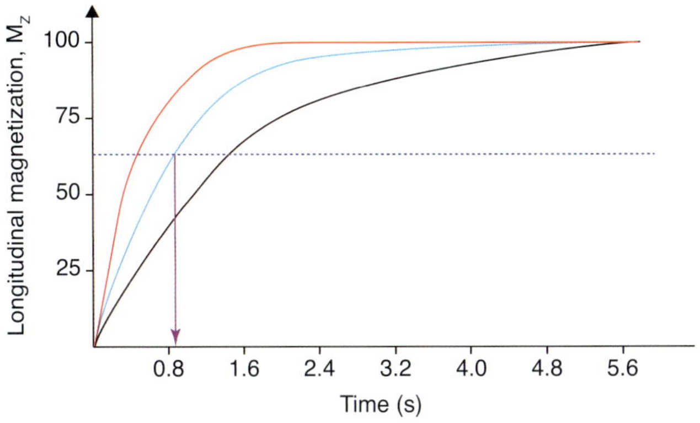

Fig. 10.5 T1 Relaxation. The behavior of T1 relaxation is different for each tissue. The T1 relaxation time is defined as the time taken for the net longitudinal magnetization vectors to return to 63% of its original value. The arrow identifies the T1 relaxation time of the tissue represented by the blue curve. An echo acquired at this time will provide contrast between the tissues based on their T1 relaxation time.

TABLE 10.2 T1 and T2 Relaxation Times in a Main Field of 1.5 T

Tissue Type	T1 Time (ms)	T2 Time (ms)
Fat	240–250	60–80
Bone marrow	550	50
White matter of cerebrum	780	90
Gray matter of cerebrum	920	100
Muscle	860–900	50
Cerebrospinal fluid (similar to water)	2200–2400	500–1400

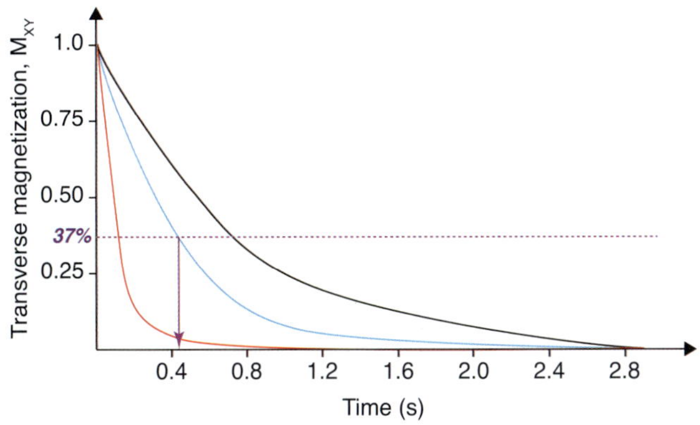

Fig. 10.6 T2 Relaxation. The behavior of T2 relaxation is different for each tissue. The T2 relaxation time is defined as the time taken for the net transverse magnetization vectors comes to decrease to 37% of its original value. The arrow identifies the T2 relaxation time of the tissue represented by the blue curve. An echo acquired around this time will provide contrast between the tissues based on their T2 relaxation time.

illustration ranges from 1.2 to 1.8 T (Fig. 10.8C). According to Larmor's formula, the frequency of the resonant radio waves is proportional to the magnetic flux density. In the illustrated example, protons in the chest region precess at 72.5 MHz, whereas the protons in the knee region precess at a frequency of 55.5 MHz.

When a 55.5 MHz radio waves is applied, only the protons in the tomographic plane of the knee resonate, acquire energy, and align in phase (Fig. 10.8D). However, there is no resonance of protons in other locations, and this provides specificity of slice selection. Likewise, when

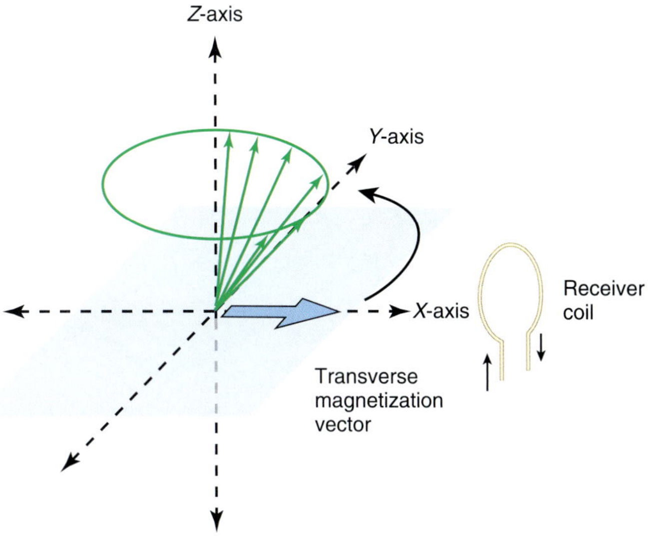

Fig. 10.7 Receiver Coil. The precession of the net transverse magnetic vector in the *XY* plane induces a current flow in a receiver coil, the magnetic resonance signal. The frequency of this induced alternating current signal matches the frequency of the radiofrequency pulse and the Larmor frequency of hydrogen nuclei.

a radio wave with a frequency of 72.5 MHz is applied, only protons in the chest region will respond and generate MR signals. This method of tomographic imaging with MRI was invented by Sir Peter Mansfield.

B. Phase and Frequency Encoding

Although the Z-axis section identification is complete, the "image blackboard" will display a uniform signal because the X–Y coordinates of individual signals are unknown. To assign spatial locations of signals from different areas of the imaged tissue volume, the image matrix needs a grid with vertical columns and horizontal rows so that signals can be assigned to appropriate pixels within the image matrix. To accomplish this, a gradient magnetic field is transiently applied along the Y-axis, causing a phase difference. Finally, a gradient in the X-axis direction changes frequency of precession to provide spatial encoding in the third dimension. Signals can now be assigned to spatial locations using three coordinates (Fig. 10.9).

i. Phase Encoding

A gradient magnetic field is applied in the Y-axis direction (anteroposterior), which is typically the shortest dimension. The gradient is applied for a short period and then turned off. To understand phase encoding, consider the transverse magnetization M_{XY} (see Fig. 10.7). When viewed from above, the transverse magnetization vector is analogous to a clock hand rotating around the face of a clock. Before the phase gradient is applied, the magnetization vectors from different Y-axis locations rotate around the face of the clock synchronously. When the Y-axis gradient is applied, it alters the precession, causing protons to precess faster or slower relative to protons in the adjacent areas along the Y-axis. The Y-gradient is transient, so when the gradient is removed, proton precessions return to their original frequency. However, the relative positions of the M_{XY} vectors—the hands across the clock face—are now in different phases and can be detected independently by the receiving coils permitting separation of signals along the Y-axis (Fig. 10.9).

ii. Frequency Encoding

For this step a gradient magnetic field is applied along the X-axis (left to right), which is usually the longest dimension of the anatomy.

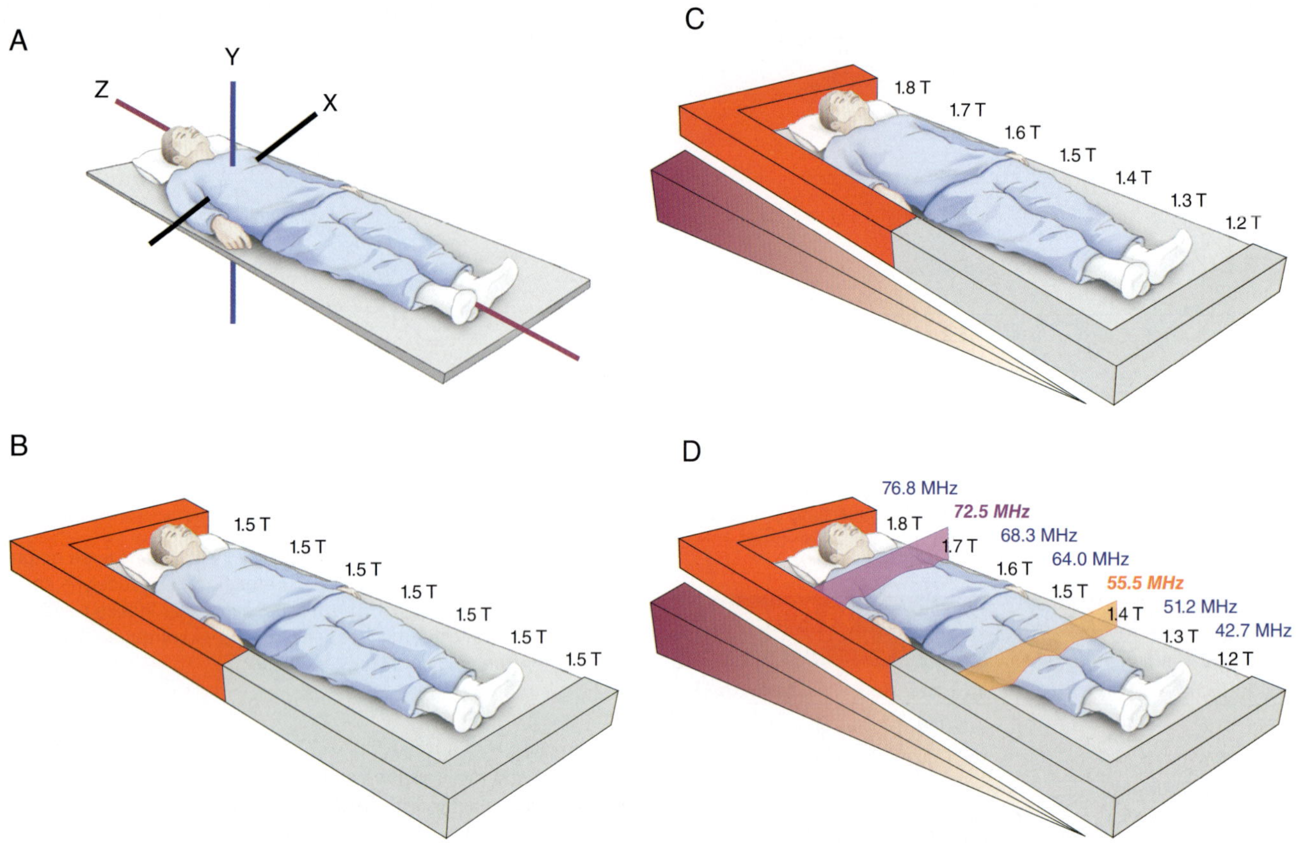

Fig. 10.8 (A) Reference coordinates used in magnetic resonance imaging. (B) Graphic representation of patient placed in a uniform 1.5 T external magnetic field. All protons will experience a 1.5 T field. (C) When a magnetic field gradient is applied, the magnetic flux density felt by protons in different parts of the human body differs. In this example, the magnetic flux ranges between 1.2 and 1.8 T. (D) The frequency of proton precession can be determined with Larmor's equation. In this illustration, when a 55.5 MHz radio wave is applied, only protons in the tomographic plane of the knee are excited. Likewise, a 72.5 MHz radio wave will only excite protons in the chest.

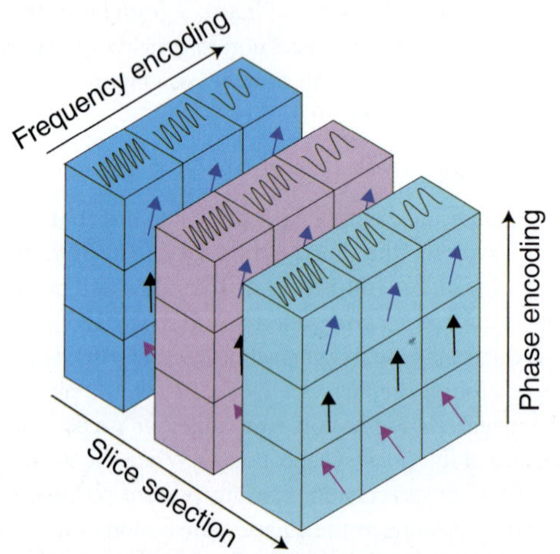

Fig. 10.9 Spatial encoding of information in magnetic resonance imaging. The slice selection, frequency encoding and phase encoding gradients.

Protons within each tomographic slice experience a different magnetic field and precess at different frequencies in the X-axis direction (Fig. 10.9). Consider a left–right width of 15 cm—if the frequency is divided into 300 steps, the width of one matrix element will be 0.5 mm. Such encoding is quick and performed in milliseconds.

C. k-Space

MRI signals cannot be placed directly into a matrix within an MR image. Analog MRI signals are digitized into discrete numbers through analog-to-digital conversion. The data from each repetition time (TR)'s acquisition are stored in the *k-space* (Fig. 10.10). Each point within the k-space matrix represents a unique combination of frequency and phase encoding values. Each line in the matrix corresponds to a specific phase-encoding value. During MR acquisition, multiple lines are acquired, one for each phase encoding gradient step. The k-space is not a simple mathematical abstraction of data. Rather it represents active encoding of spatial information during the acquisition process. An MR image is then created by performing a two-dimensional Fourier transform of the k-space, a method invented by Richard Ernst. An MR image is created only after all the data is embedded in k-space. Sequentially filling multiple rows increase scan time, so methods such as fast spin echo (FSE) and echo planar imaging (EPI) were developed to quickly embed acquired data into the k-space.

To better understand k-space, it is important to recognize the significance of the "center" and "edge" of k-space, both of which are important for image reconstruction. The center of the k-space contains low spatial frequency information and represents the overall structure and contrast. The edges of the k-space contain high spatial frequency information. These correspond to the fine details and transitions

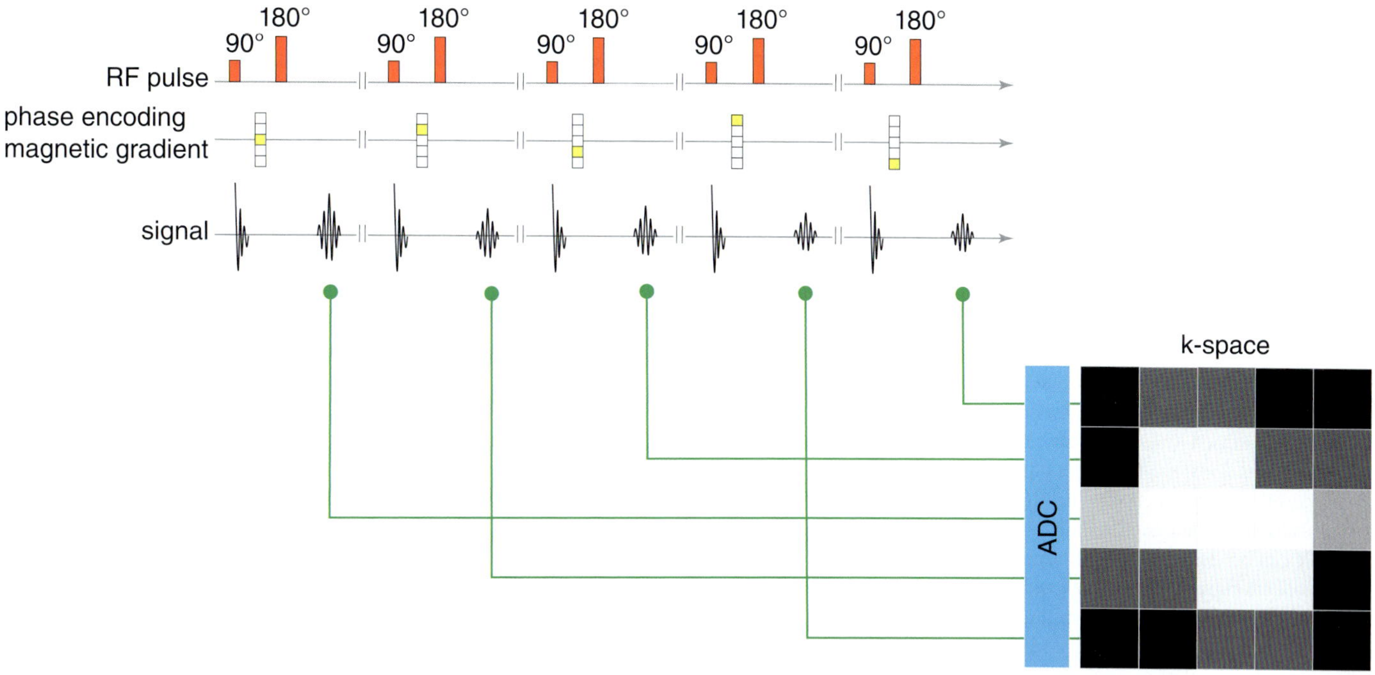

Fig. 10.10 Overview of k-space filling to create a 5 × 5 matrix magnetic resonance imaging (MRI) image. Stepwise phase encoding is performed after each 90-degree excitation radio frequency (RF) pulse to obtain the signal. This signal is digitized by an analog-to-digital converter (ADC) and filled in k-space line by line. Once the five lines have been filled, an MRI image can be created by performing a two-dimensional Fourier transformation on this k-space.

between tissues. The center of the k-space is acquired first to allow a coarse representation of the anatomic structures. Acquiring data for the edges of the k-space is more time-consuming but provides detailed information.

D. Pulse Sequences

The net longitudinal magnetization vector is parallel to and precesses around the Z-axis. An RF pulse applied along the Y-axis will displace the magnetization vector by 90 degrees toward the X-axis (see Fig. 10.7). To detect the magnetization along the XY-plane, a receiving coil is placed in the X-axis direction—as the magnetization vector moves past the receiving coil, it generates an electric current that is measured as the signal. The spin echo (SE) and gradient echo (GRE) are the two principal sequences used in clinical MRI. These methods differ in the timing and magnitude of the application of the RF pulses and the time of recording the data. The TR and the echo time (TE) are the two principal parameters adjusted in these various sequences.

i. Spin Echo

In the SE method, a 90-degree excitation pulse is first applied along the Y-axis to tilt the longitudinal magnetization vector by 90 degrees into the XY plane. When the 90-degree excitation pulse stops, the magnetization vector starts to undergo transverse relaxation. Individual proton magnetization vectors undergo transverse relaxation differently, influenced by other protons in their immediate environment. After a certain amount of time (t) passes, a 180-degree inversion pulse is applied and removed. This causes the protons to reverse the direction of precession, after which they start to return to their original state. At time $2t$, the transverse magnetization vectors of individual protons converge again (see Fig. 10.11). This process is called is called coherence. During the rephasing, there is a detectable echo that is measured to produce the MR signal.

ii. Gradient Echo

Instead of the 180-degree inversion pulse used in the SE method, the GRE method applies a pair of gradient magnetic fields. After the 90-degree excitation pulse, a magnetic field gradient is briefly applied in one direction. The gradient changes proton precession frequency and the signal is generated directly from these spins. Then, a gradient magnetic field is applied for a short time in the opposite direction (readout gradient) to acquire echo signals. The readout signal will be small. The GRE method was initially developed to decrease scan times.

iii. Fast Spin Echo

In conventional SE imaging, echo signals are acquired one at a time. FSE, also called turbo SE or fast/turbo SE, shortens the imaging time by acquiring multiple echoes in one TR to fill the k-space. In this technique, multiple 180-degree pulses are used within a single TR to create a train of echoes. The number of echoes to be acquired is called the echo train length (ETL). Filling all k-space in one repetition is called a "single shot."

In FSE, the TE that fills the center of the k-space is called the effective TE, which is a measure of contrast. A T1-weighted image with a short TR will not have many echoes, whereas a T2-weighted image with a long TR will have many echoes. For example, using an SE sequence with a TR of 3000 ms and 256 phase encoded, the imaging time will be 768,000 ms (3000 × 256) or 12.8 minutes. When an FSE sequence with 24 ETL is applied, the imaging time will be reduced to 32,000 ms (768,000 ÷ 24) or 32 seconds. The interval between echoes when acquiring multiple TEs is called echo space. If the echo space is

10 ms and the echo train is 9, the first TE will be 10 ms and subsequently 20, 30, … , 90 ms.

The disadvantage of FSE is that the image is blurry. Also, because the refocusing pulse is applied continuously, energy absorbed may lead to tissue heating, resulting in a higher specific absorption rate (SAR), especially noticeable at 3T. FSE is commonly used for T2-weighted imaging. In FSE T2-weighted images, fat produces high-intensity signals, whereas in SE T2-weighted images, only water has a high signal (see Fig. 10.16). Thus, fat suppression techniques are often applied to FSE T2-weighted images.

iv. Echo Planar Imaging

EPI is the fastest imaging technique in MRI, making it valuable for functional MRI (fMRI) and diffusion-weighted imaging (DWI) studies. Unlike traditional MR image reconstruction, data acquisition from multiple slices is performed in a single scan. With fast and repeated switching of gradient directions, multiple lines of the k-space can be encoded during a single TR. All data necessary for image reconstruction is acquired during this time, so the imaging time per slice is equal to the TR.

EPI can be classified into SE type and GRE type. SE-EPI completes data collection by reversing the gradient field after applying 90-degree and 180-degree pulses. In contrast, GRE-EPI completes data collection by applying an α-degree pulse and then reversing the gradient field. The impact of magnetic susceptibility artifacts influences the choice between SE-EPI and GRE-EPI. SE-EPI uses a refocusing RF pulse and thus, magnetic susceptibility artifacts are less. However, SE-EPI has a longer ETL compared to GRE-EPI and thus, the likelihood of patient motion increases. In contrast, GRE-EPI is more sensitive to magnetic susceptibility artifacts. However, due to a shorter ETL, the chances for patient motion are less. GRE-EPI is used for fMRI, which requires high temporal resolution.

4. PULSE SEQUENCE DIAGRAM

Pulse sequence diagrams (PSDs) are graphical representations of the timing and sequence of RF pulses, gradient pulses, and the resulting echoes during an MRI scan.

A. Pulse Sequence Diagram of the Spin Echo Method

Fig. 10.11 shows a pulse sequence diagram of the SE method. The horizontal direction of PSD represents the time course.

- The first row represents the timing of RF pulse delivery. For the SE method, a 90-degree RF pulse is applied first to excite protons and an inverted 180-degree RF pulse is subsequently applied to converge the out-of-phase magnetization vectors. The 90- and 180-degree RF pulses are repeated for each phase encoding step. The interval between two successive 90-degree RF pulse is called the *time of repetition* (*TR*). Twice the time interval between the 90-degree RF pulse and the 180-degree RF pulse is called the *time of echo* (*TE*).
- The second row is the slice selection gradient magnetic field in the Z-axis direction. The magnetic gradient for slice selection is applied for about 10 ms when delivering the 90-degree RF pulse and the 180-degree RF pulse. No other gradient can be applied at this time.
- The third row is the gradient magnetic field in the Y-axis direction and indicates the timing of applying phase encoding gradients. It takes 1–5 ms and can be applied at any time after 90-degree RF pulse irradiation but before obtaining an echo signal. At each repetition, the strength of the gradient is varied. Typically, 256 different magnetic field strengths are applied, so the signal acquisition process is repeated 256 times.
- The fourth row is the gradient magnetic field in the X-axis direction, which is applied throughout the time of echo signal acquisition. It takes about 10 ms.

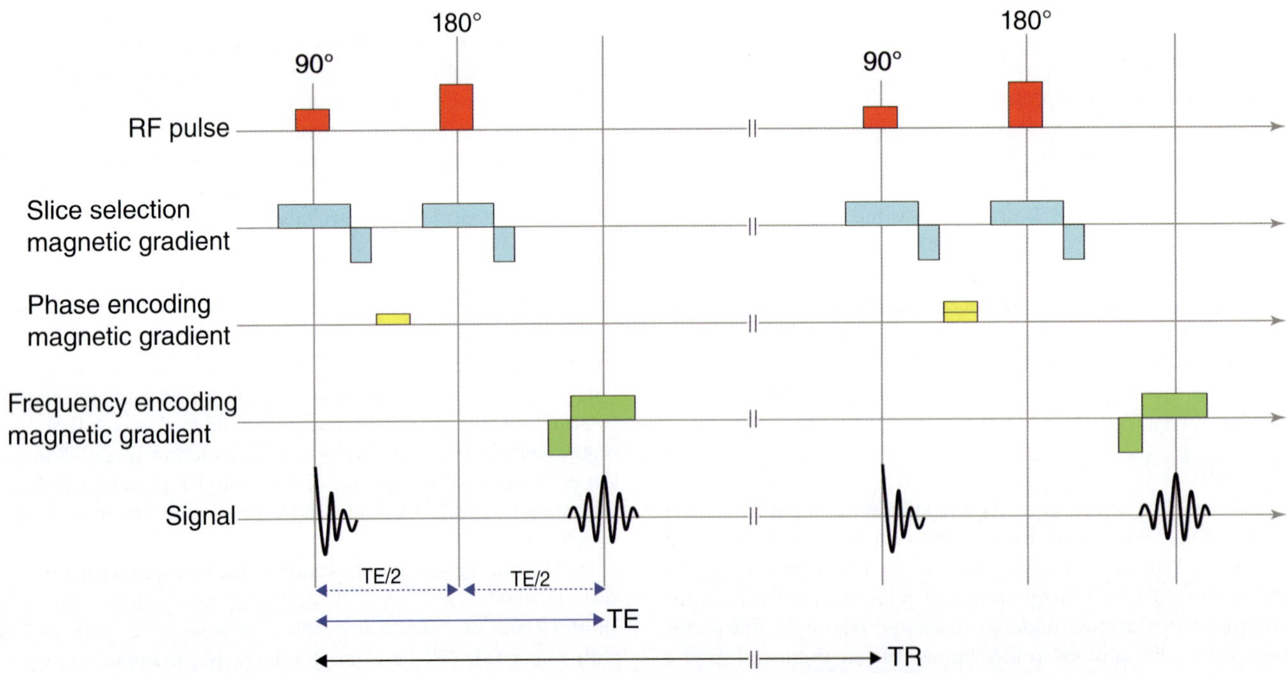

Fig. 10.11 In the spin echo method, an echo signal is generated using a combination of 90-degree and 180-degree radio frequency (RF) pulses. Select the desired slice during this pulse irradiation. Phase encoding is repeated step by step according to the image matrix size. Frequency encoding is applied during each signal acquisition. The interval between 90-degree pulses is called time of repetition (TR). Twice the time between the 90-degree pulse and the 180-degree pulse is called time of echo (TE).

- The fifth row represents the time at which the receiver coils receive signals. First, a *free induction decay* signal is generated by a 90-degree RF pulse but is not recorded. The echo signals are recorded at TE. The TR and TE are indicated at the bottom of the PSD.

B. Pulse Sequence Diagram of the Gradient Echo Method

PSD of the GRE method is similar to the SE method, except there is no 180-degree RF pulse for inversion in the first row. In addition, a pulse with a partial FA of α degrees is given as an excitation pulse rather than the standard 90-degree RF pulse. Since the time it takes to obtain an echo signal is short, TR can be shortened, reducing the imaging time.

5. MRI TISSUE CONTRAST

MRI is characterized by high contrast between soft tissues. Compared to other imaging modalities, MR image contrast is more diverse and complex. Tissue-specific factors that contribute to MRI contrast include T1 relaxation time, T2 relaxation time, mobility of and the number of protons in tissue, and their diffusion. Depending on what parameters are emphasized, MR images are called T1-weighted images, T2-weighted images, proton density–weighted images, or diffusion-weighted images (DWI).

The formula for signal strength in the SE method is shown as follows:

$$SI = \kappa \times \rho \times \{1 - e^{(-TR/T1)}\} \times \{e^{(-TE/T2)}\}$$

where ρ = proton density, T1 = T1 relaxation time, T2 = T2 relaxation time, TR = time of repetition, and TE = time of echo.

The critical parameters controlled by the operator are TR and TE. TR, the duration between repeated 90-degree RF pulses, determines the amount of T1 relaxation that occurs when the signal is collected. TE, the time between the center of the 90-degree RF pulse and the center of the echo measurement, controls the amount of T2 relaxation that occurs when the signal is collected. Clinical MRI protocols adjust TR and TE to emphasize tissue differences based on T1 relaxation time, T2 relaxation time, or proton density, producing images with different tissue contrasts (Box 10.2). Fig. 10.12 illustrates the supremacy of MRI to generate different contrasts that provide valuable information on the tissue properties.

BOX 10.2 Proton Density–Weighted MRI

- Long TR and short TE
- TR > 2000 ms, TE < 20 ms
- Neglect T1-time, neglect T2-time
- Fat and water yield high-intensity signals and appear bright (white)

T1-Weighted MRI

- Short TR and short TE
- TR < 600 ms, TE < 20 ms
- Emphasize T1-time, neglect T2-time
- Fat yields high-intensity signals and appears bright (white)

T2-Weighted MRI

- Long TR and long TE
- TR > 2000 ms, TE > 60 ms
- Neglect T1-time, emphasize T2-time
- Water yields high-intensity signals and appears bright (white)

A. Proton Density–Weighted Image

The combination of long TR and short TE produces a proton density–weighted image.

Consider the equation for signal intensity with SE sequences:

$$SI = \kappa \times \rho \times \{1 - e^{(-TR/T1)}\} \times \{e^{(-TE/T2)}\}$$

Note that TR and TE are the numerators, whereas T1 and T2 times are denominators. If the TR is set to be long, the relative differences in tissue T1 times can be ignored. Likewise, if TE is set to be short, the relative differences in tissue T2 times contribute less to image contrast. Thus, when using a long TR and short TE, NMR signal intensity represents the magnitude of the proton density.

B. T1-Weighted Image

The combination of short TR and short TE produces a T1-weighted image.

Consider the equation for signal intensity with SE sequences:

$$SI = \kappa \times \rho \times \{1 - e^{(-TR/T1)}\} \times \{e^{(-TE/T2)}\}$$

When TR is set to be short, the relative differences in tissue T1 are principal contributors to image contrast. However, if TE is set very short, relative differences in magnitude of T2 times can be ignored. The signal intensity thus represents the proton density and the T1 time.

Tissues with short T1 time yield strong signals, whereas tissues with long T1 time will produce weak signals. A typical example of a tissue with a short T1 time is adipose tissue—subcutaneous fat and lipoma appear bright on MR images. On the other hand, water, which has a long T1 relaxation time, appears dark on T1-weighted MR images. In bone, the water content is low and hydrogen nuclei are tightly bound to the hydroxyapatite crystal yielding weak, undetectable signals. Thus, bone appears dark on MR images. Gadolinium is paramagnetic and shortens tissue T1 time, making them appear bright on T1-weighted MR images and is thus used as a contrast agent in MRI.

C. T2-Weighted Image

The combination of a long TR and long TE produces a T2-weighted image.

Consider the equation for signal intensity with SE sequences:

$$SI = \kappa \times \rho \times \{1 - e^{(-TR/T1)}\} \times \{e^{(-TE/T2)}\}$$

When TR is set to be long, the relative differences between tissue T1 times contribute less to image contrast. However, if TE is also set very long, image contrast will depend on differences in tissue T2 relaxation times. The signal intensity thus represents the proton density and the T2 time. Tissues with long T2 relaxation times will result in strong signals, whereas tissues with a short T2 relaxation time will produce weak signals. Water has a long T2 time, and most malignant tumors, cysts, abscesses, and inflammations appear bright on MR images.

D. Diffusion-Weighted Image

Diffusion-weighted MR imaging (DWI) makes it possible to understand the molecular motions of protons within normal and diseased tissues. The principle of DWI is to apply strong magnetic field gradients with an SE-EPI sequence. This strong magnetic gradient, called *motion probing gradient* (MPG), is briefly superimposed on the main magnetic field.

The MPG is applied before and after the 90-degree and 180-degree RF pulses. When applied, protons in water will experience a shift in their magnetic field, depending on their motion. When diffusion is restricted, for example, within cellular structure, the effect of the gradient is more pronounced. This results in a high signal (bright) in regions where diffusion is limited, indicating presence of cellular structures and barriers to diffusion. In contrast, areas where diffusion is not

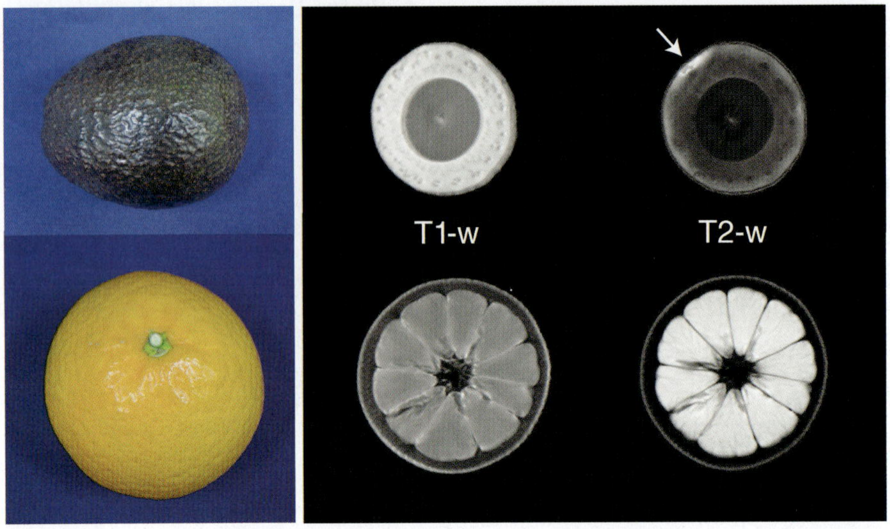

Fig. 10.12 Tissue contrast in magnetic resonance imaging. An avocado and an orange were imaged in a 3 T magnet with T1- and T2-weighted spin echo sequences. The mesocarp (the creamy edible flesh) of the avocado contains fat, which creates a bright signal on T1-weighted images. The juice-filled, individual segments of the orange appear bright on T2-weighted images. The arrow points to a rotten part of the avocado, creating a bright signal on T2-weighted images like a malignant tumor!

limited, for example, with edema or necrosis, produce low signals and appear dark. The *apparent diffusion coefficient* (ADC) is one parameter derived from DWI data. It reflects the rate of diffusion of water and is expressed in units of square millimeters per second. High ADC values indicate rapid diffusion, indicating free, unrestricted water motion, as in cysts and fluid-filled pathoses. Low ADC values suggest restricted diffusion. Malignant tumors typically have low ADC values, reflecting restriction of diffusion due to increased cellularity and complexity of the tissue architecture.

6. FAT SUPPRESSION

In SE T1-weighted images, fat appears bright because the T1 time of fat is short and the T1 time of water is long. In FSE T2-weighted images, not only water but also fat appears bright. The high signal intensity of fat may obscure details. Fat suppression techniques selectively eliminate or reduce the signals from adipose tissue. Practical applications for maxillofacial imaging include detection and characterization of tumors, postcontrast MRI, evaluation of the orbit and optic nerve, and evaluation of the parotid gland. The three principal methods of fat suppression are discussed as follows.

A. Chemical Shift Selective

The resonance frequencies of protons in water and protons in fat are slightly different. In fat, the hydrogen atoms are surrounded by carbon atoms, which create a shielding effect and lower the resonance frequency of the hydrogen nuclei. This difference is about 3.5 parts per million at 1.5 and 3 T and is called the *chemical shift*. With a 1.5 T device, the resonance frequency of fat and water differ by about 224 Hz. In chemical shift selective (CHESS), the sequence starts with a frequency-selective RF pulse, tuned to the resonance frequency of fat protons. Next, an excitation pulse is applied to tip the net magnetization vectors of both fat and water. At the same time, an inversion pulse is applied to invert the net magnetization of protons. In the subsequent time delay, water and fat protons start to return to align with the external magnetic field. Data acquisition is timed such that the magnetization of protons in water is mostly recovered, while the magnetization vector of fat remains inverted and does not yield a signal. Thus, fat signals are selectively suppressed.

B. Dixon's Method

The precession frequency of protons in fat is lower than in water. Therefore, after the excitation RF pulse, the phase of the transverse magnetization of protons in fat lags behind the transverse magnetization of protons in water. At 2.25 ms, the fat and water signals are in opposite phase but at 4.5 ms, the two phases align (Fig. 10.13A). The Dixon method acquires two echoes specifically at the in-phase and out-of-phase time points to mathematically emphasize or suppress signals from fat and water (Fig. 10.13B). Thus, signal intensity from fat and water can be calculated and separately suppressed. Because two sets of echoes are recorded, the examination time is twice as long.

C. Short Tau (T1) Inversion Recovery

The T1 time of protons in fat is shorter than in water. The short tau (T1) inversion recovery (STIR) pulse sequence starts with an inversion pulse to flip the net magnetization vector by 180 degrees. The inversion pulse is followed by a short time interval (inversion time [TI]), timed to allow the net magnetization of protons in fat to become zero and is typically less than 200 ms. At this null point, a 90-degree excitation pulse is applied to generate transverse magnetization. Because the net magnetization vector from fat is zero at this time, there is no magnetization vector from fat protons, and thus, no signal from adipose tissue. Likewise, it is also possible to lengthen the TI such that signals from water can be selectively suppressed, a technique called the fluid-attenuated inversion recovery (FLAIR) method.

7. CONTRAST AGENTS FOR MRI

Contrast agents, most commonly the aqueous solution of gadolinium chelate, may be administered intravenously to improve tissue contrast. Gadolinium is paramagnetic and shortens the T1 relaxation times of tissues, generating brighter signals on T1-weighted images. The contrast agent is administered intravenously and accumulates in tissues with increased vascularity. Highly vascularized normal tissues such as

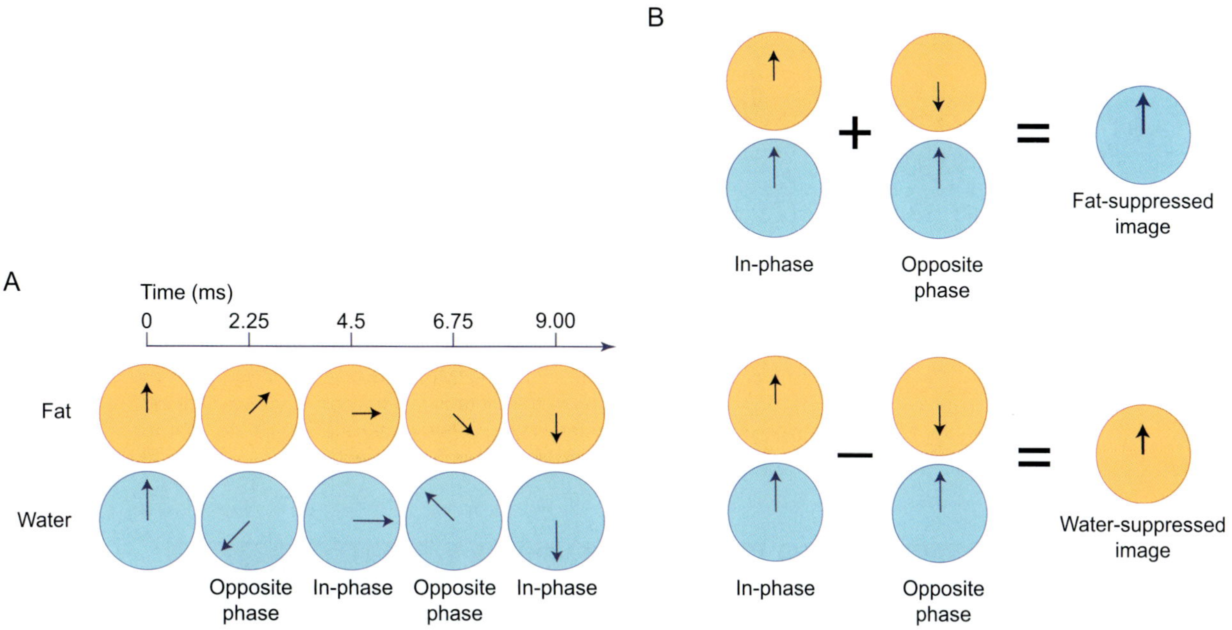

Fig. 10.13 Dixon method to suppress fat and water signals. (A) The phase of the transverse magnetization vector in fat and water is shown at the indicated times following the excitation radio frequency pulse. The phases of precession are in phase at 4.5 and 9 ms, and in exactly opposite phases at 2.25 and 6.75 ms. (B) Signals acquired when precession is in phase and in exactly opposite phases are mathematically manipulated to selectively subtract fat signals (fat-suppressed image) or water signals (water-suppressed image).

the nasal turbinates, sinus mucosa, and the tonsils accumulate contrast agents and appear bright on postcontrast images. Diseased tissues, including malignant tumors and inflammations, enhance following contrast. This allows better demarcation from surrounding normal tissue compared to the precontrast image.

8. ADVANTAGES OF MRI

The advantages of MRI are as follows:

- *No exposure to ionizing radiation*: Examinations can be prescribed or repeated without risk of harm.
- *High soft tissue contrast*: MRI displays lesions that may not be apparent with other imaging modalities.
- *Perform tomographic imaging in any plane*: It is possible to image in coronal, sagittal, and axial planes to better understand the three-dimensional extent of pathoses.
- *Generate images with multiple contrast combinations*: By using different imaging sequences, we can display tissues with different contrasts and gather more information on the nature of the pathologic changes, for example, cyst versus benign tumor and lipoma versus a nonadipose tissue mass.
- *Advanced MRI techniques*: The principles of MRI and NMR can be applied to provide additional data beyond morphologic information: magnetic resonance angiography (MRA), magnetic resonance spectroscopy (MRS), and fMRI are MR-based imaging techniques that complement information from standard T1-, T2-, and proton density–weighted images.

9. LIMITATIONS OF MRI

- *Long imaging times*: This limits use in patients who cannot hold still for extended periods.
- *Patients with claustrophobia*: The gantry of most MRI machines is a confined space, and patients may not be able to tolerate the procedure, especially considering the length of the imaging examinations.
- *Ferromagnetic substances*: The presence of ferromagnetic substances within the patient's body poses potential hazards—the strong magnetic fields can move these objects, cause excessive heating, or induce strong electrical currents, which may harm the patient. These include embedded ferrous foreign bodies, such as shrapnel or bullets.
- *Implanted electronic medical devices*: MRI is contraindicated in patients with implanted electronic medical devices, such as cardiac pacemakers and some cerebral aneurysm clips.
- *Dental restorative material and prostheses*: Metals used in dental restorations are not dislodged by the external magnetic field. However, their presence alters the local magnetic field, and as a consequence, changes the Larmor frequency of protons in the vicinity, which makes protons unresponsive to the applied RF pulses. This creates a signal void in the region, called a *magnetic susceptibility artifact* (Fig. 10.14). Depending on their location, these artifacts may interfere with diagnostic evaluation. Removable dental appliances must be removed before MRI scanning. Orthodontic wires containing stainless steel create extensive artifacts, including signal voids and image distortion (Fig. 10.15). Stainless steel wires produce more artifacts than chromium–cobalt alloys or nickel–titanium wires. Thus, when the jaws are the primary region of interest for MRI, orthodontic wires may need to be removed.

10. MRI vs. CT (TABLE 10.3)

- MRI and CT are both modalities that generate tomographic images. Both modalities use electromagnetic radiation. MRI uses radio waves, which are long wavelength. In contrast, CT uses X-rays, which are short wavelength, and thus, exposure to ionizing radiation is unavoidable. MRI examinations do not pose a risk from

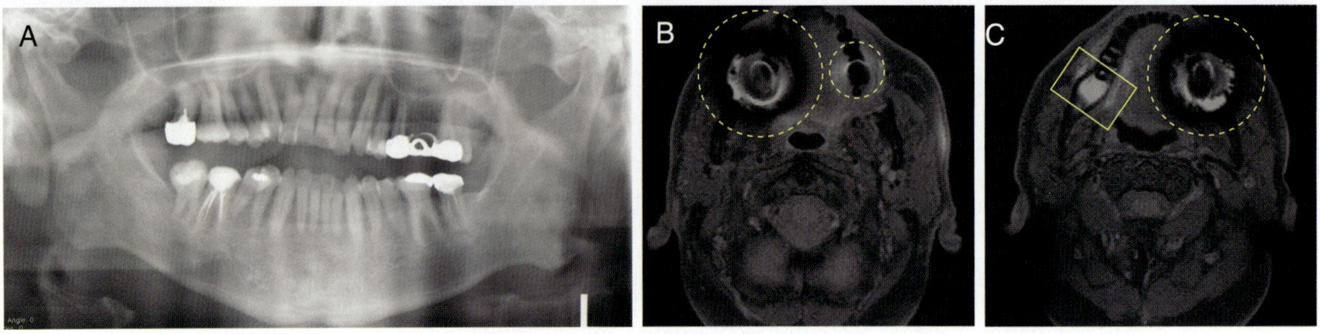

Fig. 10.14 Magnetic susceptibility artifacts. (A) Panoramic radiograph shows metallic restorations and prosthesis in the maxillary teeth. (B) T1-weighted magnetic resonance imaging (MRI) shows artifacts *(dashed circles)* manifesting as dark and bright areas adjacent to the region of the metallic restorations. (C) T1-weighted MRI shows artifacts adjacent to the region of the metallic restorations *(dashed circle)* and also in the right third molar region, outside the immediate vicinity of the right maxillary molars *(yellow rectangle)*.

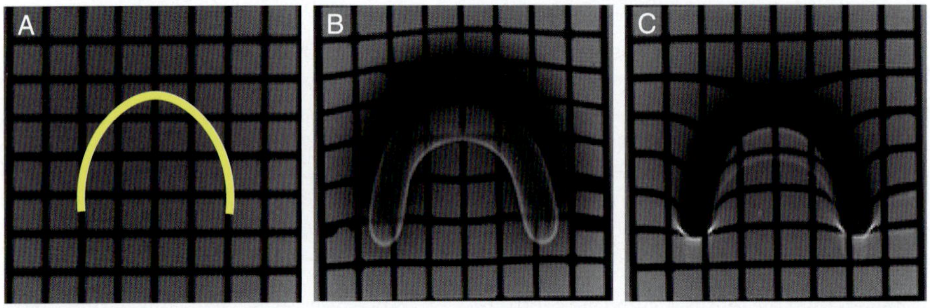

Fig. 10.15 Images Illustrating Artifacts Caused Orthodontic Wire. (A) A stainless-steel orthodontic wire (represented by the *curved yellow line*) was placed onto a plastic grid immersed in a solution of gadolinium pentetate. (B) T1-weighted MRI shows bright and dark artifacts due to the orthodontic wire. (C) T1-weighted MRI shows distortion of the image of the grid due to the presence of the orthodontic arch wire. The images illustrate that artifacts and distortion may limit MRI of the jaws in patients with fixed orthodontic appliances.

TABLE 10.3 Comparison of Magnetic Resonance Imaging and Computed Tomography

	MRI	CT
Radiation exposure	No	Yes
Contrast between soft tissues	High	Low
Contrast between hard tissues	Low	High
Primary tomographic plane	Selectable	Axial or coronal
Scan time	Long	Short
Artifact from tooth or bone	No	Yes
Artifact from magnetic metals	Large	Yes
Artifact from nonmagnetic metals	No	Yes
Imaging contraindications	Yes	No

ionizing radiation but is limited by the presence of ferromagnetic materials within the human body.

- Relative to multidetector CT (MDCT) and cone beam CT (CBCT), MRI scan times are significantly longer, increasing the potential of motion artifacts.
- Metals produce artifacts on both CT and MRI. These include dental restorations, implants, surgical hardware, and orthodontic wires. On CT, metals and other highly attenuating structures such as teeth and cortical bone produce *beam hardening artifacts* (see Chapter 9). On MRI, certain ferromagnetic metals and alloys, such as stainless steel, cobalt–chromium, and nickel–titanium, produce magnetic susceptibility artifacts, which may degrade image quality and decrease diagnostic value.
- CT data is represented as a three-dimensional array of voxels, each with a *CT number* that describes the gray value to be displayed. MDCT numbers are more reliable indicators of attenuation than CBCT numbers. These MDCT numbers serve as a parameter to assess soft tissue and osseous pathoses. However, MRI has no such absolute parameter.
- CT numbers represent attenuation by tissues with high atomic number or with high density but are unable to discriminate between these two factors. X-ray attenuation coefficients of soft tissues may vary by no more than 1%, limiting radiographic contrast that can be achieved. However, T1 and T2 relaxation times may vary by up to 40%, providing rich contrast with the MR images using different sequences (Fig. 10.16).

11. CLINICAL APPLICATIONS OF MRI IN ORAL AND MAXILLOFACIAL DIAGNOSIS

A. Practical Considerations in Prescribing Maxillofacial MRI

Most dental diseases affect the teeth and jawbones, and thus, conventional X-ray examinations, CBCT, and MDCT are the most widely used diagnostic imaging techniques.

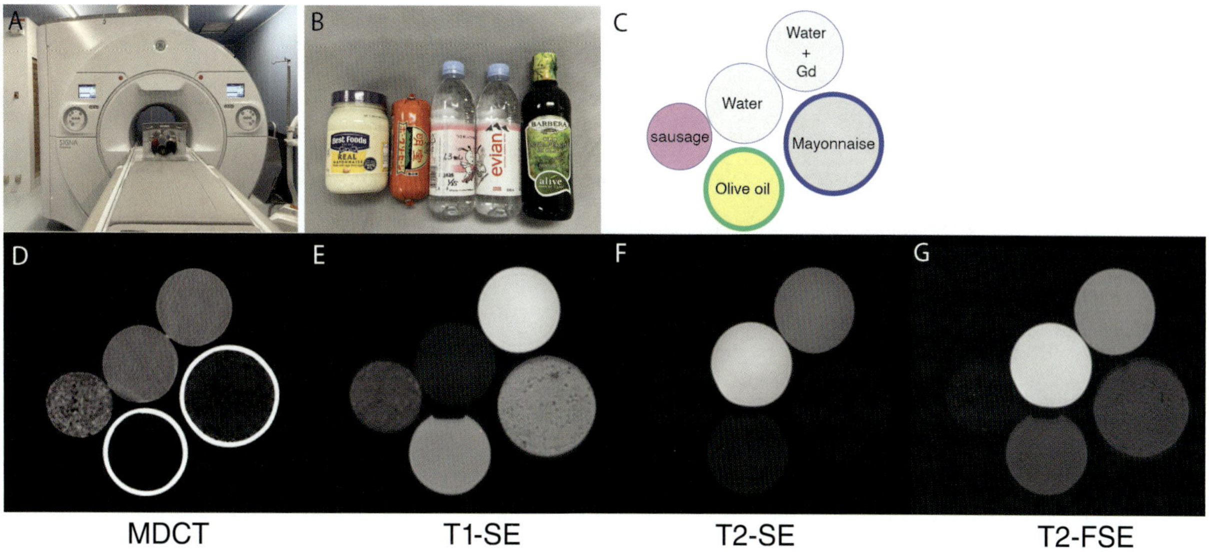

Fig. 10.16 Magnetic resonance (MR) image contrast illustrated through imaging of food substances. (A) A 3 T MRI scanner. (B) Food substances imaged: mayonnaise, sausage, water, water with gadolinium pentetate, and olive oil. (C) Schematic of the orientation of the food substances in the computed tomography (CT) and MR scanners. (D) Multidetector CT (MDCT) scan. (E) T1-weighted MRI with spin echo (SE) sequence. (F) T2-weighted MRI with SE sequence. (G) T2-weighted MRI with fast spin echo (FSE) sequence. Note changes to contrast in water and oil between the different MRI sequences.

However, for diseases of soft tissues, such as benign and malignant tumors and cysts, MRI provides valuable information to decipher the nature of the lesion and its extent. MRI is the gold standard to evaluate the position of the temporomandibular joint (TMJ) disk, which may be displaced in patients with TMJ disorders (see Chapter 28). Practically, the application of maxillofacial MRI is limited by metallic restorative materials and prostheses and orthodontic appliances. Metals used in many dental restorative materials may not cause artifacts if their magnetic susceptibility is small. However, metallic prosthesis and restorations pose significant limitations to use of MRI to image adjacent regions. These metals induce local inhomogeneity in the magnetic field, and the image of tissues within this region will be distorted or appear as signal voids (see Figs. 10.14 and 10.15). Ferromagnetic or conductive metals may be heated, leading to discomfort, or in rare extreme cases, local tissue injury. Patients with certain types of metallic implants, such as aneurysm clips or cochlear implants, cannot be imaged with MRI.

B. How to Evaluate Maxillofacial MR Images

An image on a CT scan represents attenuation of photons by tissues and materials via photoelectric absorption and Compton scatter. The tissue elements that contribute to attenuation include atomic number and physical density (see Chapter 1). With MRI, tissue contrasts vary with the specific pulse sequence used, and thus, knowledge of the scan sequence and its options are important.

First, determine whether the MR image is T1-weighted or T2-weighted, based on the TR and TE (Box 10.2). Determine whether options, for example, fat suppression or fast scan technique, were applied. Then, assess whether the scan was performed before or after injecting the contrast agent. Knowledge of signal intensities of different tissues and substances is fundamental to interpretation of MR images (see Fig. 10.16). As with any other image interpretation, knowledge of normal anatomy is the basis for assessing pathologic change (Fig. 10.17).

C. Clinical Applications

Infections: MRI provides value in evaluating patients with suspected osteomyelitis. In early osteomyelitis, there is insufficient demineralization of bone, and changes are not apparent on panoramic or CT images. MRI allows detection of early changes in the bone marrow, even before changes are seen on radiographs. The edema caused by inflammation results in loss of bone marrow signal with low signal intensity on T1-weighted images and high signal intensity on T2-weighted images (Fig. 10.18).

Cysts: Cysts are fluid filled and produce bright images on T2-weighted images. On T1-weighted images, they appear as well-demarcated low-intensity signals areas with no internal contrast (Fig. 10.19).

Benign neoplasms: Benign neoplasms of the soft tissues are well suited to MRI, which can identify the composition and nature of the tissue. Lesions of adipose tissue such as lipoma are well depicted due to their inherent high contrast on T1-weighted images and the ability to identify presence of fat via fat suppression or enhancement pulse sequences (Fig. 10.20). Because odontogenic neoplasms are intraosseous, CT imaging is performed to assess changes to teeth and bone. However, MRI provides insight on the nature of the neoplasm and its internal contents (Fig. 10.21). For example, ameloblastoma, the most common odontogenic tumor, often has cystic components, which is hyperintense on T2-weighted images.

Malignant neoplasms: MRI plays an important role in detection and management of malignant neoplasms of the oral cavity. The extent of the neoplasm into adjacent tissues, metastases to regional lymph nodes, and intracranial extent of maxillary lesions all require high tissue contrast (Fig. 10.22), which is provided via the various MR pulse sequences. Most malignancies in the oral cavity are squamous cell carcinomas (SCC) arising on the oral mucosal surfaces or tongue. The tongue, with intrinsic tissue contrasts of muscle and fat, is well suited for MRI. Because the tongue contains significant fat, a T2-weighted image with fat suppression is desirable when

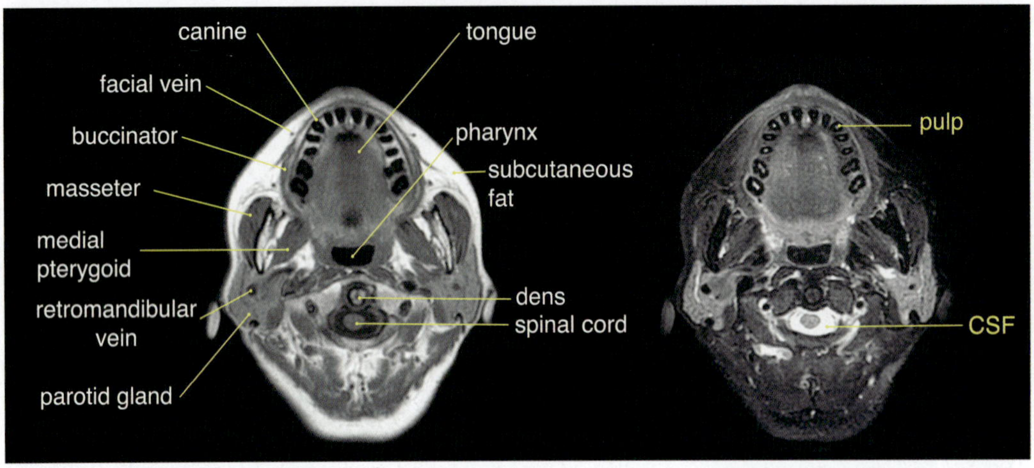

T1-weighted MRI

T2-weighted MRI with fat suppression

Fig. 10.17 Basic anatomic structures identified on T1-weighted and T2-weighted, fat-suppressed magnetic resonance (MR) images. Anatomy is best viewed on T1-weighted images. Note that bone does not yield a signal and appears black, unlike in computed tomography images. Note bright signal from subcutaneous fat on T1-weighted images and attenuation of this signal intensity on the fat-suppressed T2-weighted MR image. Note that fluid in cerebrospinal fluid (CSF) and pulp yields bright signals on T2-weighted MR images.

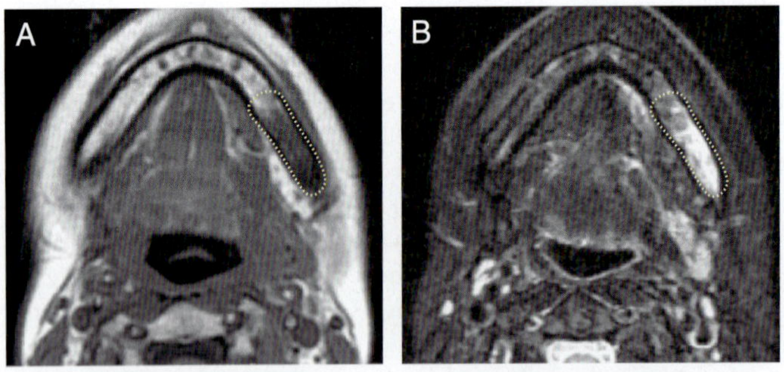

T1-weighted MRI

T2-weighted MRI
Fat suppression

Fig. 10.18 Magnetic resonance (MR) image contrast in disease detection: osteomyelitis. (A) T1-weighted MR image shows an axial section of the mandible with loss of bone marrow signal in the left posterior body, as outlined by the *dashed line*. Note robust signal from subcutaneous fat and fat in the marrow through the remainder of the mandible. (B) T2-weighted fat-suppressed MR image shows high signal intensity from edema within that same region, as outlined by the *dashed line*. Note suppression of fat signals to better outline the edema.

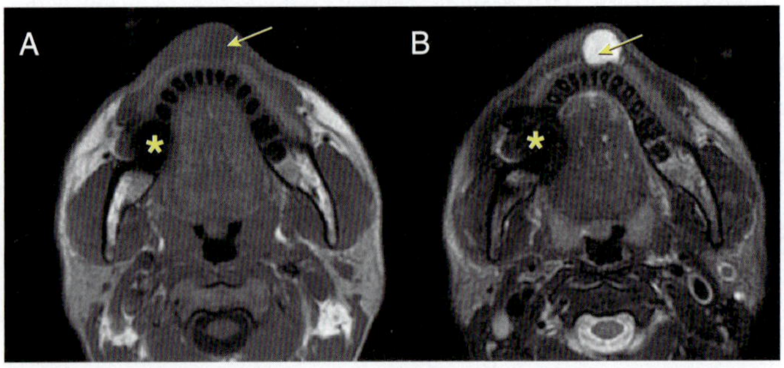

Fig. 10.19 Magnetic resonance (MR) image contrast in disease detection: mucocele. (A) T1-weighted MR image shows an axial section of the mandible with an oval intermediate signal intensity in the labial vestibule *(arrow)*. (B) T2-weighted MR image shows high signal intensity indicating fluid within the lesion. Note artifacts from dental restorations *(asterisk)*.

evaluating tongue SCC. With high intrinsic contrast, tongue carcinomas are clearly depicted without need for contrast enhancement (Fig. 10.23). When imaging potentially malignant lesions, gadolinium-contrast enhancement provides additional contrast to assess tumor invasion and extent (Fig. 10.24).

Temporomandibular disorders: MRI is the gold standard to determining the position and configuration of the TMJ articular disc and the presence or absence of reduction with mouth opening (Fig. 10.25). Joint space effusion can be seen on T2-weighted images and typically corresponds to a painful click.

12. OTHER APPLICATIONS OF MRI

Beyond providing morphologic information, the principles of NMR and MRI are applied to diverse diagnostic tasks.

A. Magnetic Resonance Angiography

MRA encompasses contrast and noncontrast techniques. In contrast-enhanced MRA, gadolinium-based contrast is injected intravenously to view the vascular system (Fig. 10.26).

Time-of-flight MRA is a noncontrast technique that uses flow velocities of blood to generate contrast. In this technique, the stationary

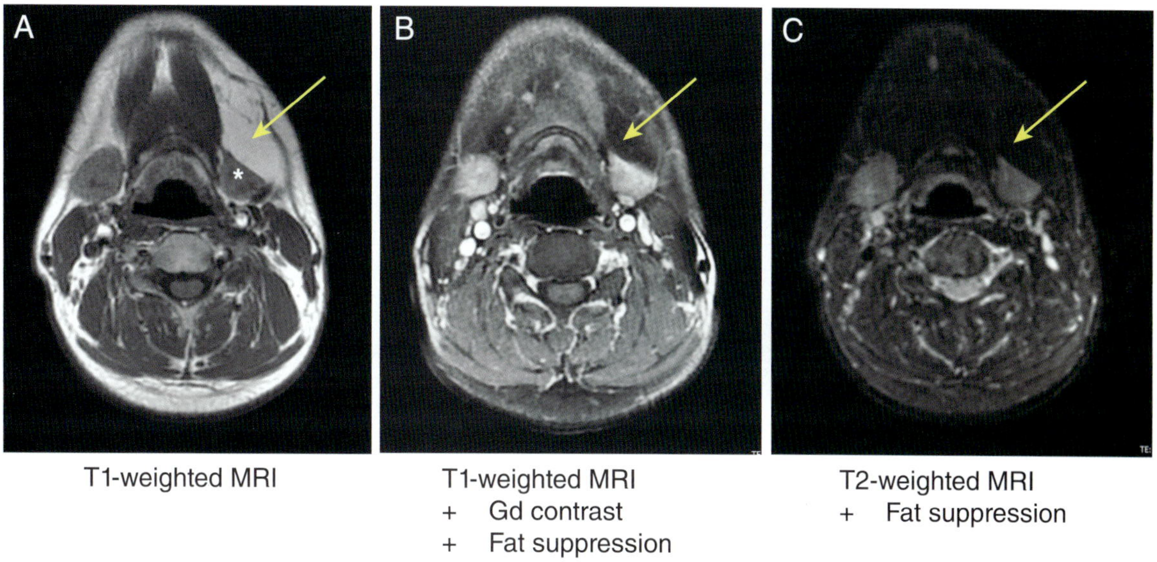

Fig. 10.20 Magnetic resonance (MR) image contrast in disease detection: benign neoplasms. (A) T1-weighted MR image shows an axial section in the suprahyoid neck. Note a bright mass occupying the submandibular space that displaces the left submandibular salivary gland *(asterisk).* (B) Postcontrast T1-weighted MR image with fat suppression shows elimination of the bright signal, indicating that the mass is composed of fat. (C) T2-weighted MR images with fat suppression now shows low signals, unlike malignant neoplasms, which will be bright on T2-weighted images.

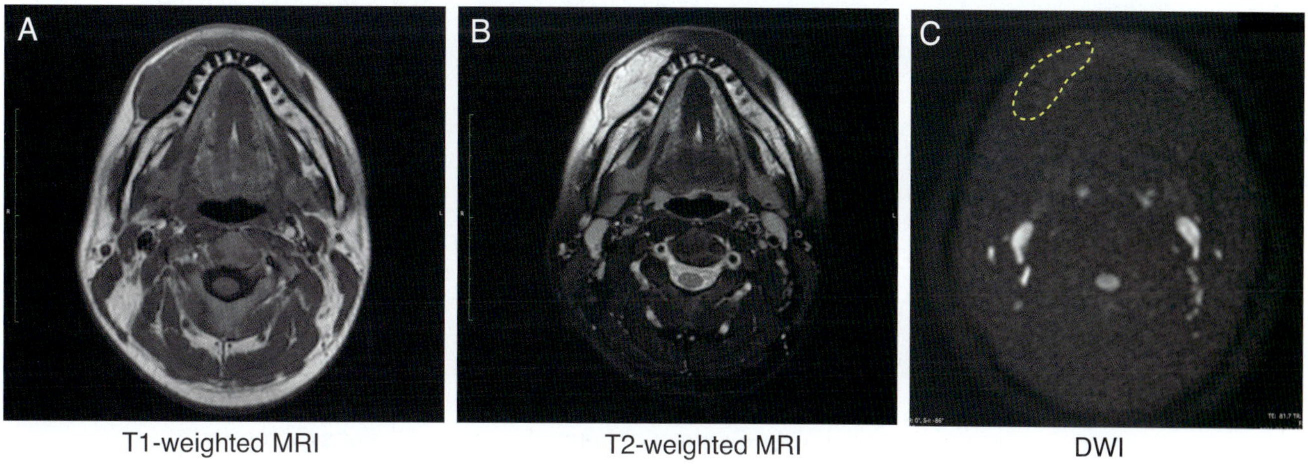

Fig. 10.21 Magnetic resonance (MR) image contrast in disease detection: Diffusion-weighted imaging (DWI). (A) T1-weighted MRI shows a relatively well-defined low signal intensity lesion on the buccal aspects of the right mandibular body. (B) T2-weighted MRI shows a bright signal suggesting a neoplastic or vascular lesion. (C) However, on diffusion-weighted imaging, the lesion is dark *(dashed outline),* suggesting unrestricted diffusion. The lesion was an arteriovenous malformation.

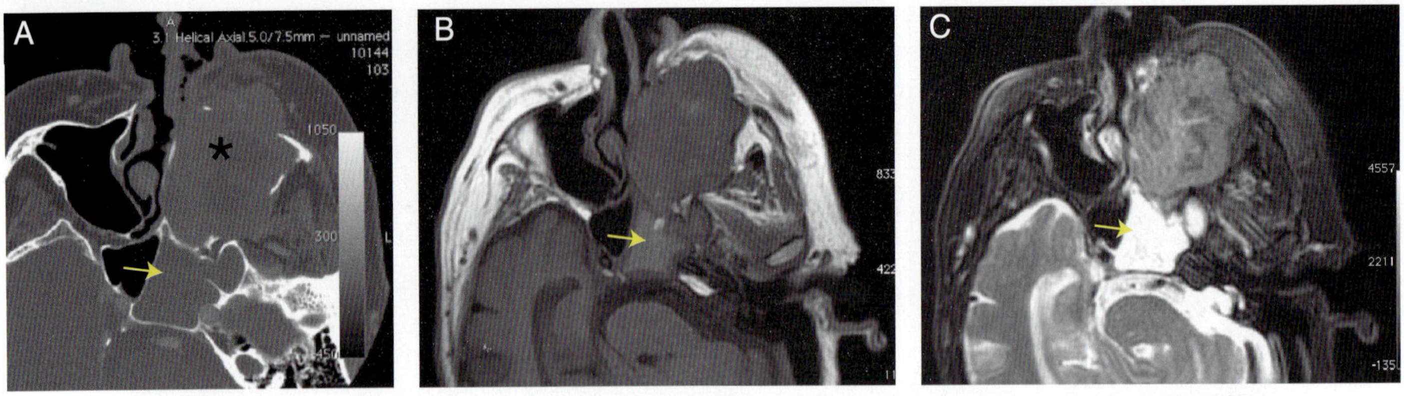

MDCT T1-weighted MRI T2-weighted MRI + Fat suppression

Fig. 10.22 Magnetic resonance (MR) image contrast in disease detection: malignant neoplasms. (A) Multidetector CT scan (MDCT, bone kernel reconstruction) shows an expansile mass in the left maxilla with disruption of sinus walls and soft tissue extension *(asterisk)*. The sphenoid sinus is opacified *(yellow arrow)*. Due to the patient's renal disease, iodinated contrast was not administered. (B) T1-weighted magnetic resonance (MR) image shows difference in signal intensity within sinus *(yellow arrow)*, relative to the neoplasm. (C) T2-weighted MR image with fat suppression shows increased signal intensity of the lesion, suggesting a malignant neoplasm. Note bright signal in the sphenoid sinus *(yellow arrow)*, suggesting presence of sinus inflammation rather than tumor invasion. The neoplastic lesion was diagnosed as an osteosarcoma at histopathology.

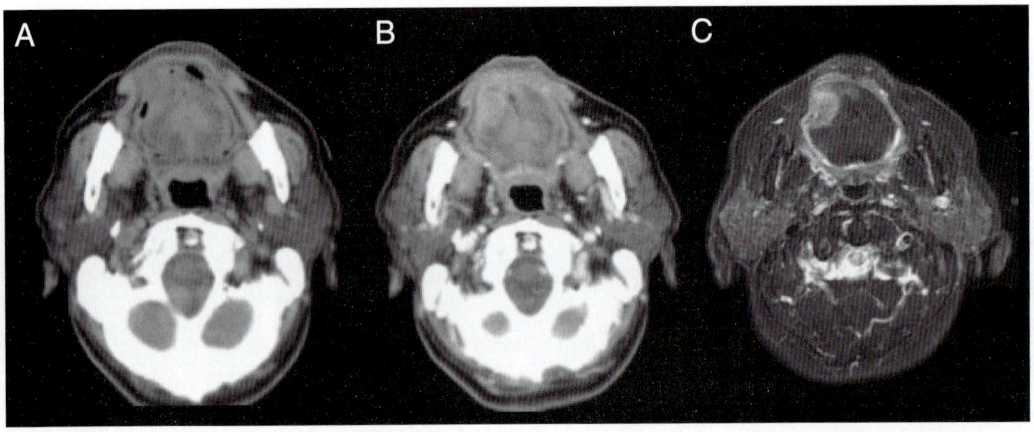

MDCT MDCT Contrast-enhanced T2-weighted MRI + Fat suppression

Fig. 10.23 Magnetic resonance (MR) image contrast in disease detection: malignant neoplasms of the tongue. (A) Multidetector CT (MDCT) scan through the tongue. There is little contrast between the tumor and the tongue muscles. (B) Contrast-enhanced MDCT scan demarcates the lesion due to enhancement from increased vascularity. (C) T2-weighted MR image with fat suppression shows increased signal intensity of the tongue neoplasm and clearly delineated from the tongue muscles.

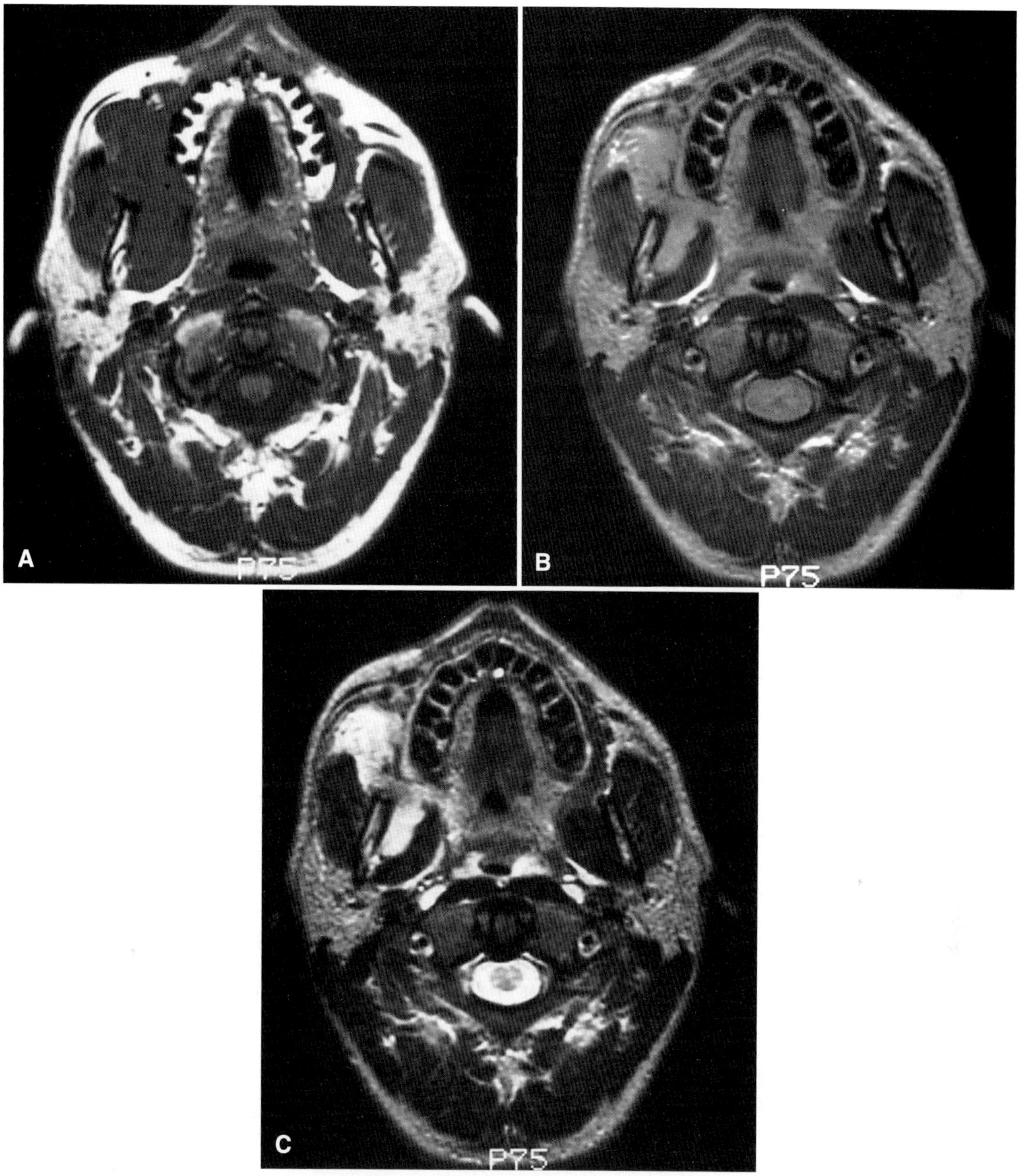

Fig. 10.24 Magnetic resonance (MR) image contrast in disease detection: gadolinium enhancement of malignant tumors. (A) Axial T1 MR image of a rhabdomyosarcoma involving the soft tissues of the right face. The tumor cannot be distinguished from the adjacent masseter and pterygoid muscles because both have the same tissue signal. (B) Axial T1 postgadolinium MR image. The tumor now has a brighter signal (lighter) than the adjacent muscles because of its greater vascularity, enhanced by gadolinium. (C) Axial T2 MR image. The tumor has a brighter signal than adjacent muscles because of greater fluid content of the tumor.

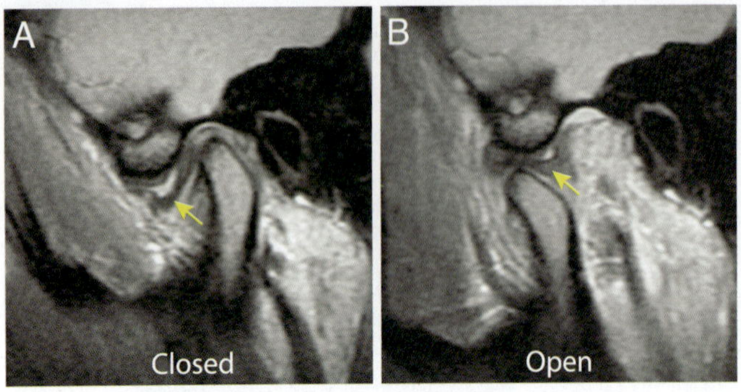

Fig. 10.25 Magnetic resonance (MR) image contrast in disease detection: temporomandibular joint (TMJ) articular disk. (A) T1-weighted MR image shows a sagittal section through the TMJ in the closed position. Due to its low proton density, the disc is seen as a low-intensity image *(arrow)* anterior to the condyle indicating disc displacement. (B) Same patient as in panel A, with the mouth open. Note the low signal intensity disc *(arrow)* now reduced back into normal position. The TMJ articular disk is not seen on computed tomography (CT) images, and MR contrast is necessary to evaluate disc abnormalities.

spins in the tomographic slice are saturated, yielding low-intensity signals. Blood flowing into that tomographic slice has unsaturated spins and thus produces higher signal intensity relative to the tissue. The technique is noninvasive and does not require contrast injection, reducing risks associated with gadolinium contrast agents (see section on Magnetic Resonance Imaging Safety). *Phase contrast angiography (PCA)* directly measures the phase shift of moving spins in flowing blood. The technique applies two gradients of equal magnitude and opposite directions. The stationary spins do not change phase, whereas moving spins (such as in blood) acquire a phase shift, directly proportional to the velocity of the flow. PCA is used to determine blood flow velocities and generate MR images of blood vessels.

B. Magnetic Resonance Spectroscopy

MRS analyzes specific metabolites. MRI produces images based on signals from water protons. MRS detects signals from nuclei in a specific metabolite. Proton MRS detects protons found in N-acetyl aspartate (NAA), creatine, choline, myo-inositol, glutamate, and lactic acid rather than muscle or fat. Monitoring NAA and lactic acid levels provides insight on tumor recurrence and necrosis.

C. Functional Magnetic Resonance Imaging

fMRI measures and maps brain activity depending on changes in blood flow in real time. The hemoglobin in red blood cells can be oxygenated (oxyhemoglobin) or unoxygenated (deoxyhemoglobin). The technique uses the difference in the magnetic properties of oxyhemoglobin (diamagnetic) and deoxyhemoglobin (paramagnetic).

In active brain areas, oxygen consumption is high and the deoxyhemoglobin concentration increases. The increased oxygen consumption also causes a significant rise in oxyhemoglobin-rich regional cerebral blood flow. The second effect is much more significant, decreasing the deoxyhemoglobin/oxyhemoglobin ratio. Deoxyhemoglobin is a paramagnetic substance, so a decrease in its concentration causes a slight increase in the T2*-weighted signal in the active region. This is the principle behind blood oxygen level–dependent (BOLD) contrast. Therefore, deoxyhemoglobin can be considered an endogenous contrast agent. Deoxyhemoglobin is the origin of the contrast between active and surrounding brain areas. fMR images are obtained by statistically comparing images acquired during resting and activation periods. This data is then superimposed on an anatomical image acquired during the same examination. Of relevance to dentistry, fMRI has been used to study neural control of swallowing, mastication, taste, and parafunctional jaw movements (Fig. 10.27).

13. MRI SAFETY

Unlike X-ray–based imaging, MRI does not expose the patient to ionizing radiation. Thus, there is no concern for cancer induction. Potential adverse events from MRI are discussed as follows.

A. Tissue Heating

A potential effect from MRI is tissue heating from deposition of RF pulse energy, especially with longer duration examinations. The average temperature increase during an MRI examination is less than 1°C

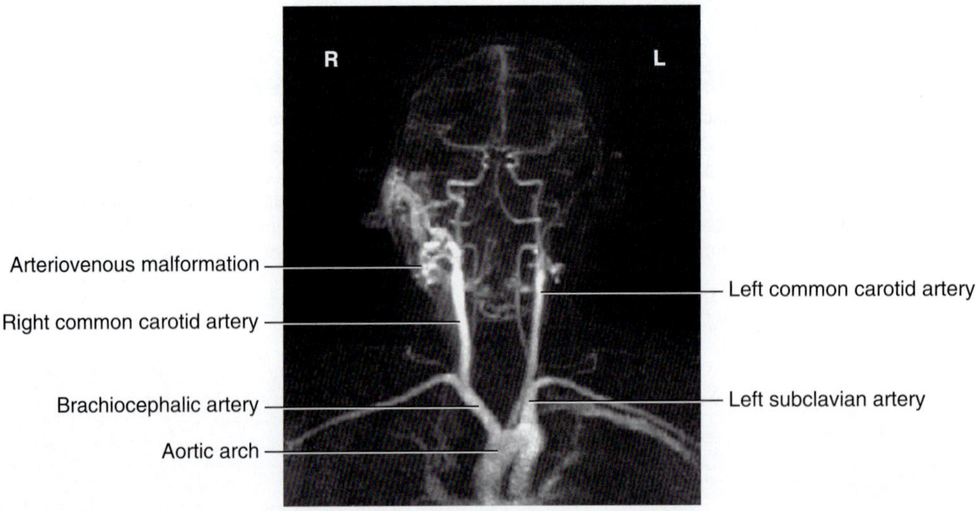

Fig. 10.26 Magnetic resonance angiography of the head and neck. This image, made with gadolinium as a contrast agent, demonstrates an arteriovenous malformation in the region of the right face. Note the widened carotid artery and rich vasculature supply in the right midfacial region. This is a maximum intensity image made from a stack of individual slices. (Image courtesy Dr. Susan White, UCLA School of Dentistry.)

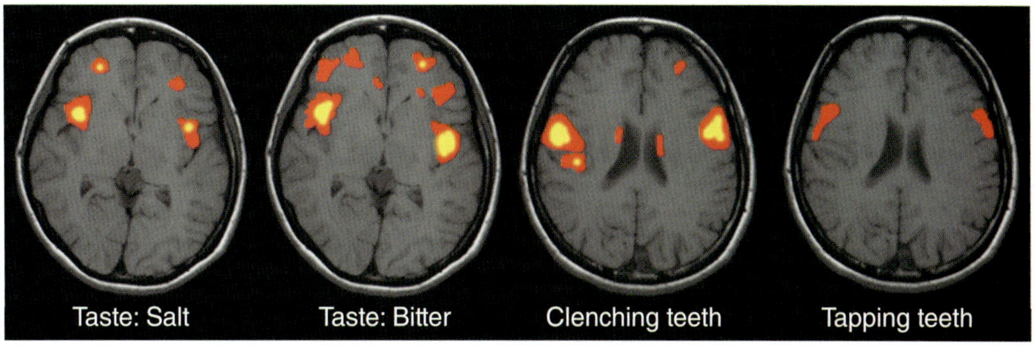

Fig. 10.27 Functional magnetic resonance imaging. Regions of activity within the brain with taste stimulation and with parafunctional habits are shown.

and is mitigated by physiologic thermoregulation. The specific absorption rate *(SAR)* is a measure of the rate of energy absorption by the tissues and is measured in watts per kilogram (W/kg). As an approximation, a SAR of 1 W/kg will elevate tissue temperature by 1°C per hour. To mitigate this patient risk, SAR limits have been established by the International Electrotechnical Commission (IEC) and the United States Food and Drug Administration (FDA). For MR imaging of the head, the recommended limits are 3.2 W/kg averaged over 6 minutes (IEC) and 3 W/kg averaged over 10 minutes (FDA).

B. Peripheral Nerve Stimulation

Rapid switching of magnetic gradients can induce tingling or twitching sensations in patients causing discomfort. This is more common with echo planar and turbo spin-echo sequences and can occur in 2% to 5% of MRI examinations. The varying magnetic field induces an electric current that can stimulate nerves and muscles. The perceived sensation may be tolerable but may surprise the patient or cause involuntary twitching and result in motion.

C. Metal Heating and Conduction

Placing metals within the magnetic field can induce an electrical current, which may cause local heating. Titanium dental implants, dental amalgam, and metal crowns are MR compatible and do not get heated within the magnetic field. Orthodontic wires are also made of nonferromagnetic substances such as stainless steel or titanium. Screening for MRI eligibility should query the patient for presence of metallic implants, cardiac pacemakers, surgical interventions that may indicate presence of surgical clips, transdermal medication patches and foreign bodies. Before entering the MRI suite, patients should remove any metal jewelry or clothing with metallic components. Certain athletic clothing contains metal fibers which pose a risk for inducing thermal skin burns.

D. Contrast Agents

Gadolinium-based contrast agents are used to identify blood vessels and enhance vascular areas. However, use of these contrast agents is associated with nephrogenic systemic fibrosis (NSF), in particular in patients with impaired renal function. It is standard practice to evaluate the patient's renal function prior to gadolinium contrast administration. Gadolinium contrast is considered safe when the estimated glomerular filtration rate (eGFR) is 30 mL/min/1.73 m^2 or higher. At this eGFR range, the risk of NSF and other adverse effects is low. The American College of Radiology recognizes three groups of gadolinium-based contrast agents. Group I agents are associated with the most NSF cases.

11

Nuclear Medicine

Hiroaki Shimamoto and Sanjay M. Mallya

RADIOPHARMACEUTICALS AND RADIATION DETECTORS

Radiopharmaceuticals

Radiopharmaceuticals are radiolabeled compounds used for *in vivo* diagnosis or radiation therapy. This chapter focuses on radiopharmaceuticals used in diagnostic nuclear medicine. A radiopharmaceutical has two components of relevance to imaging: (1) a molecule to target a biologic tissue or organ of interest and (2) a radioactive element to track the biodistribution of the targeting molecule. Table 11.1 lists the radiopharmaceuticals of relevance to imaging oral and maxillofacial diseases.

Radiopharmaceuticals are delivered directly into the circulation by intravenous injection. The targeting molecule is recognized by the body, similar to its nonlabeled physiologic equivalent and is transported to the tissue or organ of interest. The kinetics of radiopharmaceutical concentration within tissues of interest and its subsequent clearance provides information on the functional activity of the tissue imaged. To improve the signal-to-noise ratio, the targeting molecule should be specific, with a high uptake in the tissues of interest with minimal nontarget uptake. The half-life of the radionuclide should be long enough to allow adequate and specific biodistribution but short enough to minimize postprocedure patient radiation exposure.

Radiation Detectors

Nuclear medicine imaging uses radiopharmaceuticals that emit γ (gamma) rays or positrons. In this imaging modality, the patient's tissues serve as the source of radiation and the image represents the pattern of radiopharmaceutical's biodistribution at a point in time. The intensity and location of the signal are the key parameters in interpretation of nuclear medicine studies.

When using γ-emitting radiopharmaceuticals, projection images are made and the image density at a location represents the magnitude of the photon flux from radiopharmaceutical accumulation. Because radionuclides emit radiation in all directions, collimators are used to make projection images with photons emitted along a specific trajectory. Likewise, the source of radiation (tissue of interest) is placed closest to the receptor to enhance signal. For example, when performing bone scintigraphy to evaluate the temporomandibular joints, separate right and left lateral views and anterior and posterior views are often done to enhance subjective and objective assessment. The projection images are made with a *gamma camera*, which is composed of scintillation crystals coupled with photomultiplier tubes, and is the source of the term *scintigraphy* for this technique.

In planar scintigraphy, the signal represents net photon flux at a particular point, and contributions to this signal from structures at different depths are not differentiated. Tomographic imaging overcomes this limitation. Single photon emission computed tomography (SPECT) and positron emission tomography (PET) are nuclear medicine techniques that generate tomographic views, and this functional information is often superimposed onto the morphological information from multidetector computed tomography (MDCT) examinations.

TABLE 11.1 Radiopharmaceuticals Used to Image Maxillofacial Disease

Radiopharmaceutical	Target Tissue
^{99m}Tc-methylene diphosphonate	Bone
^{99m}Tc-hydroxymethylene diphosphonate	
^{99m}Tc-pertechnetate	Salivary glands
2-[^{18}F] fluoro-2-deoxy-D-glucose	Metabolically active cells (malignant neoplastic cells)

NUCLEAR MEDICINE IMAGING OF MAXILLOFACIAL DISEASES

Bone Scintigraphy

Bone scintigraphy is a two-dimensional imaging technique that depicts the locations of active bone turnover. It uses the radionuclide technetium 99m (^{99m}Tc). ^{99m}Tc has a half-life of 6 hours and emits primarily 140 keV γ-photons. To image bone, ^{99m}Tc is bound to methylene diphosphonate (MDP) or hydroxymethylene diphosphonate (HMDP), a pyrophosphate analog. The compound is stable, is not metabolized in the body, and is rapidly cleared from plasma by renal excretion, with more than 70% of the administered radioactivity cleared within 6 hours. Bone scintigraphy has a high sensitivity and can detect as low as 5% to 10% demineralization in bone. These drugs accumulate in bone by chemical adsorption onto hydroxyapatite on the bone surface. Its location to bone depends on the local vascularity and the degree of osteoblastic activity. Approximately 30% of the administered radionuclide is adsorbed onto bone, with the maximal uptake occurring within the first hour.

Although the protocol for bone scintigraphy is usually one phase 3–4 hours after intravenous administration, the three-phase bone scintigraphy is a useful protocol to evaluate osteomyelitis and primary bone tumors. A dose of 555 to 1110 megabecquerels (MBq, approximately 20 to 30 mCi) is administered by intravenous injection. Subsequently, images are acquired with a gamma camera. The effective dose from bone scintigraphy is approximately 3 to 6 mSv (see Chapter 3).

TABLE 11.2 Three-Phase Skeletal Scintigraphy

Phase	Description	Time After Injection	Functional Information
1	Blood flow	30–60 s	Reflects vascularity
2	Blood pool	Within 10 min	Reflects soft tissue involvement
3	Delayed	2–6 h	Reflects osteoblastic activity

The three phases are described in Table 11.2. Both blood flow and osteoblastic activity influence uptake. Radionuclide uptake is more in trabecular bone and in areas that have a larger mineralization surface such as the spine. In children, growth-associated osteoblastic activity causes increased uptake in the physes and facial bones. The low-level bone turnover associated with periodontal disease or healing of an extraction socket also manifests as increased uptake.

Single Photon Emission Computed Tomography

SPECT is a tomographic nuclear medicine technique. In this technique, the gamma camera is rotated 180 degrees to 360 degrees around the patient and acquires images at several angles, typically 120 or more. These projections may be acquired with a single detector or with multiple detectors. At each projection, data is collected for 20 to 30 seconds and total image acquisition takes about 30 to 45 minutes. Minor patient motion degrades image quality. The acquired data are processed by mathematical reconstruction algorithms into contiguous axial slices, similar to the process in CT image reconstruction. The tomographic imaging minimizes superimposition and increases the contrast and spatial resolution. SPECT images can be fused with CT images to combine the functional and morphological information allowing better resolution of the location and extent of pathologic changes (see Figs. 11.1D and E and 11.2C and D).

Applications of Bone Scintigraphy and Single Photon Emission Computed Tomography

Bone scintigraphy and SPECT have the following applications in diagnosis and treatment planning of maxillofacial disease, and capitalize on the high sensitivity of this technique.

- Osteomyelitis and osteonecrosis of the jaws (Figs. 11.1–11.3)
- Temporomandibular joint osseous abnormalities, such as condylar hyperplasia (Fig. 11.4) and condylar resorption (Fig. 11.5)
- Skeletal dysplasias, for example, fibrous dysplasia (Fig. 11.6) and Paget disease
- Primary and metastatic neoplasms that originate in or involve bone (Fig. 11.7)
- Bone fracture

Salivary Gland Scintigraphy

The radiopharmaceutical technetium-99m-pertechnetate ($^{99m}TcO_4^-$) is localized to the salivary and thyroid glands. $^{99m}TcO_4^-$ (185–370 MBq) is administered intravenously and imaging is started immediately. Data collection for functional assessment is continued for 40 minutes. The administered $^{99m}TcO_4^-$ quickly migrates from the vasculature to the salivary glands, where it is ingested by excretory duct epithelial cells in the gland body and concentrated, accumulating in the salivary glands and saliva. In general, the concentration is higher in the parotid gland than in the submandibular gland and the sublingual gland is not depicted. To assess secretory capability, salivary stimulation with ascorbic acid or citric acid is performed 20 minutes after the start of the scan and the relative decrease in accumulated radioactivity in the salivary glands is measured (Fig. 11.8). In Sjögren's syndrome, the radiopharmaceutical uptake is decreased due to decreased salivary gland function and radionuclide accumulation is virtually unaffected by acid stimulation (Fig. 11.9). Warthin's tumor and oncocytoma are known to show high accumulation of $^{99m}TcO_4^-$. These tumors do not show a decrease in accumulation upon salivary stimulation.

Positron Emission Tomographic Imaging

PET imaging is a tomographic diagnostic technique in nuclear medicine that uses positron-emitting radionuclides, which are almost 100 times more sensitive than gamma cameras. The radiopharmaceutical emits a positron, which interacts with a free electron and mutual annihilation occurs, resulting in the production of two 551 keV photons emitted at 180 degrees to each other. The PET scanner consists of a ring of many detectors in a circle around the patient (Fig. 11.10). Electronically coupled opposing detectors simultaneously identify the pair of γ-photons and this is the basis of spatial location of the signal origin. PET is superior to SPECT in terms of sensitivity, spatial resolution, and quantitation. Contemporary PET-CT and PET-MRI scanners sequentially acquire the PET image and the CT or MRI image and superimpose morphological and functional information (Fig. 11.11).

Various PET preparations labeled with positron-emitting radionuclides such as ^{11}C, ^{13}N, ^{15}O, and ^{18}F are used in clinical nuclear medicine. In particular, 2-[^{18}F] fluoro-2-deoxy-D-glucose (FDG), a glucose-like agent labeled with ^{18}F (half-life of 109.8 minutes), is widely used for the diagnosis and treatment planning of malignant tumors including in the oral and maxillofacial region. Malignant tumor cells undergo frequent cell division, resulting in increased glucose metabolism. Glucose transporters on the plasma membrane of malignant cells are overexpressed compared to normal cells and more glucose or FDG is taken up into malignant cells. Intracellular glucose or FDG is phosphorylated by hexokinase and converted to glucose-6-phosphate and FDG-6-phosphate, respectively. Glucose-6-phosphate proceeds through the glycolytic system and is finally broken down into water and carbon dioxide, but FDG-6-phosphate is not further metabolized and accumulates in cells over time (metabolic trapping). As a result, tissues with higher glucose metabolism have higher radioactivity, which is detected by PET as a high accumulated image of FDG. In other words, PET scanner detects the degree of accumulation of FDG in the body and provides a functional image reflecting tissue glucose metabolism.

If the examination is performed immediately after a meal or in a hyperglycemic state, such as in patients with diabetes, FDG antagonizes glucose and its uptake into malignant tumor cells is relatively decreased, making accurate diagnosis difficult. Therefore, fasting for 4–5 hours prior to testing and restriction of beverages with sugar are necessary. Then, 2–5 MBq/kg of FDG is administered intravenously, and after 60 minutes of resting and waiting after administration, PET imaging is performed for 30 minutes. In the PET-CT scanner, CT imaging is performed first for 10 seconds. This provides the distribution data of linear absorption coefficients throughout the whole body, enabling correction of attenuation of annihilation γ-rays due to living organisms, thereby improving image quality and quantifying radioactivity.

To semiquantitatively express the FDG accumulation, the standardized uptake value (SUV), which is the accumulation ratio per unit body weight to the administered dose, is used. If there is uniform distribution throughout the body and no excretion, SUV = 1.00. An SUV_{max} (maximum SUV in the region of interest) of 2.5 or greater is commonly used as the cut-off value for qualitative diagnosis of benign versus malignant disease.

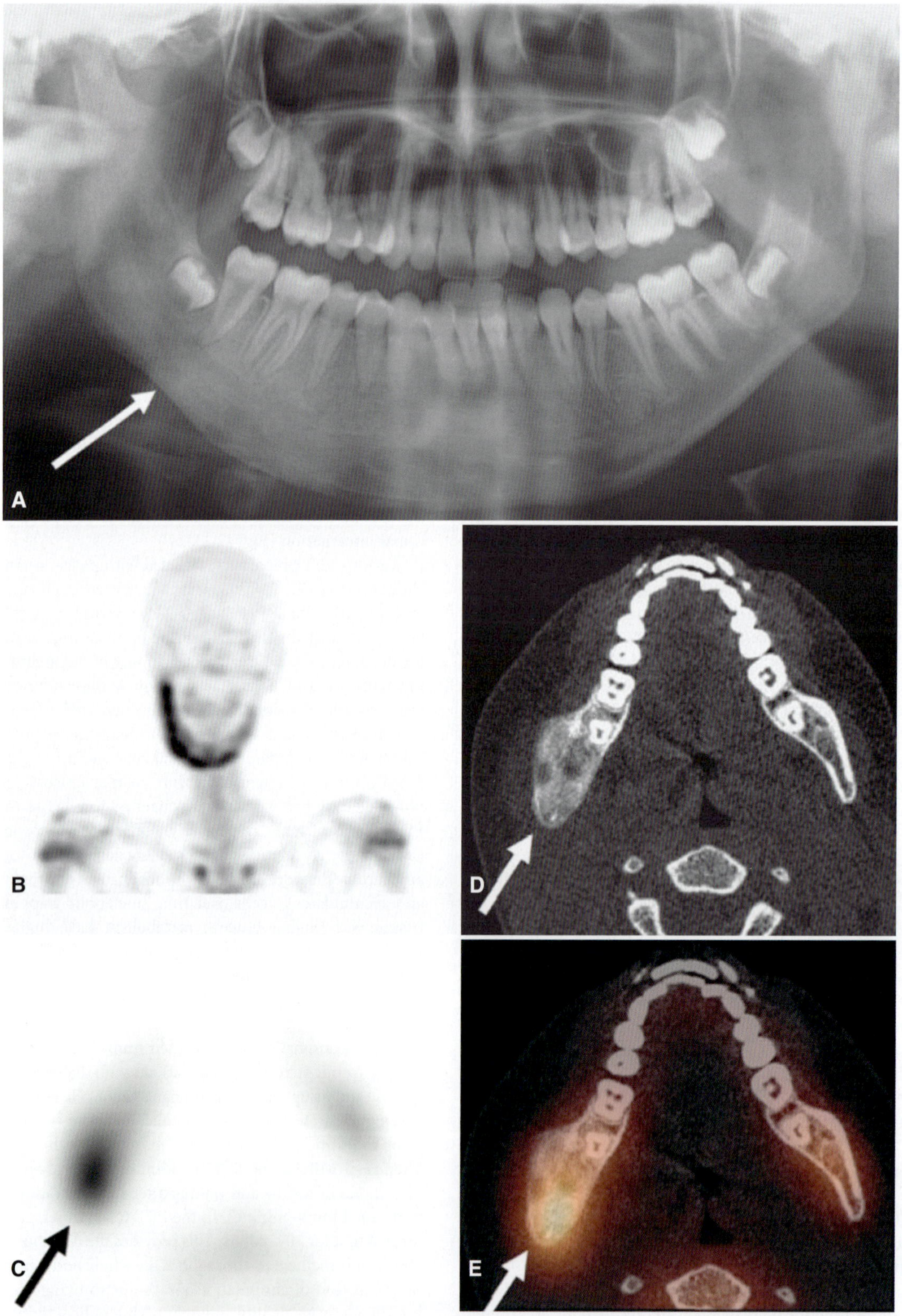

Fig. 11.1 Single photon emission computed tomography (SPECT)/computed tomography (CT) imaging of a 14-year-old girl with chronic osteomyelitis of the mandible. (A) Panoramic view showing expansion and sclerosis of the right mandible *(arrow)*. (B) Planar radionuclide image showing uptake throughout the mandible and especially on the right side. (C) SPECT axial image showing increased activity in the posterior regions of both sides of the mandible and especially on the right side *(arrow)*. (D) CT axial image at the same level as the image in C. Note periosteal expansion and lytic areas in the right mandible *(arrow)*. (E) SPECT/CT fusion image shows the area of highest accumulation in the right mandible *(arrow)*. (Modified from Strobel K, Merwald M, Huellner MW, et al.: [Importance of SPECT/CT for resolving diseases of the jaw] [in German]. *Radiologe.* 2012;52:638–645.)

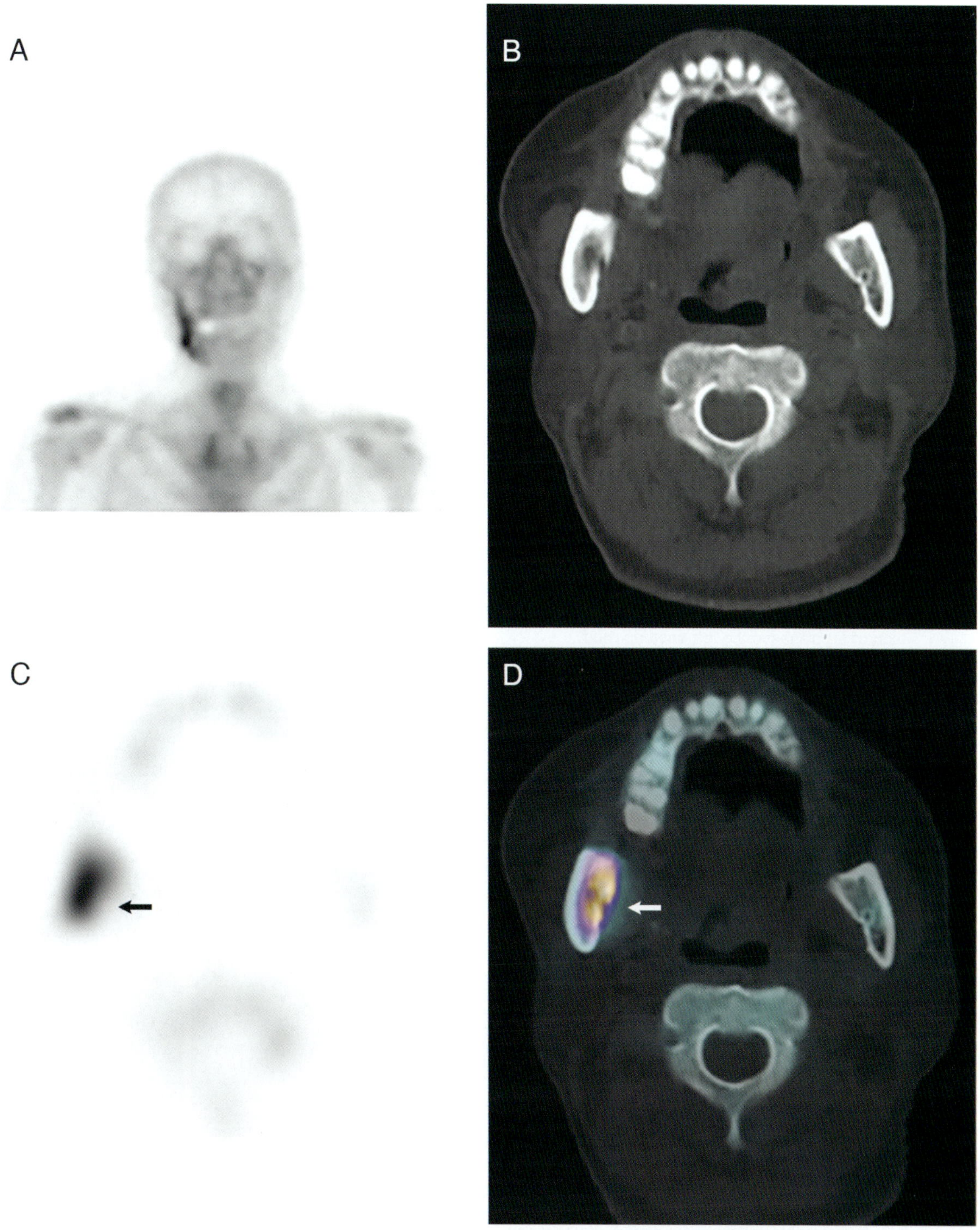

Fig. 11.2 Single photon emission computed tomographic (SPECT)/computed tomography (CT) imaging of chronic osteomyelitis of the mandible. (A) Planar radionuclide image showing uptake in the mandible posterior body and ascending ramus. (B) Axial section from multidetector CT examination shows altered radiodensity of right ramus, relative to the contralateral side. Note facial swelling on the right side. (C) SPECT axial image showing increased uptake in the right ramus *(arrow)*. (D) SPECT/CT fusion image shows the area of highest accumulation in the right mandible *(arrow)*.

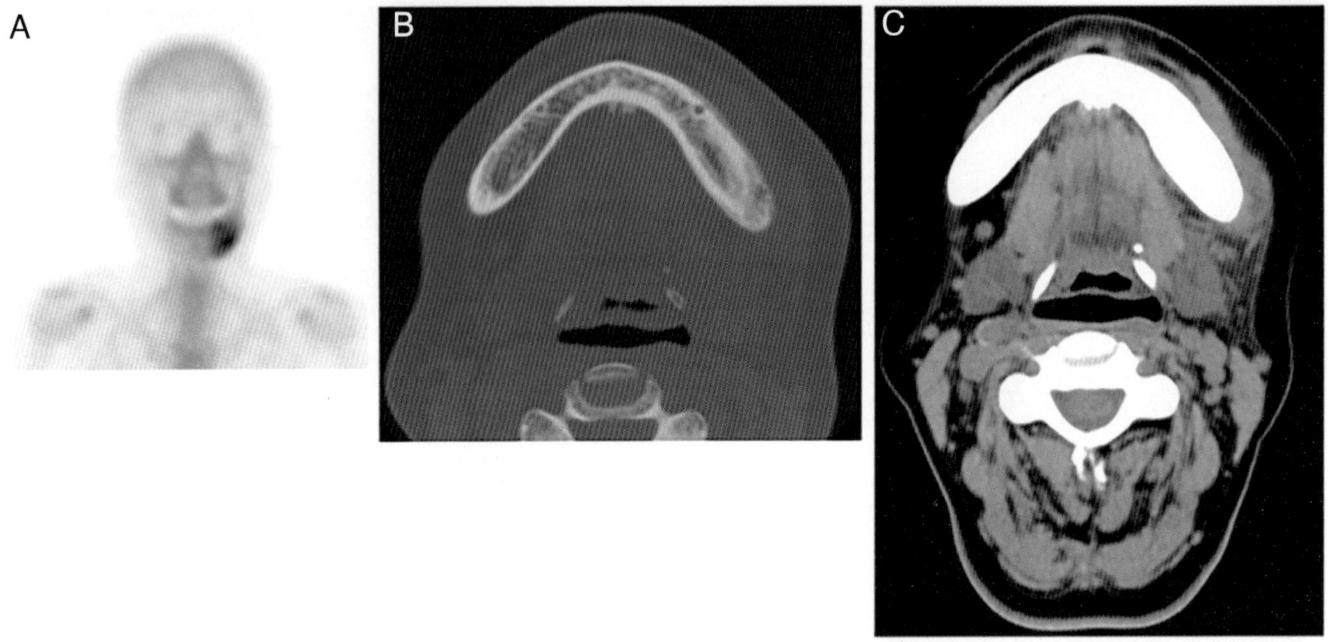

Fig. 11.3 Skeletal scintigraphy to evaluate osteomyelitis. (A) Planar radionuclide image showing uptake in the left mandibular body. (B) Axial multidetector computed tomography (MDCT, bone kernel) shows diffuse trabeculation in the left body of the mandible. (C) Axial MDCT section (soft tissue kernel) shows minimal disruption of fat planes in the left posterior body.

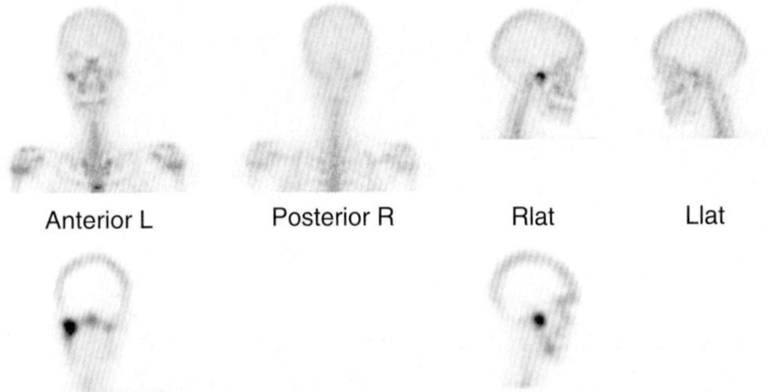

Fig. 11.4 Skeletal scintigraphy shows increased uptake of ^{99m}Tc-methylene diphosphonate in the region of the right temporomandibular joint. The planar images in the top row were captured with a gamma camera. The lower two tomographic images were captured with single photon emission computed tomographic imaging.

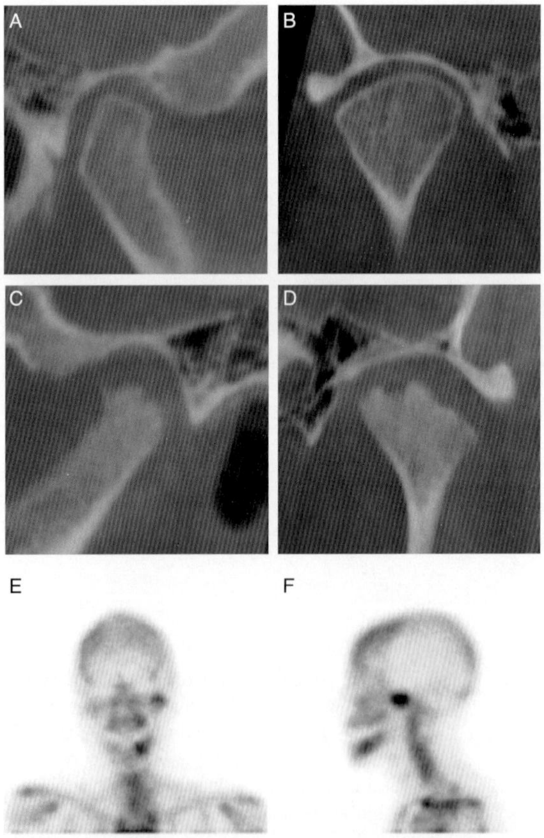

Fig. 11.5 Skeletal scintigraphy to evaluate a patient with unilateral progressive condylar resorption. (A and B) Corrected sagittal and frontal sections through the normal, right temporomandibular joint. (C and D) Corrected sagittal and frontal sections through the left temporomandibular joint. The condyle is irregular in shape with loss or articular cortication and trabecular sclerosis. (E and F) Anterior and left lateral projections of the bone scan showing increased uptake of ^{99m}Tc-methylene diphosphonate in the left condyle. Increased uptake in the left mandibular body reflects a recent extraction of the mandibular left first molar.

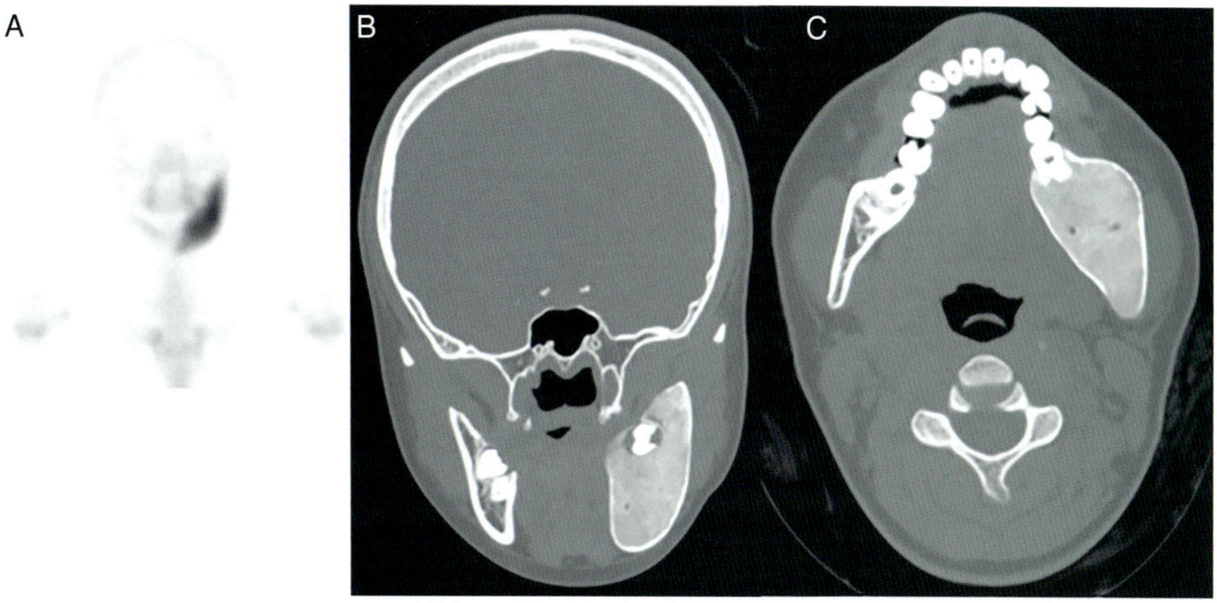

Fig. 11.6 Bone scintigraphy to evaluate fibrous dysplasia. (A) Planar bone scan shows localized increased accumulation of ^{99m}Tc-methylene diphosphonate in the left mandible. Quantitative comparison of uptake relative to prior scans provides information on status of lesion growth. (B and C) Coronal and axial multidetector computed tomography sections show an expansile radiodensity with granular trabeculation characteristic of fibrous dysplasia.

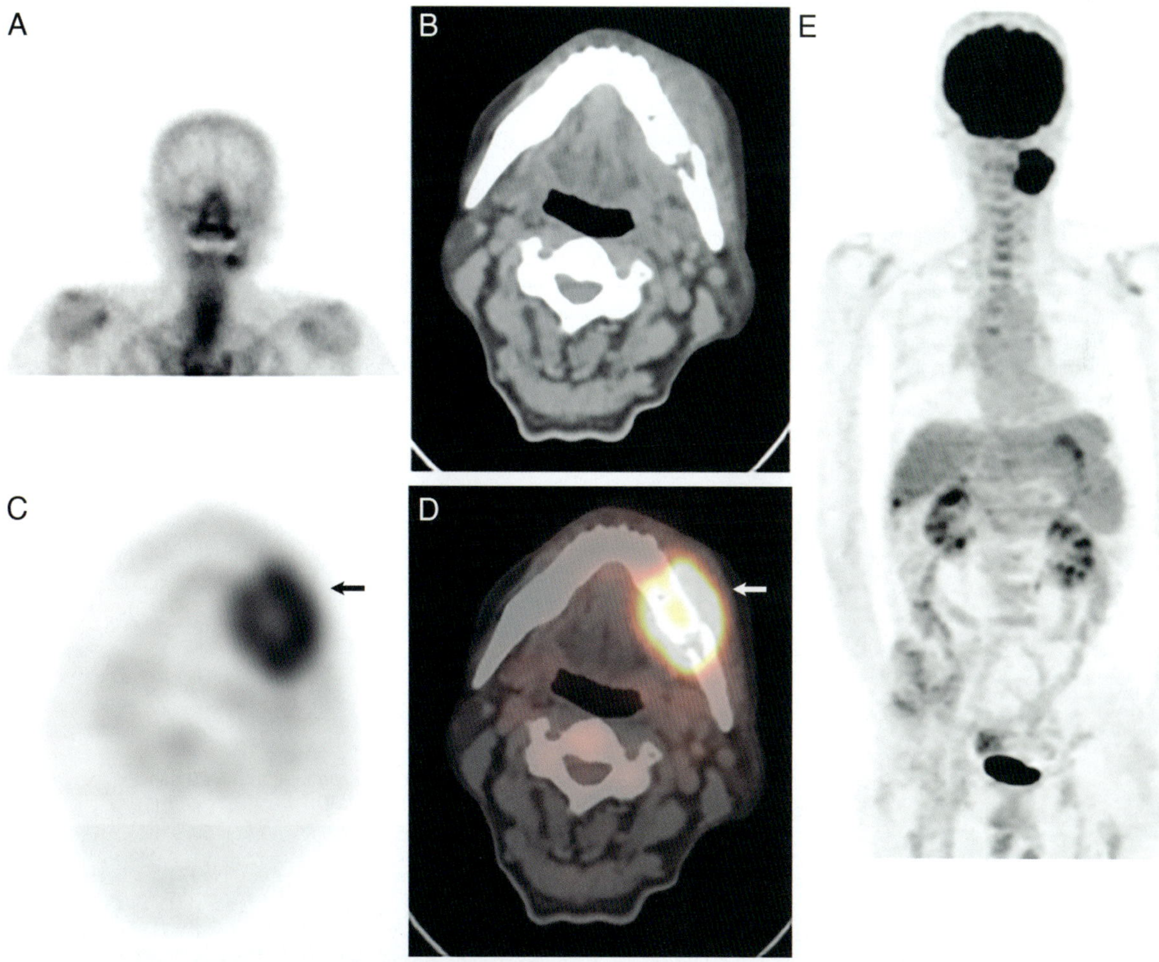

Fig. 11.7 Bone scintigraphy and ^{18}F-fluoro-2-deoxy-D-glucose (FDG)-positron emission tomography (PET)/computed tomography (CT) imaging of gingival cancer. (A) Planar bone scintigraph showing uptake in the left mandibular body. (B) Axial multidetector CT section shows a soft tissue mass with lytic changes in the mandible. (C) FDG-PET axial image showing increased radiopharmaceutical uptake in the body of the left mandible and surrounding soft tissues *(arrow)*. (D) PET/CT fusion image shows an area of high accumulation superimposed over the neoplasm *(arrow)*. The spatial location of the neoplasm is improved relative to planar bone scintigraphy. (E) FDG-PET maximum intensity projection. Note physiologic accumulation in the brain, spleen, kidneys, and bladder, with absence of areas of increased uptake in the regional lymph nodes, lungs, or distal sites in the skeleton.

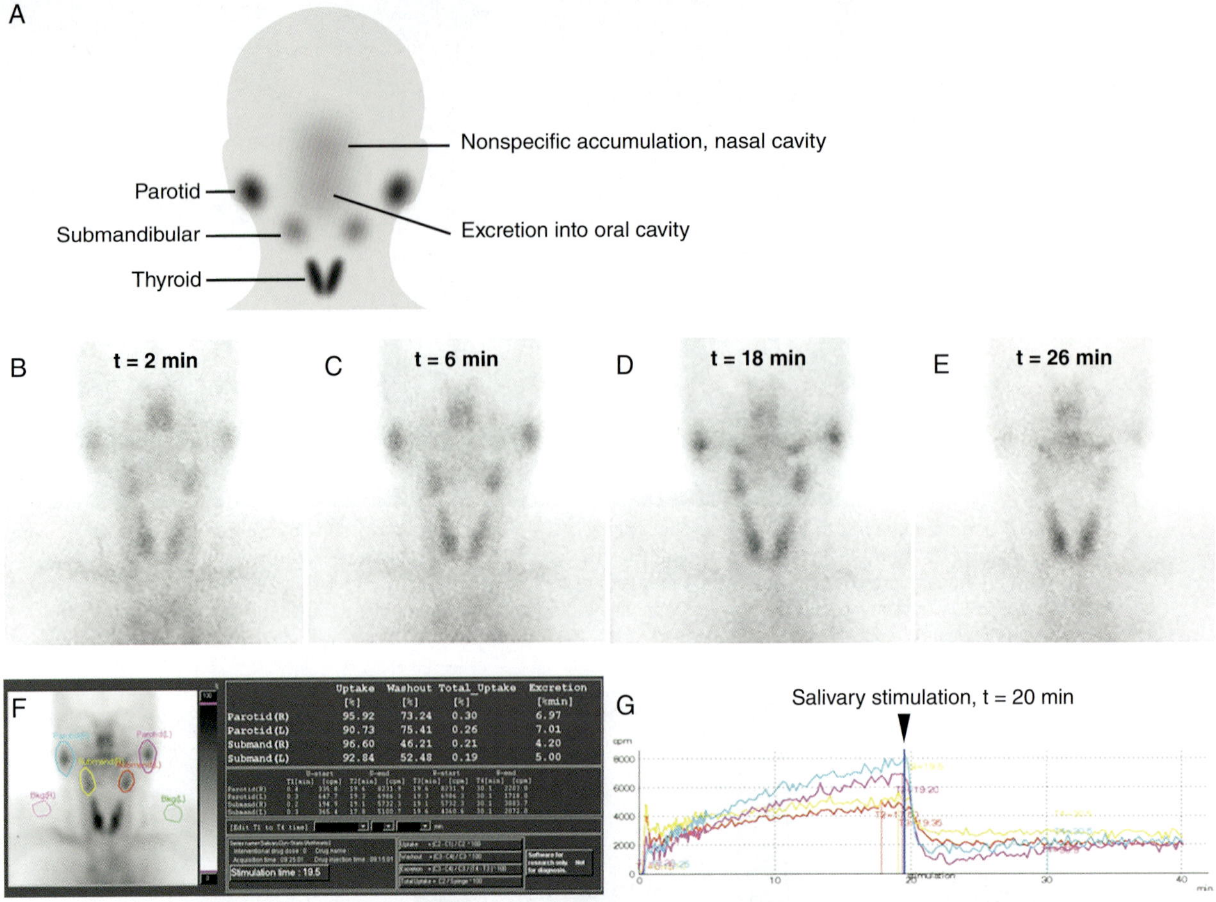

Fig. 11.8 Normal salivary gland scintigraphy. (A–E) Accumulation of radiopharmaceutical in the salivary glands at 2, 6, 18, and 26 minutes following administration of $^{99m}TcO_4^-$. (F) Quantitative evaluation of salivary function. Signals within regions of interest (ROI) to include the parotid and submandibular glands are measured, relative to background. (G) Time-activity curve radioactivity measured within the regions of right and left parotid and submandibular glands at various times following radiopharmaceutical administration. Note rapid decrease of radionuclide from the parotid and submandibular glands after salivary stimulation at t = 20 minutes.

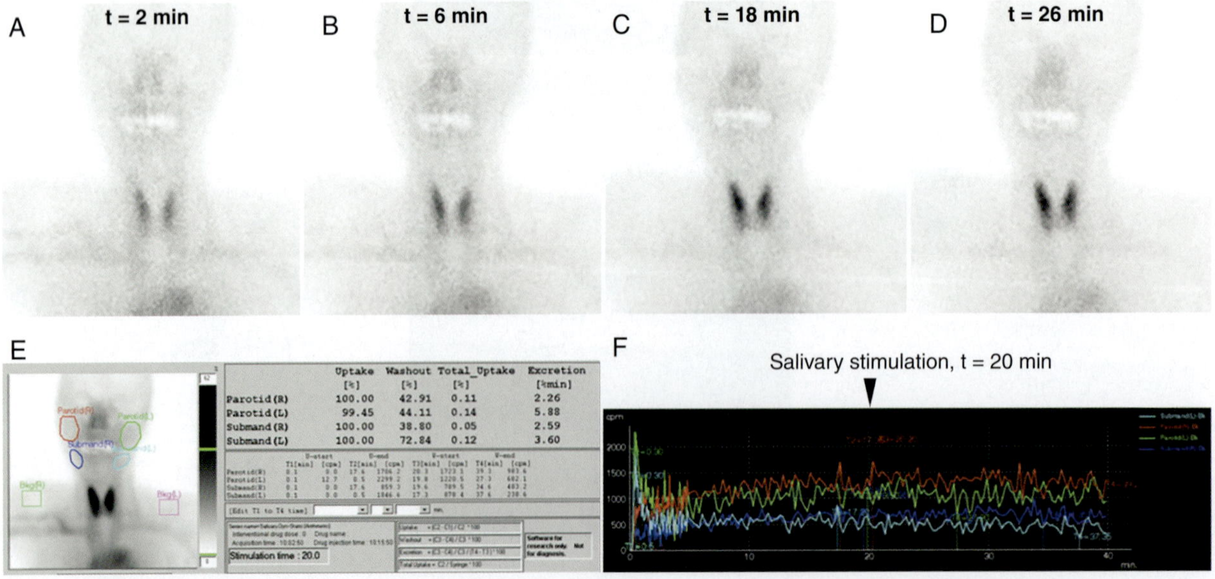

Fig. 11.9 Salivary gland scintigraphy in a patient with Sjögren's syndrome. (A–D). Accumulation of radiopharmaceutical in the salivary glands at 2, 6, 18, and 26 minutes following administration of $^{99m}TcO_4^-$. Note lack of radionuclide accumulation in parotid and submandibular glands. (E) Quantitative evaluation of salivary function. Signals within regions of interest (ROI) to include the parotid and submandibular glands are measured, relative to background. (F) Graph of radioactivity measured within the regions of right and left parotid and submandibular glands at various times following radiopharmaceutical administration. Radiopharmaceutical accumulation within the salivary glands is mostly less than 1500 counts per minute (cpm) with no change after salivary stimulation at t = 20 minutes.

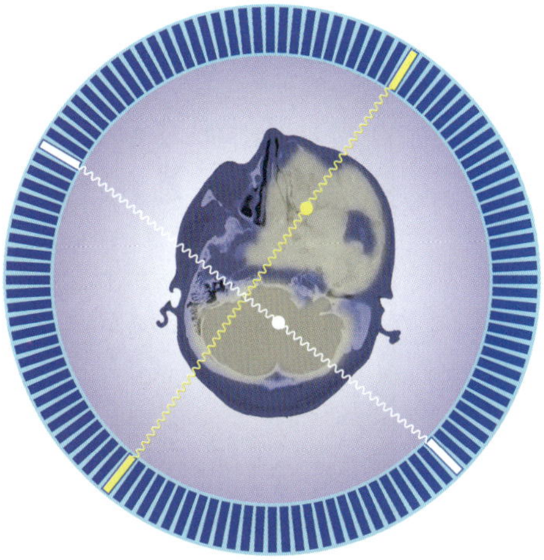

Fig. 11.10 Positron emission tomography scanner consists of a ring of detectors that measure pairs of 511 keV γ-rays traveling in opposite directions from positron annihilation. Each pair is recorded and the location of the radionuclide can be determined as the intersection of the pairs of detectors recording simultaneous events.

In the oral and maxillofacial diagnosis, FDG-PET/CT is suitable for (1) staging of malignancies, by evaluating the primary tumor and presence or absence of regional lymph node metastasis or distant metastasis; (2) qualitative diagnosis of benign versus malignant disease; (3) evaluation of the effect of radiotherapy and chemotherapy on tumor size and appearance of new lesions; and (4) monitoring for posttreatment disease recurrence (Figs. 11.11–11.17).

However, FDG also accumulates in nonmalignant tumors. In salivary gland tumors, not only malignant neoplasms but also benign neoplasms show strong accumulation, making differentiation between benign and malignant salivary gland tumors difficult (Fig. 11.17). Physiologic accumulation in the oral and maxillofacial region includes the major salivary glands (Fig. 11.18) and the palatine tonsils (Figs. 11.18 and 11.19). FDG is increased in muscle after exercise and in brown adipose tissue. FDG is also taken up by macrophages and juvenile granulation tissue and thus, shows accumulation in inflammatory lesions such as abscesses, osteomyelitis, tooth extraction sockets, severe marginal periodontitis (Fig. 11.20), apical periodontitis, osteoarthritis, and sinusitis. Other sites of accumulation include carotid plaques, mucositis due to radiotherapy, and wounds immediately after tooth extraction or biopsies.

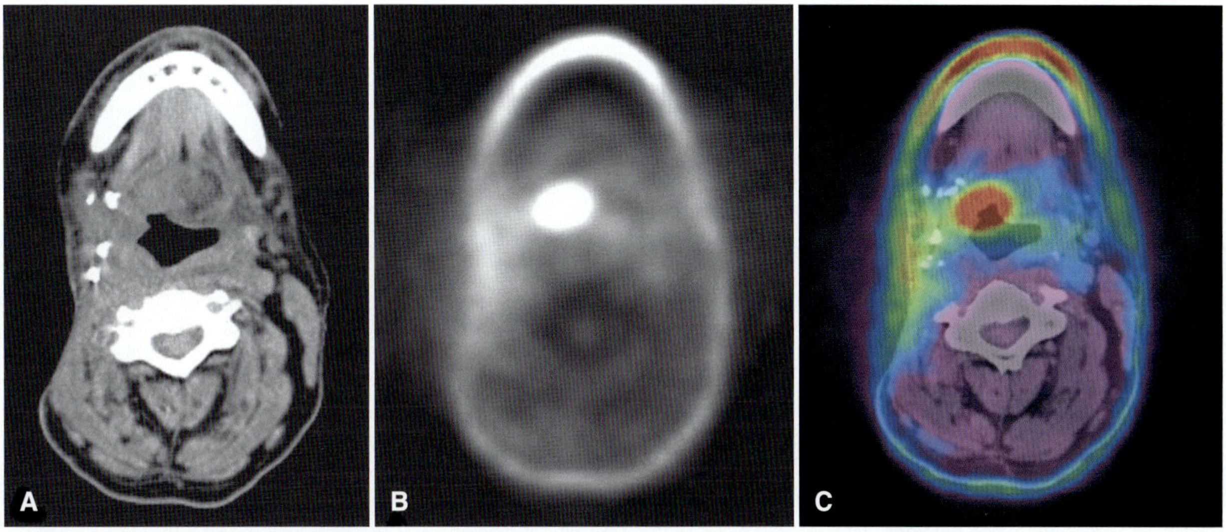

Fig. 11.11 Positron emission tomography (PET) scan and fusion of PET with computed tomography (CT). This patient has a known recurrent carcinoma at the base of the tongue. (A) Soft tissue kernel CT image at the level of the inferior border of the mandible. The four metallic objects on the patient's right side, posterior to the mandible represent vascular clips from prior surgery. (B) Fluoro-2-deoxy-D-glucose (FDG)-PET scan showing an *oval-shaped* region of high metabolic activity of tumor at the right tongue base. The FDG activity in the anterior mandible is related to low-level metabolic activity in the vicinity of a reconstruction plate. (C) Fused images A and B demonstrating the region of high metabolic activity superimposed on the CT anatomy. The intensity of the FDG activity has been color-coded with *red* being the highest intensity and *purple* being the lowest. Images were acquired on a combined PET/CT scanner. (Courtesy Dr. Todd W. Stultz, Cleveland Clinic, OH.)

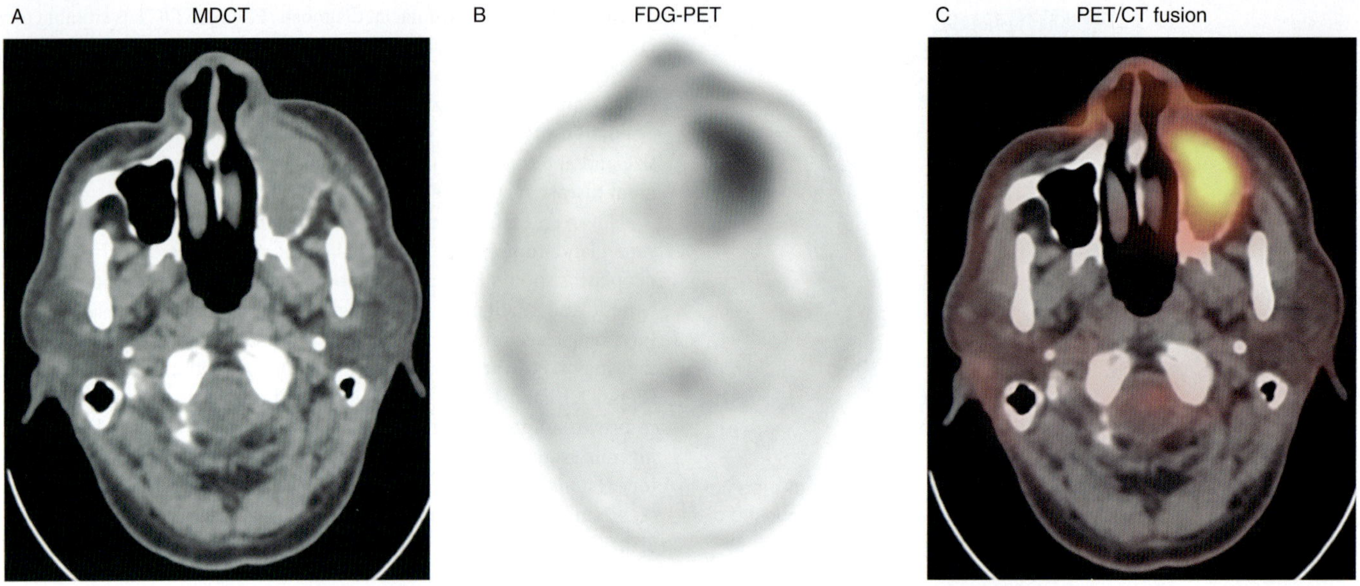

Fig. 11.12 Fluoro-2-deoxy-D-glucose (FDG)-positron emission tomography (PET)/computed tomography (CT) imaging of an adenoid cystic carcinoma in the left maxillary sins. (A) Axial multidetector CT (MDCT) section through the level of the maxillary sinuses and pterygoid plates. The left maxillary sinus is expanded and opacified with loss of the anterolateral wall. (B) Corresponding axial PET image shows increased uptake of FDG in the left maxillary sinus. (C) Superimposition of the PET and CT examinations provides anatomic boundaries relative to the areas of increased uptake. The intensity of the FDG activity has been color-coded to facilitate visual evaluation.

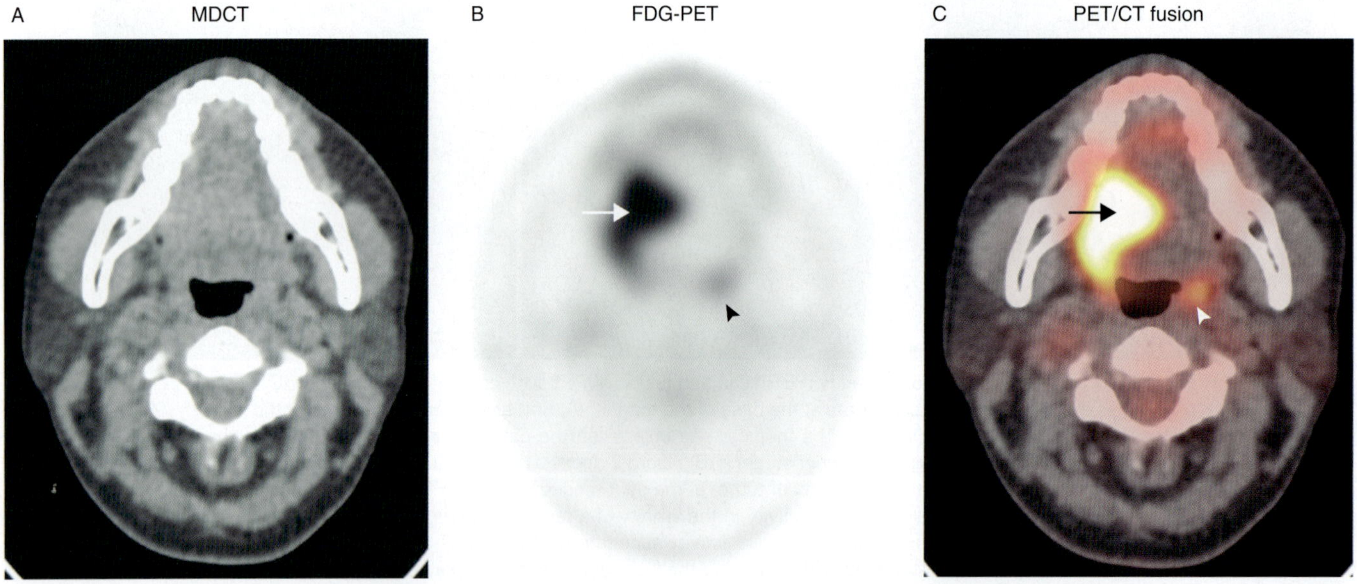

Fig. 11.13 Fluoro-2-deoxy-D-glucose (FDG)-positron emission tomography (PET)/computed tomography (CT) imaging of a squamous cell carcinoma on the tongue. (A) Axial multidetector CT (MDCT) section through the tongue. (B) Corresponding axial PET image shows increased uptake of FDG in the tongue *(white arrow)*. Note physiologic uptake in the left palatine tonsil *(black arrowhead)*. (C) Superimposition of the PET and CT examinations provides anatomic boundaries relative to the areas of increased uptake. The intensity of the FDG activity has been color-coded *(black arrow)*. Note uptake in the left palatine tonsil, a physiological false positive *(white arrowhead)*.

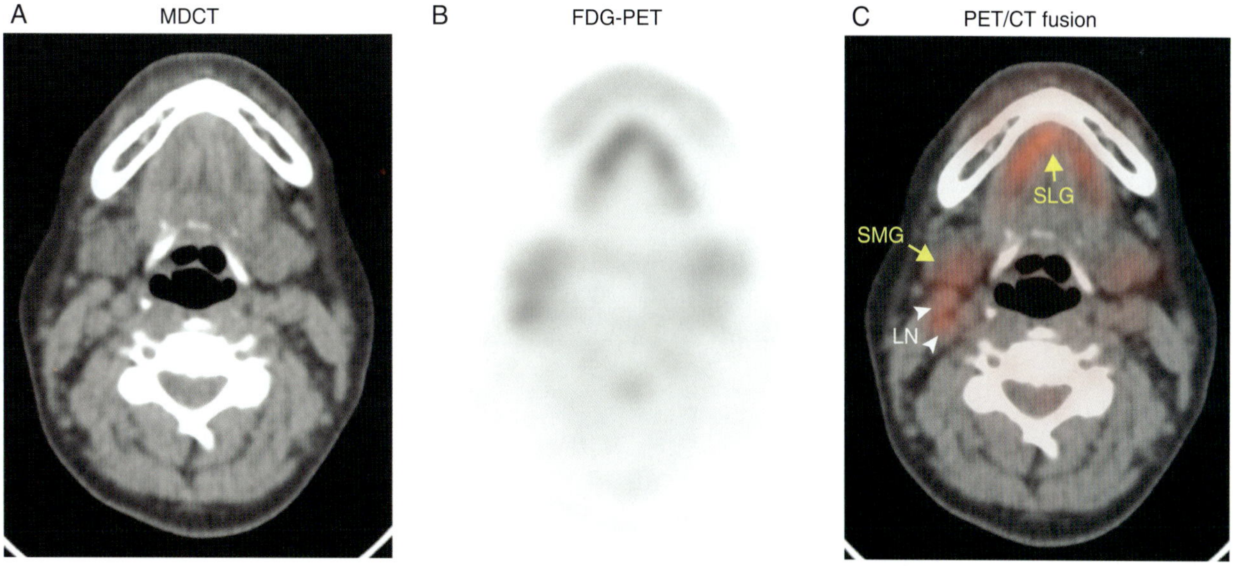

Fig. 11.14 Fluoro-2-deoxy-D-glucose (FDG)-positron emission tomography (PET)/computed tomography (CT) imaging to evaluate a squamous cell carcinoma on the tongue. (A) Axial multidetector CT (MDCT) section through the floor of the mouth. (B) Corresponding axial PET image shows increased uptake of FDG in the right neck. (C) Superimposition of the PET and CT examinations identifies metastasis to the regional lymph nodes (*white arrowheads*, LN). Note nonspecific uptake *(yellow arrows)* in the submandibular (SMG) and sublingual (SLG) salivary glands.

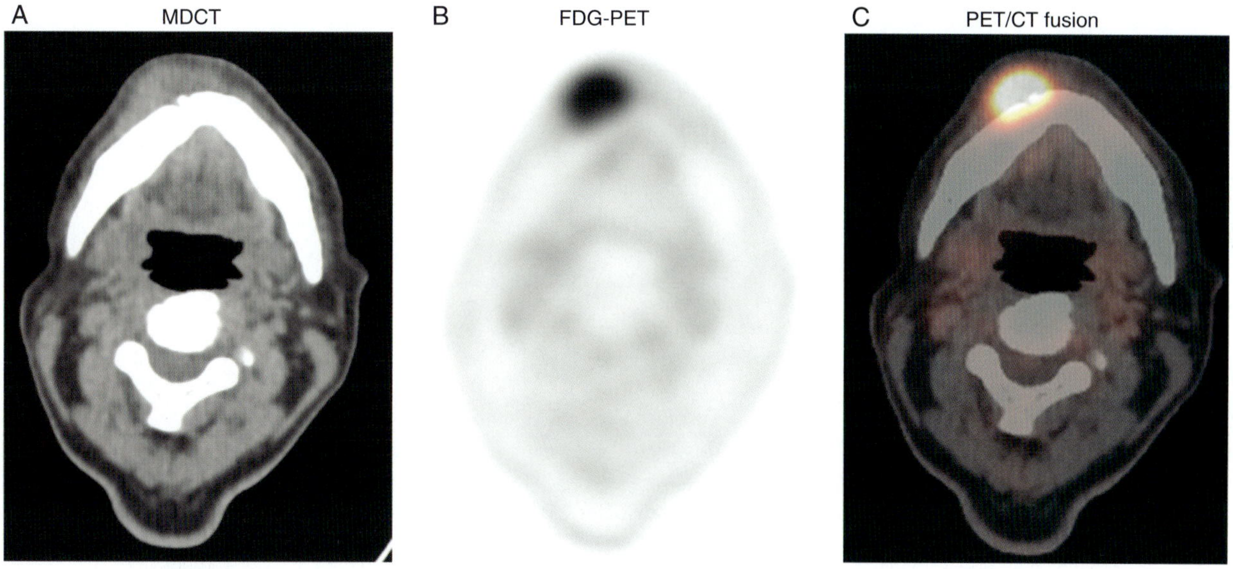

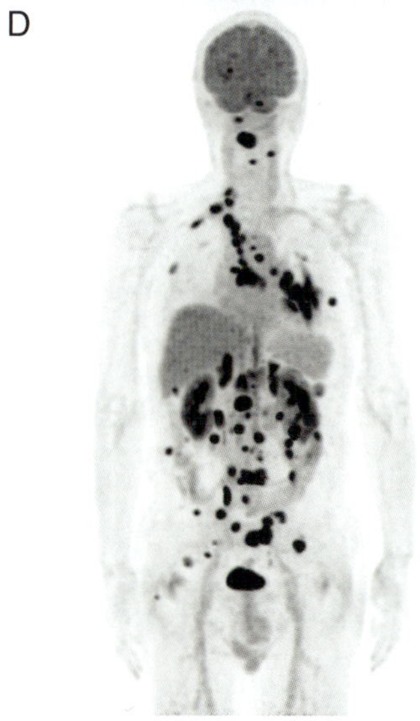

Fig. 11.15 Fluoro-2-deoxy-D-glucose (FDG)-positron emission tomography (PET)/computed tomography (CT) imaging of a metastatic malignancy in the oral cavity. (A) Axial multidetector CT (MDCT) section through the basal body of the mandible showing a soft tissue swelling in the right anterior buccal vestibule. (B) Corresponding axial PET image shows increased uptake of FDG in the soft tissue mass. (C) Superimposition of the PET and CT examinations shows avid uptake in the soft tissue mass and adjacent mandible. (D) Whole body PET maximum intensity projection shows numerous areas of uptake in the bone and soft tissue indicating a metastatic malignancy with poor prognosis.

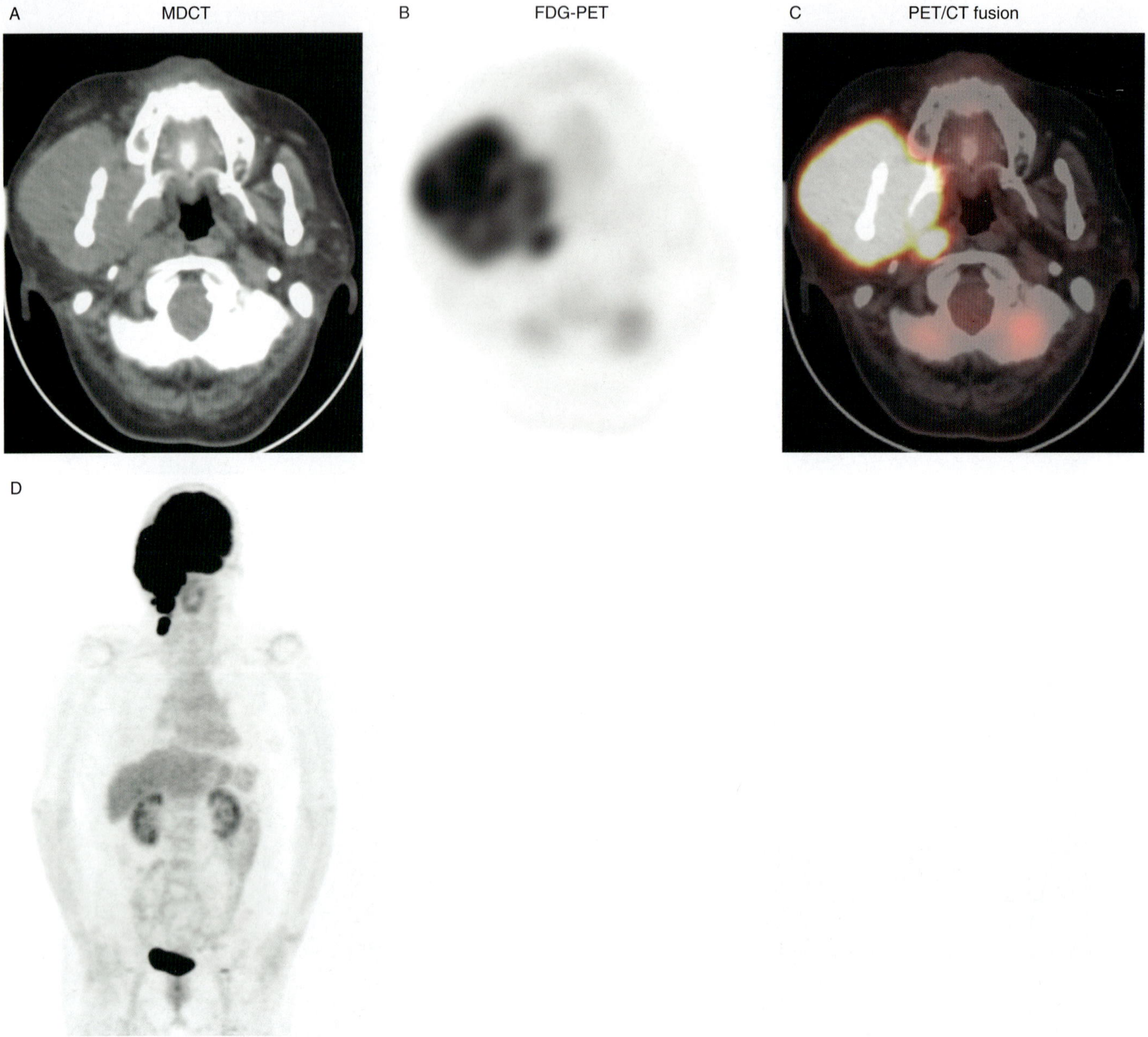

Fig. 11.16 Fluoro-2-deoxy-D-glucose (FDG)-positron emission tomography (PET)/computed tomography (CT) imaging of a malignant lymphoma. (A) Axial multidetector CT (MDCT) section through mid-ramus shows a prominent mass in the right masticator space with displacement of the parapharyngeal space. (B) Corresponding axial PET image shows avid FDG uptake in the right masticator space region. (C) Superimposition of the PET and CT examinations shows avid uptake within the right masticator space. (D) PET maximum intensity projection shows specific uptake within the right parotid region.

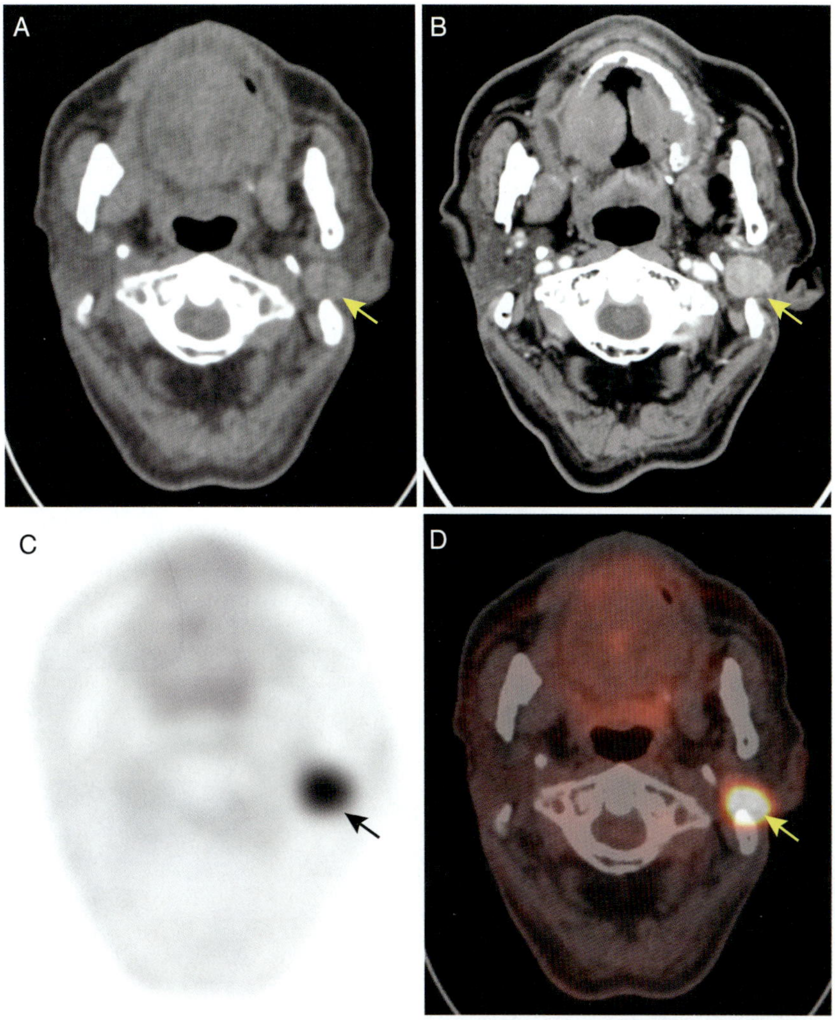

Fig. 11.17 Fluoro-2-deoxy-D-glucose (FDG)-positron emission tomography (PET)/computed tomography (CT) imaging to evaluate a pleomorphic adenoma. (A) Axial multidetector CT (MDCT) section shows an oval mass in the deep lobe of the parotid gland *(yellow arrow)*. (B) Contrast-enhanced CT shows uniform enhancement of the mass. (C) Corresponding axial PET image shows localized increased uptake in the left parotid region. (D) Superimposition of PET and CT examinations shows avid uptake in the deep lobe of the left parotid gland.

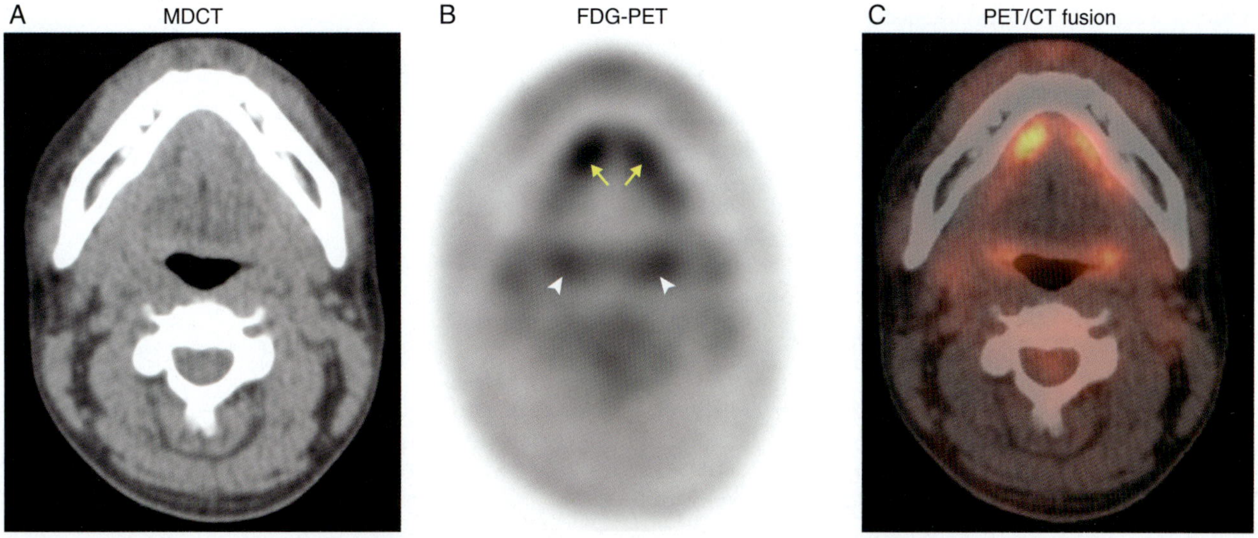

Fig. 11.18 Physiologic uptake of fluoro-2-deoxy-D-glucose (FDG) in the sublingual salivary glands and palatine tonsils. (A) Axial multidetector computed tomography (MDCT) section through the floor of the mouth. (B) Corresponding axial positron emission tomography (PET) section shows increased uptake in the sublingual salivary glands *(yellow arrows)* and the palatine tonsil *(white arrowheads)*. (C) Superimposition of the PET and CT examinations shows increased uptake in the sublingual salivary glands, bilaterally.

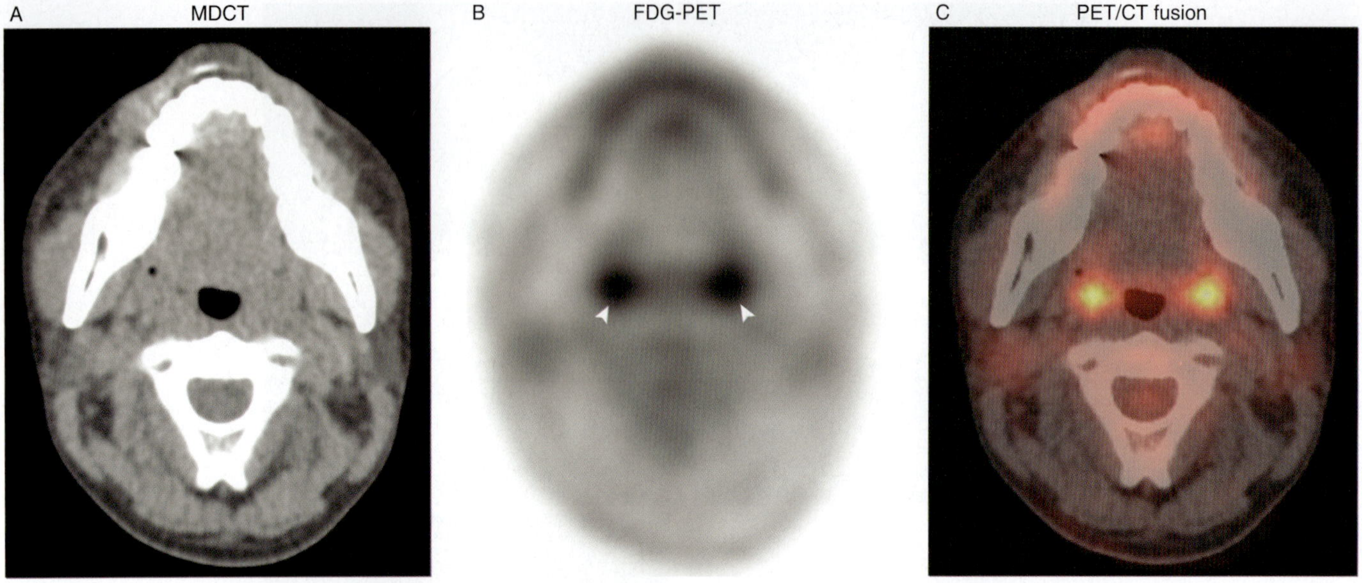

Fig. 11.19 Physiologic uptake of fluoro-2-deoxy-D-glucose (FDG) in the palatine tonsils. (A) Axial multidetector computed tomography (MDCT) section through the palatine tonsils. (B) Corresponding axial positron emission tomography (PET) section shows increased uptake in the tonsil region, bilaterally *(white arrowheads).* (C) Superimposition of the PET and CT examinations shows increased uptake in the palatine tonsils, bilaterally, adjacent to the oropharynx.

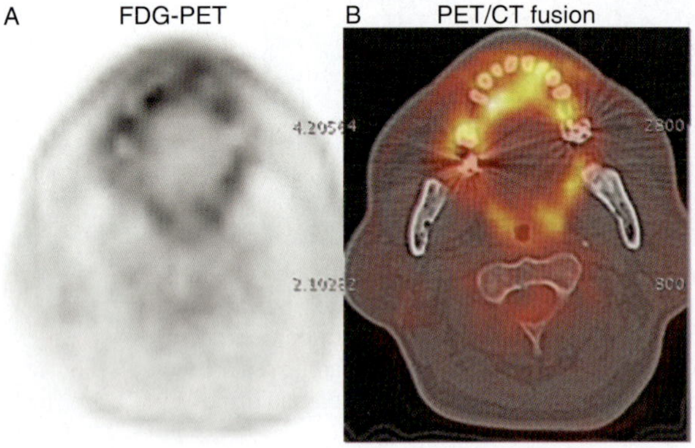

Fig. 11.20 Nonspecific uptake of fluoro-2-deoxy-D-glucose (FDG) in areas of periodontal inflammation. (A) Axial positron emission tomography (PET) section shows increased uptake in the dentoalveolar region. (B) Superimposition of the PET and computed tomography (CT) examinations shows localization of uptake to the dentoalveolus, reflecting increased uptake in areas of periodontal inflammation.

12 Ultrasound Imaging

Sanjay M. Mallya

Ultrasound imaging, or *sonography*, is an imaging modality that uses high-frequency sound waves to generate images of biological tissues in real time without the use of ionizing radiation. Ultrasound provides morphologic imaging as well as functional imaging that examines the blood flow in vessels in a region of interest. Ultrasound imaging has become more versatile and widely available. Ultrasound imaging equipment is mobile and relatively less expensive than computed tomography and magnetic resonance imaging. Portable point-of-care ultrasound imaging has become more popular in primary and specialty medical care offices, both for diagnosis and to guide interventional procedures.

ULTRASOUND PHYSICS AND TECHNOLOGY

Physical Characteristics of Sound

The phenomenon perceived as sound is the result of periodic changes in the pressure of air against the eardrum. Humans can perceive sound between the frequencies of 20 and 20,000 Hz, with the average upper limit of approximately 15,000 to 17,000 Hz in adults. By definition, ultrasound has a frequency greater than 20 kHz, which is greater than the audible range of humans. Diagnostic ultrasonography, the clinical application of ultrasound, uses vibratory frequencies between 2 and 20 MHz.

Imaging Equipment

The user must understand the features and settings on ultrasound equipment and their modulation to make diagnostically useful ultrasound images. The choice of an appropriate transducer and the frequency of sound produced are important determinants of image depth and resolution. When these parameters are not optimal, the examination will be technically difficult and the diagnostic information compromised.

Ultrasound imaging uses a pulse-echo approach to image generation. The core hardware of the imaging device is the *transducer* (Fig. 12.1). The transducer is placed on the skin surface over the region to be examined and produces a localized pulse of ultrasound that is transmitted into the patient. The transducer also records ultrasound echoes back from the tissues to provide the signals for image generation. An aqueous-based polymer gel is used to facilitate transmission of sound from the probe to the tissues and eliminates the air gap between the probe and the skin surface. The principal component of the transducer is a *piezoelectric* crystal. When an electric field is applied, the material will deform and the resultant stresses generate sound waves. Conversely, when a mechanical stress is applied, an electric field is generated within the piezoelectric crystal. These properties of piezoelectric crystals are used to produce and measure sound within the ultrasound range. Transducers are categorized based on the layout of the array of piezoelectric crystals and the range of frequencies of sound generated.

- *Linear transducers* use high frequency sound waves (6 to 15 MHz). The individual piezoelectric elements are arranged in a linear array to generate a parallel field of sound that penetrates into the superficial tissues, typically to a depth of approximately 4 cm. Image resolution adjacent to the transducer at the skin surface *(near field)* and at the depth of the imaged field *(far field)* are the same. Linear transducers are used to image superficial tissues and organs.
- *Curvilinear transducers* use a lower frequency (1 to 5 MHz) and image deeper tissues, for example, abdominal organs. The individual piezoelectric elements are in a curvilinear array. Because of its shape, the imaged field is wider in deeper far-field regions. However, the number of signal-receiving elements is the same and thus, the resolution of images in the far-field region is less than that at near field.
- *Phased array transducers* use a lower frequency (2 to 8 MHz), providing depth of imaging. The individual piezoelectric elements are controlled independently to modulate the amplitude and timing of the ultrasound pulse. This provides flexibility in imaging depth and resolution without having to change the transducer.

A contemporary approach to generate ultrasound uses *capacitive micromachined ultrasound transducers (CMUTs)* instead of piezoelectric crystals. The basic unit of a CMUT transducer is a parallel-plate capacitor, where one plate is fixed and the other is a flexible membrane. Applying alternating voltage across the capacitor causes the membrane to vibrate and produce ultrasound. Likewise, returning echoes cause the membrane to vibrate inducing a change in capacitance that serves as a measurable signal. The frequency range of CMUT transducers ranges from 500 kHz to 50 MHz. Notably, a two-dimensional CMUT array can be programmed to provide linear, curvilinear, or phased waveforms. Thus, a single transducer provides whole body imaging. CMUT technology can be integrated with associated solid-state electronic circuits that control the transducer and receive signals from the individual capacitors. This provides flexibility to manufacture custom ultrasound transducers.

Imaging Modes

Echoes from tissue interfaces constitute signals for ultrasound imaging. These signals can be manipulated and displayed to provide a variety of information. Current techniques permit echoes to be processed at a sufficiently rapid rate to allow perception of motion; this is referred to as *real-time imaging*.

A-mode or *amplitude mode* measures the amplitude of returning echoes to decipher the depth of structures. Other scanning modes have replaced the use of A-mode ultrasound imaging.

B-mode or *brightness mode* measures the amplitude of returning echoes and represents the signal intensity as shades of gray, yielding a two-dimensional grayscale image. Structures that reflect more sound appear relatively brighter.

M-mode or *motion mode* measures the amplitude of returning echoes from moving tissues planes to allow dynamic evaluation of structures such as the heart.

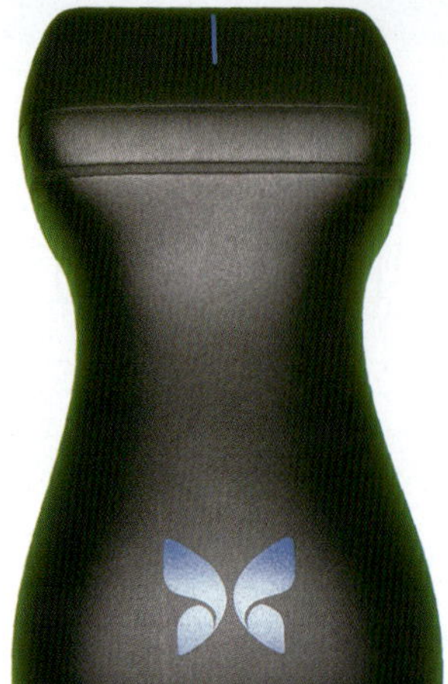

Fig. 12.1 A portable handheld transducer (Butterfly Network, Inc.) that connects to a smartphone or tablet.

Doppler-mode uses the Doppler effect to quantitatively assess velocity of moving blood in vessels. Often, the system will color pixels based on the blood flow to provide a graphic representation and semiquantitative evaluation of blood flow. In dentistry, it is used to image blood vessels in the neck near metastatic lymph nodes and vascular malformations.

Ultrasound Beam Parameters

Wavelength and *frequency* are primary parameters used to describe sound. Wavelength is inversely proportional to frequency—as wavelength decreases, frequency increases. The relationship between wavelength and frequency is expressed as follows:

$$c \text{ (velocity of sound in tissue)} = f \text{ (frequency)} \times \lambda \text{ (wavelength)}$$

Shorter wavelengths provide better spatial resolution. However, shorter wavelengths are attenuated more in tissues and the depth of penetration of the beam is less, and may be inadequate to image deeper tissues and organs.

The strength of the ultrasound beam is described in terms of its *amplitude, power,* and *intensity*. Amplitude defines the maximum displacement of particles by a sound wave traveling through a medium. The higher the amplitude of the returning echo, the brighter the image signal. Power is the rate of transmission of sound energy from the transducer and impacts the depth of penetration. Intensity is the power per unit area. A high intensity may cause tissue heating and potential biologic damage.

Ultrasound Beam Interactions With Tissues

The fraction of the beam that is reflected to the transducer depends on the tissue *acoustic impedance* defined as follows:

$$Z \text{ (acoustic impedance)} = p \text{ (tissue density)} \times c \text{ (velocity of sound in tissue)}$$

Table 12.1 lists tissue density, velocity of sound in medium and the acoustic impedance of tissues and materials relevant to maxillofacial ultrasound imaging. When the ultrasound wave crosses a smooth extended interface between tissues of different acoustic impedance, the ultrasound pulse is partly reflected back to the transducer and the remainder sound waves will penetrate deeper into the tissue. This is referred to as *specular reflection*. When the beam is perpendicular to the tissue interface, the intensity of the reflected pulse is dependent on the acoustic impedance of the two tissues expressed as follows:

$$IR \text{ (Reflected pulse intensity)} = (Z_2 - Z_1)^2 \div (Z_2 + Z_1)^2$$

When the acoustic impedance of the two tissues is the same ($Z_2 = Z_1$), $I_R = 0$, and there is no echo, and the tissue interface is not recorded. When the difference between the acoustic impedance of two tissues is marked, for example, between soft tissue and bone, the intensity of the echo is high and the interface appears bright. If the angle of the incident ultrasound beam is not perpendicular to the tissue interface, the echo is reflected back at an angle and may not be recorded by the transducer.

The intensity of the incident beam is *attenuated by* reflection, refraction, and scatter. When an ultrasound beam traverses an interface between two tissues that transmit sound with different velocity, the beam is deflected by *refraction*. When the sound wave interacts with structures that are smaller than dimension of its wavelength, the beam is scattered and the intensity of the returning echo is low. Energy losses from attenuation interactions are transferred to the tissue in the form of heat.

Tissue Signals

Because of its acoustic impedance, a tissue has a characteristic internal echo pattern. This pattern is used to distinguish between different tissues and boundaries, and can be correlated with pathologic changes within a tissue. Thus, interpretation of sonograms relies on knowledge of both the physical properties of ultrasound and the anatomy of the tissues being scanned.

TABLE 12.1 Physical Density, Velocity of Sound and Acoustic Impedance

Tissue	Density (g/cm³)	Velocity of Sound (m/s)	Z (rayls)
Air	0.0012	330	3.96×10^2
Fat	0.95	1450	1.34×10^6
Water	1	1480	1.48×10^6
*Soft tissue**	*1050*	*1540*	*1.62×10^6*
Muscle	1.1	1600	1.71×10^6
Skull bone	1.9	4080	7.8×10^6

*Mathematical algorithms that generate ultrasound images assume a sound velocity of 1540 m/s in soft tissue.

Tissue signals in ultrasound imaging are described as follows:

- **Anechoic:** Tissues that do not produce signals appear black, for example, fluid-filled cysts.
- **Hyperechoic:** These tissues and materials produce intense signals and appear bright, for example, ligaments, skin, bone, needles, and catheters.
- **Hypoechoic:** These tissues produce a weak signal and appear relatively less bright.

CLINICAL APPLICATIONS OF MAXILLOFACIAL ULTRASONOGRAPHY

There are established ultrasound imaging protocols to evaluate the salivary glands, lymph nodes, and other soft tissue masses in the maxillofacial region. Application of diagnostic ultrasonography for specific organ imaging is discussed.

Salivary Glands

Salivary gland ultrasonography can provide valuable information in addition to the clinical evaluation. Salivary glands should be evaluated in at least two orthogonal planes. A lower frequency pulse may be needed to assess the deep lobe of the parotid gland. The glands must be examined bilaterally for comparison. The major salivary glands' ultrasound echoes are homogenous and hyperechoic to adjacent muscle (Fig. 12.2A–D). The presence of intraglandular fat in the parotid gland makes the appearance brighter. Intraparotid lymph nodes appear hypoechoic (Fig. 12.2C). Acute inflammations of the salivary

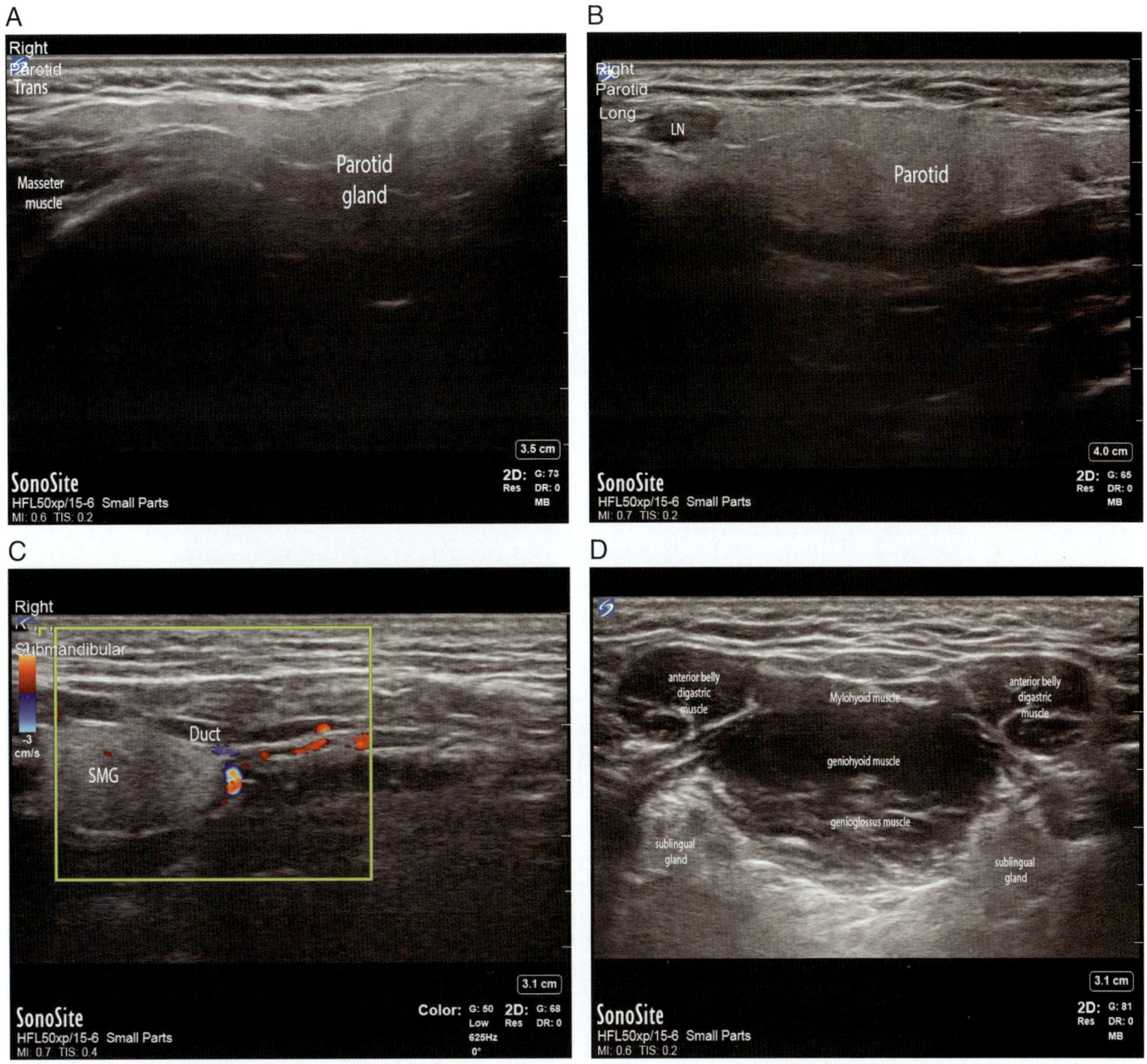

Fig. 12.2 Normal salivary glands. (A) B-mode ultrasound image shows the normal parotid gland as uniformly hyperechoic relative to the adjacent masseter muscle. (B) Intraparotid lymph node (LN) appears as hypoechoic signal within the uniform hyperechoic signal of the normal parotid gland. (C) Submandibular gland (SMG) appears as a uniform hyperechoic signal. The submandibular duct is anechoic and differentiated from the adjacent blood vessels by Doppler ultrasound. (D) B-mode ultrasound image through the floor of the mouth shows the submandibular glands, which are hyperechoic to the adjacent muscles. (Images courtesy of Dr. Anita Gohel and Dr. Almas Binnal, Oral and Maxillofacial Diagnostic Sciences, University of Florida College of Dentistry, Florida, USA.)

glands manifest as heterogeneous and hypoechoic gland enlargement, with increased blood flow on Doppler imaging. With chronic inflammation and obstruction, the gland is atrophic, and relatively isoechoic to muscle. Sialoliths yield hyperechoic curved lines. Normal ducts are not usually seen on ultrasound. Dilated ducts are seen as anechoic bands and can be differentiated from blood vessels by the absence of blood flow (Fig. 12.2C). In patients with Sjögren's syndrome, the imaged glands are heterogeneous with multiple hypoechoic regions (Fig. 12.3). It has been suggested that this characteristic appearance may be a valuable aid to establish the diagnosis of Sjögren's syndrome. Both benign and malignant tumors of the salivary glands appear hypoechoic, and ultrasonography does not adequately distinguish between these tumor types.

Indications for ultrasonographic evaluation of the salivary glands include the following:

- Inflammatory sialadenitis
- Sjögren's disease (Fig. 12.3)
- Recurrent swelling suggestive of salivary gland obstruction
- Solitary masses suggestive of benign and malignant neoplasms
- Salivary gland cysts
- Cystic enlargement due to human immunodeficiency virus infection
- Lesions in the anterior floor of the mouth
- Evaluation of radioactive iodine–induced sialadenitis

Lymph Nodes

A palpable cervical lymph node is well suited for ultrasound evaluation. Although the clinical presentation may involve a single node or group of nodes, the ultrasound examination should comprehensively evaluate all cervical lymph node levels. Normal lymph nodes are ovoid and hypoechoic relative to muscle. The hilum of the node appears echogenic due to fat (Fig. 12.4A). Malignant lymph nodes tend to be more than 1 cm and round, typically with a ratio of the long and short dimensions less than two (Fig. 12.4B). Malignant lymph nodes have irregular contours and are internally heterogenous with loss of the

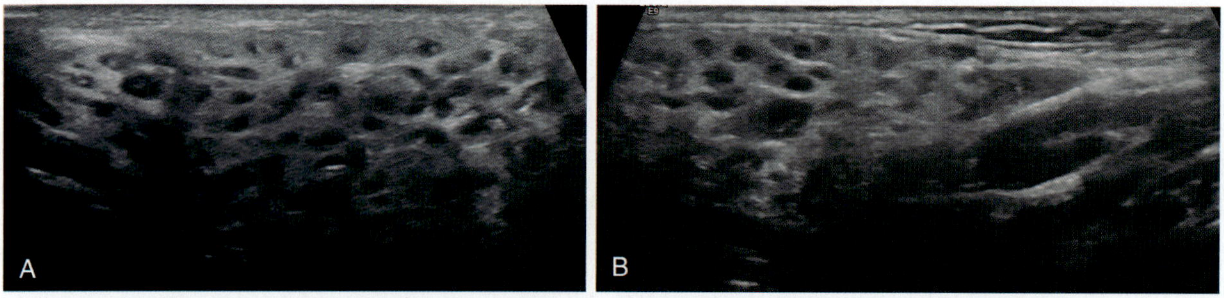

Fig. 12.3 B-mode ultrasound image of a patient with Sjögren's syndrome. (A) Parotid gland. (B) Submandibular gland. Note heterogenous echogenicity with multiple anechoic areas through the glands. (From Wang KY, Wintermark M, Penta M. Imaging characteristics of Sjögren's syndrome. *Clin Imaging*. 2022;92:7-18.)

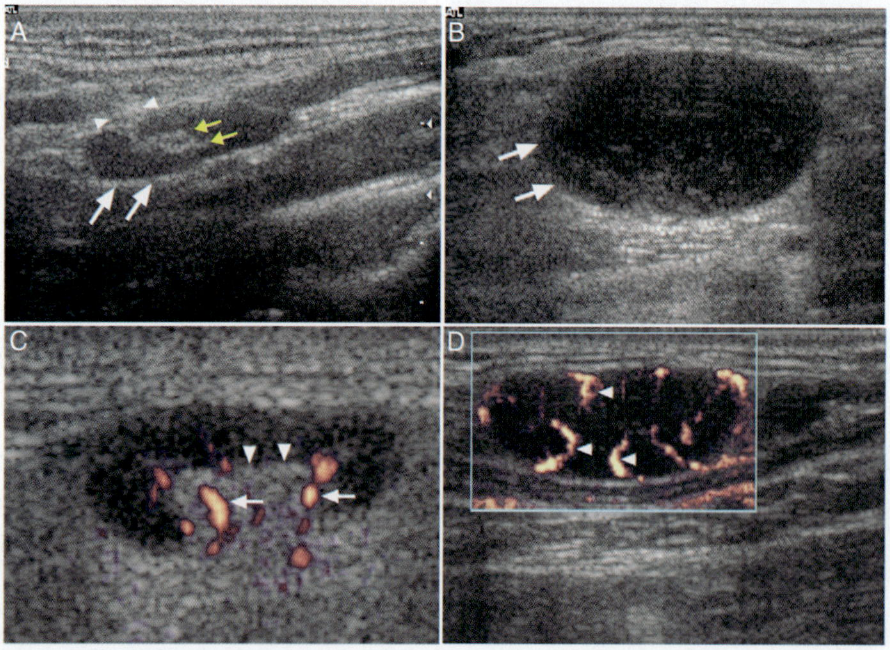

Fig. 12.4 B-mode ultrasound evaluation of cervical lymph nodes. (A) Longitudinal ultrasound section through a cervical lymph node shown as an oval, hypoechoic image *(white arrows)* with an echogenic hilum *(yellow arrows)*. The arrowheads indicate the adjacent soft tissues. (B). Metastatic submandibular lymph node. Note round, hypoechoic gland *(arrows)* with loss of echogenic hilum. (C) Doppler ultrasound image of a lymph node. The hilum is echogenic *(arrowheads)* and vascular *(arrows)*. (D) Doppler ultrasound image of a metastatic lymph node showing peripheral vascularity *(arrowheads)*. (Images from Ying M, Ahuja AT. Ultrasound of neck lymph nodes: How to do it and how do they look? *Radiography*. 2006;12(2):105-117.)

bright hilum signal (Fig. 12.4B). Doppler imaging shows eccentric hilar vascularity, aberrant internal vascularity, and peripheral subcapsular vascularity (Fig. 12.4C and D). Indications for ultrasonographic evaluation of cervical lymph nodes include the following:

- Evaluate inflammatory and obstructive lymphadenitis
- Detect lymph node metastases and describe their anatomic location to guide surgical management
- Detect and evaluate lymph node malignancies
- Image-guided fine-needle aspiration biopsy for cytology
- Image-guided core biopsy for lymphoma

Soft Tissue Masses in the Oral and Maxillofacial Region

Ultrasonography can be used to examine soft tissue masses in the maxillofacial region. These include congenital lesions, developmental malformations, and soft tissue neoplasms. Indications for ultrasonographic evaluation of maxillofacial soft tissue masses include the following:

- Congenital lesions such as lymphangiomas and vascular malformations
- Branchial cleft cyst
- Thyroglossal duct cyst
- Lipoma
- Neurovascular tumors

Temporomandibular Joint

B-mode ultrasound imaging has been suggested as a potential alternative to magnetic resonance imaging to evaluate the articular disc of the temporomandibular joint (TMJ). The surface of the condyle is hyperechoic. The lateral pterygoid muscle, joint capsule, and the articular disc are isogenic. However, the attachment of the capsule is seen as a hyperechoic line (Fig. 12.5). Clinical application of ultrasound for evaluation of TMJ disc displacement has been limited. Protocols for imaging are not established and criteria for interpretation are not well defined. When displaced medially, the disc is deeper with the tissues and less visible on ultrasound due to the overlying condyle and eminence. Nevertheless, the convenience and lower cost of a point-of-care evaluation to assess synovial effusion and disc displacement make ultrasound an attractive option for future consideration as protocols and diagnostic criteria are developed and validated.

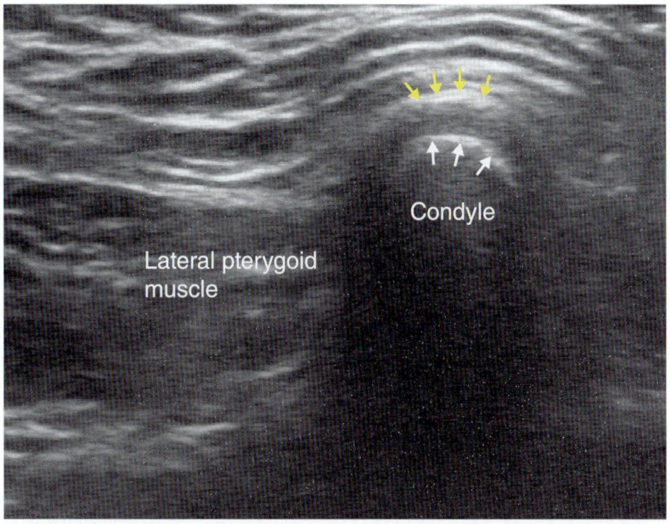

Fig. 12.5 B-mode ultrasound of the temporomandibular joint. Transverse ultrasound section through the temporomandibular joint region in the open position. The condyle is hypoechoic and its articular surface is hyperechoic *(white arrows)*. The attachment of the capsule to the glenoid fossa is seen as a curved hyperechoic line *(yellow arrows)*. *(Images courtesy of Dr. Anita Gohel and Dr. Almas Binnal, Oral and Maxillofacial Diagnostic Sciences, University of Florida College of Dentistry, Florida, USA.)*

BIOLOGIC EFFECTS OF DIAGNOSTIC ULTRASOUND

Unlike X-rays, diagnostic ultrasound imaging does not use ionizing radiation and thus does not pose any cancer risks. As sound waves traverse through tissue, they lose energy that is converted to heat, which is dissipated by conduction through tissues and by adjacent blood flow. Exposure to high-intensity sound waves for prolonged periods of time can cause a localized increase in tissue temperature. However, diagnostic ultrasound imaging uses low sound intensities and the temperature rise is less than 1°C. Using ultrasound equipment within the established guidelines ensures the safety from this procedure.

Besides heating, ultrasound may induce tissue cavitation. In this process, ultrasound induces tiny air bubbles that enlarge and coalesce to cause cavitation within a tissue. To prevent this effect, the frequency and intensity of sound and the time of exposure are carefully adjusted to ensure safety of imaging.

In summary, the power of the diagnostic ultrasound beam and the duration of imaging are both below the threshold to cause adverse effects. In general, ultrasound imaging and Doppler evaluations are both safe procedures that can be used as effective point-of-care diagnostic aids.

BIBLIOGRAPHY

AIUM-ACR-SPR-SRU practice parameter for the performance and interpretation of a diagnostic ultrasound examination of the extracranial head and neck. *J Ultrasound Med*. 2018;37(11):E6-E12.

Bhatia KSS, Dai YL. Routine and advanced ultrasound of major salivary glands. *Neuroimaging Clin N Am*. 2018;28(2):273-293.

Bukhari AF, Farag A, Papas A, et al. Salivary glands ultrasonography as a diagnostic aid in Sjögren syndrome: a prospective pilot investigation. *Oral Surg Oral Med Oral Pathol Oral Radiol*. 2021;132(2):172-181.

Hoffman HT, Pagedar NA. Ultrasound-guided salivary gland techniques and interpretations. *Atlas Oral Maxillofac Surg Clin North Am*. 2018;26(2):119-132.

Kremkau FW. *Sonography: Principles and Instruments*. 10th ed. Saunders; 2020.

Rumack CM, Wilson SR, Charboneau JW, et al. *Diagnostic Ultrasound*. 4th ed. Mosby; 2011.

Shimizu M, Okamura K, Yoshiura K, et al. Sonographic diagnostic criteria for screening Sjögren's syndrome. *Oral Surg Oral Med Oral Pathol Oral Radiol Endod*. 2006;102:85-93.

Straughan AJ, Badger CD, Benito DA, Joshi AS. Salivary gland ultrasound training: improving anatomic identification in residents. *Am J Otolaryngol*. 2020;41(6):102734.

Tempkin B. *Ultrasound Scanning: Principles and Protocols*. 3rd ed. Saunders; 2009.

Tognini F, Manfredini D, Melchiorre D, Bosco M. Comparison of ultrasonography and magnetic resonance imaging in the evaluation of temporomandibular joint disc displacement. *J Oral Rehabil*. 2005;32:248-253.

Xu MJ, Chang JL. Practical salivary ultrasound imaging tips and pearls. *Otolaryngol Clin North Am*. 2021;54(3):471-487.

Ying M, Ahuja AT. Ultrasound of neck lymph nodes: how to do it and how do they look? *Radiography*. 2006;12(2):105-117.

13

Radiographic Anatomy

Sanjay M. Mallya

Knowledge of the radiographic appearances of normal structures is the foundation of radiologic interpretation. Proficient radiologic diagnosis requires an appreciation of the wide variation in the appearances of normal anatomic structures. Often the ranges of normal radiographic appearance overlap with the radiographic appearance of disease. Such equivocal findings pose challenges to decision making for further investigation and management.

GENERAL PRINCIPLES OF RADIOLOGIC EVALUATION

- The radiographic appearance of structures reflects the pattern of x-ray photon attenuation. Tissues that attenuate more photons appear more radiopaque (brighter), whereas low-attenuation tissues appear radiolucent (darker). This pattern of radiodensity is the basis of all x-ray–based imaging, including intraoral, panoramic, cephalometric, and computed tomographic (CT).
- On two-dimensional projections, the anatomic structures along the path of the beam are superimposed onto the same region on the image (Fig. 13.1 and Fig. 13.2). In viewing these images, the clinician should combine information on the x-ray beam angulation with knowledge of anatomy and decipher the positions and projections of individual structures.
- CT images depict the imaged anatomy in three dimensions, without superimposition. Cone beam CT (CBCT) and multidetector CT (MDCT) are typically displayed as multiplanar reconstructions of the imaged structures in three orthogonal planes (Fig. 13.3). To facilitate evaluation, the imaged volume is typically reoriented with tools within the CBCT software. The reorientation of the image volume is guided by the diagnostic task. For example, to examine the skull base, the axial plane is reoriented parallel to the Frankfort plane. When viewing the dentoalveolar region, the axial plane is set to be parallel to the occlusal plane. Likewise, when examining individual teeth, the image may be reoriented along the long axis of individual roots. Sometimes it may be necessary to make additional custom reconstructions in specific planes, referred to as cross sections, to evaluate the teeth and dentoalveolar ridges. Be aware that in any single section, the plane of section may be oblique and incomplete through an anatomic site and may cause the structure to appear abnormal.
- Although the region of immediate diagnostic interest may be limited to a specific site, it is important to evaluate all structures imaged. Often, disease is an incidental finding—that is, located typically in part of the image unrelated to the reason for which the image was made. Accordingly it is critical to systematically evaluate the entire image or imaged volume.

TEETH

Hard Tissues

Teeth are composed primarily of dentin, with an enamel cap over the coronal portion and a thin layer of cementum over the root surface (see Fig. 13.1). The enamel cap characteristically appears more radiopaque than the other tissues because it is the most dense naturally occurring substance in the body. Because it is about 96% mineral, it causes the greatest attenuation of x-ray photons. Its radiographic appearance is uniformly opaque and without evidence of the fine structure. Only the occlusal surface reflects the complex gross anatomy. The dentin is about 75% mineralized and because of its lower mineral content, its radiodensity is similar to that of bone. Dentin is homogeneous on radiographs because of its uniform morphologic features. The junction between enamel and dentin appears as a distinct interface that separates these two structures. The thin layer of cementum on the root surface has a mineral content (50%–60%) comparable to dentin. Cementum is not usually apparent radiographically because the contrast between it and dentin is so low and the cementum layer is so thin. On periapical and bitewing radiographs, diffuse radiolucent areas with ill-defined borders may be apparent radiographically on the mesial or distal aspects of teeth in the cervical regions between the edge of the enamel cap and the crest of the alveolar ridge (see Fig. 13.2). This phenomenon is called *cervical burnout* (Box 13.1).

For most diagnostic tasks, the radiographic anatomy of teeth as displayed on intraoral radiographs is adequate to detect and evaluate dental hard tissue abnormalities. The radiographic appearance of teeth on CBCT images is similar to that on intraoral radiographs. Detailed anatomy of the teeth and the supporting periodontium is depicted better on limited field-of-view (FOV) scans than on medium- and full-FOV scans. Similar to intraoral radiographs, the teeth demonstrate a radiopaque enamel cap and a homogeneously radiopaque dentin (Fig. 13.3). As in periapical radiographs, cementum is typically not radiographically apparent because of the lack of radiographic contrast between cementum and dentin. However, unlike intraoral radiographs, CBCT also shows the buccal and lingual surfaces of the tooth. Thus morphologic variations, such as root dilacerations in the buccolingual dimension that are not apparent on periapical radiographs, are well demonstrated on CBCT examinations (Fig. 13.4).

Pulp

The pulp of normal teeth is composed of soft tissue and consequently appears radiolucent. The chambers and root canals containing the pulp extend from the interior of the crown to the apices of the roots. Although the shape of most pulp chambers is fairly uniform within tooth groups, variations exist among individuals in the size of the

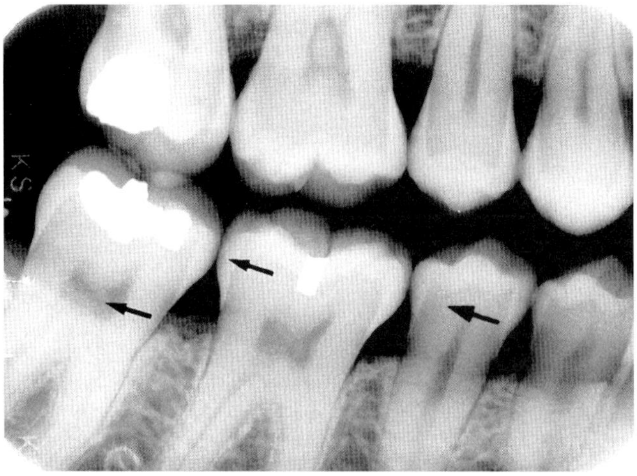

Fig. 13.1 Teeth are composed of pulp (*arrow* on the second molar), enamel (*arrow* on the first molar), dentin (*arrow* on the second premolar), and cementum (usually not visible radiographically).

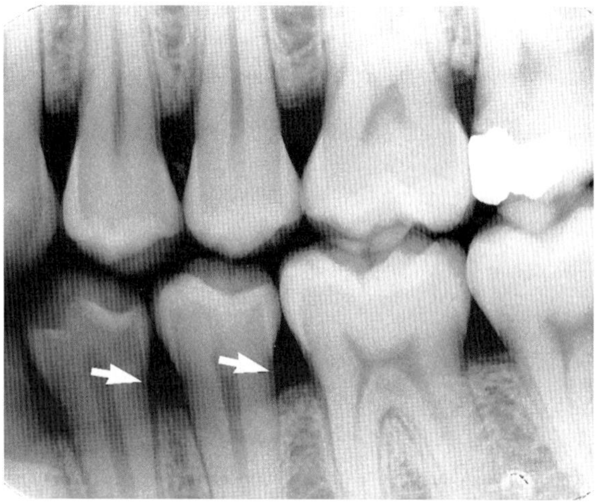

Fig. 13.2 Cervical burnout is caused by overexposure of the lateral portion of roots between the enamel and the alveolar crest and results in an ill-defined radiolucent zone *(arrows)*.

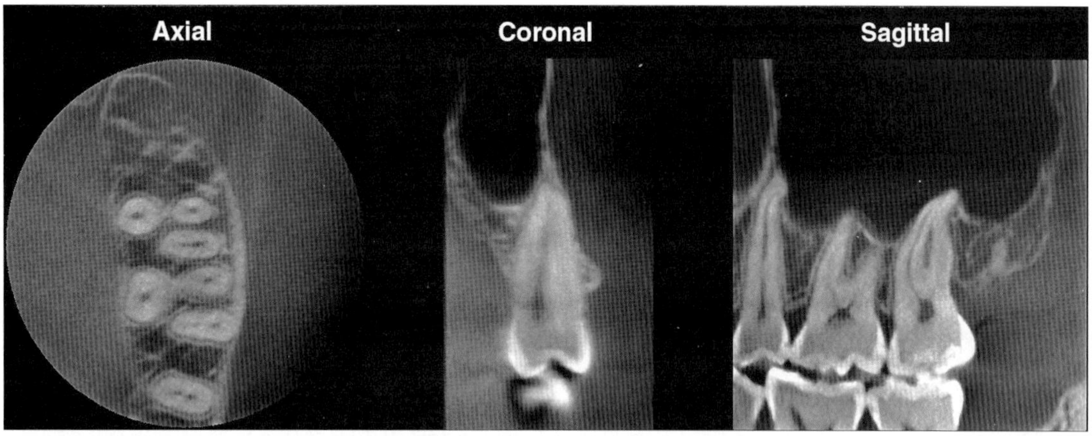

Fig. 13.3 Multiplanar reconstructions with a limited field-of-view cone beam computed tomography scan showing high-resolution axial, coronal, and sagittal sections through the dentoalveolar region of the posterior maxilla.

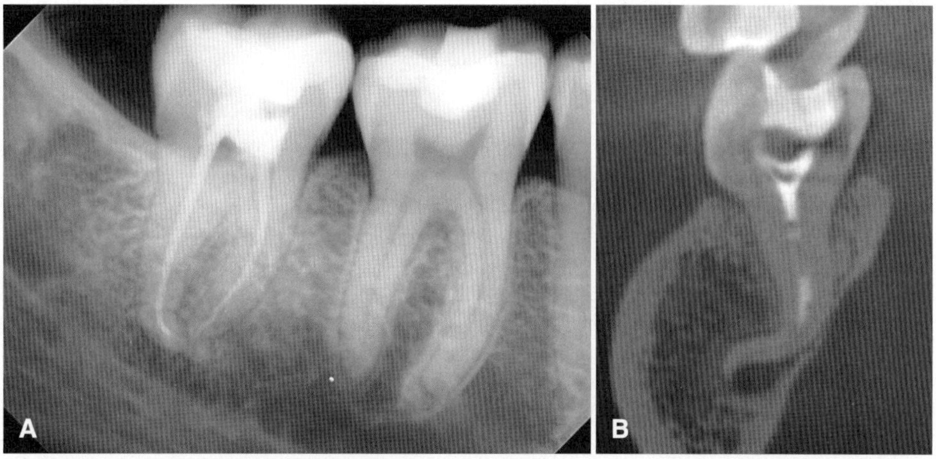

Fig. 13.4 (A) Periapical radiograph of the mandibular right posterior region showing close proximity of the root apices to the inferior alveolar canal. (B) Cross section through the distal root demonstrates marked dilaceration, which was not apparent on the periapical radiograph.

BOX 13.1 Radiographic Phenomenon: Cervical Burnout

Cervical burnout is caused by the normal configuration of the teeth, which results in decreased x-ray absorption in the areas in question (see Fig. 13.2). Close inspection reveals intact edges of the proximal surfaces. The perception of these radiolucent areas results from contrast with the adjacent, relatively opaque enamel and alveolar bone. Such radiolucencies should be anticipated in almost all teeth and should not be confused with root surface caries, which frequently have a similar appearance.

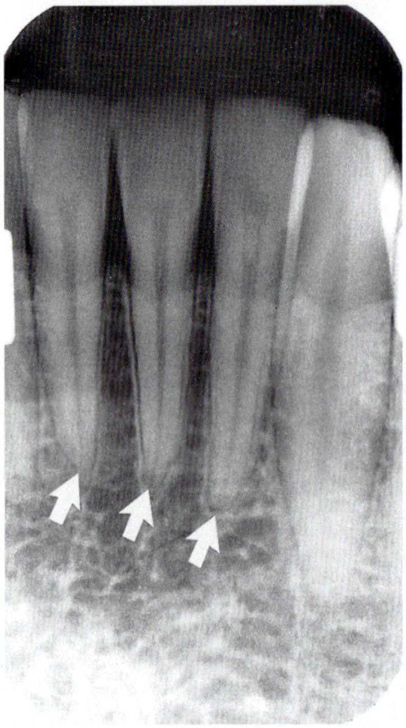

Fig. 13.5 Root canals open at the apices of adult incisors *(arrows)*.

pulp chambers and the extent of pulp horns. Such variations must be evaluated on the radiographs, especially when planning restorative procedures.

In normal, fully formed teeth, the pulp canal may be apparent, extending from the pulp chamber to the apex of the root. An apical foramen is usually recognizable (Fig. 13.5). In other normal teeth, the canal may appear constricted in the region of the apex and not discernible in the last 1 mm or so of its length (Fig. 13.6). In this case, the canal may occasionally exit on the side of the tooth, just short of the radiographic apex. Lateral canals may occur as branches of an otherwise normal root canal. They may extend to the apex and end in a normal, discernible foramen or may exit the side of the root. In either case, two or more terminal foramina might cause endodontic treatment to fail if they are not identified.

In periapical radiographs, there may be superimposition of two pulp canals within the same root, for example, in the mesiobuccal root of the maxillary molar. Radiographs taken at different horizontal angulations may be needed to separate the images of these canals. Identification of individual pulp canals and their morphology is important for endodontic treatment planning. Despite these limitations, periapical radiographs provide adequate information for the initial evaluation of pulpal and periapical disease.

CBCT scans portray the three-dimensional morphology of the roots, pulp chambers, and pulp canals more accurately than intraoral radiographs. A pulp canal that is not evident in periapical radiographs due to

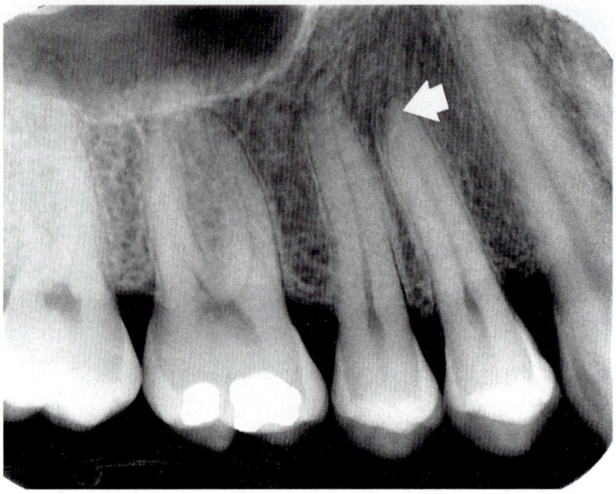

Fig. 13.6 Although the root canal is typically not radiographically visible in the apical 2 mm of a tooth, anatomically it is present and contains the vascular and neural supply to the pulp *(arrow)*.

superimposition may be clearly depicted on CBCT scans. CBCT imaging is particularly useful to evaluate anatomy of multirooted teeth and roots with multiple pulp canals. The number and morphology of pulp canals and their course through the roots in all three planes can be examined. Reconstruction of the image volume along the long axis of each root may also be required. Individual canals are best identified on axial sections, whereas the course of the canal through the length of the root and its exit through the apex are typically assessed on coronal and sagittal sections (Fig. 13.7). When periapical radiographic findings suggest potential extra canals or complex morphology in a tooth being evaluated for endodontic treatment, limited FOV CBCT scans should be made to provide additional diagnostic information (see Box 15.3, Chapter 15).

In a mature tooth, the shape of the pulp chamber and canal may change. A gradual deposition of secondary dentin occurs with aging. This process begins apically, proceeds coronally, and may lead to pulp obliteration. Trauma to the tooth (e.g., from caries, a blow, restorations, attrition, or erosion) also may stimulate dentin production, leading to a reduction in size of the pulp chamber and canals. Such cases usually include evidence of the source of the pathologic stimulus. However, in the case of a minor trauma to the teeth, only the patient's recollection may suggest the true reason for the reduced pulp chamber size.

Developing Teeth

At the end of a developing tooth root, the pulp canal diverges, and the walls of the root rapidly taper to a knife edge (Fig. 13.8). In the recess formed by the root walls and extending a short distance beyond is a small, rounded, radiolucent area in the trabecular bone, surrounded by a thin layer of cortical bone. This is the dental papilla bounded by its bony crypt. The papilla forms the dentin and the primordium of the pulp. When the tooth reaches maturity, the pulpal walls in the apical region begin to constrict and finally come into close apposition. Awareness of this sequence and its radiographic pattern is often useful in evaluating the stage of maturation of the developing tooth; it also helps avoid misidentifying the apical radiolucency as a periapical lesion.

SUPPORTING DENTOALVEOLAR STRUCTURES

Lamina Dura

A radiograph of sound teeth in a normal dental arch demonstrates that the tooth sockets are bounded by a thin radiopaque layer of dense bone

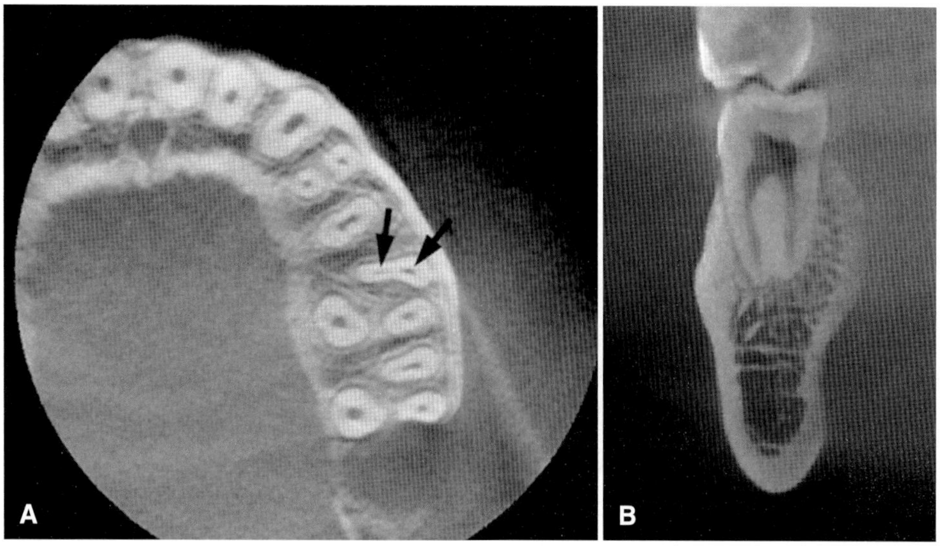

Fig. 13.7 Limited cone beam computed tomography scans demonstrate pulpal morphology. (A) Axial section through the roots of the maxillary teeth. Two pulp canals *(arrows)* are visible in the mesiobuccal root of the first molar. (B) Cross-sectional slice through the long axis of the mesial root of the mandibular first molar demonstrates the course of two pulp canals, with independent apical foramina. Also, the lingual location of the inferior alveolar canal relative to the root apex is evident.

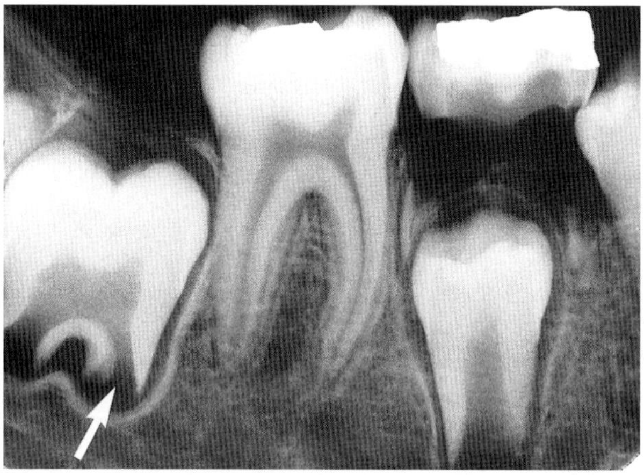

Fig. 13.8 A developing root shown by a divergent apex around the dental papilla *(arrow)*, which is enclosed by an opaque bony crypt. The apices of the first molar are still open but nearing closure.

BOX 13.2 Radiographic Projection of the Lamina Dura

The radiographic appearance of the lamina dura is determined by the angulation of the x-ray beam relative to the tooth root. When the x-ray beam is directed through a relatively long expanse of the structure, the lamina dura appears radiopaque and well defined. When the beam is directed more obliquely, the lamina dura appears more diffuse and may not be discernible. In fact, even if the supporting bone in a healthy arch is intact, identification of a lamina dura completely surrounding every root on each film is frequently difficult, although it is usually evident to some extent about the roots on each image (Fig. 13.10).

The appearance of the lamina dura is a valuable diagnostic feature. The presence of an intact lamina dura around the apex of a tooth strongly suggests a vital pulp. However, because of the variable appearance of the lamina dura, the absence of its image around an apex on a radiograph may be normal. Rarely, the lamina dura may be absent from a molar root extending into the maxillary sinus in the absence of disease. Therefore, when establishing a diagnosis and treatment, the clinician should consider other signs and symptoms as well as the integrity of the lamina dura.

(Fig. 13.9). Its name, **lamina dura** ("hard layer"), is derived from its radiographic appearance. This layer is continuous with the shadow of the cortical bone at the alveolar crest. It is only slightly thicker and with the same radiodensity as the trabeculae of cancellous bone in the area. Its radiographic appearance is caused by the fact that the x-ray beam passes tangentially through many times the thickness of the thin bony wall, which results in its observed attenuation (the eggshell effect). Developmentally, the lamina dura is an extension of the lining of the bony crypt that surrounds each tooth during development.

The appearance of the lamina dura on radiographs may vary, depending on the direction of the x-ray beam relative to the cortical bone thickness (Box 13.2). In addition, small variations and disruptions in the continuity of the lamina dura may result from superimpositions of cancellous bone and small nutrient canals passing from the marrow spaces to the periodontal ligament (PDL). The thickness and density of the lamina dura on the radiograph vary with the amount of occlusal stress to which the tooth is subjected. The lamina dura is thicker and more radiopaque around the roots of teeth in heavy occlusion and thinner and less dense around teeth not subjected to occlusal function.

Alveolar Crest

The gingival margin of the alveolar process that extends between the teeth is apparent on radiographs as a radiopaque line—the alveolar crest (Fig. 13.11). The level of this bony crest is considered normal when it is 0.5–2 mm apical to the cementoenamel junction of the adjacent teeth. The alveolar crest may recede apically with age and show marked resorption with periodontal disease. Radiographs can demonstrate only the position of the crest; determining the significance of its level is primarily a clinical decision (see Chapter 18).

The length of the normal alveolar crest in a particular region depends on the distance between the teeth in question. In the anterior region, the crest is reduced to only a point of bone between the close-set incisors. Posteriorly it is flat, aligned parallel with and slightly below a

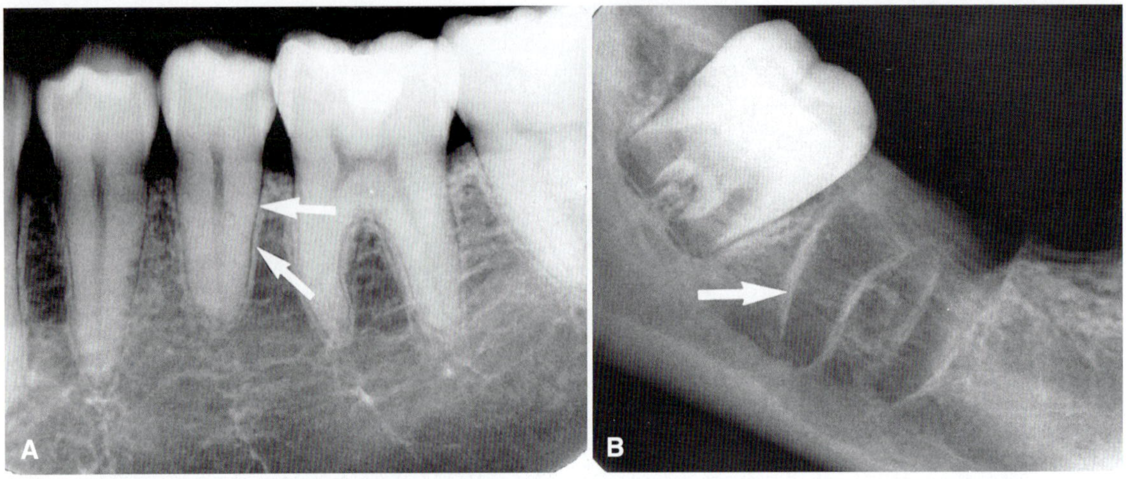

Fig. 13.9 The lamina dura *(arrows)* appears as a thin opaque layer of bone around teeth (A) and around a recent extraction socket (B).

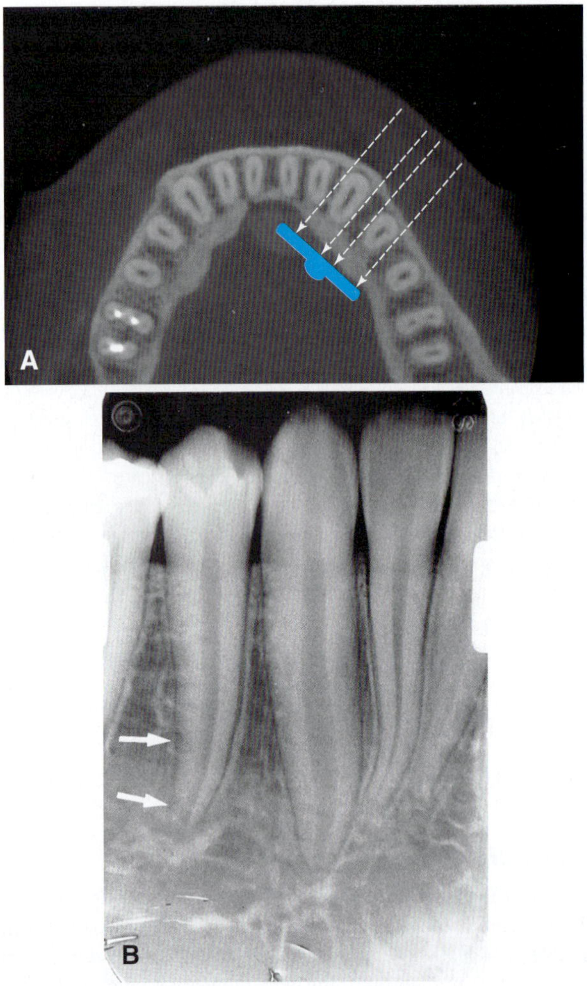

Fig. 13.10 (A) Representation of the position of the image receptor for a periapical projection of the mandibular canine and premolar. Note how the x-ray beam *(dashed arrows)* traverses through partial thicknesses of the lamina dura on the mesial surface of the canine and distal surface of the first premolar. (B) The lamina dura is poorly visualized on the distal surface of this premolar *(arrows)* but is clearly seen on the mesial surface. A broad, flat lamina dura oriented parallel to the x-ray beam produces a prominent lamina dura, whereas a curved narrow lamina dura is less visible.

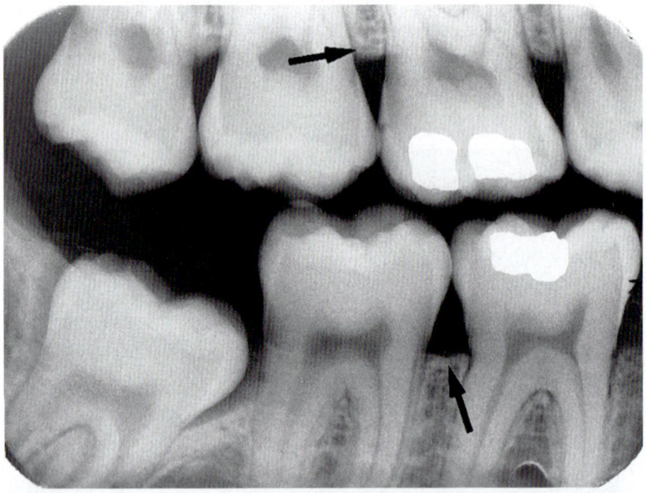

Fig. 13.11 The alveolar crests *(arrows)* are seen as cortical borders of the alveolar bone. The alveolar crest is continuous with the lamina dura.

line connecting the cementoenamel junctions of the adjacent teeth. The crest of the bone is continuous with the lamina dura and forms a sharp angle with it. Rounding of these sharp junctions is indicative of periodontal disease.

The image of the crest varies from a dense layer of cortical bone to a smooth surface without cortical bone. In the latter case, the trabeculae at the surface are of normal size and density. In the posterior regions, this range of radiodensity of the crest is presumed to be normal if the bone is at a proper level in relation to the teeth. However, the absence of an image of cortex between the incisors is considered by many to be an indication of incipient disease, even if the level of the bone is not abnormal.

Periodontal Ligament Space

Because the PDL is composed primarily of collagen, it appears as a radiolucent space between the tooth root and the lamina dura. This space begins at the alveolar crest, extends around the portions of the tooth roots within the alveolus, and returns to the alveolar crest on the opposite side of the tooth (Fig. 13.12).

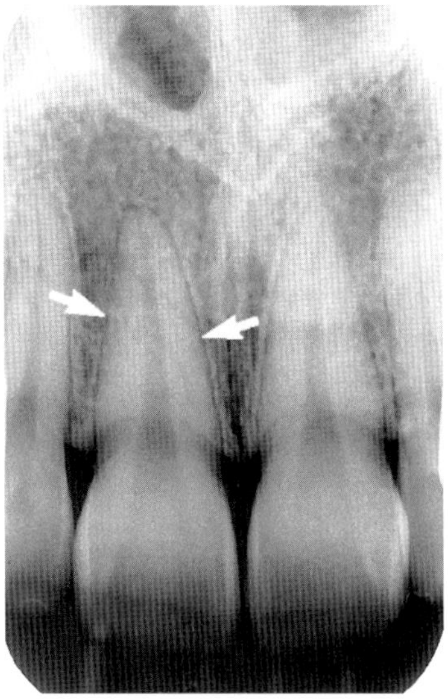

Fig. 13.12 The periodontal ligament space *(arrows)* is seen as a narrow radiolucency between the tooth root and the lamina dura.

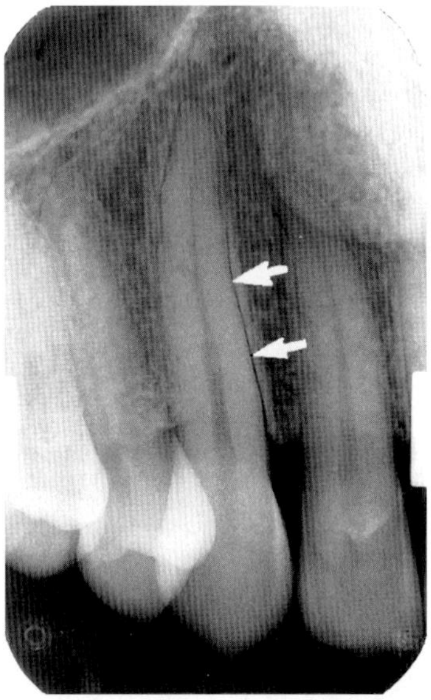

Fig. 13.13 The periodontal ligament space appears wide on the mesial surface of this canine *(arrows)* and thin on the distal surface.

The PDL width varies between individuals, from tooth to tooth in the same individual and even from location to location around one tooth (Fig. 13.13). It is usually thinner in the middle of the root and slightly wider near the alveolar crest and root apex, suggesting that the fulcrum of physiologic movement is in the region where the PDL is thinnest. The thickness of the ligament relates to the degree of function because the PDL is thinnest around the roots of embedded teeth and teeth that have lost their antagonists. The reverse is not true, however, because an appreciably wider space is not regularly observed in persons with especially heavy occlusion or bruxism.

The shape of the tooth may create the appearance of a double PDL space. When the x-ray beam is directed so that two convexities of a root surface appear on a film, a double PDL space is seen (Fig. 13.14). A common example of this double PDL space is seen on the buccal and lingual eminences on the mesial surface of mandibular first and second molar roots.

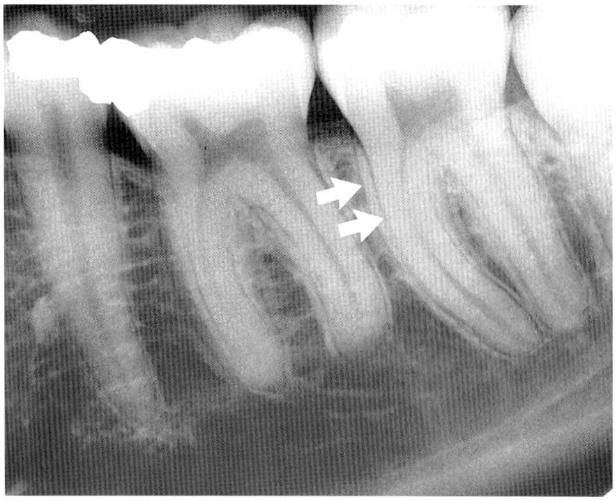

Fig. 13.14 A double periodontal ligament space and lamina dura *(arrows)* may be seen when there is a convexity of the proximal surface of the root resulting in two heights of contour. Double periodontal ligament spaces may also be seen on the mesial surfaces of both roots of the first molar.

Cancellous Bone

The cancellous bone (also called trabecular bone or spongiosa) lies between the cortical plates in both jaws. It is composed of thin radiopaque plates and rods (trabeculae) surrounding many small radiolucent pockets of marrow. On two-dimensional radiographs, the radiographic pattern of the trabeculae comes from two anatomic sources. The first is the cancellous bone itself. The second is the endosteal surface of the outer cortical bone where the cancellous bone fuses with the cortical bone. At this surface, trabecular plates are relatively thick and make a significant contribution to the radiographic image. There is wide variation in the trabecular pattern among individuals and between different anatomic sites in the same patient. It is important to recognize the limits of this variation so that it is not confused with disease. To evaluate the trabecular pattern in a specific area, the practitioner should examine the trabecular distribution, size, and density and compare them throughout both jaws and especially with the corresponding region on the opposite side. This comparison allows the clinician to assess whether a particularly suspect region is anatomic or pathologic in nature.

The trabeculae in the anterior maxilla are typically thin and numerous, forming a fine, granular, dense pattern (Fig. 13.15), and the marrow spaces are consequently small and relatively numerous. In the posterior maxilla, the trabecular pattern is usually quite similar to the pattern in the anterior maxilla, although the marrow spaces may be slightly larger.

In the anterior mandible, the trabeculae are thicker than in the maxilla, resulting in a coarser pattern (Fig. 13.16), with trabecular plates that are oriented more horizontally. The trabecular plates are also fewer than in the maxilla, and the marrow spaces are correspondingly larger. In the posterior mandible, the periradicular trabeculae and marrow spaces may be similar to those in the anterior mandible but are usually larger (Fig. 13.17). The trabecular plates are also oriented mainly horizontally in this region. Below the apices of the mandibular molars, the number of trabeculae dwindles still more. In some cases, the area from just below the molar roots to the inferior border of the mandible may appear to be almost devoid of trabeculae. The distribution and size of the trabeculae throughout both jaws show a relationship to the thickness (and strength) of the adjacent cortical plates. It may be speculated

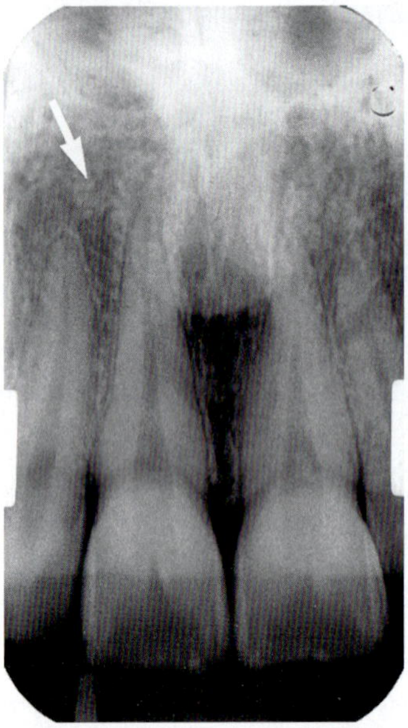

Fig. 13.15 The trabecular pattern in the anterior maxilla is characterized by fine trabecular plates and multiple small trabecular spaces *(arrow)*.

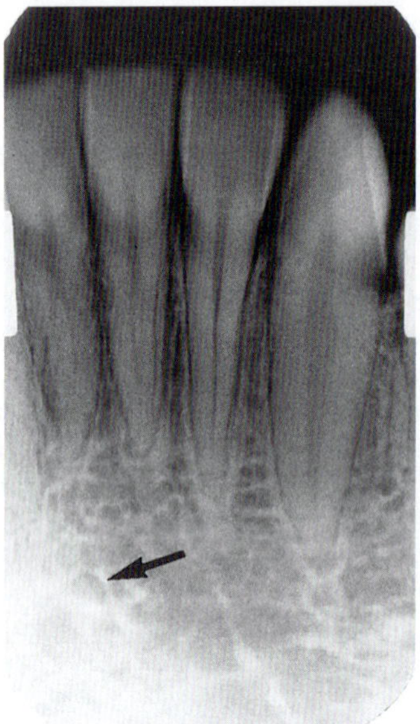

Fig. 13.16 The trabecular pattern in the anterior mandible is characterized by coarser trabecular plates *(arrow)* and larger marrow spaces than in the anterior maxilla.

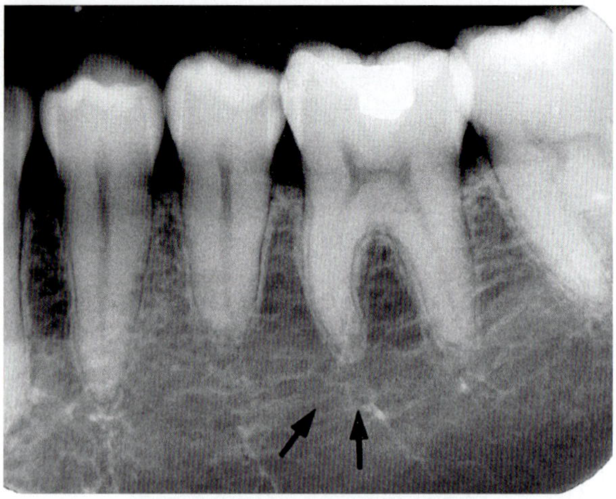

Fig. 13.17 The trabecular pattern in the posterior mandible is quite variable, generally showing large marrow spaces and sparse trabeculation, especially inferiorly *(arrows)*.

that where the cortical plates are thick (e.g., in the posterior region of the mandibular body), internal bracing by the trabeculae is not required, so there are relatively few except where required to support the alveoli. By contrast, in the maxilla and anterior region of the mandible, where the cortical plates are relatively thin and less rigid, trabeculae are more numerous and lend internal bolstering to the jaw. Occasionally, the trabecular spaces in this region are very irregular, with some so large that they mimic pathologic lesions. This finding may be diagnostically challenging (Box 13.3).

Cortical Bone

Buccal and lingual cortical plates of the mandible and maxilla do not cast a discernible image on periapical, bitewing, and panoramic radiographs. They are well depicted on CBCT images and best visualized on the axial, coronal, or cross-sectional images (see Figs. 13.7 and 13.18). Cortical bone has higher mineral content than the adjacent cancellous bone and appears more radiopaque. The endosteal surface of the cortex is smooth and merges with the trabeculae of the cancellous bone. The thickness of the cortical bone varies with anatomic location. In particular, buccal bone adjacent to teeth is often thin and barely discerned on radiographs. CBCT images reveal the proximity of the root surface to the cortical plates of the alveolar bone and detect anatomic variations, such as fenestrations or dehiscence defects (see Fig. 13.18).

BOX 13.3 Trabecular Sparseness: Anatomic Variation Versus Disease

Sparseness or apparent absence of trabeculae may suggest the presence of disease in an otherwise asymptomatic patient.

- Considerable variation may exist in trabecular patterns among patients, so it is important to examine other regions of the jaws, preferably on the contralateral side, to assess the general trabecular pattern for that individual. Assess whether the area of trabecular sparseness deviates appreciably from that norm.
- Compare with previous radiographs of the region in question to determine whether the current appearance represents a change from a prior condition. An abnormality is more likely when the comparison indicates a change in the trabecular pattern.
- If prior films are unavailable, it is frequently useful to repeat the radiographic examination at a reduced exposure because this may demonstrate the presence of a sparse trabecular pattern that was overexposed and "burned out" in the initial projection.
- In an asymptomatic patient, it may be appropriate to expose another radiograph at a later time to monitor for interval changes.

MAXILLA AND MIDFACIAL BONES

The maxilla and palatine bones form the upper jaw. The maxilla comprises a pyramidal-shaped body and four processes—alveolar, palatine, zygomatic, and frontal.

Intermaxillary Suture

The alveolar and palatine processes articulate in the midline to form the intermaxillary suture between the central incisors. On intraoral

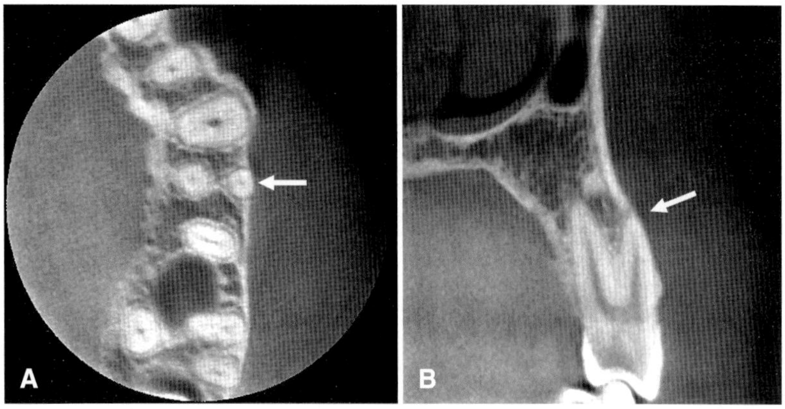

Fig. 13.18 Axial (A) and coronal (B) cone beam computed tomography sections demonstrating the proximity of the roots of the first premolar to the buccal cortical plate. Note the fenestration defect adjacent to the buccal root of the first premolar *(arrows)*.

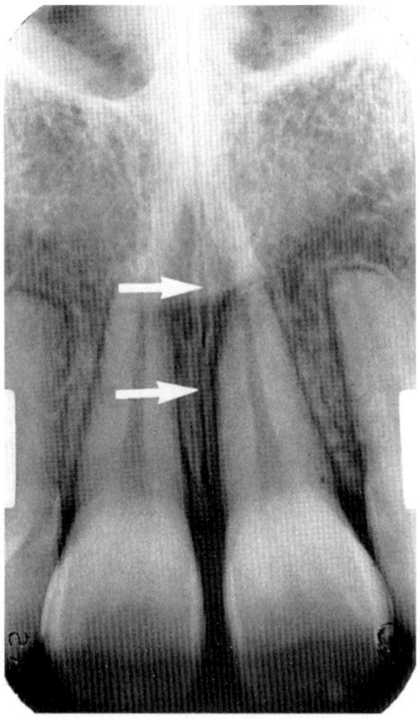

Fig. 13.19 The intermaxillary suture *(arrows)* appears as a curved radiolucency in the midline of the maxilla.

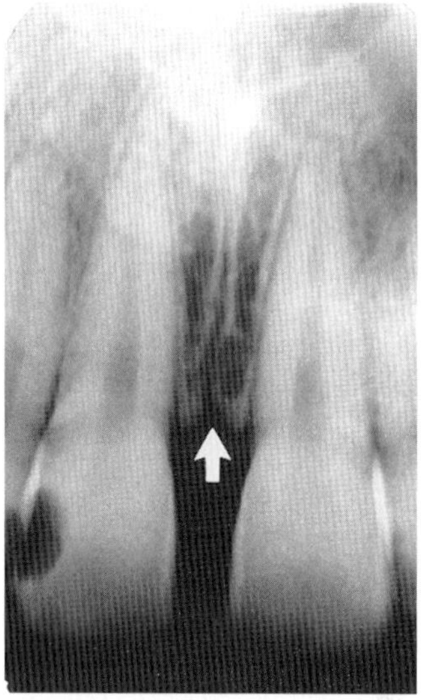

Fig. 13.20 The intermaxillary suture may terminate in a V-shaped widening *(arrow)* at the alveolar crest. This is a normal variation and should not be confused with alveolar bone loss associated with periodontal disease.

periapical radiographs, this suture appears as a thin radiolucent line in the midline between the two portions of the premaxilla (Fig. 13.19). It extends from the alveolar crest between the central incisors superiorly through the anterior nasal spine and continues posteriorly between the maxillary palatine processes to the posterior aspect of the hard palate. It is not unusual for this narrow radiolucent suture to terminate at the alveolar crest in a small rounded or V-shaped enlargement (Fig. 13.20).

On CBCT images, the intermaxillary suture is best evaluated on coronal and axial sections (Plate 13.2). The suture is limited by two parallel radiopaque borders of thin cortical bone on each side of the maxilla. The radiolucent region is usually of uniform width. The adjacent cortical margins may be either smooth or slightly irregular. The appearance of the intermaxillary suture depends on both anatomic variability and, in the case of periapical radiography, on the angulation of the x-ray beam through the suture. Evaluation of the intermaxillary suture is important in planning for orthodontic expansion of the palate.

Anterior Nasal Spine

The anterior nasal spine is frequently demonstrated on periapical radiographs of the maxillary central incisors (Fig. 13.21). Located in the

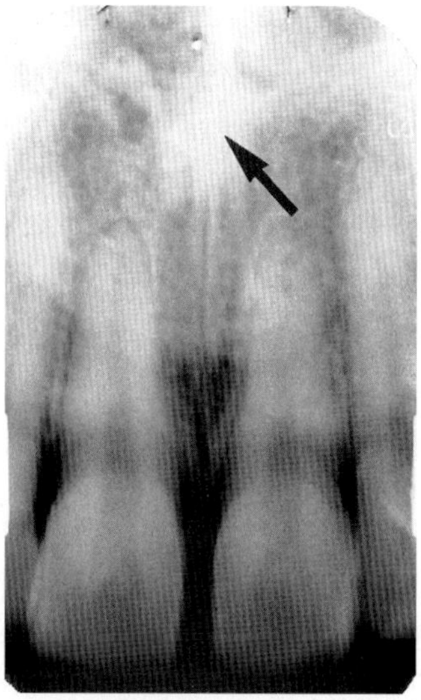

Fig. 13.21 The anterior nasal spine is seen as an opaque, irregular, or V-shaped projection from the floor of the nasal aperture in the midline *(arrow)*.

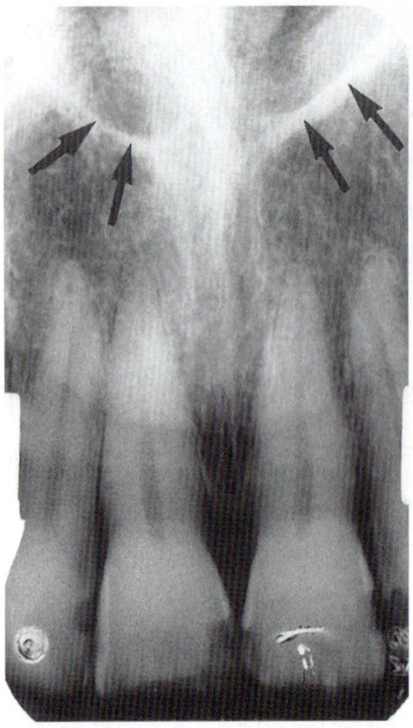

Fig. 13.22 The anterior floor of the nasal aperture *(arrows)* appears as opaque lines extending laterally from the anterior nasal spine.

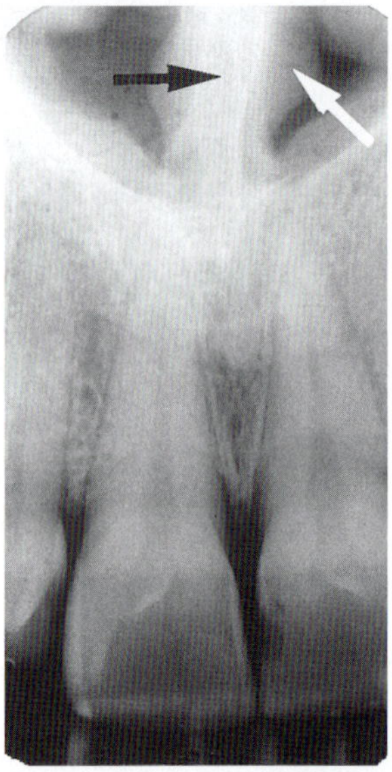

Fig. 13.23 The nasal septum *(black arrow)* arises directly above the anterior nasal spine and is covered on each side by mucosa *(white arrow)*.

midline, it lies approximately 1.5–2 cm above the alveolar crest, usually at or just below the junction of the inferior end of the nasal septum and the inferior outline of the nasal aperture. It is radiopaque because of its bony composition and is usually V shaped. On CBCT images, the anterior nasal spine is best observed on axial and sagittal sections as a triangular projection from the anterior surface of the maxilla at the level of the nasal floor (Plates 13.2 and 13.7).

Nasal Aperture and Nasal Cavity

Because the air-filled nasal aperture and cavity lie just above the oral cavity, its radiolucent image may be apparent on intraoral radiographs of the maxillary teeth, especially in central incisor projections. On maxillary incisor periapical views, the inferior border of the fossa aperture appears as a radiopaque line extending bilaterally away from the base of the anterior nasal spine (Fig. 13.22). Above this line is the radiolucent space of the inferior portion of the nasal cavity. The relatively radiopaque nasal septum is seen arising in the midline from the anterior nasal spine (Fig. 13.23). The shadow of the septum may appear wider than anticipated and not sharply defined because the image is a superimposition of septal cartilage and vomer bone. Also, the septum frequently deviates slightly from the midline, and its plate of bone (the vomer) is curved.

Depending on the field of view, CBCT scans may encompass the full extent of the nasal cavity. The boundaries of the nasal cavity may be evaluated in the coronal, sagittal, and axial planes. The cribriform plate of the ethmoid bone and the ethmoidal air cells form the roof of the nasal cavity. The hard palate forms the floor (see Plates 13.2, 13.4, and 13.5).

Nasal Conchae and Nasal Turbinates

The lateral walls contain thin bony projections called **conchae.** The conchae plus their mucosal covering are called **turbinates** (see Plates 13.2, 13.4, and 13.5). There are three nasal turbinates—superior, middle, and inferior—which define spaces termed superior, middle, and inferior meati (see Plate 13.4). Pneumatization of the concha is termed **concha bullosa** and is a common variant with a reported frequency of 14%–53% (Fig. 13.24).

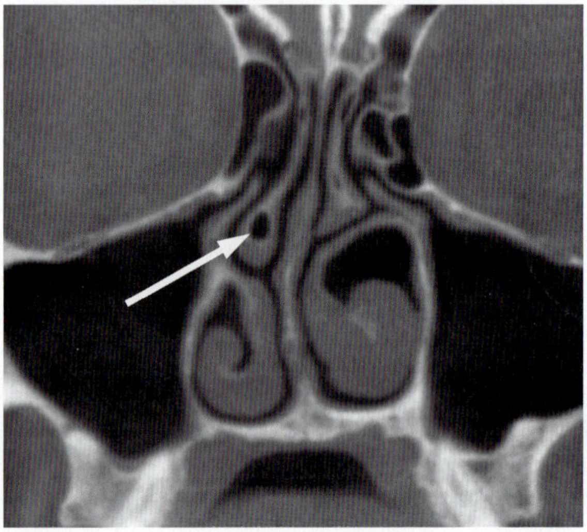

Fig. 13.24 Concha bullosa. Coronal section through the nasal turbinates showing pneumatization of the middle concha *(arrow)* or concha bullosa.

On periapical radiographs of the maxillary incisor and canine regions, the inferior nasal conchae is often visualized, extending from the right and left lateral walls for varying distances toward the septum. These conchae fill varying amounts of the lateral portions of the cavity (Fig. 13.25).

Nasal Floor and Hard Palate

The palatine processes are thick horizontal bony projections that form the anterior three-fourths of the hard palate and the floor of the nasal cavity. On periapical radiographs, the floor of the nasal aperture and a small segment of the nasal cavity are occasionally projected high onto a maxillary canine radiograph (Fig. 13.26). In the posterior maxillary region, the floor of the nasal cavity may be seen in the region of the maxillary sinus. It may falsely convey the impression of a septum in the sinus or a limiting superior sinus wall (Fig. 13.27).

Medium- and full-FOV CBCT scans may show the entire extent of the nasal floor (hard palate), best displayed on coronal and sagittal sections (see Plates 13.4, 13.5, and 13.7). Disruption of the hard palate

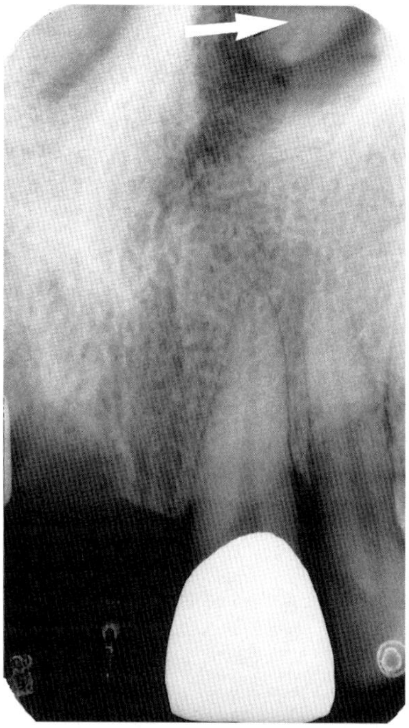

Fig. 13.25 The mucosal covering of the inferior concha *(arrow)* is occasionally visualized in the nasal cavity.

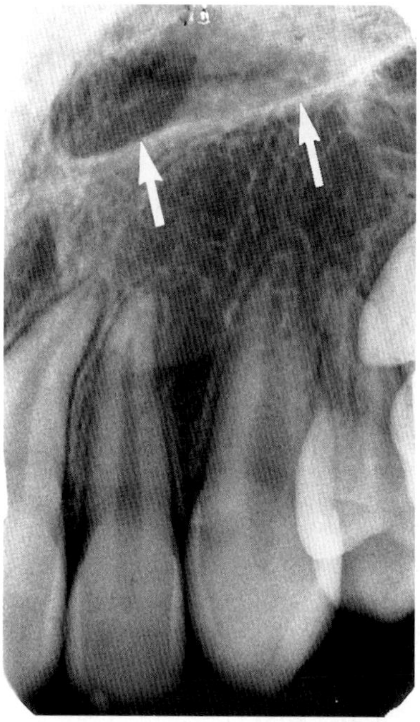

Fig. 13.26 The floor of the nasal aperture *(arrows)* often may be seen extending posteriorly from the anterior nasal spine above the maxillary lateral incisor and canine.

suggests developmental disturbances, such as a cleft palate. Areas of bony protuberance or tori are frequently noted, especially in the midline. Numerous nutrient canals also may be observed perforating the cortical outline of the hard palate on high-resolution scans.

Nasopalatine Canal and Incisive Foramen

The nasopalatine canal originates in the anterior floor of the nasal cavity and exits on the anterior maxilla as the incisive foramen, located in the midline on the anterior aspect of the palatine process immediately

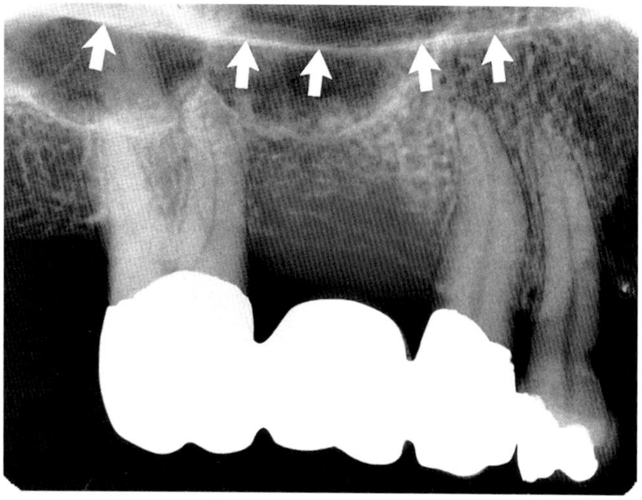

Fig. 13.27 The floor of the nasal cavity, or hard palate *(arrows)*, extends posteriorly, superimposed over the maxillary sinus.

palatal to the maxillary central incisors. Within this foramen are two lateral canals—the incisive canals or foramina of Stensen—that transmit the terminal branch of the descending palatine artery and the nasopalatine nerve. Occasionally, there may be two additional midline canals—the foramina of Scarpa, which transmit the nasopalatine nerves.

On intraoral and panoramic radiographs, the incisive foramen is usually projected between the roots and in the region of the middle and apical thirds of the central incisors (Fig. 13.28). It appears as an ovoid radiolucency, often with diffuse borders. Occasionally, the lateral walls of the nasopalatine canal are seen as a pair of radiopaque lines running vertically from the floor of the nasal aperture to the incisive foramen (Fig. 13.29A). When an exaggerated vertical angle is used, as in anterior maxillary occlusal projections, the openings of the foramina of Stensen at the nasal floor may be seen (Fig. 13.30).

There is wide variation in the appearance of the incisive foramen on periapical radiographs. The foramen varies markedly in its radiographic shape, size, and sharpness. It may appear smoothly symmetric or very irregular, and its borders may be well demarcated or ill-defined. The position of the foramen's image is also variable and may be recognized at the apices of the central incisor roots, near the alveolar crest, anywhere in between, or extending over the entire distance. The great variability of its radiographic image is primarily the result of (1) the differing angles at which the x-ray beam is directed for the maxillary central incisors and (2) some variability in its anatomic size. Often, a large incisive foramen may mimic disease (Box 13.4).

CBCT images better demonstrate the anatomy of the nasopalatine canal and incisive foramen (see Fig. 13.29B and C). The shape and size of the incisive foramen is best assessed on axial sections (see Fig. 13.29B and Plates 13.2 and 13.3). The variation in the size of the nasopalatine canal is recognized on sagittal sections (Fig. 13.31 and Plate 13.7). Evaluation of the locations of the foramen and canal is important in planning implant placement in the anterior maxilla (see Chapter 31).

Lateral Fossa

The lateral fossa (also called the incisive fossa) is a gentle depression in the maxilla near the apex of the lateral incisor (Fig. 13.32A). It may appear diffusely radiolucent on periapical projections of this region, superimposed over the root of the lateral incisor (see Fig. 13.32B). An intact lamina dura around the root of the lateral incisor coupled with absence of clinical symptoms will indicate absence of periapical disease.

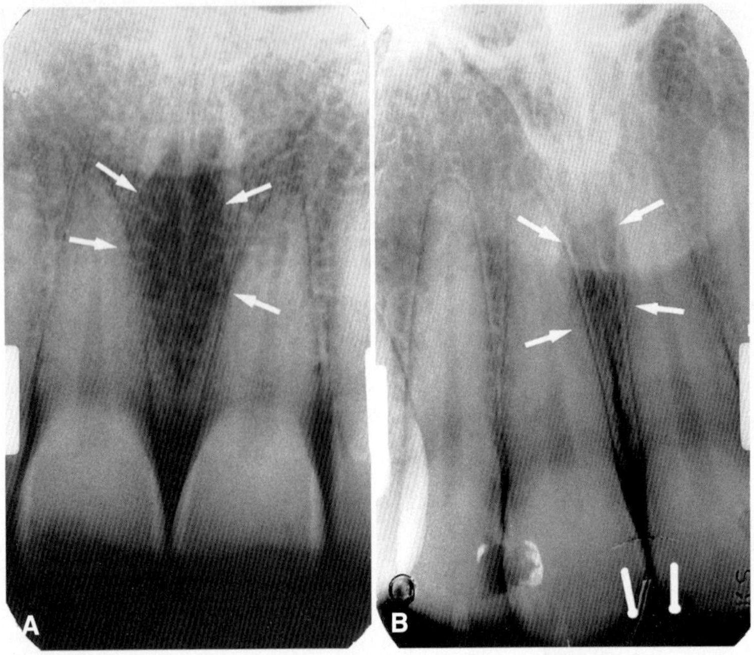

Fig. 13.28 (A) The incisive foramen appears as an ovoid radiolucency *(arrows)* between the roots of the central incisors. (B) Note its borders, which are diffuse but within normal limits.

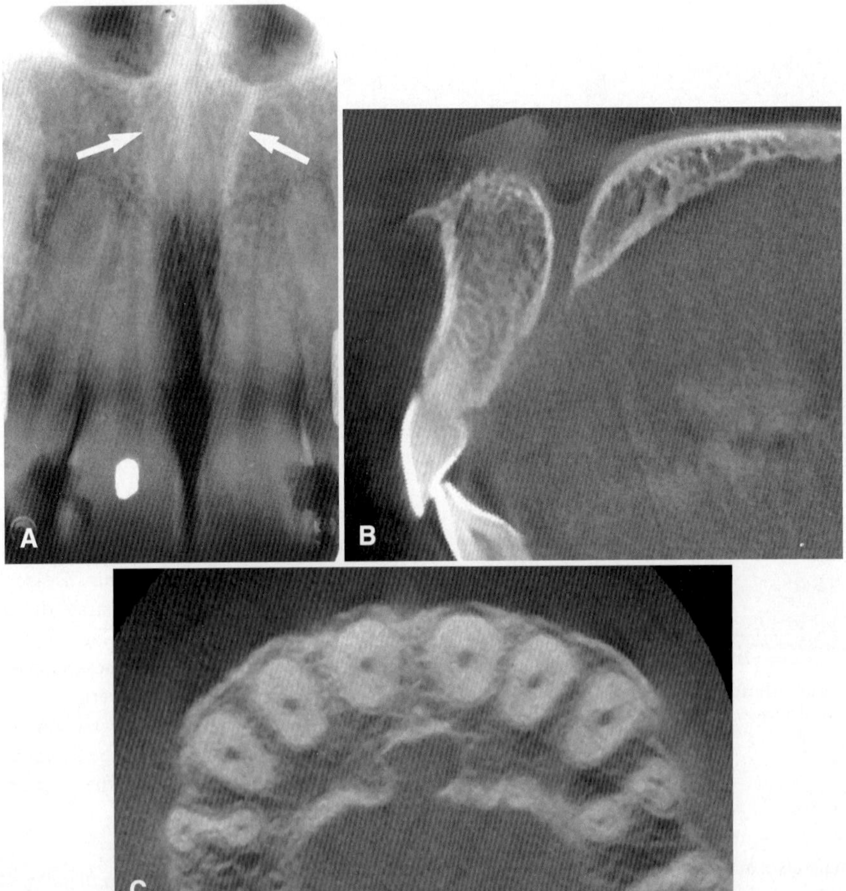

Fig. 13.29 Nasopalatine canal. (A) The lateral walls of the nasopalatine canal *(arrows)* extend from the incisive foramen to the floor of the nasal fossa. (B) Cone beam image in the sagittal plane shows superior foramina in the floor of the nasal fossa, the anterior and posterior borders of the canal, and the incisive foramen opening onto the hard palate. (C) Cone beam image in the axial plane at the level of the incisive foramen shows anterior and lateral borders of the incisive canal lying palatal to the incisor roots seen in cross section.

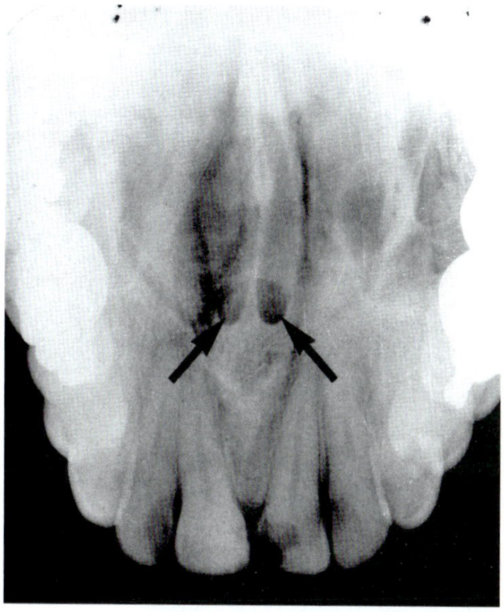

Fig. 13.30 The superior foramina of the nasopalatine canal *(arrows)* appear just lateral to the nasal septum and posterior to the anterior nasal spine.

BOX 13.4 Nasopalatine Canal—Anatomic Variation Versus Disease

- The nasopalatine canal is a potential site of cyst formation. A nasopalatine canal cyst is radiographically discernible because it frequently causes enlargement of the foramen and canal. Often the appearance of a large incisive foramen may mimic a cyst. The presence of a cyst is presumed if the width of the foramen exceeds 1 cm or if enlargement can be demonstrated on successive radiographs.
- On a periapical radiograph, the radiolucency of the normal incisive foramen may be projected over the apex of one central incisor to mimic a periapical radiolucency. The presence of an intact lamina dura around the central incisor in question and a lack of clinical symptoms will indicate absence of periapical disease.

Nose

The soft tissue of the tip of the nose is frequently seen in projections of the maxillary central and lateral incisors, superimposed over the roots of these teeth. The image of the nose has a uniform, slightly opaque appearance with a sharp border (Fig. 13.33). Occasionally, the radiolucent nares can be identified, especially when a steep vertical angle is used.

Nasolacrimal Canal

The nasal and maxillary bones form the nasolacrimal canal. It runs from the medial aspect of the anteroinferior border of the orbit inferiorly to drain under the inferior concha into the nasal cavity. The anatomy of the nasolacrimal canal is distinct on CBCT and best evaluated in the axial and coronal planes (see Plates 13.2 and 13.4). Occasionally, it can be visualized on periapical radiographs in the region above the apex of the canine, especially when a steep vertical angulation is used (Fig. 13.34). The nasolacrimal canals are usually seen on maxillary occlusal projections (see Chapter 7) in the region of the molars (Fig. 13.35).

Paranasal Sinuses

The paranasal sinuses consist of four pairs of air-filled cavities—the maxillary, frontal, sphenoid sinuses, and ethmoid air cells—and drain into the nasal cavity via ostia. The sinuses are lined by mucous membrane. Only the maxillary sinuses are visualized on periapical radiographs. CBCT scans encompass the sinuses to different extents depending on the FOV and the region being imaged. Limited- and medium-FOV CBCT imaging of the posterior maxillary arch will image some portion of the maxillary sinuses and often the ethmoid air cells. Full-FOV CBCT scans will encompass all paranasal sinuses. The intricate anatomy of the sinus boundaries and its drainage routes into the nasal cavity are the basis of radiologic sinus evaluation.

Maxillary Sinus

The maxillary sinus develops by the invagination of mucous membrane from the nasal cavity. The largest of the paranasal sinuses, it normally occupies virtually the entire body of the maxilla. Its function is unknown. The maxillary sinus may be considered as a three-sided pyramid,

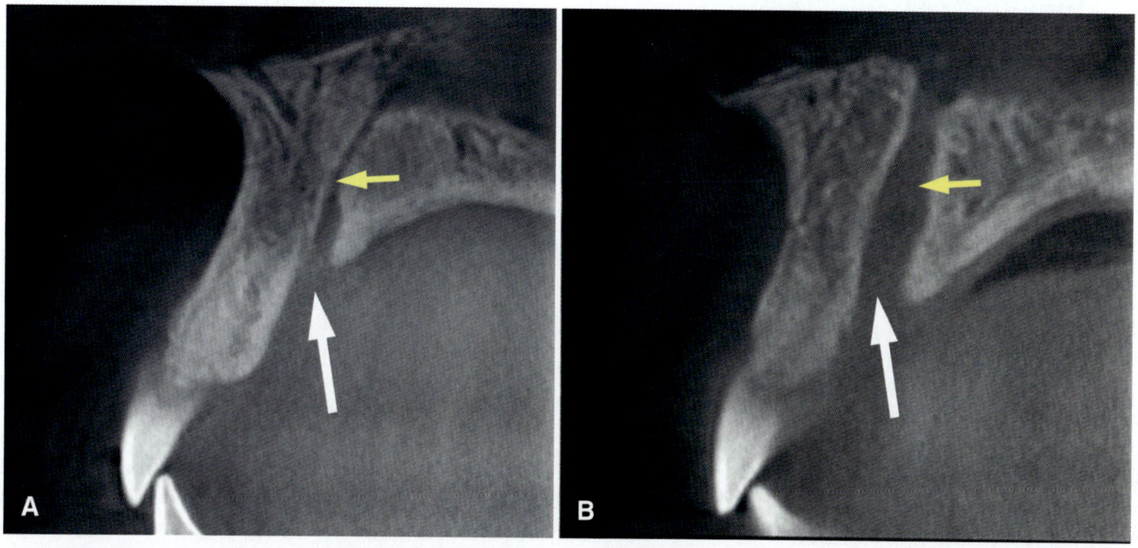

Fig. 13.31 (A) and (B) Sagittal cone beam computed tomography sections through the midsagittal plane showing the course of the nasopalatine canal *(yellow arrow)* and the opening of the incisive foramen *(white arrow)*. Note the range of normal variation in the size of these structures.

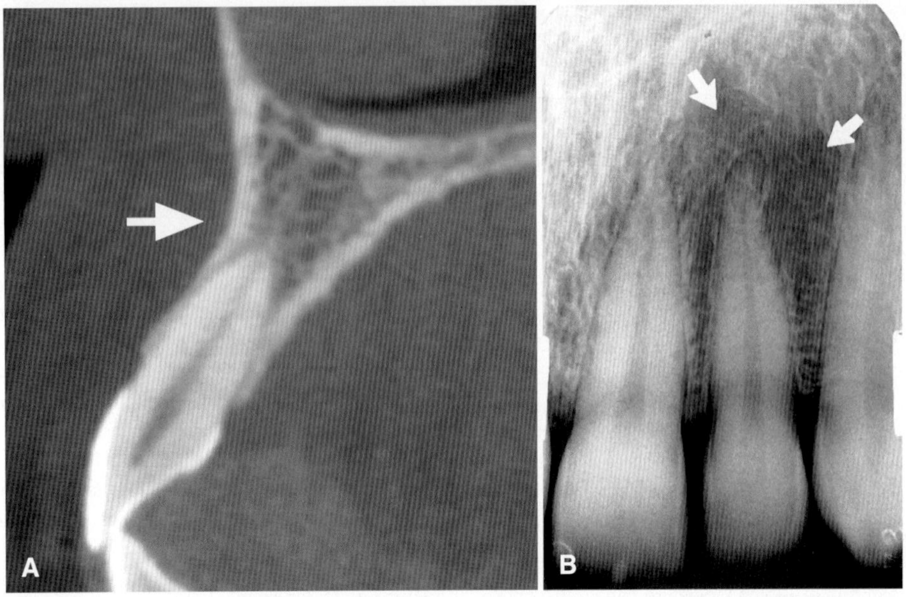

Fig. 13.32 (A) Cone beam computed tomography section through the long axis of a maxillary lateral incisor showing the lateral fossa as a depression on the buccal surface *(arrow)*. (B) The lateral fossa is a diffuse radiolucency *(arrows)* in the region of the apex of the lateral incisor.

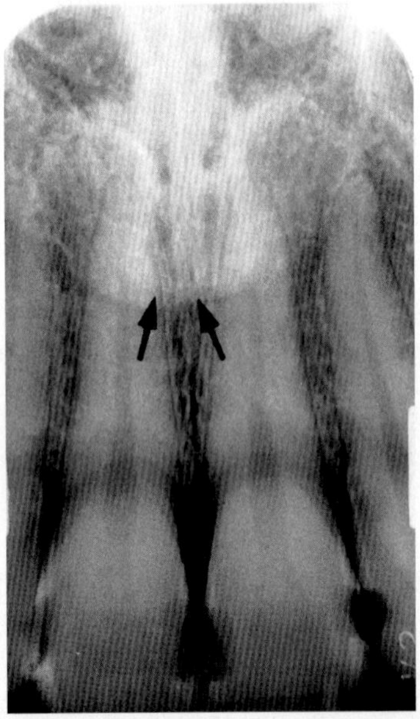

Fig. 13.33 The soft tissue outline of the nose *(arrows)* is superimposed on the anterior maxilla.

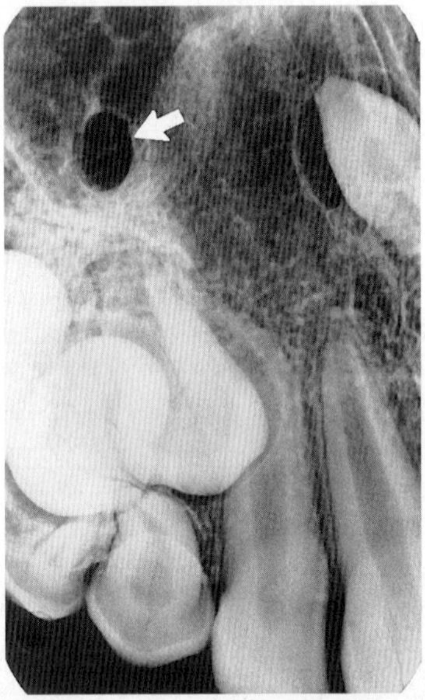

Fig. 13.34 The nasolacrimal canal *(arrow)* is occasionally seen near the apex of the canine when steep vertical angulation is used. Note the mesiodens (supernumerary tooth) in the midline superior to the central incisor.

with its base, the medial wall, adjacent to the nasal cavity and its apex extending laterally into the zygomatic process of the maxilla. Its three sides are (1) the superior wall forming the floor of the orbit, (2) the anterior wall extending above the premolars, and (3) the posterior wall bulging above the molar teeth and maxillary tuberosity. The sinus communicates with the nasal cavity by the ostium, approximately 3–6 mm in diameter and positioned under the posterior aspect of the middle concha of the ethmoid bone (see Plates 13.2, 13.4, 13.5, and 13.7).

Periapical radiographs show the inferior portion of the maxillary sinus. The maxillary sinus floor is a thin layer of cortical bone and appears as a thin radiopaque line (Fig. 13.36). In adults, the sinuses are usually seen to extend from the distal aspect of the canine to the posterior wall of the maxilla above the tuberosity. In the absence of disease, it appears continuous, but on close examination, it can be seen to have small interruptions in its continuity or radiodensity. When viewed on periapical radiographs, these discontinuities are probably illusions caused by superimposition of small marrow spaces.

The maxillary sinuses show considerable variation in size. They enlarge during childhood, achieving mature size by age 15–18 years. They may change during adult life in response to environmental factors. The right and left sinuses usually appear similar in shape and size, although marked asymmetry is occasionally present. The floors of the maxillary sinus and nasal cavity are seen on periapical radiographs at approximately the same level around the age of puberty. In older individuals,

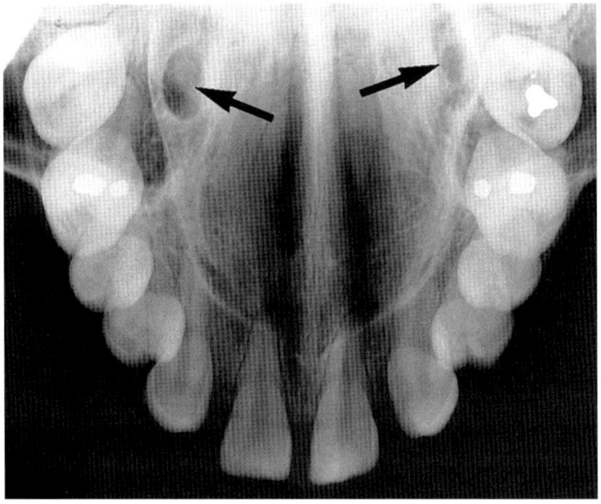

Fig. 13.35 The nasolacrimal canals are commonly seen as ovoid radiolucencies *(arrows)* on maxillary occlusal projections. They should not be confused with the greater palatine foramina, which are not apparent on maxillary occlusal projections.

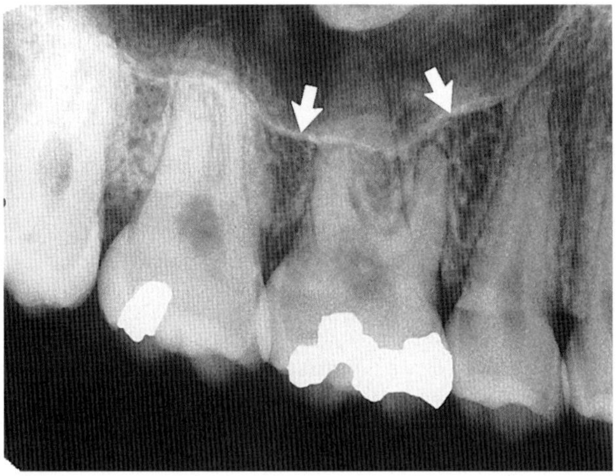

Fig. 13.36 The inferior border of the maxillary sinus *(arrows)* appears as a thin radiopaque line near the apices of the maxillary premolars and molars.

the sinus may extend farther into the alveolar process; in the posterior region of the maxilla, its floor may appear considerably below the level of the floor of the nasal cavity. Anteriorly, each sinus is restricted by the canine fossa and is usually seen to sweep superiorly, crossing the level of the floor of the nasal cavity in the premolar or canine region. Consequently, on periapical radiographs of the canine, the floors of the sinus and nasal cavity are superimposed and seen crossing one another, forming an inverted "Y" in the area (Fig. 13.37).

The degree of extension of the maxillary sinus into the alveolar process is extremely variable. In some periapical projections, the floor of the sinus is well above the apices of the posterior teeth; in others, it may extend well beyond the apices toward the alveolar ridge. In response to a loss of function (associated with the loss of posterior teeth), the sinus may expand farther into the alveolar bone, occasionally extending to the alveolar ridge (Fig. 13.38). The roots of the molars usually lie in close apposition to the maxillary sinus. Root apices may project anatomically into the floor of the sinus, causing small elevations or prominences along the maxillary sinus floor. Periapical images may convey the impression that the roots project into the sinus

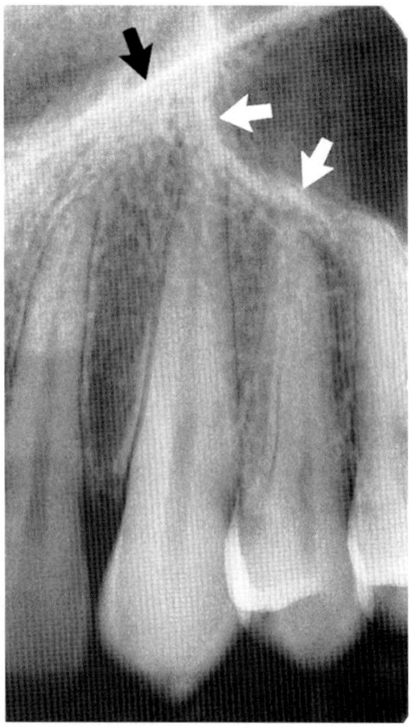

Fig. 13.37 The anterior border of the maxillary sinus *(white arrows)* crosses the floor of the nasal fossa *(black arrow)*.

BOX 13.5 Relationship Between Teeth and the Maxillary Sinus

The close relationship between the maxillary sinus and teeth leads to the possibility that clinical symptoms originating in the sinus may be perceived in the teeth and vice versa.

- Canals that carry the superior alveolar nerves traverse the anterolateral and posterolateral walls of the sinus (Fig. 13.40). The nerves are in intimate contact with the membrane lining the sinus. As a result, an acute inflammation of the sinus is frequently accompanied by pain in the maxillary teeth innervated by the portion of the nerve proximal to the area of sinus inflammation. Careful clinical evaluation of the maxillary posterior teeth to rule out dental disease is important to differentiate true odontogenic pain from sinus-related pain.
- Occasionally, periapical and periodontal inflammation from the maxillary molar teeth may extend to cause inflammation of the maxillary sinus mucosa, referred to as odontogenic maxillary sinusitis. Unlike chronic rhinosinusitis, odontogenic maxillary sinusitis is usually unilateral. Approximately 10% of maxillary sinusitis is due to odontogenic causes.

cavity, which is an illusion. The intimate relationship between the tooth roots and the maxillary sinus is evaluated better with CBCT (Fig. 13.39), and this is the modality of choice when critical evaluation of the maxillary sinus floor is clinically indicated. The thin layer of bone covering the root is seen as a fusion of the lamina dura and the floor of the sinus. Rarely, defects may be present in the bony covering of the root apices in the sinus floor, and the apical lamina dura may be indistinct. Due to this close relationship, manifestations of odontogenic disease and maxillary sinus disease are often diagnostically challenging (Box 13.5).

Frequently, thin radiolucent lines of uniform width are found within the periapical image of the maxillary sinus (see Fig. 13.40). These are the shadows of neurovascular canals or grooves in the lateral sinus walls that accommodate the posterior superior alveolar vessels, their branches, and the accompanying superior alveolar nerves. Although

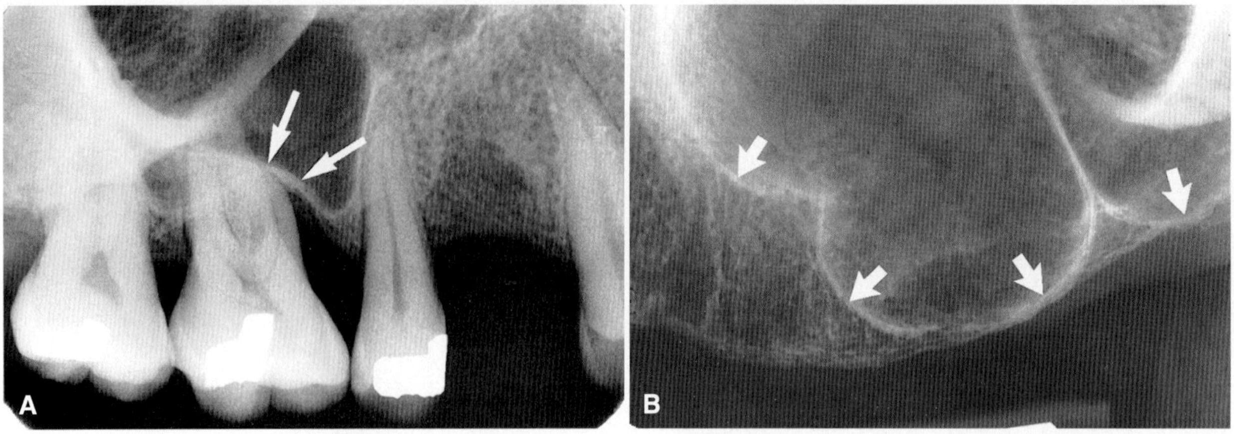

Fig. 13.38 (A and B) The floor of the maxillary sinus *(arrows)* often extends toward the crest of the alveolar ridge in response to missing teeth.

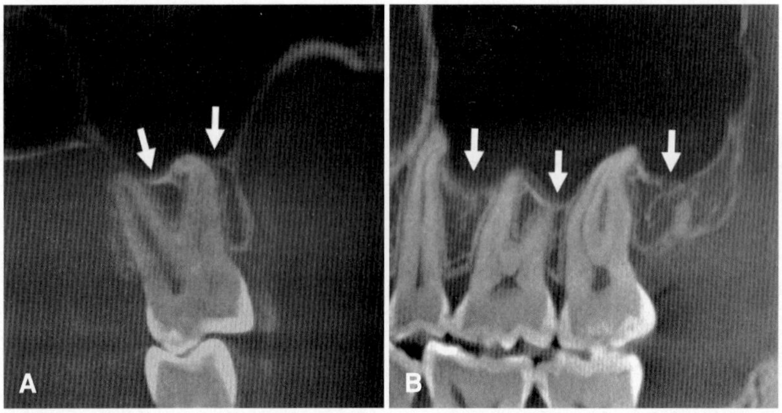

Fig. 13.39 Coronal (A) and sagittal (B) cone beam computed tomography sections through the maxillary posterior region demonstrating the relationship between the teeth and the maxillary sinus floor *(arrows)*. The corticated border of the sinus dips in between the tooth roots. Dilaceration of the mesiobuccal root of the maxillary molar is depicted on the coronal image.

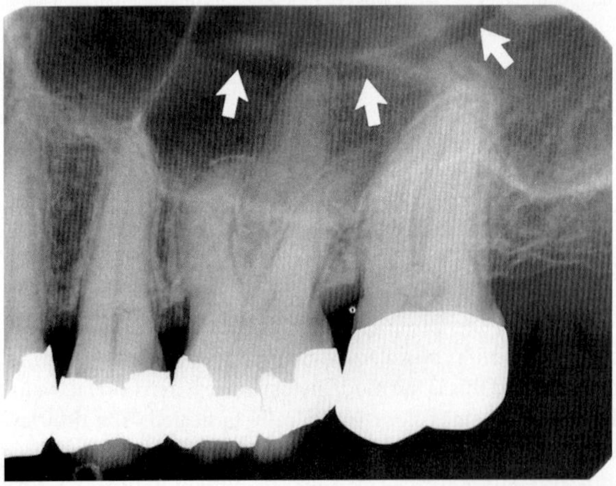

Fig. 13.40 Neurovascular canals *(arrows)* in the lateral wall of the maxillary sinus. Such vascular canals, although typically less prominent, are commonly seen in the walls of the normal maxillary sinus.

they may be found coursing in any direction (including vertically), they are usually seen running a curved posteroanterior course that is convex toward the alveolar process.

Often one or several radiopaque lines traverse the image of the maxillary sinus (Fig. 13.41). These opaque lines are called septa. They are thin folds of cortical bone that project a few millimeters away from the floor and wall of the antrum, or they may extend across the sinus. They are usually oriented vertically and vary in number, thickness, and length. Although septa appear to separate the sinuses into distinct compartments, this is seldom the case. Rather, the septa typically extend only a few millimeters into the central volume of the sinus. Septa warrant attention because they sometimes mimic periapical disease, and the chambers they create in the alveolar recess may complicate the search for a root fragment displaced into the sinus. In these clinical situations, CBCT is the modality of choice in performing this anatomic evaluation.

The floor of the maxillary sinus occasionally shows small radiopaque projections, which are nodules of bone (Fig. 13.42). These must be differentiated from root tips, which they resemble in shape. In contrast to a root fragment, which is quite homogeneous in appearance, the bony nodules often show trabeculation; although they may be quite well defined, at certain points on their surface, they blend with the trabecular pattern of adjacent bone. A root fragment may also be recognized by the presence of a root canal.

On periapical radiographs, it is common to see the floor of the nasal fossa in periapical views of the posterior teeth superimposed on the maxillary sinus (see Fig. 13.27). The floor of the nasal fossa is usually oriented more or less horizontally, depending on film placement, and is superimposed high on maxillary views. The image, a solid opaque line, frequently appears thicker than the adjacent sinus walls and septa.

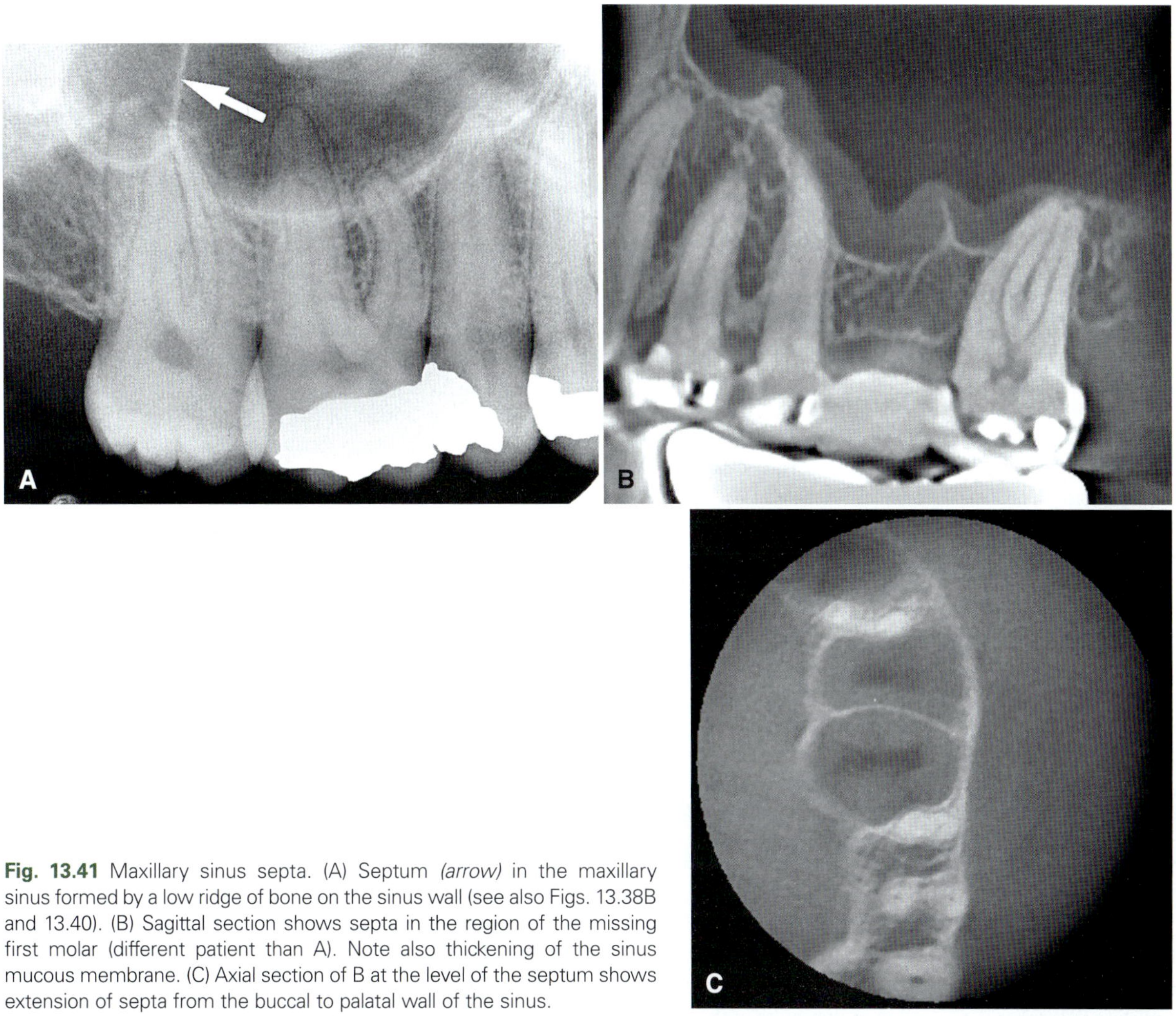

Fig. 13.41 Maxillary sinus septa. (A) Septum *(arrow)* in the maxillary sinus formed by a low ridge of bone on the sinus wall (see also Figs. 13.38B and 13.40). (B) Sagittal section shows septa in the region of the missing first molar (different patient than A). Note also thickening of the sinus mucous membrane. (C) Axial section of B at the level of the septum shows extension of septa from the buccal to palatal wall of the sinus.

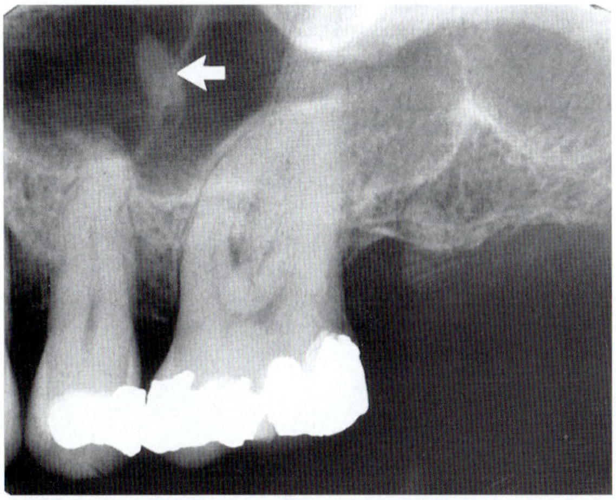

Fig. 13.42 This bony mass *(arrow)* may represent a bony nodule, a normal variant of the floor of the maxillary sinus, but is most likely a retained root fragment from a prior extraction.

Ethmoid, Sphenoid, and Frontal Sinuses

The ethmoid, sphenoid, and frontal sinuses are not in the imaging field for periapical radiography. However, these sinuses are well visualized on CBCT scans and on panoramic and cephalometric radiographs. When the paranasal sinuses are imaged on CBCT scans, the anatomic boundaries and drainage patterns of the sinus must be systematically examined (Box 13.6).

The ethmoidal sinuses are divided into the anterior and posterior ethmoidal air cells by the basal lamella—the attachment of the middle concha to the lamina paprecea. The number of air cells per side ranges from 3 to 18. Frequently extramural air cells—air cells outside of the ethmoid bone—can be visualized. These include agger nasi air cells, causing pneumatization of the lacrimal bone, and Haller cells, which cause pneumatization of the orbital floor. Occasionally Haller cells are seen on panoramic images (see Chapter 8).

The sphenoid sinuses are midline structures in the body of the sphenoid bone and start to develop at approximately 4 months in utero. The sinuses vary considerably in size, and the right and left sphenoid sinuses are often asymmetric and separated by a bony septum. Often multiple septa are present, giving the sinus a "locular" appearance. The sphenoid sinuses may extend inferiorly, resulting in pneumatization of the pterygoid bones. The sphenoid sinuses are not visualized on periapical images but are well demonstrated on CBCT scans and on lateral cephalometric radiographs (see Chapter 7).

The frontal sinuses are the last paranasal sinuses to develop, usually starting at approximately 6–7 years of age. Hypoplasia of the frontal sinus is a common normal variant, and aplasia of the frontal sinuses is noted in approximately 4% of the population. The frontal sinuses are well demonstrated on CBCT scans and on cephalometric radiographs (see Chapter 7).

BOX 13.6 Systematic Evaluation of Paranasal Sinuses on Computed Tomography Scans

In a normal paranasal sinus, the epithelial lining is relatively thin and barely visible on radiographs. Thus the sinuses appear radiolucent, with a well-corticated bony outline. Inflammatory and neoplastic changes in the sinus lining appear as a soft tissue density contrasted against the air-filled cavity. Sinuses are evaluated for the presence of soft tissue thickening, the integrity of the borders, and the patency of the drainage paths of the paranasal sinuses. Evaluation of the paranasal sinuses should include a critical examination of the following anatomic structures:

- *Osteomeatal complex*: The maxillary sinus drains via the ostium into the infundibulum—a channel between the uncinate process of the ethmoid bone and the inferomedial wall of the orbit (see Plates 13.1, 13.2, 13.4, and 13.5). The infundibulum channels drain into the hiatus semilunaris (see Plate 13.4) and then into the middle meatus. The complex of the maxillary ostium, infundibulum, uncinate process, hiatus semilunaris, ethmoidal bulla, and middle meatus is referred to as the osteomeatal complex. This region is the common drainage path for the frontal and maxillary sinuses and anterior ethmoidal air cells and thus must be carefully inspected for patency. This complex is best visualized on the coronal and axial sections.
- *Frontal recess*: This is the path for the drainage of the frontal sinus into the middle meatus. This recess is best visualized on sagittal and coronal sections (see Plate 13.4).
- *Sphenoethmoidal recess:* This is the drainage path for the sphenoid sinus and posterior ethmoidal air cells in the superior meatus at the posterior region of the nasal cavity. This recess is located between the posterior ethmoidal cells and the sphenoid sinus (see Plate 13.1). It is best appreciated in axial and sagittal sections.

Zygomatic Process and Zygoma

The zygomatic process of the maxilla is an extension of the lateral maxillary surface that arises in the region of the apices of the first and second molars and articulates with the maxillary process of the zygoma. On periapical radiographs, the zygomatic process appears as a U-shaped radiopaque line with its open end directed superiorly. The enclosed rounded end is projected in the apical region of the first and second molars (Fig. 13.43). The size, width, and definition of the zygomatic process are quite variable, and its image may be large, depending on the angle at which the beam was projected. The maxillary antrum may expand laterally into the zygomatic process of the maxilla (and into the zygomatic bone after the maxillozygomatic suture has fused), resulting in a relatively increased radiolucent region within the U-shaped image of the process.

When the sinus is recessed deep within the process, as in Fig. 13.43B (and perhaps into the zygoma), the image of the air space within the process is dark. Typically, the walls of the process are thin and well defined (in contrast to the very dark radiolucent air space). When the sinus exhibits relatively little penetration of the maxillary process, as in Fig. 13.43A (usually in younger individuals or individuals who have maintained their posterior teeth and vigorous masticatory function), the image of the walls of the zygomatic process of the maxilla tends to be thicker, and the appearance of the sinus in this region is smaller and more opaque.

The inferior border of the zygoma extends posteriorly from the inferior border of the zygomatic process of the maxilla to the zygomatic process of the temporal bone. It can be identified as a uniform radiopacity over the apices of the molars (Fig. 13.44). The zygomatic process of the temporal bone and the body of the zygoma compose the zygomatic arch. The prominence of the molar apices superimposed on the shadow of the zygoma and the amount of periapical detail supplied by the radiograph depend primarily on the extent of aeration (pneumatization) of the zygoma by the maxillary sinus and on the orientation of the x-ray beam.

The zygomatic processes of the maxilla articulate posteriorly with the maxillary process of the zygoma. These two processes form the anterior segment of the zygomatic arch (see Plates 13.2 and 13.5). The zygomaticomaxillary suture is visualized as a thin, radiolucent, and jagged line in this portion of the arch. Disruptions of the integrity or symmetry of the arch may be associated with craniofacial developmental abnormalities or facial trauma.

Nasolabial Fold

An oblique line demarcating a region that appears to be covered by a veil of slight radiopacity frequently traverses periapical radiographs of the premolar region (Fig. 13.45). The line of contrast is sharp, and the area of increased radiopacity is posterior to the line. The line is the nasolabial fold, and the opaque veil is the thick cheek tissue superimposed on the teeth and the alveolar process. The image of the fold becomes more evident with age, as the repeated creasing of the skin along the line (where the elevator of the lip, zygomatic head, and orbicularis all insert into the skin) and the degeneration of the elastic fibers finally lead to the formation and deepening of permanent folds. The image of the

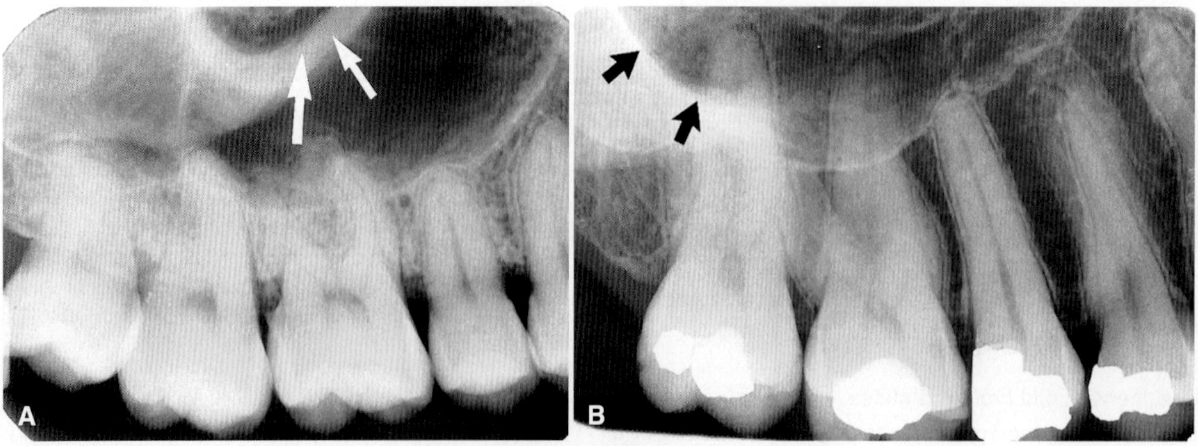

Fig. 13.43 The zygomatic process of the maxilla *(arrows)* protrudes laterally from the maxillary wall. Its size may be quite variable: small with thick borders (A) or large with thin borders (B).

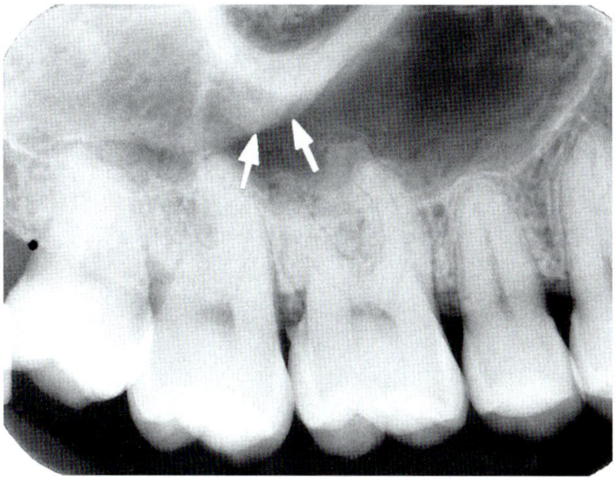

Fig. 13.44 The inferior border of the zygoma *(arrows)* extends posteriorly from the inferior portion of the zygomatic process of the maxilla.

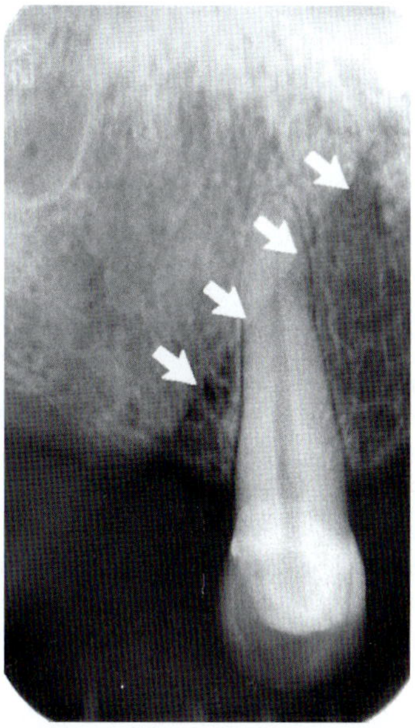

Fig. 13.45 The nasolabial soft tissue fold *(arrows)* extends across the canine-premolar region.

nasolabial fold courses inferior and posterior. This helps to decipher the anterior and posterior orientation of radiographs of an edentulous maxillary ridge.

Pterygoid Plates

The medial and lateral pterygoid plates lie immediately posterior to the maxilla. These structures are best visualized on coronal and axial CT sections (see Plates 13.2 and 13.5) and must be carefully evaluated when assessing a patient with facial trauma. Involvement of the pterygoid plates is an essential feature of Le Fort fractures (see Chapter 25). The images on these two plates are extremely variable, and they do not appear at all on many intraoral radiographs of the third molar area. When they are apparent, they almost always cast a single radiopaque homogeneous shadow without any evidence of trabeculation (Fig. 13.46). Extending inferiorly from the medial pterygoid plate is the hamular process (Fig. 13.47), which on close inspection can show trabeculae.

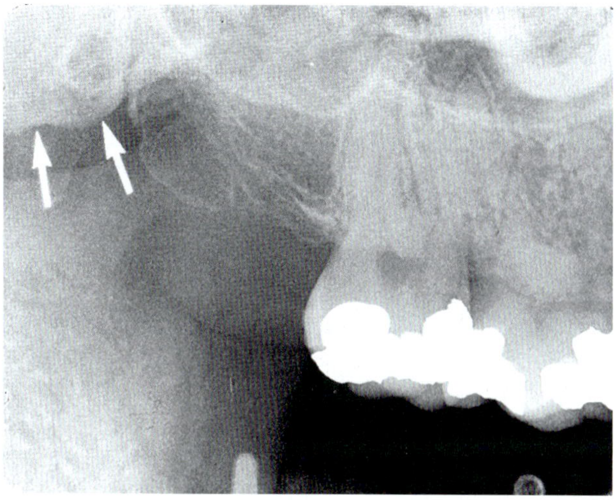

Fig. 13.46 Pterygoid plates *(arrows)* located posterior to the maxillary tuberosity.

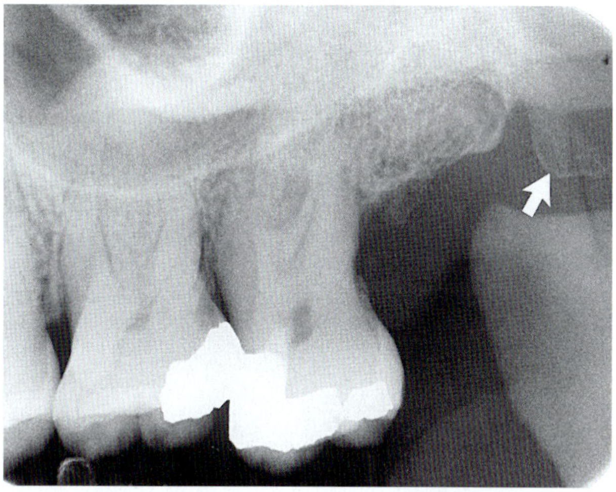

Fig. 13.47 The hamular process *(arrow)* extends inferiorly from the medial pterygoid plate.

MANDIBLE

Symphysis

Radiographs of the region of the mandibular symphysis in infants demonstrate a radiolucent line through the midline of the jaw between the images of the forming deciduous central incisors (Fig. 13.48). This suture usually fuses by the end of the first year of life, after which it is no longer radiographically apparent. It is not frequently encountered on dental radiographs because few young patients have cause to be examined radiographically. If this radiolucency is found in older individuals, it is abnormal and may suggest a fracture or a cleft.

Genial Tubercles

The genial tubercles (also called the mental spine) are located on the lingual surface of the mandible slightly above the inferior border and in the midline. They are bony protuberances, more or less spine shaped, that are often divided into a right and left prominence and a superior and inferior prominence. They attach the genioglossus muscles (at the superior tubercles) and the geniohyoid muscles (at the inferior tubercles) to the mandible. They are well visualized on mandibular occlusal radiographs as one or more small projections (Fig. 13.49). Their appearance

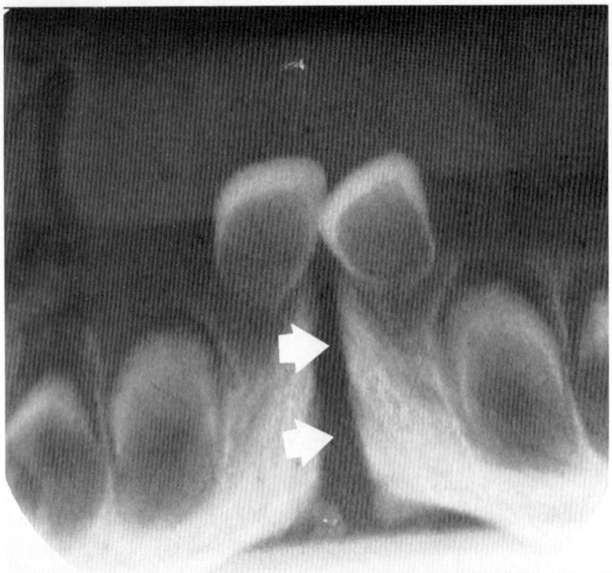

Fig. 13.48 Mandibular symphysis *(arrows)* in a newborn infant. This suture closed within the first year. Note the erupted bilateral supernumerary primary incisors.

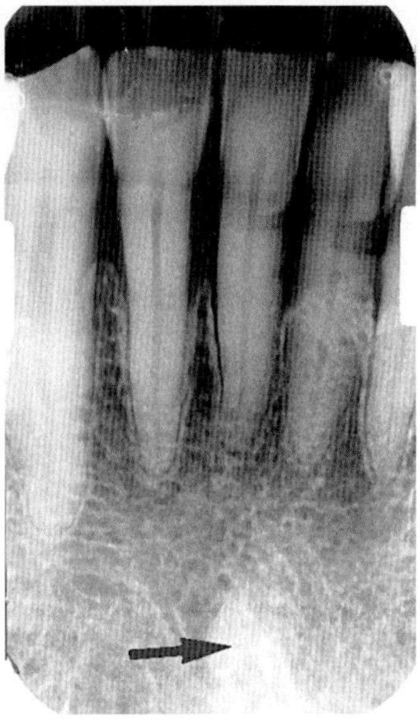

Fig. 13.50 The genial tubercles *(arrow)* appear as a radiopaque mass, in this case without evidence of the lingual foramen.

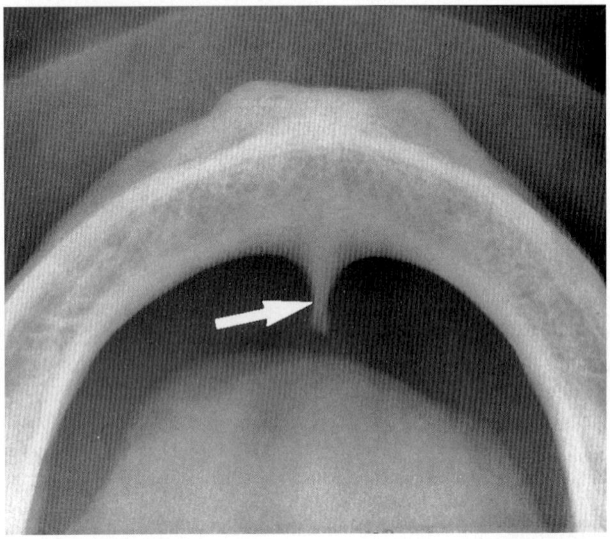

Fig. 13.49 Genial tubercle *(arrow)* on the lingual surface of the mandible in this cross-sectional mandibular occlusal view. This tubercle is unusually prominent.

on periapical radiographs of the mandibular incisor region is variable; often they appear as a radiopaque mass (3–4 mm in diameter) in the midline below the incisor roots (Fig. 13.50). They may also not be apparent at all.

Lingual Foramen

Midline lingual foramina are present in 96%–100% of individuals, located in the region of the genial tubercles (see Plate 13.8B). The superior foramen contains a neurovascular bundle from the lingual arteries and nerve, whereas the inferior foramen is supplied from the sublingual or submental arteries and from the mylohyoid nerve. On periapical radiographs, the lingual foramen (Fig. 13.51) is typically visualized as a single round radiolucent canal with a well-defined opaque border lying in the midline below the level of the apices of the incisors.

The anatomic location is essential in presurgical treatment planning because damage to the neurovascular bundle in the course of implant bed preparation, for example, may lead to excessive bleeding.

Mental Ridge

On periapical radiographs of the mandibular central incisors, the mental ridge (protuberance) may occasionally be seen as two radiopaque lines sweeping bilaterally forward and upward toward the midline (Fig. 13.52). They are of variable width and density and may be found to extend from low in the premolar area on each side up to the midline, where they lie just inferior to or are superimposed on the mandibular incisor tooth roots. The image of the mental ridge is most prominent when the beam is directed parallel with the surface of the mental tubercle (as in using the bisecting-angle technique).

Mental Fossa

The mental fossa is a depression on the labial aspect of the mandible extending laterally from the midline and above the mental ridge. Because of the resulting thinness of jawbone in this area, the image of this depression may be similar to that of the submandibular fossa (see later) and likewise may be mistaken for periapical disease involving the incisors (Fig. 13.53).

Mental Foramen

The mental foramen is usually the anterior limit of the inferior dental canal that is apparent on periapical radiographs (Fig. 13.54). Its image is quite variable, and it may be identified on periapical radiographs only about half the time because the opening of the mental canal is directed superiorly and posteriorly. As a result, the usual view of the premolars is not projected through the long axis of the canal opening. This circumstance is responsible for the variable appearance of the mental foramen. Although the wall of the foramen consists of cortical bone, the density of the image of the foramen varies, as does the shape and definition of its border. It may be round, oblong, slit-like, or very irregular and partially or completely corticated. The foramen is seen about halfway between the lower border of the mandible and the crest of the alveolar process, usually in the region of the apex of the second premolar. Also, because it lies on the surface of the mandible, the

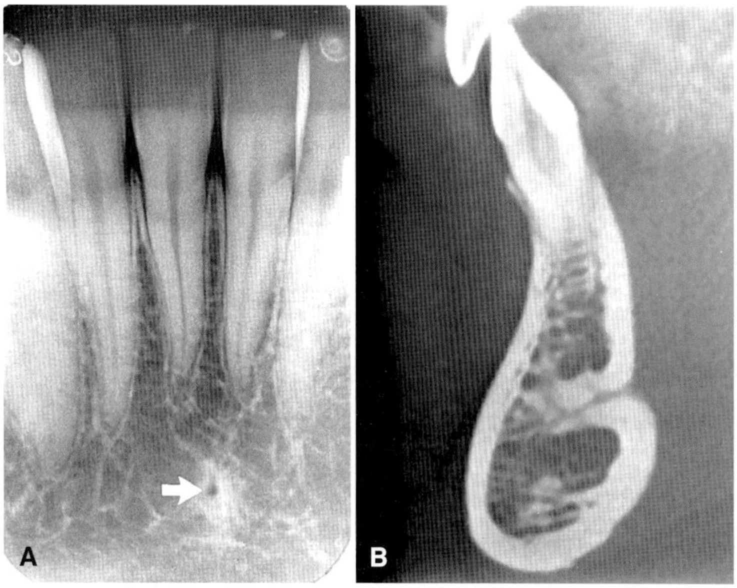

Fig. 13.51 Lingual foramen. (A) Lingual foramen on a periapical view *(arrow)*, with a sclerotic border, in the symphyseal region of the mandible. (B) Cone beam sagittal section through mandibular midline shows superior lingual foramen extending deep into the mandible from the lingual surface.

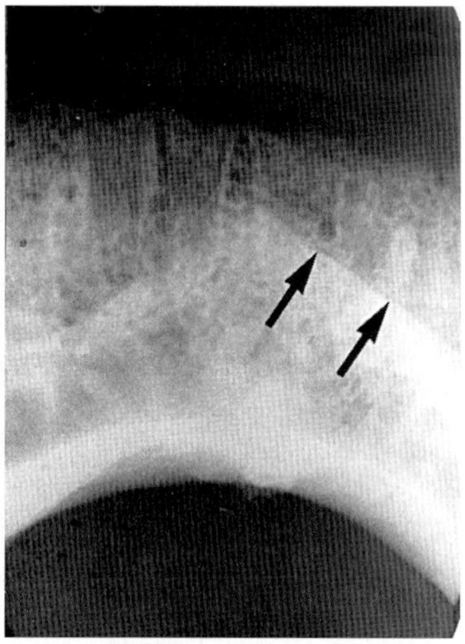

Fig. 13.52 Mental ridge *(arrows)* on the anterior surface of the mandible, seen as a radiopaque ridge. The mental ridge is most prominent when the beam is angled from well below the occlusal plane.

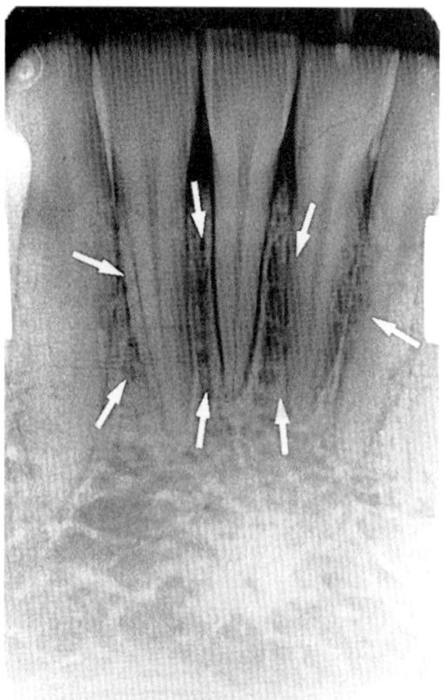

Fig. 13.53 The mental fossa is a depression on the anterior surface of the mandible and is seen as a radiolucent area with ill-defined borders *(arrows)* in the region of the incisor roots.

position of its image in relation to the tooth roots is influenced by projection angulation. It may be projected anywhere from just mesial of the permanent first molar roots to as far anterior as mesial of the first premolar root.

The location and size of the mental foramen is better evaluated on CT sections (Fig. 13.55 and Plate 13.3). When visualization of the mental foramen is critical to the treatment plan, as in implant placement, CBCT is the modality of choice. An important anatomic variation to detect when placing implants in the premolar region is the anterior loop, where the inferior alveolar canal extends anterior to the mental foramen before it loops posteriorly to exit through the mental foramen. The incidence of an accessory mental foramen is about 7%.

When the mental foramen is projected over one of the premolar apices, it may mimic periapical disease (Fig. 13.56). In such cases, evidence of the inferior alveolar canal extending to the suspect radiolucency or a detectable lamina dura in the area would suggest the true

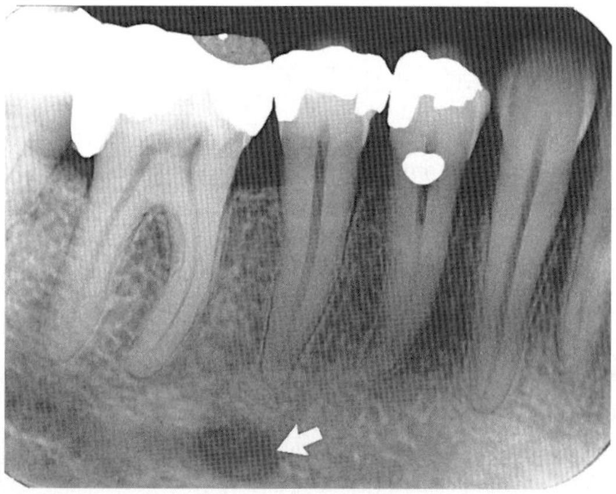

Fig. 13.54 The mental foramen *(arrow)* appears as an oval radiolucency typically near the apex of the second premolar.

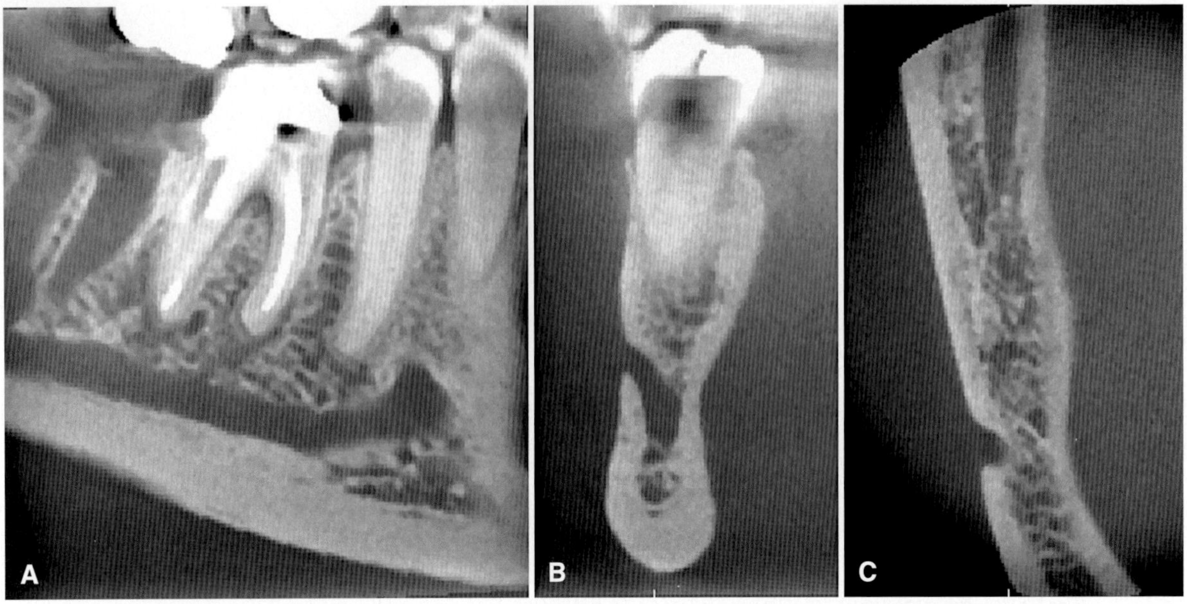

Fig. 13.55 Cone beam images through the mental foramen. (A) Sagittal section through the body of the mandible shows the inferior alveolar canal rising toward the mental foramen, which lies anterior to the apex of the second premolar. (B) Coronal section through the mental foramen shows how the inferior alveolar canal ascends to exit through the buccal cortex at the mental foramen. A clear understanding of this anatomy is important when implants are placed in this region. (C) Axial section through the mental foramen demonstrates posterior inclination of the opening of the mental foramen on the mandibular buccal surface. Note also the section of the inferior alveolar canal lying more posteriorly, inferior to the molars, and adjacent to the lingual cortex *(top of image)*.

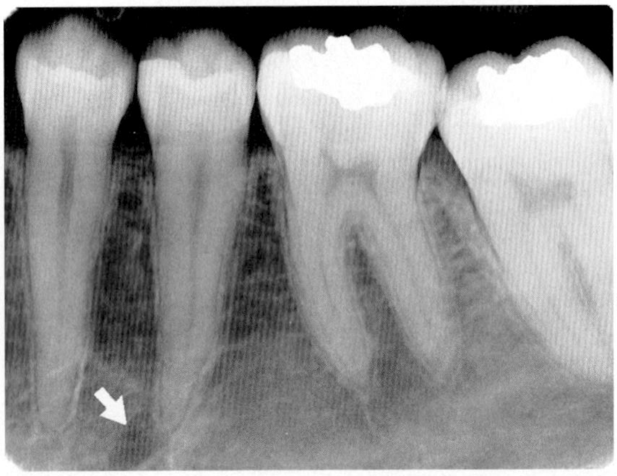

Fig. 13.56 The mental foramen *(arrow)* (over the apex of the second premolar) may simulate periapical disease. However, continuity of the lamina dura around the apex indicates the absence of periapical abnormality.

nature of the dark shadow. However, the relative thinness of the lamina dura superimposed with the radiolucent foramen may result in considerable "burnout" of the lamina dura image, which complicates its recognition. Nevertheless, a second radiograph from another angle is likely to show the lamina dura clearly as well as some shift in position of the radiolucent foramen relative to the apex.

Inferior Alveolar Canal

The radiographic image of the inferior alveolar canal is a dark linear shadow with thin radiopaque superior and inferior borders cast by the lamella of bone that bounds the canal (Fig. 13.57). Sometimes the borders are seen only partially or not at all. The width of the canal shows some interpatient variability but is usually constant anterior to the third molar region. The canal's course may be apparent between the mandibular and mental foramina. Only rarely is the image of its anterior continuation toward the midline discernible on the radiograph.

The relationship of the inferior alveolar canal to the roots of the lower teeth may vary from one in which there is close contact with all molars and the second premolar to one in which the canal has no intimate relationship to any of the posterior teeth. In the usual picture, however, the canal is in contact with the apex of the third molar, and the distance between it and the other roots increases as it progresses anteriorly. When the apices of the molars are projected over the canal, the lamina dura may be overexposed, conveying the impression of a missing lamina or a thickened PDL space that is more radiolucent than apparently normal for the patient (Fig. 13.58). To ensure the soundness of such a tooth, other clinical testing procedures must be used (e.g., vitality testing). Because the canal is usually located just inferior to the apices of the posterior teeth, altering the vertical angle for a second periapical radiograph of the area is not likely to separate the images of the apices and canal.

The course of the inferior alveolar canal is well demonstrated on CT scans (Fig. 13.59 and Plate 13.8C and F). In cross-sectional and coronal slices, the inferior alveolar canal is typically seen as an oval or round radiolucency with corticated borders (see Fig. 13.59). Sometimes the cortication may be thin or imperceptible. The relationship of the canal to the tooth roots should be assessed. This relationship varies greatly among patients, especially in the molar region, with the inferior alveolar canal occupying a position from close to the root apices to adjacent to the inferior border of the mandible. Other variations include bifid inferior alveolar canal with a reported frequency of about 15%; these can be seen on panoramic and cone beam images (see Fig. 13.59). Patients with bifid canals are at greater risk of inadequate anesthesia or surgical complications, for example, from implant placement.

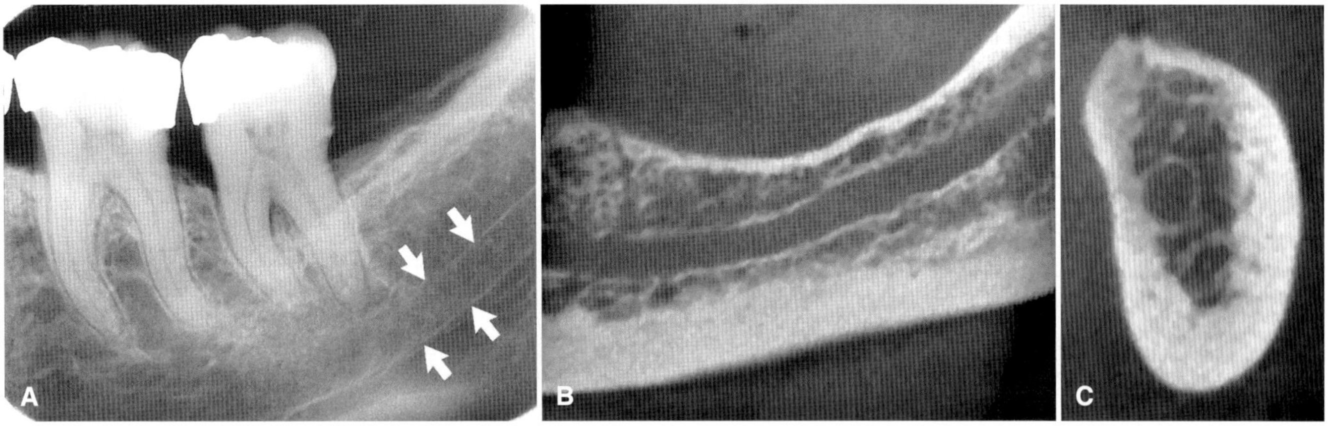

Fig. 13.57 Inferior alveolar canal. (A) On periapical view, *arrows* denote radiopaque superior and inferior cortical borders. (B) Cone beam section through the body of the mandible (different patient) shows corticated borders of the inferior alveolar canal. (C) Cone beam cross-sectional view shows the circular inferior alveolar canal with corticated borders lying adjacent to the lingual plate.

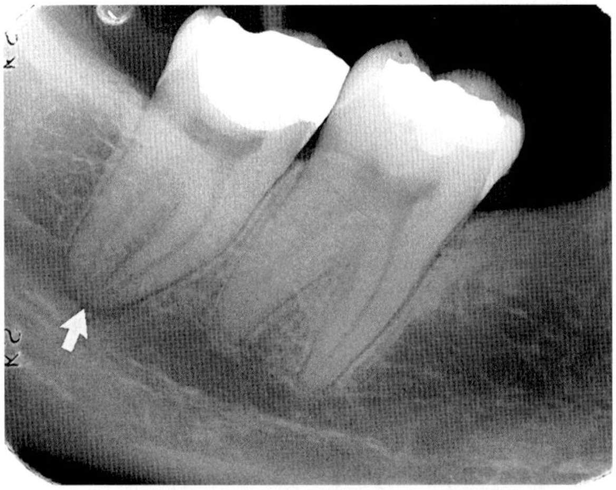

Fig. 13.58 Superimposition of the inferior alveolar canal over the apex of a molar causes the image of the periodontal ligament space to appear wider *(arrow)*. However, the presence of an intact lamina dura indicates that there is no periapical disease.

Nutrient Canals

Nutrient canals carry a neurovascular bundle and appear as radiolucent lines of fairly uniform width. They are most often seen on mandibular periapical radiographs running vertically from the inferior dental canal directly to the apex of a tooth (Fig. 13.60) or into the interdental space between the mandibular incisors (Fig. 13.61). They are visible in about 5%–40% of all patients and are more frequent in Black patients, male patients, older patients, and patients with high blood pressure, diabetes mellitus, or advanced periodontal disease. They may be accentuated in a thin ridge. Because they are anatomic spaces with walls of cortical bone, their images occasionally have hyperostotic borders. Sometimes a nutrient canal is oriented perpendicular to the cortex and appears as a small round radiolucency simulating a pathologic radiolucency.

Mylohyoid Ridge

The mylohyoid ridge (also called the internal oblique ridge) is a slightly irregular crest of bone on the lingual surface of the mandibular body. Its anterior margin lies about 10 mm inferior to the alveolar ridge lingual to the second premolar and extends posteriorly to the area of the third molar about 5 mm below the alveolar crest. This ridge serves as an attachment for the mylohyoid muscle. On a periapical radiograph, its image runs diagonally downward and forward from the area of the third molars to the premolar region at approximately the level of the apices of the posterior teeth (Fig. 13.62). This image is sometimes superimposed on the images of the molar roots. The margins of the image are not usually well defined but appear quite diffuse and of variable width. Occasionally, the ridge is relatively dense with sharply demarcated borders (Fig. 13.63). It is more evident on periapical radiographs when the beam is positioned with excessive negative angulation. Generally, as the ridge becomes less defined, its anterior and posterior limits blend gradually with the surrounding bone.

Submandibular Gland Fossa

On the lingual surface of the mandibular body, immediately below the mylohyoid ridge in the molar area, there is frequently a depression in the bone. This concavity accommodates the submandibular gland and often appears as a radiolucent area with the sparse trabecular pattern characteristic of the region (Fig. 13.64). This trabecular pattern is even less defined on periapical and panoramic radiographs of the area because it is superimposed on the relatively reduced mass of the concavity. The radiographic image of the fossa is sharply limited superiorly by the mylohyoid ridge and inferiorly by the lower border of the mandible but is poorly defined anteriorly (in the premolar region) and posteriorly (at about the ascending ramus). Although the image may appear strikingly radiolucent, accentuated as it is by the dense mylohyoid ridge and inferior border of the mandible, awareness of its possible presence should preclude its being confused with a bony lesion by inexperienced clinicians.

CBCT scans allow assessment of the submandibular fossa region in the coronal and axial planes. The extent and depth of this concavity, or undercut, varies greatly (see Plate 13.8D). The identification of this anatomic feature is crucial in examining mandibular anatomy for implant treatment planning.

External Oblique Ridge

The external oblique ridge is a continuation of the anterior border of the mandibular ramus. It follows an anteroinferior course lateral to the alveolar process and is relatively prominent in its upper part; it juts considerably on the outer surface of the mandible in the region of the third molar (Fig. 13.65). This bony elevation gradually flattens and usually disappears at about where the alveolar process and mandible

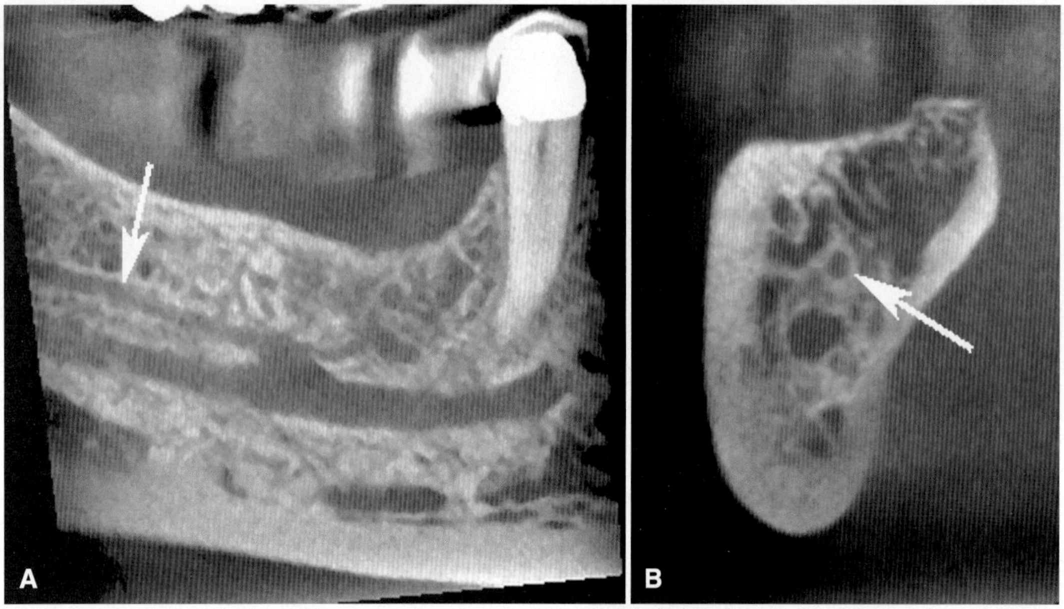

Fig. 13.59 Bifid inferior alveolar canal. (A) Cone beam sagittal section through the body of the mandible shows a bifid inferior alveolar canal. The superior branch has a smaller diameter than the primary canal *(arrow)*. (B) Cross-sectional image shows primary canal and superior secondary canal *(arrow)*.

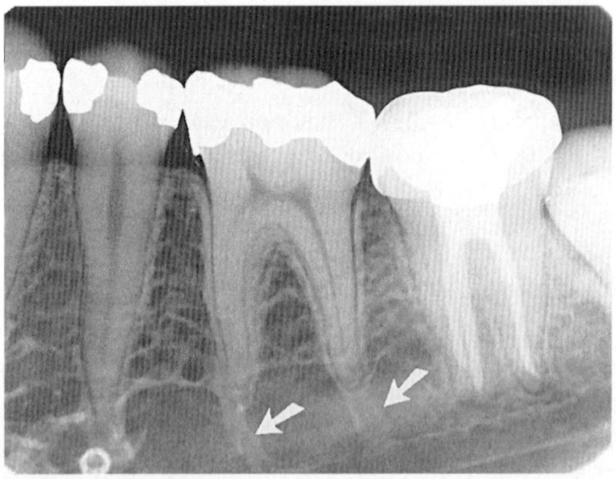

Fig. 13.60 Nutrient canals *(arrows)*, demonstrated by radiopaque cortical borders, descend from the mandibular first molar. Nutrient canals at this location are a common finding.

join below the first molar. The ridge is a line of attachment of the buccinator muscle. Characteristically, it is projected onto posterior periapical radiographs superior to the mylohyoid ridge, with which it runs an almost parallel course. It appears as a radiopaque line of varying width, density, and length, blending at its anterior end with the shadow of the alveolar bone.

Inferior Border of the Mandible

Occasionally, the inferior mandibular border is seen on periapical projections (Fig. 13.66) as a characteristically dense, broad, and radiopaque band of bone.

Coronoid Process

The image of the coronoid process of the mandible is frequently apparent on periapical radiographs of the maxillary molar region as a triangular radiopacity, with its apex directed superiorly and anteriorly, superimposed on the region of the third molar (Fig. 13.67). In some cases, it may appear as far forward as the second molar and be projected above, over, or below these molars, depending on the position of the jaw and the projection of the x-ray beam. Usually the shadow of the coronoid process is homogeneous, although internal trabeculation can be seen in some cases. Its appearance on maxillary molar radiographs results from the downward and forward movement of the mandible when the mouth is open. Consequently, if the opacity reduces the diagnostic value of the image, the radiograph must be remade, and the second view should be

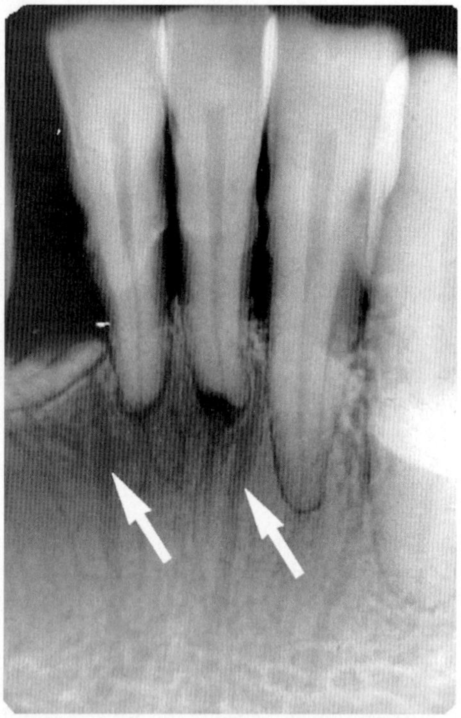

Fig. 13.61 Nutrient canals seen as vertical radiolucent structures *(arrows)* in the anterior mandible are often associated with periodontal disease as in this patient.

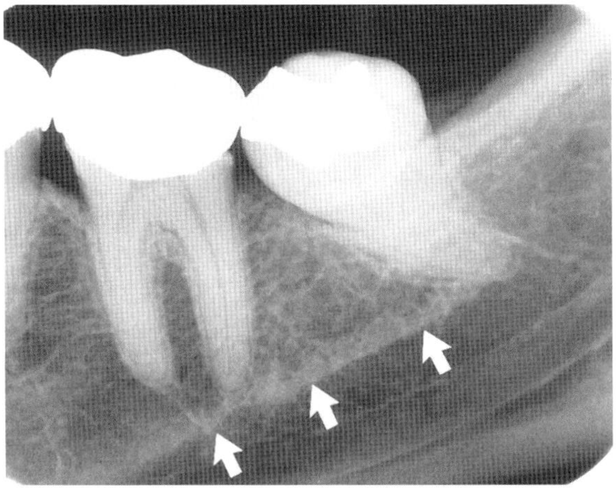

Fig. 13.62 Mylohyoid ridge *(arrows)* running at the level of the molar apices and above the inferior alveolar canal.

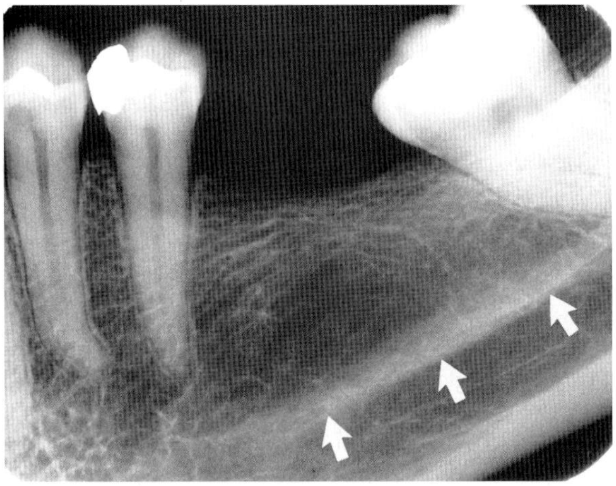

Fig. 13.63 The mylohyoid ridge *(arrows)* may be dense, especially when a radiograph is exposed with excessive negative angulation.

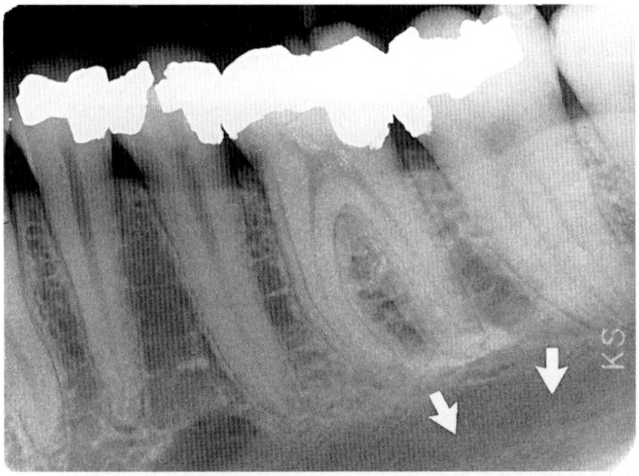

Fig. 13.64 Submandibular gland fossa *(arrows)*, indicated by a radiolucent region with ill-defined borders and sparse trabecular bone lying inferiorly to the mandibular molars.

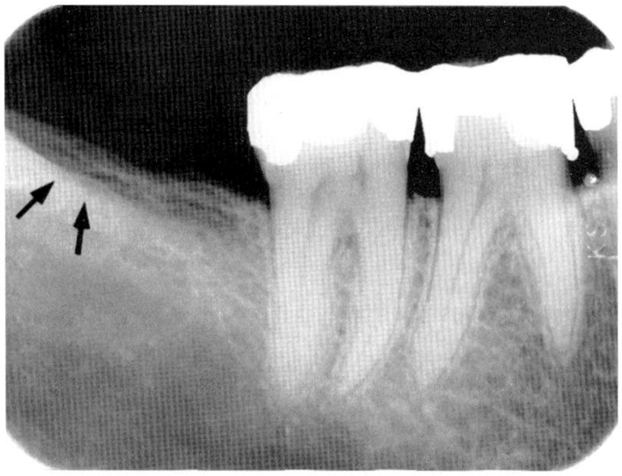

Fig. 13.65 External oblique ridge *(arrows)* on the buccal surface of the mandible, seen as a radiopaque line near the alveolar crest in the mandibular third molar region.

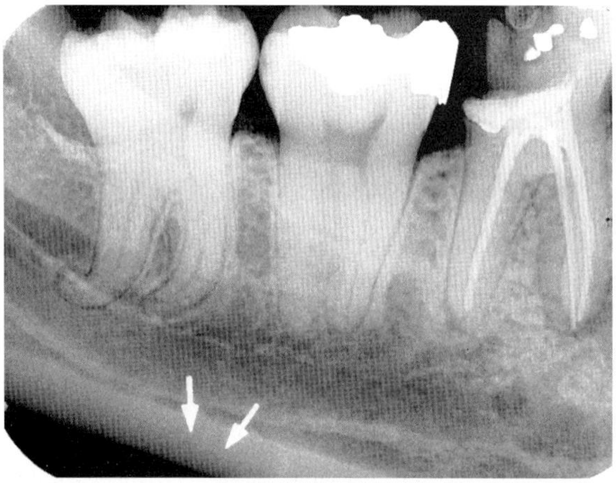

Fig. 13.66 The inferior border of the mandible *(arrows)* is seen as a dense, broad radiopaque band.

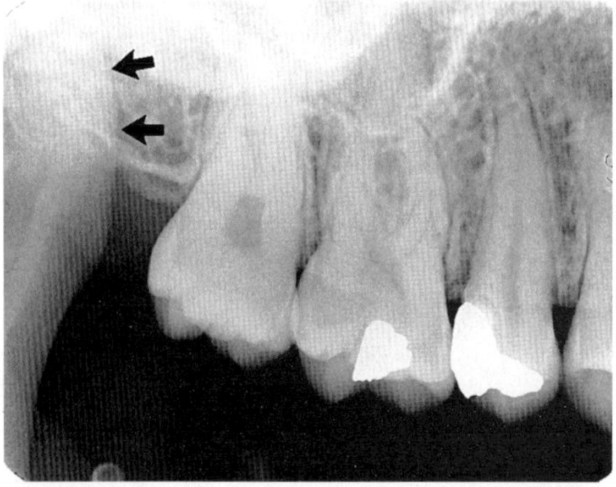

Fig. 13.67 Coronoid process of the mandible *(arrows)* superimposed on the maxillary tuberosity.

acquired with the mouth minimally open. (This contingency must be considered whenever this area is radiographically examined.) Occasionally, especially when its shadow is dense and homogeneous, the coronoid process is mistaken for a root fragment. The true nature of the shadow can be easily demonstrated by obtaining two radiographs with the mouth in different positions and noting the change in position of the suspect shadow.

The coronoid process is viewed free of superimposition on CT images (see Plates 13.2 and 13.5). When the primary diagnostic task is evaluation of the coronoid process—for example, to assess coronoid hyperplasia—CT imaging, preferably CBCT, should be the modality of choice.

TEMPOROMANDIBULAR JOINT

The temporomandibular joint (TMJ) region is imaged on panoramic, cephalometric, and CBCT imaging. The TMJ is the articulation between the glenoid fossa of the temporal bone and the condyle of the mandible. The glenoid fossa is a concave depression located in the squamous portion of the temporal bone (see Plates 13.6 and 13.7). It is bordered anteriorly by the articular eminence and posteriorly by the squamotympanic and petrotympanic fissures. The articular eminence is usually described as a posterior slope adjacent to the fossa and the crest, which is the inferiormost tip of the eminence. The condyle is typically ellipsoid and is longer in the mediolateral dimension than in the anteroposterior dimension. The condyle is angulated with the medial pole being positioned posterior to the lateral pole, typically forming an angle of 15–30 degrees with the sagittal plane. When viewing sections through the TMJ, it is useful to make custom reconstructions through the axial long axis of the condylar head. The resulting oblique sections are referred to as "corrected" sagittal and frontal sections (Fig. 13.68).

- In the sagittal view, the fossa and eminence form an inverted "S" shape, characteristically seen as a smooth radiopaque line (see Fig. 13.68B). The angle of the posterior slope of the eminence can vary considerably and is typically 30–60 degrees to the Frankfort plane. Anatomic variation that forms a steep eminence (angle >60 degrees) is suggested to predispose to TMJ internal derangements.
- The superior surface of the condylar head is usually rounded or convex (see Fig. 13.68C), but anatomic variations, such as slight flattening or marked convexity, are frequently observed. The size and shape of the right and left condylar heads should be compared. When an asymmetry is observed, the symmetry of the entire mandible should be assessed, including the intercuspation of the teeth and any deviation of the mandible on opening.
- In adults, the articular surfaces of the condyle, glenoid fossa, and articular eminence have a corticated border. Pathologic conditions, such as osteoarthritis, often cause a thinning or loss of this normal cortication. However, this corticated border is not visualized during periods of condylar growth and thus is not seen until approximately age 18 years.
- With the teeth in maximal intercuspation, the condyle is normally seated concentrically within the glenoid fossa. Although considerable deviation from this position is observed in radiographs of asymptomatic individuals, the condyle is frequently retruded in individuals with TMJ dysfunction.

BASE OF THE SKULL

A full- and often medium-FOV CBCT scan encompasses the region of the skull base; the anatomy of this region is best evaluated on axial and coronal sections. To facilitate viewing, it is useful to orient the CBCT volume to the Frankfort plane, with the axial slices parallel to this plane and coronal slices perpendicular to it. Five bones form the skull base: ethmoid, sphenoid, occipital, frontal (paired), and temporal (paired).

The entire cranial base is evaluated for symmetry, integrity, and continuity. For example, infections or neoplasms may extend from the ethmoid air cells into the cranial fossa through the cribriform plate, disrupting this anatomic structure. Furthermore, it is important to be familiar with the various foramina and canals in the skull base.

The anterior cranial base is formed by the frontal bones (laterally), the cribriform plate and crista galli of the ethmoid bone (medially), and the lesser wing of the sphenoid bone (posteriorly). These bones also contribute to the roof of the nasal cavity, ethmoid air cells, and orbits. The anterior cranial base is best visualized on coronal and sagittal sections (see Plates 13.4, 13.5, and 13.7).

The middle cranial base is formed by the body and greater wings of the sphenoid bone and the petrous and squamous portions of the temporal bones; it overlies the sphenoid sinuses and the mastoid air cells, middle and inner ears, and infratemporal fossae (see Plates 13.5–13.7). The sella turcica is a depression in the body of the sphenoid that contains the pituitary gland. This depression, together with the anterior and posterior clinoid processes, forms a U-shaped corticated line on sagittal sections and is saddle shaped on coronal sections. There is a broad range in the dimensions of the sella turcica, with the anteroposterior dimension ranging from 5 to 16 mm and the depth ranging from 4 to 12 mm (see Fig. 13.68). On either side of the sella turcica is the carotid groove, seen extending posteriorly to the carotid canal, which passes vertically through the petrous portion of the temporal bone (see Plate 13.2). The clivus is a triangular bone formed by the union of the basisphenoid and basiocciput bones and extends posteriorly and caudally from the sella turcica (Fig. 13.69). The union between these

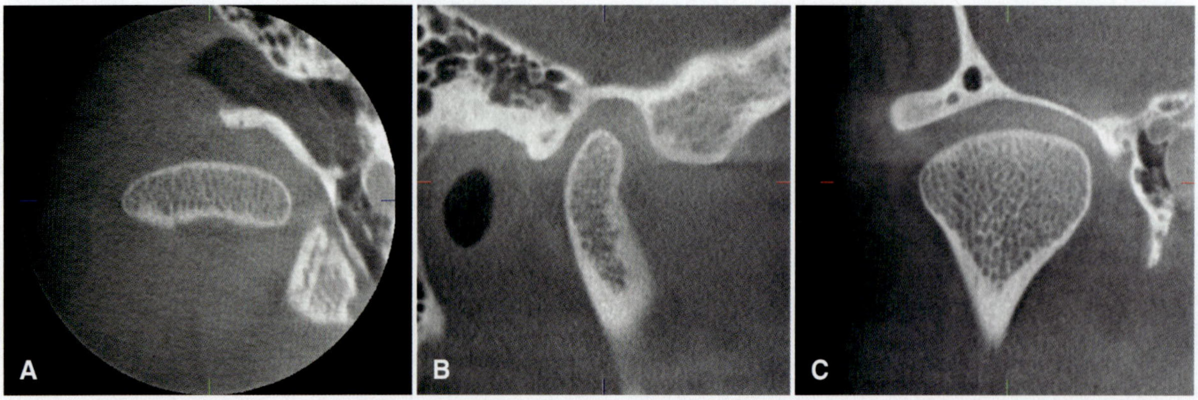

Fig. 13.68 Limited field-of-view cone beam computed tomography image of the temporomandibular joint. Axial (A), corrected sagittal (B), and frontal (C) sections. Note intact cortical borders on all articular surfaces.

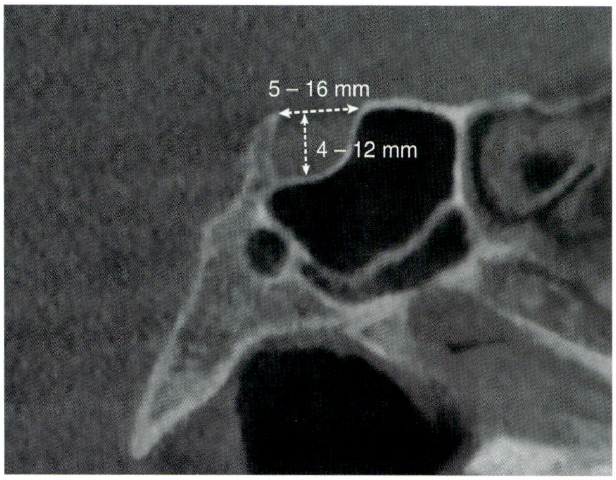

Fig. 13.69 Cone beam computed tomography section through the midsagittal plane showing the sella turcica. The range of variation in its anteroposterior and vertical dimensions is indicated.

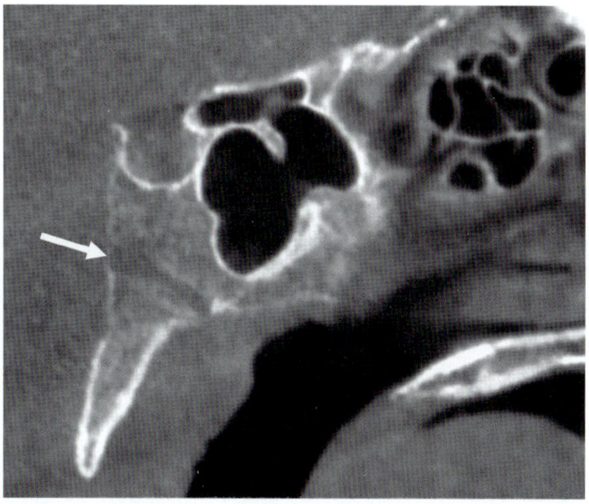

Fig. 13.70 Clivus showing incomplete spheno-occipital synchondrosis *(arrow)*. This is a normal appearance until the synchondrosis is completed, typically by 16–20 years. Note appearance of a completed synchondrosis in Fig. 13.69.

bones—the spheno-occipital synchondrosis—is completed by 16–20 years. Thus, an open synchondrosis, seen as a gap in the clivus, is a normal appearance for children younger than 16 years of age (Fig. 13.70).

There are several key communications between the middle cranial fossa and the extracranial space, as follows:

- *Superior orbital fissure* (see Plate 13.1): Located lateral to the sphenoid body and immediately below the anterior clinoid processes, it transmits cranial nerves III, IV, V, and VI and the superior ophthalmic vein.
- *Foramen rotundum*: A canal that traverses the greater wing of the sphenoid bone and transmits the maxillary division of the trigeminal nerve to the pterygopalatine fossa. The course of this canal is best visualized on coronal sections (see Plate 13.5).
- *Foramen ovale*: Located in the sphenoid body, it transmits the mandibular division of the trigeminal nerve to the infratemporal fossa. It is adequately visualized on axial and coronal sections (see Plates 13.2 and 13.5). There is considerable variation in the size of this foramen.
- *Foramen spinosum*: Located posterior and lateral to the foramen ovale, it is best visualized on axial sections (see Plate 13.2).

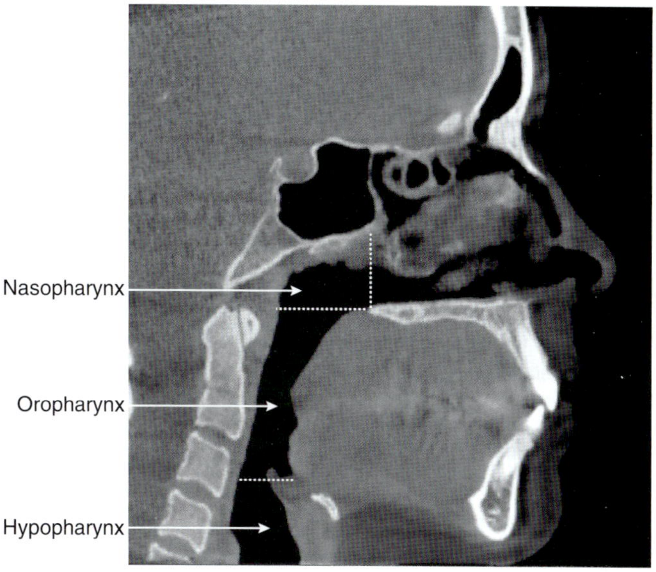

Fig. 13.71 Cone beam computed tomography image through the midsagittal plane showing the pharyngeal airway. The *dotted lines* indicate the boundaries of the nasopharynx, oropharynx, and hypopharynx.

An important anatomic region to examine is the pterygopalatine fossa. This is a funnel-shaped fossa located below the skull base that has communications with the middle cranial fossa, nasal cavity, orbit, infratemporal fossa, and oral cavity (Plate 13.6). This fossa is bordered anteriorly by the posterior wall of the maxilla and posteriorly by the pterygoid process of the sphenoid bone. The opening to the pterygopalatine fossa from the lateral aspect is the pterygomaxillary fissure. On sagittal sections, the fossa is seen as an inverted pear-shaped radiolucency (see Plate 13.7); on axial and coronal sections, it appears as a rectangular area (see Plates 13.1 and 13.5).

The styloid process is noted as a bony projection from the inferior surface of the petrous temporal bone adjacent to the stylomastoid foramen. The length of this process ranges from 5 to 50 mm. The stylohyoid ligament is often calcified, with reported frequencies of up to 30%. The mastoid process is another protuberance from the inferior surface of the temporal bone. Pneumatization of this bony process by the mastoid air cells occurs starting at age 3–5 years. As a result of the presence of air, the mastoid air cells appear as radiolucent air spaces, and opacification of these air cells often indicates disease. Sometimes pneumatization may extend anteriorly into the articular eminence and even into the zygoma or the occipital bone adjacent to the mastoid process.

AIRWAY

Medium- to full-FOV CBCT scans often encompass the airway space from the nasal cavity to the pharynx. The pharynx is typically considered in three zones: the nasopharynx, oropharynx, and hypopharynx (Fig. 13.71 and Plate 13.7). The nasopharynx lies behind the nasal cavity and extends to the level of the hard palate. The oropharynx spans the region between the tongue and the pharyngeal wall, extending from the level of the hard palate to the base of the epiglottis. The region posterior to the soft palate from the level of the hard palate to the caudal tip of the uvula is sometimes referred to as the velopharynx. The hypopharynx is the most caudal part of the pharynx, below the epiglottis. Anatomic variations in the size of the soft palate or tongue or pathologic enlargements of the palatine tonsils can cause narrowing of the airway dimensions.

RESTORATIVE MATERIALS

Restorative materials vary in their radiographic appearance, depending principally on their atomic number and also influenced by their thickness and density. A variety of restorative materials may be recognized on projection radiographs and CT scans.

- Silver amalgam is completely radiopaque (Fig. 13.72).
- Gold is equally opaque to x-rays, whether cast as a crown (Fig. 13.73) or an inlay or condensed as gold foil.
- Stainless steel pins (Fig. 13.74) and stainless steel crowns (Fig. 13.75) appear highly radiopaque.
- A calcium hydroxide base is placed in a deep cavity to protect the pulp. Such base material is typically composed to be radiopaque (Fig. 13.76) so that the development of recurrent caries (radiolucent) can be identified.
- Gutta-percha, a rubber-like substance used to fill pulp canals during endodontic therapy, is also radiopaque, but lower in radiodensity than amalgam (Fig. 13.77).
- Silver points, previously used to obliterate pulp canals during endodontic therapy, are highly radiopaque (Fig. 13.78).
- Composite restorations are typically partially radiopaque, as are porcelain restorations, which are usually fused to a metallic coping (Fig. 13.79).
- Orthodontic appliances around teeth (Fig. 13.80) are relatively radiopaque, although less than stainless steel crowns.

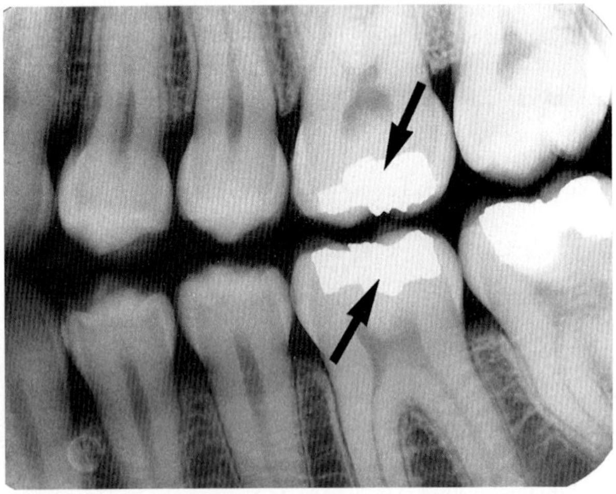

Fig. 13.72 Amalgam restorations appear completely radiopaque *(arrows)*.

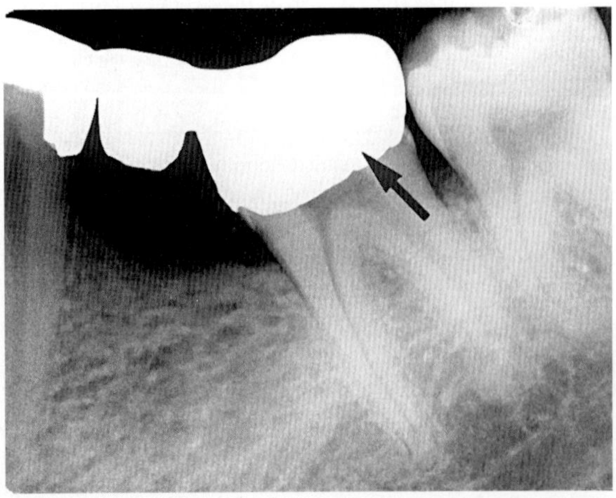

Fig. 13.73 A cast gold crown, appearing completely radiopaque *(arrow)*, serves as the terminal abutment of a bridge.

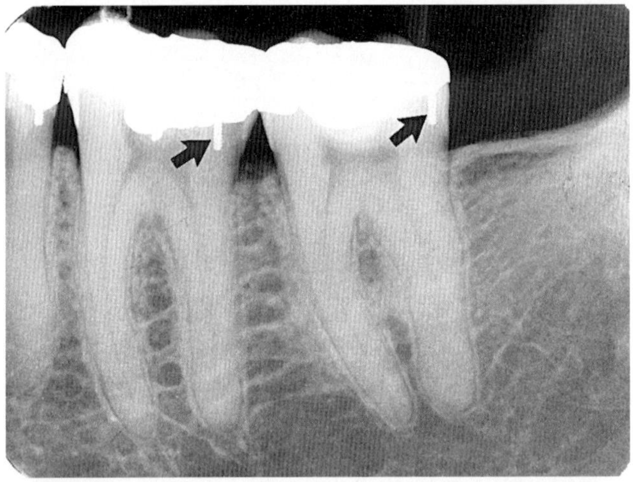

Fig. 13.74 Stainless steel pins *(arrows)* provide retention for amalgam restorations.

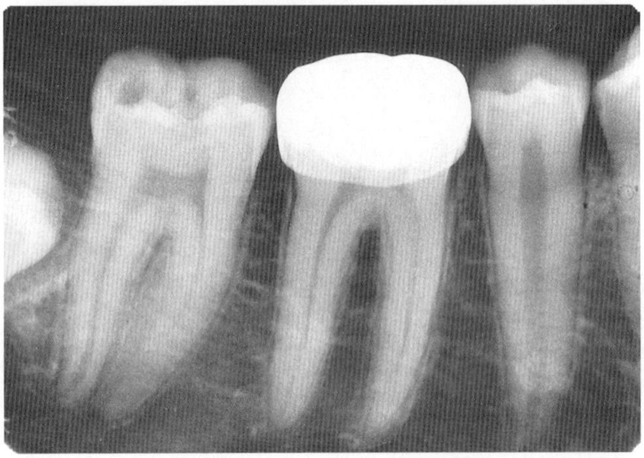

Fig. 13.75 Stainless steel crowns appear mostly radiopaque.

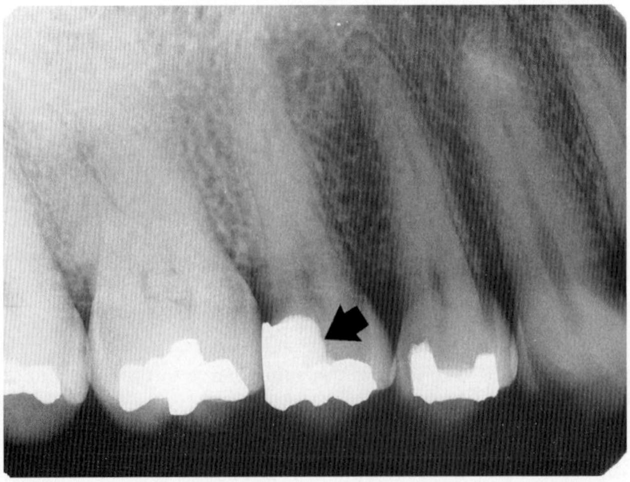

Fig. 13.76 Base material *(arrow)* is usually radiopaque but less opaque than the amalgam restoration.

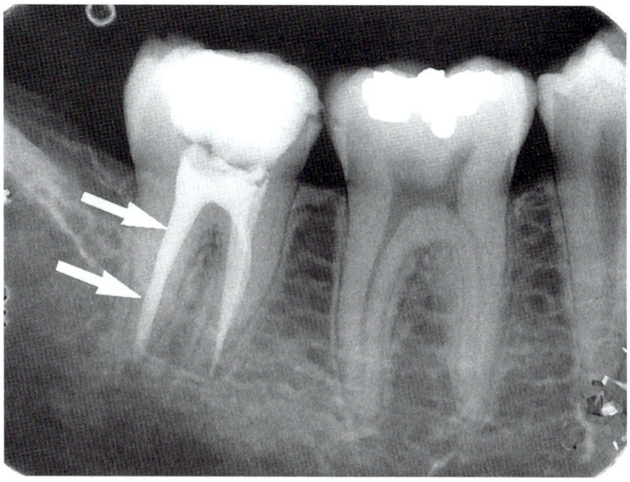

Fig. 13.77 Gutta-percha *(arrows)* is a radiopaque rubber-like material used in endodontic therapy.

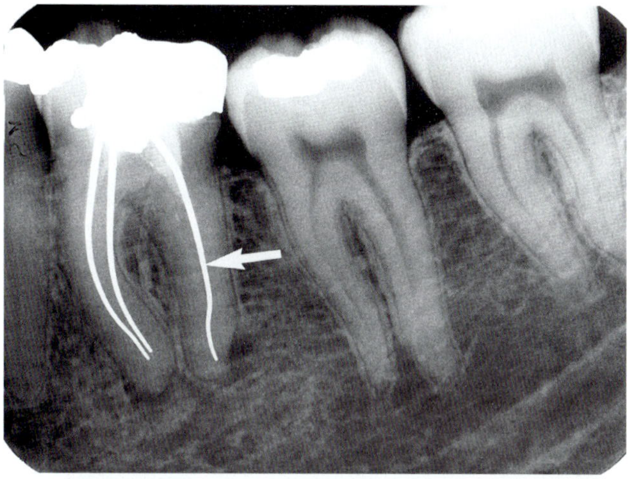

Fig. 13.78 Silver points *(arrow)* were used to fill the root canals in this patient.

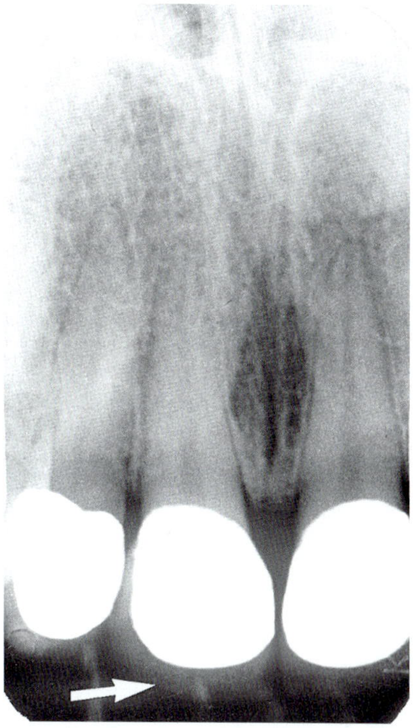

Fig. 13.79 Porcelain appears radiolucent *(arrow)* over a metal coping.

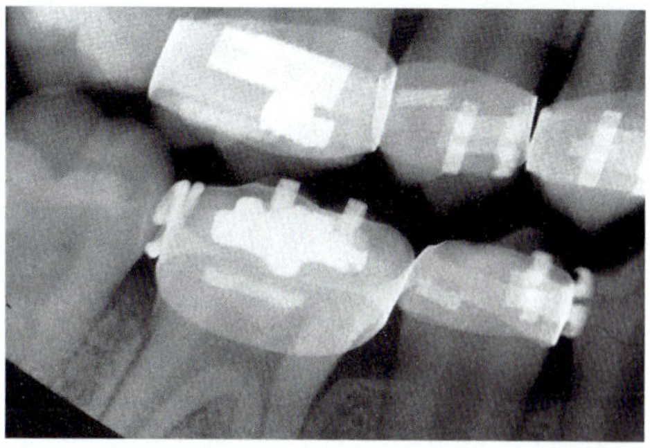

Fig. 13.80 Orthodontic appliances have a characteristic radiopaque appearance.

BIBLIOGRAPHY

Berkovitz BKB, Holland GR, Moxham BL. *Oral Anatomy, Histology and Embryology*. 4th ed. Mosby; 2009.

Claeys V, Waskens G. Bifid mandibular canal: literature review and case report. *Dentomaxillofac Radiol*. 2005;34:55-58.

Harnesberger HR, Osborn AG, Ross J, et al., eds. *Diagnostic and Surgical Imaging Anatomy: brain, Head and Neck, Spine*. Amirsys; 2006.

Jacobs R, Mraiwa N, van Steenberghe D, et al. Appearance, location, course, and morphology of the mandibular incisive canal: an assessment on spiral CT scan. *Dentomaxillofac Radiol*. 2002;31:322-327.

Kasle MJ. *An Atlas of Dental Radiographic Anatomy*. 4th ed. Saunders; 1994.

Liang X, Jacobs R, Lambrichts I, et al. Lingual foramina on the mandibular midline revisited: a macroanatomical study. *Clin Anat*. 2007;20:246-251.

Lusting JP, London D, Dor BL, et al. Ultrasound identification and quantitative measurement of blood supply to the anterior part of the mandible. *Oral Surg Oral Med Oral Pathol Oral Radiol Endod*. 2003;96:625-629.

Mraiwa N, Jacobs R, van Steenberghe D, et al. Clinical assessment and surgical implications of anatomic challenges in the anterior mandible. *Clin Implant Dent Relat Res*. 2003;5:219-225.

Naitoh M, Hiraiwa Y, Aimiya H, et al. Accessory mental foramen assessment using cone-beam computed tomography. *Oral Surg Oral Med Oral Pathol Oral Radiol Endod*. 2009;107:289-294.

Von Arx T, Matter D, Buser D, et al. Evaluation of the location and dimensions of lingual foramina using limited cone-beam computed tomography. *J Oral Maxillofac Surg*. 2011;69:2777-2785.

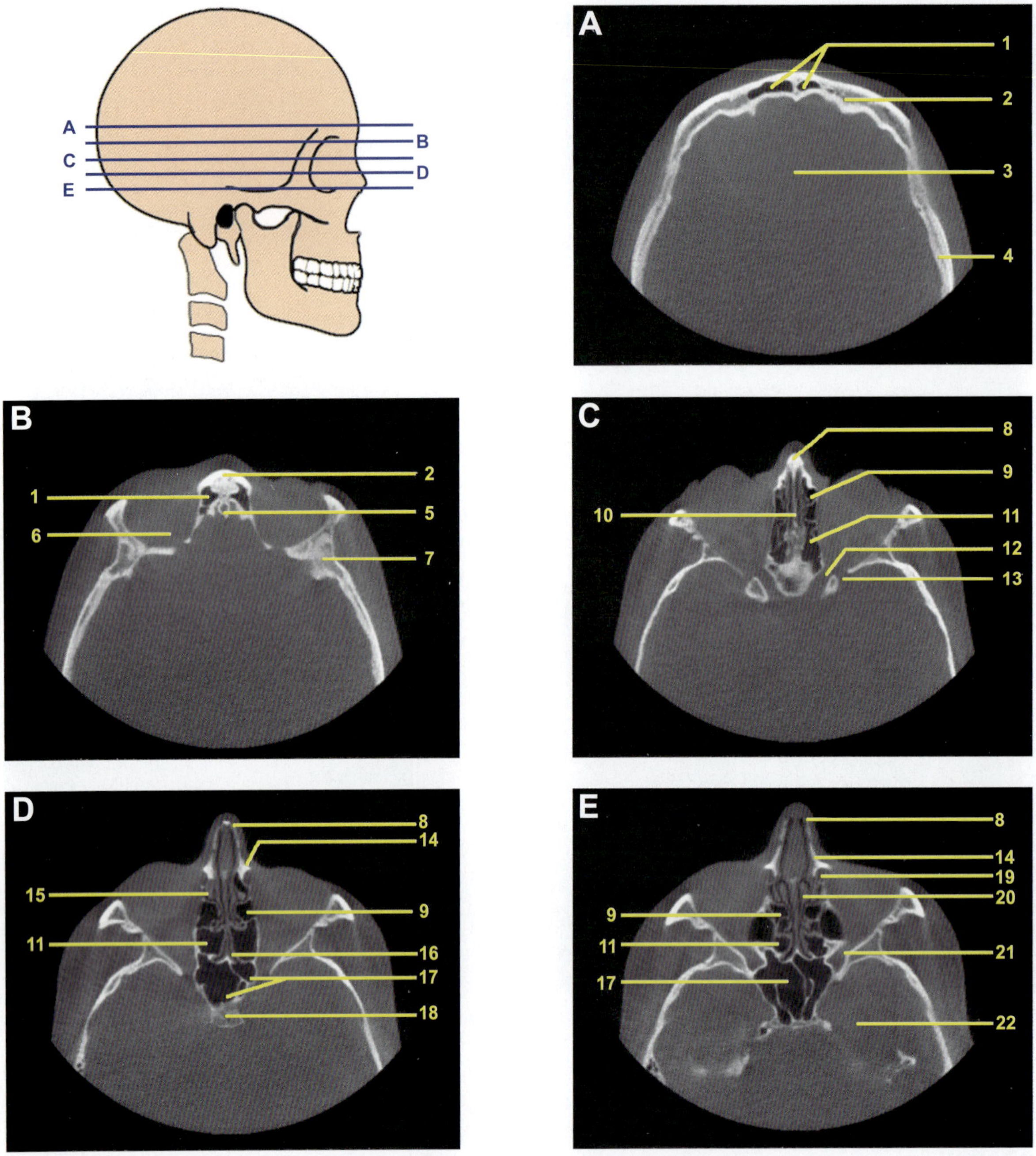

1. Frontal sinus
2. Frontal bone
3. Anterior cranial fossa
4. Squamous portion of temporal bone
5. Crista galli
6. Orbit
7. Greater wing of sphenoid bone
8. Nasal bone
9. Anterior ethmoid air cells
10. Perpendicular plate of ethmoid bone
11. Posterior ethmoid air cells
12. Optic canal
13. Superior orbital fissure
14. Nasal process of maxillary bone
15. Uncinate process
16. Sphenoethmoid recess
17. Sphenoid sinus
18. Floor of sella turcica
19. Nasolacrimal duct
20. Superior turbinate
21. Inferior orbital fissure
22. Middle cranial fossa

PLATE 13.1

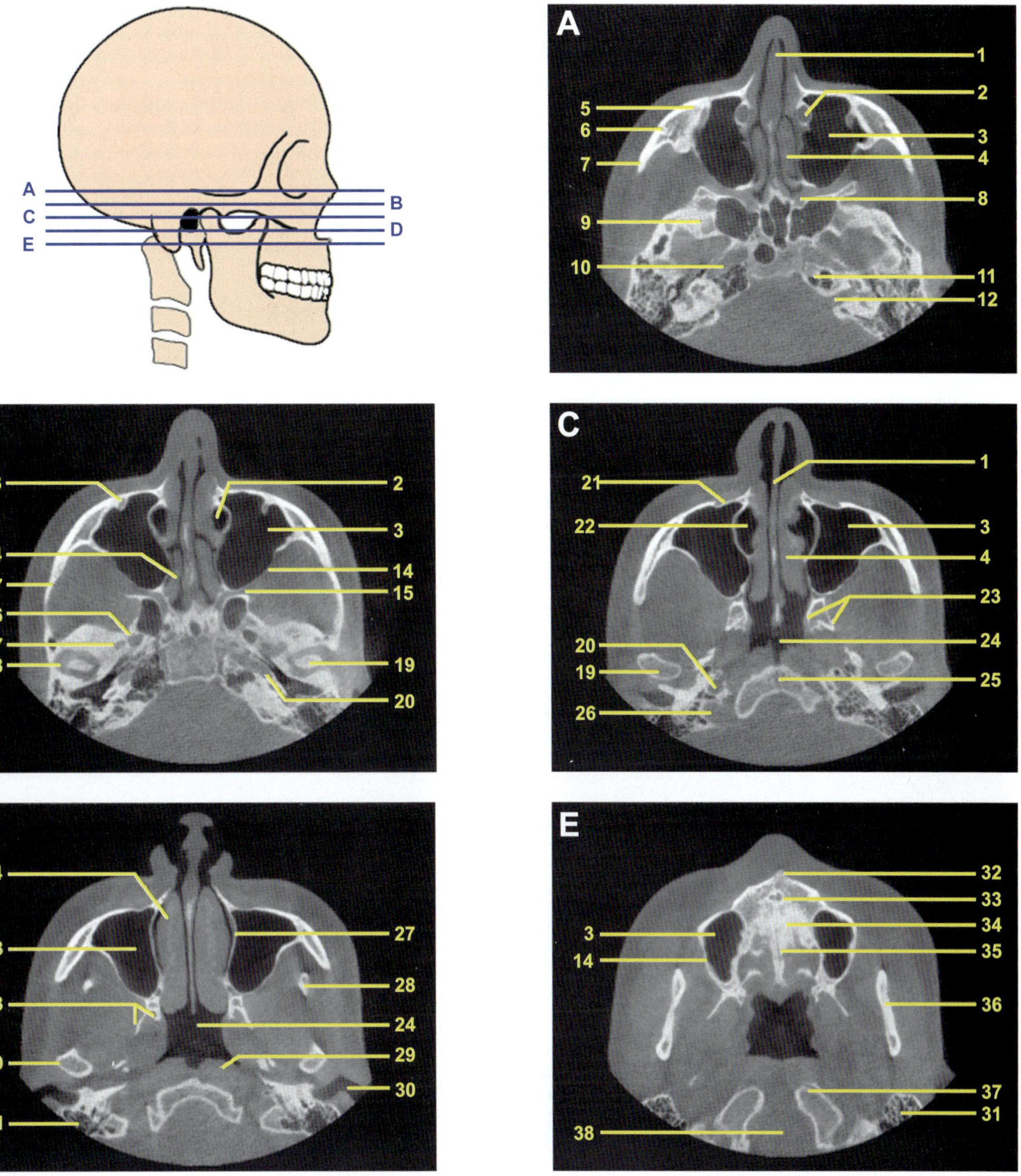

1. Nasal septum
2. Nasolacrimal duct
3. Maxillary sinus
4. Nasal turbinate
5. Zygomatic process of maxilla
6. Zygomatico-maxillary suture
7. Zygomatic arch
8. Pterygopalatine fossa
9. Greater wing of sphenoid bone
10. Carotid canal
11. Petrous portion of temporal bone
12. Internal auditory canal
13. Infraorbital canal
14. Lateral wall of maxillary sinus
15. Pterygomaxillary fissure
16. Foramen ovale
17. Foramen spinosum
18. Glenoid fossa
19. Mandibular condyle
20. Carotid canal
21. Infraorbital foramen
22. Nasal cavity
23. Pterygoid plates
24. Nasopharyngeal airway
25. Occipital bone
26. Jugular foramen
27. Medial wall of maxillary sinus
28. Coronoid process
29. Pharyngeal wall
30. External auditory meatus
31. Mastoid process
32. Anterior nasal spine
33. Nasopalatine canal
34. Hard palate
35. Intermaxillary suture
36. Ramus of mandible
37. Anterior arch of atlas (C1)
38. Foramen magnum

PLATE 13.2

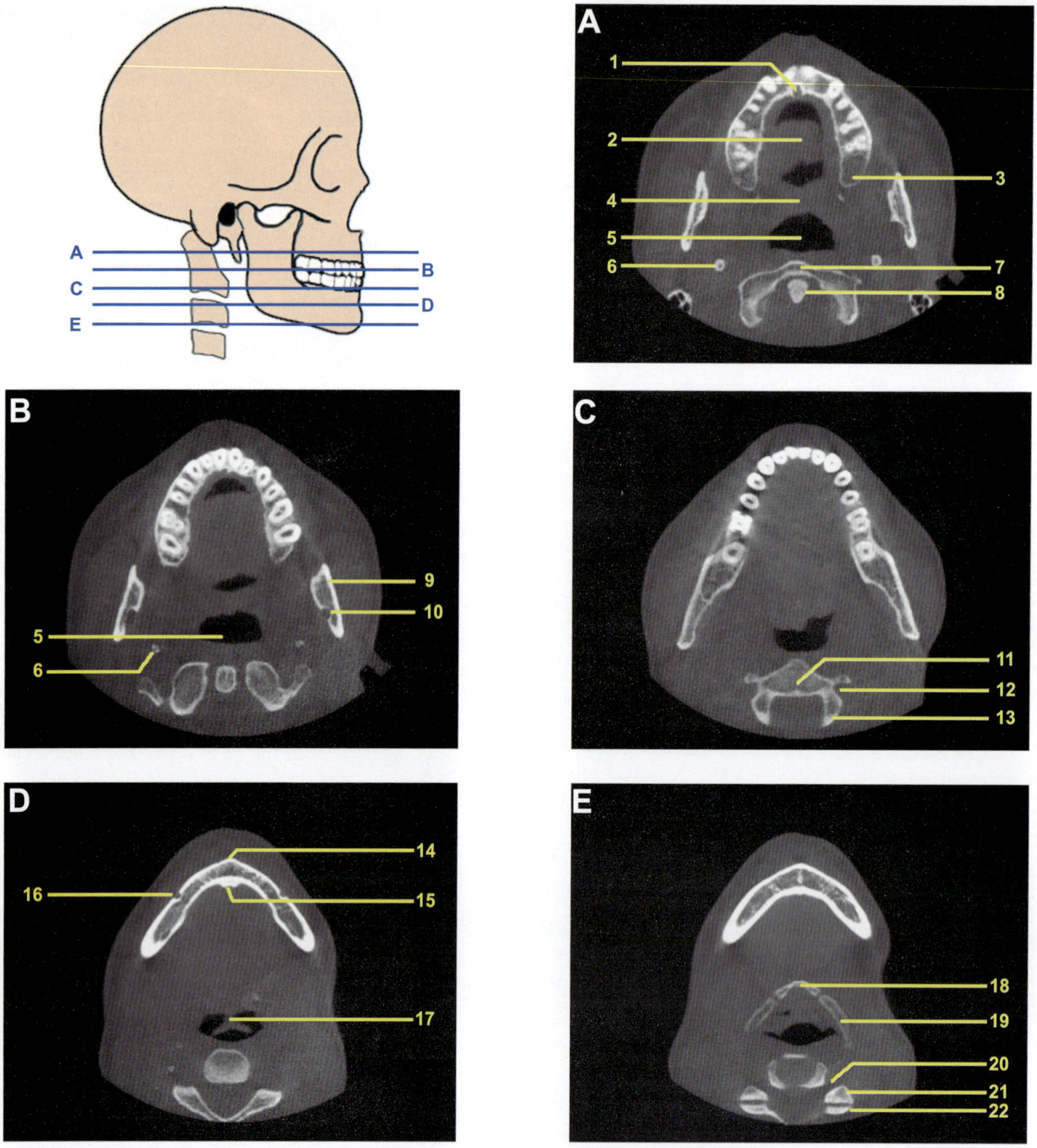

1. Incisive foramen
2. Tongue
3. Maxillary tuberosity
4. Soft palate
5. Oropharyngeal airway
6. Styloid process
7. Anterior arch of atlas (C1)
8. Odontoid process of C2
9. Ramus of mandible
10. Mandibular foramen
11. Inferior body of C2
12. Transverse foramen
13. Lamina of C2
14. Mandibular symphysis
15. Genial tubercles
16. Mental foramen
17. Epiglottis
18. Body of hyoid bone
19. Greater cornu of hyoid bone
20. C2-C3 neural foramen
21. Superior articular process of C3
22. Inferior articular process of C2

PLATE 13.3

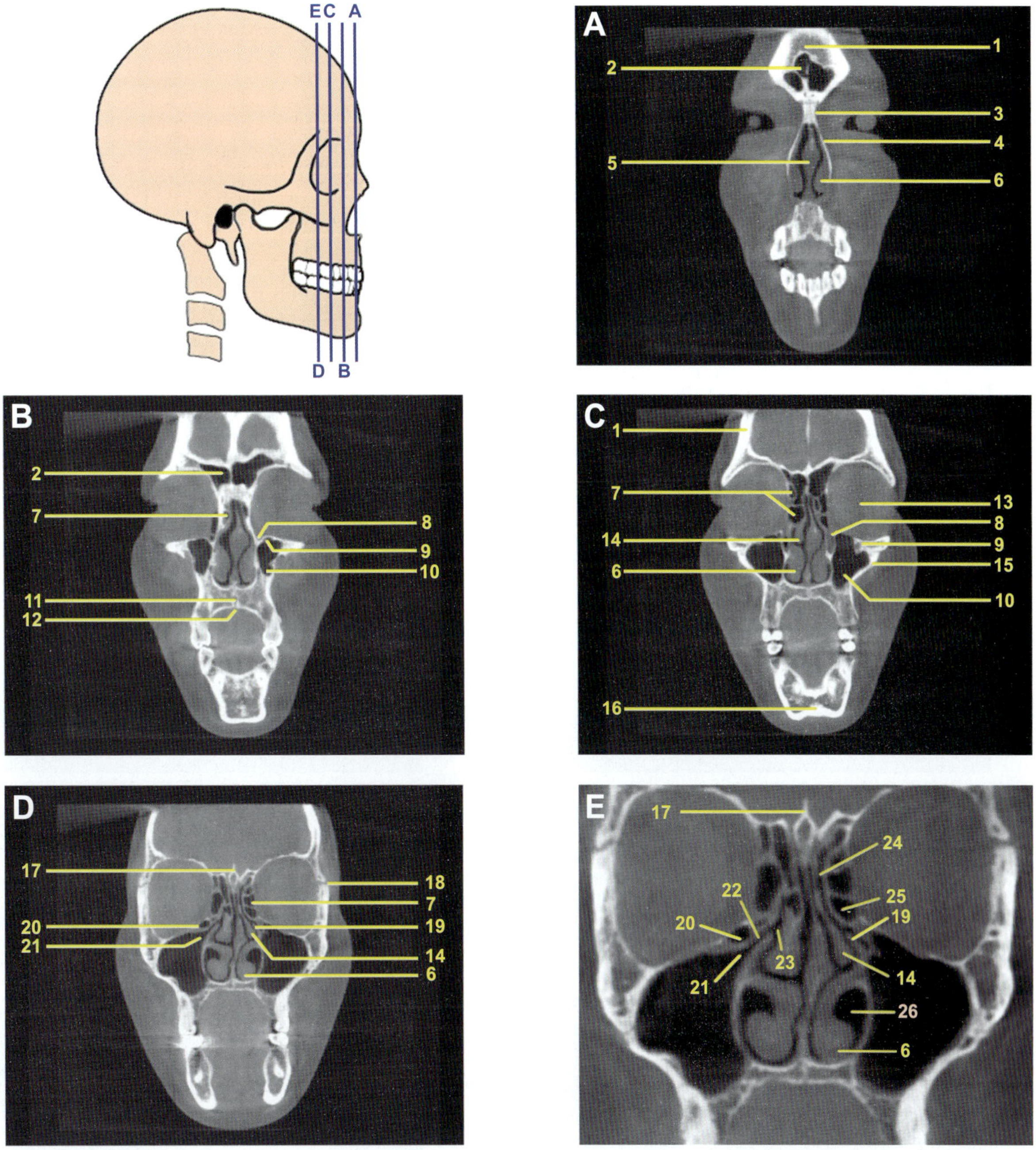

1. Frontal bone
2. Frontal sinus
3. Nasal bone
4. Maxillary bone
5. Nasal septum
6. Inferior nasal turbinate
7. Ethmoid air cells
8. Nasolacrimal duct
9. Infraorbital canal
10. Maxillary sinus
11. Nasopalatine canal
12. Incisive foramen
13. Orbit
14. Middle nasal turbinate
15. Zygomatic process of the maxilla
16. Mandible
17. Crista galli of ethmoid bone
18. Fronto-zygomatic suture
19. Uncinate process
20. Infraorbital ethmoid air cells (Haller cells)
21. Ostium of maxillary sinus
22. Infundibulum
23. Hiatus semilunaris
24. Frontal recess
25. Ethmoid bulla
26. Inferior meatus

PLATE 13.4

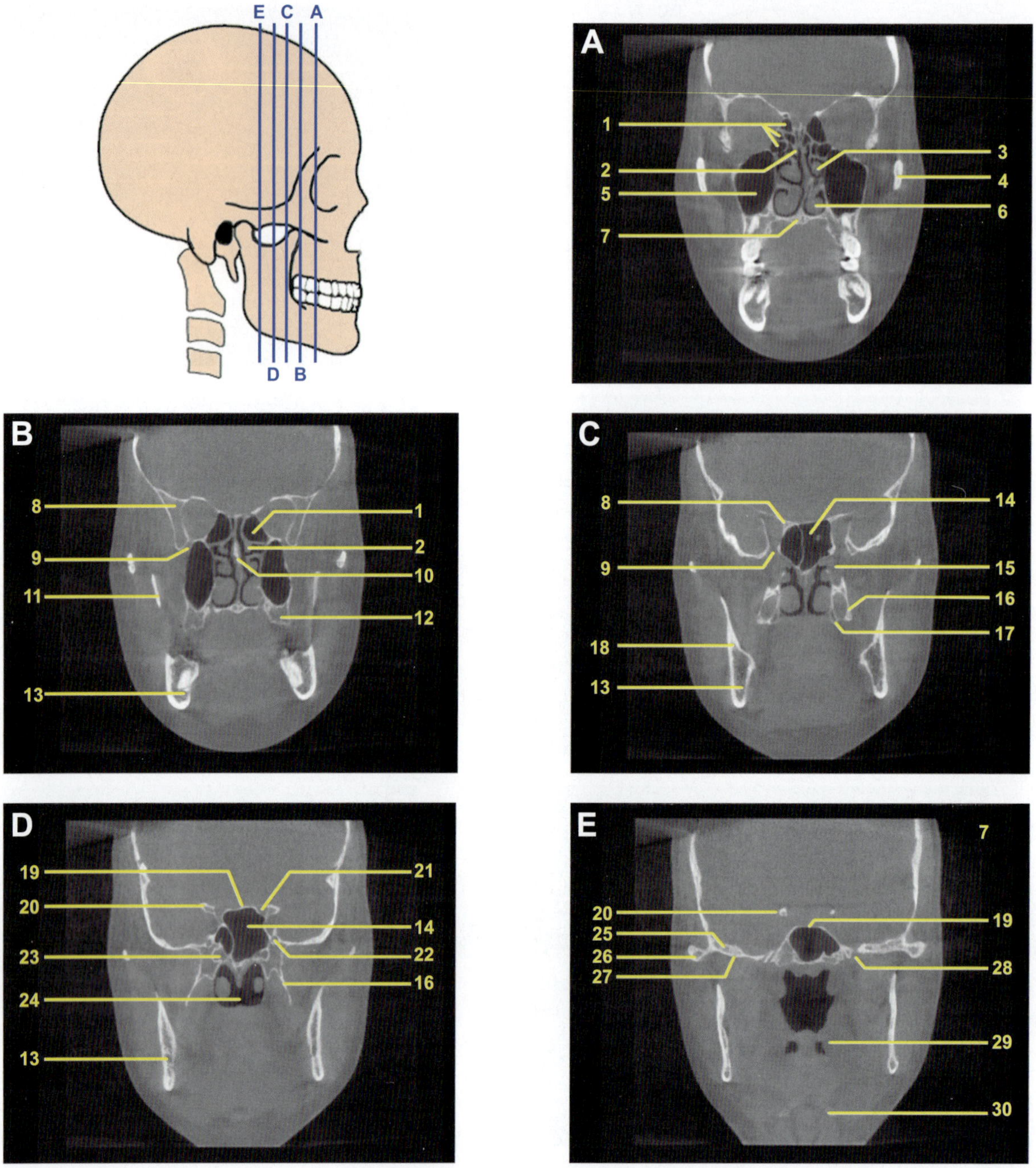

1. Ethmoid air cells
2. Superior nasal turbinate
3. Middle nasal turbinate
4. Zygomatic arch
5. Maxillary sinus
6. Inferior nasal turbinate
7. Hard palate (floor of nasal cavity)
8. Sphenoid bone
9. Inferior orbital fissure
10. Perpendicular plate of ethmoid bone
11. Coronoid process of mandible
12. Maxillary tuberosity
13. Inferior alveolar canal
14. Sphenoid sinus
15. Pterygopalatine fossa
16. Lateral pterygoid plate
17. Medial pterygoid plate
18. Mandibular ramus
19. Floor of sella turcica
20. Anterior clinoid process
21. Optic canal
22. Foramen rotundum
23. Pterygoid (vidian) canal
24. Nasopharyngeal airway
25. Squamous temporal bone
26. Zygomatic process of temporoal bone
27. Sphenosquamousal suture
28. Foramen ovale
29. Palatine tonsils
30. Hyoid bone

PLATE 13.5

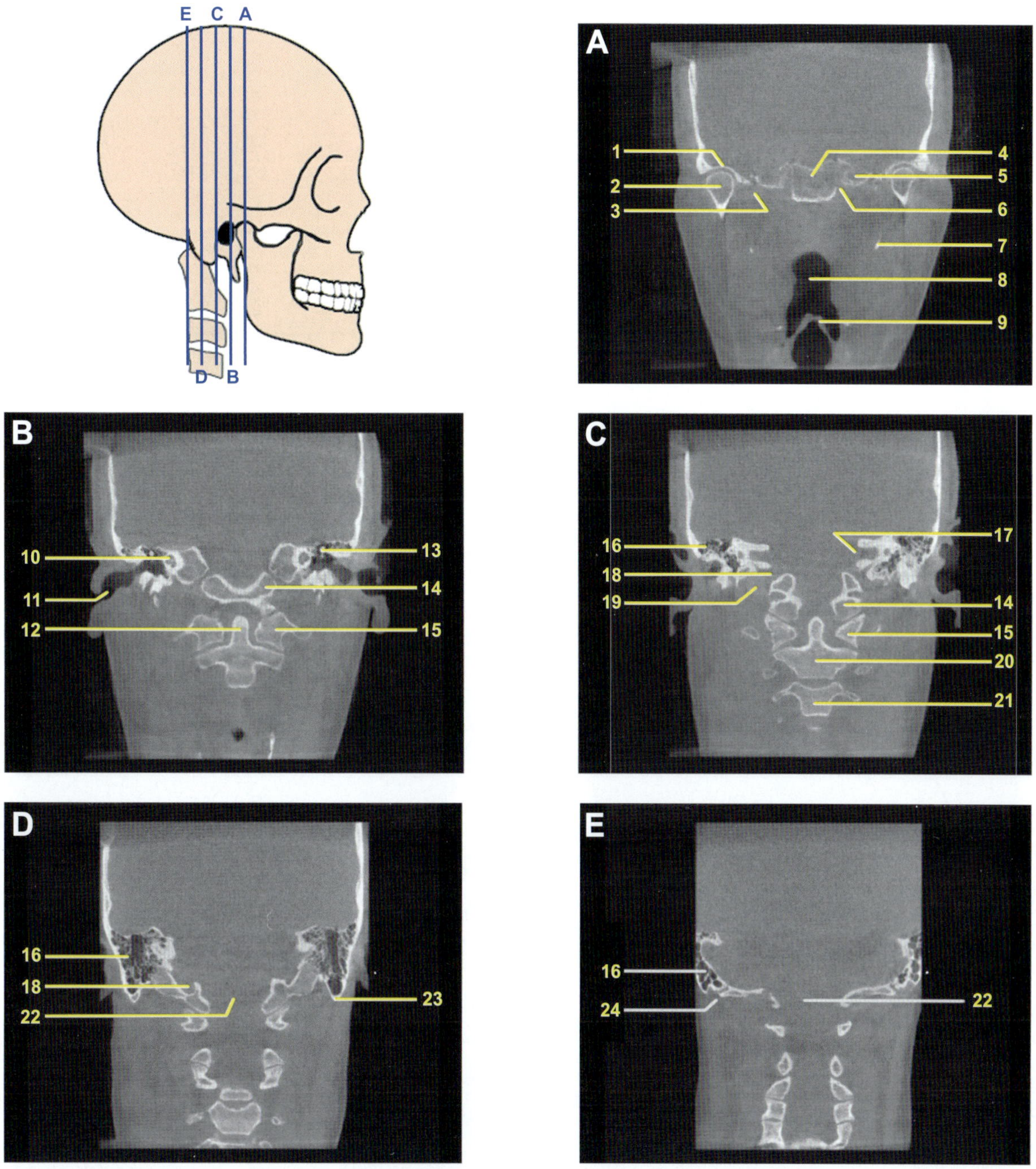

1. Glenoid fossa
2. Mandibular condyle
3. Foramen spinosum
4. Basiocciput
5. Carotid canal
6. Petrooccipital suture
7. Styloid process
8. Oropharnygeal airway
9. Epiglottis
10. Semicircular canal
11. External auditory meatus
12. Odontoid process of C2
13. Ossicles of ear
14. Occipital condyles
15. Lateral mass of C1
16. Mastoid air cells
17. Internal auditory meatus
18. Jugular foramen
19. Jugular bulb
20. Body of C2
21. Body of C3
22. Foramen magnum
23. Mastoid process
24. Occipito-mastoid suture

PLATE 13.6

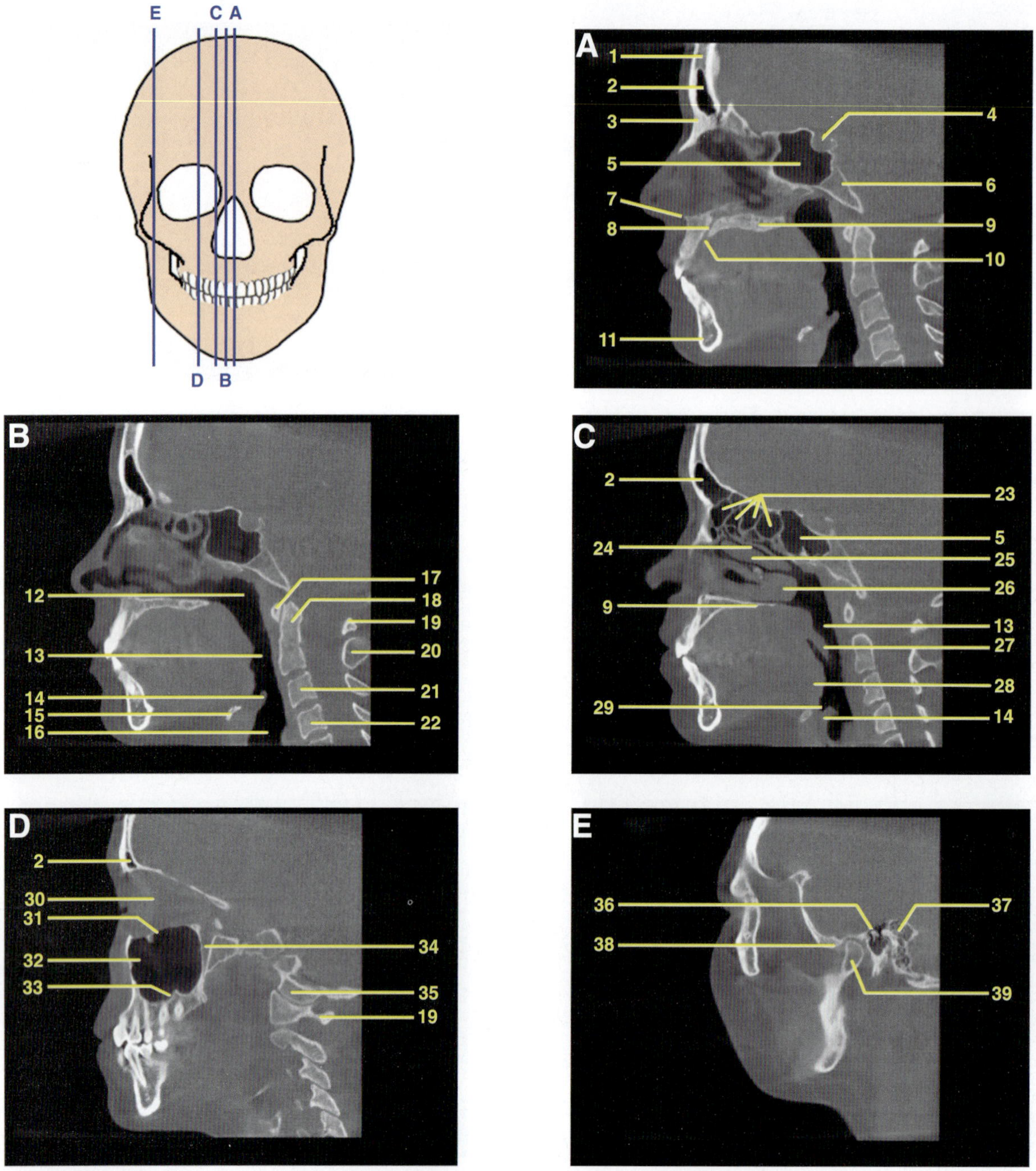

1. Frontal bone
2. Frontal sinus
3. Nasal bone
4. Sella turcica
5. Sphenoid sinus
6. Clivus
7. Anterior nasal spine
8. Nasopalatine canal
9. Hard palate
10. Incisive foramen
11. Mandibular symphysis
12. Nasopharyngeal airway
13. Oropharyngeal airway
14. Epiglottis
15. Hyoid bone
16. Hypopharynx
17. Anterior arch of C1
18. Odontoid process of C2
19. Posterior arch of C1
20. Spinous process of C2
21. Body of C3
22. Body of C4
23. Ethmoid air cells
24. Hiatus semilunaris
25. Middle turbinate
26. Inferior turbinate
27. Soft palate
28. Base of tongue
29. Vallecula
30. Orbit
31. Floor of orbit/Roof of maxillary sinus
32. Maxillary sinus
33. Floor of maxillary sinus
34. Pterygopalatine fossa
35. Occipital condyle
36. Ossicle of middle ear
37. Mastoid process
38. Articular eminence
39. Mandibular condyle

PLATE 13.7

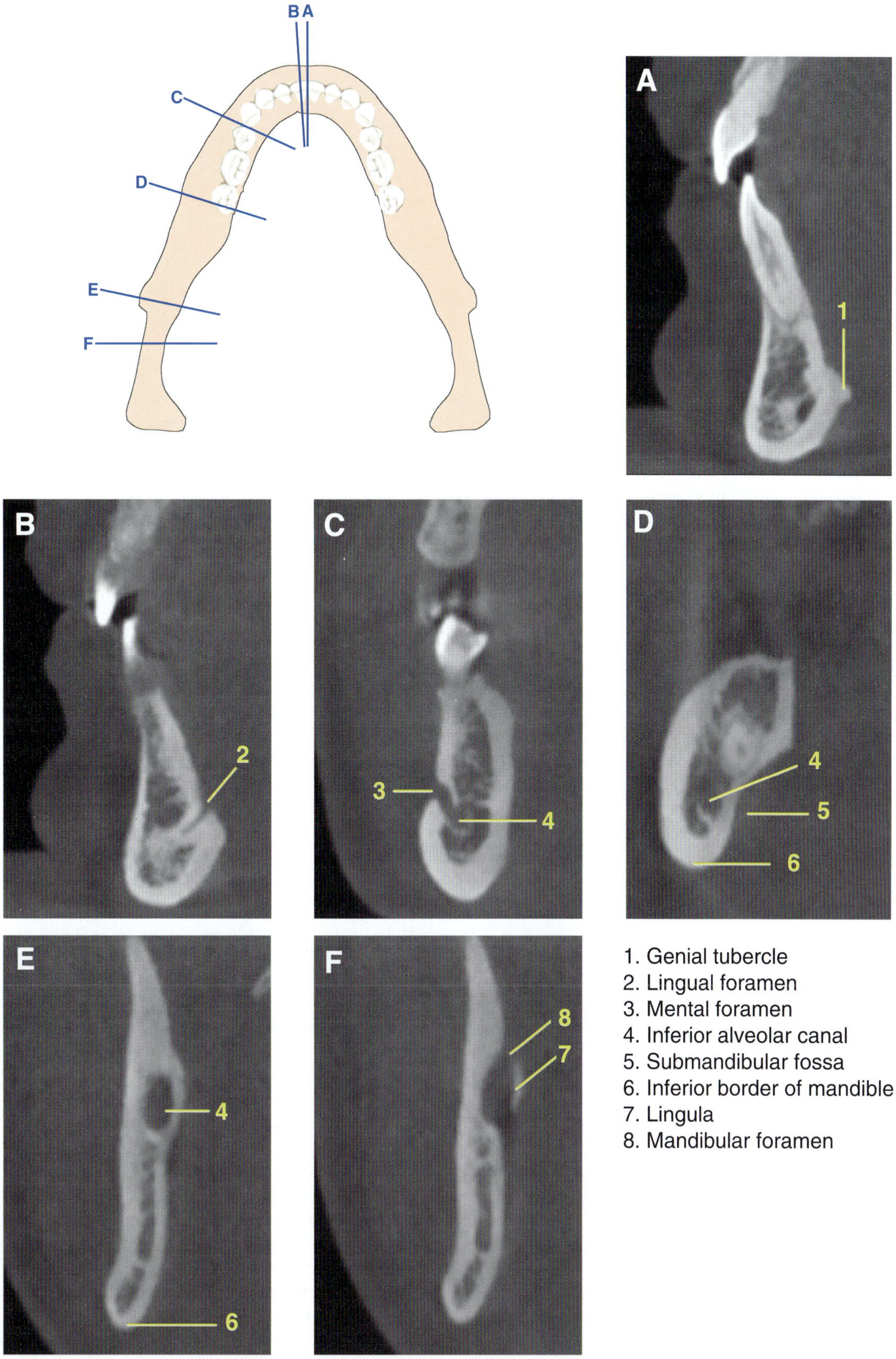

1. Genial tubercle
2. Lingual foramen
3. Mental foramen
4. Inferior alveolar canal
5. Submandibular fossa
6. Inferior border of mandible
7. Lingula
8. Mandibular foramen

PLATE 13.8

14

Quality Assurance and Infection Control

Sanjay M. Mallya

A quality assurance program in radiology is a series of procedures designed to ensure optimal and consistent operation of each component in the imaging chain. When all components function properly, the result is consistently high-quality radiographs and reduced radiation dose to patients and office personnel.

The goal of an infection control program in radiology is to avoid cross contamination among patients and between patients and the dental staff in the course of imaging.

RADIOGRAPHIC QUALITY ASSURANCE

Diagnostic quality radiographs are indispensable for patient diagnosis. To continuously maintain image quality, a quality assurance program evaluates the performance of x-ray machines, image receptors, manual and automatic film processing procedures, and viewing media and conditions. Optimization of all steps in the imaging chain maximizes diagnostic yield and decreases radiation dose to patients. Examples of common faults in digital sensor handling and problems with film processing are presented in Chapter 4.

To effectively manage a quality assurance program, a dental office should identify one individual to assume the primary responsibility to implement the quality assurance program and to coordinate corrective action when indicated. Most quality assurance procedures are quickly accomplished and can have a significant influence on radiographic quality. The quality assurance procedures described in this section address intraoral, panoramic, cephalometric, and cone beam computed tomography (CBCT) imaging. Table 14.1 summarizes the tasks and their frequency.

X-Ray Sources

The x-ray source is the core component of a radiographic device. The accuracy and consistency of the radiation output is key to consistently make diagnostic quality radiographs. This set of quality assurance procedures verify safe and consistent production of x-rays that accurately reflects the exposure parameters set by the operator.

Acceptance Tests

When a new x-ray machine is purchased, it should be installed by a qualified expert, following federal and state regulations. Before its clinical use, the qualified expert performs acceptance tests. *Acceptance testing* refers to a formal group of tests that inspect the x-ray unit and confirm that the x-ray unit functions according to vendor-specific and industry standards. The United States Code of Federal Regulations Title 21, Part 1020 specifies the performance standards for ionizing radiation-emitting products. Details of acceptance tests for dental x-ray devices are described in the American Association of Physicists in Medicine (AAPM) Report No. 175 and include all elements of the daily, monthly, and annual test procedures.

When in use, intraoral x-ray machines are generally quite stable, and only infrequently is a malfunction of the machine the cause of poor radiographs. Panoramic, cephalometric, and CBCT radiographic devices include multiple mechanical and electrical components in addition to x-ray source, including the C-arm to rotate the source and receptor and head-holder assemblies. Malfunction of these components could result in poor image quality. Thus components of the acceptance tests should be performed at periodic intervals to ensure continued optimal function.

Establish Exposure Settings

The dental office must develop exposure settings for each x-ray device. For intraoral radiography, separate settings must be established for each x-ray source-receptor combination used in the practice. Separate exposure settings must be established for adult and pediatric patients. A radiographic exposure chart should be maintained, preferably adjacent to the x-ray unit control panel where these parameters are selected. The chart should specify the x-ray source and receptor used and indicate the proper peak kilovoltage (kVp), milliamperes (mA), and exposure times(s) for making radiographs of each region of the oral cavity (Fig. 14.1). These charts help ensure that all operators use the same optimal range of exposure factors. Each month, this chart should be inspected to verify that the information is legible and accurate.

The American National Standard/American Dental Association Standard Number 1094 provides guidance to establish optimal exposure factors for intraoral radiography. This is done using phantom test objects to measure spatial resolution, contrast resolution, and dynamic range. To establish optimal exposure factors, images of the test object are made with multiple exposure settings. For intraoral radiography, a beam energy of 60–70 kVp is used. The highest mA setting available on the x-ray device is selected and multiple exposures are made with different exposure times. The parameters of spatial resolution, contrast resolution and dynamic range, and image uniformity are visually examined on the resultant images. Spatial resolution is measured using a line-pair gauge. Contrast resolution is measured by examining radiolucent circles created by wells of varying depth or width within a block of plexiglass. Dynamic range is determined using a lead step wedge to demonstrate a range of radiodensities. The digital dental quality assurance (DDQA) phantom (Dental Imaging Consultants, LLC, Fig. 14.2) provides assessment of spatial resolution, dynamic range, and contrast resolution on a single image. The phantom is designed to provide clinically relevant source-object and source-receptor distances. Leeds Test Objects (North Yorkshire, United Kingdom) manufactures multiple phantoms to

TABLE 14.1 Schedule of Radiographic Quality Assurance Procedures

	Task	At Purchase	Daily	Weekly	Monthly	Yearly
X-ray sources	Acceptance tests	✓				
	Establish optimal exposure settings	✓				
	Inspect function		✓			
	Calibration and preventive maintenance					✓
Radiographic technique	Log retakes		✓			
	Review retake log			✓		
	Check exposure charts				✓	
Digital receptor systems	Acceptance tests	✓				
	Establish optimal exposure settings	✓				
	System start-up and shut-down		✓			
	Calibrate image displays				✓	
	Inspect PSP plates				✓	
	Inspect solid-state sensors				✓	
	Check image quality (intraoral, panoramic, and cephalometric)					✓
	Preventive maintenance of PSP plate readers					✓
Film-based radiography	Replenish processing solutions		✓			
	Check temperature of processing solutions		✓			
	Compare radiographs with reference film		✓			
	Replace processing solutions			✓		
	Clean processing equipment			✓		
	Clean viewboxes			✓		
	Check darkroom safelight				✓	
	Clean intensifying screens				✓	
	Rotate film stock				✓	
CBCT	Acceptance tests	✓				
	System start-up and shut-down		✓			
	Detector calibration	✓	✓[a]			✓
	CT contrast phantom	✓	✓			✓
	Image uniformity and noise	✓	✓			✓
	Spatial resolution for high-contrast and low-contrast objects				✓	✓
	Geometric accuracy					✓
	Preventive maintenance					✓

[a]Varies depending on manufacturer recommendation.

CBCT, Cone beam computed tomography; *CCD,* charge-coupled device; *CMOS,* complementary semiconductor metal oxide; *PSP,* photostimulable phosphor.

examine intraoral, panoramic, and cephalometric digital imaging systems and CBCT devices.

The optimal exposure time is the lowest exposure time that provides the necessary diagnostic information. Optimal exposure settings must be re-established when any component of the imaging system is changed, for example, a new x-ray source, switching from film to digital imaging, and using a different brand of digital receptor.

Diagnostic reference levels (DRLs) are a measure of optimal exposure conditions and serve as a benchmark that can be achieved by practices for a specific imaging procedure. Typically, 75% of facilities will use a dose at or below the DRL and provides the motivation for practices that uses doses above the DRL for that procedure. Thus DRLs provide the first step toward establishing optimal exposure settings. Achievable dose (AD) provides the second step and represents the dose used by 50% of the facilities, providing further motivation to achieve dose reduction without compromising image quality. The National Council of Radiation Protection and Measurements Report No. 172 recommends DRLs and ADs for intraoral, panoramic, and cephalometric imaging. DRLs and ADs for CBCT have yet to be developed.

Procedure	Diagnostic Reference Level	Achievable Dose
Intraoral radiograph	1.6 mGy	1.2 mGy
Panoramic radiograph	100 mGy/cm^2	76 mGy/cm^2
Cephalometric radiograph	0.14 mGy	0.09 mGy

Daily Tasks

Daily inspection. Typically, the power to an x-ray machine is switched on at the start of each workday. A quick inspection of the unit should confirm active equipment indicators with no error messages on the control panel and to ensure general mechanical safety. Handheld dental x-ray devices should be examined to confirm adequate battery charge and to ensure the integrity and position of the radiation shield. Intraoral, panoramic, and cephalometric devices need no additional preparation before clinical imaging. In contrast, image reconstruction steps in CBCT are more complex and may require daily testing to ensure operation within the manufacturer's specifications. Procedures for monitoring quality of CBCT images are described in a separate section.

Room No 4

X-ray source	Image receptor
Planmeca ProX	XDR Clarity
Source-object: 30 cm	Sensor holder
kVp: 66 mA: 8	Rectangular collimation

Projection	Exposure time (s)
Adult, Periapical	
Incisor	0.160
Canine-Premolar	0.200
Molar	0.300
Adult, Bitewing	
Premolar	0.200
Molar	0.300
Edentulous, Periapical	
Incisor	0.160
Canine-Premolar	0.160
Molar	0.200
Child	
Anterior	0.160
Posterior	0.160
Bitewing	0.160

Fig. 14.1 Sample wall chart showing identification information for x-ray machine, receptor type, milliamperage (mA) and peak kilovoltage (kVp) settings, and appropriate exposure times for various anatomic locations and patient sizes. The optimal exposure times must be determined empirically in each office because they vary with the machine settings used, source-to-skin distance, and other factors.

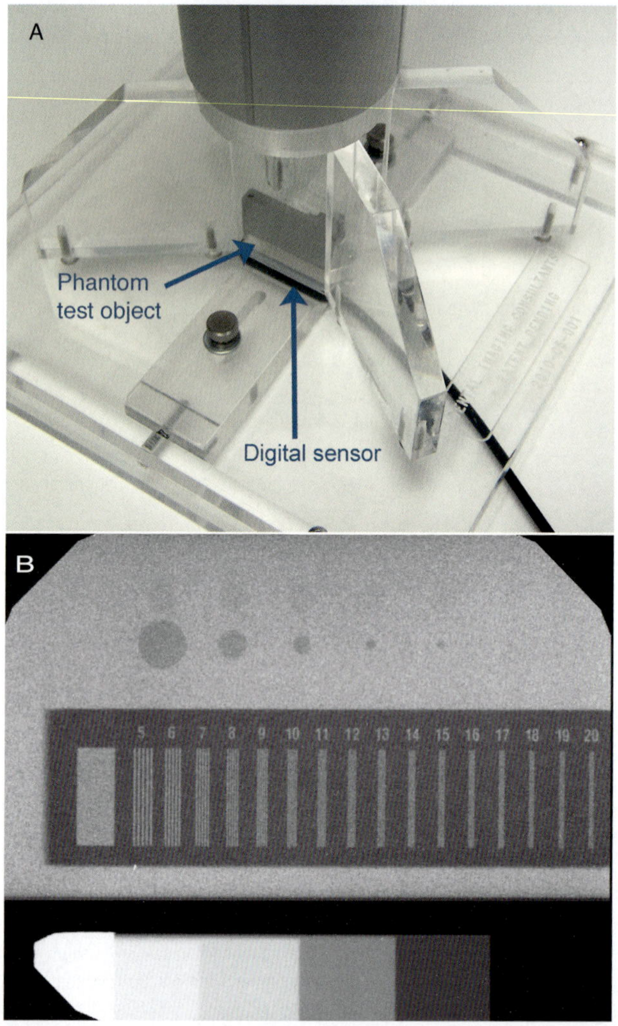

Fig. 14.2 Phantom for measuring image quality performance of digital dental x-ray systems. (A) Plastic stand allows positioning of the aiming tube of the x-ray machine over the test device, which is positioned over the digital sensor. (B) Resulting image of test device, showing from the *top*, two rows of wells of varying diameter and depth in an acrylic background for measuring contrast detail, an etched pattern of slits in a metallic background for measuring the spatial resolution in line pairs per millimeter, and a calibrated step wedge for measuring dynamic range. (Images courtesy Dr. Peter K. Mah: www.dentalimagingconsultants.com.)

At the end of the workday, power to x-ray devices is switched off to prevent accidental exposure. The battery of handheld x-ray devices should be disconnected from the x-ray source unit and connected to the charging unit to prepare for use for the next day.

Yearly Tasks

Inspect and calibrate x-ray unit. X-ray machines should be calibrated annually, or earlier, when a specific problem is identified or substantive repair is necessary that may affect operation. A qualified expert, typically vendor service personnel, qualified medical physicists, or qualified oral and maxillofacial radiologists, should make these radiation dose measurements because of the specialized equipment and knowledge required. The AAPM Report No. 175 describes these procedures in detail and specifies the limits of tolerance for variance for the various parameters. Radiation detectors designed to meet the need of dental offices provide a relatively simple approach to measure kVp, half-value layer (HVL), air kerma, and exposure time (Fig. 14.3).

- Tube head stability: The tube head should be stable when placed around the patient's head, and it should not drift during the exposure. When the tube head is unstable, service is necessary to adjust the suspension mechanism. The drift should be 0.5 cm or less.
- Leakage radiation: A high-sensitivity radiation detector should be used to detect leakage radiation from the tube housing. No leakage radiation should be detected.
- Beam quality: The HVL of the beam should be measured to ensure that the beam meets regulatory requirements. This is done using a dosimeter and aluminum sheets of specific thickness. Some devices will calculate and display the measured HVL directly (Fig. 14.3). The regulatory requirements of the US Food and Drug Administration, 21 CFR 20 are listed as follows.

Minimum Half-Value Layer (mm of Aluminum)

Peak Kilovoltage (kVp)	Intraoral X-Ray Devices	Panoramic and Cephalometric Devices
60	1.5	1.5
70	1.5	1.8
71	2.1	2.5
80	2.3	2.9
90	2.5	3.2

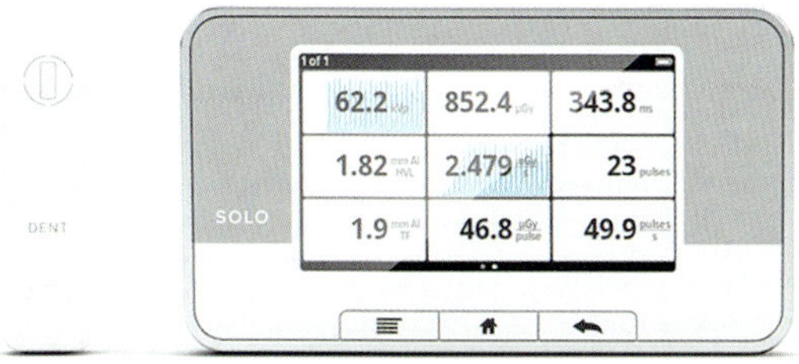

Fig. 14.3 The RaySafe X2 Solo DENT device is designed for dental offices and measures dose, dose rate, kVp, exposure time, pulses, and pulse rate. The sensor can be used for intraoral, panoramic, cephalometric, and cone beam computed tomography applications. (Courtesy Fluke Biomedical, www.flukebiomedical.com.)

- kVp accuracy: The measured kVp of the beam should be accurate and reproducible. Measurement of kVp requires specialized equipment (Fig. 14.3). Measurements should be made across the full spectrum of kVp values used for that unit. The anticipated variation is specified by the manufacturer and should be no more than 10%.
- Exposure reproducibility: A radiation dosimeter should be used to evaluate the reproducibility of radiation output (Fig. 14.3). Make at least three air kerma measurements and calculate the coefficient of variation (COV = standard deviation divided by mean). The COV should not exceed 5%.
- Timer accuracy: For intraoral and cephalometric devices, the exposure times can be manually selected. The accuracy and reproducibility of timer settings should be verified. Deviation should not exceed 10% for timer settings greater than 10 ms.
- mA and milliampere-second (mAs): For intraoral and cephalometric devices, the linearity of the mA control should be verified if two or more mA settings are available on the machine. Typically, the air kerma is measured using the adult bitewing setting. The mA setting is then reduced to the next lower mA value, and the exposure time is increased to yield the same mAs (product of the mA and exposure time in seconds). A discrepancy in measured air kerma implies nonlinearity in the mA control or a fault in the timer. This variation should not exceed 10%. An example of acceptable variance is illustrated below.

	Milliamperes (mA)	Exposure Time (seconds)	Calculated Milliamperes × Seconds (mAs)	Measured Air Kerma (mGy)
Exposure setting 1	10	0.2	2	1.5
Exposure setting 2	5	0.4	2	1.4

Variance = 1.5 − 1.4 = 0.1 mGy

Maximum variance = ± 10% = ± 0.15 mGy

- Collimation and beam alignment, intraoral radiography: The field diameter for dental intraoral x-ray machines should be no greater than 2.75 inches (7 cm). The edge of the position-indicating device (PID), or aiming cylinder, should be closely aligned with the x-ray beam.
- Collimation and beam alignment, panoramic radiography: For panoramic machines, the beam is collimated at the source and before it strikes the receptor. The two collimators should be aligned and the beam should be congruent with receptor area exposed. The beam width should be within the collimator aperture and should not extend beyond the receptor height.

In a panoramic x-ray device, the relative speeds of the x-ray beam and the movement of the receptor past the collimator determine the position and shape of the image layer (focal trough). Most manufacturers provide a radiographic phantom to confirm image layer position and symmetry of x-ray beam rotation.

- Collimation and beam alignment, cephalometric radiography: The alignment of the x-ray beam and the cephalostat assembly should be verified. Confirm position of the ear rods in the vertical and horizontal planes, such that the beam is perpendicular to both ear support rods and the receptor plane. Check integrity and stability of the nasion pointer. Many manufacturers provide metal markers on the ear rods to easily detect ear rod misalignment.
- Collimation and beam alignment, CBCT: The alignment of the x-ray beam and field size are verified.
- Focal spot size: The size of the focal spot may become enlarged with excessive heat buildup within an x-ray machine. An enlarged focal spot contributes to unsharpness in the resultant image. A specialized piece of equipment is required for this test. This is not part of the routine quality assurance process and may need to be performed to troubleshoot geometric unsharpness.

Radiographic Technique

This set of quality improvement procedures allows the office to identify a broad range of errors that impact image quality including technical errors and x-ray source and receptor malfunction. The procedures focus on the radiographic technique, are the same for digital- and film-based radiography, and can be applied to intraoral, panoramic, cephalometric, and CBCT examinations. The processes help to (1) minimize errors in radiographic technique, including patient positioning and exposure settings, and (2) identify systematic errors related to equipment malfunction.

Daily Tasks

Enter findings in retake log. A simple and effective means to reduce the number of faulty radiographs is to maintain a retake log to record errors that require retaking the radiograph. The log should identify the operator, the specific equipment used, and a description or indication of the nature of the error that required correction. This process quickly reveals the source of recurring problems and facilitates early resolution. Errors that impact diagnostic quality or interpretation should be included in the radiology report.

Weekly Tasks

Review retake log. The retake record should be reviewed weekly to identify any recurring problems, for example, with specific operators, specific radiographic projections, defective receptors, and film processing conditions. This information can be used to initiate corrective actions, including staff education.

Monthly Tasks

Check exposure charts. Verify that the information is legible and accurate.

Digital Radiographic Receptor Systems

This section describes quality assurance and periodic maintenance of digital receptors for intraoral, panoramic, and cephalometric radiography. These include solid-state sensors (charge-coupled device [CCD], complementary metal oxide semiconductor [CMOS]) and photostimulable phosphor (PSP) systems. Essential elements of quality assurance programs for digital dental radiography are described in the American National Standards Institute/American Dental Association Standard No. 1094 and Standard No. 1099 and the AAPM Report No. 175.

Acceptance Tests for Image Detector Performance

Before using solid-state sensors and PSP systems for intraoral imaging, the dental team must establish exposure settings as described in the section on x-ray source. This provides an opportunity to ensure that the product is received undamaged without any detector defects. A study found image discrepancies in approximately 24% of new solid-state intraoral receptors, which may be due to manufacturing defects or damage that may have occurred in transit. Close evaluation of phantom images used to establish optimal exposure settings images will help identify these defects before they are accepted for clinical use.

Daily Tasks

System start-up and shut-down. Digital radiographic devices comprise the physical imaging device, receptor, and associated computer hardware with software applications to interact with the radiographic device. The system is powered on at the start of the workday. Typically, the associated software application linked to the device will display warnings and error messages when equipment start-up checks malfunction or fail. Ensure intact connections from the computer to the radiographic devices and intraoral receptors and to local or cloud-based data servers.

Monthly Tasks

Calibrate image displays. Interpretation of digital images is performed on a computer display. The same digital file may have different appearances when viewed on two different computer displays with an impact on diagnostic quality. Calibration of the display seeks to provide consistency in viewing a digital image. Digital Imaging and Communication in Medicine (DICOM) standards specify how grayscale values in a radiographic image are mapped into the range of luminance of human perception. *Medical-grade displays* conform to DICOM standards and are designed specifically to meet the needs of medical imaging. More often, high-end consumer-grade displays—liquid crystal displays or light-emitting diode displays—are used in dental clinics and hospitals. Irrespective of type, displays used for radiologic diagnosis should be checked and calibrated on a monthly basis. Test pattern images, such as the Society for Motion Picture and Television Engineers (SMPTE, pronounced *SIMP-tee*) Medical Diagnostic Imaging Test Pattern (Fig. 14.4A) or the AAPM TG18-QC image (Fig. 14.4B) should be used to guide brightness and contrast adjustments and to identify defects in the display. These test pattern images are publicly available via the internet and require minimal training to use. The image display adjustments can be completed in a few minutes by the dentist or allied staff. To perform the assessment, the digital test pattern image is displayed on a computer display in a room with minimal ambient light. Both test patterns include a low contrast feature (gray square within a black square) that should be visible when the display brightness is optimal. If the low contrast features are not perceptible, the display brightness may need to be adjusted. A display that is too bright will not depict high contrast features (gray square within a white square). The outcome from the monthly calibration should be recorded, including any corrective adjustments.

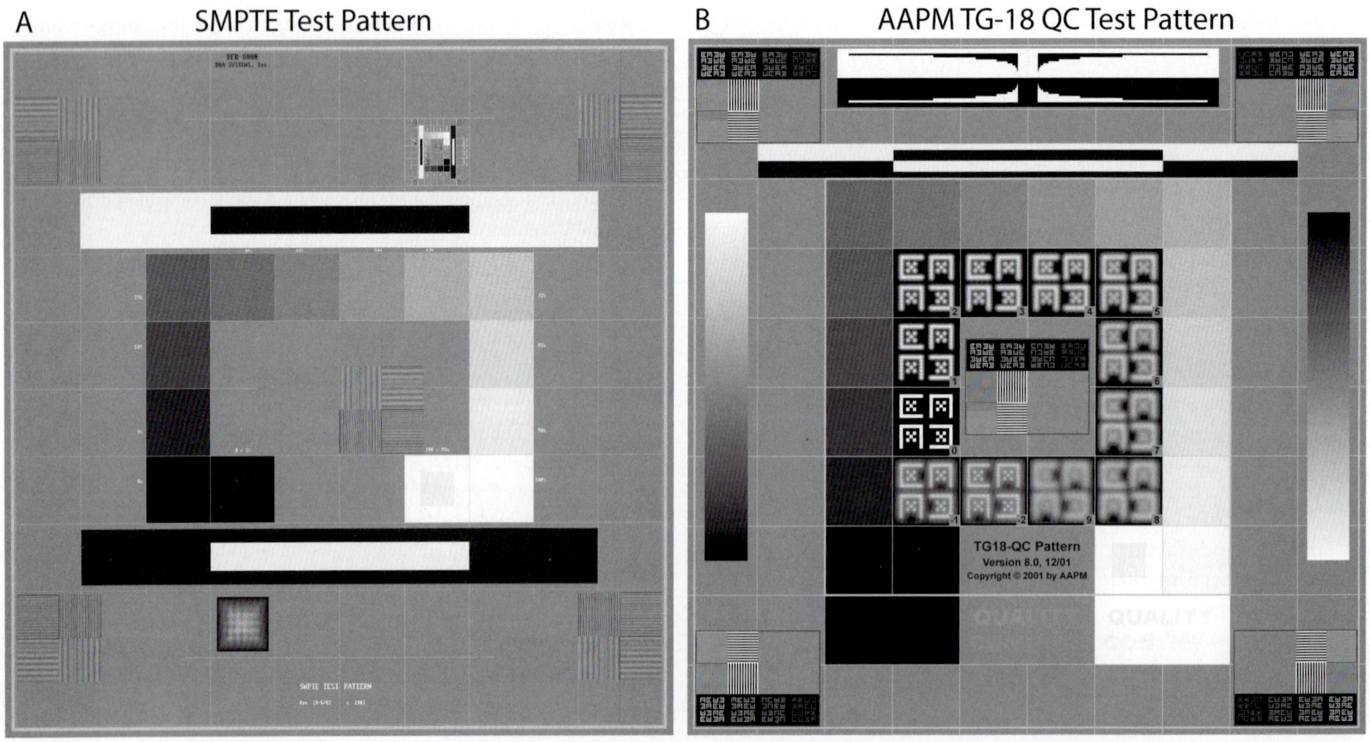

Fig. 14.4 (A) The Society for Motion Pictures and Television Engineers (SMPTE) test pattern. (B) The American Association of Physicists in Medicine TG-18 QC test pattern. Both patterns contain regions of low and high contrast to guide setting image display brightness and contrast. (Image source for SMPTE Pattern. Rich Franzen 1987, https://commons.wikimedia.org/wiki/File:SMPTE_RP-133.png.)

Computer hardware will need additional maintenance so that operating system and the software applications are current.

Inspect photostimulable phosphor plates. PSP plates may become scratched in the course of use. These scratches may be seen as light streaks on processed images (see Figs. 4.22A and 4.23) and may compromise diagnostic quality and mimic pathology or foreign objects. PSP plates should be inspected monthly and removed from service when such defects are found.

Inspect charge-coupled device and complementary metal oxide semiconductor sensors. CCD and CMOS sensors should be inspected monthly to confirm that the plastic housing and cable connections to the sensor and Universal Serial Bus are intact. Although the sensor may be functional with signs of damage to these components, it may indicate an impending failure. When damage is visible, images made using that sensor should be evaluated for potential image artifact. Some of these damages, for example, cord connections, may be repairable.

Yearly Tasks

Check image quality, intraoral digital sensors. The ANSI/ADA Standard No. 1094 recommends that intraoral digital sensors be checked yearly for signs of image degradation. Ideally, the test object images used for acceptance testing should be used for annual quality evaluation to detect change in image quality. The periodical evaluation should test spatial resolution, contrast resolution, dynamic range, and receptor uniformity. Defects within the CMOS sensor can cause artifacts, for example, *delamination* artifacts, which may be discovered on tests of receptor uniformity.

Check image quality, solid-state receptor-based panoramic and cephalometric radiographic devices. The ANSI/ADA Standard No. 1099 recommends at least annual testing of image quality of digital panoramic and cephalometric machines that use solid-state receptors. The inspection and calibration of the x-ray output, the verification of the imaging layer position for panoramic devices, and the verification of integrity and alignment of cephalostat components are described in the section on the x-ray source.

Many machines have removable sensors and the sensor should be visually inspected for integrity of electrical contacts. The CCD and CMOS detectors should be evaluated for image uniformity and artifacts. Phantoms are usually provided by the manufacturer. The Leeds Test Objects TOR DEN digital phantom can be used for this purpose.

Preventive maintenance of photostimulable phosphor readers. The latent image on PSP plates is converted to a digital image in a PSP scanner. These scanners must be calibrated and tested at initial installation and at periodic intervals to ensure proper function and production of images that meet vendor system specifications and industry standards. Following the initial acceptance testing, yearly preventive maintenance should be performed to evaluate the entire PSP system. Improper functioning of mechanical and electronic components that control the laser beam and collect signal could yield dimensional inaccuracies in the image, which may impact cephalometric analysis. Annual quality assurance and preventive maintenance should confirm proper functioning of these processes.

The AAPM Report No. 93 describes procedures for acceptance testing and quality control of PSP imaging systems. The measures of quality and function include dark noise and uniformity, system linearity and autoranging, image geometric uniformity, spatial resolution, and laser jitter.

Film-Based Radiography

Quality assurance tasks for film-based imaging are primarily directed to ensuring consistent and optimal conditions for film processing. These conditions, including processing chemical strength and temperature, can fluctuate rapidly; daily checks are necessary. Quality assurance tasks for film-based imaging are more frequent and typically require more time than quality assurance for digital receptors.

Daily Tasks

Replenish processing solutions. At the beginning of each workday, check the levels of the processing solutions and replenish with fresh developing solution and fresh fixing solution, as necessary. The most common cause of poor film radiographs is poor processing in the darkroom, in particular, the use of depleted solutions.

Check temperature of processing solutions. At the beginning of each workday, check the temperature of the processing solutions. The solutions must reach the optimal temperature before use—68°F (20°C) for manual processing and 82°F (28°C) for heated automatic processors. The instructions accompanying the film and processor verify the optimal temperature. Unheated automatic processors should be located away from windows or heaters that may cause their temperature to vary during the day. Proper temperature regulation is required for accurate time-temperature processing.

Compare film radiographs with reference film. A simple and effective means to routinely monitor the quality of images produced in an office is to check daily films against a reference film. A reference film provides a visual standard for optimal film processing. Comparison of daily images with the reference film may reveal problems before they interfere with the diagnostic quality of the images. When a problem is identified, it is important to determine the probable source and to take corrective action. For example, if the processing solutions have become depleted, the resultant radiographs are light and have reduced contrast. Both developer and fixer should be changed when degradation of the image quality is evident. Light images may also result from cold solutions or insufficient developing time. Dark images may be caused by excessive developing time, developer that is too warm, or light leaks.

Reference films may be:

- *Patient images:* Soon after film processing solutions are replaced, a patient's radiograph that has been properly exposed and processed with exact time-temperature technique is mounted on a corner of the viewbox. This image, with optimal density and contrast, serves as a reference for the radiographs made in the following days and weeks (Fig. 14.5).
- *Radiographs of a standard test object:* This is the most accurate and rigorous method of testing film processing solutions but requires

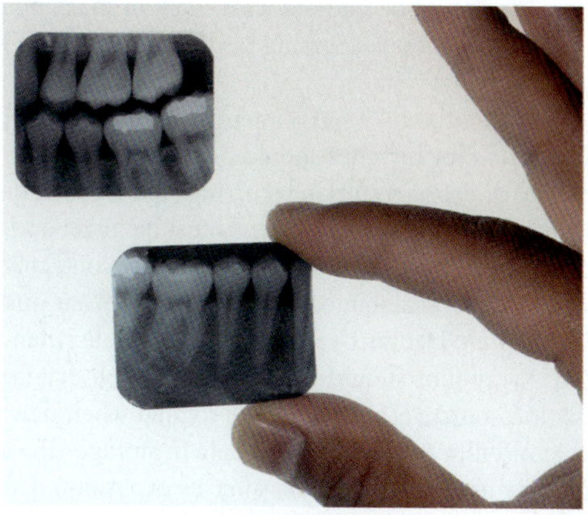

Fig. 14.5 Radiographs should be checked daily against a reference film made with fresh solutions. As processing solutions become exhausted, the daily images become increasingly light and lose contrast. When these changes are apparent, both the developer and the fixer should be changed.

additional equipment and more time to perform. An aluminum step wedge serves as a test object that provides a consistent range of gray shades (see Figs. 4.22 and 4.24). A step wedge can be fabricated using few overlapping sheets of lead foils, staggered to create "steps" with multiple thicknesses of lead. The step wedge is placed on the film and exposed to make the reference image. The DDQA phantom, described later, can also be used to provide a reliable test object. Daily reference images should be made with the same set of exposure settings (kVp and mAs) and source-film distance. Standard images can also be made using a sensitometer to expose film to a calibrated light pattern. After processing, a densitometer is used to measure the optical density of each region of the image pattern on the film. A change in the density readings from day to day indicates a problem in film processing.

Weekly Tasks

Replace processing solutions. How frequently processing solutions are replaced depends primarily on the rate of use of the solutions and also on the size of tanks, whether a cover is used, and the temperature of the solutions. In most offices, the solutions should be changed weekly or every 2 weeks. The results of the step-wedge test help determine the proper frequency.

Clean processing equipment. Regular cleaning of the processing equipment is necessary for optimal operation. The solution tanks of manual and automatic processing equipment should be cleaned when the solutions are changed. The rollers of automatic film processors should be cleaned weekly according to the manufacturer's instructions. After cleaning, the tanks and rollers should be rinsed as the manufacturer recommends to prevent the cleaner from interfering with the action of the film processing solutions.

Clean viewboxes. Viewboxes should be cleaned weekly to remove any particles or defects that may interfere with film interpretation.

Monthly Tasks

Check darkroom safelight. Film becomes fogged in the darkroom because of inappropriate safelight filters, excessive exposure to safelights, and stray light from other sources. These films are dark, show low contrast, and have a muddy gray appearance. The darkroom should be inspected monthly to assess the integrity of the safelights (preferably GBX-2 filters with 15-W bulbs). The glass filter should be intact, with no cracks. To check for light leaks in a darkroom, all lights are turned off; the individual allows his or her vision to accommodate to the dark and checks for light leaks, especially around doors and vents. Light leaks should be marked with chalk or masking tape to facilitate correction. Weather stripping is useful for sealing light leaks under doors.

Clean intensifying screens. All intensifying screens in panoramic and cephalometric film cassettes should be cleaned monthly. The presence of scratches or debris results in recurring light areas on the resultant images. The foam supporting the screens must be intact and capable of holding both screens closely against the film. If close contact between the film and screens is not maintained, the image will appear unsharp.

Rotate film stock. Dental x-ray film is quite stable when it is properly handled. X-ray film should be stored in a cool, dry facility away from a radiation source. Stock should be rotated when new film is received so that old film does not accumulate in storage. The oldest film always should be used first but never after its expiration date.

Cone Beam Computed Tomography

In-office CBCT imaging is used in dental clinics, hospitals, and imaging centers. Although quality assurance protocols for multidetector computed tomography are well established, CBCT quality assurance protocols are less well developed. The International Commission on Radiation Protection Publication 129, the Intersocietal Accreditation Commission (IAC) Standards for Dental CT accreditation, and the European Commission Radiation Protection Report No. 172 (SEDENTEXCT) have published guidance on acceptance and periodic testing for dental CBCT devices. Testing protocols and frequencies vary by manufacturer, and the manufacturer's instructions should be strictly followed, including when the manufacturer recommendations exceed guidance provided by national agencies and professional organizations.

Acceptance Tests

CBCT devices must be installed by a qualified expert, and acceptance tests should include evaluation of the x-ray output parameters, beam alignment and collimation, and mechanical and electronic controls of the equipment. The acceptance tests should verify that the device functions as per the manufacturer's specifications and are described in detail in the section on *x-ray sources*. Routine procedures to calibrate detectors and to assess image quality are described in this section.

Many CBCT device vendors provide proprietary phantoms to conduct these periodic tests. Phantoms are also available from third-party vendors for measurement of image uniformity, spatial resolution, contrast resolution, image noise, and geometric accuracy (Fig. 14.6).

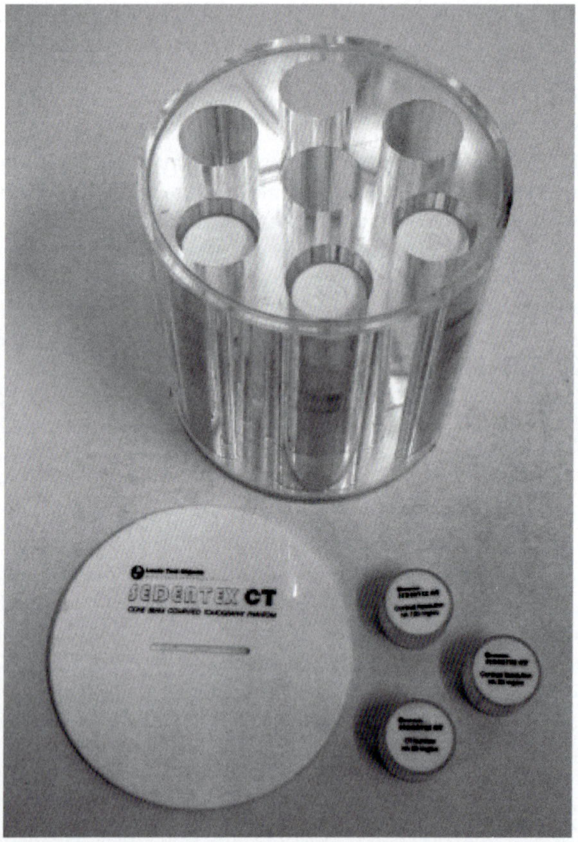

Fig. 14.6 The SEDENTEXCT IQ phantom for cone beam computed tomography image quality measurement. The insert holder is 16 cm in diameter. Attenuation in the body of the insert holder provides assessment of image uniformity and image noise. Individual inserts allow measurement of spatial resolution, contrast resolution, pixel intensity, and beam hardening artifacts. (From Pauwels R, Beinsberger J, Stamatakis H, et al. Comparison of spatial and contrast resolution for cone-beam computed tomography scanners. *Oral Surg Oral Med Oral Pathol Oral Radiol.* 2012;114(1):127-135.)

Daily Tasks

Daily system start-up and shut-down. After powering on the CBCT device, confirm that the equipment function indicators and other safety checks are active. For most CBCT devices, the software application that controls the CBCT device will provide warning and error messages when equipment start-up checks malfunction or fail.

Daily calibration and image quality assessment. Follow the manufacturer's instructions for daily equipment calibration and system checks.

Some manufacturers require an air calibration to be performed, for example, daily to weekly. For this process, a CT scan is made without a phantom or a subject in the imaging field, exposing the detector to an unattenuated x-ray beam. The attenuation data serve to normalize detector response for patient scans.

The IAC Dental CT Standards require daily image quality evaluation that includes measurement of the mean CT number for water and other reference materials, image uniformity and noise, and assessment of artifacts (Figs. 14.7 and 14.8).

Monthly Tasks

Image quality measurement. The IAC Dental CT standards recommend periodic evaluation of spatial resolution for high and low contrast objects and image uniformity. The SEDENTEXCT report recommends monthly measurement of image density values with an acceptable variation of ±10% from the baseline value measured during the acceptance tests.

Annual Tasks

Preventive maintenance. Most CBCT manufacturers recommend preventive maintenance of CBCT units, typically on an annual basis. This is usually performed by a qualified service technician or a qualified expert. The maintenance tasks include evaluation of the x-ray output, beam collimation, electrical and mechanical components controlling the gantry and C-arm, detector response, and image quality. These include tests to align laser beams used for patient positioning and for accuracy of the slice position.

Image quality measurement. In addition to image quality parameters evaluated on a daily and monthly basis, the SEDENTEXCT report recommends annual measurement of image noise, limiting resolution, contrast detail, and geometric accuracy.

INFECTION CONTROL

Dental personnel and patients are at increased risk for acquiring tuberculosis, herpes viruses, upper respiratory infections, and hepatitis strains A through E. After the recognition of acquired immunodeficiency syndrome in the 1980s, rigorous hygienic procedures were introduced in dental offices. The primary goal of infection control procedures is to prevent cross contamination and disease transmission from patient to staff, from staff to patient, and from patient to patient. The potential for cross contamination in dental radiography is great. In the course of making radiographs, an operator's hands become contaminated by contact with a patient's mouth and saliva-contaminated films and film holders. The operator also must adjust the x-ray tube head and x-ray machine control panel settings to make the exposure. These actions lead to the possibility of cross contamination. Cross contamination also may occur when an operator handles digital sensors or opens film packets to process the films in the darkroom. The procedures described in the following sections minimize or eliminate such cross contamination (Box 14.1). Each dental office or practice

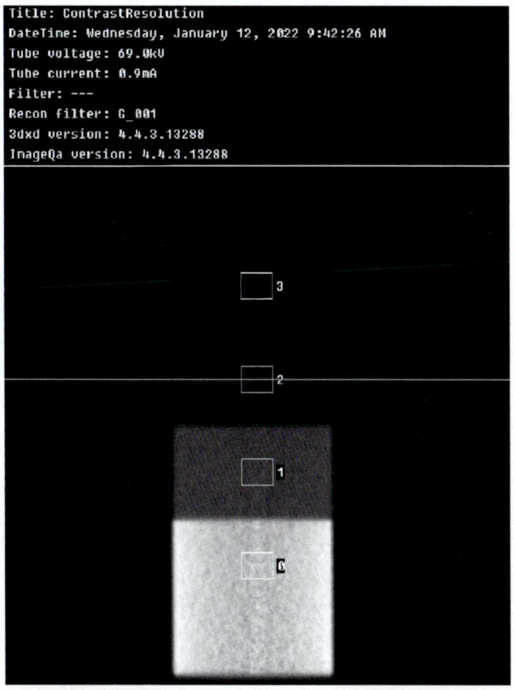

TestMode	ContrastResolution		
DateTime	Wednesday	January 12	2022 9:42:26 AM
Tube voltage	69.0	kV	
Tube current	0.9	mA	
Filter			
Recon filter	G_001		
3dxd version	4.4.3.13288		
ImageQa version	4.4.3.13288		
Position	Value	SD	
0	214.937	6.46279	
1	105.845	3.18371	
2	47.9742	2.39232	
3	5.86452	1.44257	

Fig. 14.7 Test of contrast resolution. Image of the contrast resolution phantom with four discrete materials representing aluminum *(bottom)*, bone, water, and air *(top)*. Regions of interest 3 mm × 3 mm in dimension are defined (boxes labeled 0, 1, 2, and 3) within each radiodensity. The test report indicates the date, exposure settings, reconstruction filter applied, and versions of the software used to acquire and assess the image. The gray values measured in each ROI (mean ± standard deviations) are listed. There should be no overlap between gray values measured in the bone- and water-equivalent regions of the phantom. (Images courtesy J Morita, USA.)

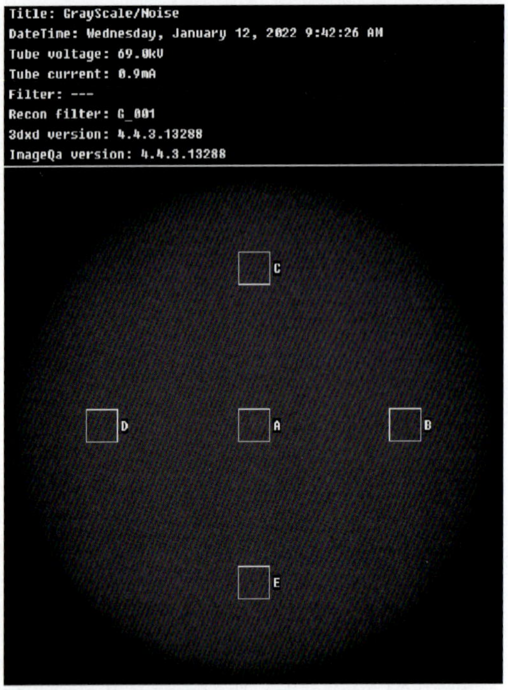

TestMode	GrayScale/Noise		
DateTime	Wednesday	January 12	2022 9:42:26 AM
Tube voltage	69.0	kV	
Tube current	0.9	mA	
Filter			
Recon filter	G_001		
3dxd version	4.4.3.13288		
ImageQa version	4.4.3.13288		
Position	Value	SD	
A	47.4048	2.16959	
B	41.8959	2.28955	
C	42.3652	2.13313	
D	41.9792	1.91755	
E	42.1904	2.10894	

Fig. 14.8 Test of image uniformity and noise. Using the contrast resolution phantom, an axial image is made through the acrylic portion of the phantom to represent attenuation of water. Five discrete regions of interest 3mm × 3mm in dimension are defined (boxes labeled A through E) in the center and in the periphery of the phantom at 3-, 6-, 9-, and 12-o'clock positions. The test report indicates the date, exposure settings, reconstruction filter applied, and versions of the software used to acquire and assess the image. The gray values measured in each ROI (mean ± standard deviations) are listed. When the standard deviations of the five means are less than 6.4, the image is considered uniform. For image noise, the standard deviation of the gray value measured in the center should be less than 6.4. (Images courtesy J Morita, USA.)

BOX 14.1 Key Steps in Radiographic Infection Control

- Apply standard precautions
- Wear personal protective equipment during all radiographic procedures
- Disinfect and cover x-ray machine, working surfaces, chair, and apron
- Sterilize nondisposable instruments
- Use barrier-protected film (sensor) or disposable container
- Prevent contamination of processing equipment

should have a written policy describing its infection control practices. It is best if one individual in a practice, usually the dentist, assumes responsibility for implementing these procedures. This person also educates other members of the practice.

Standard Precautions

Standard precautions are infection control practices designed to protect healthcare workers and patients from disease pathogens spread by blood or any other body fluid, excretion, or secretion. Standard precautions apply when there is exposure to blood; any body fluids, secretions, and excretions (except sweat), regardless of whether they contain blood; nonintact skin; and mucous membranes. Under standard precautions, all human blood and saliva are treated as if known to be infectious for human immunodeficiency virus (HIV) and hepatitis B virus. Accordingly, the means used to protect against cross contamination are used for all individuals. The ADA and the US Centers for Disease Control and Prevention (CDC) stress the use of standard precautions because many patients are unaware that they are carriers of infectious disease or choose not to reveal this information.

Wear Personal Protective Equipment During All Radiographic Procedures

Personal protective equipment is an effective means to shield the operator from exposure to potentially infectious material, including blood and saliva.

- Hand hygiene is considered the most critical measure that can reduce transmission of disease pathogens in healthcare environments. After the patient is seated, the practitioner should wash their hands using plain or antimicrobial soap for a minimum of 15 seconds. An alcohol-based hand rub may be adequate when the hands are not visibly soiled. Many healthcare personnel use hand lotions to manage skin irritation or dryness caused by frequent handwashing or glove use. Petroleum-based formulations degrade latex gloves and should not be used during the work period.
- Disposable gloves should be worn in sight of the patient if the operatory arrangement permits. The operator should always wear gloves when making radiographs or handling contaminated receptor barriers or associated materials such as cotton rolls and receptor-holding instruments or when removing barrier protections from surfaces and radiographic equipment. Operators should remove hand jewelry when it interferes with wearing gloves or could compromise the integrity of the glove.
- Operators should wear protective clothing (e.g., disposable gown or laboratory coat) that covers clothes and skin to protect against potential contamination. Eyewear, a mask, or a face shield must be worn if splash exposure to blood or saliva or other body fluids is anticipated.

Disinfect and Cover Clinical Contact Surfaces

Clinical contact surfaces are surfaces that might be touched by gloved hands or instruments that go into the mouth. These include the x-ray machine and control panel, chair-side computer, beam alignment device, dental chair and headrest, protective apron, thyroid collar, and surfaces on which the receptor is placed. The CDC classifies these as noncritical items. These are objects that may come in contact with saliva, blood, or intact skin but not oral mucous membranes. The goal of preventing cross contamination is addressed by disinfecting all such surfaces and by using barriers to isolate equipment from direct contact.

Working surfaces should be cleaned and disinfected, and covered with a barrier made of clear plastic wrap. Barriers protect the underlying surface from becoming contaminated and should be changed when damaged and disposed routinely after each patient. Although barriers greatly aid infection control, they do not replace the need for effective surface cleaning and disinfection. Experience has demonstrated that failure of mechanical barriers is common during the daily activity of treatment. Whenever this happens, surfaces that become accidentally exposed must be cleaned and disinfected. Operators should avoid touching walls and other surfaces with contaminated gloves.

Any clinical contact surface that is contaminated or potentially contaminated should be disinfected. Table 14.2 lists intermediate- and low-level activity disinfectants recommended for use on clinical contact surfaces. Intermediate-level disinfectants are Environmental Protection Agency (EPA)-registered agents and are tuberculocidal—an effective killer of tuberculosis—and capable of preventing other infectious diseases, including hepatitis B virus and HIV. Low-level disinfectants are EPA registered without tuberculocidal activity but inactivate hepatitis B virus and HIV. High-level disinfectants are used for chemical sterilization and should never be used on clinical contact surfaces.

- Countertops and the x-ray control console should be covered with a plastic barrier. When covering the x-ray control console, the operator should be sure to include the exposure switch and the exposure time control, if they are integral parts of the unit (Fig. 14.9). An x-ray exposure switch that is separate from the console should be covered with a plastic barrier.
- The dental chair headrest, headrest adjustments, and chair back may be easily covered with a plastic bag (Fig. 14.10). The x-ray tube head, PID, and yoke should be covered while they are still wet with disinfectant with a barrier to stop any dripping (Fig. 14.11). The bag should be secured by tying a knot in the open end or by placing a heavy rubber band over the x-ray tube head just proximal to the swivel.
- Exposure charts should be kept away from sources of contamination and not handled during the radiographic examination.

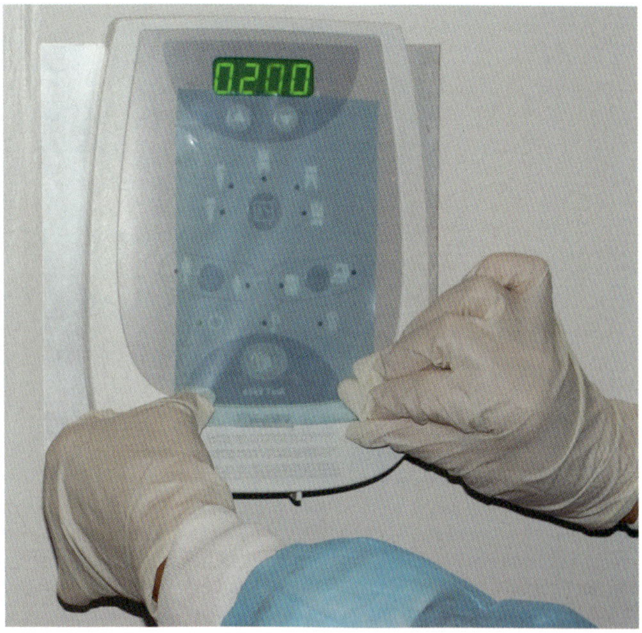

Fig. 14.9 The exposure control console should be covered with a clean barrier and changed after every patient.

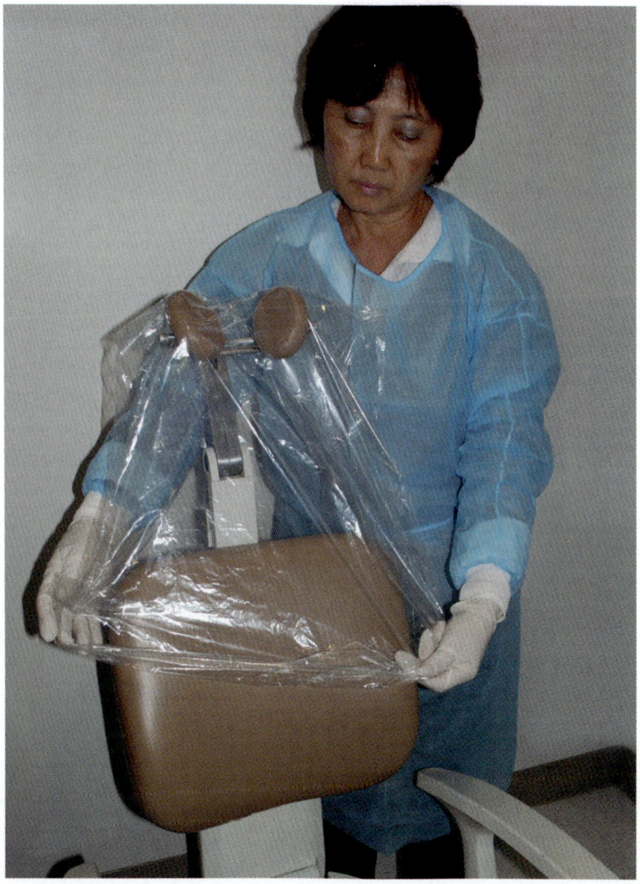

Fig. 14.10 A new plastic bag is placed over the chair and headrest for each patient.

TABLE 14.2 Disinfectants for Clinical Contact Surfaces

Activity	Disinfectant Agent	Concentration
Low	Quaternary ammonium compounds	
Low to intermediate	Phenolic compounds	0.5%–3%
	Iodophor compounds[a]	0.1%–0.2%
Intermediate	Ethyl alcohol, isopropyl alcohol	70%
	Sodium hypochlorite	1000 ppm[b]

[a]Only iodophors that are Environmental Protection Agency–registered disinfectants.

[b]5.25%–6% household bleach diluted 1:50 provides >1000 ppm available chlorine.

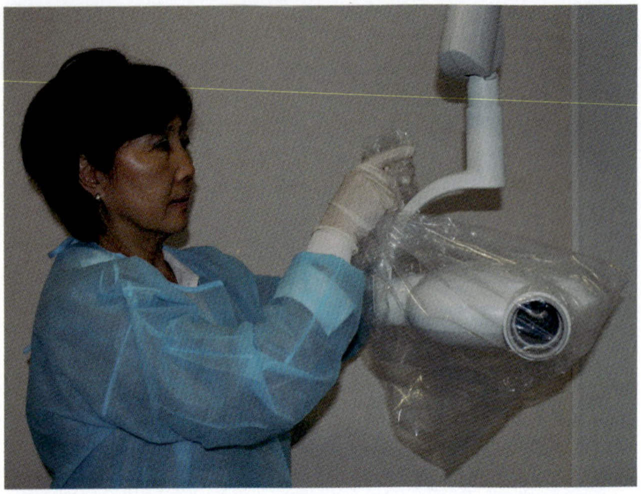

Fig. 14.11 A plastic bag is slipped over the x-ray tube head with a large rubber band just proximal to the swivel or tie ends, as shown here. The plastic is pulled tight over the position-indicating device (PID) and secured with a light rubber band slipped over the PID and placed next to the head.

- Panoramic chin rest and patient handgrips should be cleaned with a low-level disinfectant. Disposable bite blocks may be used. The head-positioning guides, control panel, and exposure switch should be carefully wiped with a paper towel that is well moistened with disinfectant. The radiographer should wear disposable gloves while positioning and exposing the patient. The gloves should be removed before the cassette is removed from the machine for processing because the cassette and film remain extraoral and should not be handled with contaminated disposable gloves.
- Cephalostat ear posts, ear post brackets, and forehead support or nasion pointer should be cleaned and disinfected.
- After patient exposures are completed, the barriers should be removed, and contaminated working surfaces (including surfaces in the darkroom) should be sprayed with disinfectant and wiped as described previously. The barriers should be replaced in preparation for the next patient.

Sterilize Nondisposable Instruments

Receptor-holding instruments are classified by the CDC as semicritical items—instruments that are not used to penetrate soft tissue or bone but do come in contact with the oral mucous membrane. It is best to use receptor-holding instruments that can be sterilized, preferably by steam under pressure (autoclave). After using these instruments, disassemble the aiming ring, support arm, and bite block. Each instrument should be cleaned with hot water and soap to remove saliva and debris. The cleaned components are then loaded into plastic or paper pouches and sterilized in an autoclave. After sterilization, the instruments should be kept in pouches for storage and subsequent transport to the radiography area. When the instruments are taken to the radiography area, it is good practice to keep them in the pouch until immediately before use. After use, instruments should be replaced in the pouch to reinforce cleanliness in the area. The same sterilization pouch should be used to transport the contaminated instruments back to the cleaning and sterilizing areas.

Use Barriers With Digital Sensors

Sensors for digital imaging cannot be sterilized by heat, so it is important to use a barrier to protect them from contamination when placed in the patient's mouth (Fig. 14.12). Typically, the manufacturers of these sensors recommend the use of plastic barrier sheaths that extend a few inches along the sensor cord. However, such barriers fail approximately 40% of the time. Supplemental latex finger cots provide significant added protection. Because such barriers may fail, the sensors should be cleaned and disinfected with an EPA-registered, intermediate-level hospital disinfectant after every patient. The manufacturer of such equipment should be consulted for the proper disinfectant. Some manufacturers have designed solid-state sensors that can be immersed into a cold sterilant (a high-level EPA-registered disinfectant).

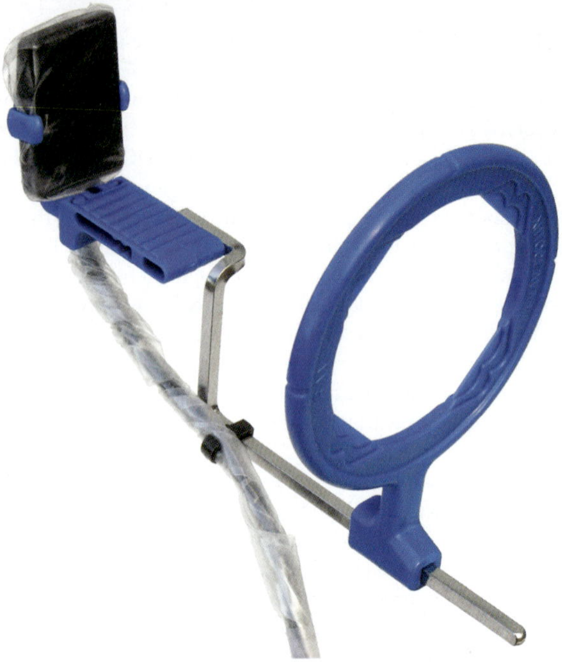

Fig. 14.12 Receptor-holding instrument with barrier wrapping to protect sensor and cord from saliva. (Image courtesy Dentsply Rinn: www.rinncorp.com.)

PSP sensors are placed in disposable plastic bags with a folded seal for use in the mouth. Because the entire plastic bag goes into the mouth with PSP sensors, these plates may become contaminated with saliva when removed from the plastic bags for processing. This contamination could lead to cross contamination of other plates and the processing equipment. To minimize this problem, PSP plates should be disinfected between patients, using a method recommended by the manufacturer. PSP plates may be gas sterilized with ethylene oxide.

Use Barrier-Protected Film (Sensor) or Disposable Container

To prevent contamination of bulk supplies of film, they should be dispensed in procedure quantities. The required number of films for a full-mouth or interproximal series should be prepackaged in coin envelopes or paper cups in the central preparation room. These envelopes of films should be dispensed with the film-holding instruments. For unanticipated occasions in which an unusual number of films are required, a small container of films can be on hand in the central preparation and sterilizing room. No one wearing contaminated gloves should retrieve a film from this supply. Films should be dispensed only by staff members with clean hands or wearing clean gloves.

Film packets may be prepackaged in a plastic envelope (Fig. 14.13), which protects the film from contact with saliva and blood during exposure. Barrier-protected film fits in most film-holding instruments. An attractive feature of the protective envelopes is the ease with which

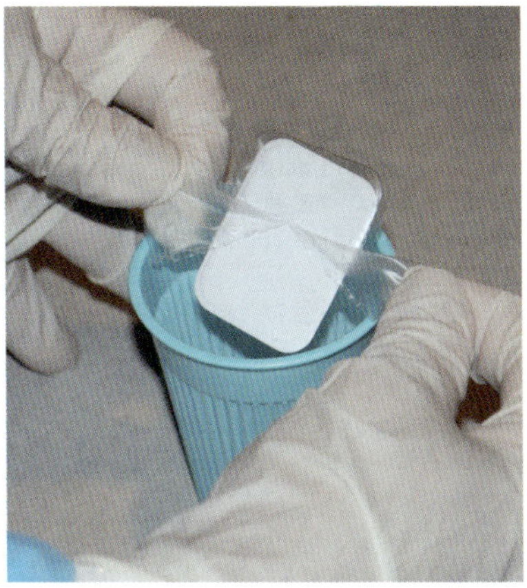

Fig. 14.13 Dental film with a plastic barrier to protect film from contact with saliva. During opening, the plastic is removed and the clean film is allowed to drop into a container.

they may be opened and the film extracted. For best results, the packet should be immersed in a disinfectant after the films have been exposed in the patient's mouth. Then the packet should be dried and opened, allowing the film to drop out. The barrier envelopes can be conveniently opened in a lighted area, the film can be dropped onto a clean work area or into a clean paper or plastic cup, and the film can be transferred to the daylight loader or darkroom for processing.

If barrier-protected film is not used, the exposed film should be placed in a disposable container for later transport to the darkroom for processing. Paper film packets are exposed to saliva and possibly blood during exposure in the patient's mouth. To prevent saliva from seeping into a paper film packet, a paper towel should be placed beside the container for exposed films. The practitioner should use this towel to wipe each film as it is removed from the patient's mouth and before it is placed with the other exposed films. This problem may also be avoided by using film packaged in vinyl.

Prevent Contamination of Processing Equipment

After all film exposures are made, the operator should remove his or her gloves and take the container of contaminated films to the darkroom. The goal in the darkroom is to break the infection chain so that only clean films are placed into processing solutions. Two towels should be placed on the darkroom working surface. The container of contaminated films should be placed on one of these towels. After the exposed film is removed from its packet, it should be placed on the second towel. The film packaging is discarded on the first towel with the container.

The procedure to remove film from a packet without touching (contaminating) is simple. Fig. 14.14 illustrates the method for opening a contaminated film packet while wearing contaminated gloves without touching the film. The practitioner dons a clean pair of gloves, picks up the film packet by the color-coded end, and pulls the tab upward and away from the packet to reveal the black paper tab wrapped over the end of the film. Holding the film over a cup, the practitioner carefully grasps the black paper tab that wraps the film and pulls the film from the packet. When the film is pulled from the packet, it falls from the paper wrapping into the cup. The paper wrapper may need to be shaken lightly to cause the film to fall free. The packaging materials should be placed on the first paper towel. After all films are opened, the practitioner gathers the contaminated packaging and container and discards them along with the contaminated gloves. The clean films are processed in the usual manner. It is not necessary to wear gloves when handling processed films, film mounts, or patient charts.

An alternative procedure when exposing films in vinyl packaging is to place the exposed film, still in the protective plastic envelope, in an approved disinfecting solution when it is removed from the mouth and

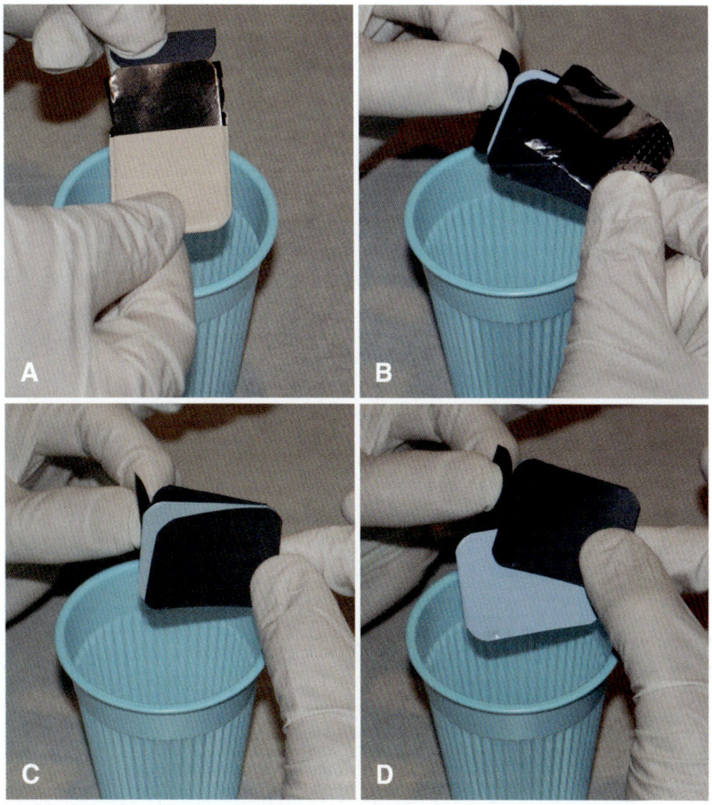

Fig. 14.14 Method for removing films from packet without touching them with contaminated gloves. (A) Packet tab is opened, and lead foil and black interleaf paper are slid from wrapping. (B) Foil is rotated away from black paper and discarded. (C) Paper wrapping is opened. (D) Film is allowed to fall into a clean cup.

after wiping it with a paper towel. It should remain in the disinfectant after the exposure of the last film for the recommended time. Immersion for 30 seconds in a 5.25% solution of sodium hypochlorite is effective.

Automatic film processors with daylight loaders present a special problem because of the risk for contaminating the sleeves with contaminated gloves or film packets. One approach is to clean the films by immersion in a disinfectant, with or without a plastic envelope, as previously described. With this method, the operator cleans the films, puts on clean gloves, and takes only cleaned film packets into the daylight loader. An alternative approach is to open the top of the loader, place a clean barrier on the bottom, and insert the cup of exposed film packets into a clean cup. The operator closes the top, puts on clean gloves, pushes his or her hands through the sleeve, and opens the film packets, allowing the film to drop into the clean cup. After all film packets have been opened, the contaminated gloves are removed, the films are loaded into the developer, and hands are removed. The top of the loader may be removed, and the contaminated materials are then removed.

BIBLIOGRAPHY

Quality Assurance

American Dental Association Council on Scientific Affairs. The use of dental radiographs: update and recommendations. *J Am Dent Assoc.* 2006;137: 1304-1312.

American Dental Association Council on Scientific Affairs. Dental radiographic examinations: recommendations for patient selection and limiting radiation exposure. Revised 2012. https://www.fda.gov/media/84818/download.

American National Standard/American Dental Association. *Standard. No. 1094. Quality Assurance for Digital Intraoral Radiographic Systems.* 2020. https://engage.ada.org/p/eg/ada-standard-no-1094-quality-assurance-for-digital-intra-oral-radiographic-e-book-1235. Accessed July 22, 2024.

American National Standard/American Dental Association. *Standard. No. 1099. Quality Assurance for Digital Panoramic and Cephalometric Radiographic Systems.* 2020. https://engage.ada.org/p/eg/ansiada-standard-no-1099-quality-assurance-for-digital-panoramic-and-cephalometric-e-book-1389. Acessed July 22, 2024.

Buchanan A, Benton B, Carraway A, et al. Perception versus reality-findings from a phosphor plate quality assurance study. *Oral Surg Oral Med Oral Pathol Oral Radiol.* 2017;123(4):496-501.

Code of Federal Regulations Title 21, Chapter I: Food and drug administration, Department of Health and Human services, subchapter J – radiological health. Performance standards for ionizing radiating emitting products. https://www.accessdata.fda.gov/scripts/cdrh/cfdocs/cfcfr/CFRSearch.cfm?CFRPart=1020.

Kwan AL, Ching H, Gray JE, et al. Acceptance testing and quality control of dental imaging Equipment. The Report of AAPM Task Group 175. 2016. http://www.aapm.org/pubs/reports/RPT_175.pdf.

Mah P, McDavid WD, Dove SB. Quality assurance phantom for digital dental imaging. *Oral Surg Oral Med Oral Pathol Oral Radiol Endod.* 2011;112: 632-639.

National Council for Radiation Protection and Measurements. *Radiation Protection in Dentistry, NCRP Report No. 145.* National Council on Radiation Protection and Measurement; 2003.

National Council for Radiation Protection and Measurements. *Reference Levels and Achievable Doses in Medical and Dental Imaging: Recommendations for the United States, NCRP Report No. 172.* National Council on Radiation Protection and Measurement; 2003.

National Radiological Protection Board. *Guidance Notes for Dental Practitioners on the Safe Use of X-Ray Equipment.* 2020. https://www.rqia.org.uk/RQIA/files/44/449bdd1c-ccb0-4322-b0df-616a0de88fe4.pdf. Accessed July 22, 2024.

Pauwels R, Beinsberger J, Stamatakis H, et al. Comparison of spatial and contrast resolution for cone-beam computed tomography scanners. *Oral Surg Oral Med Oral Pathol Oral Radiol.* 2012;114(1):127-135.

IAEA. *Handbook of Basic Quality Control Tests for Diagnostic Radiology.* 2023. https://www.iaea.org/publications/14890/handbook-of-basic-quality-control-tests-for-diagnostic-radiology. Accessed 22 July, 2024.

Quality Assurance in Radiology and Medicine. *Dental Conebeam CT Phantoms.* http://www.qrm.de/index.htm.

Samei E, Badano A, Chakraborty D, et al. *Assessment of Display Performance for Medical Imaging Systems, Report of the American Association of Physicists in Medicine (AAPM) Task Group 18.* Medical Physics Publishing; 2005. https://www.aapm.org/pubs/reports/OR_03.pdf.

Seibert J, Bogucki T, Ciona T, et al. Acceptance testing and quality control of photostimulable storage phosphor imaging systems. The report of AAPM Task Group 93. 2006. http://www.aapm.org/pubs/reports/RPT_93.pdf.

SMPTE RP-133: Specifications for Medical Diagnostic Imaging Test Pattern for Television Monitors. 1991. https://pub.smpte.org/pub/rp133/rp0133-1991_stable2010.pdf. Accessed 22 July 2024.

U.S. Department of Health and Human Services, Food and Drug Administration. *Performance Standards for Ionizing Radiation Emitting Products. 21 CFR 1020.30: Diagnostic X-Ray Systems and Their Major Components.* U.S. Food and Drug Administration; 2014. https://www.accessdata.fda.gov/scripts/cdrh/cfdocs/cfcfr/CFRSearch.cfm?fr=1020.30.

Infection Control

American Academy of Oral and Maxillofacial Radiology infection control guidelines for dental radiographic procedures. *Oral Surg Oral Med Oral Pathol.* 1992;73:248-249.

American Dental Association Council on Scientific Affairs and American Dental Association Council on Dental Practice. Infection control recommendations for the dental office and the dental laboratory. *J Am Dent Assoc.* 1996;127:672-680.

Centers for Disease Control and Prevention. *Summary of Infection Prevention Practices in Dental Settings: Basic Expectations for Safe Care.* October 2016. https://www.cdc.gov/dental-infection-control/hcp/summary/index.html. Accessed 22 July 2024.

Kalathingal S, Youngpeter A, Minton J, et al. An evaluation of microbiologic contamination on a phosphor plate system: is weekly gas sterilization enough? *Oral Surg Oral Med Oral Pathol Oral Radiol Endod.* 2010;109: 457-462.

MacDonald DS, Waterfield JD. Infection control in digital intraoral radiography: evaluation of microbiological contamination of photostimulable phosphor plates in barrier envelopes. *J Can Dent Assoc.* 2011;77:b93.

U.S. Department of Labor, Occupational Safety and Health Administration. Occupational exposure to bloodborne pathogens, needlestick and other sharp injuries, final rule. *Fed Regist.* 2001;66:5317-5325. https://www.osha.gov/pls/oshaweb/owadisp.show_document?p_id=16265&p_table=FEDERAL_REGISTER.

15

Prescribing Diagnostic Imaging

Ernest W.N. Lam and Sanjay M. Mallya

Oral and maxillofacial imaging is one of the most important tools in the diagnostic armamentarium of the dentist. Unfortunately, some dentists use imaging as a shortcut in lieu of taking the time to acquire a comprehensive patient history or conduct a thorough clinical examination. But as with other diagnostic evaluations, the imaging examination should be informed by and ultimately designed on the basis of findings identified in the patient's medical and dental histories, the clinical presentation, and the results of a physical examination. Moreover, when other diagnostic evaluations yield unclear or equivocal results, imaging may be required to support or refute other diagnostic test results. The specific diagnostic imaging procedure that is prescribed should be guided by the results of these evaluations and tailored specifically to the patient's needs and treatment goals. Because most oral and maxillofacial imaging uses ionizing radiation, the dentist must ensure that potential diagnostic and treatment planning benefits associated with imaging outweigh the risks associated with the radiation dose delivered to the patient (Chapters 2 and 3).

RADIOLOGIC EXAMINATIONS

The effectiveness of the imaging examination refers to the likelihood that the procedure will meet the diagnostic objectives. To this end, the design of the type and scope of the imaging examination should be guided by:

- The perceived nature or severity of an abnormality (including its size and accessibility);
- The efficacy of the imaging technique (see Box 15.1 and Table 15.1) to accurately reveal the characteristic radiologic features of the abnormality;
- The amount of image detail required (density, contrast and spatial resolution);
- The radiation dose to the patient.

In some instances, planar imaging (i.e., intraoral) or panoramic imaging may be entirely appropriate and may be the only radiologic examination required. Other cases may require more sophisticated imaging approaches such as computed tomography (CT), magnetic resonance imaging (MRI), nuclear medicine, or ultrasound. Intraoral imaging produces images of high spatial resolution and is the best choice for critically evaluating the effects of diseases involving the teeth and their supporting structures. In contrast, panoramic imaging may allow the clinician to examine more extensive disease involving a larger area, but with lower image resolution and more image artifacts. Advanced imaging techniques such as cone beam computed tomography (CBCT) and multidetector computed tomography (MDCT) may be required when there is a need to evaluate patient anatomy in multiple dimensions without the limitations of anatomical superimposition, while MRI and ultrasound are better suited to demonstrate the soft tissues. When the metabolic activity of an abnormality has to be assessed, nuclear medicine may be useful. Imaging with MDCT and nuclear medicine will deliver substantially higher radiation doses to a patient than will planar imaging or CBCT. Thus, it is important that dentists develop decision-making skills to select the most appropriate examination(s) considering the diagnostic task, radiation dose, and cost of the imaging procedure.

Intraoral Images

Intraoral images offer the clinician the highest spatial resolution relative to other radiographic imaging modalities used in dentistry. Therefore, when fine detail is important or imaging is required to investigate a possible abnormality involving a tooth or its supporting structures, intraoral imaging is the best choice.

The geometry of the incident x-ray beam and the position of the receptor relative to the x-ray beam determine the area imaged. Periapical images, where the image receptor is positioned parallel to the long axis of the teeth and the alveolar process, are optimal to demonstrate the tooth root or roots, the supporting structures (the periodontal ligament and lamina dura), and the periradicular alveolar process. A

BOX 15.1 Parameters of Diagnostic Efficacy

Sensitivity *(true positive ratio)* is the ability of a test to detect disease when the disease is present. A test with a high sensitivity has few false negatives (i.e., fewer cases of a disease, when present, are missed).

$$\text{Sensitivity} = \text{True positive} \div (\text{True positive} + \text{False negative})$$

Specificity *(true negative ratio)* is the ability of a test to detect the absence of disease when the disease is absent. A test with a high specificity has few false positives (i.e., fewer cases of a nonexistent disease are identified as being present).

$$\text{Specificity} = \text{True negative} \div (\text{True negative} + \text{False positive})$$

Positive predictive value (PPV) is the fraction of positive test outcomes that are truly positive.

$$\text{PPV} = \text{True positive} \div (\text{True positive} + \text{False positive})$$

Negative predictive value (NPV) is the fraction of negative test outcomes that are truly negative.

$$\text{NPV} = \text{True negative} \div (\text{True negative} + \text{False negative})$$

	Disease Present	Disease Absent
Radiograph positive	True positive	False positive
Radiograph negative	False negative	True negative

TABLE 15.1 American Dental Association/United States Food and Drug Administration Guidelines for Prescribing Dental Radiographs

	PATIENT AGE AND DENTAL DEVELOPMENTAL STAGE	
Type of Encounter	**Child with Primary Dentition (Before Eruption of First Permanent Tooth)**	**Child with Transitional Dentition (After Eruption of First Permanent Tooth)**
New patient[a] being evaluated for oral diseases	Individualized radiographic exam consisting of selected periapical/occlusal views and/or posterior bitewings if proximal surfaces cannot be visualized or probed. Patients without evidence of disease and with open proximal contacts may not require a radiographic examination at this time	Individualized radiographic exam consisting of posterior bitewings with panoramic exam or posterior bitewings and selected periapical images
Recall patient[a] with clinical caries or at increased risk for caries[b]	Posterior bitewing exam at 6- to 12-month intervals if proximal surfaces cannot be examined visually or with a probe	
Recall patient[a] with no clinical caries and not at increased risk of developing caries[b]	Posterior bitewing examination at 12- to 24-month intervals if proximal surfaces cannot be examined visually or with a probe	
Recall patient[a] with periodontal disease	Clinical judgment as to the need for and type of radiographic images for the evaluation of periodontal disease. Imaging may consist of but is not limited to selected bitewing and/or periapical images of areas in which periodontal disease (other than nonspecific gingivitis) can be demonstrated clinically	
Patient (new and recall) for monitoring of dentofacial growth and development and/or assessment of dental/skeletal relationships	Clinical judgment as to need for and type of radiographic images for evaluation and/or monitoring of dentofacial growth and development or assessment of dental and skeletal relationships	
Patient with other circumstances, including but not limited to proposed or existing implants, other dental and craniofacial pathosis, restorative/endodontic needs, treated periodontal disease, and caries remineralization	Clinical judgment as to need for and type of radiographic images for evaluation and/or monitoring of these conditions	

PATIENT AGE AND DENTAL DEVELOPMENTAL STAGE		
Adolescent with Permanent Dentition (Before Eruption of Third Molars)	**Adult, Dentate or Partially Edentulous**	**Adult, Edentulous**
Individualized radiographic exam consisting of posterior bitewings with panoramic exam or posterior bitewings and selected periapical images; full-mouth intraoral radiographic exam is preferred when patient has clinical evidence of generalized dental disease or a history of extensive dental treatment		Individualized radiographic exam based on clinical signs and symptoms
Posterior bitewing exam at 6- to 12-month intervals if proximal surfaces cannot be examined visually or with a probe	Posterior bitewing examination at 6- to 18-month intervals	Not applicable
Posterior bitewing exam at 18- to 36-month intervals	Posterior bitewing exam at 24- to 36-month intervals	Not applicable
Clinical judgment as to the need for and type of radiographic images for the evaluation of periodontal disease. Imaging may consist of, but is not limited to, selected bitewing and/or periapical images of areas in which periodontal disease (other than nonspecific gingivitis) can be demonstrated clinically		Not applicable
Clinical judgment as to need for and type of radiographic images for evaluation and/or monitoring of dentofacial growth and development or assessment of dental and skeletal relationships. Panoramic or periapical exam to assess developing third molars	Usually not indicated for monitoring of growth and development. Clinical judgment as to the need for and type of radiographic images for evaluation of dental and skeletal relationships	
Clinical judgment as to need for and type of radiographic images for evaluation and/or monitoring of these conditions		

[a]Refer to Box 15.2.
[b]Factors increasing risk for caries may be assessed using the American Dental Association Caries Risk Assessment forms (0–6 years of age) and (greater than 6 years of age), available at http://www.ada.org.
Note. The recommendations in this table are subject to clinical judgment and may not apply to every patient. They are to be used by dentists only after reviewing the patient's medical and dental histories, and completing a clinical examination. Because every precaution should be taken to minimize radiation exposure, protective thyroid collars and aprons should be used whenever possible.
From Dental Radiographic Examinations: Recommendations for patient selection and limiting radiation exposure; 2012.

limitation of periapical imaging is geometric distortion, which occurs if the incident x-ray beam is not oriented perpendicular to the long axis of a tooth root or the crest of the alveolar process.

Bitewing images are made with the receptor positioned adjacent to the crowns of a sextant of the dentition and the crests of the alveolar processes of the maxilla and mandible. In the instance where there has been resorption of the alveolar process in either or both arches, perhaps due to periodontal disease, the image receptor may be rotated so that its longer dimension is vertically oriented; this is the so-called vertical bitewing. Bitewing images are optimal for revealing interproximal caries. These images are made with a 5- to 10-degree downward inclination of the incident x-ray beam to project the crests of the alveolar processes relative to the adjacent teeth with minimal distortion. This orientation also minimizes overlapping of the opposing cusps onto the occlusal surface and may potentially improve the probability of detecting early occlusal caries at the dentinoenamel junction.

Occlusal images are made with the image receptor located between the occlusal surfaces of the teeth in the closed mouth position. In children who may have shallow vestibular depths, occlusal images can be made in place of periapical images, and smaller (American National Standards Institute [ANSI] number 2) receptors are typically used. In adults, occlusal images may supplement periapical and bitewing images, and these are commonly made with larger receptors (ANSI number 4) so that larger areas of the jaws can be imaged without compromising spatial resolution. For digital imaging options, the ANSI number 4 format is only available with photostimulable phosphor plates.

Extraoral Images

Extraoral images allow the clinician to visualize a larger region of anatomy than intraoral images, but with much lower spatial resolution. As the term implies, extraoral images are made with the image receptor located outside the mouth. Depending on the positions of the incident x-ray beam and receptor, numerous views of the face and jaws can be made to specifically depict various anatomic structures. The most commonly used extraoral imaging techniques in dentistry are panoramic imaging (Chapter 8) and lateral skull cephalometric imaging (Chapter 7). Less commonly, planar projection images of the skull, midface, and jaws may be made using lateral oblique, posterior-anterior (Caldwell), occipitomental (Waters), fronto-occipital (Towne), or submentovertex (basal) projections (Chapter 7). However, with increasing availability of CT (particularly CBCT), these planar skull images are made less often.

Panoramic imaging is a form of thin body-section imaging that creates a broad view of the midface and jaws achieved by a single partial rotation of the x-ray source and image receptor around the patient's head. Panoramic imaging has lower spatial resolution than intraoral imaging, and x-ray beam angulation and improper patient positioning can result in image distortion. Furthermore, panoramic imaging is susceptible to patient movement during acquisition, and the complex pattern of superimposition of anatomic structures complicate its interpretation. So while a broad depiction of the anatomy is advantageous, the disadvantages of lower resolution, anatomical superimposition, image distortion, and potential patient movement during image acquisition may make panoramic imaging less optimal than intraoral imaging.

Advanced Imaging

The investigation of many oral and maxillofacial pathoses may require the use of three-dimensional advanced imaging modalities that may include CBCT, MDCT, and MRI. In particular, this is often the case if intraoral, panoramic, or planar skull imaging does not yield the necessary information for patient diagnosis or management. Importantly, the dentist should recognize that these advanced imaging techniques may produce images with lower spatial resolution than intraoral and panoramic images, and that CBCT and MDCT deliver substantially higher radiation doses (these advanced imaging techniques are discussed in Chapters 9, 12). Although these advanced imaging modalities have become more widely available in recent years, it is important to recognize that the decision to employ them should be carefully guided by an understanding of their advantages and limitations. When conventional two-dimensional planar imaging is considered inadequate, prescribing three-dimensional imaging may be appropriate. Dentists who choose to operate their own advanced imaging systems must be well versed in all aspects of that imaging technology, including imaging physics, image artifact generation, image reconstruction, and most importantly, the interpretation of any abnormalities present. In general, these topics require specialized knowledge and training; hence dentists should consider referring their patients to a specialist in oral and maxillofacial radiology for these procedures.

GUIDELINES FOR ORDERING IMAGING

Guidelines are frameworks for professional practice. In oral and maxillofacial radiology, such guidelines inform the image ordering practices of dentists, including the appropriateness of the imaging examination to provide the necessary diagnostic information, and radiation-associated risks. Guidelines are not hard and fast rules. Rather, they should be used to help direct dentists in their decision making. It is important to note that the dentist may use their own clinical experience and judgment to override these guidelines. Nonetheless, guidelines assist the dentist in enhancing their quality of care and provide the justification to use ionizing radiation for the patient's benefit. The appropriate selection of patients and the scope of imaging are effective ways to reduce unnecessary patient radiation exposure.

Previous Diagnostic Images

Many patients may have already been seen by another dentist, and images may have already been made. Such images may be helpful, regardless of when they were made. Even when prior imaging does not reflect the current clinical condition of the patient, it may be of value to demonstrate whether a condition (e.g., caries, periodontal disease) has remained unchanged, worsened, or has shown resolution or healing. Images made relatively more recently may be adequate for the current diagnostic task, thus precluding the need to make additional images during a current visit. For all new patients, the dentist must review the patient's prior imaging history as part of the initial visit and attempt to obtain these images from the office of the patient's previous dentist.

Administrative Images

Administrative images are those that are made for reasons other than diagnosis or treatment planning; these may include images made for an insurance company to approve a treatment or for a dental examining board beyond what might be required for diagnosis. Images made for administrative purposes typically do not benefit the patient, be it the patient's diagnosis or treatment plan; therefore making such images must be avoided. The National Council on Radiation Protection and Measurements Report No. 177 provides specific guidance: "*Administrative use of radiation to provide information that is not necessary for the treatment or diagnosis of the patient shall not be permitted. Students or candidates for licensure shall not be compelled or permitted to perform radiographic exposures of humans solely for purposes of education, licensure, credentialing, or other certification.*"

Guidelines for Ordering Dental Radiographic Examinations

The following general clinical situations may indicate a need for imaging:

- Where there is clinical evidence of an abnormality that cannot be fully assessed by physical examination alone;
- Where there is a high probability of disease that is asymptomatic and not clinically evident.

In the first situation, a patient may have a hard swelling in the premolar region of the mandible with expansion of the buccal and lingual surfaces. This clinical presentation alerts the dentist to the need for a diagnostic image to investigate the nature of the swelling. In the second situation, a patient may seek general dental care after not having seen a dentist for many years, although clinical examination may reveal no evidence of caries. Nonetheless, bitewing images may be indicated. Because the patient has not had bitewing images for many years, it is reasonable to assume that there may be potential benefits for the patient in the detection of interproximal caries that is either not clinically evident, or detectable through other means. In the absence of clinical indicators of early caries, the dentist must rely on their knowledge of caries prevalence and epidemiology (i.e., the sensitivity and specificity of caries detection) (Box 15.1), as well as the patient's risk factors in order to decide whether bitewing imaging may yield a potential diagnostic benefit.

In the mid-1980s, a panel of experts was convened by the United States Food and Drug Administration (FDA) to develop practice guidelines for prescribing dental imaging. These guidelines were developed, in part, as a radiation protection measure to reduce x-ray exposure to patients without compromising the quality of their general dental care. The guidelines were revised in 2004 and again in 2012 in collaboration with the American Dental Association (ADA). It is important to appreciate that since the first document was published in 1987, there has been no change in the philosophy underpinning the original guidelines.

The selection criteria that are a part of the FDA/ADA guidelines describe clinical findings that could benefit from diagnostic imaging (Table 15.1). These circumstances include the identification of positive medical or dental historical findings, or clinical signs or symptoms. The 2012 revised guidelines recognize 6 positive historical findings and 23 positive clinical signs or symptoms for which imaging may be warranted (Box 15.2). In many instances, the selection criteria can become known to the dentist only after an interview and/or clinical examination of the patient. The identification of selection criteria suggests the type of imaging examination most likely to benefit the patient by yielding a positive diagnostic result. Although these guidelines provide the dentist with the principles underlying the ordering of diagnostic imaging, their application relies heavily on the dentist's own clinical judgment. As the practitioner may be the only individual who knows the patient's medical and dental histories, and their susceptibility to oral disease, they must make the ultimate decision to order images using the guidelines as a resource rather than a regulation. The ADA was an equal partner with the FDA in the revision of the guidelines and recommends their use. These guidelines therefore form the basis of the recommendations on intraoral and panoramic imaging in this chapter.

The guidelines underscore the importance of balancing diagnostic benefit with patient risk. Therefore, dentists should expose patients to radiation only when there is a reasonable expectation that the diagnostic image will benefit patient care. A key concept in the use of the selection criteria and the application of the guidelines is recognition of the need to consider each patient as an individual. In other words, the images that a dentist chooses to make are a prescription based on individual need in the same way that medication drugs are prescribed on the basis of individual need. In some jurisdictions, this practice is called prescription radiology. Without some specific indication, it is inappropriate to irradiate the patient "just to see if there is something there." The major exception to this rule is the example we used earlier; that of bitewing images for the detection of interproximal caries when no clinical signs exist of even early carious lesions. The probability of finding occult disease in a patient with all permanent teeth erupted and no clinical or historical evidence of an abnormality or risk factors is so low that making any image just to look for such disease is not indicated. The decision to prescribe imaging to a patient without having obtained a dental or medical history or having completed a clinical examination is not considered responsible.

BOX 15.2 American Dental Association Selection Criteria for Prescribing Dental Radiographs

Positive Historical Findings	Positive Clinical Signs or Symptoms
1. Previous periodontal or endodontic treatment	1. Clinical evidence of periodontal disease
2. History of pain or trauma	2. Large or deep restorations
3. Familial history of dental anomalies	3. Deep carious lesions
4. Postoperative evaluation of healing	4. Malposed or clinically impacted teeth
5. Remineralization monitoring	5. Swelling
6. Presence of implants or evaluation for implant placement	6. Evidence of dental/facial trauma
	7. Mobility of teeth
	8. Sinus tract ("fistula")
	9. Clinically suspected sinus pathology
	10. Growth abnormalities
	11. Oral involvement in known or suspected systemic disease
	12. Positive neurologic findings in the head and neck
	13. Evidence of foreign objects
	14. Pain and/or dysfunction of the temporomandibular joint
	15. Facial asymmetry
	16. Abutment teeth for fixed or removable partial prosthesis
	17. Unexplained bleeding
	18. Unexplained sensitivity of teeth
	19. Unusual eruption, spacing, or migration of teeth
	20. Unusual tooth morphology, calcification, or color
	21. Unexplained absence of teeth
	22. Clinical tooth erosion
	23. Peri-implantitis

From Dental Radiographic Examinations: Recommendations for patient selection and limiting radiation exposure; 2012.

Applying these guidelines to the specific circumstances with each patient requires both discipline and clinical judgment, bringing together the dentist's knowledge, experience, and concern for the well-being of the patient. Clinical judgment is also required to recognize situations that are not described by the guidelines but may be appropriate for ordering diagnostic images nonetheless.

Initial Visit

For a child in the primary dentition who is cooperative and has closed posterior contacts, only bitewing images are required to detect interproximal caries. Additional imaging is recommended only when the medical or dental history or the clinical examination reveals cause. Children without evidence of abnormality or with open proximal contacts may not require a radiologic examination at this time.

For a child in the mixed dentition following the eruption of a permanent first molar tooth, the guidelines recommend bitewing images to detect interproximal caries and a panoramic image or selected periapical or occlusal images to detect abnormalities that may arise during growth and development.

For partially or fully dentate adolescents and adults, the guidelines recommend individualized radiologic examinations based on the patient's medical or dental history, or if the clinical examination reveals cause for additional imaging. The presence of widespread disease (e.g., generalized caries or periodontal disease) may indicate a need for a full-mouth series of bitewing and periapical images. Alternatively, if disease is localized, a more limited examination consisting of a subset of these images may be completed. In a circumstance with no evidence of past or current dental disease, only bitewing images may be necessary to investigate the patient for interproximal caries.

For an edentulous patient requesting prosthodontic care, the guidelines recommend an individualized examination that is based on the patient's medical or dental history, or if the clinical examination reveals cause for additional imaging. This may include selected periapical, occlusal, or panoramic images, and CBCT if dental implants are being considered.

Recall Visit

Patients who return after their initial treatment is completed require careful examination before determining the need for additional diagnostic images. As with the initial examination, images should be obtained if there has been an update to the patient's medical or dental history, or if the clinical examination reveals cause for further evaluation and imaging.

The guidelines recommend bitewing images for recall patients to detect interproximal caries. The optimal frequency for these images depends on the age of the patient and the probability of detecting caries as it relates to caries risk (Box 15.4). If the patient has high risk factors for dental caries (e.g., cariogenic diet, poor oral hygiene) or clinically demonstrable caries, bitewing images may be made at intervals as short as 6–12 months for children and adolescents and 6–18 months for adults until no carious lesions are clinically evident. The recommended intervals are longer for patients not at a high risk for caries: 12–24 months for a child, 18–36 months for an adolescent, and 24–36 months for an adult. Because an individual's risk category can change, the interval between imaging can also change. Apart from bitewing imaging, the guidelines do not recommend that other forms of imaging, including panoramic imaging, be ordered at predetermined, regular time intervals without clinical indication (Table 15.1).

The 2012 FDA/ADA guidelines also include a section related to evaluation and monitoring of bone loss due to periodontal disease. Some form of periodontal disease may affect older adults, and this disease is responsible for a substantial portion of tooth loss. Radiologic imaging plays an important role in the evaluation of patients with periodontal disease after the disease is initially detected on clinical examination, and for monitoring of disease progression. Imaging may assist in the demonstration of bone support for the dentition as well as the presence of local irritation factors that may contribute to the disease, including the presence of calculus or faulty restorations. Occasionally the length and morphologic features of the tooth roots, visible on periapical images, may also be crucial factors in the prognosis of the disease. These observations suggest that when clinical evidence of periodontal disease exists, it is appropriate to make intraoral images, generally a combination of periapical and bitewing images, to help establish and monitor the severity of the periodontal bone loss.

Guidelines for Ordering Cone Beam Computed Tomography Examinations

Unlike the guidelines for dental imaging, guidelines for ordering CBCT imaging are relatively new, and their selection criteria are largely untested. SEDENTEXCT, a European consortium of researchers and clinical oral and maxillofacial radiologists, has published a comprehensive document that addresses selection criteria, quality assurance, and approaches to minimize patient radiation dose. The SEDENTEXCT consortium extensively reviewed the literature for evidence for CBCT use in a wide range of clinical scenarios in dentistry. Among the broad topics addressed is imaging of the developing dentition (e.g., impacted teeth), imaging requirements for assisting in the restoration of the dentition (e.g., the assessment of periapical disease, endodontics, trauma), and oral and maxillofacial surgical applications (e.g., tooth extraction, dental implant placement, orthognathic surgery, treatment of the temporomandibular joint). The document is a comprehensive resource that guides practitioners in the CBCT decision-making process. The approach taken by this group is appropriately conservative in the use of ionizing radiation.

Along the same lines as the guidelines for ordering dental radiographic examinations, the SEDENTEXCT consortium recommends that CBCT examinations:

- Must not be prescribed unless a history and clinical examination have been performed;
- Must be justified for each patient to ensure that the benefits outweigh the risks;
- Should potentially add new information to aid in patient diagnosis and/or management.

Of the many applications discussed in the SEDENTEXCT document, two general themes emerge as best practices for CBCT imaging examinations. First, if, in the past, MDCT has been the imaging modality of choice for a particular investigation of hard tissues, CBCT should now be used. This statement recognizes that radiation doses from CBCT are generally lower than doses from MDCT for similar examinations. Second, the size of the imaging field should be limited to only the area of interest and not go beyond. In keeping with the first theme, smaller imaging field sizes deliver lower radiation doses than do larger imaging field sizes.

Guidelines for CBCT use in specific clinical disciplines have been developed by several professional organizations. The American Academy of Oral and Maxillofacial Radiology (AAOMR) and the American Association of Endodontists jointly developed a position statement to guide clinicians on the use of CBCT for specific diagnostic tasks in endodontics. These evidence-based guidelines consider the diagnostic efficacy of CBCT and its impact on guiding decision making in endodontic treatment; they provide 11 recommendations that address CBCT use in nonsurgical and surgical endodontic management (Box 15.3). Studies have shown that the guidelines when appropriately applied have a positive impact on endodontic diagnostic and treatment decisions.

To provide guidance on the use of CBCT in orthodontic diagnosis and treatment planning, the AAOMR convened a panel of oral and maxillofacial radiologists and orthodontists to develop clinical recommendations. The panel identified several specific clinical situations that could potentially benefit from CBCT imaging beyond that provided by two-dimensional imaging with panoramic and lateral cephalometric skull imaging (Box 15.4).

A joint position statement from the AAOMR and the American Academy of Orofacial Pain provides recommendations for imaging of the temporomandibular joint (Box 15.5).

Several professional organizations throughout the world have developed guidelines for CBCT use in dental implantology. The AAOMR

BOX 15.3 Recommendations for the Use of Cone Beam Computed Tomography in Endodontic Diagnosis and Treatment Planning

1. Intraoral radiographs should be considered the imaging modality of choice in the evaluation of the endodontic patient.
2. Limited field-of-view (FOV) cone beam computed tomography (CBCT) should be considered the imaging modality of choice for diagnosis in patients who present with contradictory or nonspecific clinical signs and symptoms associated with untreated or previously endodontically treated teeth.
3. Limited FOV CBCT should be considered the imaging modality of choice for initial treatment of teeth with the potential for extra canals and suspected complex morphology, such as mandibular anterior teeth, maxillary and mandibular premolars and molars, and dental anomalies.
4. If a preoperative CBCT has not been taken, limited FOV CBCT should be considered as the imaging modality of choice for intra-appointment identification and localization of calcified canals.
5. Intraoral radiographs should be considered the imaging modality of choice for immediate postoperative imaging.
6. Limited FOV CBCT should be considered the imaging modality of choice if clinical examination and two-dimensional intraoral radiography are inconclusive in the detection of vertical root fracture (VRF).
7. Limited FOV CBCT should be the imaging modality of choice in evaluating the nonhealing of previous endodontic treatment to help determine the need for further treatment, such as nonsurgical or surgical treatment or extraction.
8. Limited FOV CBCT should be the imaging modality of choice for nonsurgical re-treatment to assess endodontic treatment complications, such as overextended root canal obturation material, separated endodontic instruments, and localization of perforations.
9. Limited FOV CBCT should be considered as the imaging modality of choice for presurgical treatment planning to localize root apex/apices and to evaluate the proximity to adjacent anatomic structures.
10. Limited FOV CBCT should be considered as the imaging modality of choice for surgical placement of implants.
11. Limited FOV CBCT should be considered the imaging modality of choice for diagnosis and management of limited dentoalveolar trauma, root fractures, luxation, and/or displacement of teeth and localized alveolar fractures in the absence of other maxillofacial or soft tissue injury that may require other advanced imaging modalities.
12. Limited FOV CBCT is the imaging modality of choice in the localization and differentiation of external and internal resorptive defects and the determination of appropriate treatment and prognosis.
13. In the absence of clinical signs or symptoms, intraoral radiographs should be considered the imaging modality of choice for the evaluation of healing following nonsurgical and surgical endodontic treatment.
14. In the absence of signs and symptoms, if limited FOV CBCT was the imaging modality of choice at the time of evaluation and treatment, it may be the modality of choice for follow-up evaluation. In the presence of signs and symptoms, refer to Recommendation #7.

From AAE-AAOMR Joint Position Statement. Use of cone beam computed tomography in endodontics. *Oral Surg Oral Med Oral Pathol Oral Radiol Endod.* 2015;120:508-512.

BOX 15.4 Clinical Indications for the Use of Cone Beam Computed Tomography in Orthodontic Diagnosis and Treatment Planning

1. To assess anomalies in the structure and eruption of teeth
2. To evaluate dental-alveolar boundaries
3. To assess craniofacial skeletal asymmetry
4. To assess maxillomandibular discrepancies
5. To evaluate the temporomandibular joints
6. To assess airway morphology
7. To plan for combined orthodontic and orthognathic surgical management
8. To identify optimal locations for temporary anchorage devices
9. To assess skeletal and dental changes produced by maxillary expanders

From AAOMR. Clinical recommendations regarding use of cone beam computed tomography in orthodontic treatment. *Oral Surg Oral Med Oral Pathol Oral Radiol.* 2013;116(2):238-257.

position statement provides active recommendations to guide presurgical evaluation of potential implant sites and postsurgical assessment of implant placement and related complications. These recommendations are discussed in more detail in Chapter 31 (see Box 31.1).

IMAGING CONSIDERATIONS IN THE ABSENCE OF A POSITIVE SELECTION CRITERIA FINDING

In the absence of a historical finding, or a clinical sign or symptom, the dentist must consider four factors before ordering imaging: the prevalence of an abnormality in the jaws, the probability that such an

BOX 15.5 Recommendations for Imaging of the Temporomandibular Joint (TMJ)

1. Intraoral radiographs/panoramic radiographs should be used to evaluate patients with suspected odontogenic pain. In complex odontogenic pathoses, a limited FOV CBCT scan may be required.
2. CT imaging, preferably CBCT, should be used to evaluate osseous changes in patients with suspected TMJ arthritis. Panoramic radiography has a limited role in establishing arthritic changes.
3. Panoramic radiography should be used for the initial radiologic assessment of a suspected TMJ developmental disorder. CBCT imaging should be acquired for the pre- and postoperative analysis of the TMJ complex.
4. Proton density – or T1-weighted MRI (PDWI or T1WI) of the TMJ, acquired in the closed and open mouth positions, should be used to evaluate the patient with suspected disk displacement. When joint space effusion is suspected, T2-weighted MRI (T2WI) should be acquired.
5. Panoramic radiography can be used as the initial imaging examination of a patient with trauma limited to the mandible. CBCT imaging, with three-dimensional reconstruction, should be used to evaluate patients with known or suspected fractures of the mandibular condyle.
6. CT imaging should be used to evaluate patients with known or suspected cysts and benign tumors in TMJ regions.
7. CT imaging/MRI should be used to evaluate patients with known or suspected malignant tumors in TMJ regions.

From Mallya SM, Ahmad M, Cohen JR, Kaspo G, Ramesh A. Recommendations for imaging of the temporomandibular joint. Position statement from the American Academy of Oral and Maxillofacial Radiology and the American Academy of Orofacial Pain. *Oral Surg Oral Med Oral Pathol Oral Radiol.* 2022;134(5):639-648.

abnormality would not produce a clinically detectable sign or symptom, the ability of the imaging modality to detect the disease, and whether the detection of such an abnormality would influence the management of the patient.

There is, unfortunately, little prevalence data for abnormalities of the jaws. Most of the information is biased toward data reported by academic oral and maxillofacial pathology services that archive data from biopsy submissions. However, because a majority of abnormalities are never biopsied and only noted in the records of patients, it is difficult to obtain reliable information. Abnormalities developing centrally within the jaw bones have an approximately 85% likelihood of occurring in the periapical areas of the teeth and are primarily odontogenic in origin. Approximately 7% are reported to be developmental in origin; the remaining 8% are said to form the basis of the decision-making process. Despite the dearth of data, it is reasonable to question whether imaging would be appropriate for this 8% of cases. As a group, odontogenic neoplasms are rare. Data from various oral and maxillofacial pathology biopsy services report their incidences to range from approximately 0.7% to 2.7% of all accessions—a very small number. Odontogenic cysts are more common with an incidence of approximately 17%, the largest percentage of which are diagnosed by oral and maxillofacial pathologists as radicular cysts. Nonodontogenic cysts by comparison are even more rare, representing approximately 1% of accessions, with the incisive canal or nasopalatine duct cyst being the most common.

In the United States, a review of approximately 30 million health insurance records determined that attempting to detect quiescent disease (disease without any clinical sign or symptom) is not justified on the basis of economic and radiobiologic costs, and the morbidity and mortality to patients. In patient-based studies, where the ADA/FDA selection criteria have been carefully applied to dental patients, only a small number of entities are missed: resorbed roots, retained primary tooth roots, hypercementosis, and dense bone islands. Typically, these entities require no treatment.

Some dentists establish standard operating procedures in their practices so that new or recall patients are seen by a dental assistant or hygienist who makes a predetermined set of diagnostic images at the beginning of the appointment, even before the dentist has had a chance to examine the patient. Although this may be perceived as making more efficient use of the dentist's time, it is contrary to best clinical practices whereby the selection of images is based on the findings of the medical or dental history, or the clinical examination. Conducting a thorough patient interview and examination before ordering images should be the standard protocol in any dental practice.

Radiation doses from diagnostic oral and maxillofacial imaging are typically very low, and realistically, there is negligible risk of harm for any individual patient from one set of images. However, there is a large societal cost, both in terms of health care costs and radiation risk, if millions of dental patients receive examinations without a diagnostic yield. Certainly, this would be the case if widespread routine or screening examinations were conducted. Furthermore, there is now growing concern among the public and the health professionals about the increasing use of ionizing radiation in health care in general, and the risks of this to the public. In dentistry, this concern has come to the fore most recently with the application of large field-of-view CBCT systems.

In summary, there is insufficient evidence to justify imaging, periodic or otherwise, solely to detect quiescent jaw pathoses. Often, dentists take a "defensive approach" to ordering imaging, and perform imaging to reduce their exposure to malpractice liability. Although lawsuits can be filed for many reasons, it is unlikely that they will be successful if the dentist can demonstrate that they have practiced within the accepted standards of care, documenting a thorough medical and dental history, a clinical examination, and that they have carefully considered the guidelines for ordering diagnostic imaging when clinically indicated.

SPECIAL CONSIDERATIONS

Pregnancy

Occasionally it is necessary to obtain diagnostic images of a pregnant patient. Although imaging is not contraindicated in a pregnant patient, many dentists and expectant mothers have concerns about irradiating the developing fetus. When radiation protection practices are followed (see Chapter 3), including rectangular collimation, digital receptors, and protective shielding, the doses from diagnostic oral and maxillofacial radiology are negligible (see Table 3.2 and Fig. 3.4). Indeed, doses from oral and maxillofacial imaging are approximately 30,000-fold lower than the threshold doses necessary to damage embryonic or fetal tissue (see Chapter 2 and Fig. 2.7). Because radiologic imaging in all patients is predicated on there being a diagnostic need, the guidelines apply equally to pregnant patients and to women who are not pregnant.

Radiation Therapy

Patients with a diagnosed malignancy in the head and neck may receive radiation therapy for their disease. During treatment, oral tissues may receive 50 Gy or more, and although such patients are often apprehensive about receiving diagnostic imaging, radiation doses from imaging procedures in dentistry are relatively insignificant compared with the therapeutic doses they have already received. Patients who have received radiation therapy may have radiation-induced xerostomia and are at a high risk for the development of caries, which may produce serious consequences if extractions are needed in the future. Patients who have undergone radiation therapy to areas in or around the oral cavity should be carefully monitored because they are at special risk for dental disease.

EXAMPLES OF USE OF THE GUIDELINES

In the following examples, consider the ways in which the guidelines can be applied to different clinical situations:

- The first visit of a 5-year-old boy to a dental office. The patient's parent reports no known medical conditions, and the patient is cooperative. Clinical examination of the child reveals that there are open contacts between all the primary teeth and there is no evidence of caries. The child has also grown up in a community that has a fluoridated water supply. As a reasonably good diet is being observed, and the parent seems well motivated to promote good oral hygiene, no radiologic examination is required at this time. Images for the detection of developmental abnormalities are not appropriate at this age because a complete appraisal cannot be made at age 5 years. Even if it could be made, it may be too early to initiate treatment for such abnormalities.
- The first visit of a 10-year-old girl in the mixed dentition to the dental office. The patient's first visit to the dentist occurred when she was 6, and her family has recently moved to your community from one that does not have water fluoridation. Unfortunately, you were unable to obtain previous images of the patient. The parent reports no known medical conditions, and the patient is cooperative. The patient has stainless steel crowns on the two remaining deciduous molar teeth and some conservatively placed two-surface resin-based restorations on a single deciduous maxillary molar.

Clinical examination of the child reveals that there is no evidence of decay, and where adjacent teeth are present, there are contacts between them. At this time, it may be reasonable to image the posterior teeth for interproximal decay with two bitewing images. If pulpotomies have been identified in the remaining deciduous molar teeth, it may be useful to make selected periapical images of the teeth if the periapical areas cannot be reasonably evaluated on the bitewing images. A panoramic image of this patient may also be made to evaluate the developing dentition, as this will allow the dentist to identify the presence (or absence) of any permanent teeth and any developing dental anomalies.

- The recall visit of a 17-year-old adolescent male to a dental office. You have seen this patient since he was 4 years old. When the patient was a child, he was allowed to drink juice before bedtime; you were able to bring a stop to this practice by the patient's parents but not before extensive treatment of the patient's deciduous dentition was performed. Fortunately, your efforts to enforce good oral hygiene practices have worked out well, and the 17-year-old has a caries-free permanent dentition. In the past, you placed fissure sealants in all of the permanent premolar and molar teeth. The patient's last bitewing images were made approximately 26 months ago. At this time, it may be reasonable to image the posterior teeth for interproximal decay with two bitewing images. In addition, it may be useful to make a panoramic image of this patient to evaluate the presence of developing third molars.
- A 25-year-old woman receiving a 6-month checkup after her last treatment for a fractured incisor involving both enamel and dentin, but not the pulp. The patient does not have high-risk factors for caries, there are no clinical signs of caries, and no caries is evident on bitewing images made 6 months ago. In addition, the patient shows no evidence of periodontal disease or other remarkable signs or symptoms in general or associated with the recently fractured tooth. As long as the fractured incisor pulp responds normally to vitality testing, no images are recommended for this patient. If the tooth becomes symptomatic, or if the pulp becomes nonvital, a periapical image of this tooth should be made.
- A 45-year-old man returning to the dentist's office after 1 year. At his last visit, two three-surface resin-based restorations were placed on the maxillary right first and second premolars, and root canal treatment was performed on the mandibular right first molar. Also at this time, the patient is found to have a 5-mm pocket in the buccal furcation of the maxillary left first molar but no other evidence of periodontitis. The guidelines recommend that this patient receive bitewing images to determine if he still has active caries and to evaluate the extent of the periodontal disease. Depending on the periodontal charting in other parts of the mouth, consideration should be made for vertical rather than horizontal bitewing images. A periapical image of the mandibular right first molar should be made to evaluate resolution of the periapical inflammatory disease.
- A 65-year-old woman coming to the office for the first time. No previous radiologic images are available. The patient has a history of root canal therapy in two teeth, although she does not know which teeth were treated. Clinical examination reveals multiple carious teeth, multiple missing teeth, and periodontal pockets of between 3 and 7 mm involving most of the remaining teeth. The guidelines recommend a full-mouth series examination including vertical bitewing images for this patient because of the high probability of finding caries, periodontal disease, and periapical inflammatory disease.

BIBLIOGRAPHY

Guidelines for Ordering Imaging

American Academy of Oral and Maxillofacial Radiology Position Statement. Selection criteria for the use of radiology in dental implantology with emphasis on cone beam computed tomography. *Oral Surg Oral Med Oral Pathol Oral Radiol.* 2012;1113:817-826.

American Academy of Oral and Maxillofacial Radiology. Clinical recommendations regarding use of cone beam computed tomography in orthodontic treatment. *Oral Surg Oral Med Oral Pathol Oral Radiol.* 2013;116(2):238-257.

American Association of Endodontists, American Academy of Oral and Maxillofacial Radiology Joint Position Statement. Use of cone beam computed tomography in endodontics. *Oral Surg Oral Med Oral Pathol Oral Radiol Endod.* 2015;120:508-512.

American Dental Association Council on Scientific Affairs. Dental radiographic examinations: recommendations for patient selection and limiting radiation exposure. Revised 2012. https://www.fda.gov/media/84818/download.

American Dental Association Council on Scientific Affairs. The use of cone-beam computed tomography in dentistry. An advisory statement from the American Dental Association Council on Scientific Affairs. *J Am Dent Assoc.* 2012;143:899-902.

Kim DM, Bassir SH. When is cone-beam computed tomography imaging appropriate for diagnostic inquiry in the management of inflammatory periodontitis? An American Academy of Periodontology Best Evidence Review. *J Periodontol.* 2017;88(10):978-998.

Mallya SM, Ahmad M, Cohen JR, Kaspo G, Ramesh A. Recommendations for imaging of the temporomandibular joint. Position statement from the American Academy of Oral and Maxillofacial Radiology and the American Academy of Orofacial Pain. *Oral Surg Oral Med Oral Pathol Oral Radiol.* 2022;134(5):639-648.

Mandelaris GA, Neiva R, Chambrone L. Cone-beam computed tomography and interdisciplinary dentofacial therapy: an American Academy of Periodontology Best Evidence Review focusing on risk assessment of the dentoalveolar bone changes influenced by tooth movement. *J Periodontol.* 2017;88(10):960-977.

Mandelaris GA, Scheyer ET, Evans M, et al. American Academy of Periodontology Best Evidence consensus statement on selected oral applications for cone-beam computed tomography. *J Periodontol.* 2017;88(10):939-945.

McClean PM, Miller JW. Recommendations on administratively required radiographs. *J Am Dent Assoc.* 1983;107:61-63.

National Council on Radiation Protection and Measurements. *Radiation Protection in Dentistry and Oral and Maxillofacial Imaging. NCRP Report Number 177.* National Council on Radiation Protection and Measurements; 2019.

Rios HF, Borgnakke WS, Benavides E. The use of cone-beam computed tomography in management of patients requiring dental implants: an American Academy of Periodontology Best Evidence Review. *J Periodontol.* 2017;88(10):946-959.

SEDENTEXCT. Radiation Protection Number 172, Cone beam CT for dental and maxillofacial radiology (Evidence-based guidelines). http://www.sedentexct.eu/files/radiation_protection_172.pdf. Accessed August 23, 2023.

Tyndall DA, Price JB, Tetradis S, et al. Position statement of the American Academy of Oral and Maxillofacial Radiology on selection criteria for the use of radiology in dental implantology with emphasis on cone beam computed tomography. *Oral Surg Oral Med Oral Pathol Oral Radiol.* 2012;113:817-826.

U.S. Department of Health and Human Services, Public Health Service, Food and Drug Administration, American Dental Association, Council on Dental Benefit Programs, Council on Scientific Affairs. The selection of patients for dental radiographic examinations. Revised 2012. http://www.fda.gov/Radiation-EmittingProducts/RadiationEmittingProductsandProcedures/MedicalImaging/MedicalX-Rays/ucm116504.htm.

Application of Guidelines for Ordering Imaging

Atchison KA, White SC, Flack VF, et al. Efficacy of the FDA selection criteria for radiographic assessment of the periodontium. *J Dent Res.* 1995;74:1424-1432.

Atchison KA, White SC, Flack VF, et al. Assessing the FDA guidelines for ordering dental radiographs. *J Am Dent Assoc.* 1995;126:1372-1383.

Bohay RN, Stephens RG, Kogon SL. A study of the impact of screening or selective radiography on the treatment and post delivery outcome for edentulous patients. *Oral Surg Oral Med Oral Pathol Oral Radiol Endod.* 1998; 86:353-359.

Brooks SL. A study of selection criteria for intraoral dental radiography. *Oral Surg Oral Med Oral Pathol.* 1986;62:234-239.

Chugal N, Assad H, Markovic D, Mallya SM. Applying the American Association of Endodontists and American Academy of Oral and Maxillofacial Radiology guidelines for cone-beam computed tomography prescription: impact on endodontic clinical decisions. *J Am Dent Assoc.* 2024;155(1):48-58. https://doi.org/10.1016/j.adaj.2023.09.007. Accessed July 19, 2024.

Fontana M, Yepes JF, Eckert GJ, Hale KJ, Benavides E. Patterns of radiograph use in a population of commercially insured children. *J Am Dent Assoc.* 2022;153(5):405-413.

Gillies RC, Quiñonez C, Wood RE, et al. Radiographic prescription practices of dentists in Ontario, Canada. *J Am Dent Assoc.* 2021;52:284-292.

Kantor ML. Longitudinal trends in the use of individualized radiographic examinations at dental schools in the United States and Canada. *J Dent Educ.* 2006;70(2):160-168.

Menaker NH, Yepes JF, Vinson LA, et al. Prescription of bite-wing and panoramic radiographs in pediatric dental patients: An assessment of current trends and provider compliance. *J Am Dent Assoc.* 2022;153(1): 23-30.

Rushton VE, Horner K, Worthington HV. Routine panoramic radiography of new adult patients in general dental practice: relevance of diagnostic yield to treatment and identification of radiographic selection criteria. *Oral Surg Oral Med Oral Pathol Oral Radiol Endod.* 2002;93:488-495.

Disease Detection

Reia VCB, de Toledo Telles-Araujo G, Peralta-Mamani M, et al. Diagnostic accuracy of CBCT compared to panoramic radiography in predicting IAN exposure: a systematic review and meta-analysis. *Clin Oral Investig.* 2021;25(8):4721-4733.

Corbet EF, Ho DK, Lai SM. Radiographs in periodontal disease diagnosis and management. *Aust Dent J.* 2009;54(suppl 1):S27-S43.

Daley TD, Wysocki GP, Pringle GA. Relative incidence of odontogenic tumors and oral and jaw cysts in a Canadian population. *Oral Surg Oral Med Oral Pathol.* 1994;77:276-280.

Devereux L, Moles D, Cunningham SJ, et al. How important are lateral cephalometric radiographs in orthodontic treatment planning? *Am J Orthod Dentofacial Orthop.* 2011;139:e175-e181.

Jing W, Xuan M, Lin Y, et al. Odontogenic tumours: a retrospective study of 1642 cases in a Chinese population. *Int J Oral Maxillofac Surg.* 2007;36:20-25.

Madden RP, Hodges JS, Salmen CW, et al. Utility of panoramic radiographs in detecting cervical calcified carotid atheroma. *Oral Surg Oral Med Oral Pathol Oral Radiol Endod.* 2007;103:543-548.

Masood F, Robinson W, Beavers KS, et al. Findings from panoramic radiographs of the edentulous population and review of the literature. *Quintessence Int.* 2007;38:e298-e305.

Moles DR, Downer MC. Optimum bitewing examination recall intervals assessed by computer simulation. *Community Dent Health.* 2000;17:14-19.

Osterne RLV, de Matos Brito RG, Nues Alves APV, et al. Odontogenic tumors: a 5-year retrospective study in a Brazilian population and analysis of 3406 cases reported in the literature. *Oral Surg Oral Med Oral Pathol Oral Radiol Endod.* 2011;111:474-481.

Reddy MS, Geurs NC, Jeffcoat RL, et al. Periodontal disease progression. *J Periodontol.* 2000;71:1583-1590.

Schiffman E, Ohrbach R, Truelove E, et al. Diagnostic criteria for temporomandibular disorders (DC/TMD) for clinical and research applications: recommendations of the International RDC/TMD Consortium Network and the Orofacial Pain Special Interest Group. *J Oral facial Pain Headache.* 2014;28:6-27.

Senel B, Kamburoglu K, Ucok O, et al. Diagnostic accuracy of different imaging modalities in detection of proximal caries. *Dentomaxillofac Radiol.* 2010;39:501-511.

Tawfik MA, Zyada MM. Odontogenic tumors in Dakahlia, Egypt: analysis of 82 cases. *Oral Surg Oral Med Oral Pathol Oral Radiol Endod.* 2010;198:e67-e73.

White SC, Atchison KA, Hewlett ER, et al. Efficacy of FDA guidelines for ordering radiographs for caries detection. *Oral Surg Oral Med Oral Pathol.* 1994;77:531-540.

White SC, Atchison KA, Hewlett ER, et al. Clinical and historical predictors of dental caries on radiographs. *Dentomaxillofac Radiol.* 1995;24:121-127.

Yoon SJ, Yoon W, Kim OS, et al. Diagnostic accuracy of panoramic radiographs in the detection of calcified carotid arteries. *Dentomaxillofac Radiol.* 2008;37:104-108.

Zeichner SJ, Ruttimann UE, Webber RL. Dental radiography: efficacy in the assessment of intraosseous lesions of the face and jaws in asymptomatic patients. *Radiology.* 1987;162:691-695.

Radiation Dose and Effects

Benavides E, Bhula A, Gohel A, et al. Patient shielding during dentomaxillofacial radiography: Recommendations from the American Academy of Oral and Maxillofacial Radiology. *J Am Dent Assoc.* 2023;154(9):826-835.e2. https://doi.org/10.1016/j.adaj.2023.06.015. Accessed July 19. 2024.

Goske MJ, Applegate KE, Boylan J, et al. The "Image Gently" campaign: increasing CT radiation dose awareness through a national education and awareness program. *Pediatr Radiol.* 2008;38:265-269.

Ludlow JB, Timothy R, Walker C, et al. Effective dose of dental CBCT - a meta analysis of published data and additional data for nine CBCT units. *Dentomaxillofac Radiol.* 2015;44:20140197.

Ludlow JB, Davies-Ludlow LE, White SC. Patient risk related to common dental radiographic examinations: the impact of 2007 International Commission on Radiological Protection recommendations regarding dose calculation. *J Am Dent Assoc.* 2008;139:1237-1243.

16

Principles of Radiographic Interpretation

Mariam T. Baghdady

Dentists must have basic skills in interpreting the radiologic images they acquire in their dental practices. This ability requires the mastery of two identifiable and inseparable components of visual diagnosis: perception, the ability to recognize abnormal patterns in the image; and cognition, the ability to interpret abnormal patterns. The following chapter provides an overview of diagnostic reasoning in oral and maxillofacial radiology and an analytic framework to aid in interpreting diagnostic images. The framework will equip the reader with a systematic strategy for image analysis.

ADEQUATE DIAGNOSTIC IMAGES

Any method of image analysis is limited by the information contained in the available diagnostic images. An essential first step is ensuring an adequate number of images of diagnostic quality displaying the region of interest in its entirety. When conventional two-dimensional planar images are being used, multiple images at different projection angles as well as images made at right angles often provide significant additional information. When appropriate, advanced forms of diagnostic imaging can also provide valuable information (see Chapters 9 to 12).

VISUAL SEARCH STRATEGIES

Finding and identifying abnormal patterns in the diagnostic image first involves a visual search of the entire image. Recognizing an abnormal pattern requires both an appreciation and an in-depth knowledge of the variations of appearances of normal anatomy. This is especially true when searching panoramic images. Recent research has shown that the employment of a systematic search strategy by novice clinicians improves their ability to detect abnormalities in panoramic images.

A systematic search strategy involves the identification of a list of normal anatomic structures that would be contained within that particular image. In a periapical image, the list might include the crown, root structure, pulp chamber and root canal system, periodontal ligament (PDL) space, and lamina dura. In a panoramic image, this strategy might involve identifying the posterior border of the maxilla, the floor of the maxillary sinus, the zygomatic process of the maxilla, and the infraorbital rim. In a set of cone beam computed tomography (CBCT) images, normal anatomy would be reviewed through the entire image volume in the axial, coronal, and sagittal imaging planes. In the face of a complex assortment of anatomic structures, using a systematic search strategy will enable the novice clinician to search the complete image more meaningfully. A thorough appreciation of normal anatomy and its variants on two-dimensional images and cross-sectional images is a vital first step in image interpretation. When an abnormality is detected in an image, the clinician must then focus on formulating an interpretation or diagnosis.

DIAGNOSTIC REASONING IN ORAL AND MAXILLOFACIAL RADIOLOGY

Clinical reasoning in diagnostic oral and maxillofacial radiology can be considered unique. The initial task requires the dentist to engage in a complex perceptual phase that involves differentiating normal and abnormal anatomic structures on two-dimensional images of three-dimensional structures. After the visual search process, if a finding is deemed abnormal, the clinician forms a mental three-dimensional representation of the abnormality, including the precise location, size, internal structure, and how the abnormality affects the surrounding normal structures. This complex perceptual step is a method of identifying those features of the abnormality that will assist in arriving at a plausible interpretation or diagnosis.

Frequently, the novice clinician may memorize specific features associated with each type of abnormality and then attempt to use this information to interpret images. This approach has been shown to be ineffective with respect to the correct or accurate interpretation of radiologic abnormalities. Alternatively, it has been found that understanding the basic mechanisms of disease that underpin the changes that each type of abnormality can produce in the diagnostic image is more effective in enhancing a novice clinician's diagnostic accuracy.

Worth, a pioneer in diagnostic oral and maxillofacial radiology, stated, "Radiographic appearances are governed by anatomic and physiologic changes in the presence of disease processes. Radiologic diagnosis is founded on knowledge of these alterations, the prerequisite being awareness of disease mechanisms." In this chapter, the term *disease mechanism* will be used interchangeably with the term *basic science* to describe the pathophysiology of abnormalities at the biochemical, cellular, tissue, and organ levels. Our own work and that of others suggests that understanding disease mechanisms is essential in improving diagnostic accuracy in novice clinicians. Such an approach may assist the novice in creating a firmer understanding of diagnostic entities and their features by creating coherent mental representations of different disease categories. Hence, when clinicians understand why certain features occur, they are better able to make an interpretation or diagnosis that makes sense, rather than simply focusing on radiologic feature counting and rote memory. Furthermore, teaching disease mechanisms and radiographic feature identification in an integrated fashion produces a higher level of diagnostic accuracy in the novice clinician than when instruction is provided in a more segregated manner.

ANALYSIS OF ABNORMAL FINDINGS

There are two main forms of diagnostic processing in radiology; the first is the analytic or systematic strategy, which we have already mentioned. This approach relies on a step-by-step analysis of all the imaging features of an abnormal finding so that an interpretation or diagnosis can be made based on these findings (Fig. 16.1). This type of approach is believed to reduce bias and premature ending of the decision-making process.

The second form, a nonanalytic strategy, assumes that viewing an abnormality in its entirety on a more global level can automatically lead to a more holistic diagnostic hypothesis. This hypothesis is then tested by initiating a deliberate search for features that support the hypothesis. This nonanalytic approach suggests that the clinician can make a more automatic decision regarding the diagnosis without a thorough feature analysis of the image. The expert oral and maxillofacial radiologist may rely on "pattern recognition" as a nonanalytic diagnostic strategy. There is, however, some empirical evidence that novice clinicians can successfully employ nonanalytic reasoning. Critics of teaching novices to rely on nonanalytic processing argue that the success of this diagnostic strategy is limited by the novice's minimal experience and the varied appearances of both normal anatomy and pathologic entities in images. Although analytic and nonanalytic reasoning may be viewed as separate and distinct processes, research has demonstrated that they may be complementary. Students learning oral and maxillofacial radiology could potentially benefit from specific training in combining nonanalytic and analytic diagnostic strategies.

An analytic tool for the identification of abnormal findings is presented in the next section. The main function of this tool is to collect all the available imaging characteristics of the abnormal finding. Once the information is assembled, it is used in the diagnostic process. As imaging characteristics are being collected, it is important to integrate the disease mechanism that has given rise to these characteristics when possible. For instance, Fig. 16.2 depicts the maturation of cemento-osseous dysplasia. In the early stage (see Fig. 16.2A), the periapical bone is resorbed and replaced with a fibrous connective tissue matrix; therefore, it appears radiolucent in the image compared with the normal adjacent bone. In a later, more mature stage, the abnormality begins to produce immature bone in the center (see Fig. 16.2B), resulting in the appearance of a radiopaque focus located at the center of the radiolucency. Knowledge of the disease mechanism underlying the development of cemento-osseous dysplasia allows the dentist to make the correct diagnosis even though the lesion is in an unusual location (the maxilla) and in an edentulous site where the associated tooth has been extracted (see Fig. 16.2C).

ANALYTIC (SYSTEMATIC) STRATEGY

Step 1: Localize the Abnormality

Localized or Generalized

The anatomic location of the abnormality and its extent should be described. If an abnormal appearance affects all the osseous structures of the maxillofacial region uniformly, generalized disease processes, such as metabolic or endocrine abnormalities of bone, should be considered. If the abnormality is localized, is the abnormality unilateral or bilateral? Abnormal conditions such as fibrous dysplasia are more commonly unilateral, whereas Paget disease of bone and cherubism are always seen bilaterally in the jaws (Fig. 16.3). It is also worth noting that many variations of normal anatomy tend to appear bilateral. For example, deep submandibular gland fossa and mandibular tori are often bilateral.

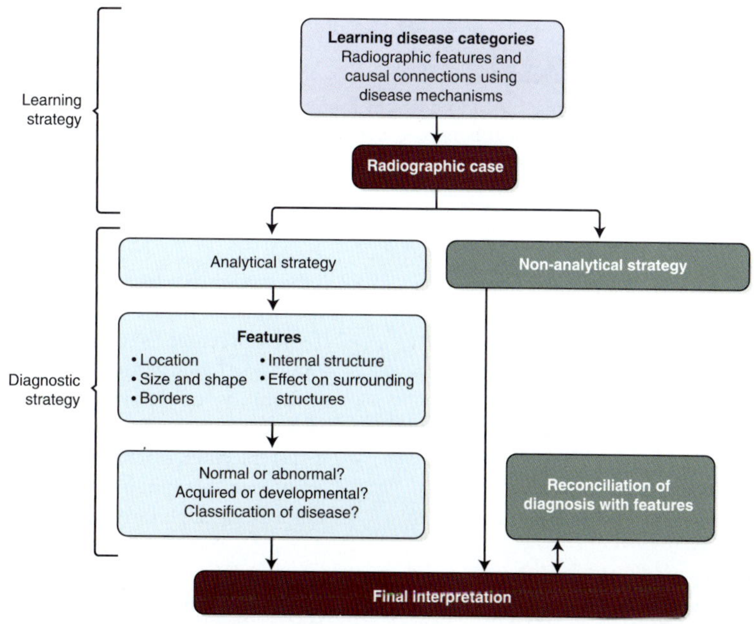

Fig. 16.1 Diagrammatic illustration of the diagnostic process in oral and maxillofacial radiology. The learning strategy phase is the stage in which a novice learns about disease, disease mechanisms, and disease categories. The diagnostic strategy phase is the stage in which diagnostic techniques are used by the clinician to investigate and collect the imaging features of an abnormality.

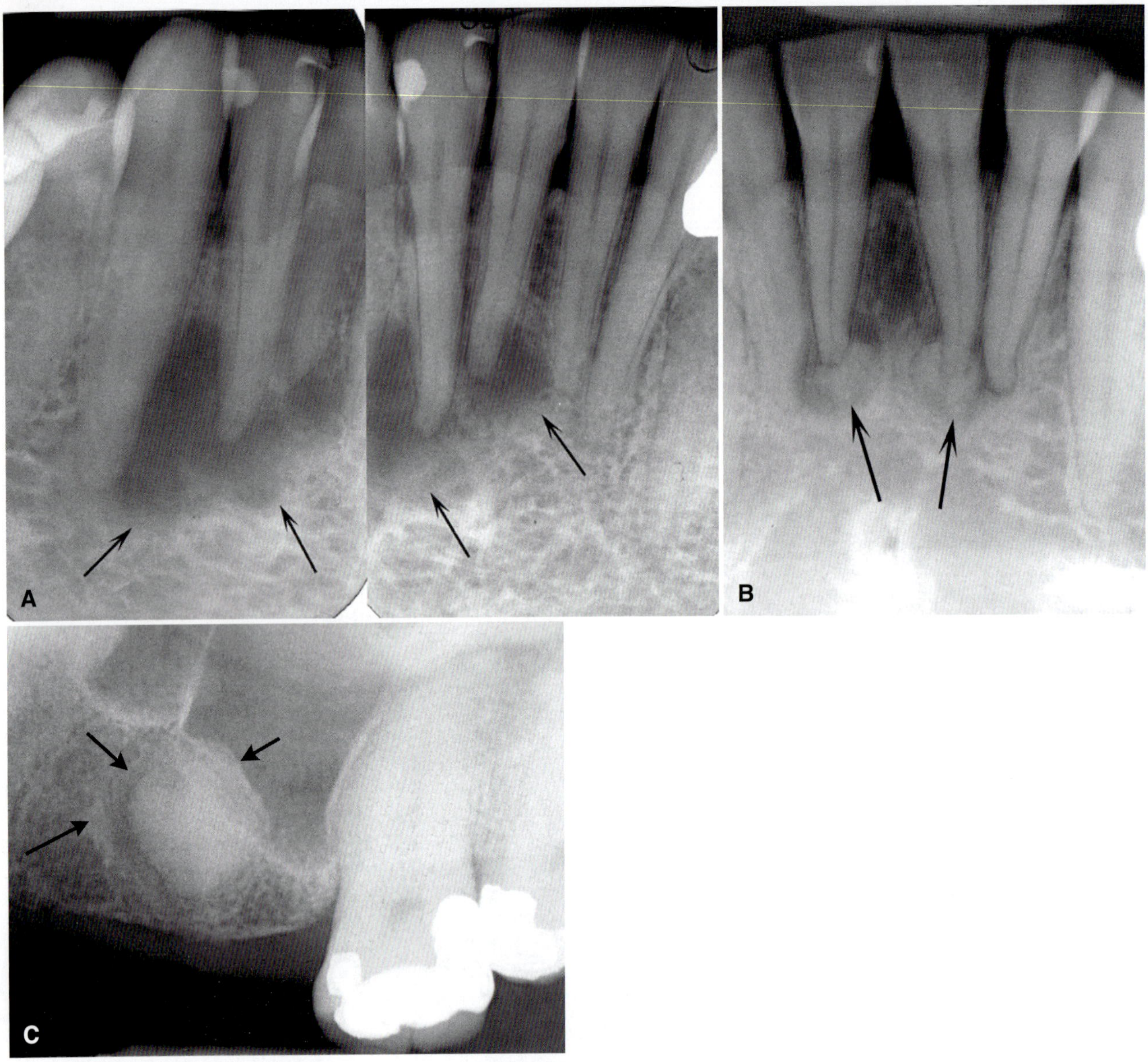

Fig. 16.2 Series of periapical images showing different maturation phases of cemento-osseous dysplasia. (A) Early radiolucent phase after periapical bone has been resorbed and replaced with a connective tissue matrix. (B) Late maturation phase *(arrows)* showing central amorphous bone (radiopaque) surrounded by a radiolucent internal border. (C) Mature phase *(arrows)* of cemento-osseous dysplasia in an unusual location and after the associated tooth has been extracted.

Position in the Jaws

Identification of the geometric center or *epicenter* of a lesion may assist in determining the cell or tissue types contained within the abnormality in question. The epicenter can be estimated by identifying the midpoint of the mesial-distal, superior-inferior, and buccal-lingual extensions of the abnormality. This estimation may become less accurate with very large lesions or lesions with poorly defined borders. The following are a few examples of relating the epicenter of the lesion to the tissue of origin:

- If the epicenter is located coronal to a tooth, the lesion is likely to be odontogenic in origin (Fig. 16.4).
- If the epicenter is located superior to the inferior alveolar canal (IAC), the likelihood is greater that the lesion is of odontogenic origin (Fig. 16.5).
- If the epicenter is located inferior to the IAC, a lesion is unlikely to be odontogenic in origin (Fig. 16.6); rather, it is more likely to have arisen from nonodontogenic sources.
- If the epicenter is located within the IAC, the lesion is likely neural or vascular in nature (Fig. 16.7).
- If the epicenter is in the region of the temporomandibular joint, particularly the condylar head, the lesion has a high probability of arising from either bone or cartilaginous sources.
- If the epicenter is within the maxillary sinus, the lesion is not of odontogenic origin, as opposed to a lesion that has displaced the antral floor superiorly from the alveolar process of the maxilla (Figs. 16.8 and 16.9).

It has also been generally accepted that some abnormalities may arise in very specific locations within the jaws. Although this form of disease localization is often used, it is often unreliable. Therefore, this form of location should never be used as the principal or sole characteristic feature when abnormalities are being interpreted. Rather, it may be considered in the final analysis as a means of validating

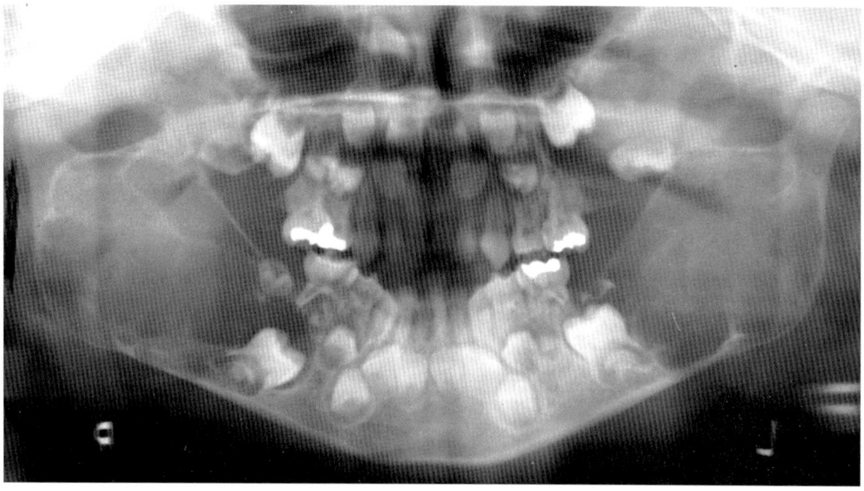

Fig. 16.3 This lesion, called *cherubism,* is bilateral, manifesting in both the left and the right mandibular rami. Because the origin of the lesion is in the midramus region, the mandibular molars have been bodily displaced mesially toward the anatomical midline on both sides.

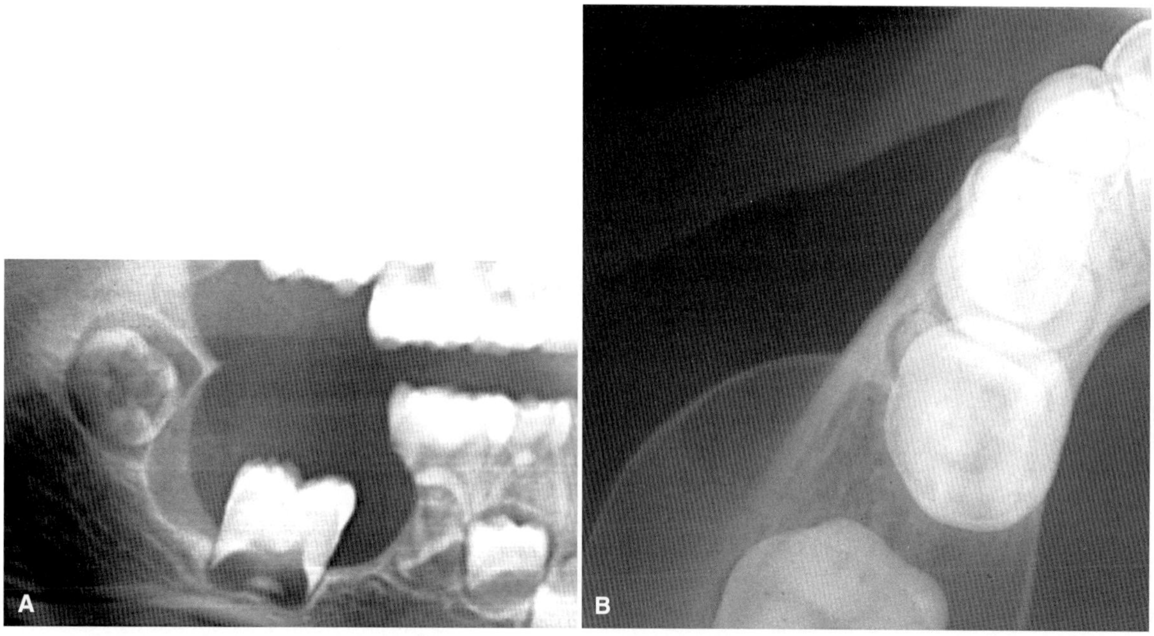

Fig. 16.4 (A) Cropped panoramic image of a lesion where the epicenter is located coronal to the unerupted mandibular first molar. (B) Occlusal projection providing a right-angle view of the same lesion.

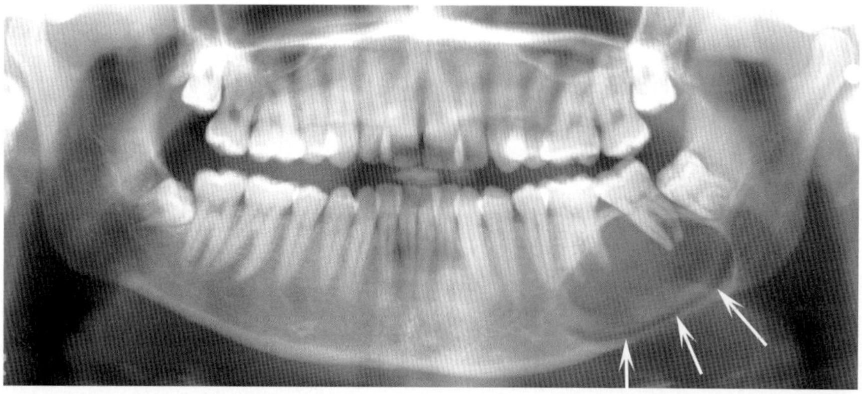

Fig. 16.5 Panoramic image of an ameloblastoma in the body of the left mandible. The inferior alveolar nerve canal has been displaced inferiorly to the inferior cortex *(arrows),* indicating that the lesion started superior to the canal.

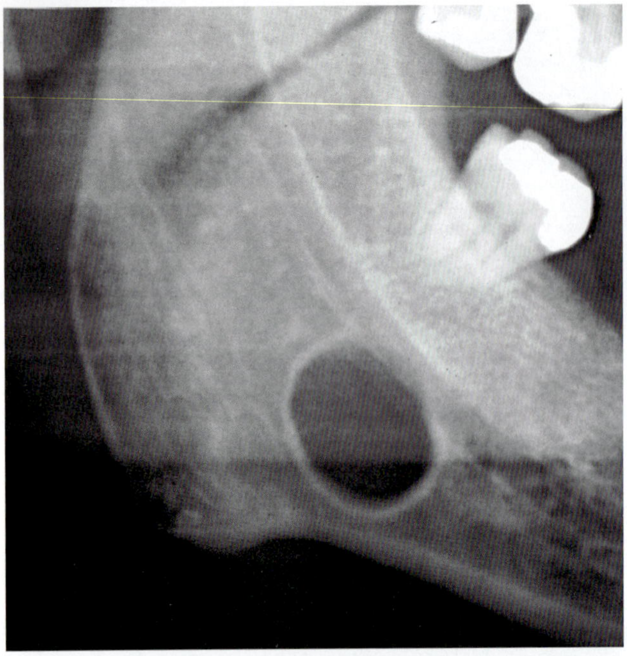

Fig. 16.6 Cropped panoramic image displaying a lesion (a submandibular salivary gland or Stafne defect) with an epicenter located inferior to the inferior alveolar canal. This characteristic is unlikely to be associated with an odontogenic origin.

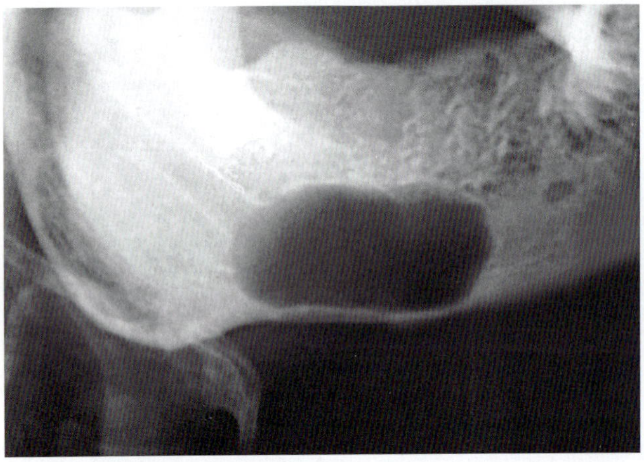

Fig. 16.7 Lateral oblique image of the mandible revealing a lesion within the inferior alveolar canal. The smooth fusiform expansion of the canal suggests a neural lesion.

potential diagnoses. The following disease processes are a few examples of when this approach is used:

- The epicenters of central giant cell lesions are commonly located mesial to the first molar teeth in the mandible and mesial to the canine teeth in the maxilla.
- Osteomyelitis occurs more commonly in the mandible and rarely in the maxilla.
- Periapical osseous dysplasia occurs in the periapical regions of teeth (see Fig. 16.2).

Single or Multiple

Establishing whether an abnormality is solitary or multiple aids in understanding the disease mechanism of the abnormality. Additionally, the list of possible multiple, similarly appearing abnormalities in the jaws is relatively short. Examples of lesions that can be multifocal

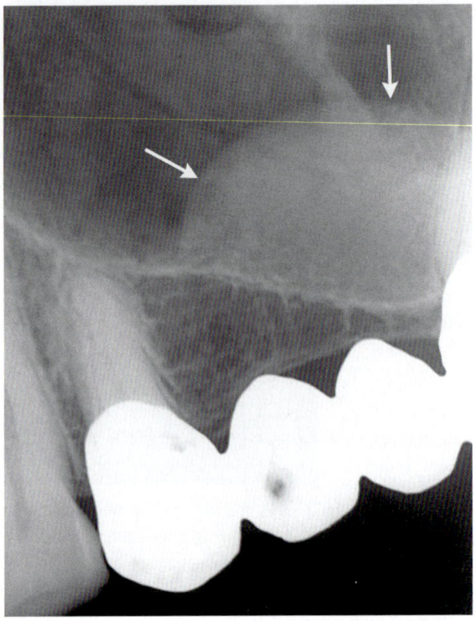

Fig. 16.8 The lack of a peripheral cortex *(arrows)* on this retention pseudocyst indicates that it originated from within the sinus and not in the alveolar process. Therefore it is unlikely to be of odontogenic origin.

in the jaws are cemento-osseous dysplasia, odontogenic keratocysts, metastatic malignant lesions, multiple myeloma (Fig. 16.10), and leukemic infiltrates. Exceptions, of course, may occur, but these general criteria serve as a guide to an accurate interpretation or diagnosis.

Step 2: Assess the Periphery and Shape of the Abnormality

Is the periphery well or poorly defined? If an imaginary pencil can be used to reproducibly and confidently trace the border of a lesion, the border is likely well defined (Fig. 16.11). The clinician should not become overly concerned if some areas are poorly defined; this may be due to the shape of the lesion or direction of the x-ray beam at that particular location. A well-defined lesion is one in which most of the periphery is well defined. In contrast, a poorly defined periphery is one that is difficult to exactly and reproducibly delineate (Fig. 16.12).

The manner in which the normal bone pattern transitions to the abnormal bone pattern of a lesion, and vice versa, is another important feature of the periphery to consider. This is referred to as the "zone of transition." For example, a lesion with a thin radiopaque cortex at its periphery displays a narrow zone of transition; that is, the change in the bone pattern associated with the abnormal lesion across the cortex to the normal adjacent bone is narrow. In contrast, lesions with a sclerotic border exhibit a relatively wide zone of transition.

Well-Defined Borders

Punched-out border. A punched-out border is one that has a sharp and very narrow zone of transition; there is no bone reaction immediately adjacent to the abnormality. The term *punched out* is an appearance that is akin to a device creating a hole in a piece of film or paper with a hole punch. The border of the resulting hole is well defined, and the adjacent bone has a normal appearance up to the edge of the hole. This type of border is sometimes seen in multiple myeloma (see Fig. 16.10).

Corticated border. A corticated border is one that displays a thin, uniform, radiopaque line of bone at the periphery of a lesion. This is commonly seen with cysts and benign neoplasms or tumors (see Fig. 16.4). The presence of a cortical border is usually indicative of a benign and slow-growing biologic process.

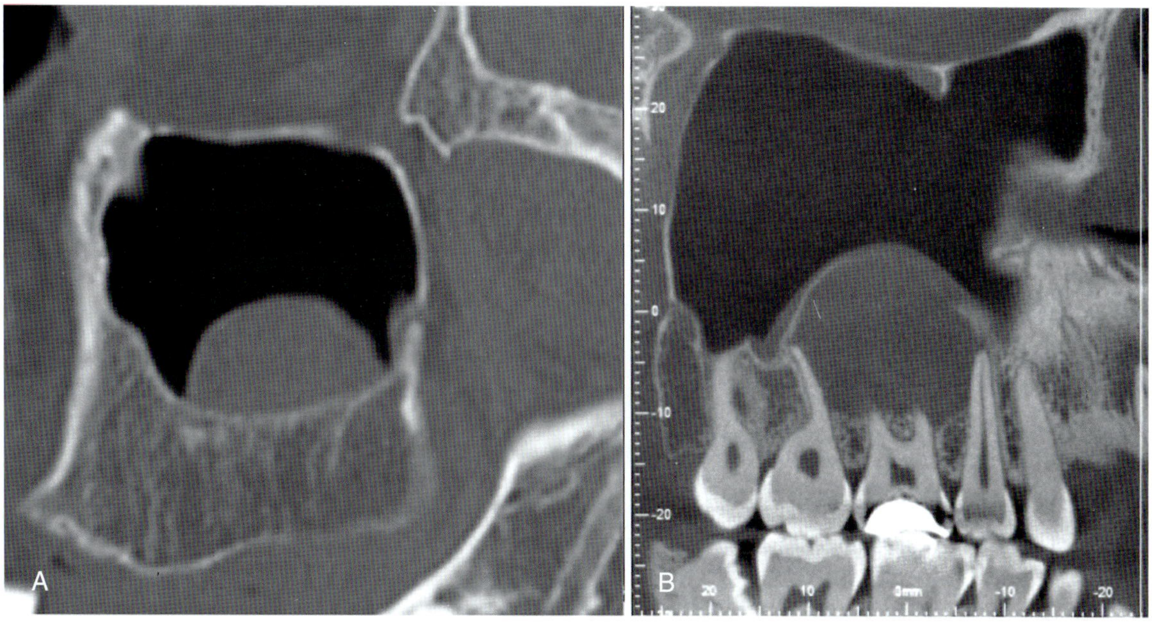

Fig. 16.9 (A) Sagittal cone beam computed tomographic image of the maxillary sinus. The lack of a peripheral cortex on this retention pseudocyst and the preservation of the floor of the sinus indicates that it has originated in the sinus and not the alveolar process. (B) In comparison, an odontogenic cyst originating in the alveolar process, displacing the floor of the maxillary sinus superiorly, exhibits a cortex surrounding the lesion.

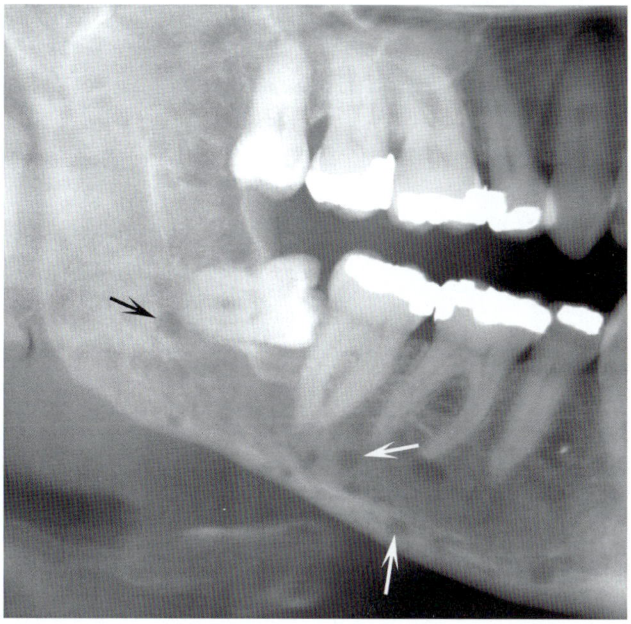

Fig. 16.10 Cropped panoramic image revealing several small punched-out lesions of multiple myeloma (a few are indicated by *arrows*) involving the body and ramus of the mandible.

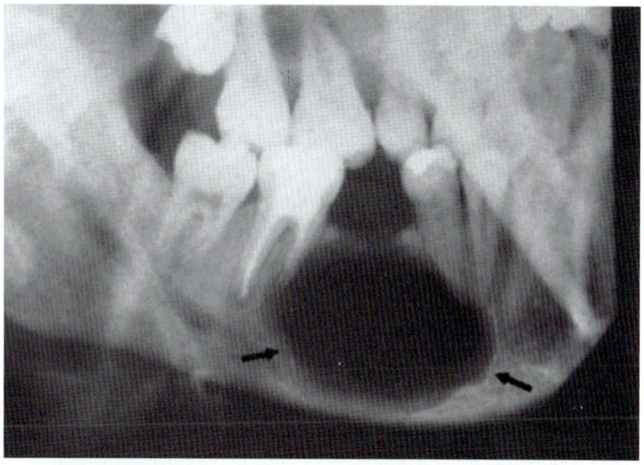

Fig. 16.11 Lateral oblique image of the mandible showing the well-defined border *(arrows)* of a residual cyst.

Sclerotic border. A sclerotic border is one that shows a wider, more diffuse zone of transition between the lesion and the normal surrounding bone. The radiopaque border represents reactive bone that is usually not uniform in width. This border may be seen in periapical cemento-osseous dysplasia and reflects the ability of the lesion to stimulate the production of bone in the surrounding tissues (see Fig. 16.2).

Internal radiolucent "soft tissue" periphery. A centrally located radiopaque lesion may be surrounded by a radiolucent rim of variable width. These lesions are described as having a mixed radiolucent and radiopaque internal structure. Histopathologically, the radiolucent rim represents nonmineralized connective tissue and is sometimes referred to as a "soft tissue capsule." This radiolucent rim may be seen in conjunction with a corticated periphery, as is observed with odontomas and cementoblastomas (Figs. 16.13 and 16.14). A well-encapsulated "soft tissue capsule" is also indicative of a benign and slow-growing lesion.

Poorly Defined Borders

Blending border. A poorly defined border is one that is difficult to resolve. The zone of transition is often more gradual and wider between the adjacent normal bone pattern and the abnormal-appearing pattern of the lesion. The focus of this observation is on the trabeculae rather than the radiolucent marrow spaces. Examples of conditions with this type of margin are sclerosing osteitis (Fig. 16.15) and fibrous dysplasia.

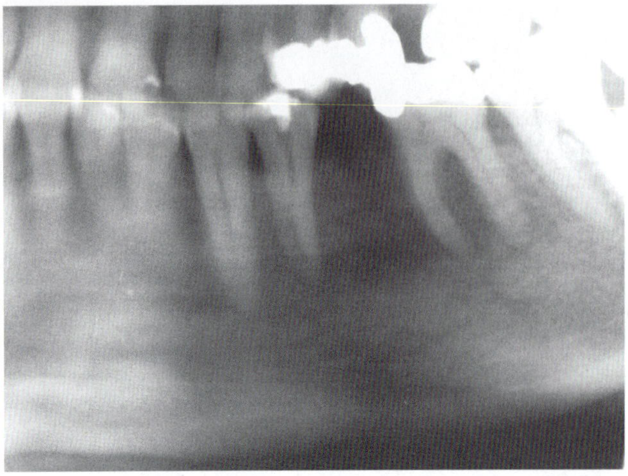

Fig. 16.12 Cropped panoramic image showing the poorly defined border of a malignant neoplasm that has destroyed bone between the first molar and the first bicuspid.

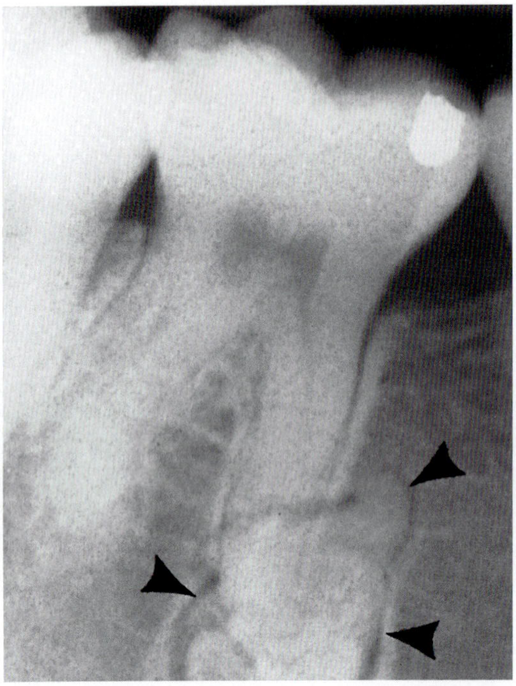

Fig. 16.13 Thin, radiolucent periphery indicates a connective tissue capsule positioned between the internal radiopaque structure of this odontoma and the radiopaque outer cortical boundary *(arrows)*.

Invasive border. An invasive border is one in which there are few or no trabeculae between the periphery of the lesion and the normal bone. Furthermore, the zone of transition is typically wide (Fig. 16.16). In contrast to the blending border described earlier, the focus of this observation is on the enlarging radiolucency at the expense of adjacent normal bone trabeculae. These borders have also been described as permeative because the lesion appears to grow around or through existing trabeculae, producing radiolucent, finger-like, or bay-type extensions into the adjacent normal bone. This growth may result in enlargement of marrow spaces at the periphery (Fig. 16.17). Invasive borders are usually associated with rapid growth and can be seen with malignant lesions.

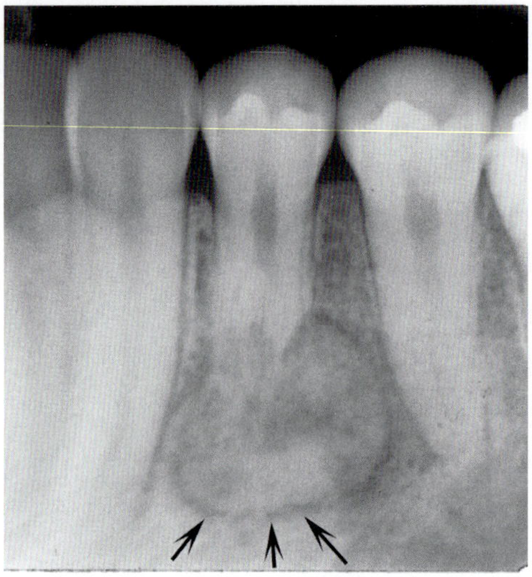

Fig. 16.14 Periapical image revealing a radiopaque mass associated with the root of the first premolar. The prominent radiolucent periphery *(arrows)* is characteristic of a connective tissue capsule of this cementoblastoma.

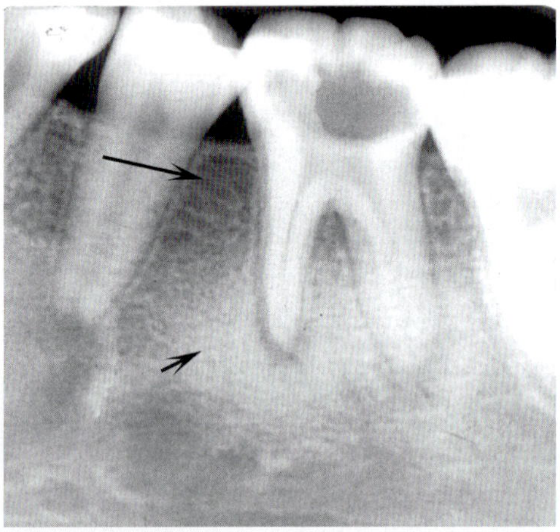

Fig. 16.15 Periapical image shows a gradual transition from the dense trabeculae of sclerosing osteitis *(short arrow)* to the normal trabecular pattern near the crest of the alveolar process *(long arrow)*. This is an example of a poorly defined blending border.

Shape

The lesion may have a particular shape, or it may be irregular. Two examples follow:

- A circular or "hydraulic" shape, similar to an inflated or water-filled balloon, is characteristic of a cyst (see Fig. 16.4).
- Scalloping describes a series of contiguous arcs or semicircles that may develop around the roots of teeth or within adjacent bone or bone cortices. Scalloping may reflect the mechanism of a lesion's growth (Fig. 16.18). This shape may be seen in cysts (e.g., odontogenic keratocyst), pseudocysts (e.g., simple bone cavity), and some benign neoplasms. Occasionally, a lesion with a scalloped periphery is referred to as multilocular; however, the term *multilocular* is reserved for the description of the internal structure in this text.

Step 3: Assess the Internal Structure

The internal appearance of a lesion can be classified into one of three basic categories: entirely radiolucent, entirely radiopaque, or mixed

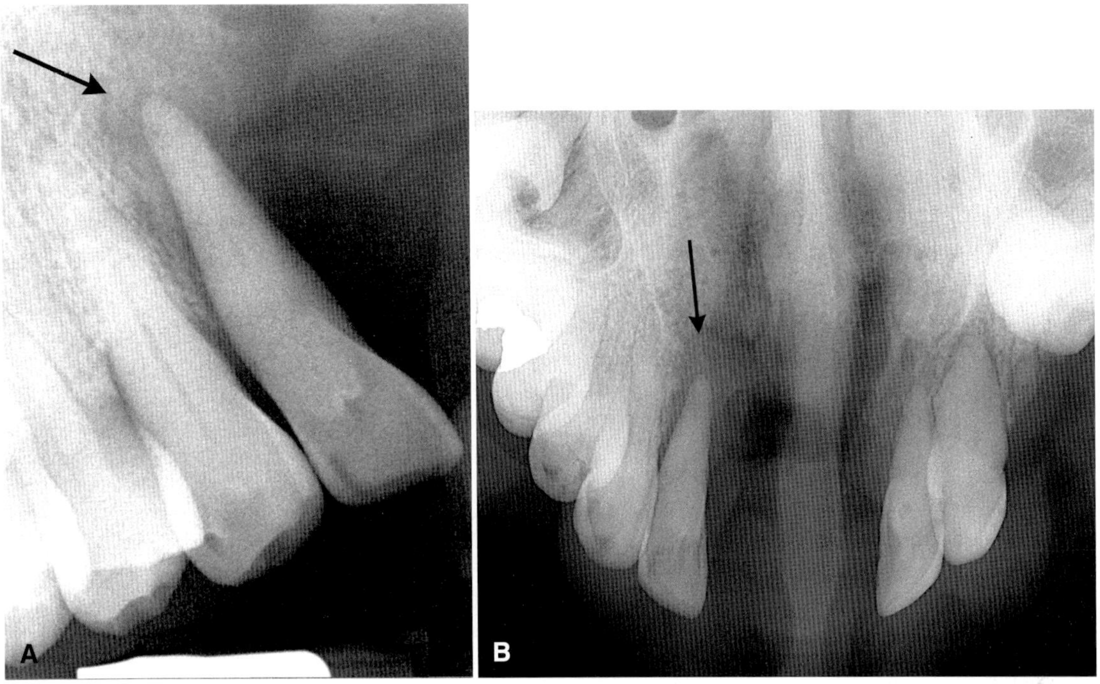

Fig. 16.16 Periapical (A) and occlusal (B) images reveal a squamous cell carcinoma in the anterior maxilla. The invasive margin extends beyond the lateral incisor *(arrow)*, and the radiolucent region with no apparent trabeculae represents bone destruction behind this margin.

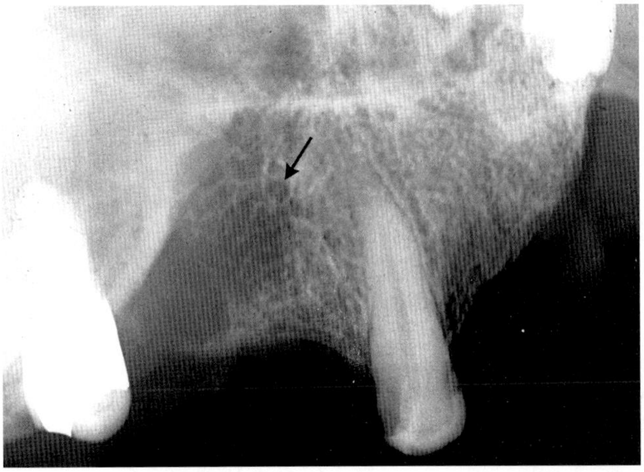

Fig. 16.17 Lateral occlusal image of a lesion revealing an ill-defined periphery with enlargement of the small marrow spaces at the margin *(arrow)*. This is characteristic of a malignant neoplasm; in this case, lymphoma.

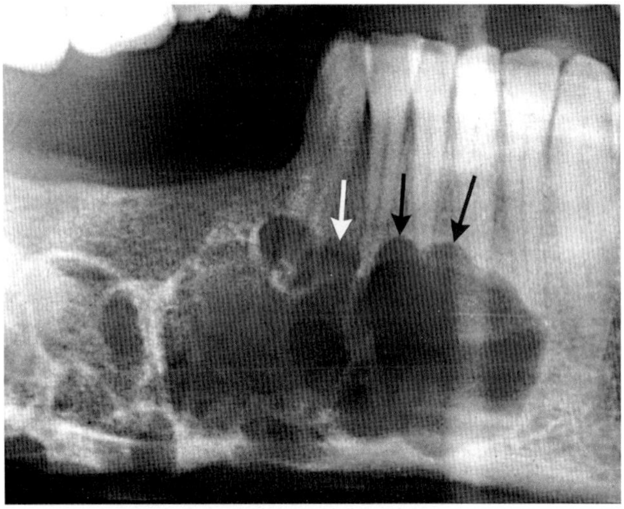

Fig. 16.18 Cropped panoramic image of an odontogenic keratocyst displaying a scalloped border, especially around the apex of the associated teeth *(arrows)*.

radiolucent and radiopaque ("mixed density"). Entirely radiolucent is characteristic of a lesion where the normal bone has been completely resorbed. This is commonly seen in cysts (see Fig. 16.4A). In contrast, entirely radiopaque implies that the lesion is filled with some sort of mineralized matrix; this is observed in osteomas. Mixed radiolucent and radiopaque lesions are those in which calcified material (radiopaque) is deposited against a radiolucent background. A challenging part of this analysis may be deciding whether the perceived calcified material is located within the lesion itself or is located buccal or lingual to the lesion; this difficulty is inherent to using two-dimensional images to represent three-dimensional structures. The shape, size, pattern, and density of the calcified material should be examined. For example, bone can be identified by the presence of a trabecular pattern. Also, the degree of radiopacity may help. For instance, enamel is more radiopaque than bone. The following is a list of the most radiolucent to most radiopaque material seen in plain radiographs:

- Air, fat, and gas
- Fluid
- Soft tissue
- Bone marrow
- Trabecular bone
- Cortical bone and dentin
- Enamel
- Metal

This list is useful, but the amount of tissue or material in the area can affect the degree of radiolucency or radiopacity. For example, a large amount of cortical bone may be as radiopaque as enamel.

The following section describes possible internal structures that may be seen in mixed radiolucent and radiopaque lesions.

Abnormal Trabecular Patterns

Abnormal bone may exhibit various trabecular patterns that are different from those that are seen in normal bone. These variations result from a difference in the numbers, lengths, thicknesses, and orientations of the trabeculae. For instance, in fibrous dysplasia, the trabeculae are usually greater in number, shorter, and not aligned in a manner that may respond to applied forces to the bone. Rather, they are randomly oriented, resulting in patterns described as having orange peel- or ground glass-like appearances (Fig. 16.19). Another example of an abnormal trabecular pattern is the one that develops as a result of stimulation of new bone formation on existing trabeculae in response to inflammation. The change results in the formation of thick trabeculae, giving an area a more radiopaque appearance (see Fig. 16.15).

Internal Septation

Septations represent striations of bone found within a lesion that appear to divide the lesion into two or more compartments. The term *multilocular* is used to describe the resultant compartments. The origin of this internal bone may be trapped normal bone, such as in ameloblastomas. In other lesions, such as central giant cell lesions, cells within the tumor can manufacture bone in a recognizable linear pattern. The length, thickness, and orientation of a septum should be assessed. The appearance of the septa can inform the clinician about the nature and pathogenesis of the lesion. For instance, septa that are curved and coarse may be seen in ameloblastoma, giving rise to an internal pattern that is multilocular or "soap bubble" in appearance. This pattern reflects small nests of tumor cells or cyst-like formations within the tumor at the histopathologic level within the ameloblastoma. The small tumor nests or cyst-like areas entrap and remodel the bone around them as they increase in size (Fig. 16.20A and B). This pattern may also be observed in odontogenic keratocysts. Odontogenic myxomas also exhibit internal septation. In some cases, this tumor contains a few straight, thin septa. In central giant cell lesions, reactive bone in the form of poorly calcified osteoid may develop and appear as low-density and wispy or granular septations in the image.

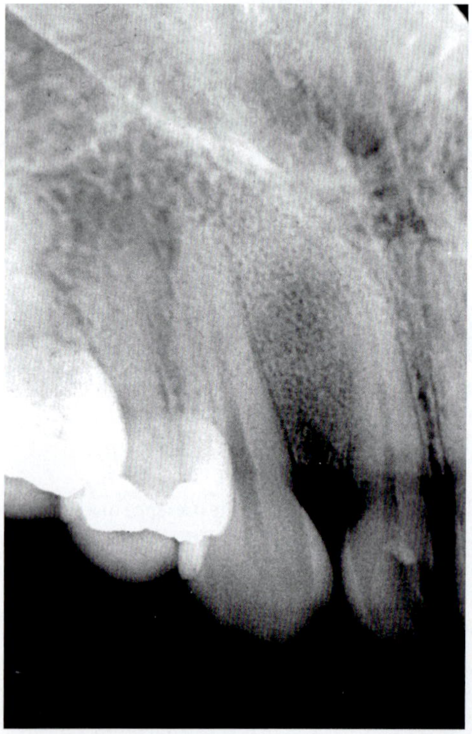

Fig. 16.19 Periapical image of a small lesion of fibrous dysplasia between the lateral incisor and canine demonstrates a change in bone pattern. A greater number of trabeculae per unit area are present; they are small and thin and randomly oriented in an orange peel-like pattern.

Dystrophic Calcification

Dystrophic calcification is mineralization that occurs in damaged soft tissue. It is most commonly seen in calcified lymph nodes that appear as dense, cauliflower-like masses in the soft tissue. In chronically inflamed cysts, the calcification may have a very delicate, particulate appearance without a recognizable pattern.

Amorphous Bone

This type of dystrophic bone has a homogeneous, dense, but poorly organized form. These may sometimes appear round or oval in shape, or flocculant like clouds (see Fig. 16.2). Amorphous bone is commonly seen in bone-forming lesions like the cemento-osseous dysplasias and cemento-ossifying fibroma.

Tooth Structure

Tooth structure can be identified by the presence of enamel, dentin, and pulp chambers. Also, the density of this material is equivalent to the normal density of tooth structure and is of greater density than the surrounding bone (see Fig. 16.13). The most common lesions that demonstrate these changes are compound and complex odontomas.

Step 4: Assess the Effects of the Lesion on Adjacent Structures

Evaluating the effects of a lesion on adjacent structures allows the dentist to infer biologic behavior, and this behavior may aid in the diagnosis of the disease. However, understanding the disease mechanisms that gives rise to these changes is required. For instance, periapical inflammatory disease can stimulate bone resorption (rarefaction) or formation (sclerosis). Bone formation may occur on the surface of existing trabeculae, resulting in thickened trabeculae, and this may be reflected in an overall increase in the radiopacity of the bone (see Fig. 16.15). A space-occupying lesion, such as a cyst or a benign neoplasm or tumor, slowly creates its own space by displacing teeth and other adjacent structures (see Fig. 16.4). The following sections give examples of effects on surrounding structures and the conclusions that may be inferred from the behavior of the lesions.

Teeth, Lamina Dura, and Periodontal Ligament Space

Displacement of teeth is seen more commonly with benign, slower-growing, space-occupying lesions. The direction of tooth displacement is significant. Lesions with an epicenter above the crown of a tooth (i.e., dentigerous cysts and occasionally odontomas) will displace the tooth apically (see Fig. 16.4A). Central giant cell lesions arising in cherubism have a propensity to bodily displace teeth in a mesial (anterior) direction given the epicenters of these lesions (see Fig. 16.3). Some lesions (e.g., lymphoma, leukemia) can develop in the papillae of developing teeth and may push a developing tooth in a coronal direction (Fig. 16.21).

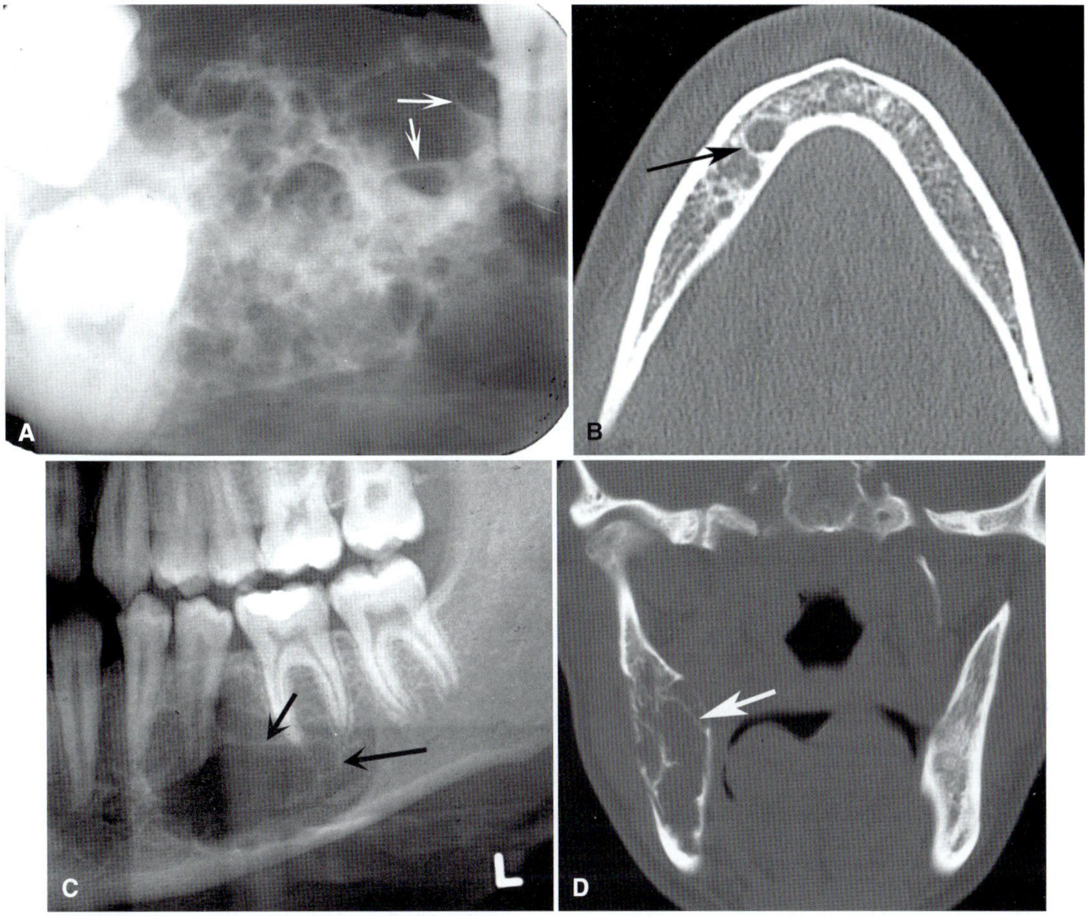

Fig. 16.20 (A) Periapical image of an ameloblastoma. The multilocular pattern created by septa *(arrows)* divides the internal structure into smaller, soap bubble-like compartments. (B) Axial multidetector computed tomography image of an ameloblastoma has typically curved septa *(arrow)*. (C) A cropped panoramic image of a central giant cell lesion with faint septations *(arrows)*. (D) Coronal computed tomography image of an odontogenic myxoma with typically straight septa *(arrow)*.

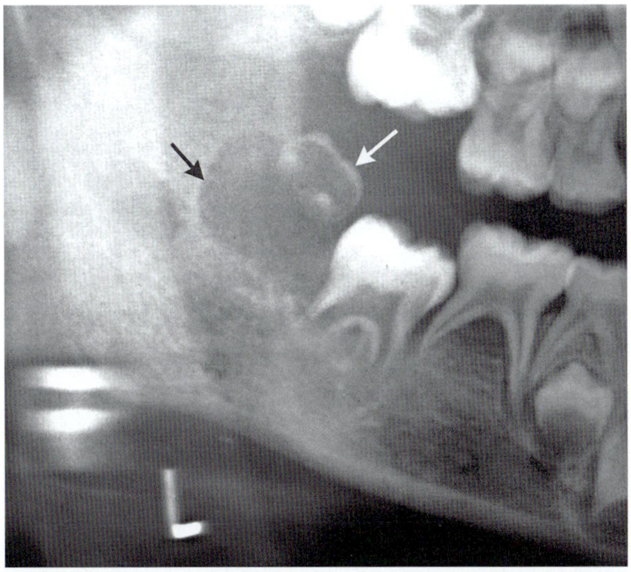

Fig. 16.21 Leukemic infiltration of the mandible shows coronal displacement of the developing second molar *(white arrow)* from the remnants of its crypt *(black arrow)*. There is a lack of a lamina dura around the apex of the first molar and widening of the periodontal ligament space around the second deciduous molar.

Resorption of teeth usually occurs with slow-growing processes (see Fig. 16.4A). It may also result from chronic inflammation. Although tooth resorption is more commonly related to benign processes, some malignant tumors, particularly sarcomas, can occasionally resorb teeth.

Widening of the PDL space may be seen with a number of abnormalities. It is important to observe whether the widening is localized or generalized, irregular or uniform, as well as the epicenter of the widening. The adjacent lamina dura should also be simultaneously assessed to determine its condition. For instance, orthodontic movement of teeth results in generalized but uniform widening of the PDL space around the entirety of the tooth roots, but the lamina dura remains intact. Malignant lesions can rapidly grow into and invade the PDL space resulting in irregular widening with destruction of the lamina dura (Fig. 16.22). The epicenter of the widening may also aid in determining the behavior of a lesion. If the widening of the PDL space has an epicenter located at the apex of the tooth (e.g., in rarefying osteitis), then the source of inflammation will most probably be from the pulp chamber and the root canal of the tooth. If the epicenter of the widening is coronal, near the bone crest, then the source of inflammation is most probably periodontal in nature.

Surrounding Bone Reaction

Some abnormalities can stimulate a bone reaction at the periphery. An example is the cortex of a cyst or the sclerotic border that is often seen

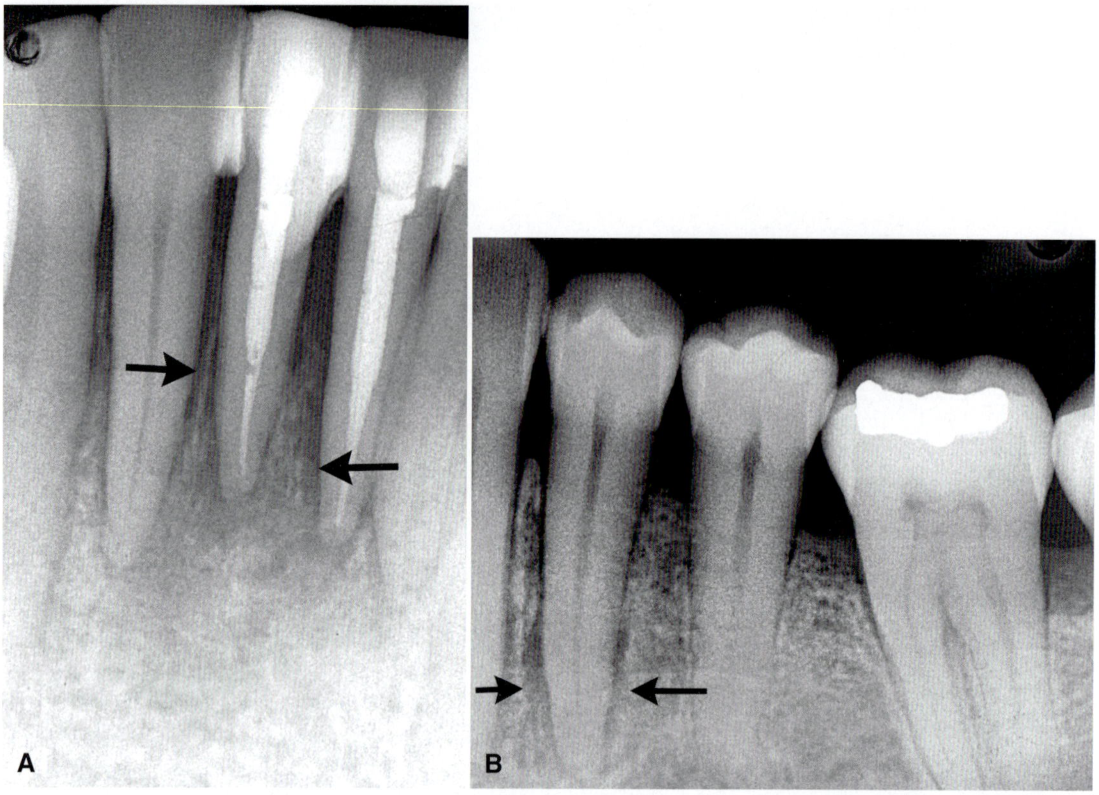

Fig. 16.22 (A and B) Periapical images revealing a lymphoma that has invaded the mandible. There is irregular widening of the periodontal ligament spaces *(arrows)*.

in the cemento-osseous dysplasias, as previously described. The corticated border of a cyst is not actually part of the cyst; rather, it is a bone reaction that develops in response to the cyst as it enlarges. Identification of peripheral bone formation provides a behavioral characteristic suggesting that the abnormality has the ability to stimulate an osteoblastic reaction. Periapical rarefying osteitis can also stimulate a sclerotic bone reaction (see Fig. 16.15), as can some metastatic prostate and breast lesions.

Inferior Alveolar Canal and Mental Foramen

Changes to the IAC can be characteristic of specific disease processes. Superior displacement of the IAC is strongly associated with fibrous dysplasia when the epicenter of the abnormality is located inferior to the canal. Widening of the IAC with the maintenance of a cortical boundary may indicate the presence of a benign lesion of vascular or neural origin within the canal (see Fig. 16.7). Irregular widening with cortical destruction may indicate the presence of a malignant neoplasm growing within the canal along its length.

Cortical Bone and Periosteal Reactions

The cortical boundaries of bone may remodel in response to the growth of a lesion within the maxilla or mandible. A slowly growing lesion may allow time for the surface periosteum to manufacture new bone so that the resulting expanded bone surface is intact and the outer cortex maintained (see Fig. 16.4B). In contrast, a rapidly growing lesion outstrips the ability of the periosteum to respond, and the cortex may be lost (Fig. 16.23). The remodeled external shape of the mandible or maxilla can provide information about the way in which the entity is growing. For instance, a tumor such as ossifying fibroma often has a concentric growth pattern with a clear epicenter. In contrast, bone dysplasias such as fibrous dysplasia, will enlarge the bone along its length without an obvious epicenter (Fig. 16.24). The amount of expansion may also hint at the type of lesion. For example, some lesions tend to grow along the bone with minimal expansion; for example, odontogenic keratocysts, myxomas, and simple bone cavities. On the other hand, dentigerous cysts and ameloblastomas tend to cause marked expansion of the involved cortical boundaries.

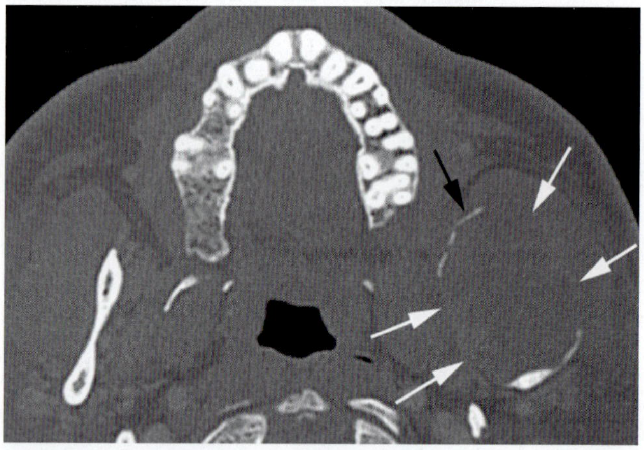

Fig. 16.23 Axial computed tomography image of an ameloblastoma involving the left mandibular ramus shows significant expansion of the ramus with displacement of the bone border *(black arrow)*. In some areas *(white arrows)*, the speed of growth of the tumor has exceeded the ability of the bone to keep it confined.

Exudate from an inflammatory lesion can stimulate the periosteum to lay down new bone (Fig. 16.25). When this process occurs more than once, a layering of new bone commonly referred to as an "onionskin"

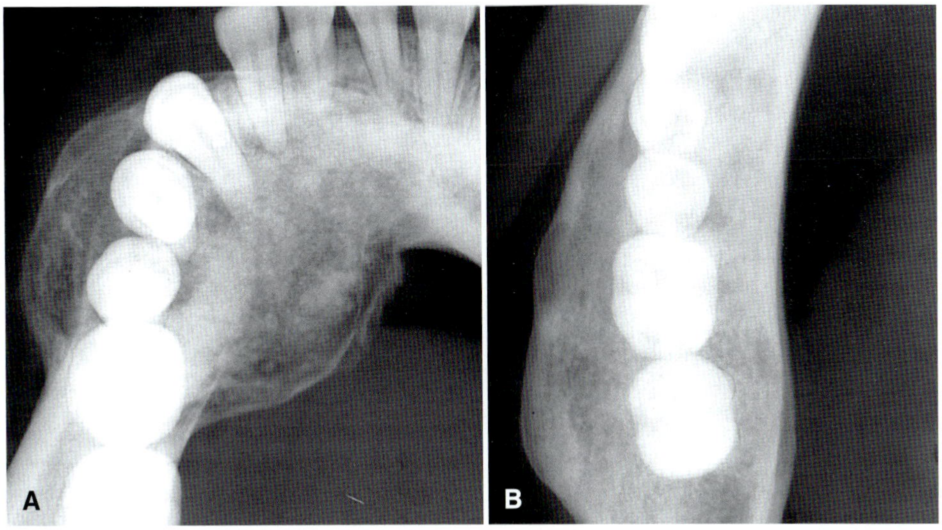

Fig. 16.24 (A) Occlusal image of a cemento-ossifying fibroma. The concentric expansion of the mandible is characteristic of a benign tumor. (B) Occlusal image of fibrous dysplasia with enlargement of bone along the length of the mandibular body without an obvious epicenter.

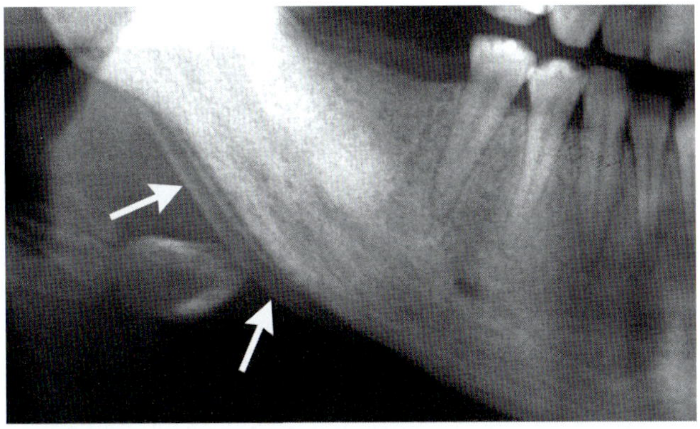

Fig. 16.25 Panoramic image of osteomyelitis revealing at least two layers of new bone *(arrows)* produced by the periosteum at the inferior border of the mandible.

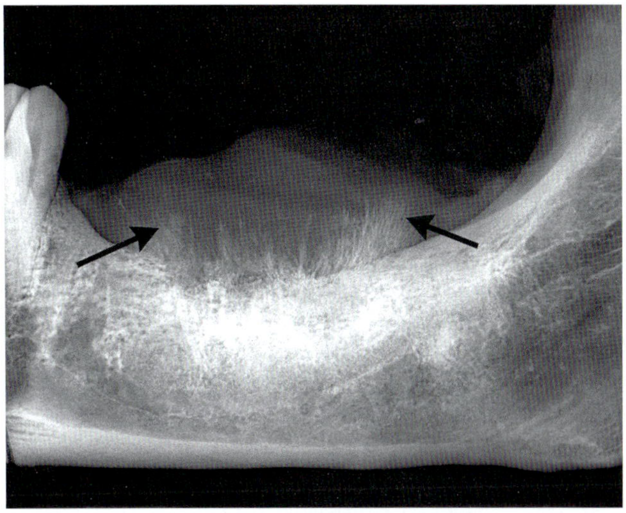

Fig. 16.26 Specimen image of a resected mandible with an osteosarcoma. Note the fine linear spicules of bone at the superior margin of the alveolar process *(arrows)*.

type of pattern can be seen. This pattern is most commonly encountered in inflammatory lesions and more rarely in tumors such as leukemia and Langerhans cell histiocytosis. Other examples of patterns of reactive periosteal bone formation include a spiculated bone pattern formed at right angles to the surface cortex. This type of pattern is seen with metastatic lesions of the prostate gland, or in a more exuberant radiating pattern of bone otherwise known as a "sunburst" pattern seen in osteosarcoma (Fig. 16.26) or a hemangioma.

Step 5: Formulate an Interpretation

The preceding steps enable the dentist to collect or catalog a series of radiologic findings in an organized and systematic fashion (Box 16.1 presents the process in abbreviated form). Now, the significance of each observation must be determined and weighted. The ability to give more significance weighting to some observations over others comes with experience.

After an initial working interpretation has been reached, ambiguities are resolved either by searching for more features or by putting more weight on one feature over another. For instance, in the analysis of a hypothetical lesion, observations of tooth movement, tooth resorption, and an invasive, destructive border are made. The effects on the teeth in this example may indicate a benign process; however, the invasive border and bone destruction are more important characteristics and indicate a malignant process. In the analytic approach (see Fig. 16.1), all these accumulated characteristics are used to make a diagnostic decision. A diagnostic algorithm such as that shown in Fig. 16.27 can aid in this decision-making process. Following this algorithm, the observer makes decisions regarding which general disease category the proposed diagnosis aligns with, and then proceeds to smaller, more specific categories. This is not an infallible method because any algorithm may occasionally fail since lesions sometimes do not behave as expected.

Decision 1: Normal or Abnormal

The clinician should determine whether the entity of interest is a variation of normal or an abnormality. This is a crucial decision because variations of normal do not require treatment or further investigation. Therefore, the clinician must develop an in-depth knowledge and appreciation for the variations in the appearance of normal anatomy. The importance of this cannot be overstated.

BOX 16.1 Analysis of Intraosseous Lesions

Step 1: Localize the Abnormality

- Anatomic position (epicenter)
- Localized or generalized
- Unilateral or bilateral
- Single or multifocal

Step 2: Assess Periphery and Shape of the Abnormality

Periphery

- Well defined
- Punched out
- Corticated
- Sclerotic
- Soft tissue capsule
- Poorly defined
- Blending
- Invasive

Shape

- Circular
- Scalloped
- Irregular

Step 3: Analyze the Internal Structure

- Totally radiolucent
- Totally radiopaque
- Mixed radiolucent and radiopaque (describe pattern)

Step 4: Assess the Effects of Lesion on Surrounding Structures

- Teeth, lamina dura, periodontal ligament space
- Inferior alveolar nerve canal and mental foramen
- Maxillary antrum
- Surrounding bone density and trabecular pattern
- Outer cortical bone and periosteal reactions

Step 5: Formulate an Interpretation

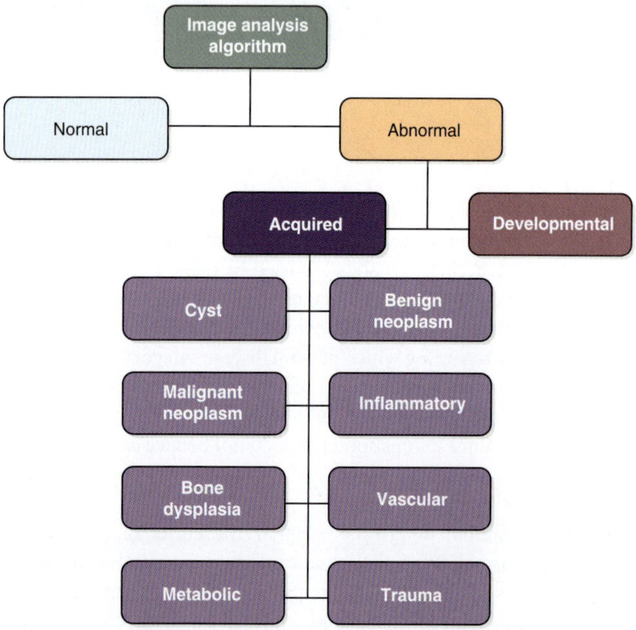

Fig. 16.27 Algorithm representing the diagnostic process that follows evaluation of the radiographic features of an abnormality.

Decision 2: Developmental or Acquired

If the area of interest is abnormal, the next step is to decide whether the radiographic characteristics represent a developmental abnormality or an acquired change. For example, the observation that a tooth has an abnormally short root leads to the pertinent question, "Did the tooth develop with a short root, or did the root develop to a normal length and then become shorter?" If the answer is the latter, the process must be external root resorption (an acquired abnormality). If the tooth merely developed a short root, the root canal should not be visible to the apex of the root because of normal apex development. In contrast, external root resorption may shorten the root, but the canal remains visible to the root apex (Fig. 16.28).

Decision 3: Disease Classification

If the abnormality is acquired, the next step is to select the most likely disease category for the acquired abnormality. The disease category can be determined by analyzing the way in which the features reflect a particular disease mechanism. The categories may include inflammation, cysts, benign neoplasia, malignant neoplasia, bone dysplasia, vascular abnormalities, metabolic disease, or physical changes such as fracture (i.e., trauma). The following chapters describe the characteristic radiologic features of diseases in these categories based on the mechanisms that may give rise to these abnormalities. The analysis should strive to narrow the interpretation to one of these disease categories; this directs the next course of action for continued investigation, referral, and treatment. This may also be a good time to add any relevant clinical information (i.e., patient history, and clinical signs and symptoms) into the decision-making process. The additional information may help the clinician to refine the interpretation to a short list (a differential interpretation) of diseases within the category. When possible, considering clinical information at the end helps avoid the problem of short cutting or performing an incomplete search of the images, or trying to make the radiologic characteristics conform to a preconceived diagnosis.

Decision 4: Ways to Proceed

After a disease category or a differential interpretation of diseases is determined, the clinician must decide how to proceed. This decision may require further imaging, biopsy, observation (watchful waiting), or definitive treatment. For example, if a lesion fits into the category of malignant neoplasia, the patient first should be referred to an oral and maxillofacial radiologist or a medical radiologist for possible advanced imaging to thoroughly characterize and stage the lesion. Advanced imaging may also help determine an optimal site for biopsy. Some entities, such as periapical cemento-osseous dysplasia may not require any

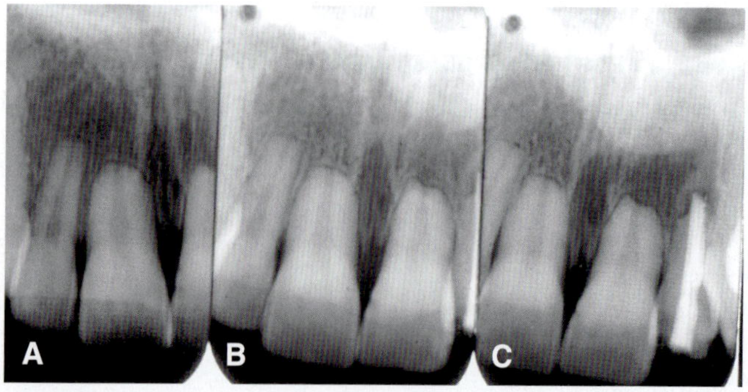

Fig. 16.28 (A–C) Periapical images revealing external resorption of the maxillary incisors, which is an acquired abnormality because of the presence of the wide pulp chambers at the apex of the roots of the teeth.

further investigation or treatment. In other instances, a period of watchful waiting followed by reexamination in a few weeks or months may be indicated if the abnormality appears benign and there is no clear need for immediate treatment.

With advanced training or additional experience in diagnostic imaging, the dentist may be better able to name one specific abnormality or at least create a short list of abnormalities from one or two disease categories. It is important to recognize, however, that imaging is but one diagnostic test available to the dentist, and it is not infallible. It is therefore important for the dentist to understand the limitations of imaging, and recognize its value alongside other clinical information that may be available and diagnostic testing that may be ordered.

WRITING A DIAGNOSTIC IMAGING REPORT

When analyzing diagnostic images, it is advisable to create a formal report for the purposes of documentation and communication with other clinicians. The radiographic report can be divided into the following subsections.

General Patient Information

The patient's information section should appear at the beginning of the report and include the patient's name, age, sex, and any alphanumeric patient identifier such as a clinic or medical registration number. The name of the referring clinician (if applicable) and the date of report are also included.

Imaging Procedure

This section summarizes the imaging procedures provided along with the date of the examination. Specific information should be provided regarding CBCT. For example, field-of-view size, slice thickness, distance between slices, and a comment on image quality. An example for reporting imaging procedure could be the following: "The imaging examination consists of panoramic and intraoral maxillary standard occlusal images, and contrast-enhanced axial and coronal multidetector computed tomographic images of the mandible conducted on February 20, 2024. The images are of diagnostic quality."

Clinical Information

Clinical information is an optional section that includes pertinent clinical information regarding the patient's condition provided by the referring clinician or by the clinician dictating the report if a clinical examination was made before the radiologic examination. The clinical information should be brief and should summarize the information pertaining to the abnormality in question. For example, "Clinical examination revealed a mass in the floor of the mouth, possibly a ranula. The patient has a history of lymphoma."

Findings

The findings section is an objective, detailed list of observations made from the diagnostic images. The findings may be described following the previously presented step-by-step analysis of the anatomic location, extent of the lesion, periphery and shape, internal structure, and effects on surrounding structures. This section does not include a radiologic interpretation.

Interpretation

The collected observations from the radiologic image or images allow the dentist to elucidate their meaning, and this is called an interpretation. If additional information from the patient history is available or if clinical or other diagnostic information is available together with the radiologic interpretation results, a diagnosis can be made. In some instances, however, the radiologic features can be pathognomonic of a disease, in which case the interpretation is the diagnosis.

When possible, the clinician should strive to provide a definitive interpretation of the abnormality that has been imaged. When this is not possible, a short list of abnormalities or a differential interpretation (listed in order of likelihood) is acceptable. The list should not, however, be exhaustive; ideally, it should be limited to diseases within one or perhaps two disease categories at most. In some situations, advice regarding additional studies, when required, and treatment may be included. Finally, the name and signature of the clinician composing the report are included.

SELF-TEST

To practice the analytic technique presented, the reader should examine (Fig. 16.4A and B) and write down all observations and the results of the diagnostic algorithm before reading the following section.

Description

Location

The abnormality is singular and unilateral. The epicenter lies coronal to the mandibular right first molar.

Periphery and Shape

The lesion has a well-defined, corticated periphery with an attachment to the cementoenamel junction and has a round shape.

Internal Structure

The internal structure is homogeneously radiolucent.

Effects on Adjacent Structures

The occlusal radiograph reveals that the buccal cortical plate has expanded in a smooth, curved shape, and a thin cortical boundary still exists.

Effects on Adjacent Teeth

The lesion has displaced the first molar in an apical direction, which reinforces the decision that the origin was coronal to this tooth. Also, the lesion has displaced the second molar distally and the second premolar in a mesial direction. Apical resorption of the distal root of the second deciduous molar has occurred.

Analysis

Making all the observations is an important first step in the interpretation process. To accomplish this next step, further knowledge of the pathologic condition and a certain amount of experience are required. The first objective is to select the correct category of diseases (e.g., inflammation, benign neoplasia, and cyst). At this point, the clinician should not let the names of all the specific diseases be overwhelming.

These images reveal an abnormal appearance. The coronal location of the lesion suggests that the tissue making up this abnormality is probably derived from an odontogenic source; possibly a component of the dental follicle. The effects on the surrounding structures indicate that this abnormality is acquired. The displacement and resorption of teeth, intact peripheral cortex, curved shape, and radiolucent internal structure all indicate a slow-growing, benign, space-occupying lesion, most likely in the cyst category. Odontogenic tumors, such as an ameloblastic fibroma, may be considered but are less likely because of the shape. The most common type of cyst in a pericoronal location is a dentigerous cyst. Odontogenic keratocysts are occasionally seen in this location, but the tooth resorption and degree of expansion are not characteristic of that pathologic condition. Therefore, the final interpretation is a dentigerous cyst, with odontogenic keratocyst and ameloblastic fibroma as possibilities in the differential interpretation, although less likely. Treatment is usually indicated for dentigerous cysts, and such a patient should be referred for consultation with an oral and maxillofacial surgeon.

BIBLIOGRAPHY

Baghdady M, Carnahan H, Lam EW, et al. The integration of basic sciences and clinical sciences in oral radiology. *J Dent Educ*. 2013;77:757-763.

Baghdady M, Carnahan H, Lam EW, et al. Dental and dental hygiene students' diagnostic strategy and instructional method. *J Dent Educ*. 2014;8:1279-1285.

Baghdady M, Pharoah M, Regehr G, et al. The role of basic sciences in diagnostic oral radiology. *J Dent Educ*. 2009;73:1187-1193.

Eva KW, Hatala RM, LeBlanc VR, et al. Teaching from the clinical reasoning literature: combined reasoning strategies help novice diagnosticians overcome misleading information. *Med Educ*. 2007;41:1152-1158.

Woods N. Science is fundamental: the role of biomedical knowledge in clinical reasoning. *Med Educ*. 2007;41:1173-1177.

Worth HM. *Principles and Practice of Oral Radiologic Interpretation*. Year Book Medical Publishers; 1972.

17

Dental Caries

Daniel P. Turgeon

DISEASE MECHANISM

Dental caries is a multifactorial disease that develops as a result of the interaction of three factors: the tooth, the dental biofilm or plaque, and the diet. In addition, other factors may also contribute to the process; for example, saliva, the exposure to fluoride, the immune system, the duration of exposure to bacterial microorganisms, and the socioeconomic status of the patient. *Streptococcus mutans* in dental biofilm plays a pivotal role in the process of demineralization. The number of *S. mutans* present is both responsive and directly proportional to the amount of sugar consumed from the diet.

Lactic acid is produced by the fermentation of fructose by *S. mutans* in the bacterial biofilm; this, in turn, causes a reduction in the local pH and demineralization of the tooth structure. The demineralization process in early carious lesions begins beneath the enamel surface, leaving behind a thin, mineralized, intact surface layer of precipitated calcium and phosphate that may persist for some time. The caries process itself does not progress in a manner that is temporally linear. Rather, it is a continuous cycle of demineralization and remineralization in which the demineralization process eventually dominates. The cycle can, however, be modified, favoring remineralization over demineralization; for example, by reducing sugar intake, removing the dental biofilm-containing *S. mutans* through effective oral hygiene practices, and exposure to topical fluoride to strengthen mineralized tooth structures. Should these strategies prove successful, an actively demineralizing lesion can be arrested. An arrested lesion may, however, become active again if there is renewed activity in the dental biofilm.

Demineralization of tooth structure, called the carious lesion, is a reflection of the disease rather than the disease itself. Clinically, the appearance of caries will vary with time; an early, active lesion will appear as a white, chalky spot, whereas an older, arrested lesion will appear darker, either black or brown. The rate of demineralization will vary based on the factors previously mentioned but will also vary depending on the crystalline structure of the tooth. Enamel is composed mostly of closely packed mineralized acellular hydroxyapatite crystals. In comparison, dentin is composed approximately of 45% inorganic apatite crystals, 30% organic matrix, and 25% water. These differences result in a greater rate of demineralization within the dentin. Destruction of the outer enamel surface (cavitation) usually occurs after dentin involvement, and demineralization can progress to the pulp, causing necrosis and/or destruction of the mineralized tooth (Fig. 17.1).

ROLE OF IMAGING IN THE DETECTION OF CARIOUS LESIONS

A thorough clinical examination that includes imaging is needed to diagnose carious lesions. A clinical examination may be able to identify carious lesions on the occlusal and exposed smooth surfaces of the teeth. However, it is nearly impossible to clinically identify caries occurring on the proximal surfaces of teeth (i.e., interproximal caries), unless there has been cavitation. When this occurs, it usually means that the carious lesion has become large enough to be identified clinically. Unfortunately, when a caries lesion reaches this stage, the affected tooth may require a large intracoronal restoration, endodontic treatment, or, if the tooth is determined to be unrestorable, extraction.

The intraoral bitewing image is the preferred image to detect interproximal caries in posterior teeth. As long as the operator can position the image receptor correctly, the proximal surfaces should be clearly visible (Fig. 17.2). Since a carious lesion produces demineralization of the enamel and the dentin, more x-ray photons will penetrate a demineralized region of the tooth than a mineralized region, producing a relatively radiolucent (dark) region on the image receptor. Caries are sometimes visible on a panoramic image, but in these cases the caries are usually large enough to be clinically apparent. Since panoramic images have comparatively poor spatial resolution compared with intraoral receptors, they should not be relied on to detect caries (see Chapter 8).

Even when demineralization is detected on an image, this does not mean that it represents an active carious lesion. This could simply represent an older, inactive (arrested) lesion that can be described as a "scar" in the enamel. Remineralization of the surface is made possible by calcium and phosphorus in saliva that come into contact with the tooth surface but cannot penetrate into deeper tissues. No single image can differentiate active caries from arrested caries; to do so requires a second image, made at another time point, for comparison (Fig. 17.3).

Evidence-based standards of care for interval imaging examinations for dental caries can vary depending on patient age and caries risk. The decision to obtain images must therefore be tailored for each patient. The factors that increase risk are summarized in Table 17.1. For children and adolescents deemed to be at high risk for dental caries, the interval for bitewing examinations is between 6 and 12 months, and for adults, the interval for high-risk patients is 6–18 months. For patients deemed to be at low risk for caries, these intervals are 12–24 months for children, 18–36 months for adolescents, and 24–36 months for adults.

Recently some panoramic imaging systems have incorporated an "extraoral bitewing image" application (Fig. 17.4). Even though some manufacturers claim that this may be more effective than intraoral bitewing images in detecting caries, the evidence has been equivocal. We therefore continue to be of the opinion that intraoral bitewing images remain the preferred method to diagnose interproximal caries. Extraoral bitewing images may be considered when it is impossible to obtain intraoral images; for example, patients with behavioral or

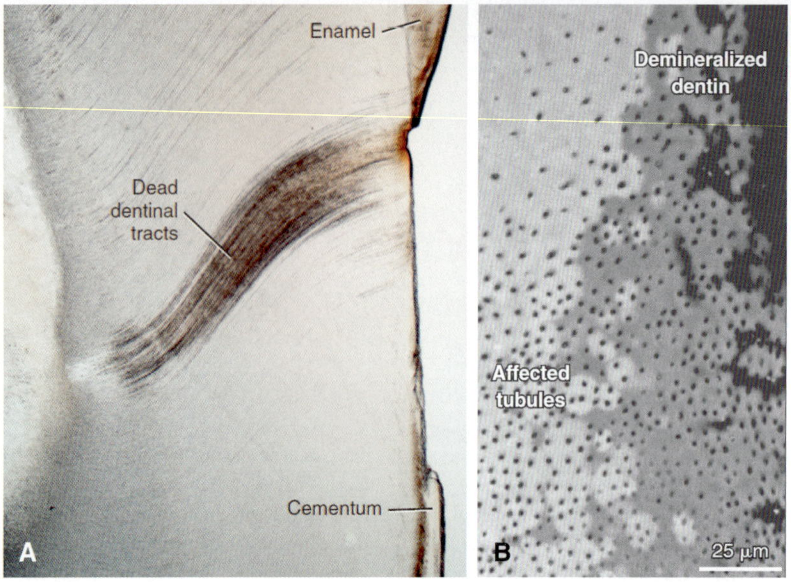

Fig. 17.1 (A) Light photomicrograph showing dead tracts in a radicular carious lesion that appear dark under transmitted light. (B) Scanning electron micrograph showing empty tubules under a carious lesion. (From Nanci A. *Ten Cate's Oral Histology: Development, Structure, and Function*. Mosby Elsevier; 2013.)

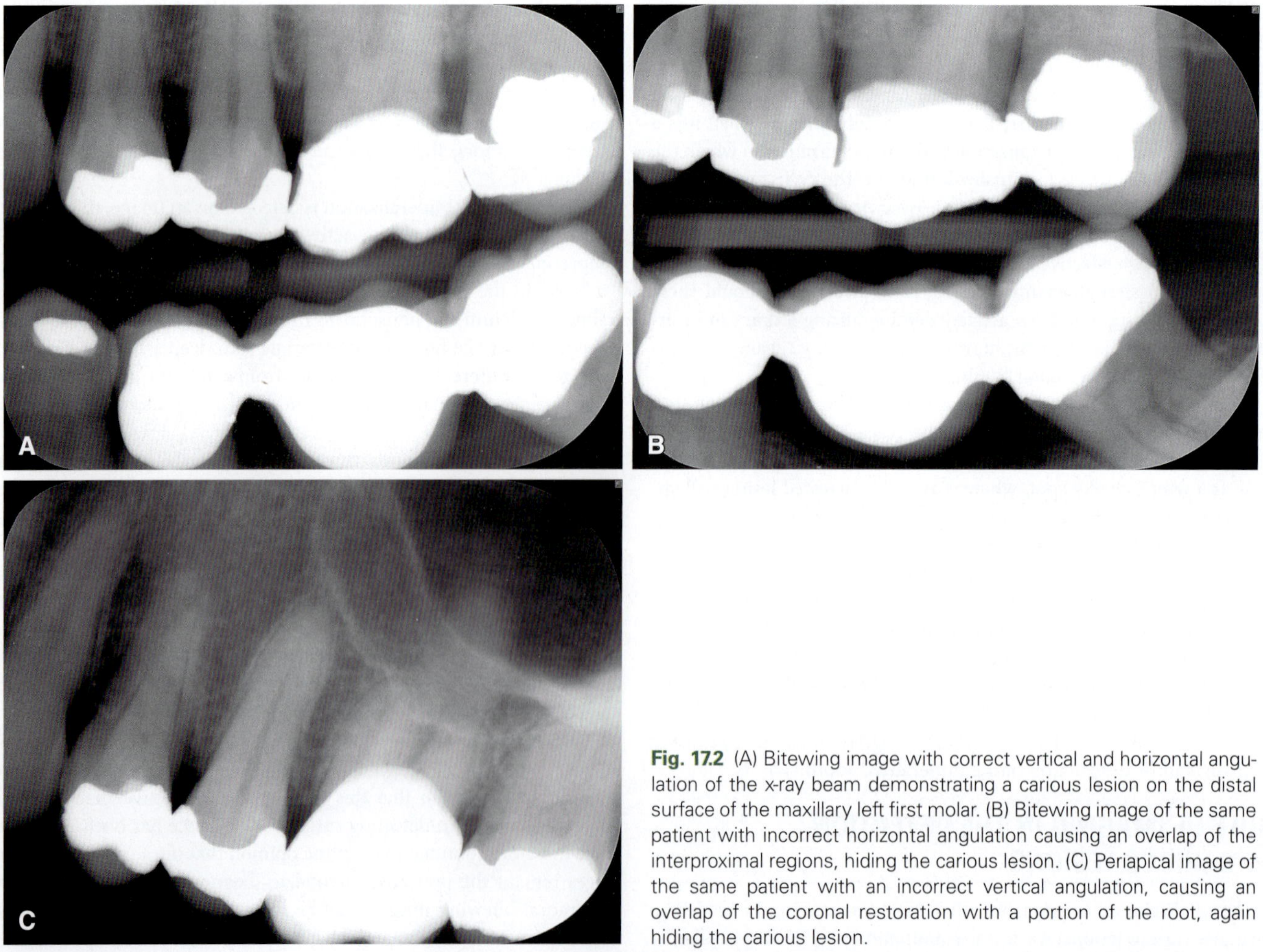

Fig. 17.2 (A) Bitewing image with correct vertical and horizontal angulation of the x-ray beam demonstrating a carious lesion on the distal surface of the maxillary left first molar. (B) Bitewing image of the same patient with incorrect horizontal angulation causing an overlap of the interproximal regions, hiding the carious lesion. (C) Periapical image of the same patient with an incorrect vertical angulation, causing an overlap of the coronal restoration with a portion of the root, again hiding the carious lesion.

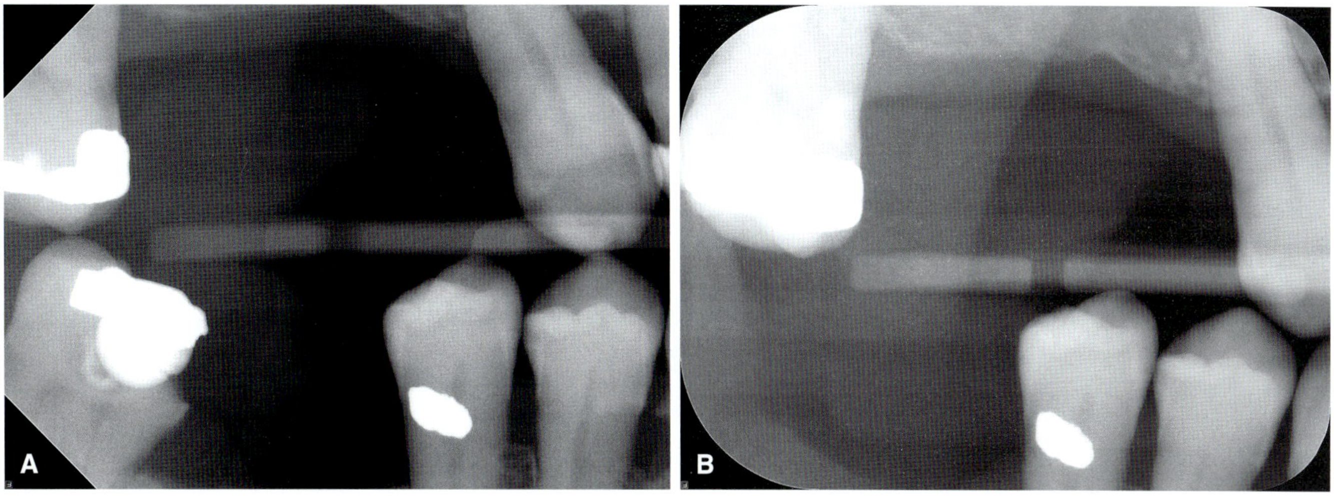

Fig. 17.3 (A) Bitewing image showing a carious lesion on the distal surface of the mandibular right first premolar. (B) Bitewing image of the same patient, obtained 5 years later. Note the absence of a size change to the carious lesion.

TABLE 17.1 Factors Increasing the Risk for Caries

1. Multiple previous caries
2. Recurrent caries
3. Existing restorations of inadequate quality
4. Poor oral hygiene
5. Insufficient fluoride exposure
6. Frequent consumption of sugary drinks (including prolonged nursing)
7. Family history of poor dental health
8. Enamel defects
9. Xerostomia
10. Inability to have proper dental hygiene (possibly from a disability)
11. Head and neck radiation therapy
12. Eating disorders (bulimia)
13. Alcohol and drug abuse
14. Irregular dental care

physical limitations, patients with a severe gag reflex, or those with anatomic constraints such as large mandibular tori.

Despite our best clinical monitoring practices, some carious lesions are not diagnosed because they may not be visible on an image. Because carious lesions progress slowly, especially in enamel, it is important for dentists to understand the factors that contribute to dental caries and caries progression, take an individualized approach for each patient, and order imaging examinations in a way that aligns with accepted clinical guidelines.

EXAMINATION WITH DIGITAL INTRAORAL SENSORS

Digital sensors have rapidly replaced film in many areas of clinical dentistry. As we saw in Chapter 4, two different sensor types are available: the solid-state sensor (CMOS) and the photostimulable phosphor plate (PSP). For some patients, solid-state sensors may be more difficult to place intraorally, and they may be uncomfortable, which is mostly due to their thickness. This may create more difficulties positioning image receptors for the dentist and their staff. That said, manufacturers are developing newer sensors that are thinner with characteristics that make them more comfortable for patients, including rounded corners. Unfortunately, the active surface area of solid-state sensors is smaller than similarly sized film, and sometimes, this leads to the need to acquire a second image to complete the examination (Fig. 17.5). Although PSPs are only minimally thicker and more rigid than film, they are similar in size and may therefore be as easy as film to position.

Holder devices for sensors are commercially available for both solid-state and PSP sensors. These position-indicating devices (PIDs) facilitate the positioning of the x-ray beam and sensor to avoid overlap of adjacent proximal tooth surfaces. Multiple studies have shown digital images to be equivalent to film-based images with respect to their sensitivity for caries detection. An exception is enamel caries detection, where film-based images have a reported higher sensitivity. For adolescents and adults, larger American National Standards Institute (ANSI) size 2 sensors are used to acquire bitewing images. Smaller ANSI size 0 or 1 sensors can be used in children. In adults with second or third molars in occlusion, there is nearly always the need for two images per side. As is the case with film-based images, digital images should be viewed on a high-quality monitor with an appropriate gray scale and in a room with subdued light.

EXAMINATION WITH INTRAORAL FILM

As with digital sensors, ANSI size 2 film is used for bitewing examinations in adolescents and adults, but it can also be used in younger patients when permanent first molar teeth have erupted. In these cases, only one image may be necessary. In smaller children, ANSI size 0 or 1 films can be used. Before being analyzed, the films should be mounted in frames with dark borders, and they should then be viewed in a room with subdued light over a light box with a magnifying glass to optimize spatial resolution of the film. The use of ANSI size 3 film should be discouraged. The length of the film in particular, when placed in the mouth, results in film bending, thus distorting the images of the teeth and bone crests.

DETECTION OF CARIOUS LESIONS

Proximal Surfaces

Typical Appearance

As enamel rods are oriented at 90 degrees to the surface of the enamel, the penetration of bacterially derived acid and therefore demineralization occurs along the long axes of the enamel rods. The resulting

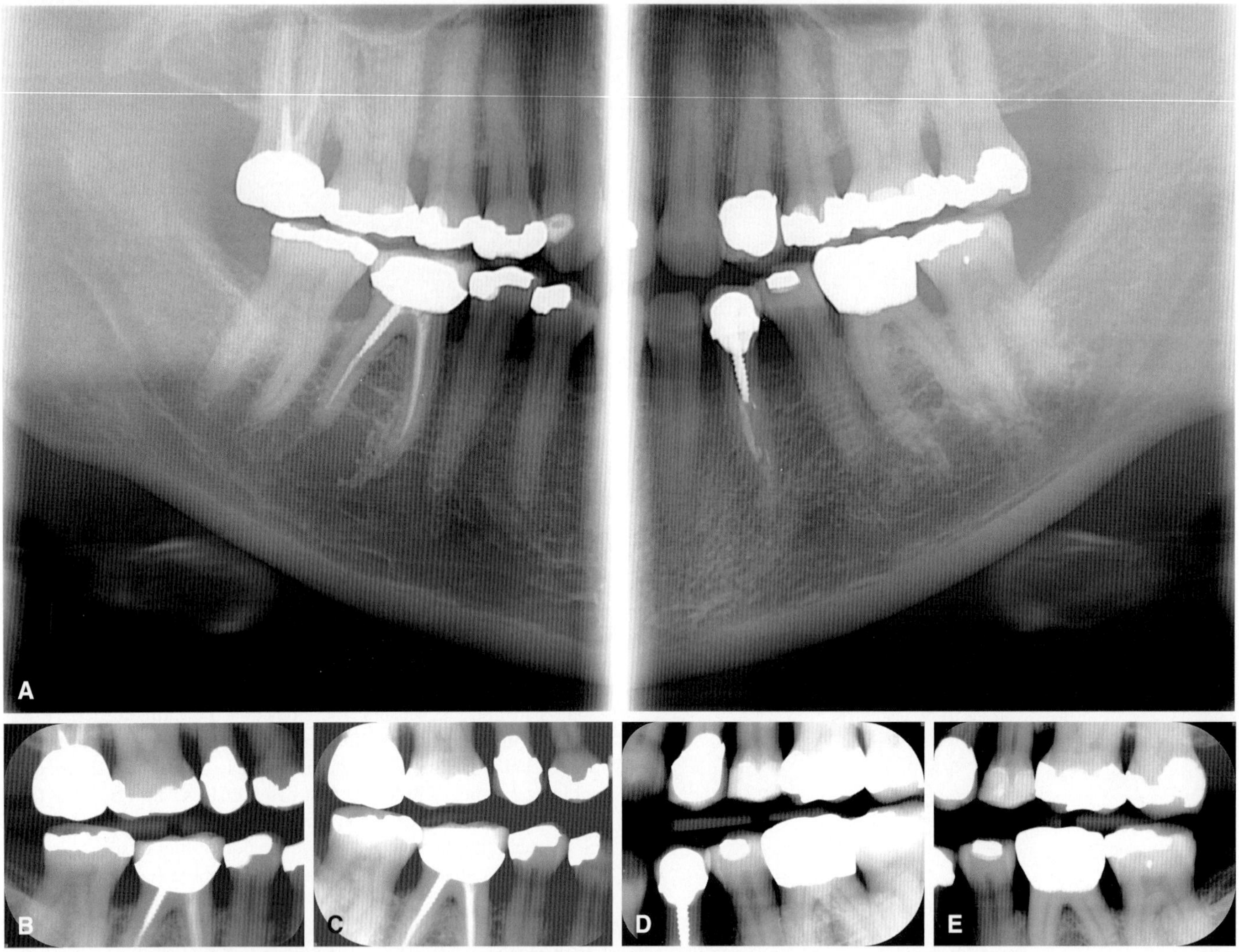

Fig. 17.4 (A) Extraoral bitewing image. (B–E) Intraoral bitewing images of the same patient. Note the better spatial resolution of the intraoral images. (Courtesy Dr. M. Michaud, Montréal, QC.)

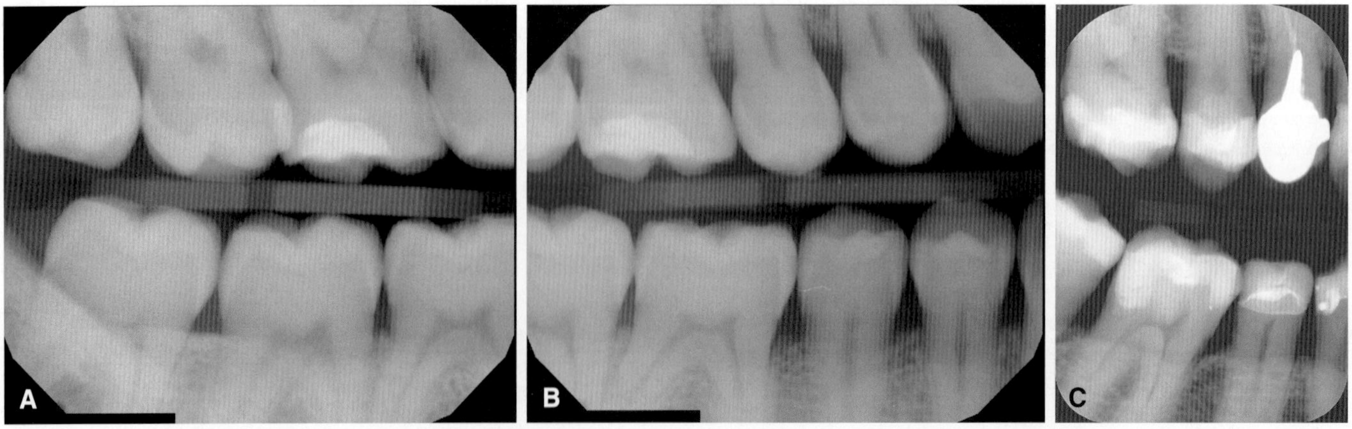

Fig. 17.5 Two bitewing images of a patient's right side (A and B) image the interproximal surfaces from the distal surface of the maxillary and mandibular canine teeth to the distal aspects of the erupted maxillary and mandibular third molar teeth. Vertical bitewing images (C) can also be obtained and are often used when the patient presents with periodontal bone loss.

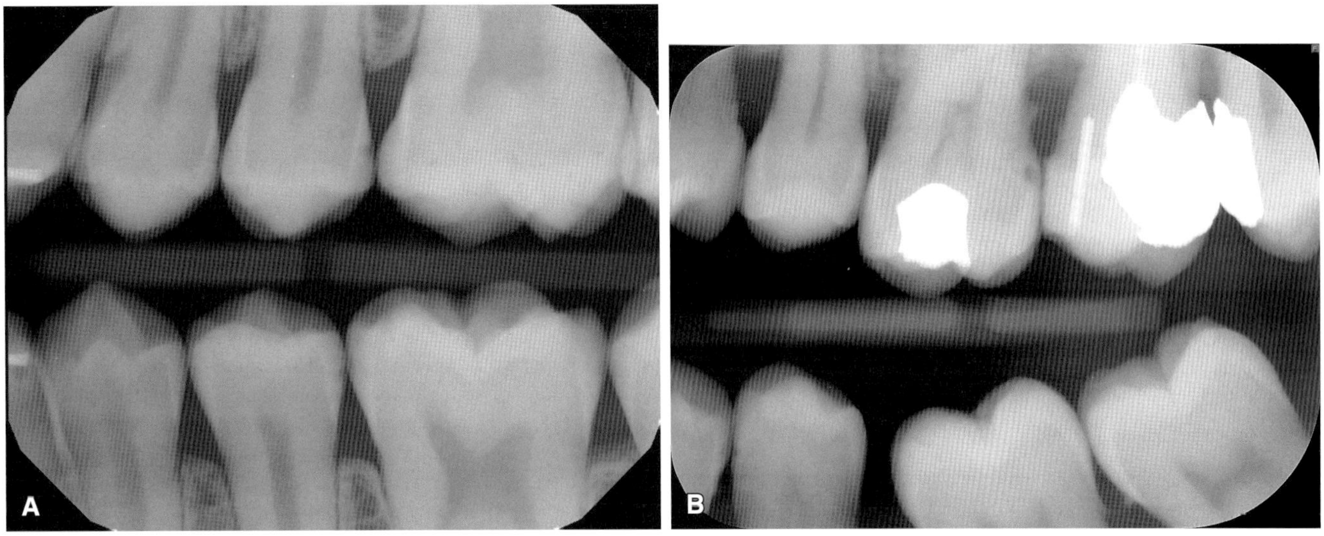

Fig. 17.6 Two bitewing images showing the triangular shape of carious lesions on the distal surfaces of the maxillary and mandibular left second premolars (A), and on the distal surface of the mandibular left first premolar and the mesial surface of the mandibular left second premolar (B). (A, Courtesy Dr. T. N. Ly, Montréal, QC.)

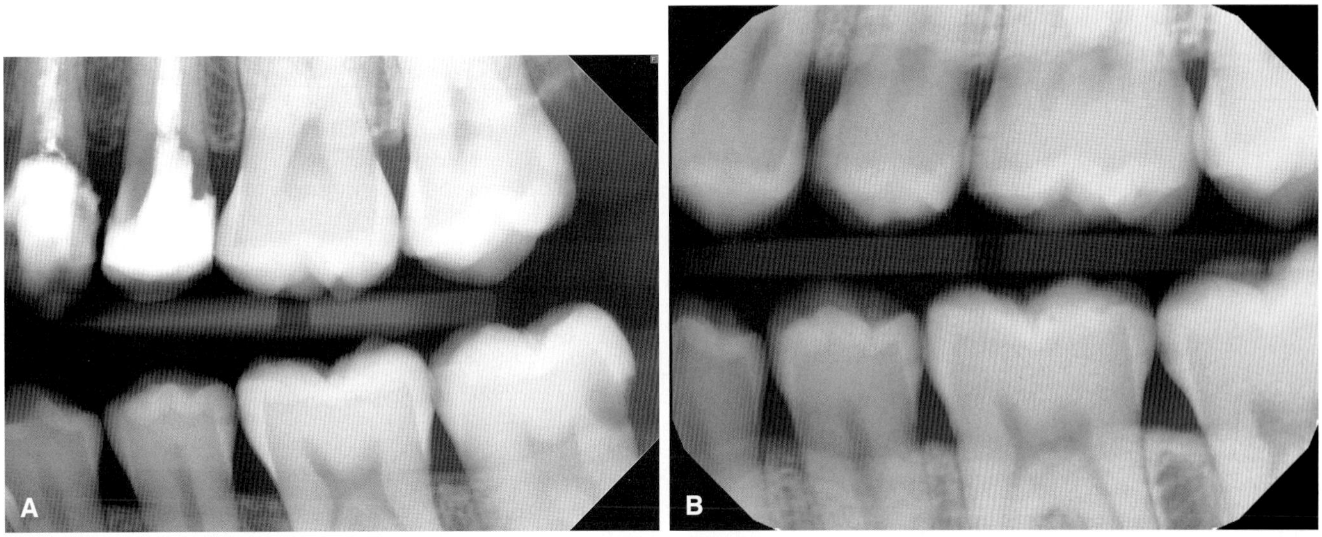

Fig. 17.7 (A) Bitewing image showing a carious lesion with a band-like appearance on the distal surface of the mandibular left second premolar. (B) Bitewing image showing a carious lesion with a rectangular shape on the mesial surface of the mandibular left second molar. Multiple other interproximal carious lesions are also visible. (B, Courtesy Dr. T. N. Ly, Montréal, QC.)

demineralization creates the classic triangular shape of an enamel carious lesion, with its broad base on the proximal surface of the tooth and its tip pointing toward the dentinoenamel junction (DEJ) (Fig. 17.6). Other shapes may also be seen, and these can include a band, a rectangle, or a semicircular notch (Fig. 17.7). When the leading edge of a carious lesion reaches the DEJ, demineralization spreads across the enamel–dentin interface and penetrates the dentin, where a second triangle forms. Here, the broad base of the triangle is located at the DEJ and its tip points toward the pulp chamber. One can expect the demineralization in the dentin to be more aggressive because of the lower mineral content, creating a triangle with a wider base than in the enamel. The carious lesion then progresses through the dentinal tubules toward the pulp chamber. Compared with enamel demineralization, once a dentinal lesion has reached a certain size, it may lose its triangular shape due to the curvilinear or "S-shaped" arrangement of the dentin tubules.

Interproximal carious lesions are most commonly found in a region that extends between the contact points of teeth apically to near the free gingival margin. The inferiormost point of this area may be most relevant in patients with periodontal bone loss (Fig. 17.8). The localization of caries in this very defined region of the tooth is of great help in differentiating caries from a common artifact of intraoral imaging termed "cervical burnout" (Fig. 17.9). There may also be a higher risk of caries developing on an interproximal surface that is in contact with either a carious lesion or a restoration. Special attention must therefore be given to the investigation of these seemingly intact surfaces.

Because of the buccal/lingual thickness of the proximal surfaces of posterior teeth, a small amount of demineralization in the middle third of the proximal surface may not be visible radiographically. It has been estimated that enamel demineralization must be greater than approximately 35% before a carious lesion can be observed on an image. This

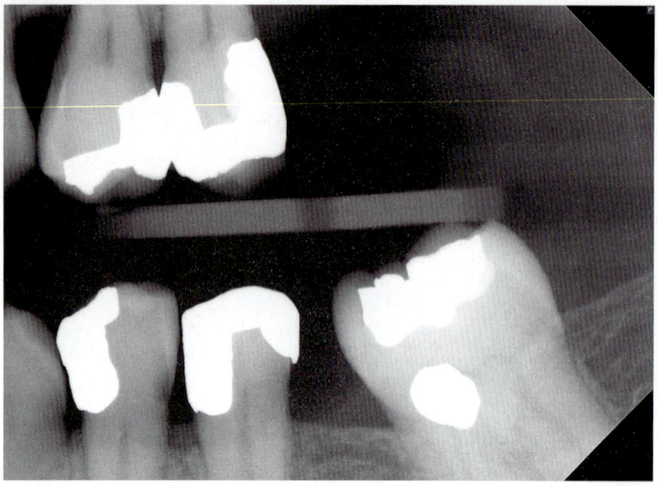

Fig. 17.8 Bitewing image of a patient with moderate horizontal bone loss and a carious lesion located at the CEJ on the distal surface of the mandibular left first premolar.

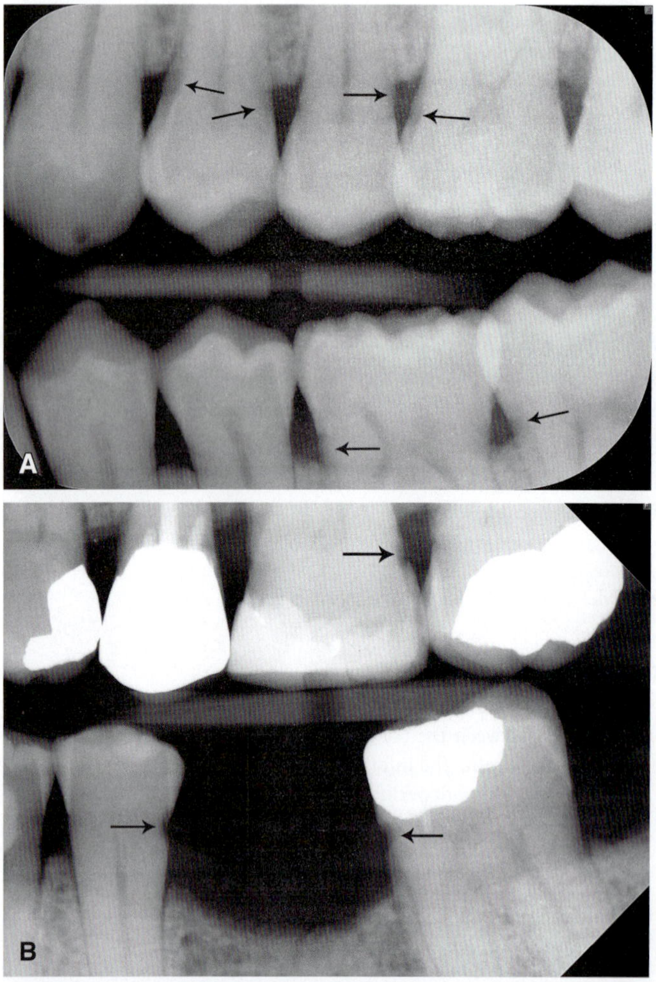

Fig. 17.9 (A) Bitewing image showing cervical burnout *(arrows)*, which mimics carious lesions. (B) Bitewing image with carious lesions *(arrows)*, which, compared with burnout, demonstrate an irregular border and a discontinuity of the tooth surface. They are often visible in patients with periodontal bone loss.

is one of the reasons why the true depth of a carious lesion (verified histologically) is most often greater than what can be seen on an image.

False-Positive Interpretations

Every published study on this subject has shown less than 100% agreement on caries diagnosis between independent observers. This is especially true with enamel caries but can also sometimes occur with caries in dentin. When a carious lesion is thought to be detected on an image but the tooth structure is in fact intact, this is referred to as a "false-positive" finding. Although such findings can be caused by variations in tooth morphology, the most common source of false-positive errors is the misinterpretation of cervical burnout as dental caries.

Cervical burnout produces an artifact that can mimic a carious lesion. As the x-ray beam meets the convex proximal surface of the tooth in this area, those x-ray photons that pass almost tangentially through the tooth surface encounter less tooth structure than those photons that pass deeper through the tooth. This area of convexity is commonly located at or just apical to the inferior border of the Cemento-enamel junction (CEJ), near the normal height of the alveolar crest. The thinner tooth structure here absorbs fewer x-rays allowing a greater number of photons to reach the receptor; consequently the area appears relatively more radiolucent on an image. In single-rooted teeth, the presence of a shallow depression or concavity on either the mesial or distal surface of the root can make the area appear more radiolucent. In multirooted teeth, cervical burnout can also be seen when roots that are more buccally positioned do not overlap perfectly with a lingual or palatal root in a mesiodistal direction (Fig. 17.9). The presence of two overlapping roots can, however, be confirmed by identifying the periodontal ligament spaces of each root.

The experience of the dentist plays a pivotal role in controlling the number of false-positive findings. Although a lack of training or experience is often the cause of false-positive findings, they can be made worse when the images used do not provide an accurate representation of the proximal surfaces of a tooth. The most common technical error in this instance is overlap between the proximal surfaces of adjacent teeth on a bitewing image. This can, however, be easily corrected by adjusting the horizontal angulation of the x-ray beam to match the plane of the sensor (see Fig. 17.2).

Staging and Cavitation

Multiple classification or scoring systems have been used over the years to categorize caries size and depth. The International Caries Classification and Management System (ICCMS) builds on the International Caries Detection and Assessment System (ICDAS) for caries staging by including important patient information, including caries risk. The merged ICDAS/ICCMS assigns caries progression to one of four stages of tooth involvement: sound surfaces (code 0), initial stage caries (RA), moderate stage caries (RB), and extensive stage caries (RC). Within each "R" stage, integer subcodes are defined, either indicating the condition of the enamel or the condition of the dentin.

With respect to radiographic scoring in the merged ICDAS/ICCMS, stage 0 is defined as no radiolucency. In stage RA (initial stage), the radiolucency is scored as appearing within the outer half of the enamel (RA1), the inner half of the enamel without or with involvement of the DEJ (RA2), and the outer third of the dentin (RA3). In the moderate stage (RB4), the radiolucency reaches the middle third of the dentin. In the extensive stage (RC), the carious lesion is scored as RC5 when it reaches the inner third of the dentin or the pulp with clinical cavitation, and RC6 when the radiolucency extends into the pulp with clinical cavitation (Fig. 17.10). On average, 32% of carious lesions extending into the outer third of the dentin also present with clinical cavitation. This

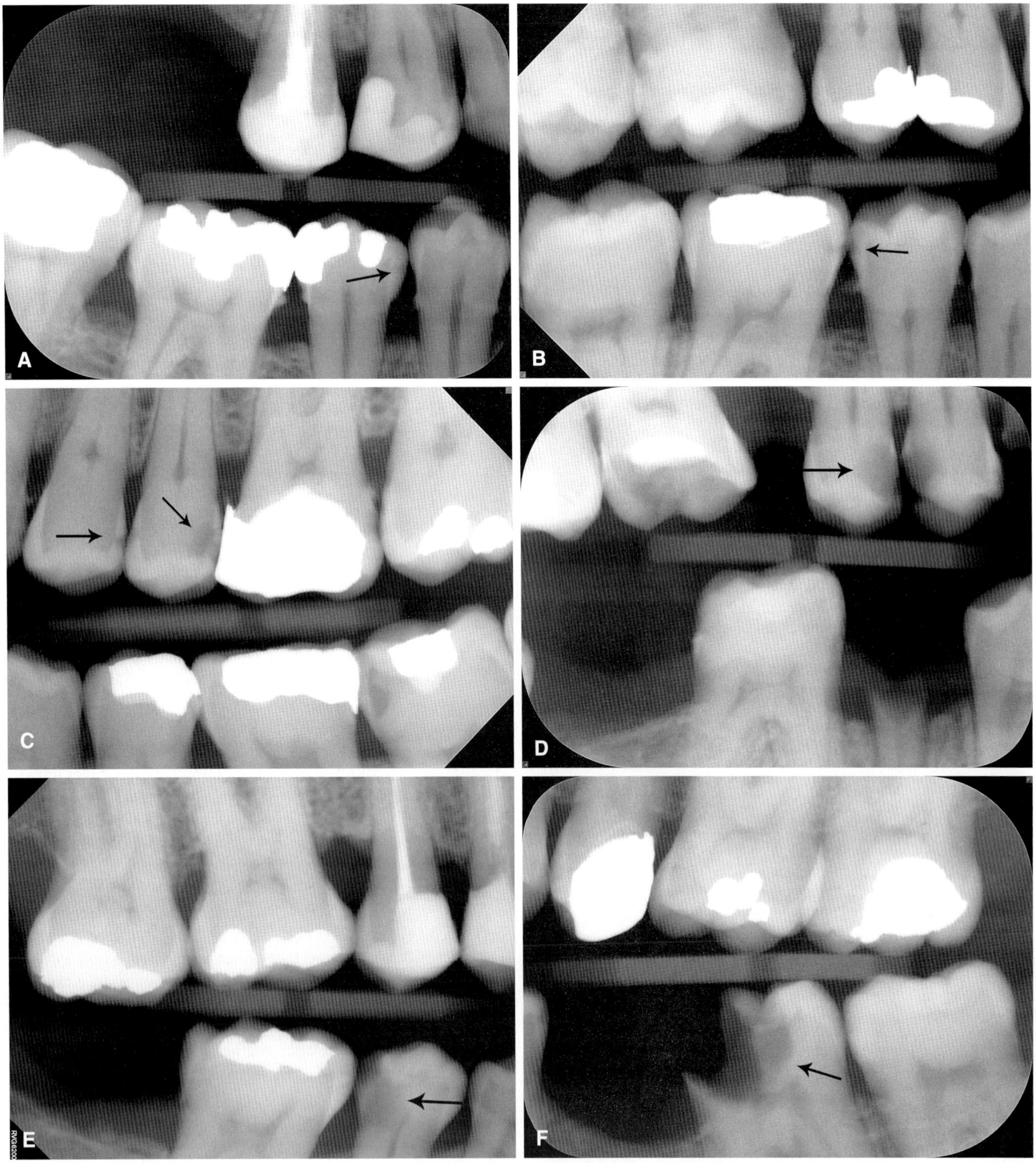

Fig. 17.10 Multiple bitewing images with different caries depth (*arrows*). (A) Caries within the outer half of the enamel (RA1). (B) Caries within the inner half of the enamel (RA2). (C) Caries within the outer third of the dentin (RA3). (D) Caries within the middle third of the dentin (RB4). (E) Caries within the inner third of the dentin (RC5). (F) Caries in contact with the pulp (RC6).

incidence climbs to 72% for lesions in the middle third of the dentin or deeper. The ability to identify or at least suspect cavitation is important, because once this occurs, the bacteria in the lesion will maintain the activity of the carious lesion unless it is managed surgically.

When there are no metallic restorations in the vicinity, some reports have maintained that a cone beam computed tomography (CBCT) examination (see Chapter 9) will be extremely accurate in determining both the depth and cavitation status of a proximal surface. However, the use of CBCT for this sole purpose is not only discouraged, but it is not evidence based. Moreover, the higher radiation dose imparted by this type of imaging examination, even utilizing a small field of view, should prohibit its use for this purpose.

When a CBCT is obtained for another reason, the entire volume should be evaluated for other anomalies and pathoses, including caries (Fig. 17.11).

Treatment Considerations

The decision to treat a carious lesion surgically is based on several factors. The dentist must take into account the caries risk status of the patient, the depth of the lesion, and whether there is cavitation. Generally speaking, conservative interventions like oral hygiene instruction and topical fluoride application can be put in place for caries in the ICCMS RA categories (involvement of the enamel or outer third of the dentin), whereas surgical management is needed when there is cavitation or when the carious lesion has reached the middle third of the dentin (RB). The differences in management strategies between patients will mostly be based on caries risk status; a patient with a higher risk for caries would benefit from a more proactive approach versus a patient with a low caries risk (see Table 17.1). When the decision is made not to manage a carious lesion surgically, a follow-up imaging schedule should be developed to monitor the lesion. The follow-up period should be based on the patient's caries risk. Ideally, when new images are made, they should be as similar as possible to the original images so that any comparisons can be as accurate as possible. The follow-up image can be compared with the original image to see if the lesion has grown (active) or not (arrested). If the lesion has progressed, the decision regarding surgical treatment may be revised.

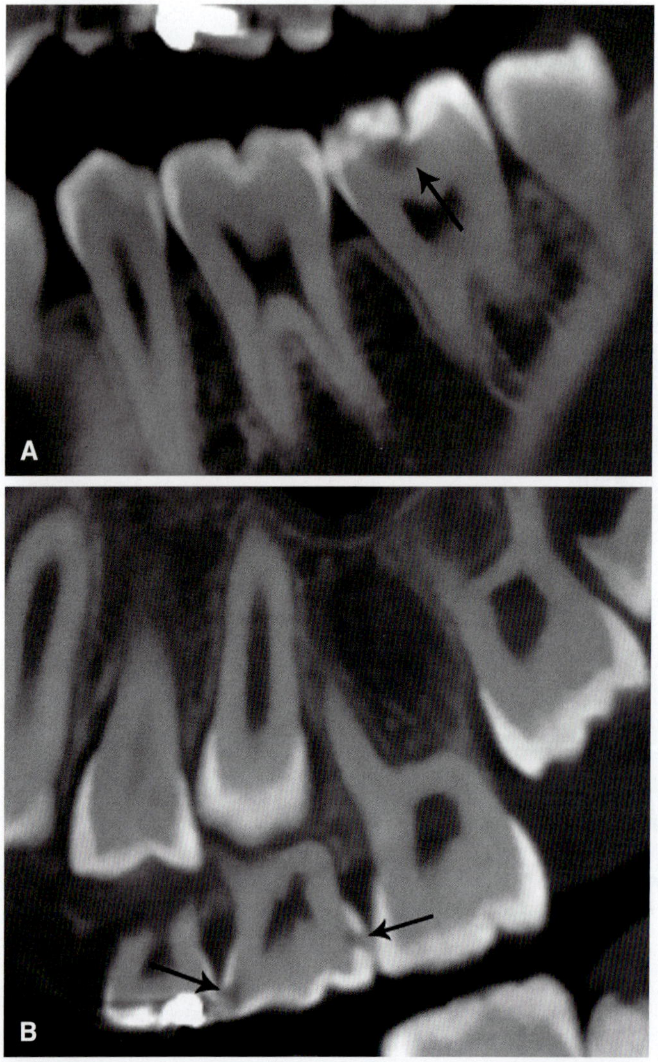

Fig. 17.11 Cone beam computed tomography images revealing carious lesions *(arrows)*. (A) A carious lesion on the occlusal surface of the second molar. (B) Carious lesions on both interproximal surfaces of the deciduous second molar.

Occlusal Surfaces

Typical Appearance

Caries can occur on the occlusal surfaces of premolar and molar teeth, most often in children and adolescents. Development and penetration of the enamel and dentin occurs in a similar way as it does on proximal surfaces. The difference lies in the radiographic appearance of occlusal caries. It is nearly impossible to detect occlusal caries limited to the enamel in a radiograph. The enamel is simply too thick for a carious lesion to be detectable. Once the lesion reaches the dentin, instead of creating a triangular shape, it will create a more semicircular shape, with the broad base of the semicircle at the DEJ.

Compared with proximal caries, clinical detection of occlusal caries is often more reliable, in particular for identifying small carious lesions. Clinically, new lesions may appear chalky white, whereas older lesions, possibly inactive, will have a darker coloration (brown or black). Once there is suspicion of occlusal caries, an image should be obtained to assess the depth of the lesion.

False-Positive Interpretations

Occlusal lesions can easily be missed, particularly those small ones that are limited to the enamel. Since occlusal lesions occur within the base of surface pits and fissures, there is often a superposition of the surrounding sound enamel, which leads to these false-negative results. This is one of the reasons why a clinical examination is vital to detect occlusal caries. Multiple studies have shown that a clinical examination is more accurate than a radiograph in detecting these small occlusal lesions.

In the same way that a carious lesion progresses through proximal enamel, occlusal caries penetrating enamel will spread along the DEJ first, before entering the underlying dentin. Within the dentin, the carious lesion will often take on a semicircular shape, centered on the occlusal pit (Fig. 17.12). With occlusal caries, the dentist may see a radiolucent line along the DEJ, which may be confused with wider spreading of the carious lesion. Although this appearance can also be seen with proximal surface caries, it is often more pronounced in this location. This artifact, which is caused by the differential contrast between the more radiopaque enamel and the less radiopaque dentin, is called the *Mach-band effect* (Fig. 17.13). First described by Ernst Mach in 1865, this optical illusion arises as a result of the differential stimulation and inhibition of neighboring receptors in the retina of the eye. When a set of retinal receptors in the eye is "overstimulated" by the perception of the very radiopaque density of enamel, adjacent receptors that perceive the more radiolucent dentin are inhibited. The result of this differential response of retinal receptors results in the perception of a radiolucent band that runs in the superficial dentin just adjacent to the DEJ. To overcome the Mach-band effect, the dentist can mask the more radiopaque enamel. If the Mach band disappears, the interpretation of this result is that caries is not present. If, however, the Mach band continues to be seen, caries is present. Should a potential lesion be perceived in this way, and is visible only on the image without clinical evidence of disease, it would be reasonable to observe and monitor the area so as to avoid unnecessary treatment.

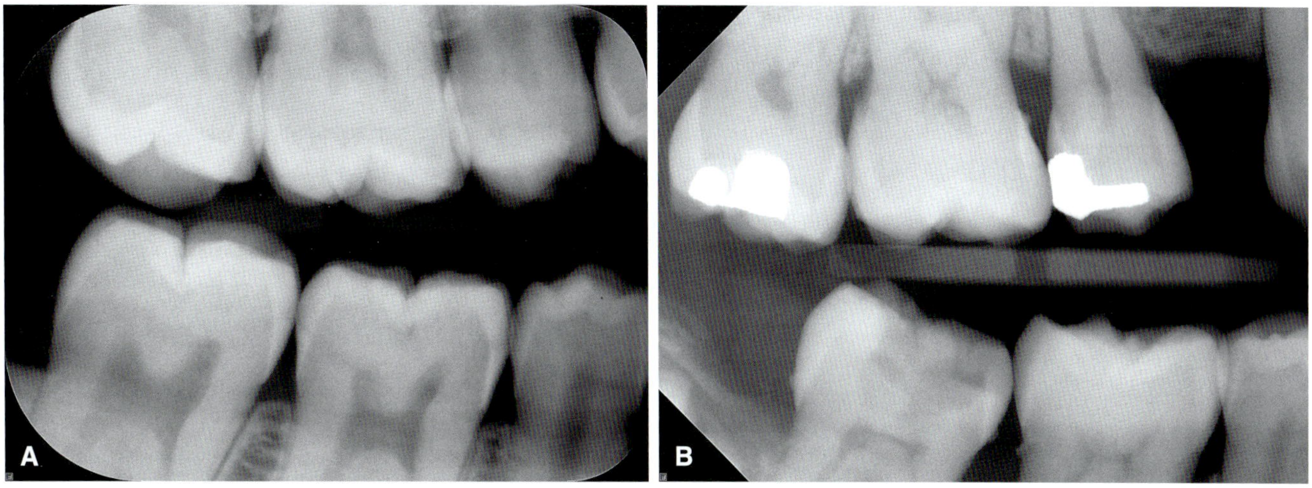

Fig. 17.12 Bitewing images with the classical appearance of occlusal caries; a small radiolucency is centered on an occlusal pit on both mandibular molars (A). If left untreated, these could cavitate and grow larger (B).

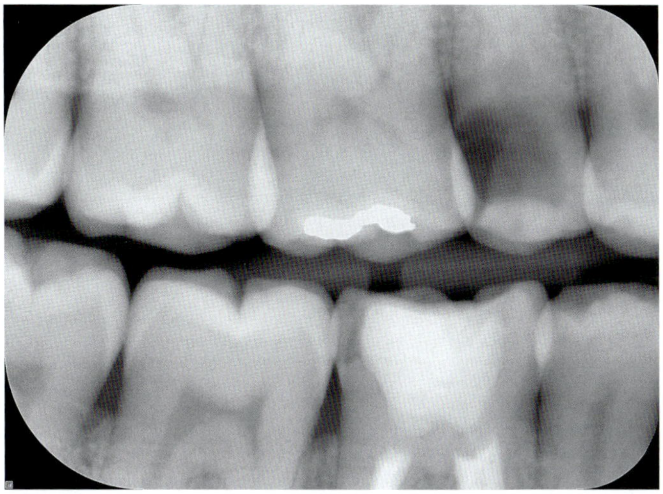

Fig. 17.13 The Mach-band effect seen as a radiolucent line is visible at the dentinal–enamel junction along the occlusal surface of the unrestored maxillary and mandibular molar teeth.

Cavitation and Treatment Considerations

As the occlusal lesion spreads into the underlying dentin, weakening the tooth, there may be insufficient dentin remaining to support masticatory forces; this may lead to cavitation of the surface. When this happens, it becomes easy to identify the carious lesion clinically. Even in these instances, it is still important to obtain images of the tooth—possibly both a bitewing image to assess the depth and a periapical image to assess the apical region (Fig. 17.14). This will allow the dentist to know beforehand the approximate depth of the carious lesion and if the pulp chamber may be involved.

If discoloration is noted in a fissure without cavitation, a bitewing image may be needed to evaluate the possibility of caries and the depth of the lesion. Even without clinical cavitation, occlusal caries reaching into the dentin will most likely require treatment.

Buccal and Lingual Surfaces

Caries arising on the buccal and lingual surfaces of the teeth can occur in the pits and fissures of these surfaces or on the smooth surfaces near the gingiva. In viewing these lesions on a single image, it is impossible

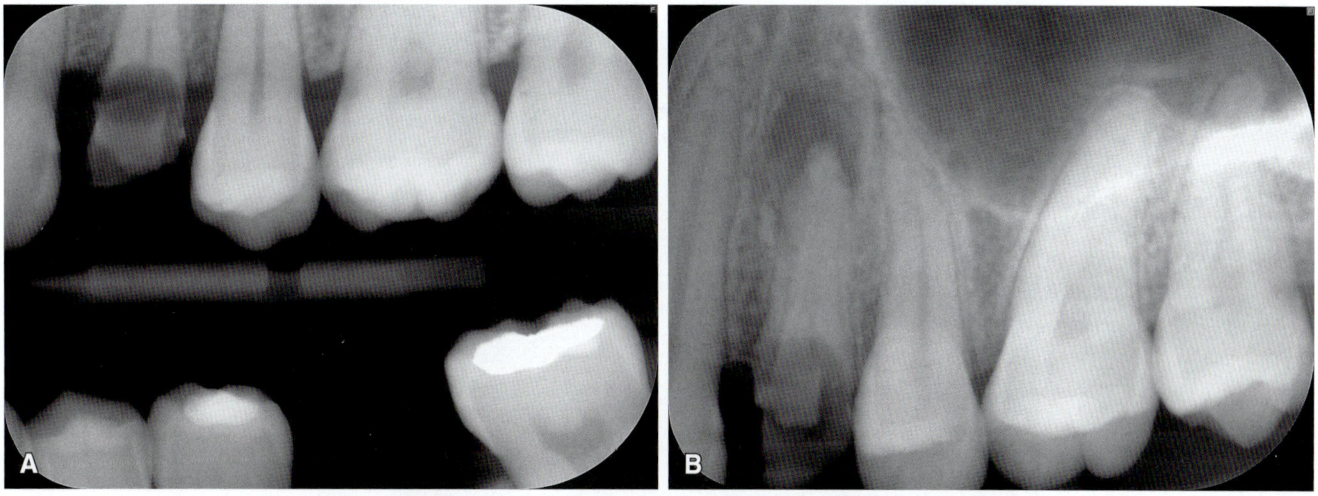

Fig. 17.14 (A) Near-complete coronal tooth destruction from caries in the maxillary left first premolar. Once a carious lesion is large enough to encroach upon or invade the pulp, a periapical image should be obtained to evaluate periapical anatomy for an inflammatory lesion (rarefying osteitis), which is the case here (B).

to localize the lesion as being on the buccal or lingual surface. A second image incorporating a different horizontal angulation can be made to aid in this determination (see the tube-shift technique or the buccal object rule in Chapter 6). Caries developing in these areas usually have a circular or oval shape and are well defined. Furthermore, the surrounding tooth structure is intact (Fig. 17.15). When a buccal or lingual carious lesion is near the occlusal surface, it can be confused with an occlusal lesion due to image superimposition. However, occlusal lesions are usually more extensive, are not as well defined, and will present a radiolucent line in the occlusal enamel. In either case, a clinical examination will confirm the diagnosis.

Root Surfaces

Caries involving the roots can be detected in patients with gingival recession or periodontal bone loss. The cementum is softer and thinner than the enamel (approximately 20–50 μm near the CEJ), causing the caries to progress more rapidly. The difficulty with a root surface carious lesions is being able to differentiate them from cervical burnout (see Fig. 17.9). Some radiographic signs can prove helpful to the practitioner. First, when there is no bone loss around a tooth, it is very likely that the radiolucency at the edge of the root is simply cervical burnout. Furthermore, with caries, clinical examination would demonstrate an irregularity or cavitation. With cervical burnout, the root surface would be intact. Finally, the shape of the radiolucency due to cervical burnout can often be explained by the anatomy of the tooth (see Fig. 17.9A). Fortunately most root lesions can and should be detected clinically, whether they are buccal, lingual, or interproximal.

Rampant Caries

Rampant caries is the term used to describe rapid progression with severe and widespread involvement. This is most often seen in young children who have poor oral hygiene habits coupled with poor dietary habits (e.g., going to sleep with a bottle of milk or juice) (Fig. 17.16). Indeed, the increased availability of fluoride in drinking water and the use of topical fluoride delivery systems have helped to control the development of caries in these patients.

Multiple carious lesions can be seen in adult patients with xerostomia. This is often the case following radiation therapy for head and neck cancers. The loss of function of the major salivary glands reduces or eliminates the ability of the glands to secrete enough saliva to buffer the effects of bacterially derived acids from oral microorganisms. Imaging examinations of these patients can demonstrate advanced, generalized caries involving smooth surfaces and teeth that usually do not present carious lesions (Fig. 17.17). These lesions, often referred to

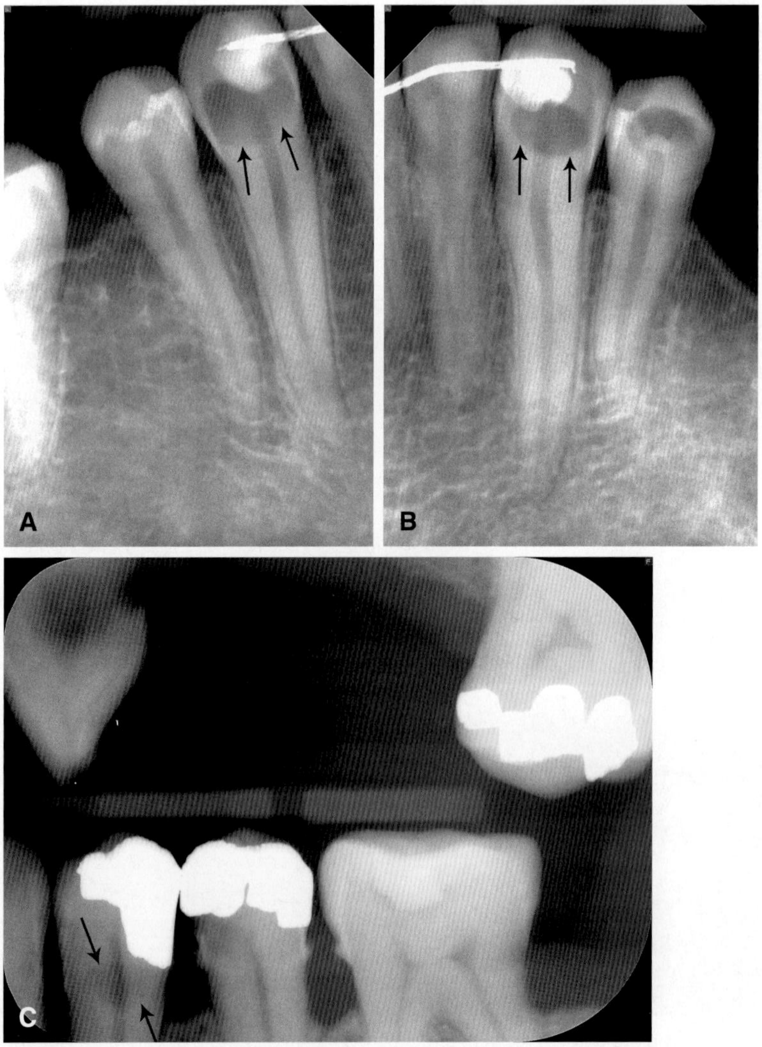

Fig. 17.15 (A–C) Buccal caries *(arrows)* usually have a circular shape, are well defined, and are in the cervical area.

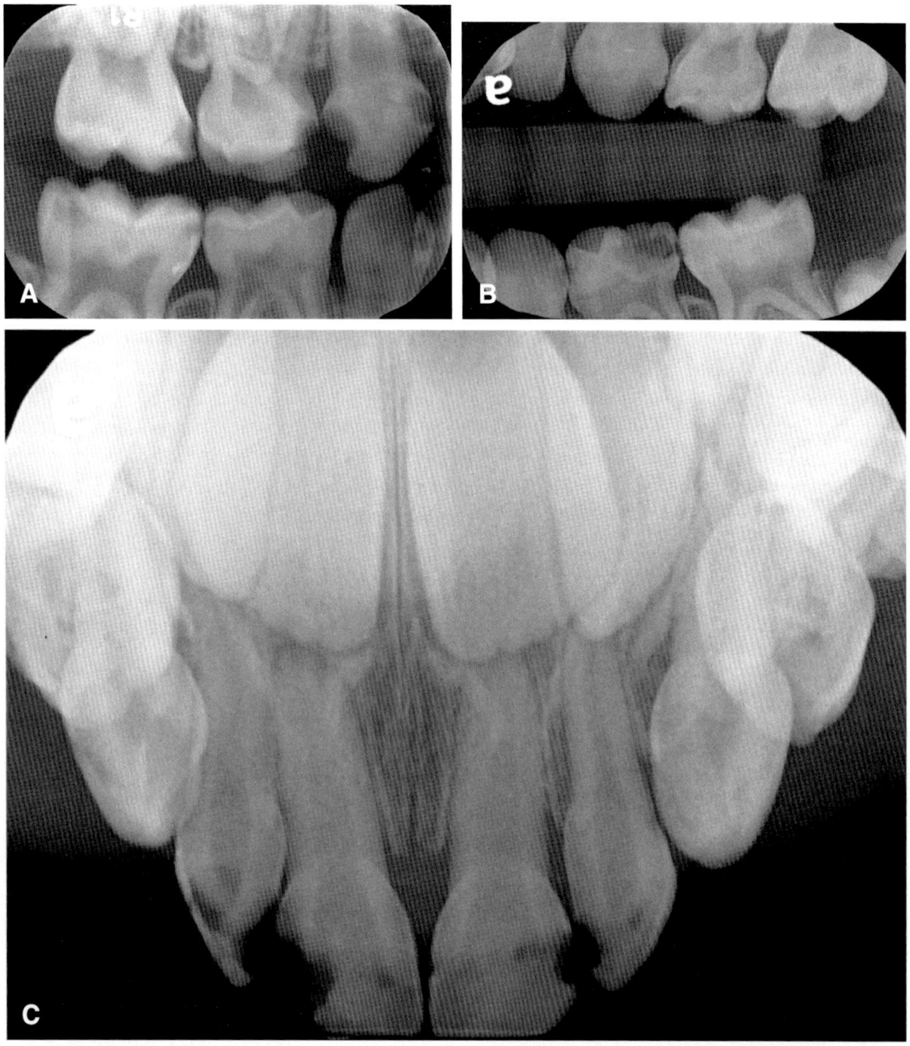

Fig. 17.16 Bitewing (A and B) and anterior occlusal (C) images of a 4-year-old patient with multiple carious lesions (rampant caries). (Courtesy Dr. C. Quach, Montréal, QC.)

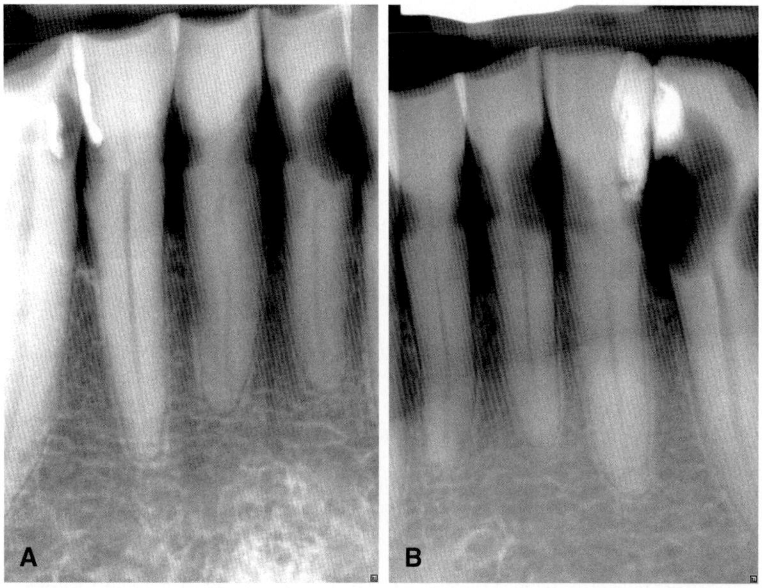

Fig. 17.17 Periapical images (A and B) showing multiple large root surface caries in a patient with xerostomia following radiation therapy of the head and neck.

as "radiation caries," are mostly smooth surface caries located near the cervical areas of the teeth. Impeccable hygiene along with topical fluoride and saliva substitutes can help negate some of the effects of xerostomia and limit the impact on the teeth.

Associated With Dental Restorations

Some carious lesions will develop at the margin of an existing restoration. These are called recurrent (or secondary) caries and represent new areas of demineralization (Fig. 17.18). These new carious lesions can be caused by either a defective restoration and/or ineffective dental hygiene. Such lesions will appear as radiolucencies in the tooth structure at the junction of the restoration and tooth. Another type of carious lesion associated with a dental restoration is called residual caries. The development of residual caries is different from that of recurrent caries in the sense that residual caries represent areas of demineralization that remain when the original carious lesion has not been completely removed. Although this can be involuntary, most often it can be purposeful when a large carious lesion encroaches on the dental pulp. A temporary restoration is placed that can stimulate the development of tertiary dentin (indirect pulp capping). A few months later, the remainder of the carious lesion is removed and a definitive restoration can be placed.

One of the difficulties in detecting interproximal recurrent caries is obtaining an image that demonstrates demineralization. Unfortunately, if the image is made at an improper vertical angulation, the restoration can mask or hide the recurrent carious lesion. Therefore it is vital to clinically examine the area thoroughly and to obtain high-quality images where the x-ray beam is optimally oriented to allow visualization of the interface between the tooth and the restoration. This is best accomplished with a bitewing image (see Figs. 17.2 and 17.19). When in doubt, a second image with a different angulation can be acquired.

Some materials used in restorative dentistry have a radiolucent appearance, and they may be confused with recurrent or residual caries. These materials are usually used as a base or liner on the prepared tooth surface beneath a restoration. The shape of the radiolucency can help the dentist differentiate between the radiolucent dental material and residual caries. The clinical history of the restorative procedure should also confirm this. Since liner and base materials should not extend to the periphery of a restoration (i.e., the cavosurface margin), they should not be confused with recurrent caries. Other types of restorative materials, including older composite materials, can also mimic carious lesions. These materials were often used for interproximal restorations in the anterior maxilla and can be differentiated from caries because of their well-defined borders, their shapes, and sometimes the radiopaque base or liner underlying them (Fig. 17.20).

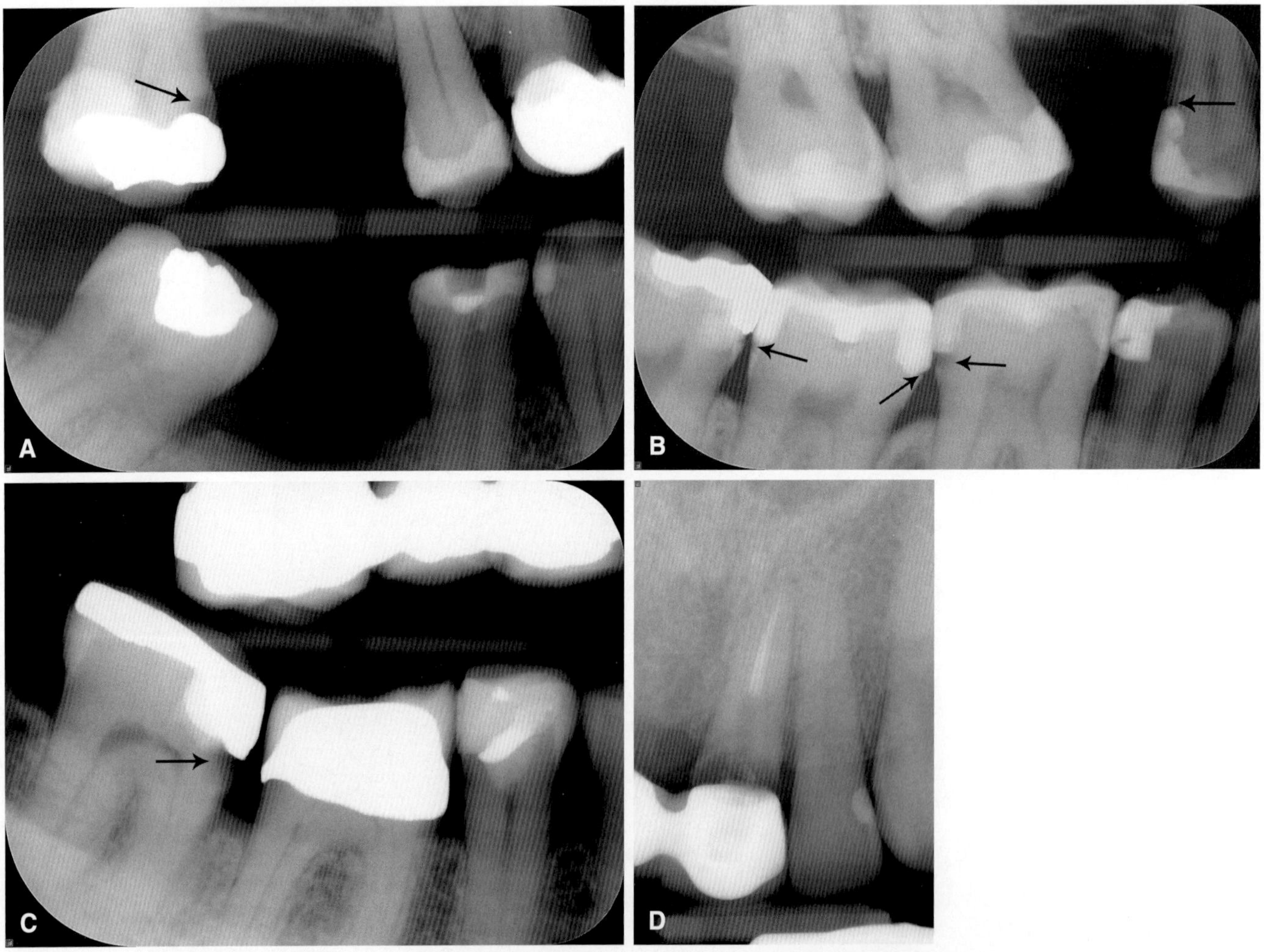

Fig. 17.18 (A) Bitewing image showing a recurrent carious lesion on the mesial surface of the maxillary right second molar *(arrow)*. (B) Bitewing image revealing multiple recurrent caries *(arrows)*. (C) Bitewing image showing a recurrent caries on the mesial surface of the mandibular right second molar *(arrow)*. (D) Anterior periapical image showing a large recurrent carious lesion on the maxillary left central incisor, which is a bridge abutment.

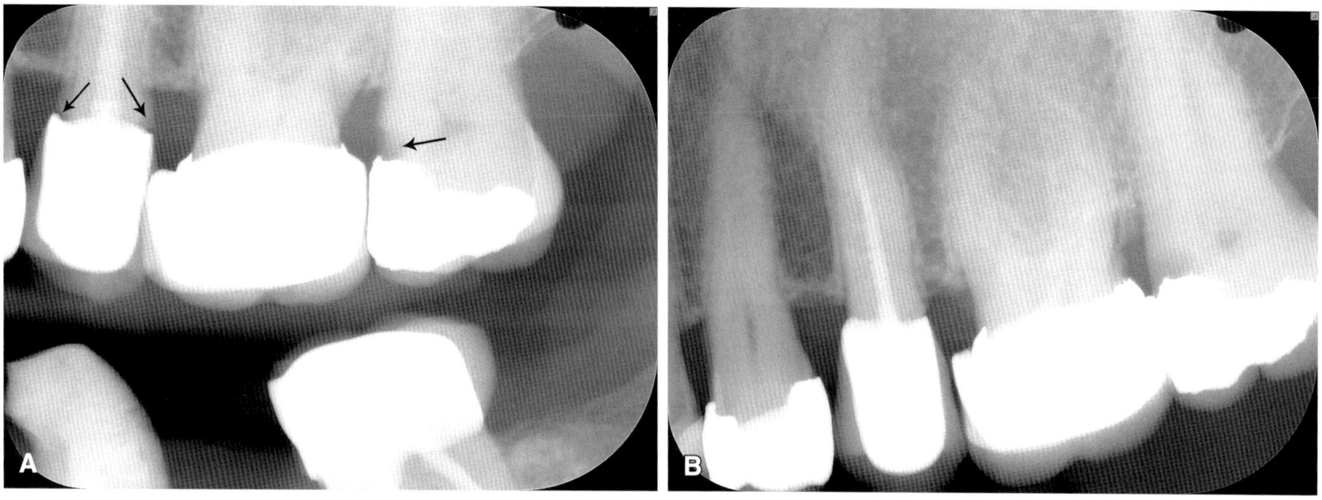

Fig. 17.19 (A) Bitewing image showing recurrent carious lesions on the mesial and distal surfaces of the maxillary left second premolar and on the mesial surface of the second molar *(arrows)*. (B) Periapical image of the same region where the recurrent lesions around the premolar are not visible because of the increased vertical angulation of the x-ray beam. The carious lesion on the second molar is still visible, but it is not as clearly visible as on the bitewing.

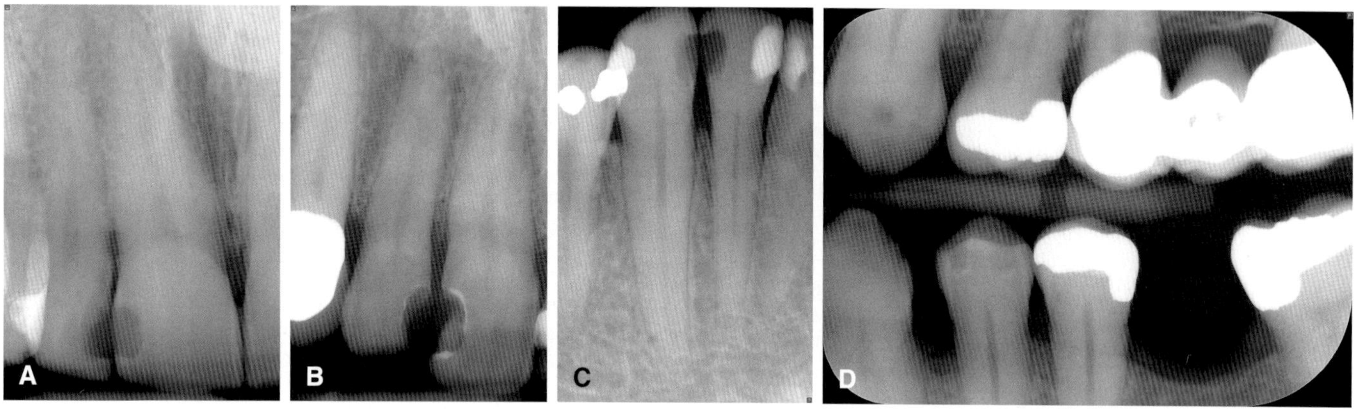

Fig. 17.20 (A) Periapical image showing radiolucent restorations placed on the distal surface of the central incisor and mesial surface of the lateral incisor. They have well-defined, almost rectangular shapes compared with true carious lesions. (B) Periapical image showing radiolucent restorations with a radiopaque liner placed beneath the composite restoration. This helps to rule out caries. (C) Periapical image with radiolucent restorations with a radiopaque liner on the distal surface of the mandibular right lateral incisor and mesial surface of the canine. (D) Bitewing image showing two occlusal radiolucent restorations with radiopaque liner material in the mandibular left first premolar.

ALTERNATIVE DIAGNOSTIC TOOLS TO DETECT DENTAL CARIES

Besides imaging, other methods have been developed to identify carious lesions. These have included light-induced fluorescence, lasers, transillumination, and electrical conductance. The light-induced fluorescence systems can be used to identify demineralization on smooth surfaces. The other systems are more commonly used on occlusal and interproximal surfaces. Such systems work by giving the dentist a number or value indicating the presence or absence of demineralization. Some of these systems may, however, have difficulty identifying carious lesions beneath and around dental restorations. For the time being, they should be used to complement imaging examinations.

The amount of research on artificial intelligence (AI) or deep learning has grown exponentially in the last few years, including its use in dentistry. Caries detection is probably where research is most active, given that caries is omnipresent sometimes difficult to diagnose accurately. Most recent studies demonstrate an improvement in diagnostic accuracy when a dentist is paired with AI compared with the dentist alone, although the long-term outcomes (described by retention of the teeth) are unclear. Like other diagnostic tools, AI should be used as an adjunctive test and should inform (but not replace) decision making by the dentist.

TREATMENT CONSIDERATIONS

The decision to treat or not to treat a carious lesion depends on a multitude of factors, including the patient's oral hygiene, their dental history, caries risk factors, and the depth and number of carious lesions. Demineralization limited to the enamel does not often require restorative treatment.

Rather, these lesions should be addressed noninvasively with topical fluoride application, more effective oral hygiene practices, and by reducing the frequency and amount of carbohydrates in the diet. Furthermore, such lesions should be followed up to confirm that they have arrested. This is also true when a lesion has just reached the dentin. In these cases, operative treatment may or may not be needed. When a carious lesion involves the deeper regions of the dentin or causes cavitation, it must be surgically removed and a restoration placed.

BIBLIOGRAPHY

Abesi F, Mirshekar A, Moudi E, et al. Diagnostic accuracy of digital and conventional imagery in the detection of non-cavitated approximal dental caries. *Iran J Radiol.* 2012;9(1):17-21.

American Dental Association Council on Scientific Affairs, US Food and Drug Administration. Dental imaging examinations: recommendations for patient selection and limiting radiation exposure. Revised 2012. https://www.fda.gov/media/84818/download.

Atchison KA, White SC, Flack VF, et al. Assessing the FDA guidelines for ordering dental images. *J Am Dent Assoc.* 1995;126(10):1372-1383.

Bahrami G, Hagstrøm C, Wenzel A. Bitewing examination with four digital receptors. *Dentomaxillofac Radiol.* 2003;32(5):317-321.

Berry HM Jr. Cervical burnout and Mach band: two shadows of doubt in radiologic interpretation of carious lesions. *J Am Dent Assoc.* 1983;106(5):622-625.

Haiter-Neto F, Wenzel A, Gotfredsen E. Diagnostic accuracy of cone beam computed tomography scans compared with intraoral image modalities for detection of caries lesions. *Dentomaxillofac Radiol.* 2008;37(1):18-22.

Kamburoglu K, Kolsuz E, Murat S, et al. Proximal caries detection accuracy using intraoral bitewing image, extraoral bitewing imagery and panoramic imagery. *Dentomaxillofac Radiol.* 2012;41(6):450-459.

NIH Consensus Development Conference on Diagnosis and Management of Dental Caries Throughout Life. Bethesda, MD, March 26–28, 2001. Conference papers. *J Dent Educ.* 2001;65(10):935-1179.

Pitts NB, Ekstrand KR, ICDAS Foundation. International Caries Detection and Assessment System (ICDAS) and its International Classification and Management System (ICCMS) - methods for staging of the caries process and enabling dentists to manage caries. *Community Dent Oral Epidemiol.* 2013;41(1):e41–52.

Pitts NB, Ismail AI, Martignon S, et al. *ICCMS Guide for Practitioners and Educators.* ICCMS Implementation Workshop; 2014.

Schwendicke F, Cjudo Grano de Oro J, Garcia Cantu A, et al. Artificial intelligence for caries detection: value of data and information. *J Dent Res.* 2022; 101(11):1350-1356.

Caries Detection

Abdinian M, Razavi SM, Faghihian R, et al. Accuracy of digital bitewing imagery versus different view of digital panoramic imagery for detection of proximal caries. *J Dent Tehran UMS.* 2015;12(4):290-297.

Akdeniz BG, Grondahl HG, Magnusson B. Accuracy of proximal caries depth measurements: comparison between limited cone beam computed tomography, storage phosphor and film imagery. *Caries Res.* 2006;40(3):202-207.

Hellén-Halme K, Petersson A, Nilsson M. Effect of ambient light and monitor brightness and contrast settings on the detection of approximal caries in digital images: an in vitro study. *Dentomaxillofac Radiol.* 2008;37(7):380-384.

Jacobsen JH, Hansen B, Wenzel A, et al. Relationship between histological and imageic caries lesion depth measured in images from four digital imagery systems. *Caries Res.* 2004;38(1):34-38.

Jørgensen PM, Wenzel A. Patient discomfort in bitewing examination with film and four digital receptors. *Dentomaxillofac Radiol.* 2012;41(4):323-327.

Mejáre I. Bitewing examination to detect caries in children and adolescents—when and how often? *Dent Update.* 2005;32(10):588-590, 593-594, 596-597.

Mejáre I, Stenlund H, Zelezny-Holmlund C. Caries incidence and lesions progression from adolescence to young adulthood: a prospective 15-year cohort study in Sweden. *Caries Res.* 2004;38(2):130-141.

Mohammad-Rahimi H, Reza Motamedian S, Hossein Rohban M, et al. Deep learning for caries detection: a systematic review. *J Dent.* 2022;122:104115.

Mjör IA, Toffenetti F. Secondary caries: a literature review with case reports. *Quintessence Int.* 2000;31(3):165-179.

Poorterman JHG, Weerheijm KL, Groen HJ, et al. Clinical and imageic judgement of occlusal caries in adolescents. *Eur J Oral Sci.* 2000;108(2):93-98.

Ratledge DK, Kidd EA, Beighton D. A clinical and microbiological study of approximal carious lesions, 1: the relationship between cavitation, imageic lesion depth, the site specific gingival index and the level of infection of the dentine. *Caries Res.* 2001;35(1):3-7.

Simon JC, Lucas S, Lee R, et al. Near-infrared imaging of secondary caries lesions around composite restorations at wavelengths from 1300-1700 nm. *Dent Mater.* 2016;32(4):587-595.

Wenzel A, Haiter-Neto F, Gotfredsen E. Risk factors for a false positive test outcome in diagnosis of caries in approximal surfaces: impact of imageic modality and observer characteristics. *Caries Res.* 2007;41(3):170-176.

Wenzel A, Hirsch E, Christensen JH, et al. Detection of cavitated approximal surfaces using cone beam CT and intraoral receptors. *Dentomaxillofac Radiol.* 2013;42(1):39458105.

Young SM, Lee JT, Hodges RJ, et al. A comparative study of high-resolution cone beam computed tomography and charge-coupled device sensors for detecting caries. *Dentomaxillofac Radiol.* 2009;38(7):445-451.

Treatment Decision

Bader JD, Shugars DA. The evidence supporting alternative management strategies for early occlusal caries and suspected occlusal dentinal caries. *J Evid Based Dent Pract.* 2006;6(1):91-100.

Bjørndal L, Kidd EA. The treatment of deep dentine caries lesions. *Dent Update.* 2005;32(7):402-404, 407-410, 413.

Evans RW, Pakdaman A, Dennison PJ, et al. The caries management system: an evidence-based preventive strategy for dental practitioners. Application for adults. *Aust Dent J.* 2008;53(1):83-92.

Evans RW, Dennison PJ. The caries management system: an evidence-based preventive strategy for dental practitioners. Application for children and adolescents. *Aust Dent J.* 2009;54(4):381-389.

Gordan VV, Garvan CW, Heft MW, et al. Restorative treatment thresholds for interproximal primary caries based on imageic images: findings from the dental practice-based research network. *Gen Dent.* 2009;57(6):654-663.

Kakudate N, Sumida F, Matsumoto Y, et al. Restorative treatment thresholds for proximal caries in dental PBRN. *J Dent Res.* 2012;91(12):1202-1208.

18

Periodontal Diseases

Trevor S.T. Thang

The periodontium supports the teeth in the jaws, and is composed of the gingiva, the periodontal ligament (PDL), cementum, and the alveolar processes of the jawbones. The periodontal diseases are a heterogeneous collection of conditions affecting these structures and are characterized by an inflammatory host response in the periodontal tissues that may lead to localized or generalized alterations in the supporting bone and soft tissues around the teeth. Left untreated, these changes may ultimately result in tooth loss.

In recent years, the health burden of the periodontal diseases has been increasing in the population, particularly among those in lower socioeconomic groups. The reported prevalence of periodontal disease worldwide varies depending on study methodologies and the thresholds used. A recent large-scale study in the United States found that 42% of adults aged 30–79 years had periodontitis, with a significant increase in prevalence with age (29.5% for ages 30–44, 46.0% for ages 45–64, and 59.8% for ages 65–79). In this study, periodontitis was defined as having both clinical attachment loss (3 mm or greater at multiple sites) and periodontal probing depths (greater than 3 mm at multiple sites OR greater than 4 mm at a single site). The identification, management, and follow-up of the periodontal diseases are important responsibilities of the dentist, and imaging plays an important role in the successful diagnosis, treatment planning, and monitoring of these conditions.

DISEASE MECHANISM

Dental plaque biofilm plays a primary role in the initiation of the periodontal diseases. Periodontal disease-implicated bacteria, predominantly gram-negative rods and spirochetes, colonize the tooth and root surfaces between the root and the gingival margin and in some cases invade into the surrounding tissues. While these bacteria can directly damage host tissues through the release of toxins, more significantly, they may also stimulate a host inflammatory reaction. The release of inflammatory mediators as part of this response is responsible for much of the damage to the surrounding soft tissues and stimulate osteoclastic bone resorption. Furthermore, the inflammatory response causes loss of and apical migration of the junctional epithelium, leading to the formation of the periodontal pocket, which further facilitates bacterial colonization.

Periodontal disease often progresses in bursts of varied severities. As with all inflammatory processes, there are cyclic periods of active inflammation and tissue destruction, followed by periods of quiescence with no appreciable changes. The relative durations of the destructive and quiescent phases depends on the form of periodontal disease, the nature of the bacterial pathogens, and the host response. Oral hygiene practices disrupt local dental plaque biofilm, and slow the development and progression of periodontal disease. The onset of disease and its progression may be modified by systemic factors that alter the host immune response. These factors may include age, stress, smoking, or systemic disease. Hormonal changes that arise during puberty, pregnancy, and menopause may also contribute to the onset and progression of periodontal disease. Greater rates of periodontal disease are also seen in lower socioeconomic populations, and those in whom dental care is neglected.

The clinical indicators of the periodontal diseases reflect the host tissue response to oral bacterial biofilm, and these manifest as signs of inflammation. Inflammation of the gingival tissues, gingivitis, is seen as gingival swelling, edema, and erythema. Progression to periodontitis occurs with pocket formation and/or gingival recession, ultimately resulting in clinical attachment loss. Other clinical signs include bleeding on probing, purulent exudate, and tooth mobility. The disease is usually painless, and most patients are unaware of its presence until tooth mobility and ultimately tooth loss occurs.

ASSESSMENT OF PERIODONTAL DISEASE

In the diagnosis of the periodontal diseases, the clinical and radiologic examinations are complementary. The clinical examination should always be conducted first and act as the foundation to justify additional testing, including the acquisition of diagnostic images.

The clinical examination for periodontal diseases may include performing periodontal probing, identifying bleeding sites, measuring gingival recession, calculating clinical attachment loss, determining tooth mobility, and evaluating the amount of attached gingiva. Radiologic images are an adjunct to this examination, and the prescription of imaging is indicated when the clinical examination suggests periodontitis. This means that prescribed radiologic images should contribute additional information about the status of the periodontium which could not be derived from the clinical examination. Images also provide a permanent record of the condition of the periosteum, which can be used to evaluate the disease longitudinally. Diagnostic images aid the clinician in identifying the extent of destruction of the alveolar process, local predisposing factors, and features of the periodontium that may influence prognosis. Radiologic images also help the dentist assess the clinical crown-to-root ratio, a factor that can influence the prognosis of the tooth and any planned prosthesis. A summary of important radiologic features related to periodontal status that may be identified in diagnostic images are listed in Box 18.1. In summary, a complete diagnosis of periodontal disease requires a thorough clinical examination of the patient, combined with evidence identified on diagnostic images.

BOX 18.1 Radiographic Assessment of Periodontal Conditions

Radiographs are especially helpful in the evaluation of the following features:

- Amount of bone present
- Condition of the alveolar crests
- Bone loss in the furcation areas
- Width of the periodontal ligament space
- Local irritating factors that increase the risk of periodontal disease
  - Calculus
  - Poorly contoured or overextended restorations
  - Root length and morphology and crown-to-root ratio
  - Open interproximal contacts, which may be sites for food impaction
- Anatomic considerations
  - Root proximity
  - Position of the maxillary sinus in relation to a periodontal deformity
  - Position of the mental foramen in relation to the alveolar crest

IMAGING MODALITIES FOR THE ASSESSMENT OF PERIODONTAL DISEASE

Intraoral Imaging

Intraoral images provide the highest spatial resolution of any imaging modality, which allows the dentist to detect fine details of the periodontium. Image detail is essential since the structures being assessed are often submillimeter in size, and many of the radiologic signs of periodontal disease are subtle, including early loss of bone, and changes to the PDL space and lamina dura. Intraoral imaging modalities used for the assessment of periodontal disease include bitewing and periapical images.

Bitewing images should be considered the primary imaging choice for characterizing the periodontal diseases. These images most accurately depict the distance between the cementoenamel junction (CEJ) and the crest of the interradicular alveolar process because the incident x-ray beam is oriented perpendicular to the long axes of the teeth. Periapical images have the benefit of demonstrating the full length of the tooth, which allows for the evaluation of the percentage of root affected by bone loss. However, periapical images often provide a distorted view of the relationship between the CEJ and the alveolar crest due to greater variations in the vertical angulation of the primary x-ray beam. This occurs most commonly in the maxilla because of anatomical limitations placed on receptor positioning by the height of the palatal vault. In such circumstances, the level of the buccal alveolar crest may be projected near or coronal to the level of the palatal CEJ, making the bone height appear greater.

The usefulness of intraoral images in the evaluation of the periodontal diseases can be optimized by making images of high technical quality. The technique for obtaining intraoral images is covered in greater detail in the chapters on projection geometry and intraoral projections (see Chapters 5 and 6), but the features that are particularly important for imaging the relationship between the teeth and the alveolar processes are emphasized here.

For patients with clinical evidence of periodontal attachment loss, standard (i.e., horizontal) bitewing images are unlikely to depict the alveolar crest because of the extent of bone loss (Fig. 18.1A). This is especially concerning when utilizing digital solid-state (direct) detectors, since these sensors have reduced active receptor areas to accommodate their thick outer housing. In these instances, the dentist must decide before the images are made to reorient the receptor 90 degrees so that a vertical bitewing image can be made. The vertical bitewing method uses the same image receptor size, but oriented in such a way that the long axis of the receptor is in a vertical orientation. Although the image geometry is unchanged compared with the standard horizontal method, this rotation provides additional receptor height and allows the dentist to visualize the crest of the alveolar process when there has been significant clinical attachment loss (Fig. 18.1B).

Limitations of Intraoral Images

Intraoral bitewing and periapical images may not provide a complete representation of the periodontium due to limitations inherent to these techniques. First, bitewing and periapical images are two-dimensional representations of three-dimensional anatomic structures. Therefore, infrabony defects may not be effectively visualized, as the buccal and/or lingual walls may superimpose themselves over the defect itself. In addition, overlapping tooth structure may superimpose over the crestal bone, masking it from being clearly seen. To overcome this limitation, multiple images can be acquired of the same site at different angulations to allow the dentist to use the buccal object

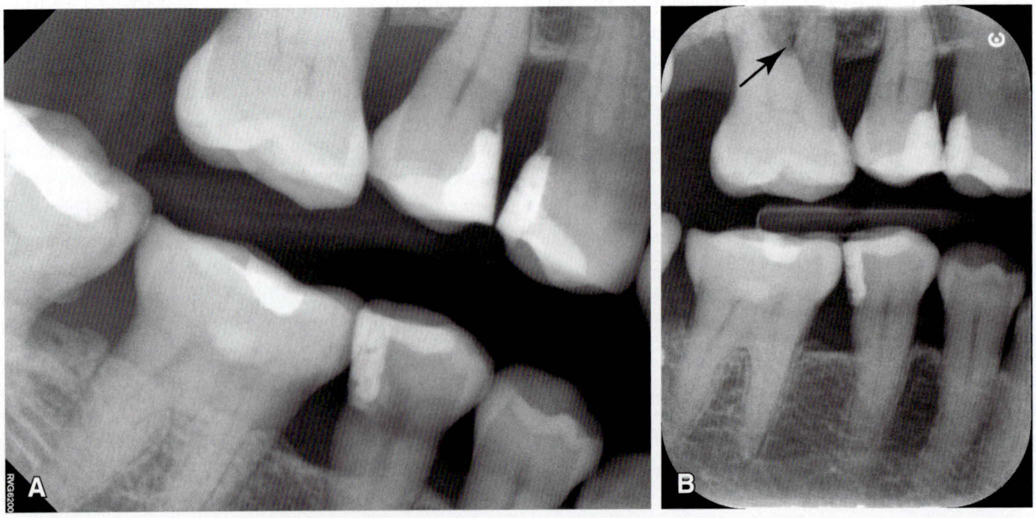

Fig. 18.1 (A) Horizontal bitewing which does not demonstrate the crestal bone levels at the distal surface of the maxillary first molar or the mesial surface of the mandibular first premolar. (B) Vertical bitewing projection in the same site captures these surfaces as well as revealing furcation involvement of the first molar *(arrow)*.

(i.e., S-L-O-B) rule to obtain additional information about the third dimension. Second, intraoral images typically underestimate the amount of bone loss, resulting in early periodontal bone lesions being indetectable radiographically. Third, intraoral images do not demonstrate soft tissue–to–hard tissue relationships, and thus, they provide no information about the depth of soft tissue pockets (which is why a complementary clinical examination is necessary). Finally, bone level is often measured relative to the position of the CEJ; however, this reference point is not valid in situations where there is supraeruption of teeth, or where there is passive eruption in patients with severe attrition. Although intraoral images play an invaluable role in the diagnosis and treatment planning of patients with periodontal disease, for these reasons, their use must be considered adjunctive to a thorough clinical examination.

Panoramic Imaging

The panoramic image has many features that are attractive for dentists. Image acquisition is relatively quick and comfortable for the patient, and the resulting image provides an overview of the teeth and jaws in a single acquisition. Despite these benefits, the use of panoramic imaging for the evaluation of periodontal bone loss is controversial. Proponents argue that high-quality panoramic images can demonstrate changes to the periodontal structures and provide comparable diagnostic information to intraoral images. These authors suggest that a panoramic image supplemented with selected intraoral images may be adequate for periodontal assessment. However, critics argue that the drawbacks outweigh these benefits. Panoramic imaging creates images with multiple superimpositions and distortions (especially in the anterior areas of the jaws). Furthermore, the lower spatial resolution of panoramic images relative to intraoral images limits image detail, making diagnosis more difficult and unreliable. Finally, the acquisition of panoramic images can be technically challenging, resulting in patient positioning errors that only add to the many compromises of this technique. Given the available evidence, a panoramic image should not be prescribed as the primary imaging tool for the characterization of the periodontal diseases. Interpretation of a panoramic image for periodontal considerations should only be considered if the image has already been acquired; and there is a low likelihood that additional intraoral imaging would present additional clinically significant findings.

Recently, some panoramic systems manufacturers have introduced extraoral bitewings as an option to the conventional intraoral bitewing. At this time, there is no evidence that supports a role for extraoral bitewing images in the characterization of periodontal bone loss.

Cone Beam Computed Tomography

Cone beam computed tomography (CBCT) has one powerful advantage: the ability to visualize the osseous supporting structures of the teeth from any angle, without anatomical superimpositions. This feature overcomes many of the limitations associated with intraoral and panoramic imaging techniques. CBCT imaging can allow better visualization of some periodontal defects that are not well depicted on conventional two-dimensional images. For example, CBCT imaging may permit a more complete assessment of the architecture of complex vertical defects, crater defects, furcations, and buccal and lingual cortical plate loss (Fig. 18.2). In addition, anatomic features, such as root morphology or cortical fenestration, and coexistent periapical inflammatory disease, which may be pertinent to diagnosis, treatment planning, and prognosis, may also be better visualized. However, CBCT imaging may be limited by image artifacts caused by metallic restorations, which greatly obscure the details of the bony architecture being examined. Current evidence does not support the use of CBCT imaging for imaging of the periodontium because it does not offer a significant advantage over intraoral imaging techniques, particularly when the additional cost, time, and radiation dose are considered. However, CBCT imaging, particularly small-volume and high-resolution systems, may be indicated in guiding the management of selected bony lesions, especially when surgery is being considered.

APPEARANCE OF NORMAL ANATOMY

The appearance of the normal alveolar processes has a characteristic appearance. A thin layer of radiopaque cortical bone often overlies the crest of the alveolar process at a level that is approximately 0.5–2.0 mm apical to the level of the CEJ. Between posterior teeth, the alveolar crest is oriented parallel to an imaginary line connecting the CEJs of adjacent teeth (Fig. 18.3), while between anterior teeth, the alveolar crest appears more peaklike (Fig. 18.4). Visualization of this corticated alveolar crest indicates the absence of periodontitis. However, the opposite is not always true; the lack of a corticated alveolar crest can be seen in both patients with and without periodontitis.

Another key region of the alveolar process to evaluate is where the alveolar crest merges with the lamina dura of adjacent anterior teeth. For posterior teeth, this transition is defined by a sharp, well-defined angle that closely approximates the root surface. In some cases, the PDL space may appear slightly wider around the cervical portions of tooth roots, particularly the premolar teeth, and in adolescents with erupting teeth. In this situation, if the lamina dura still forms a sharp, well-defined angle with the alveolar crest, the condition should be considered a variant of normal and not an indication of disease. In most instances, however, the coronal PDL space will typically appear thin and uniform in width. The buccal/lingual thickness of the alveolar crest varies widely, and it may be very thin coronally. This may appear in a two-dimensional image as an increase in bone radiolucency toward the crest. These sorts of variations in density alone are not an indication of disease. Rather, they may be a variation of normal.

IMAGING FEATURES OF PERIODONTAL DISEASES

Since gingivitis is an inflammatory condition confined to the gingival soft tissues, no associated radiographic changes to the underlying bone are seen.

The radiographic changes for all types of periodontal diseases are no different than any other inflammatory condition of bone. These changes can be broadly divided into (1) changes in the morphology of the supporting bone and (2) changes to the trabecular density and pattern. Changes in morphology become apparent by observing a loss of the interproximal crestal bone, and the bone overlapping the buccal or lingual surfaces of the tooth roots. Alterations to the trabecular pattern of the alveolar processes can manifest as a reduction in bone structure, an increase in bone structure, or a combination of both. A reduction in bone structure is seen as an increase in radiolucency (rarefaction) due to the decrease in the number and/or spatial density of existing trabeculae. An increase in bone structure is seen as an increase in radiopacity (sclerosis) as the result of an increase in the thickness and/or spatial density of trabecula. As with all inflammatory lesions of bone, periodontal disease usually involves a combination of bone loss and bone formation where acute lesions predominantly display bone loss, whereas chronic lesions have a greater component of bone sclerosis.

Changes in Morphology of Alveolar Processes

Early Bone Changes

The early bone changes that occur in periodontitis appear as areas of localized erosion of the interproximal alveolar crest (Fig. 18.5). In the

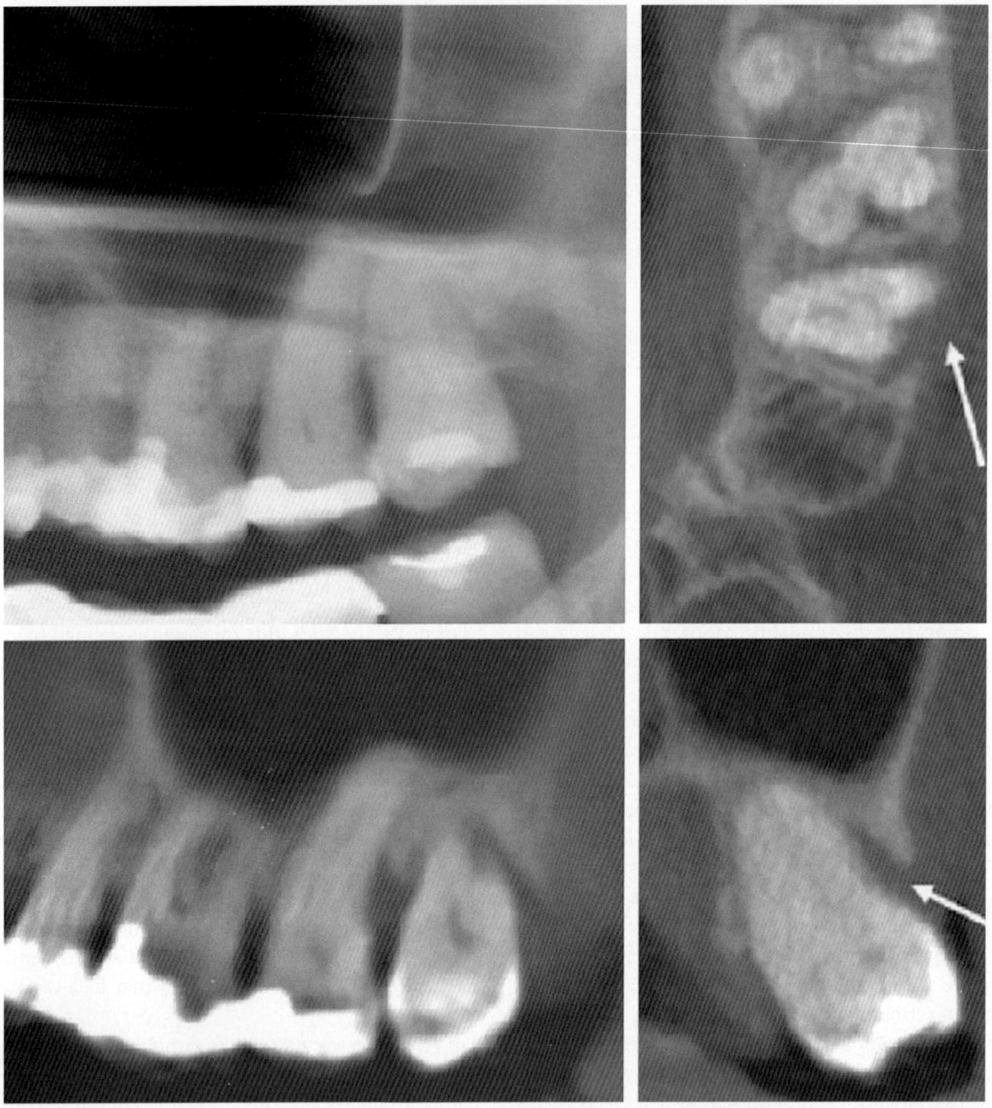

Fig. 18.2 Cropped panoramic image *(top left)* demonstrates moderate bone loss between the second and third molars. Axial *(top right)*, corrected sagittal *(bottom left)*, and coronal *(bottom right)* cone beam computed tomography images demonstrate the bone defects in this region more clearly. Periodontal bone loss adjacent to the buccal surface of the third molar is well visualized *(arrows)*, but could not be visualized on the panoramic image.

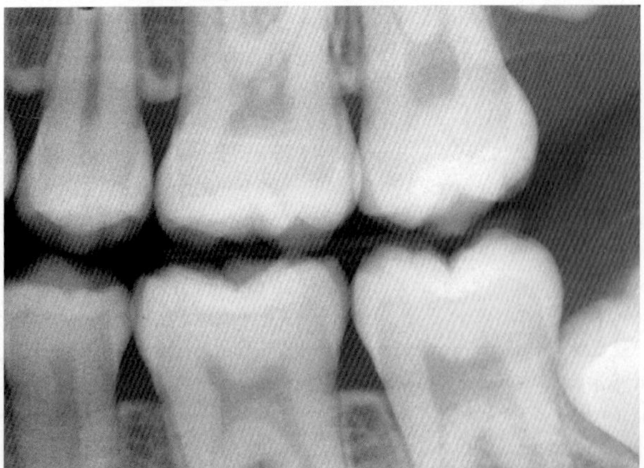

Fig. 18.3 The normal alveolar crest lies 0.5–2.0 mm apical to the adjacent cementoenamel junctions and forms a sharp angle with the lamina dura of the adjacent tooth. The crests may not always appear with a well-defined outer cortex.

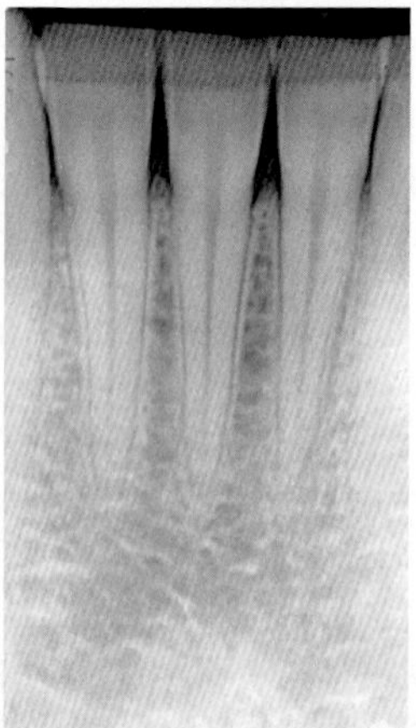

Fig. 18.4 Between the anterior teeth, the normal alveolar crest forms a peak, is well corticated, and is located within 0.5–2.0 mm of the adjacent cementoenamel junctions.

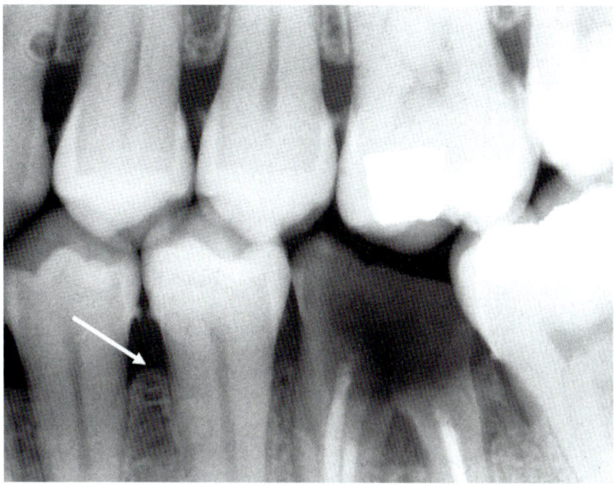

Fig. 18.5 Early periodontal disease is seen as a loss of cortical density and a rounding of the junction between the alveolar crest and the lamina dura *(arrow)*. Note also the more pronounced bone loss around the mandibular first molar and the generalized interproximal calculus.

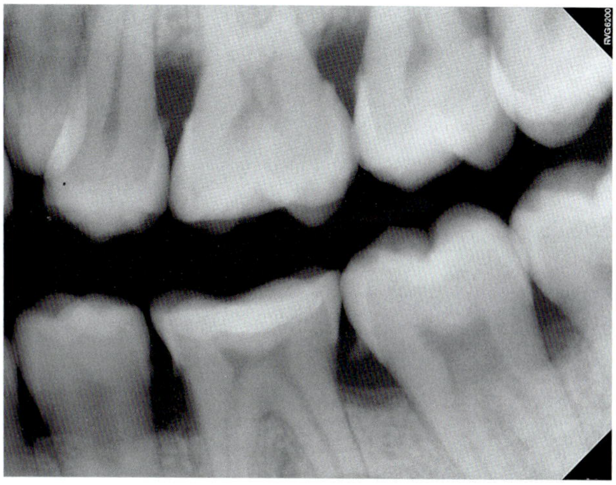

Fig. 18.7 The alveolar crest between the mandibular first and second molars appears angled but is approximately parallel to an imaginary plane created between the adjacent cementoenamel junctions, differentiating it from a vertical (angular) bone defect. There is an interproximal crater and reactive bone sclerosis present at this site.

anterior regions of the jaws, there is blunting of the alveolar crests and mild loss of alveolar crestal bone height. In the posterior regions of the jaws, there may be loss of the normally acute angle between the alveolar crest and lamina dura. In the early stages of periodontal disease, this angle may appear "rounded off," with a more irregular border. Moreover, the cortical surface of the bone edge may become more diffuse. Even if only mild changes are apparent, the onset of the disease process may not be recent, as radiographic evidence of bone loss typically follows the onset of the disease.

As periodontal disease progresses, further defects in the morphology of the alveolar process and crest may occur. These changes may include horizontal bone loss, vertical bone loss, interdental craters, furcation defects, and loss of the buccal or lingual cortical plates of bone. The presence and severity of these bone defects may vary regionally within a patient, and certainly among different patients.

Horizontal Bone Loss

Horizontal bone loss describes a loss in height of the alveolar process where the bone crest still parallels an imaginary line joining the CEJs of adjacent teeth. In horizontal bone loss, the crest of the buccal and lingual cortical plates and the intervening interdental bone have been resorbed (Fig. 18.6). The severity of radiographic horizontal bone loss is determined and characterized based on the alveolar bone level relative to the root length: (1) within the coronal 15%; (2) within the coronal 15%–33% of the root; and (3) beyond (i.e., apical to) the coronal 33% of the root length. Once evidence of horizontal bone loss is seen, categorizing its severity should be based on the entire root length (defined as the distance between the CEJ and the root apex).

When the CEJs of adjacent teeth are at different levels, the alveolar crest may have an angled appearance. Careful assessment of the imaginary line connecting the adjacent CEJs, as well as the sharp angle between the bone crest and lamina dura, should not be confused with a true vertical (angular) bone defect (Fig. 18.7). Particular care must also be taken in using the CEJ as a reference point in cases of tooth supraeruption and severe attrition (Fig. 18.8).

When teeth supraerupt, the alveolar process may not remodel to the new tooth position, resulting in apical positioning of the alveolar crest relative to the supraerupted CEJ. This situation may also occur during passive eruption of severely attrited teeth. In these cases, although the bone loss is not caused by periodontitis, there may be clinical implications due to the loss of attachment.

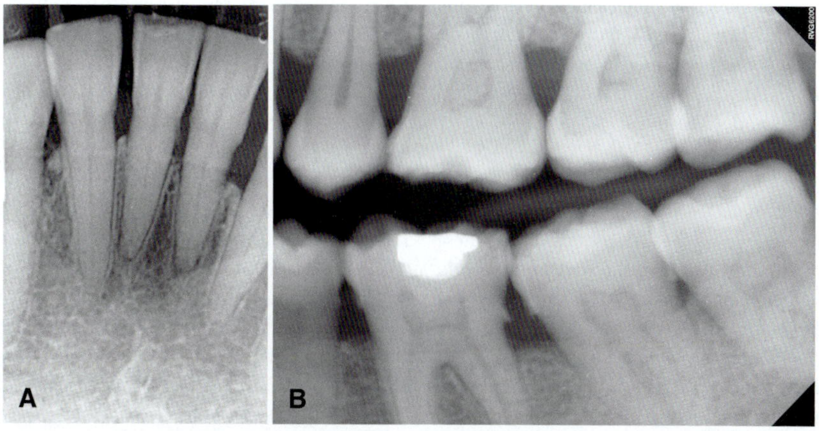

Fig. 18.6 Horizontal bone loss is seen in the anterior mandible (A) and the posterior region (B) as a loss of the buccal and lingual cortical plates and interdental alveolar bone.

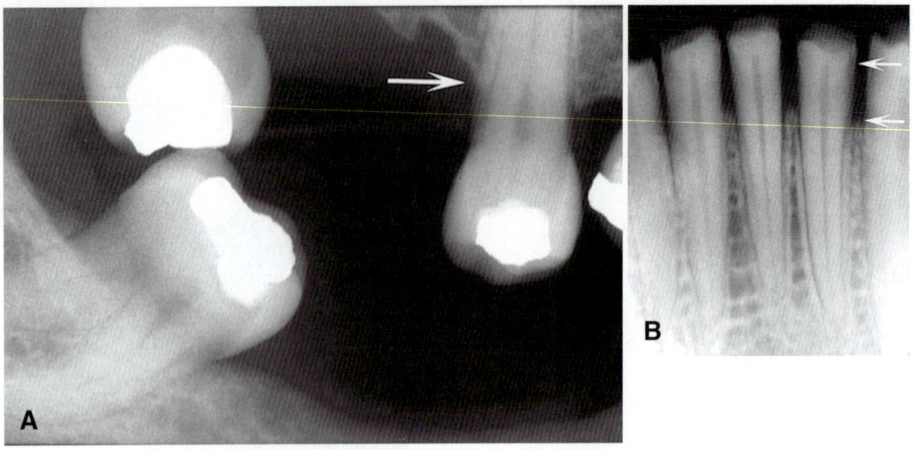

Fig. 18.8 (A) The maxillary second premolar is supraerupted; the etiology of the low bone level *(arrow)* relative to the cementoenamel junction (CEJ) is not necessarily the result of periodontal disease. (B) An example of passive eruption related to severe attrition resulting in the apparent increase in the distance from the CEJ to the bone height *(arrows)* cannot be attributed to periodontal disease. However, the resultant change in bone level relative to the CEJ still may be clinically significant.

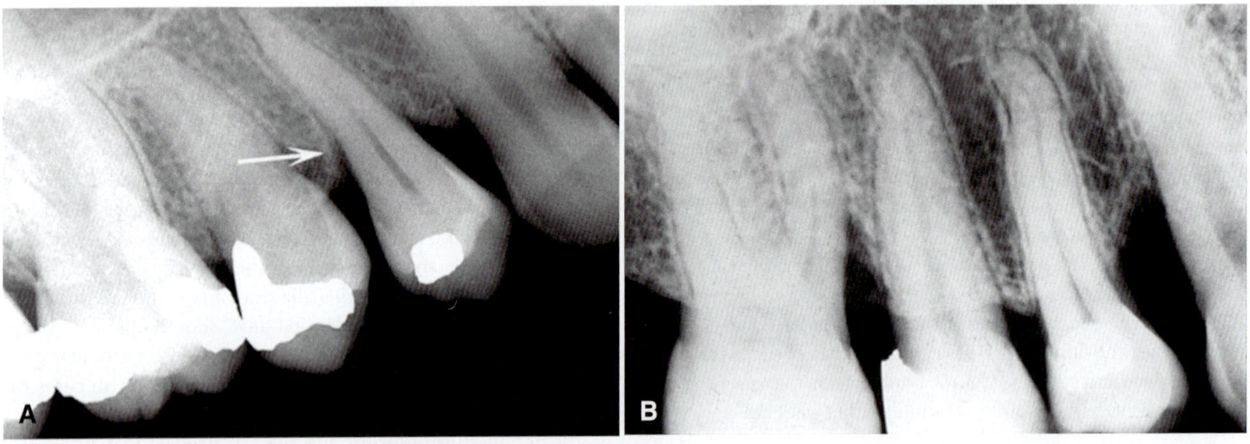

Fig. 18.9 (A) A developing vertical defect. Note the abnormal widening of the periodontal ligament space close to the crest *(arrow)*. (B) Maxillary periapical image reveals two examples of more severe vertical defects affecting the mesial surface of the first molar and the distal surface of the canine.

It is important to recognize that the extent of bone loss evident at a single examination does not indicate the current activity of the disease. For example, a patient who previously had generalized periodontal disease and subsequent successful therapy will show reduced bone height (i.e., reduced periodontium), but the bone level may remain stable. Reestablishment of the cortication of the alveolar crest is a good indicator of stabilization of the periodontium.

Vertical Bone Defects

A vertical (or angular, infrabony) defect describes the appearance of bone loss that is localized adjacent to a specific root surface. These defects develop when bone loss progresses down the root of the tooth, resulting in a deepening of the periodontal pocket. This manifests as a V- or triangular-shaped defect within the bone that extends apically along the affected root surface from the alveolar crest. Radiologically, the outline of the remaining alveolar process typically displays an angulation that is oblique to the imaginary line connecting the CEJ of the affected tooth to the adjacent tooth. In its early form, a vertical defect appears as abnormal widening of the PDL space at the alveolar crest (Fig. 18.9A).

A vertical defect is described as three walled because the defect is surrounded by three intact bony walls when both the buccal and lingual cortical plates remain intact. It is described as two walled when one of these plates has been resorbed, and as one walled when both plates have been lost (see Fig. 18.9B). Depending on the amount of bone loss, vertical bitewing images may be required to show the entire extent of the loss (Fig. 18.10). The distinctions among these groups are important in designing the treatment plan. The number of walls associated with a vertical defect is difficult or impossible to recognize on intraoral images, because one or both of the cortical bony plates may remain superimposed over the defect. Visualization of the depth of pockets may be aided by inserting a gutta-percha point into the pocket before making the intraoral image. The point appears to follow the defect because gutta-percha is relatively inflexible and radiopaque (Fig. 18.11). Clinical and surgical inspections are the best means of determining the number of remaining bony walls. CBCT imaging can also help characterize a defect more clearly, although this should not be routinely used for this purpose (Fig. 18.12).

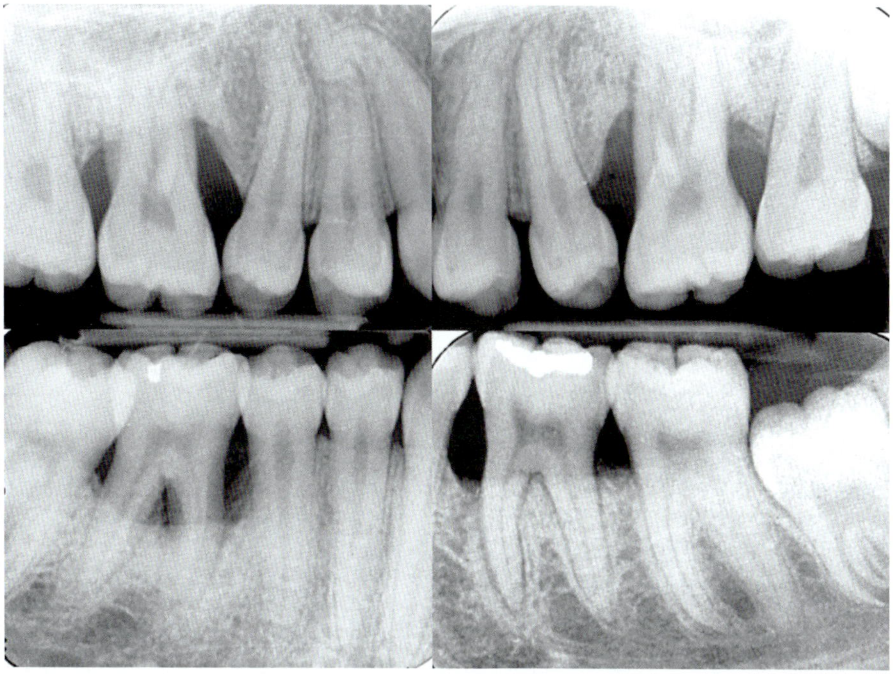

Fig. 18.10 Typical vertical bone loss in Stage IV periodontitis. Note the bone loss is confined to the region of the first molars. (Courtesy Dr. T. Charbeneau, Dallas, TX.)

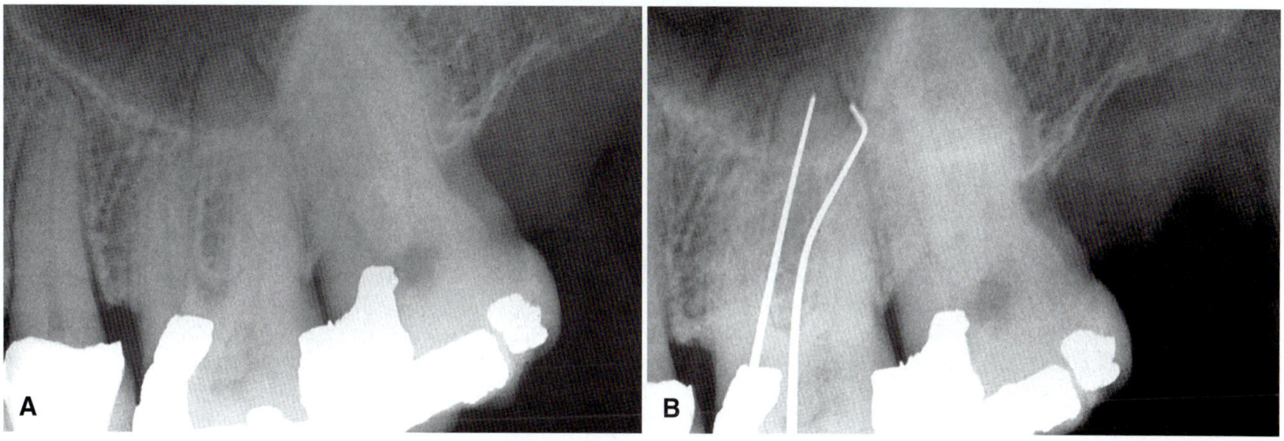

Fig. 18.11 Gutta-percha is used to visualize the depth of infrabony defects. (A) The image fails to show the osseous defect without the use of the gutta-percha points. (B) The image reveals an osseous defect extending to the region of the apex. (Courtesy Dr. H. Takei, Los Angeles, CA.)

Interdental Craters

The interproximal crater is a two walled, trough-like defect or depression that develops in the crest of the alveolar process between adjacent teeth, and the buccal and lingual outer cortical walls of the interproximal bone extend further coronally than the resorbed cancellous bone between them. In an image, this appears as a band-like or irregular region of bone with less density at the crest, immediately adjacent to the more dense normal bone apical to the base of the crater (Fig. 18.13). These defects are more common in the posterior segments of the jaws due to the broader buccal-lingual dimension of the alveolar crest in these regions.

Buccal or Lingual Cortical Plate Loss

The buccal or lingual cortical plate overlying a tooth root may resorb. Loss of a cortical plate may occur alone or with another type of bone loss, such as horizontal bone loss. This type of bone loss is seen as an increase in the radiolucency of the tooth root near the alveolar crest. The shape seen is usually semicircular, with the depth of the radiolucency directed apically in relation to the tooth (Fig. 18.14). Lack of bone loss at the interproximal region of the tooth may make this kind of defect difficult to detect on conventional images.

Osseous Deformities in the Furcations of Multirooted Teeth

Progressive periodontal disease and the associated bone loss may extend into the furcations of multirooted teeth. As bone loss extends apically along the surface of a multirooted tooth, the bone covering the root can reach the level of the furcation or more apically. Widening of the PDL space at the apex of the bony crest of the furcation is strong evidence that the periodontal disease process involves the furcation (Fig. 18.15A). If there has been sufficient loss of bone on either the

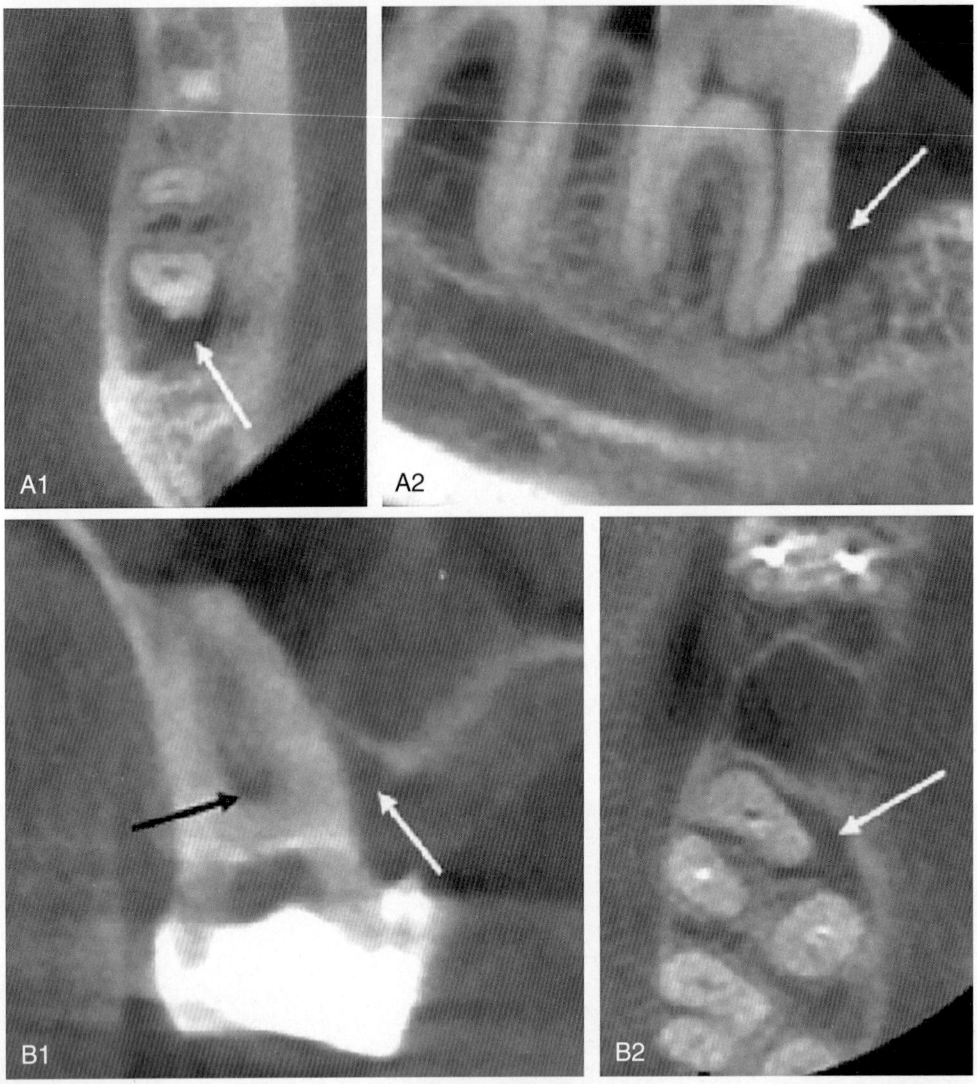

Fig. 18.12 Cone beam computed tomography images demonstrating details of the architecture of two three-walled vertical defects *(white arrows)*. Axial (A1) and corrected sagittal (A2) reconstructions show a deep vertical defect on the distal surface the distal root of the mandibular left second molar. Calculus is seen on this root surface. Corrected coronal (B1) and axial (B2) images show a three-walled defect on the palatal aspect of the mesiobuccal root of a maxillary molar. Early furcation involvement is also detected on this tooth *(black arrow)*.

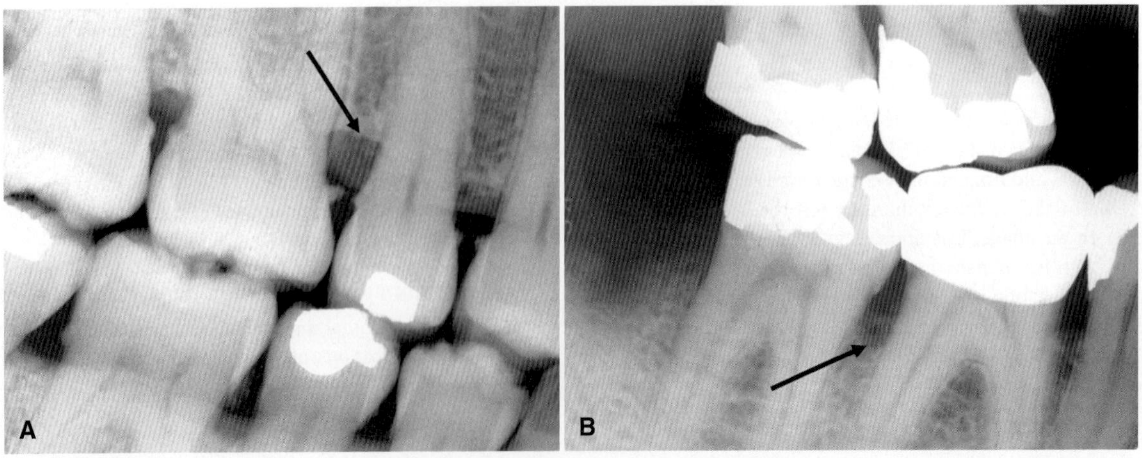

Fig. 18.13 Interproximal cratering between the buccal and lingual cortical plates, seen as a radiolucent band (A) or trough (B) apical to the level of the crestal edges. The *arrows* indicate the base of the craters.

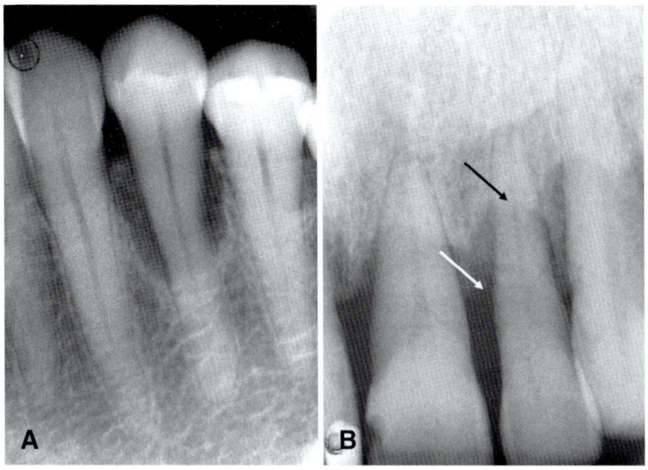

Fig. 18.14 (A) Loss of the lingual alveolar crest adjacent to this mandibular first premolar without associated interproximal bone loss. (B) Loss of the buccal cortical bone adjacent to the maxillary central and lateral incisors. The *black arrow* indicates the level of the buccal alveolar crest, which demonstrates more profound loss relative to the lingual alveolar crest *(white arrow)*.

buccal or lingual surface of a mandibular molar furcation, the radiolucent image of the furcation defect becomes prominent (Fig. 18.15B). The furcation defect may also involve only the buccal or lingual cortical plate, and extend into and apical to the roof of the furcation. In such cases, if the defect does not extend through the opposing cortical plate, involvement of the furcation may appear more irregular and radiolucent than the adjacent normal bone. In the mandible, the external oblique ridge may mask furcation involvement of the third molars (Fig. 18.15C). Convergent roots may also obscure furcation defects in maxillary and mandibular second and third molars.

The loss of interradicular bone in the furcation of a maxillary molar may originate from the buccal, mesial, or distal surfaces of the tooth. The most common route for furcation involvement of the maxillary permanent first molar is from the mesial surface of the tooth. The image of furcation involvement is not as sharply defined around maxillary molars as it is around mandibular molars, because the palatal root is superimposed over the defect (Fig. 18.15D). However, this pattern of bone destruction is occasionally prominent and appears as an inverted "J shape" radiolucency, with the hook of the "J" extending into the trifurcation (Fig. 18.15E) or as a radiolucent triangle superimposed over the roots of the involved tooth with its apex pointing toward the furcation.

A definitive diagnosis of complex furcation deformities requires careful clinical examination and sometimes surgical exploration. CBCT imaging can also be used to confirm involvement of a tooth and allow more detailed characterization of osseous furcation defects in cases where this information is necessary for treatment planning purposes.

Changes to the Internal Density and Trabecular Pattern of Bone

As with all other inflammatory lesions, the periodontal diseases may stimulate a reaction in the adjacent surrounding bone. The peripheral bone may appear more radiolucent or radiopaque, or more commonly, display a mixture of these patterns. Very rarely, no apparent change is seen in the surrounding bone. A radiolucent change reflects a loss of density and/or a reduced number of trabeculae. The trabeculae can appear very faint, which is more commonly seen in early or acute lesions (Fig. 18.16A). If the trabeculae are sufficiently decalcified, they may not clearly appear in the image, even though they are still present; this accounts for the apparent redevelopment of bone in some cases where acute inflammation resolves with successful treatment and the trabeculae remineralize. A radiopaque or sclerotic bone reaction appears because of bone deposition on existing trabeculae, resulting in thicker trabeculae. This can progress to the trabecular bone pattern being so dense it appears amorphous and radiopaque (see Fig. 18.16B). This sclerotic reaction may extend some distance from the periodontal lesion, sometimes to the inferior cortex of the mandible or to the maxillary sinus floors. Furthermore, inflammatory products from a periodontal lesion may diffuse through the cortex of the floor of the maxillary sinus to cause a regional mucositis (Fig. 18.17). In rare cases, a periosteal reaction might be seen in the adjacent alveolar process.

CLASSIFICATION OF THE PERIODONTAL DISEASES

Periodontitis

Periodontal disease classification is based on the tissue types affected (i.e., gingiva only or with involvement of the alveolar process), the staging (i.e., disease severity and complexity of management), the grading (i.e., historical rate of progression and future risk of progression), and its association with other conditions (i.e., systemic involvement, genetic conditions, or combined endodontic-periodontic lesions). A simplified overview of the classification of periodontal diseases is shown in Box 18.2 and Table 18.1.

Gingivitis is an inflammatory condition of the soft tissue surrounding the teeth, which may manifest as gingival swelling, edema, and erythema. If left unresolved, gingivitis can progress to periodontitis, resulting in clinically detectable destruction of clinical soft tissue attachment and supporting bone of the involved teeth. Although periodontitis is always preceded by gingivitis, gingivitis does not always progress to periodontitis.

Broadly speaking, periodontitis is subcategorized into the necrotizing periodontal diseases (NPDs), periodontitis, and periodontitis as a direct manifestation of systemic diseases. As with most inflammatory conditions, the radiographic appearance of all three of these subcategories of periodontitis can be similar.

Grade Modifiers of Periodontal Disease

Diabetes mellitus and cigarette smoking are well-documented risk factors which can affect the rate of progression of periodontitis (i.e., grading). Uncontrolled diabetes and periodontitis have a two-way systemic relationship, where patients with uncontrolled diabetes are predisposed to developing periodontal diseases, and increased periodontal inflammation impairs glycemic control in diabetics. Uncontrolled diabetes results in increased protein breakdown, degenerative vascular changes, lowered resistance to infection, and increased severity of infections. These systemic changes can lead to patients with uncontrolled diabetes who may present with periodontal diseases with more severe and rapid resorption of the alveolar processes, and who may also be more prone to the development of periodontal abscesses.

Similarly, cigarette smoking increases the risk of periodontal disease and hasten progression by altering the oral microflora to one that may contain more periodontal pathogens. Moreover, smoking may also impair the immune response of neutrophils.

Necrotizing Periodontal Diseases

NPD includes necrotizing gingivitis and necrotizing periodontitis. Conditions such as HIV infection, malnutrition, stress, and smoking may predispose patients to NPD. The clinical and gingival changes common to both NPD conditions include severe pain, fever and malaise with gingival erythema, bleeding, ulceration, and necrosis.

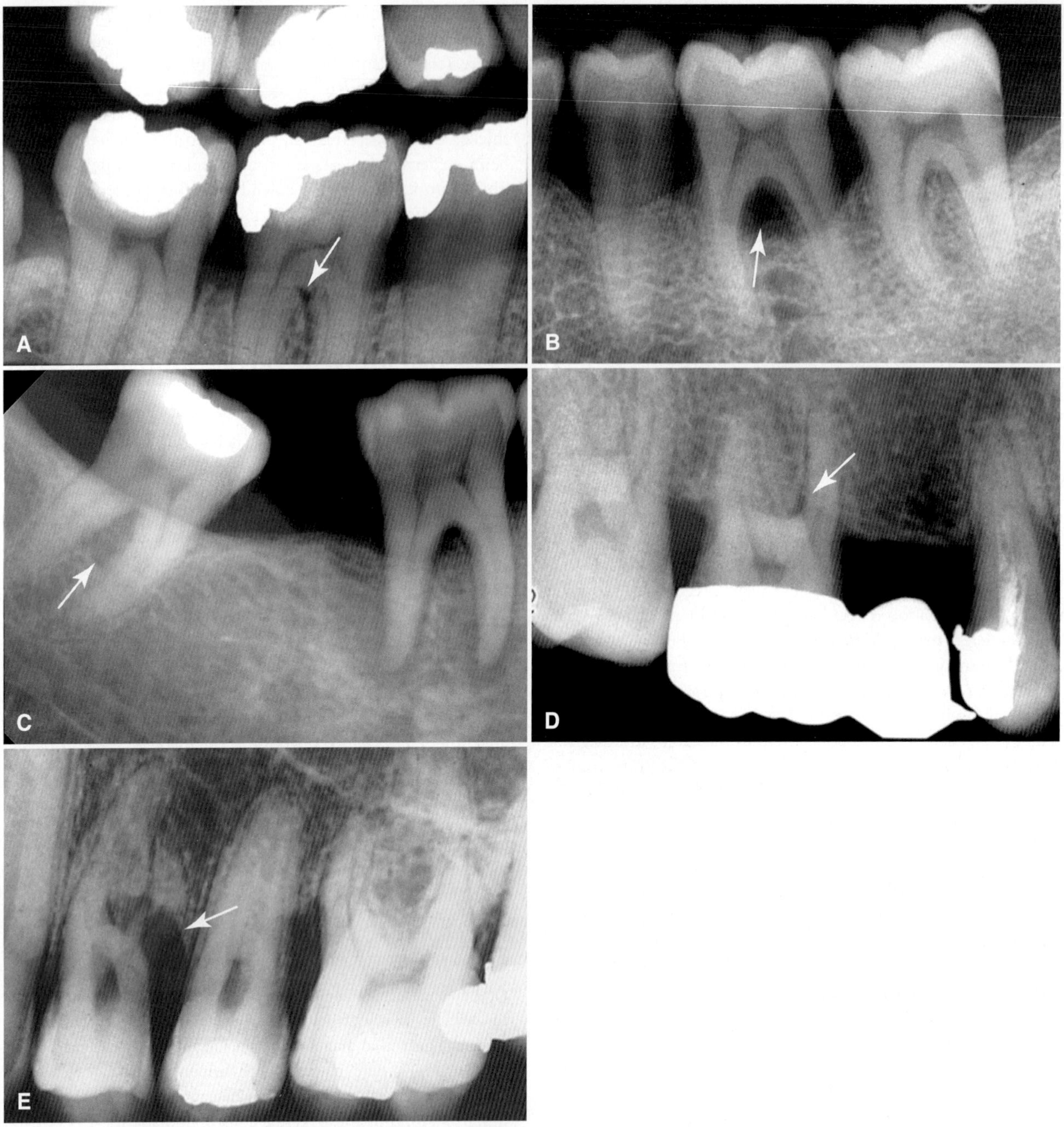

Fig. 18.15 (A) Periapical image revealing very early furcation involvement of a mandibular molar characterized by very mild widening of the periodontal ligament (PDL) space in the furcation region *(arrow)*. (B) Periapical image revealing a profound radiolucent area within the furcation *(arrow)* resulting from loss of bone in the furcation region and the buccal and lingual cortical plates. (C) Large furcation defect associated with the mandibular right third molar, which is less easily visualized due to superimposition by the external oblique ridge. There is also a combined periodontic-endodontic lesion of the first molar *(arrow)*. (D) Angulation of this periapical view of a maxillary first molar projected the palatal root away from the trifurcation region revealing early widening of the furcation PDL space *(arrow)*. (E) Example of an inverted "J shape" radiolucent lesion *(arrow)* resulting from bone destruction extending into the trifurcation region of a three-rooted maxillary first bicuspid.

Necrotizing periodontitis is diagnosed when there is also rapid loss of attachment. The diagnosis of NPD is made by clinical examination, but imaging aids in characterizing the extent of the bone loss.

Periodontitis as a Manifestation of Systemic Disease

This disease category includes diseases in which periodontal destruction is a direct result of specific systemic conditions. Examples include hematologic diseases (e.g., acquired neutropenia and leukemia) and genetic diseases (e.g., familial or cyclic neutropenia, Down syndrome, leukocyte adhesion deficiency syndrome, Papillon–Lefèvre syndrome, and Chédiak–Higashi syndrome). The oral changes in these conditions are the result of an impaired immune response to periodontal pathogens, or a connective tissue abnormality in the periodontium that results in greater destruction. Papillon–Lefèvre syndrome may be

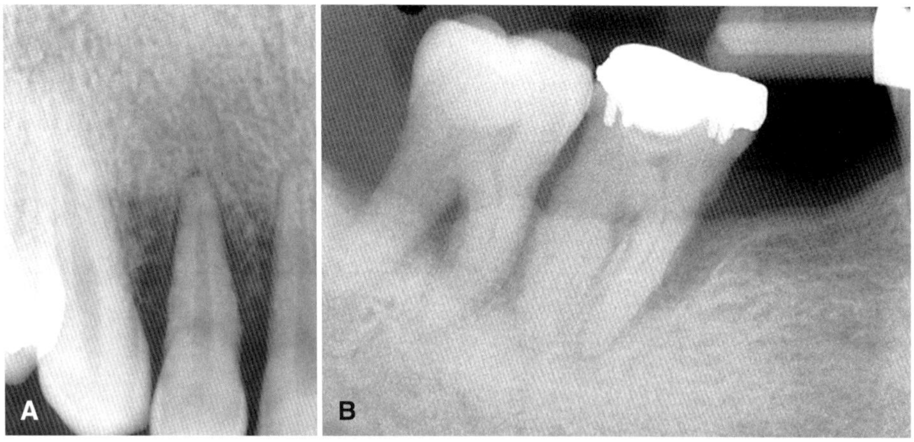

Fig. 18.16 (A) Example of a primarily radiolucent reaction around this maxillary lateral incisor. The trabeculae toward the alveolar crest on the mesial and distal aspect of the tooth are barely perceptible, and the marrow spaces are enlarged. (B) Periapical image revealing a predominantly sclerotic bone reaction resulting from periodontal disease involving the mandibular molars. The trabeculae are thickened, and the marrow spaces are barely perceptible.

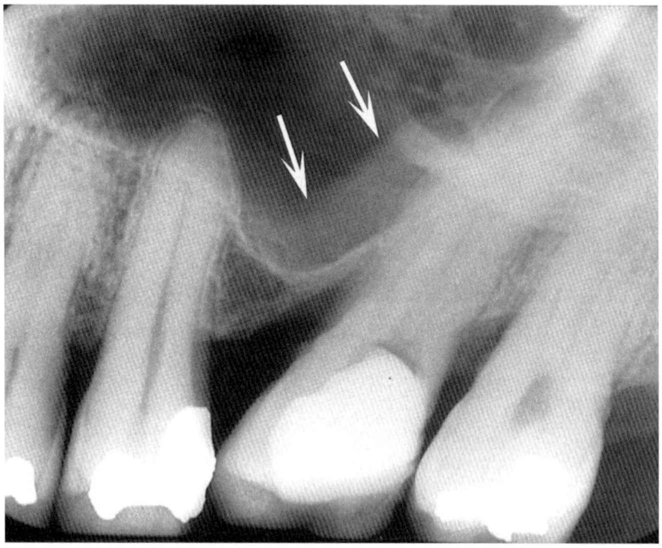

Fig. 18.17 Periapical image revealing a localized mucositis within the maxillary sinus *(arrows)* immediately adjacent to a vertical periodontal defect.

BOX 18.2 Periodontal Disease Classification

1. Periodontal health, gingival diseases and conditions
   a. Periodontal health and gingival health
   b. Gingivitis: dental biofilm induced
   c. Gingival diseases: nondental biofilm induced
2. Periodontitis
   a. Necrotizing periodontal diseases
      i. Necrotizing gingivitis
      ii. Necrotizing periodontitis
      iii. Necrotizing stomatitis
   b. Periodontitis
      i. Stages
         - Stage I: Initial periodontitis
         - Stage II: Moderate periodontitis
         - Stage III: Severe periodontitis with potential for additional tooth loss
         - Stage IV: Severe periodontitis with potential for loss of the dentition
      ii. Extent and distribution: localized; generalized; molar–incisor distribution
      iii. Grades: Evidence or risk of rapid progression, anticipated treatment response
         - Grade A: Slow rate of progression
         - Grade B: Moderate rate of progression
         - Grade C: Rapid rate of progression
   c. Periodontitis as a manifestation of systemic disease
3. Other conditions affecting the periodontium
   a. Systemic diseases or conditions affecting the periodontal support system
   b. Periodontal abscesses and endodontic-periodontic lesions
   c. Mucogingival deformities and conditions
   d. Traumatic occlusal forces
   e. Tooth and prosthesis-related factors

Modified from Canton JG, Armitage G, Berglundh T, et al. A new classification scheme for periodontal and peri-implant diseases and conditions—introduction and key changes from the 1999 classification. *J Periodontol.* 2018;89(1):S1-S8.

considered if there is a history of premature loss of deciduous teeth, and the permanent teeth are rapidly lost soon after eruption. This syndrome is usually seen with an associated hyperkeratosis of palmar and plantar surfaces.

OTHER CONDITIONS AFFECTING THE PERIODONTIUM

Periodontal Abscess

A periodontal abscess is a rapidly progressing, destructive lesion that usually originates in a deep soft tissue periodontal pocket. It occurs when the coronal portion of the pocket becomes occluded or when foreign material becomes lodged between a tooth and the gingiva. Clinically, pain and swelling, and sometimes a draining fistula, are present. If the lesion is acute, there may be no visible changes in the image. If the lesion persists, a radiolucent region appears, often superimposed over the tooth root. The radiolucency may be a focal, round area of rarefaction, with loss of the lamina dura on the involved root surface. As well, a bridge of bone may be visible over the coronal aspect of the lesion, separating it from the crest of the alveolar ridge (Fig. 18.18). After treatment, some of the lost bone may regenerate.

TABLE 18.1 **Periodontitis Classification**

Periodontitis Stage		I	II	III	IV
Severity	Radiographic bone loss	Coronal third of root (<15%)	Coronal third of root (15%–33%)	Extending to the middle third of root and beyond	Extending to the middle third of root and beyond
Complexity	Local	Maximum probing depth ≤4 mm that is mostly horizontal bone loss	Maximum probing depth ≤5 mm that is mostly horizontal bone loss	Stage II complexity and probing depth ≥6 mm; vertical bone loss ≥3 mm; Class II or III furcation; moderate ridge defect	Stage III complexity and severe ridge defect and <20 remaining teeth (10 opposing pairs)

Modified from Papapanou PN, Sanz M Buduneli N, et al. Periodontitis: consensus report of workgroup 2 of the 2017 World Workshop on the Classification of Periodontal and Peri-Implant Diseases and Conditions. *J Periodontol.* 2018;89(1):S173-S182.

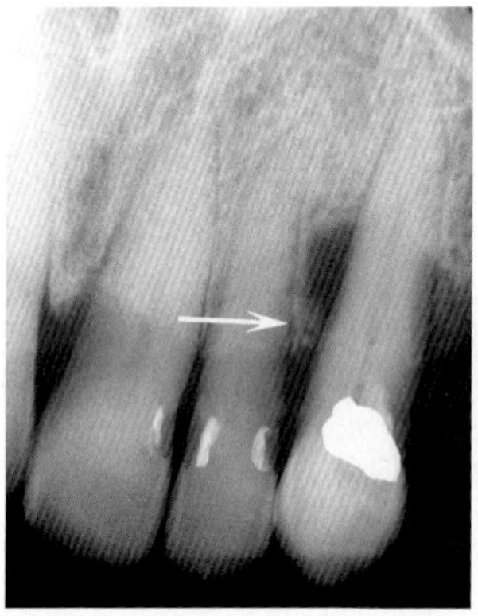

Fig. 18.18 Example of a periodontal abscess related to the maxillary canine. Note the well-defined area of bone loss over the midroot region of the tooth and extending in a mesial direction toward the lateral incisor. There appears to be a layer of bone *(arrow)* separating the area of bone destruction from the crest of the alveolar process.

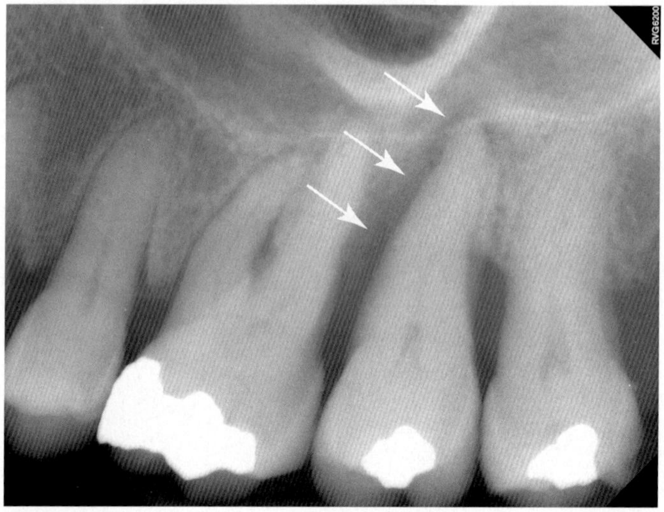

Fig. 18.19 Combined endodontic-periodontic lesion. There is an angular bone defect extending the whole length of the mesial surface of the second molar, from the crest to the apex *(arrows)*.

Endodontic-Periodontic Lesions

Inflammatory lesions from either a periodontal or pulpal origin may develop independently and merge with one another, or one lesion may induce the other. A periodontal lesion may extend to the apex of a tooth root causing secondary pulpitis, or periapical inflammatory disease may extend coronally to the bone crest causing a retrograde periodontitis. A combined periodontic-endodontic lesion appears as a deep angular bone defect on imaging, extending to the apex of a tooth and communicating with a focus of periapical rarefying osteitis (Fig. 18.19). The bone defect usually has a relatively uniform width or widens slightly at the alveolar crest, creating a funnel-like shape. Periodontic-endodontic lesions may affect one or multiple surfaces of the tooth, or they may be circumferential around the entire root. Treatment of these defects is complicated and involves both endodontic and periodontal therapy.

Occlusal Trauma

Traumatic occlusion causes degenerative changes in bone, when occlusal forces are greater than the physiologic tolerances of the tooth's supporting tissues. These degenerative changes can occur because of maladaptation to excessive occlusal forces or from normal occlusal forces on a periodontium already compromised by bone loss. In addition to clinical signs and symptoms such as increased mobility, wear facets, unusual response to percussion, and a history of contributing habits, imaging findings, such widening of the PDL space, thickening of the lamina dura, bone loss, and an increase in the number and size of trabeculae can also be seen. Other sequelae of traumatic occlusion may include hypercementosis and root fractures. Traumatic occlusion alone does not cause gingivitis or periodontitis, affect the epithelial attachment, or lead to pocket formation. However, in the presence of preexisting periodontitis, bone loss may be accelerated. Traumatic occlusion can be definitively diagnosed only by clinical evaluation and not by the imaging findings alone.

Tooth Mobility

Widening of the PDL space suggests tooth mobility, which may result from occlusal trauma or a lack of bone support arising from advanced bone loss. If the affected tooth has a single root, the socket may develop an hourglass shape. If the tooth is multirooted, it may show widening of the PDL space at the apices and in the region of the furcation. These changes can develop when the tooth moves about an axis of rotation at some point within the middle third of the root. In addition, the image of the lamina dura may appear broad and ill defined, and show increased density.

Open Contacts

When the mesial and distal surfaces of adjacent teeth are not in contact, the patient has an open contact. Open contacts are associated with sites of periodontal disease more than closed contacts. An open contact may damage the periodontium because of the potential for food impaction. Trapped food particles may damage the soft tissue and induce an inflammatory response, and

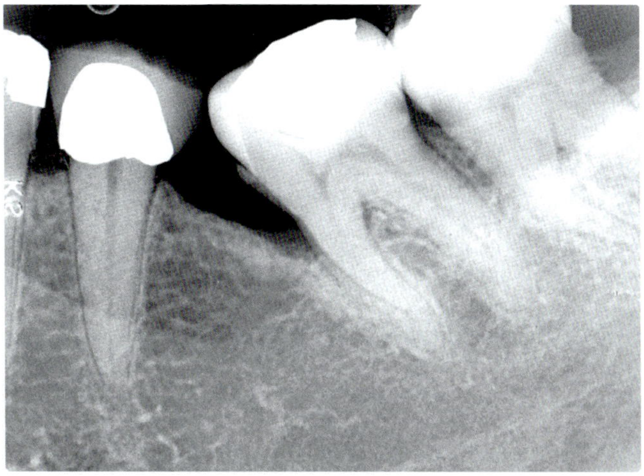

Fig. 18.20 The mandibular left second molar has tipped mesially after loss of the first molar, creating an abnormal tooth alignment that was difficult for the patient to maintain, leading to localized bone loss. Note the calculus on the mesial surface of the second molar. The crown on the second premolar was constructed with an enlarged distal contour to stop further tipping of the molar.

contribute to the development of localized bone loss. Similar potential situations in which periodontal disease may develop are discrepancies in the height of two adjacent marginal ridges or tipped teeth (Fig. 18.20). While abnormal tooth alignment does not cause periodontal disease, it can create an environment where disease may develop because of difficulties associated with maintaining good oral hygiene.

Local Irritating Factors

Other local factors may create an environment where periodontal disease may develop or aggravate existing periodontal disease. For example, deposits of calculus (Fig. 18.21) can prevent effective cleansing of a sulcus and lead to enhanced plaque formation and the progression of periodontal disease. Calculus is most commonly seen in association with the mandibular incisors but may be localized to any surface or generalized throughout the dentition. Similarly, defective

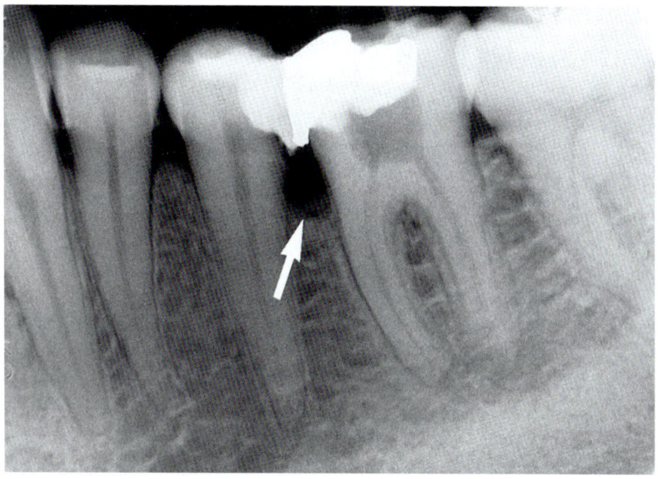

Fig. 18.22 These overhanging restorations provided an environment suitable for plaque accumulation and subsequent localized bone loss *(arrow)*.

restorations with poor contours and overhanging margins can accumulate plaque owing to the difficulty of adequately cleaning around them (Fig. 18.22). Other local tooth-related factors may include enamel pearls and cervical enamel projections, which are aberrant enamel formations commonly found in the furcation regions of multirooted teeth. These anomalies alter the periodontal attachment to the tooth and create sites prone to biofilm accumulation and periodontal breakdown.

EVALUATION OF PERIODONTAL THERAPY

Occasionally, signs of successful treatment of periodontal disease are visible in post-treatment images. Reestablishment of the interproximal crestal cortex (Fig. 18.23) and the sharp line angle between the cortex and lamina dura are good indicators of stabilization of the disease; however, these signs are not universally seen. The relatively radiolucent margins of bone that were undergoing active resorption before treatment may become more sclerotic (radiopaque) after successful therapy. In some cases, there may have been considerable

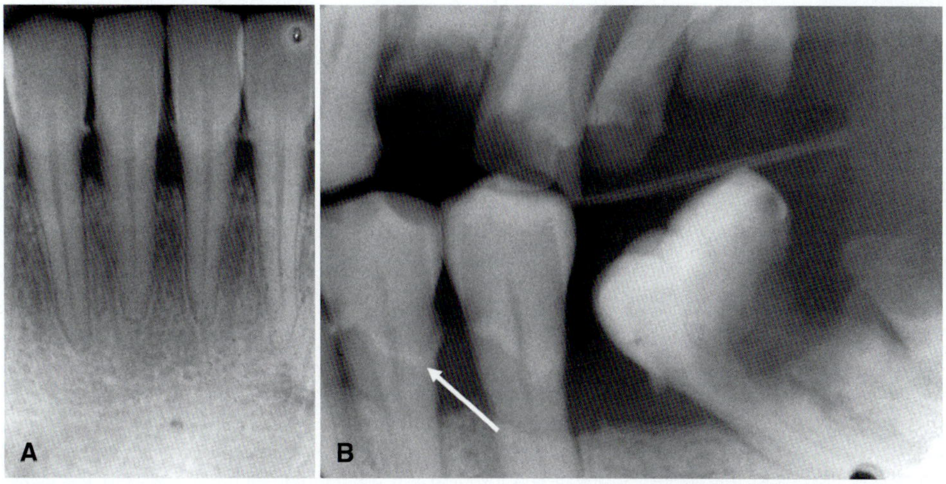

Fig. 18.21 Calculus may be seen as small angular radiopaque deposits projecting between interproximal surfaces of the teeth (A) or as radiopaque bands across the roots representing circumferential accumulation *(arrow* in B).

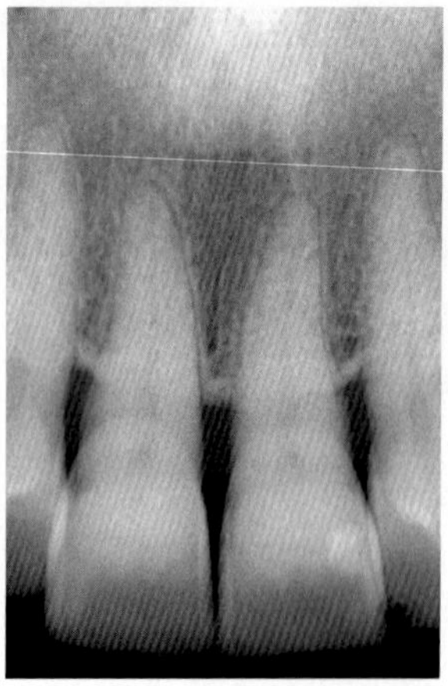

Fig. 18.23 Example of a case in which the interproximal cortex of the alveolar crest has reformed after successful periodontal therapy.

mineral loss of the cancellous bone (appearing more radiolucent), so that the bone is not visible in the image. Successful treatment may result in remineralization, causing the bone to become visible in the image. Clinicians must be conscious of the fact that x-ray beam angulation and exposure settings may affect the visibility of the alveolar crests. Sequential images made with different beam angulations or exposure settings may give the false impression that bone has regrown back into periodontal defects. Too high an x-ray exposure increases the density of the image (more black), and thin bone such as the alveolar crest may not be apparent, giving the false impression that the bone has been resorbed. Alternatively, underexposed (more light) images may give the false impression of bone growth. In many cases, there are no apparent changes in the images after successful treatment. As intraoral images do not disclose the therapeutic elimination of soft tissue periodontal pockets, healing is best assessed clinically.

DIFFERENTIAL INTERPRETATION

Most cases of bone loss around teeth are caused by the periodontal diseases. This fact can make the clinician less sensitive to other diseases with similar manifestations that should always be considered in the differential diagnosis. Occasionally, more serious diseases are missed or recognized late. The most likely clinical sign of disease other than periodontal disease is the presence of one or a few adjacent loose teeth when the rest of the mouth shows no signs of periodontal disease. Suspicion should be heightened if the bone destruction does not have the pattern or morphology normally associated with periodontal disease.

Periodontal disease originates in the gingival sulcus at the alveolar crest, and progresses along the periodontium, against the affected tooth. Thus, bone loss caused by periodontal disease, such as vertical defects, should appear larger at the coronal aspect and less severe at the leading edge apically. This appearance differs from other diseases, which may destroy the supporting bone in a more widespread or invasive pattern.

Malignant neoplasms—in particular, squamous cell carcinoma—involving the alveolar process may mimic the appearance of periodontal disease. And occasionally malignant neoplasia is treated as periodontal disease, resulting in a delay in diagnosis and treatment (Fig. 18.24A). This malignancy may display characteristics in the image that suggest its true nature, such as extensive bone destruction of a localized region beyond the periodontium, or invasive characteristics (see Chapter 24). Irregular widening of the PDL space along its entire length, with a poorly defined, ragged or irregular periphery, and destruction of the lamina dura are suggestive of infiltration by a malignancy rather than periodontal disease. In some cases, squamous cell carcinoma may mimic periodontal disease, and only the clinical characteristics of the lesion and the failure to respond to treatment indicate the presence of malignancy.

Any lesion resulting in bone destruction that has ill-defined borders and lacks a peripheral bone response (sclerosis) should be viewed with suspicion. Another disease to be considered is Langerhans cell histiocytosis (see Fig. 18.24C). Often this disease may manifest as one or more regions of bone destruction around the roots of teeth, similar to periodontal disease. The appearance of "teeth floating in space" may appear similar to periodontitis. In Langerhans cell histiocytosis, however, the epicenter of the bone destruction is at mid-root level rather than at the bone crest, which may give early lesions an "ice cream scoop" appearance, with the alveolar crest less resorbed or even intact (see Chapter 24).

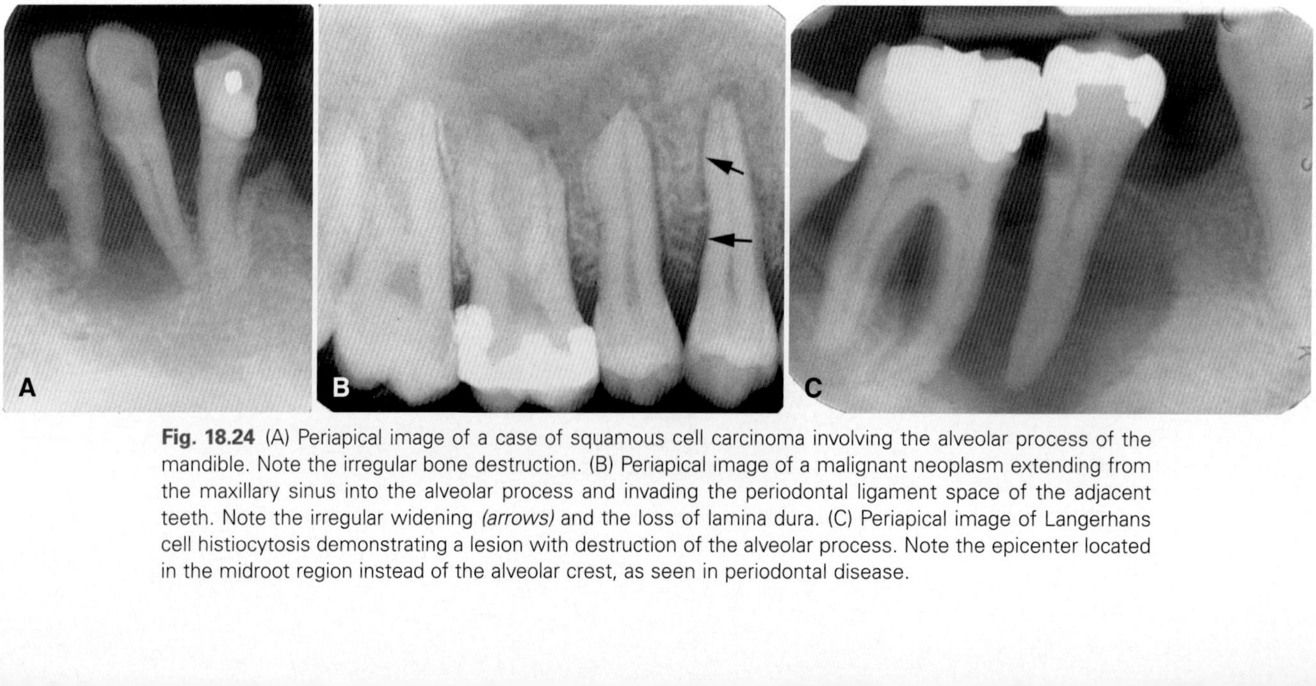

Fig. 18.24 (A) Periapical image of a case of squamous cell carcinoma involving the alveolar process of the mandible. Note the irregular bone destruction. (B) Periapical image of a malignant neoplasm extending from the maxillary sinus into the alveolar process and invading the periodontal ligament space of the adjacent teeth. Note the irregular widening *(arrows)* and the loss of lamina dura. (C) Periapical image of Langerhans cell histiocytosis demonstrating a lesion with destruction of the alveolar process. Note the epicenter located in the midroot region instead of the alveolar crest, as seen in periodontal disease.

BIBLIOGRAPHY

Classification

Canton JG, Armitage G, Berglundh T, et al. A new classification scheme for periodontal and peri-implant diseases and conditions—introduction and key changes from the 1999 classification. *J Periodontol.* 2018;89(suppl 1): S1-S8.

Papapanou PN, Sanz M, Buduneli N, et al. Periodontitis: consensus report of workgroup 2 of the 2017 World Workshop on the Classification of Periodontal and Peri-Implant Diseases and Conditions. *J Periodontol.* 2018; 89(1):S173-S182.

Kornman KS, Papapnou PN. Clinical application of the new classification of periodontal diseases: ground rules, clarifications and "gray zones". *J Periodontal.* 2020;91:352-360.

Clinical Characteristics of Periodontal Diseases

Herrera C, González I, Sanz M. The periodontal abscess (I): clinical and microbiological findings. *J Clin Periodontol.* 2000;27:387-394.

Newman MG, Takei HH, Klokkevold PR, et al. *Carranza's Clinical Periodontology.* Saunders; 2006.

Walsh TF, al-Kohail OS, Fosam EB. The relationship of bone loss observed on panoramic radiographs with clinical periodontal screening. *J Clin Periodontol.* 1997;24:153-157.

Epidemiology

Eke PI, Borgnakke WS, Genco RJ. Recent epidemiologic trends in periodontitis in the USA. *Periodontol 2000.* 2020;82(1):257-267.

Nazir M, Al-Ansari A, Al-Khalifa K, et al. Global prevalence of periodontal disease and lack of its surveillance. *ScientificWorldJournal.* 2020;2020: 2146160.

Papapanou PN. Periodontal diseases: epidemiology. *Ann Periodontol.* 1996; 1:1-36.

Position paper: epidemiology of periodontal diseases. American Academy of Periodontology. *J Periodontol.* 1996;67:935-945.

Etiology

Bimstein E, Garcia-Godoy F. The significance of age, proximal caries, gingival inflammation, probing depths, and the loss of lamina dura in the diagnosis of alveolar bone loss in the primary molars. *ASDC J Dent Child.* 1994;61: 125-128.

Page RC, Offenbacher S, Schroeder HE, et al. Advances in the pathogenesis of periodontitis: summary of developments, clinical implications and future directions. *Periodontol 2000.* 1997;14:216-248.

Salvi GE, Lawrence HP, Offenbacher S, et al. Influence of risk factors on the pathogenesis of periodontitis. *Periodontol 2000.* 1997;14:173.

Schwartz Z, Goultschin J, Dean DD, et al. Mechanisms of alveolar bone destruction in periodontitis. *Periodontol 2000.* 1997;14:158.

Van Dyke TE, Serhan CN. Resolution of inflammation: a new paradigm for the pathogenesis of periodontal diseases. *J Dent Res.* 2003;82:82-90.

Johnson GK, Guthmiller JM. The impact of cigarette smoking on periodontal disease and treatment. *Periodontol 2000.* 2007;44:178-194.

Radiographic Manifestations

Gutteridge DL. The use of radiographic techniques in the diagnosis and management of periodontal diseases. *Dentomaxillofac Radiol.* 1995;24:107-113.

Jeffcoat MK, Wang IC, Reddy MS. Radiographic diagnosis in periodontics. *Periodontol 2000.* 1995;7:54-68.

Khocht A, Zohn H, Deasy M, et al. Screening for periodontal disease: radiographs vs PSR. *J Am Dent Assoc.* 1996;127:749-756.

Koral SM, Howell TH, Jeffcoat MK. Alveolar bone loss due to open interproximal contacts in periodontal disease. *J Periodontol.* 1981;52:447-450.

Mann J, Pettigrew J, Beideman R, et al. Investigation of the relationship between clinically detected loss of attachment and radiographic changes in early periodontal disease. *J Clin Periodontol.* 1985;12:247-253.

Nielsen IM, Glavind L, Karring T. Interproximal periodontal intrabony defects: prevalence, localization, and etiological factors. *J Clin Periodontol.* 1980;7:187-198.

Rams TE, Listgarten MA, Slots J. Utility of radiographic crestal lamina dura for predicting periodontitis disease activity. *J Clin Periodontol.* 1994;21:571-576.

Waite IM, Furniss JS, Wong WM. Relationship between clinical periodontal condition and the radiological appearance at first molar sites in adolescents: a 3-year study. *J Clin Periodontol.* 1994;21:155-160.

Radiographic Technique

Scarfe WC, Azevedo B, Pinheiro LR, et al. The emerging role of maxillofacial radiology in the diagnosis and management of patients with complex periodontitis. *Periodontol 2000.* 2017;74:116-139.

Bragger I. Radiographic diagnosis of periodontal disease progression. *Curr Opin Periodontol.* 1996;3:59-67.

Gröndahl K, Gröndahl HG, Webber RL, et al. Influence of variations in projection geometry on the detectability of periodontal bone lesions: a comparison between subtraction radiography and conventional radiographic technique. *J Clin Periodontol.* 1984;11:411-420.

Pepelassi EA, Diamanti-Kipioti A. Selection of the most accurate method of conventional radiography for the assessment of periodontal osseous destruction. *J Clin Periodontol.* 1997;24:557-567.

Reed B, Polson A. Relationships between bitewing and periapical radiographs in assessing crestal alveolar bone levels. *J Periodontol.* 1984;55:22-27.

Zaki HA, Hoffmann KR, Hausmann E, et al. Is radiologic assessment of alveolar crest height useful to monitor periodontal disease activity? *Dent Clin North Am.* 2015;59:859-872.

Cone Beam Computed Tomographic Imaging

Mol A, Balasundaram A. In vitro cone beam computed tomography imaging of periodontal bone. *Dentomaxillofac Radiol.* 2008;37:319-324.

Vandenberghe B, Jacobs R, Yang J. Detection of periodontal bone loss using digital intraoral and cone beam computed tomography images: an in vitro assessment of bony and/or infrabony defects. *Dentomaxillofac Radiol.* 2008; 37:252-260.

Walter C, Weiger R, Zitzmann NU. Accuracy of three-dimensional imaging in assessing maxillary molar furcation involvement. *J Clin Periodontol.* 2010; 37:436-441.

Occlusal Trauma

Burgett FG. Trauma from occlusion: periodontal concerns. *Dent Clin North Am.* 1995;39:301-311.

Wank GS, Kroll YJ. Occlusal trauma: an evaluation of its relationship to periodontal prostheses. *Dent Clin North Am.* 1981;25:511-532.

Systemic Disease

Knight ET, Liu J, Seymour GJ, et al. Risk factors that may modify the innate and adaptive immune responses in periodontal diseases. *Periodontol 2000.* 2016;71:22-51.

Emrich LJ, Shlossman M, Genco RJ. Periodontal disease in non-insulin-dependent diabetes mellitus. *J Periodontol.* 1991;62:123-131.

Epstein JB, Lunn R, Le N, et al. Periodontal attachment loss in patients after head and neck radiation therapy. *Oral Surg Oral Med Oral Pathol Oral Radiol Endod.* 1998;86:673-677.

Farzim I, Edalat M. Periodontosis with hyperkeratosis palmaris and plantaris (the Papillon-Lefèvre syndrome): a case report. *J Periodontol.* 1974;45:316-318.

Nelson RG, Schlossman M, Budding LM, et al. Periodontal diseases and NIDDM in Pima Indians. *Diabetes Care.* 1990;13:836-840.

Rateitschak-Plüss EM, Schroeder HE. History of periodontitis in a child with Papillon-Lefèvre syndrome: a case report. *J Periodontol.* 1984;55:35-46.

Winkler JR, Grassi M, Murray PA. Clinical description and etiology of HIV-associated periodontal disease. In: Robinson PB, Greenspan JS, eds. *Prospectus on Oral Manifestations of AIDS.* PSG Publishing; 1988.

19

Dental Anomalies

Erika Benavides

Dental anomalies can develop in a variety of ways, and are broadly classified as being congenital, developmental, or acquired. Congenital abnormalities are typically genetically inherited, and developmental anomalies occur during the formation of a tooth or teeth. These anomalies may include variations in the normal number, size, morphology, or eruptive pattern of the teeth. Acquired abnormalities result from changes to teeth after normal formation. Teeth that form abnormally short roots may represent congenital or developmental anomalies, whereas the shortening of normal tooth roots by external resorption represents an acquired change.

DEVELOPMENTAL ABNORMALITIES

Number of Teeth

Supernumerary Teeth

Disease mechanism. Teeth that develop in addition to the normal complement as a result of excess dental lamina in the jaws are referred to as supernumerary or supplemental teeth, or parateeth. These additional teeth may be morphologically normal or abnormal. When supernumerary teeth have normal morphologic features, the term supplemental is sometimes also used. Supernumerary teeth that occur in the anterior maxilla are termed mesiodens. Those that occur in the premolar area are termed peridens, and those that occur in the molar area are termed distodens or, sometimes, paramolars. Recent studies in animals have suggested a genetic etiology to the development of supernumerary teeth—specifically, the roles signaling molecules such as bone morphogenetic protein (BMP) and fibroblast growth factor (FGF), and signaling pathways, that include the wingless-related (Wnt) and sonic hedgehog (SHH) pathways. The exact mechanisms through which these molecules act (e.g., up- or downregulation of pathways), however, still remain unclear.

Clinical features. Supernumerary teeth occur in 0.2%–3% of the population, and are easily identified by counting and recording all the teeth in the jaws. Supernumerary teeth may have a greater incidence in Asian and Indigenous populations, and occur twice as often in males. Although supernumerary teeth can arise in either the deciduous or the permanent dentitions, they are more common in the permanent dentition and can arise anywhere in the jaws.

Single supernumerary teeth are most common in the anterior maxilla, where they are referred to as mesiodens (Figs. 19.1 and 19.2), and in the maxillary molar region. Multiple supernumerary teeth occur most frequently in the premolar and molar regions (Figs. 19.3–19.5), usually in the mandible. In the mandible, supernumerary teeth are often positioned in the lingual aspect of the alveolar process (Fig. 19.6).

Supernumerary teeth are usually discovered on images because they interfere with normal tooth eruption (Fig. 19.7). When a supernumerary tooth does erupt, it commonly erupts outside the normal arch form because of space restrictions. Complications associated with supernumerary teeth include dental impaction, delayed eruption, ectopic eruption, overcrowding, spacing anomalies, and the formation of dentigerous cysts.

Imaging features. The imaging features of supernumerary teeth are variable. They may appear entirely normal in both size and shape, but they may also be smaller in size compared with the adjacent normal dentition or have a conical shape with the appearance of a canine tooth. In extreme cases, the supernumerary teeth may appear grossly deformed.

Images may reveal supernumerary teeth in the deciduous dentition (Fig. 19.8) after 3 or 4 years of age when the deciduous teeth have formed, or in the permanent dentitions of children between 9 and 12 years of age. Although supernumerary teeth may be identified initially in periapical, panoramic, or occlusal images, cone beam computed tomography (CBCT) may aid in determining a more precise location, reveal the number of unerupted supernumerary teeth present, associated pathosis, and any effects they may be causing on adjacent teeth and anatomical structures. In particular, care should be taken when reviewing panoramic images for supernumerary teeth, as these may be obscured in the anterior maxilla by the image of the cervical spine, or they may appear distorted if they lie outside the focal trough.

Differential interpretation. Multiple supernumerary teeth have been associated with genetic syndromes, including cleidocranial dysplasia (see Chapter 27) and familial adenomatous polyposis (Gardner syndrome) (see Chapter 22), as well as less common and more rare conditions such as trichorhinophalangeal syndrome type I, Rubinstein–Taybi syndrome, Nance–Horan syndrome, Opitz G/BBB syndrome, oculofaciocardiodental syndrome, and Robinow syndrome (autosomal dominant).

Management. The management of supernumerary teeth depends on many factors, including their potential effects on the developing normal dentition, their position and number, and the potential complications (detected clinically or radiographically) that may result from surgical intervention. No clear consensus exists as to the best time to extract unerupted supernumerary teeth. If supernumerary teeth erupt, they can cause malalignment of the normal dentition. Supernumerary teeth that remain in the jaws may cause root resorption of adjacent teeth and their follicles, may develop dentigerous cysts, or may interfere with the normal eruption sequence. All the preceding factors influence the decision to either remove a supernumerary tooth or keep it under observation. If supernumerary teeth are related to a genetic syndrome, an interdisciplinary management and treatment approach should be considered including family genetic counseling.

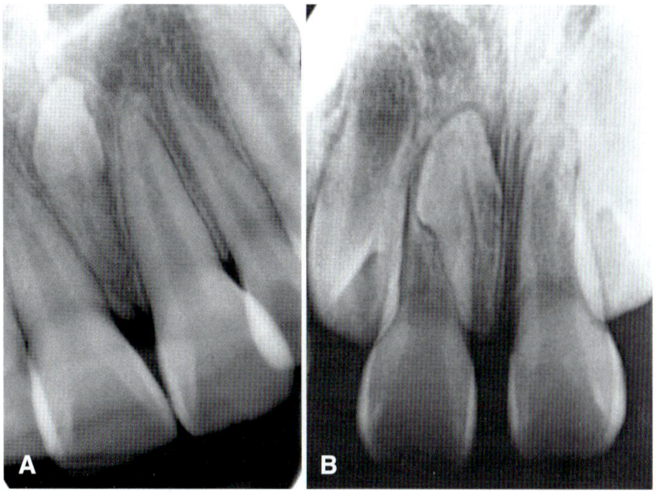

Fig. 19.1 Periapical images (A and B) of inverted mesiodens.

Missing Teeth

Disease mechanism. While it may be common for missing permanent teeth to be referred to as being congenitally absent, we have chosen to use the phrase "developmentally absent" since the permanent dentition does not develop until after birth.

Hypodontia, or tooth agenesis, is the most prevalent craniofacial malformation in humans, and refers to missing teeth other than the third molars. Oligodontia is the term used to describe the absence of more than six teeth, whereas anodontia refers to the absence of the entire dentition. Hypodontia may occur as part of a recognized genetic syndrome or as a nonsyndromic-isolated trait. Both environmental and genetic factors are involved in the etiology of hypodontia, with the latter playing a more significant role. So far, molecular genetics has revealed the genetic etiologies of only rare forms of tooth agenesis. Mutations have been identified in a diverse array of genes (e.g., *MSX1*, *PAX9*, *AXIN2*, and *EDA*) in familial severe agenesis (oligodontia), and in many other genes that have been identified in syndromes in which tooth agenesis is a regular feature. Developmentally missing teeth may

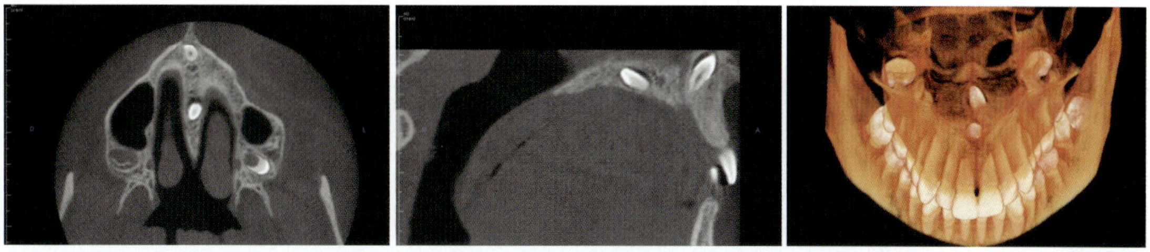

Fig. 19.2 Axial and sagittal cone beam computed tomographic image reconstructions showing two supernumerary teeth in the anterior maxilla and hard palate along the intermaxillary suture.

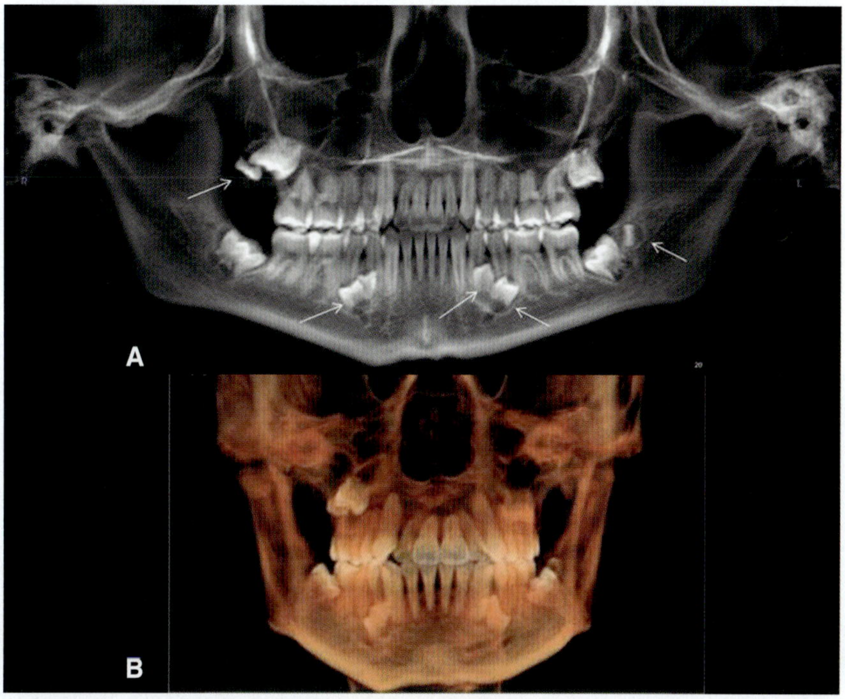

Fig. 19.3 Panoramic (A) and three-dimensional (B) reconstructions of a cone beam computed tomographic image volume showing multiple supernumerary teeth in the right maxilla and mandible *(arrows)*.

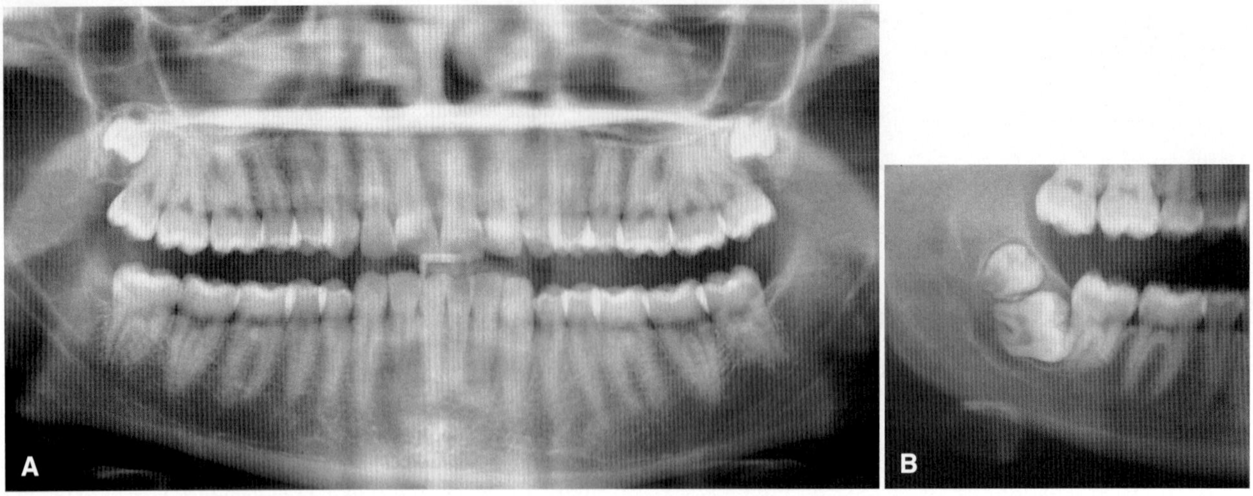

Fig. 19.4 Panoramic and cropped panoramic images of supernumerary teeth in the maxillary third molar regions (distodens) (A) and mandibular third molar region (B). (A, Courtesy Dr. H. Grubisa, Oakville, ON.)

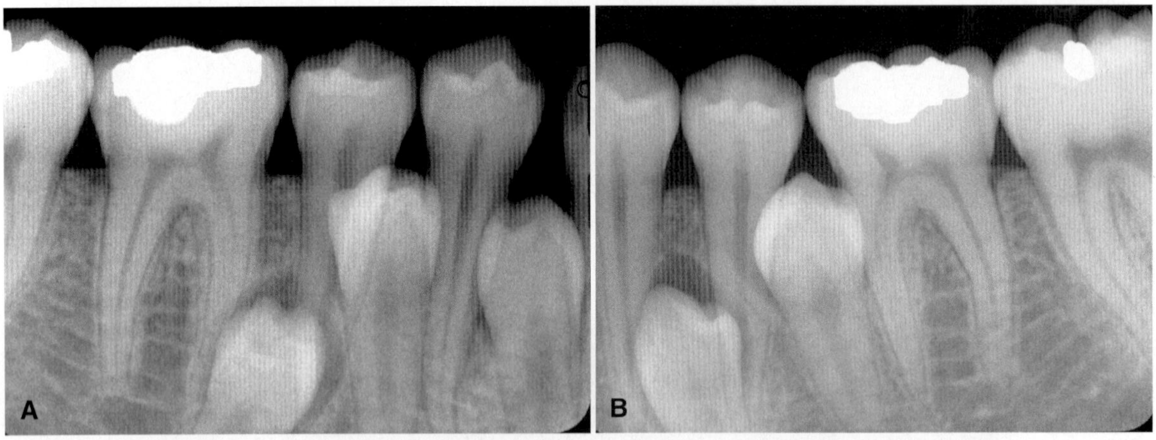

Fig. 19.5 Periapical images (A and B) show bilateral supernumerary premolar teeth (peridens).

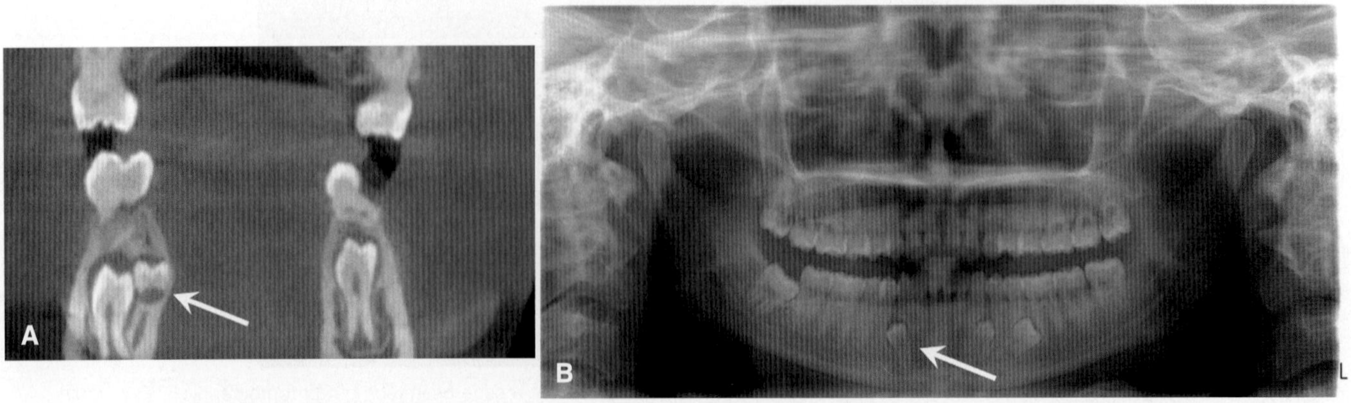

Fig. 19.6 Coronal cone beam computed tomographic (A) and panoramic (B) images of a peridens developing in the mandibular right premolar area in the lingual aspect of the body *(arrows).*

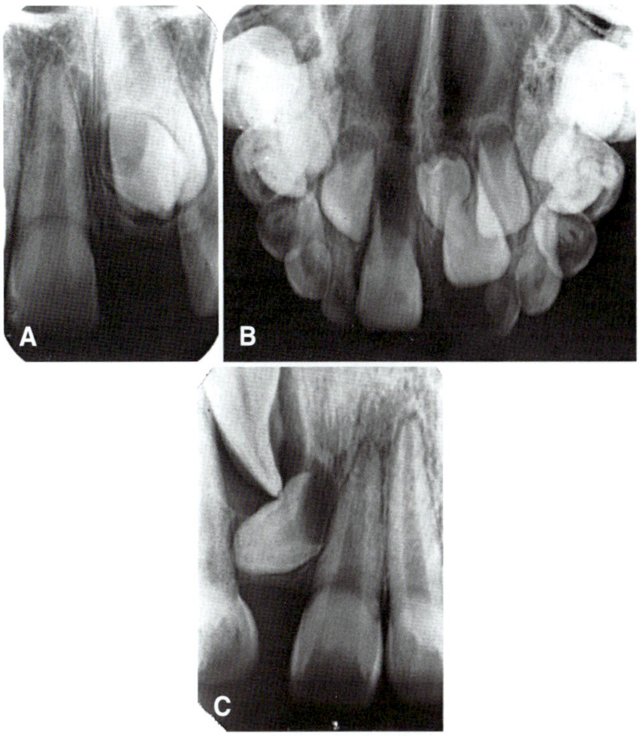

Fig. 19.7 Mesiodens (A–C) interfering with eruption of adjacent permanent teeth.

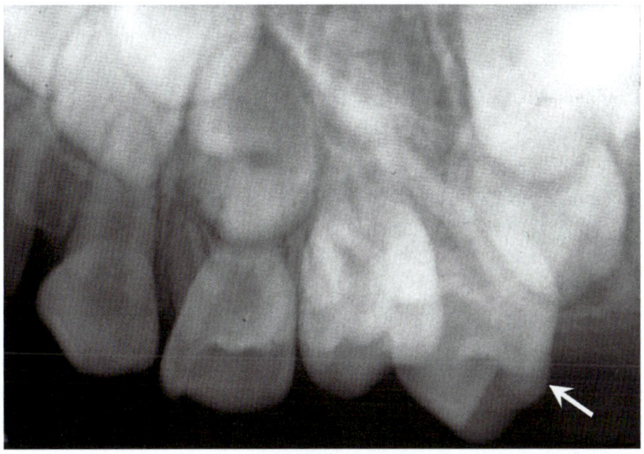

Fig. 19.8 Supernumerary deciduous molar *(arrow)*.

also be the result of numerous independent pathologic mechanisms that can affect the orderly formation of the dental lamina (e.g., orofaciodigital syndrome), failure of a tooth germ to develop at the optimal time, lack of necessary space imposed by a malformed jaw, or disproportion between tooth mass and jaw size.

Clinical features. The prevalence of hypodontia in the permanent dentition has increased in the last few decades, and ranges from 1.6% to 36.5% depending on the population studied with Asian and Indigenous populations being more commonly affected. Although missing primary teeth are relatively uncommon, when one deciduous tooth is missing, it is usually a maxillary incisor. The most commonly missing teeth are third molars, followed by mandibular second premolars and maxillary lateral and mandibular central incisors. The absence may be either unilateral (more common for mandibular second premolars) or bilateral (more common for lateral incisors). Children who have

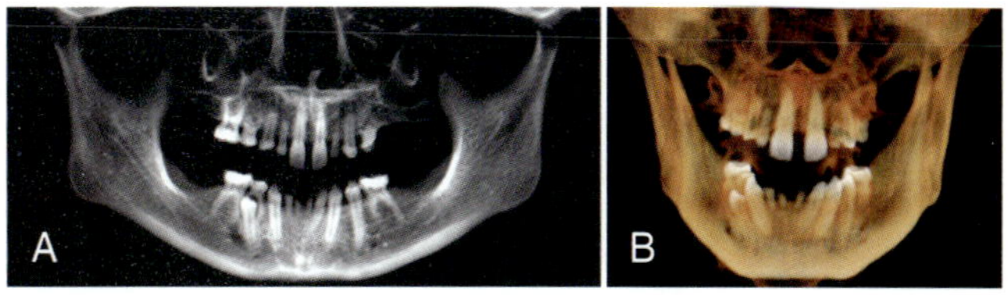

Fig. 19.9 Panoramic (A) and three-dimensional (B) cone beam computed tomographic image reconstructions of a patient with multiple missing teeth and oligodontia.

developmentally missing teeth tend to have more than one absent and more than one morphologic group (incisors, premolars, and molars) involved (Fig. 19.9).

Tooth agenesis is often nonsyndromic, but it can also be associated with cleft lip and/or palate (CLP), Down syndrome, and ectodermal dysplasia. In these conditions, there is a characteristic pattern of agenesis that is usually different from the overall population.

Hypodontia patients tend to present with lower mandibular plane angles and be associated with a smaller lower anterior face height and lip protrusion. Other features may also include smaller maxillary and mandibular arch length and a Class III skeletal relationship tendency, microdontia, ectopic positioning of the permanent teeth, transposition of teeth, enamel hypoplasia, diminutive or peg-shaped maxillary lateral incisors, primary molar infra-occlusion, and palatally inclined or impacted maxillary canines.

Imaging features. The development of teeth may vary markedly among individuals. Missing teeth may be recognized by identifying and counting the teeth present. For some individuals, the eruption of some teeth may be delayed by a number of years after the normally established eruption time (especially mandibular second premolars), whereas others may erupt up to 1 year after the contralateral tooth. Tooth agenesis, especially in its most severe forms, contributes to abnormal occlusion and is often associated with a variety of anomalies in other teeth. These include delays in development, ectopic eruption, reduction in tooth dimensions and morphology, shortened roots, taurodontia, and enamel hypoplasia.

Differential interpretation. A tooth may be considered to be developmentally absent when it cannot be identified clinically or through imaging, and no history exists of its extraction. Oligodontia or anodontia may occur in patients with several conditions that may include CLP, ectodermal dysplasia (Fig. 19.10), trisomy 21, Rieger syndrome, and Book syndrome.

The ectodermal dysplasias are a genetically diverse group of abnormalities that include 186 distinct diseases that involve 64 gene mutations. In addition to missing teeth, phenotypically, these individuals may also lack sweat glands; have thin, fine hair; thin, delicate skin; and malformed nails. When the teeth are involved, the condition may manifest with multiple missing or malformed teeth that often have a conical or canine shape, or a notable decrease in tooth size. The ectodermal dysplasias have been subdivided into two groups. Group A ectodermal dysplasia includes entities with abnormalities involving two or more of the classically involved structures previously mentioned, and group B includes abnormalities of one of these structures, and another abnormality of ectodermal origin that may include the mammary glands, thyroid gland, thymus, anterior pituitary gland, cornea, conjunctiva, lacrimal gland, lacrimal duct, or Meibomian glands.

Management. Missing teeth, abnormal occlusion, or altered facial appearance may cause some patients psychological distress. If the extent of hypodontia is mild, the associated changes may be slight and can be managed by orthodontic intervention. In more severe cases, restorative, implant, and prosthetic procedures may be considered.

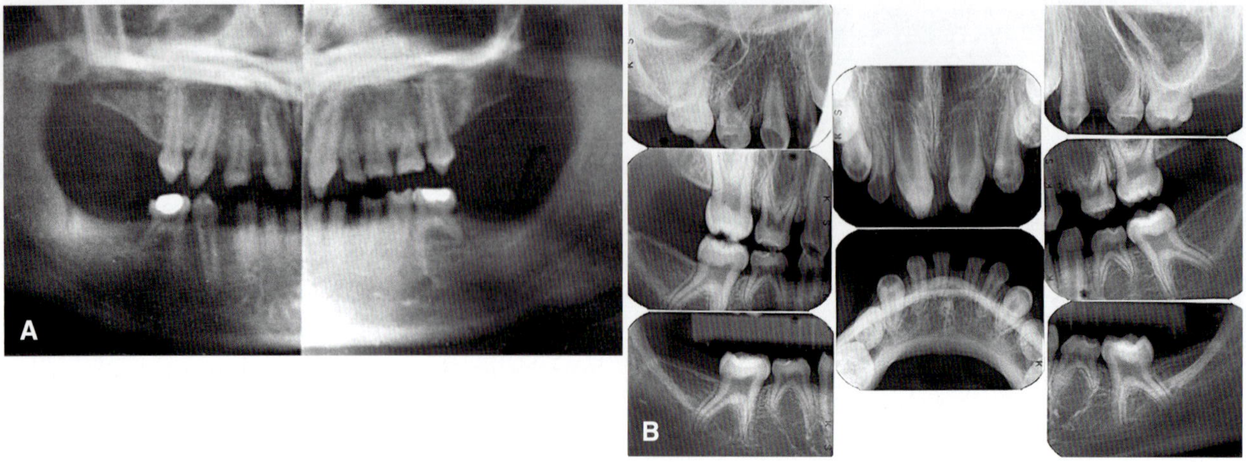

Fig. 19.10 Panoramic (A) and intraoral images (B) of a patient with multiple missing and malformed teeth in ectodermal dysplasia.

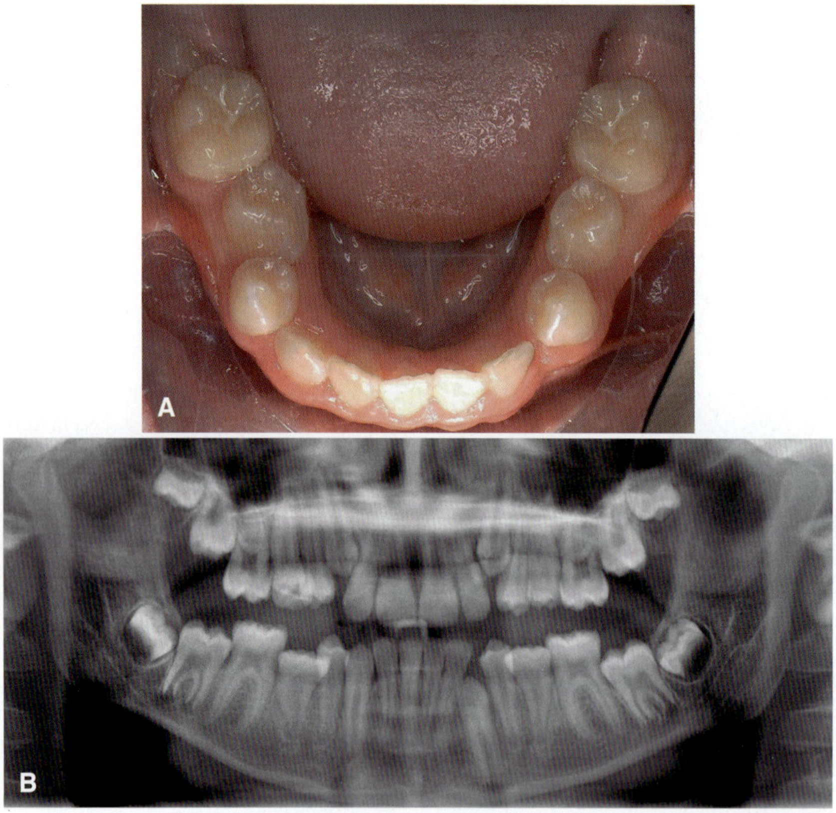

Fig. 19.11 Clinical photograph (A) and panoramic image (B) of mandibular second premolar macrodontia. Note the greater mesial/distal widths of the tooth crowns compared with their respective first premolars. (Courtesy Dr. H. Grubisa, Oakville, ON.)

Size of Teeth

A positive correlation exists between tooth size (mesiodistal or buccolingual dimension) and body height. Males also have larger primary and permanent teeth than females. Beyond these normal variations, individuals may occasionally have unusually large or small teeth.

Macrodontia

Disease mechanism. Macrodontia is a dental condition where a tooth or group of teeth are abnormally larger than average; however, macrodontia rarely affects the entire dentition. A tooth greater than two standard deviations in size from the mean size for that specific tooth is considered a macrodont in the literature. Often a single tooth, individual contralateral teeth, or a group of teeth may be involved (Fig. 19.11). Macrodontia may occur sporadically, and its cause is unknown. Vascular abnormalities such as a hemangioma (arising from within the bone or the adjacent soft tissues) can result in an increase in the size and accelerate the development of adjacent teeth. Macrodontia can also occur in hemihypertrophy of the face or in gigantism.

Clinical features. Macrodontia is thought to affect between 0.03% and 1.9% of the world population. Macrodontia is reported to have a higher incidence among men compared to women, is more frequently found in the permanent dentition than the primary dentition, and is more common in the maxilla than the mandible. Macrodontia of premolar and molar teeth is extremely rare and occurs more frequently in incisors and canines. Clinically, macrodont teeth appear large and may be associated with crowding, malocclusion, or impaction.

Imaging features. Imaging reveals the increased size of both unerupted and erupted macrodont teeth. The shape of the tooth is usually normal, but some cases may exhibit mildly distorted morphology. Crowding may cause impaction of adjacent teeth. Periapical or panoramic imaging is most commonly used to identify this condition.

Differential interpretation. Macrodontia can clinically be mistaken for other dental anomalies such as fusion—wherein two tooth germs fuse to form one tooth—or gemination—in which a single tooth germ incompletely divides to form a single tooth with a bifid crown. Concrescence refers to the union of juxtaposed teeth by cementum only. Teeth which exhibit fusion or gemination are also referred to as double teeth, double formations, joined teeth, or dental twinning. Some authors may refer to fusion as "syndontia" and to gemination as "schizodontia." When fusion occurs, a count of the teeth present reveals a missing tooth, whereas in gemination the count reveals a normal number. In gemination, however, evidence often exists of a division or cleft of the crown or root of the tooth.

Management. The differentiation between fusion, gemination, and concrescence may not influence the management, and in most cases, macrodontia does not require treatment. Orthodontic treatment may be necessary if a malocclusion is present.

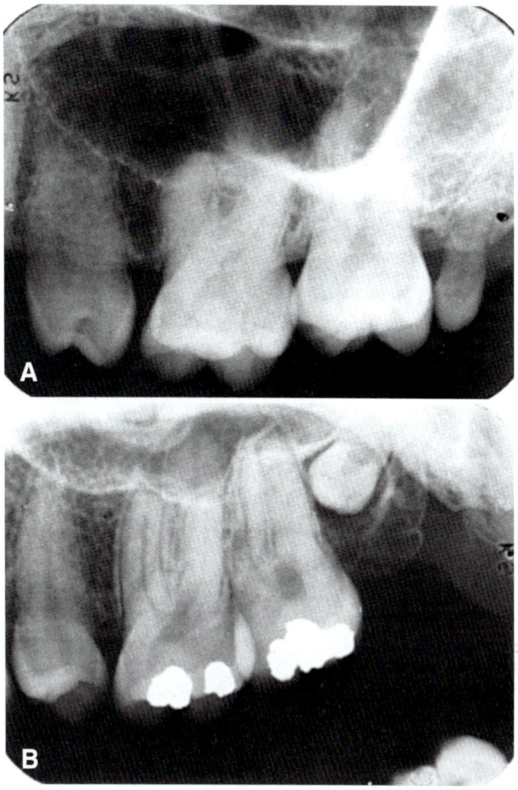

Fig. 19.12 Periapical images (A and B) show microdont maxillary third molars.

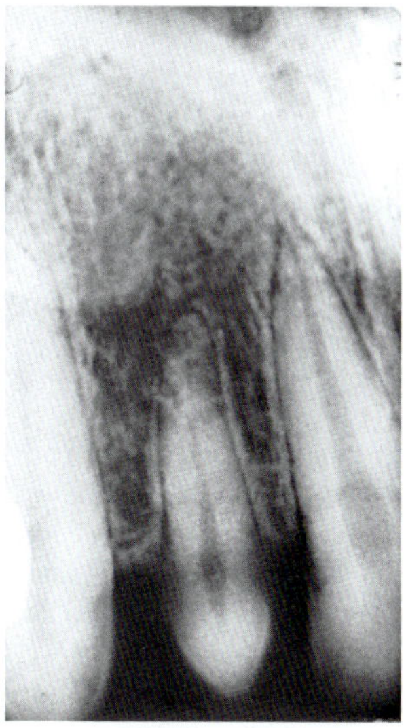

Fig. 19.13 Peg shape of a microdont maxillary lateral incisor.

Microdontia

Disease mechanism. Microdontia is a dental anomaly in which teeth are abnormally small. As with macrodontia, microdontia may involve all the teeth or be limited to a single tooth or group of teeth. Often the lateral incisors and third molars may be small. Generalized microdontia is extremely rare, although it can occur in some patients with pituitary dwarfism or as nonsyndromically. Supernumerary teeth may also be microdont teeth. Other dental anomalies such as hypodontia may also be associated with microdontia. These alterations in size may be linked to genetic factors and in particular syndromes such as pituitary dwarfism and Rieger syndrome. Microdontia can also be the result of exposure to environmental factors during dental development such as radiotherapy, chemotherapy, or persistent organic pollutants.

Clinical features. The affected teeth are noticeably small and may have an altered morphology. Microdont molars may have an altered shape. For example, mandibular molars may have four cusps rather than five, and maxillary molars may have four cusps rather than three (Fig. 19.12). Microdont lateral incisors may be peg shaped (Fig. 19.13).

Imaging features. These small teeth are frequently malformed.

Differential interpretation. The recognition of small teeth indicates the diagnosis. The number and distribution of microdont teeth may also suggest consideration of associated abnormalities (e.g., congenital heart disease, progeria).

Management. Restorative or prosthetic treatment may be considered to create a more normal-appearing tooth, especially when considering esthetic concerns in the anterior dentition.

Eruption of Teeth

Transposition

Disease mechanism. Transposition is an uncommon dental anomaly involving positional interchange of two typically adjacent teeth in the dental arch. There is strong evidence that maxillary canine—first premolar transposition, which is the most common type, is a disturbance of tooth order and eruptive position resulting from genetic influences within a multifactorial inheritance model. This transposition occurs bilaterally in approximately 25% of the cases and favors female expression (sex ratio, M:F of 1:3.8) and left-side occurrence (61% of unilateral cases). Familial occurrence has been noted with a predilection for the Caucasian population. Tooth agenesis (excluding third molars) and/or peg-shaped maxillary lateral incisors accompanies maxillary canine–first premolar transposition in 49% of the subjects, which is 4–10 times the normal rate of occurrence.

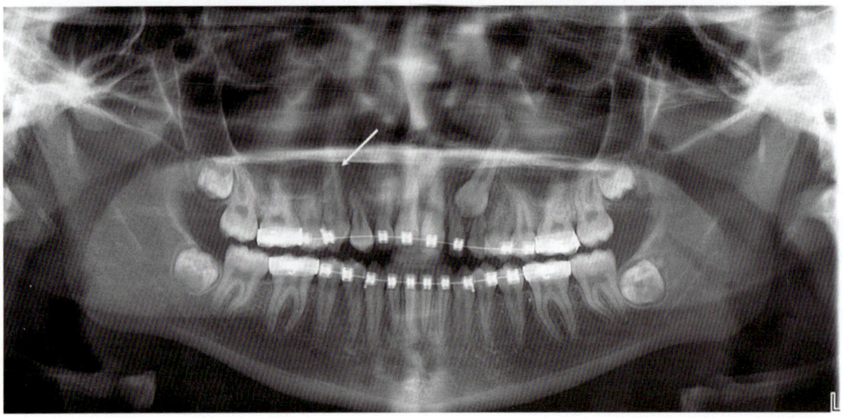

Fig. 19.14 Panoramic image demonstrating transposition of the right maxillary canine *(arrow)* and first premolar.

Clinical features. The most frequently transposed teeth are the permanent canine and the first premolar. Second premolars infrequently lie between the first and second molars. The transposition of central and lateral incisors is rare. Transposition can occur with hypodontia, supernumerary teeth, or the persistence of a deciduous predecessor. Transposition in the primary dentition has not been reported.

Imaging features. Images reveal transposition when the teeth are not in their usual positions in the dental arch (Fig. 19.14). Panoramic and CBCT imaging can aid in determining the positions and locations of these teeth.

Differential interpretation. Transposed teeth are usually easily recognized by examining the individual morphologies of the involved teeth.

Management. Transposed teeth are frequently altered prosthetically for function or esthetics, or both.

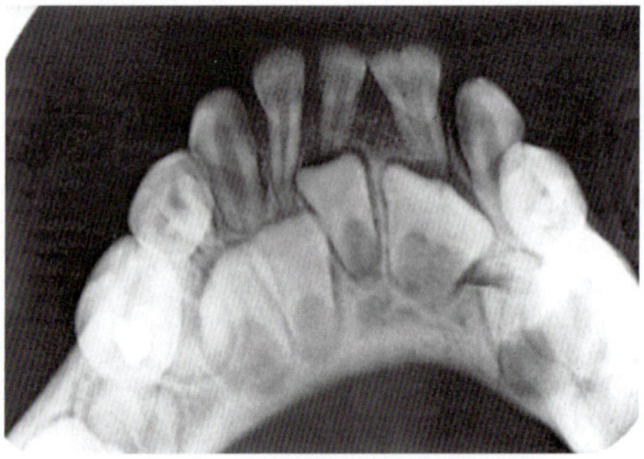

Fig. 19.15 Fusion of the mandibular left central and lateral incisors in both the primary and the permanent dentitions. Note the reduction in number of teeth and the increased width of the fused tooth mass.

Altered Morphology of Teeth

Fusion

Disease mechanism. Fusion of teeth results from the union of adjacent tooth germs of developing teeth. Some authors believe that fusion results when two tooth germs develop in such close proximity to one another that, as they grow, they contact and fuse before calcification is complete. Other authors contend that a physical force or pressure produced during development causes contact of adjacent tooth buds. Males and females experience fusion in equal numbers, and the incidence is higher in Asian and Indigenous populations.

Clinical features. Fusion results in a reduced number of teeth in the arch. Although fusion is more common in the deciduous dentition, it may also occur in the permanent dentition. When a deciduous canine and lateral incisor fuse, the corresponding permanent lateral incisor may be absent. Fusion is more common in anterior teeth of both the deciduous and permanent dentitions (Fig. 19.15). Fusion may be total or partial, depending on the stage of odontogenesis and the proximity of the developing teeth. The result can vary from a single tooth of about normal size to a tooth of nearly twice the normal size. The crowns of fused teeth usually appear to be large and single, although incisal clefts of varying depth or a bifid crown can sometimes occur. Fused teeth do not only cause problems on crowding of dentition, abnormal occlusion, and aesthetic, but can increase risks of dental caries, pulpal and periapical pathoses, and periodontal diseases. Fusion of deciduous teeth may lead to abnormalities of the succedaneous permanent teeth.

Imaging features. Periapical images, or small or limited field-of-view (FOV) CBCT, are helpful in disclosing the unusual shapes or sizes of the fused teeth. The true nature and extent of the union are frequently more evident on an image than can be determined by clinical examination. Fused teeth may also show an unusual configuration of the pulp chamber or root canal system.

Differential interpretation. The differential interpretation for fused teeth includes gemination and macrodontia. Fusion may be differentiated from gemination when the number of teeth is reduced by one, except in the unusual case in which a normal tooth and a supernumerary tooth have fused. That said, the differentiation is usually academic because little difference exists in patient management.

Management. The management of a case of fusion depends on which teeth are involved, the degree of fusion, and the morphologic result. If the affected teeth are deciduous, they may be retained as they are. If the clinician contemplates extraction, it is important to first determine whether the permanent teeth are present. In the case of fused permanent teeth, the fused crowns may be reshaped with a restoration that mimics two independent crowns. The morphology of fused teeth requires radiologic examination before the teeth are reshaped. Endodontic therapy may be necessary and perhaps may be difficult or impossible if the root canals are of unusual shape. In some cases, it is most prudent to leave the teeth as they are.

Concrescence

Disease mechanism. Concrescence occurs when the roots of two or more primary or permanent teeth are fused through cementum. Although the cause is unknown, many authorities suspect that space restriction during development, local trauma, excessive occlusal force, or local infection after development play important roles. If the condition occurs during development, it is sometimes referred to as true concrescence. If the condition occurs later, it is referred to as acquired concrescence.

Clinical features. Maxillary molars are the teeth most frequently involved, especially a third molar and a supernumerary tooth. Involved teeth may fail to erupt or may erupt incompletely. Males and females are equally affected.

Imaging features. An imaging examination may not always reveal concrescence; teeth may be in close contact or are simply superimposed (Fig. 19.16). When the condition is suspected on an image and extraction of one of the teeth is being considered, additional intraoral images made at different angles, or small FOV CBCT should be obtained to better assess the condition and possible complications.

Differential interpretation. It is usually impossible to determine with certainty whether the images of teeth whose roots appear to be superimposed are actually joined. If the roots are joined, it may be impossible to tell whether the union is through cementum or dentin (fusion). In this regard, the absence of a visible periodontal ligament space between the roots may be helpful.

Management. Concrescence affects treatment only when the decision is made to remove one or both of the involved teeth because this condition complicates the extraction. The clinician should warn the patient that an effort to remove one might result in the unintended and simultaneous removal of the other.

Gemination

Disease mechanism. Gemination or twinning is a rare anomaly that arises when a single tooth bud attempts to divide. The result may be an invagination of the crown with partial clefting or, in rare cases, complete division through the crown and root, producing identical structures. Complete twinning results in a normal tooth plus a supernumerary tooth in the arch. Although the etiology of gemination is unknown, there is some evidence that the condition may have a genetic basis with a familial tendency. Gemination is more prevalent in the anterior maxilla, whereas fusion is more commonly found in the anterior mandibular dentition.

Clinical features. Although gemination may occur in both the deciduous and the permanent dentitions, the primary teeth are more often affected. The prevalence of double teeth in the primary dentition is 0.5%–1.6%; in the permanent dentition it is approximately 0.1%–0.2%. Both sexes are affected with equal frequency. Gemination most commonly involves the anterior dentition, and the clinical manifestation of this anomaly varies considerably from a minor notch in the incisal edge of an abnormally wide incisor to the appearance of almost two separate crowns. The enamel or dentin of geminated teeth may be hypoplastic or hypocalcified.

Imaging features. Images reveal the altered shape of the hard tissue and pulp chamber of the geminated tooth. Multiple periapical images made from different angles, panoramic, or CBCT images can aid in the diagnosis. Radiopaque enamel outlines the clefts in the crowns and invaginations, and accentuates them. The pulp chamber is usually single and enlarged, and may be partially divided (Figs. 19.17 and 19.18). In the rare case of premolar gemination, the tooth image suggests a molar with an enlarged crown and two roots.

Differential interpretation. The differential interpretation of gemination includes fusion. If the malformed tooth is counted as one, individuals with gemination have a normal tooth count, whereas individuals with fusion are seen to be missing a tooth.

Management. A geminated tooth in the incisor area may compromise arch esthetics and arch length. Areas of hypoplasia, invagination lines, or areas of coronal separation represent caries-susceptible sites that may in time result in pulpal inflammation. Affected teeth can cause malocclusion and lead to the development of periodontal disease. Consequently, the affected tooth may be removed (especially if it is deciduous), the crown may be restored or reshaped, or the tooth may be left untreated and periodically monitored to preclude the development of complications. Before treatment is initiated on a primary

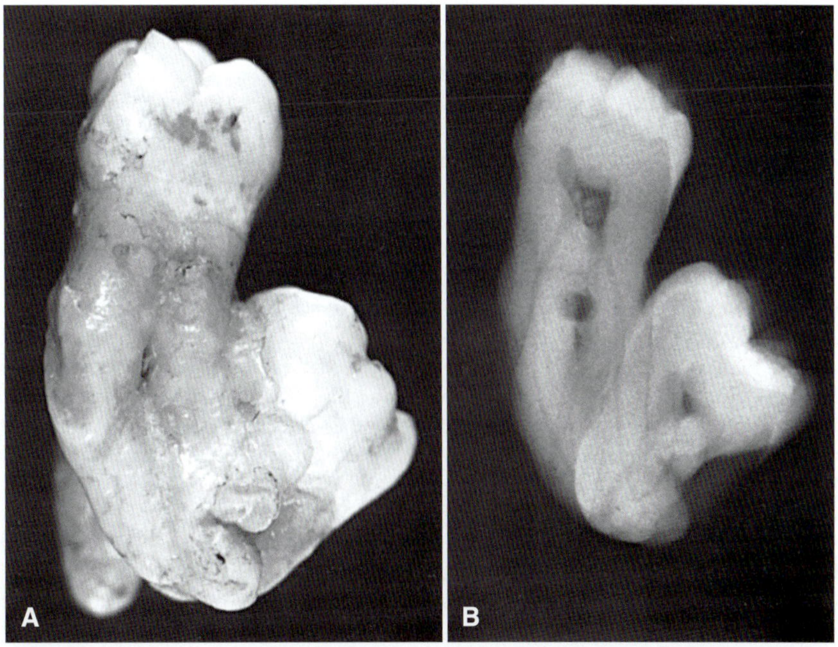

Fig. 19.16 Gross specimen (A) and planar image (B) showing concrescence between two molar teeth. Extraction of one tooth may result in the unintended removal of the second because the cementum bridge may not be well visualized. (Courtesy Dr. R. Kienholz, Dallas, TX.)

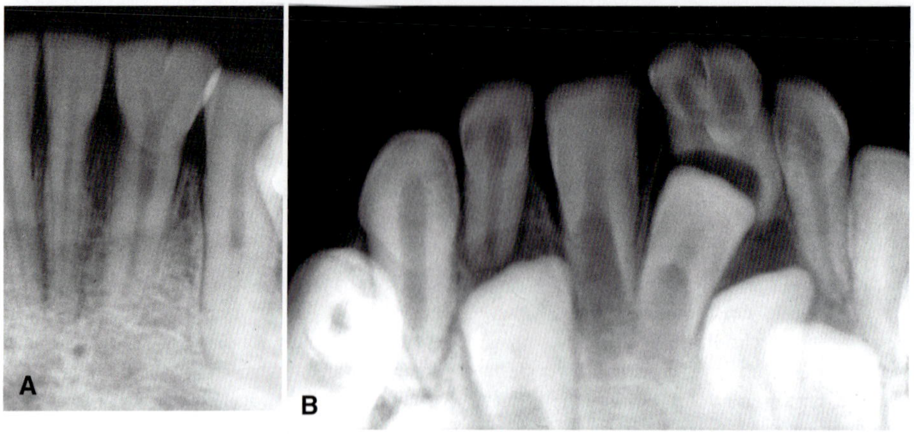

Fig. 19.17 Periapical image (A) of gemination of a mandibular left lateral incisor showing bifurcation of the crown and pulp chamber. Anterior occlusal image of the mandible (B) showing almost complete gemination of a deciduous lateral incisor.

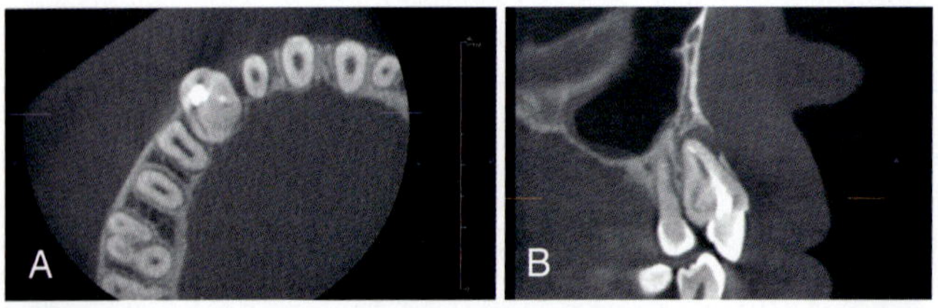

Fig. 19.18 Axial (A) and corrected coronal (B) cone beam computed tomographic image reconstructions of gemination of the maxillary right permanent canine.

tooth, the status of the permanent tooth and configuration of its root canals should be determined by imaging.

Taurodontism

Disease mechanism. Taurodontism is a morphological anomaly involving multirooted teeth that is characterized by a vertical shift of the pulp chamber floor and shortening of the roots. The pulp chamber extends from a normal position in the crown throughout the length of the elongated crown resulting in a more apically positioned pulpal floor. Single or multiple teeth may show taurodont features. Taurodontism has been reported in permanent and deciduous teeth, in premolars and molars, and it has been associated with certain syndromes, particularly those involving an ectodermal defect. With regard to genetic diseases, it has been reported that this anomaly can exist as an isolated feature. However, the majority of authors agree that taurodontism is more commonly associated with conditions such as Down syndrome, Klinefelter syndrome, CLP, hypodontia, and amelogenesis imperfecta (AI).

Clinical features. The distinguishing features of taurodont teeth are not recognizable clinically because the body and roots of these teeth are located within the bone. From a clinical standpoint, it is very important to diagnose taurodontism before dental treatment. If indicated, the endodontic treatment of a taurodont tooth is challenging due to the apical positioning of the pulpal chamber floor, the anomalous configuration of the root canal system, or the presence of additional canals. In restorative dental terms, the use of taurodont teeth as abutments is not recommended as they lack stability due to their shorter roots. The extraction of taurodont teeth can be complicated due to an apical location of the root furcation. In periodontics, taurodont teeth can have a better prognosis as there is less chance of furcation involvement. From an orthodontic point of view, it is important to note that taurodont teeth are not sufficiently embedded in the alveolar process of the bone, and have a greater tendency for root resorption.

Imaging features. The distinctive morphology of taurodont teeth is quite apparent on images. A peculiar feature is the vertically elongated pulp chamber and the more apically positioned furcation (Fig. 19.19). The shorter roots and root canals are a consequence of the long body and normal length of the tooth. The dimensions of the crown are normal. Periapical and panoramic images help with the diagnosis of this condition.

Differential interpretation. The image of the taurodont tooth is characteristic and easily recognized on imaging. The developing molar may appear similar; however, identification of the wide apical foramina and incompletely formed roots aids in the differential interpretation. Taurodontism has been reported in hypophosphatemia and with greater frequency in patients with trisomy 21.

Management. Taurodont teeth do not require treatment.

Dilaceration

Disease mechanism. Dilaceration is a disturbance in tooth formation that produces a sharp bend or increased curvature in the crown or the root. Two possible causes of dilaceration are mechanical trauma to the calcified portion of a partially formed tooth and developmental disturbances. As well, it has also been proposed that dilaceration may be associated with some developmental syndromes. Dilaceration can be seen in both the permanent and deciduous dentitions, and it is more commonly found in posterior teeth and in the maxilla.

Clinical features. Most cases of radicular dilaceration are not recognized clinically. If the dilaceration is so pronounced that the tooth does not erupt, the only clinical indication of the defect is a missing tooth. If the defect is in the crown of an erupted tooth, it may be readily recognized as an angular distortion (Fig. 19.20).

Imaging features. Imaging provides the best means of detecting a radicular dilaceration. One or more teeth may be affected, and the condition occurs most often in maxillary premolars. If the roots dilacerate mesially or distally, the condition is clearly apparent on a periapical image (Fig. 19.21). However, when the roots are dilacerated buccally (labially) or lingually, the central x-ray passes approximately parallel to the deflected portion of the root, and the apical end of the root may have the appearance of a circular or oval radiopaque area with a central radiolucency (the apical foramen and root canal), giving

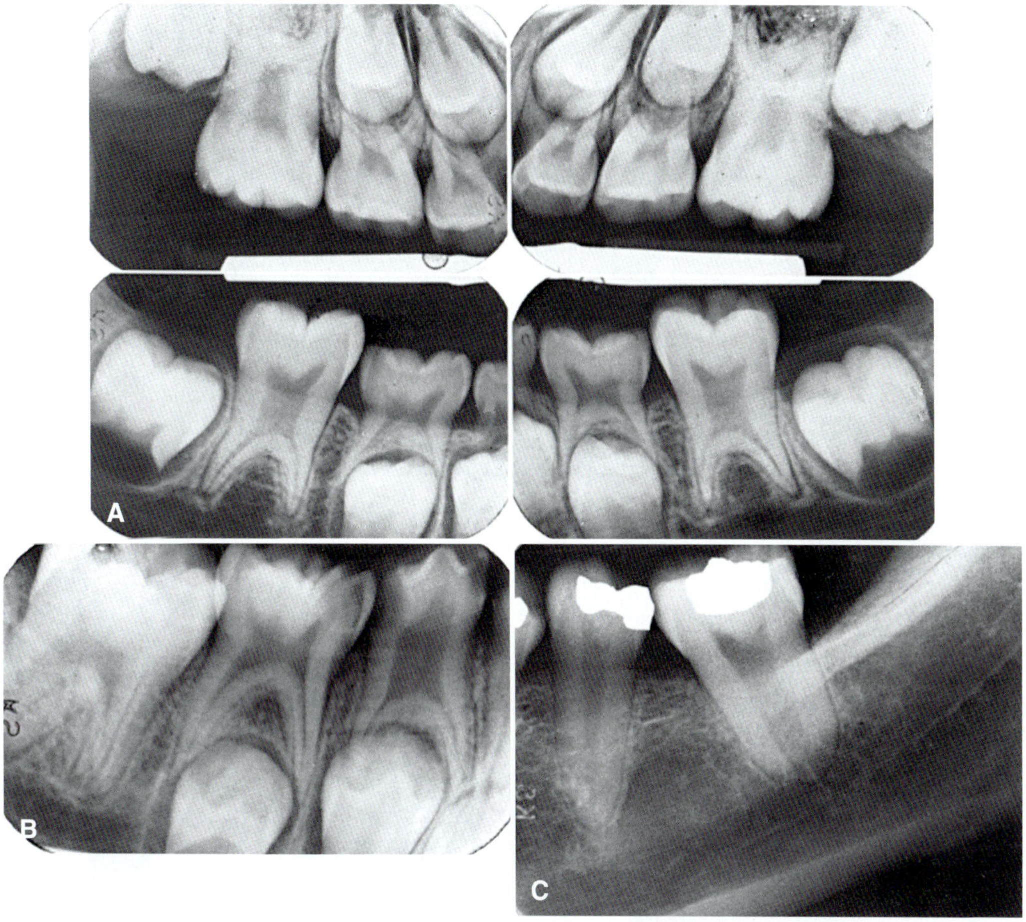

Fig. 19.19 Periapical images of taurodontism reveal enlarged pulp chambers and apically positioned furca in maxillary and mandibular permanent first molars (A), a deciduous mandibular right first molar (B), and a mandibular left permanent molar (C).

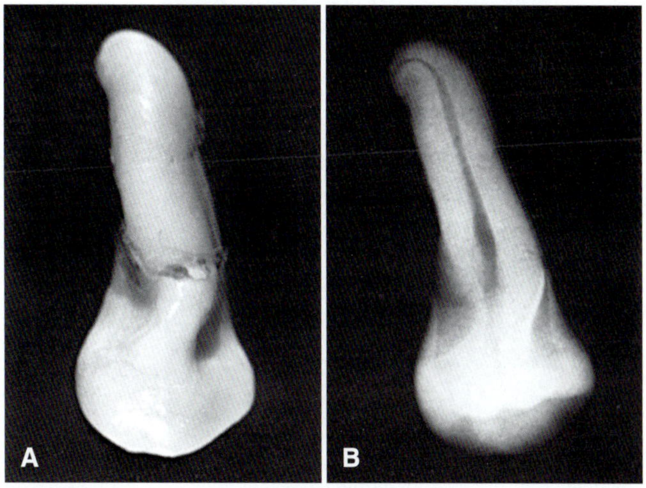

Fig. 19.20 Gross specimen (A) and planar image of the specimen in A (B) showing dilaceration of a tooth crown. (Courtesy Dr. R. Kienholz, Dallas, TX.)

the appearance of a "bull's eye." The periodontal ligament space around this dilacerated portion may be seen as a radiolucent halo encircling the radiopaque area (Fig. 19.22). In some cases, especially in the maxilla, the geometry of the projections may preclude the recognition of a dilaceration.

Differential interpretation. Occasionally, dilacerated roots may be difficult to differentiate from fused roots, hypercementosis, sclerosing osteitis, or dense bone island, particularly if the periodontal ligament space is difficult to visualize. However, these usually can be discerned by making a second image at a different angle.

Management. A dilacerated root generally does not require treatment because it provides adequate tooth support. If the tooth is to be extracted for some other reason, the removal can be complicated, especially if the clinician is not prepared with a preoperative image. Endodontic access cavity preparation, root canal preparation and filling, and other related treatments might also be complicated by the presence of a dilaceration. In contrast, dilacerated crowns are frequently restored with a prosthetic crown to improve esthetics and function.

Dens Invaginatus, Dens in Dente, and Dilated Odontome

Disease mechanism. Dens invaginatus, dens in dente, and dilated odontome represent varying degrees of invagination or infolding of the enamel surface into the interior of a tooth. The least severe form of this infolding is dens invaginatus, and the most severe form is dilated odontome. The invagination can occur in the crown or the root during tooth development. It may also involve the pulp chamber or root canal system; this may result in a deformity of either the crown or the root, although these anomalies are seen most often in tooth crowns.

Based on the severity of the invagination, Oehler classified these into three types. In type I, the invagination is confined to the crown

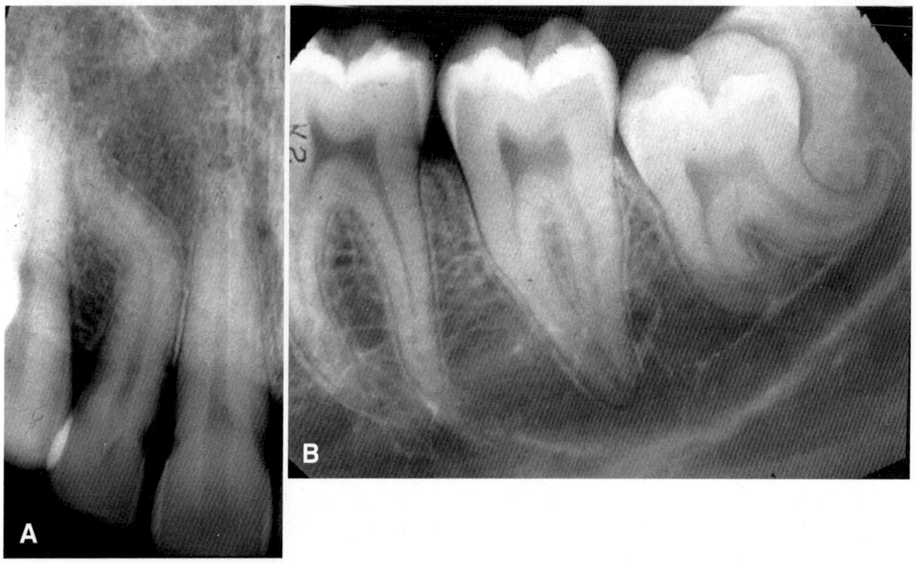

Fig. 19.21 Dilaceration of the root of a maxillary right lateral incisor (A) and mandibular left third molar (B).

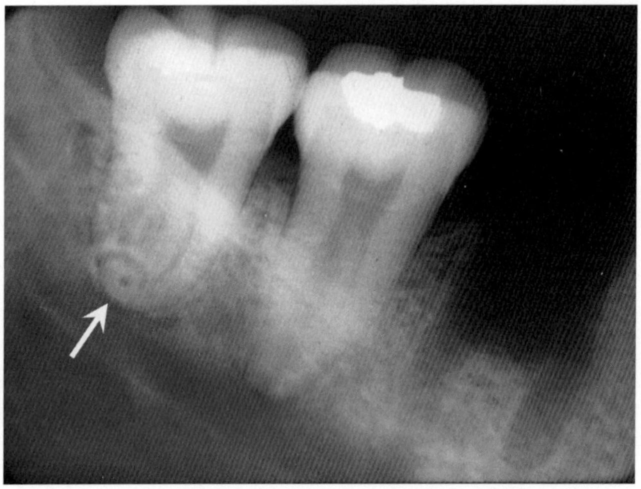

Fig. 19.22 The most apical portion of this third molar root is dilacerated in the buccal/lingual direction so that its long axis lies along the path of the x-ray beam. Note the "bull's eye" appearance of the root apex produced by the root canal, tooth root, and periodontal ligament space *(arrow)*.

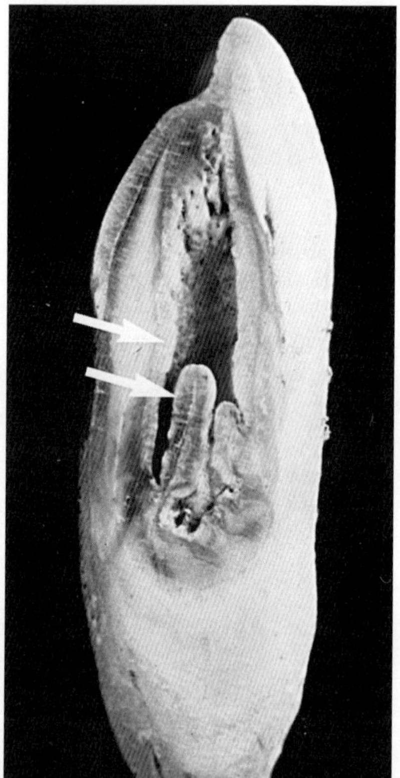

Fig. 19.23 Sectioned, extracted canine tooth with dens in dente shows the infolding of the enamel *(arrows)*.

and does not extend apical to the cementoenamel junction. In type II, the invagination extends to the pulp chamber but remains within the root canal with no communication to the periodontal ligament space. In type IIIA, the invagination extends through the root and communicates to the periodontal ligament space. And in type IIIB, the invagination extends through the root and communicates with the periodontal ligament space at the apical foramen.

Coronal invaginations usually originate from an anomalous infolding of the enamel organ into the dental papilla. In a mature tooth, the result is a fold of hard tissue within the tooth characterized by enamel lining the fold (Fig. 19.23). When the abnormality involves the root, it may be the result of an invagination of the Hertwig epithelial root sheath and produce an accentuation of the normal longitudinal root groove.

In contrast to the coronal type which is lined with enamel, the radicular type of defect is lined with cementum. If the invagination retracts and is cut off, it leaves a longitudinal structure of cementum, bone, and remnants of the periodontal ligament within the root canal. The structure often extends for most of the root length. In other cases, the root sheath may bud off a sac-like invagination that produces a circumscribed cementum defect in the root. Mandibular first premolars and second molars are especially prone to develop the radicular variety of this invagination anomaly.

Among Whites and Asians, there is little difference in frequency of occurrence. If all types of expression of invagination are included, the condition is found in approximately 5% of these two population groups. The condition appears to be rare in individuals of African descent. No sexual predilection exists. Although no specific mode of inheritance seems to fit all the data, a high degree of inheritability seems to exist.

Clinical features. Dens invaginatus may appear as nothing more than a small pit between the cingulum and the palatal surface of an incisor tooth (Fig. 19.24). In dens in dente, the pit is located at the incisal edge of the tooth, and crown morphology may appear abnormal, having the appearance of a peg-shaped microdont tooth (Fig. 19.25). A dilated odontome is the most extreme form of tooth invagination, and has roughly the shape of a doughnut with a central radiolucent soft tissue region surrounded by radiopaque dental hard tissue.

Dens invaginatus and dens in dente occur most frequently in the permanent maxillary lateral incisors, followed by (in decreasing frequency) the maxillary central incisors, premolars, and canines, and less often the posterior teeth. Invagination is rare in the crowns of mandibular teeth and in deciduous teeth. The abnormality occurs symmetrically in about half the cases, and involvement of both the central and lateral incisors may occur.

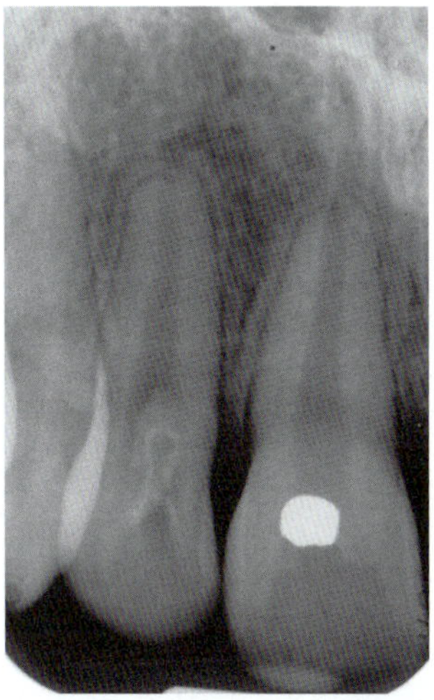

Fig. 19.24 Periapical image shows the radiopaque, inverted teardrop outline of dens invaginatus in a maxillary right lateral incisor. Note the position of the invagination in the cingulum area of the tooth crown.

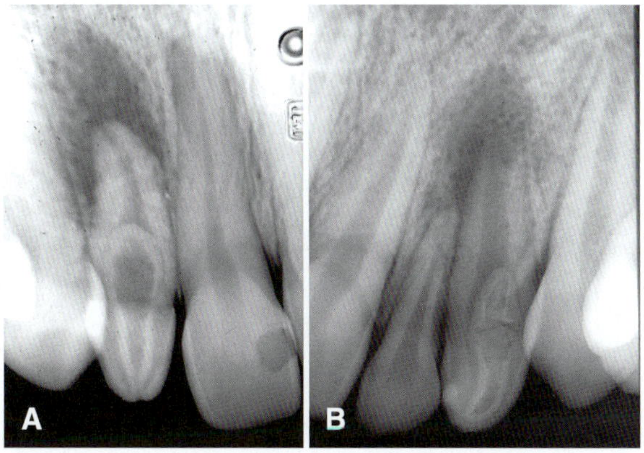

Fig. 19.25 Periapical images (A and B) showing more severe infolding of the enamel in dens in dente. The invagination begins near the incisal edge of these peg-shaped maxillary lateral incisors. Dens in dente often result in necrosis of the pulp and rarefying osteitis at the tooth apices.

The clinical importance of dens invaginatus and dens in dente is the risk of pulpal inflammation and necrosis. The base of the invagination is usually separated from the pulp chamber by a relatively thin wall of enamel and dentin that lines the base of the invagination. Here, the enamel is frequently thin, often of poor quality, and may be missing in some areas. The opening of the invagination communicates with the oral cavity through a narrow, constricted pathway. The pit that is seen clinically is often difficult if not impossible to keep clean, and consequently it offers conditions favorable for the colonization of oral microorganisms and the subsequent development of caries. Such carious lesions are difficult to detect clinically and rapidly involve the pulp. In addition, sometimes fine canals extend between the invagination and the pulp chamber, resulting in pulpal disease even in the absence of caries.

Imaging features. Most cases of dens invaginatus or dens in dente are discovered with imaging, and can be identified in the image even before the tooth erupts. The infolding of the enamel lining is more radiopaque than the surrounding tooth structure and can be identified easily as an inverted teardrop-shaped radiolucency with a radiopaque border (Fig. 19.26). Less frequently, the radicular invaginations appear as poorly defined, slightly radiolucent structures running longitudinally within the root. The defects, especially the coronal variety, may vary in size and shape from small and superficial to large and deep. If a coronal invagination is extensive, then the crown is typically malformed, and the apical foramen is usually wide (Fig. 19.26). A frequent cause of an open apical foramen is the cessation of root development that occurs as a result of pulpal necrosis. In the most severe form (dilated odontome), the tooth is severely deformed, having a circular or oval shape with a radiolucent interior (Fig. 19.27). Severe forms of invagination may require small or limited FOV CBCT to further evaluate and plan appropriate management.

Differential interpretation. The appearance and usual occurrence in incisors are so characteristic that, once recognized, little probability exists that the anomaly will be confused with another condition.

Management. Because the invagination is in communication with the oral cavity, it can retain saliva, food remnants, and bacterial microorganisms. In conditions where the enamel lining of the invagination is naturally absent or lost because of caries, bacterial microorganisms and their products can diffuse from the invagination through the dentin tubules to reach the pulp, causing inflammation and necrosis. Management of teeth with dens invaginatus includes preventive sealing or filling of the invagination, or if the pulp is affected, therapeutic options include vital pulp therapy, orthograde root canal treatment, apexogenesis, apexification, periradicular surgery, intentional replantation, or extraction.

Dens Evaginatus

Disease mechanism. In contrast to dens invaginatus or dens in dente, dens evaginatus (e.g., Leong premolar) is the result of an

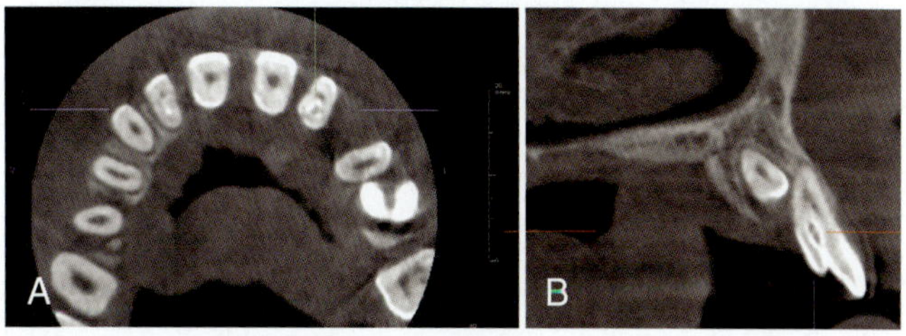

Fig. 19.26 Axial (A) cone beam computed tomographic image showing dens in dente involving the maxillary right and left lateral incisors and corrected sagittal image (B) through the maxillary left lateral incisor. Note the invagination that is lined by the higher attenuation (more radiopaque) enamel.

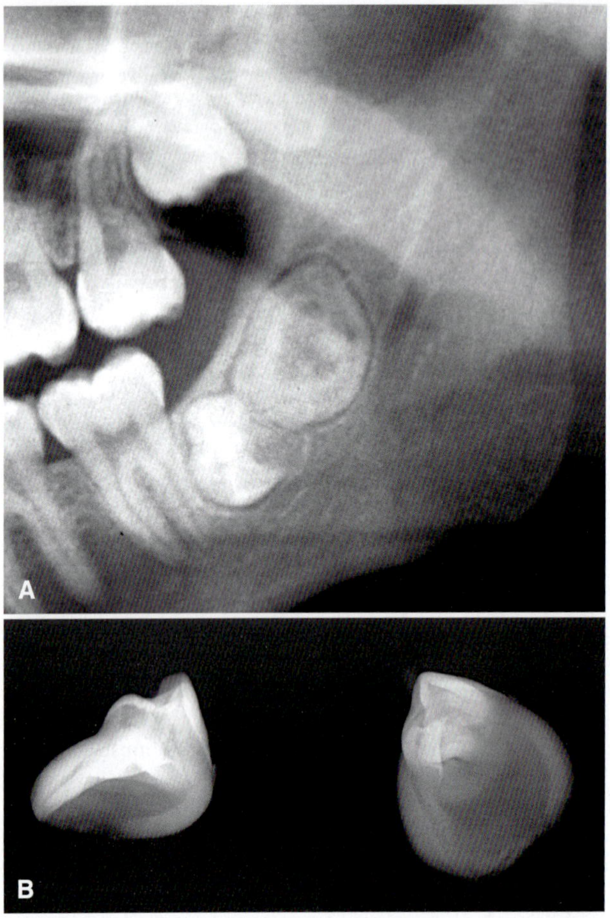

Fig. 19.27 Cropped panoramic (A) and two planar images of a gross specimen (B) of dilated odontomes; the most severe enamel invagination.

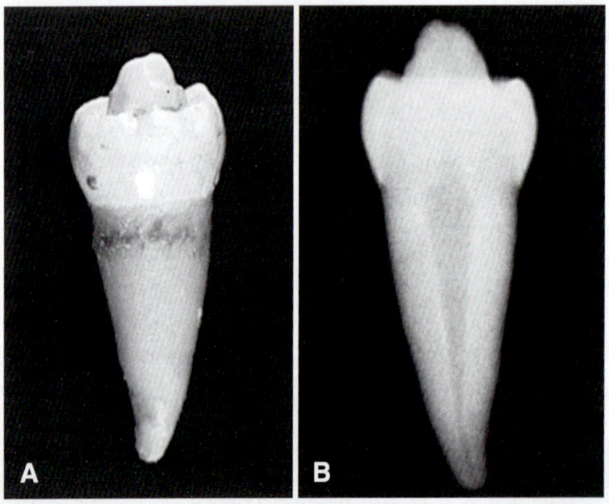

Fig. 19.28 Extracted premolar tooth (A) and planar image (B) show the occlusal tubercle of dens evaginatus. (Courtesy Dr. R. Kienholz, Dallas, TX.)

evagination or outpouching of the enamel organ. The resultant enamel-covered tubercle usually occurs in or near the middle of the occlusal surface of premolar or occasionally molar teeth (Fig. 19.28). Lateral incisors are most commonly involved, whereas canines are rarely affected. The frequency of occurrence of dens evaginatus is highest in Asian and Indigenous populations.

Clinical features. Clinically, dens evaginatus appears as a tubercle of enamel on the occlusal surface of the affected tooth. A hard, polyp-like protuberance predominantly exists in the central groove or lingual ridge of a buccal cusp of posterior teeth and in the cingulum fossa of anterior teeth. Dens evaginatus may occur bilaterally, and is usually found in mandibular teeth. The tubercle often has a dentin core, and a very slender pulp horn frequently extends into the evagination. After the tubercle is worn down by the opposing dentition, it appears as a small circular facet with a small dark pit in the center (Fig. 19.29). Wear, fracture, or indiscriminate surgical removal of this tubercle may

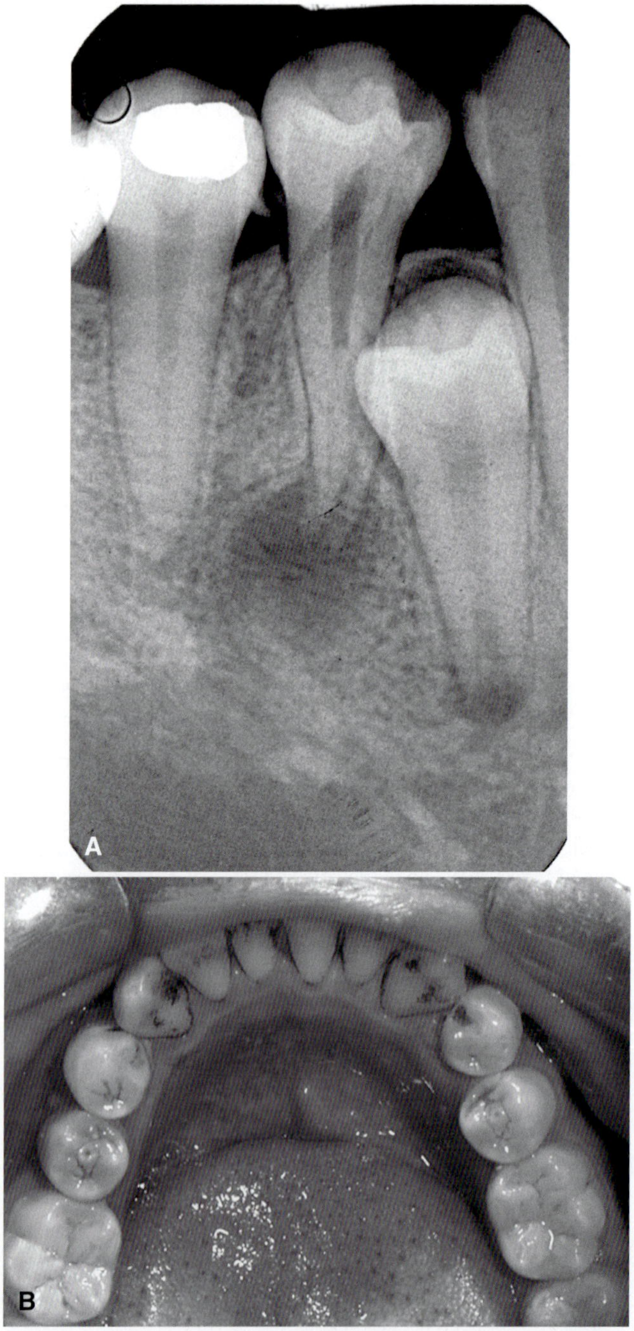

Fig. 19.29 Periapical image (A) of a mandibular right first premolar with a dens evaginatus and rarefying osteitis. Clinical photograph (B) of another case of dens evaginatus involving the mandibular second premolar teeth, bilaterally.

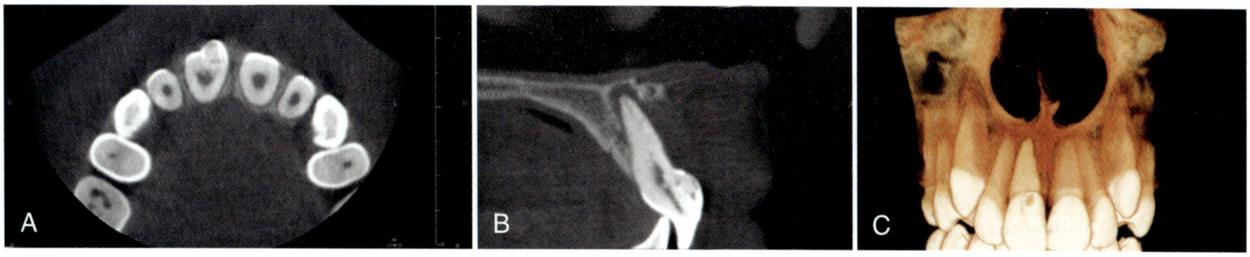

Fig. 19.30 Axial (A), corrected sagittal (B), and three-dimensional (C) cone beam computed tomographic reconstructions of a dens evaginatus in an unusual location involving the labial surface of a maxillary right central incisor.

precipitate exposure of the pulp and an inflammatory response. In rare cases, a microscopic direct communication may occur between the pulp and the oral cavity through this tubercle. In these instances, the pulp may become infected shortly after eruption.

Imaging features. Imaging shows an extension of a dentin tubercle on the occlusal surface unless the tubercle is already worn down. The dentin core is usually covered with radiopaque enamel. A fine pulp horn may extend into the tubercle, but this may not be visible in an image. If the tubercle has been worn to the point of pulpal exposure or has fractured, pulpal necrosis may result (Fig. 19.29). Necrosis is indicated by an open apical foramen and periapical radiolucency (Fig. 19.30). Multiple root formation is often associated with dens evaginatus, especially in mandibular premolars.

Differential interpretation. The clinical and imaging appearances may be characteristic or may be difficult to visualize if the tubercle has been worn down to the occlusal surface.

Management. If the tubercle causes any occlusal interference or shows evidence of marked attrition, it probably should be removed under aseptic conditions, and the pulp should be capped, if necessary. Such a precaution may preclude pulpal exposure and infection as the result of accidental fracture or advanced attrition.

Molar-Incisor Malformation

Disease mechanism. Molar-incisor malformation (MIM) or molar root-incisor malformation (MRIM) is a rare developmental dental anomaly seen in the primary second molars and permanent first molars, and sometimes the permanent maxillary central incisors. These teeth are typically identified by underdeveloped roots with a short, narrow, and spiky shape. The etiology of MIM is not fully understood at this time, although it is believed to be the result of an epigenetic factor linked to a systemic condition affecting the central nervous system when the patient is 1–2 years of age. Parents may report a history of neurological medical complications at birth or in the first 2 years of life.

Clinical features. Clinical features may include poor incisor esthetics, impactions of teeth, early exfoliation, space loss, periapical inflammatory disease, and spontaneous pain. The major manifestations are severe coronal cervical constriction of the affected molars and significant underdevelopment of one or more roots. MIM may also present with ectopic eruption of teeth.

Imaging features. The imaging features include constriction of the cervical regions of the crowns, and some patients may show an abnormal notch-like defect at the cervical enamel of the permanent maxillary central incisors. The roots of all permanent first molars may appear hypoplastic with compromised bone support, and there may also be furcation involvement.

Management. As there is often a stronger expression in the molars, identifying spontaneous ectopic eruption of permanent first molars and cervical constriction is important for management. Maintaining good periodontal health and circumferential bone is vital for adequate support to the tooth and, potentially, future implant placement. Careful planning using a team-based approach with the patient's pediatric dentist and orthodontist are key to managing this condition.

Amelogenesis Imperfecta

Disease mechanism. AI represents a group of developmental conditions, genomic in origin, which affect the structure and clinical appearance of enamel of all or nearly all the teeth in a more or less equal manner. The condition may also be associated with morphologic or biochemical changes elsewhere in the body, including the kidney (enamel renal syndrome). AI can arise from mutations that may have occurred in one or multiple genes that play some role in enamel formation including but not limited to: amelogenin *(AMELX)*, enamelin *(ENAM)*, enamelysin *(MMP20)*, kallikrein 4 *(KLK4)*, family with sequence similarity 83 member H *(FAM83H)*, FAM20A Golgi-associated secretory pathway pseudokinase *(FAM20A)*, ameloblastin *(AMBN)*, tuftelin *(TUFT1)*, amelotin *(AMELOTIN)*, and dentin sialophosphoprotein *(DSPP)*. AI can also arise in isolation or it can be associated with other abnormalities in syndromes. Inheritance may be autosomal dominant, autosomal recessive, and sex-linked, and mutations may also arise sporadically. In families with an X-linked form, the condition may result from mutations in the amelogenin gene, *AMELX*. The enamelin gene *(ENAM)* is implicated in the pathogenesis of the dominant forms of AI. Autosomal-recessive AI has been reported in families with known consanguinity. These mutations lead to changes in the enamel of teeth in both dentitions, and are not related to any time or period of enamel development or any clinically demonstrable alteration (disease or dietary abnormality) in other tissues.

In the hypoplastic and hypomineralized types of AI, the enamel may lack the normal prismatic structure and be laminated throughout its thickness or at the periphery. In these cases, the teeth have been reported to be more resistant to decay. The dentin and root form are usually normal. Eruption of the affected teeth is often delayed, and a tendency for tooth impaction exists. Many classifications of AI have evolved since the original division into hypoplastic and hypocalcified types in 1945. Some have been exclusively based on the phenotype (appearance), others have used the phenotype as the primary discriminant and the mode of inheritance as a secondary factor in diagnosis. Although as many as 23 variants of the condition have been described, with the diagnosis based on identifying the gene mutation, the family history, pedigree plotting, and meticulous clinical observation. Broadly, four general types have been delineated on the basis of their clinical or imaging appearances: a hypoplastic type, a hypomaturation type, a hypocalcified type, and a hypomaturation–hypoplastic type associated with taurodontism.

Clinical features

Hypoplastic type. The enamel of the affected teeth fails to develop to its normal thickness although the density of the enamel contrasts normally with the underlying dentin. As a consequence of the thinner enamel, the color of the underlying dentin imparts a yellow–brown color to the tooth. In addition, the enamel may be abnormal; the surface may be rough, pitted, smooth, or glossy. The crowns of the teeth may appear undersized with a roughly square shape. The reduced enamel thickness also causes either a generalized loss of interproximal contacts between adjacent teeth (Figs. 19.31 and 19.32), or broader, more elongated contacts. The occlusal surfaces of the posterior teeth are relatively flat with low cusps. This is a result of the attrition of cusp tips that were initially low and not fully formed. Hypoplastic AI is the type most easily identifiable on imaging.

Hypomaturation. In the hypomaturation form of AI, the enamel has a mottled appearance but is of normal thickness. The enamel is clinically softer than normal, and its density is comparable to dentin. Moreover, the enamel may break away from the crown. Tooth color may range from clear to cloudy white, yellow, or brown. In one form of hypomaturation AI, the teeth may be capped with white, opaque enamel. This appearance has been referred to as "snow-capped" teeth.

Hypocalcification. The hypocalcific form of AI is more common than the hypoplastic variety. The crowns of the teeth are normal in size and shape when they erupt because the enamel is of regular thickness (Fig. 19.33). However, because the enamel is poorly mineralized (it is less dense than dentin), it starts to fracture shortly after it comes into function, and this creates clinically recognizable defects. The soft enamel abrades rapidly, and the softer dentin also wears down rapidly, resulting in a grossly worn tooth, sometimes to the level of the gingiva. An explorer point under pressure can penetrate the soft enamel, yet caries in these worn teeth is unusual. The hypocalcified enamel has increased permeability and becomes stained and darkened. The teeth of a young person with generalized hypomineralization of the enamel are frequently dark brown from food stains.

Hypomaturation–hypoplastic with taurodontism. This classification indicates a combination of hypomaturation and hypoplastic with taurodontism.

Imaging features. AI is identified primarily by its clinical features, although imaging can help substantiate the clinical impression. The imaging features of hypoplastic AI include a square crown, a relatively thin radiopaque layer of enamel, low or absent cusps, and multiple open or broad-based contacts between the teeth. The anterior teeth on

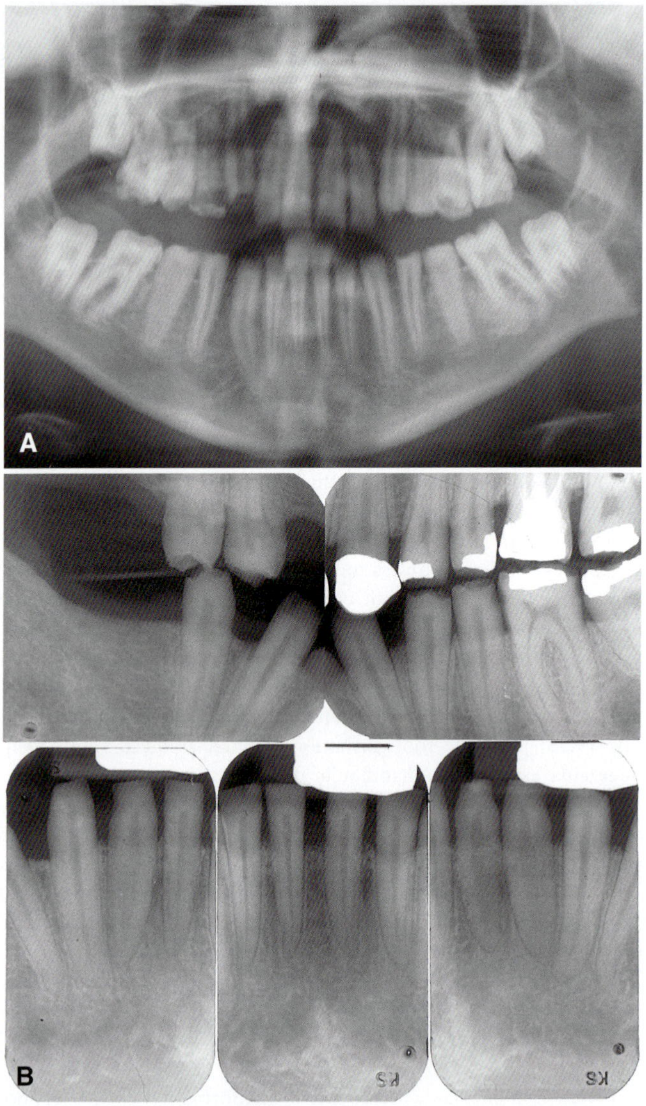

Fig. 19.31 Cropped panoramic (A) and periapical images (B) of hypoplastic amelogenesis imperfecta. Note the thin layer of enamel, the absence of interproximal contacts, and the "picket fence"–like appearance of the teeth. (A, Courtesy Dr. S. Roth, Halifax, NS.)

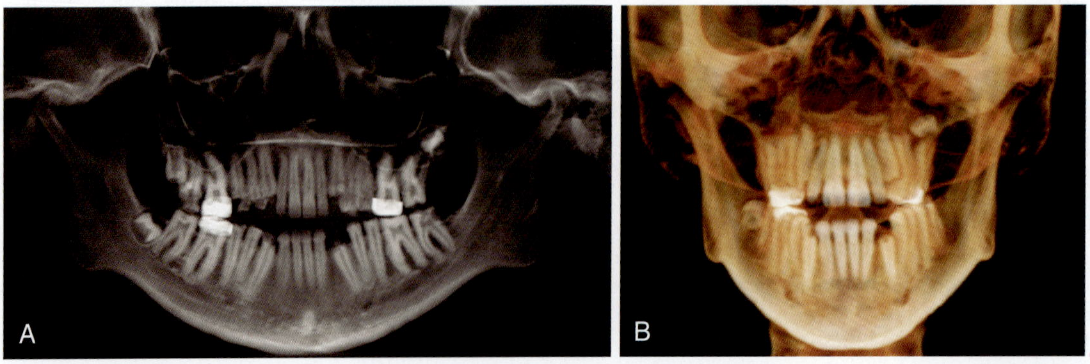

Fig. 19.32 Panoramic (A) and three-dimensional (B) reconstructions of a cone beam computed tomographic image volume demonstrating generalized loss of enamel structure and carious lesions in multiple teeth in a patient with hypoplastic amelogenesis imperfecta.

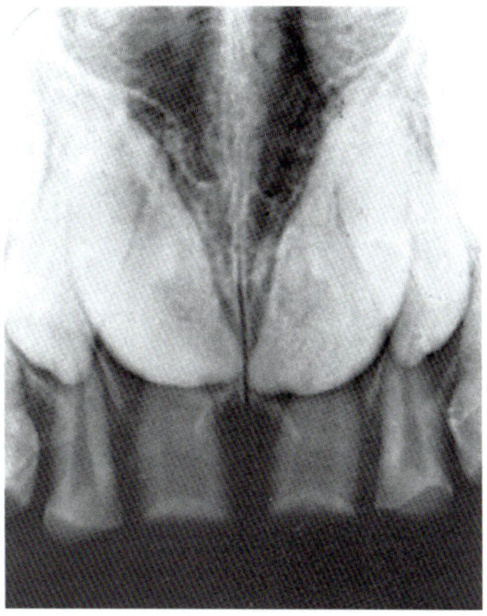

Fig. 19.33 The reduced radiopacity of the enamel and the rapid abrasion of the crowns of the primary teeth are features of hypomineralized amelogenesis imperfecta.

images are said to have a "picket fence" type of appearance. The density of the enamel contrasts normally with the underlying dentin. When the enamel is pitted, the appearance is that of sharply localized areas of mottled density, quite different from the image cast by a tooth that is normal in shape and density. The hypomaturation form exhibits a normal thickness of the enamel, but the normal density between enamel and dentin is lost. In such cases, the enamel may be very similar in density to dentin. In the hypocalcified forms, the enamel thickness is normal, but its density is even less (i.e., more radiolucent) than that of dentin. With advanced abrasion, obliteration of the pulp chambers may complicate recognition of the image.

Differential interpretation. If advanced abrasion is present and secondary dentin obliterates the pulp chambers, the imaging features of AI may appear similar to that of dentinogenesis imperfecta. However, the presence of bulbous crowns and narrow roots, the relatively normal density of any remaining enamel, and the obliteration of pulp chambers and root canals, in the absence of marked attrition, are characteristic features of dentinogenesis imperfecta (see the following section), and should distinguish it from AI.

Management. Appropriate treatment for AI is restoration of the esthetics and function of the affected teeth.

Dentinogenesis Imperfecta

Disease mechanism. Dentinogenesis imperfecta or hereditary opalescent dentin is a genetic anomaly involving primarily the dentin, although the enamel may be thinner than normal in this condition. Dentinogenesis imperfecta occurs with equal frequency in both sexes. Both the deciduous and the permanent dentition may have this defect. It follows an autosomal-dominant pattern of transmission, affecting both the formation and mineralization of dentin. Three forms of dentinogenesis imperfecta have been described, and each has been associated with a particular gene. Type I dentinogenesis imperfecta, which is associated with osteogenesis imperfecta, is caused by mutations of one of two genes involved in collagen synthesis: the collagen type I alpha 1 *(COL1A1)* and collagen type I alpha 2 *(COL1A2)* genes. Types II and III dentinogenesis imperfecta are caused by mutations of the dentin sialoprotein *(DSP)* and *DSPP* genes.

The tooth roots and pulp chambers of type I teeth are generally small and underdeveloped, and the primary dentition may be more severely affected than the permanent dentition. Type II dentinogenesis imperfecta is similar to type I but affects the dentin only without any skeletal defects. The expression of type II dentinogenesis imperfecta is variable, and occasionally individuals exhibit enlarged pulp chambers in the primary teeth. Type III dentinogenesis imperfecta, or the so-called Brandywine isolate, was described in a population of fewer than 200 persons in the Brandywine region of Maryland in the United States. There is some controversy regarding the differentiation between types II and III; however, type III teeth are said to exhibit enlarged pulp chambers, making them more susceptible to pulp exposure.

Dentinogenesis imperfecta is found in association with approximately 25% of cases of osteogenesis imperfecta, a hereditary disorder characterized by an inborn error in the synthesis of type I collagen. The abnormality is usually transmitted as an autosomal-dominant trait. Osteogenesis imperfecta results in brittle, fragile bones. In addition, patients may have blue sclerae, wormian bones (bone formation within skull sutures), skeletal deformities, and progressive osteopenia. Oral findings may also include class III malocclusions and an increased incidence of impacted first and second molars.

Clinical features. The appearance of teeth with dentinogenesis imperfecta is characteristic. The crowns exhibit a high degree of amber-like translucency and various colors from yellow to blue–gray. The colors change according to whether the teeth are observed with transmitted or reflected light. The enamel easily fractures from the teeth, and the crowns wear readily. In adults, the teeth frequently may wear down to the gingiva. The exposed dentin becomes stained. The color of the abraded teeth may change to dark brown or black. Some patients demonstrate an anterior open bite.

Imaging features. The crowns in patients with dentinogenesis imperfecta often appear bulbous or rounded, and are shorter than normal due to marked constriction of the tooth crown in the cervical area. The dentin appears abnormally thin due to increased pulp chamber size, and the layer of enamel can be almost normal in thickness but can get detached easily due to an abnormal dentino-enamel junction. Images may reveal attrition of the occlusal surface. The roots are often shorter with an enlarged pulp chamber giving a "thistle" appearance. Early in development, the teeth may appear to have large pulp chambers, but with aging these are quickly obliterated by the formation of dentin. Ultimately, the root canals may be narrow and threadlike, or obliterated (Fig. 19.34). Occasionally areas of rarefying osteitis may be seen in association with what appear to be sound teeth without evidence of pulpal involvement. These changes may occur as a result of microscopic communications between the residual pulp and the oral cavity. These lesions do not occur as frequently as in dentin dysplasia. The architecture of the bone in the maxilla and mandible is normal.

Differential interpretation. Dentin dysplasia (see the following section) is the differential interpretation.

Management. The placement of prosthetic crowns on the affected teeth is usually unsuccessful unless the teeth have good root support. The teeth should not be extracted from patients 5–15 years old. It is generally preferable to place full overdentures on the teeth to prevent alveolar resorption. In adults, extraction of the teeth and their replacement can be recommended.

Dentin Dysplasia

Disease mechanism. Dentin dysplasia is a rare genetically inherited autosomal-dominant abnormality that affects the formation of dentin in both primary and permanent teeth. In type I or radicular dentin dysplasia, the teeth have normal crowns, but the roots are short or absent with incomplete or total obliteration of the pulp chamber. In type II or coronal dentin dysplasia, changes to the crowns are most clearly seen in the altered shape of the pulp chambers. The primary teeth are discolored and translucent, and permanent teeth may appear normal or with amber discoloration. The specific genetic cause has been difficult to pinpoint due to the rarity and complexity of the

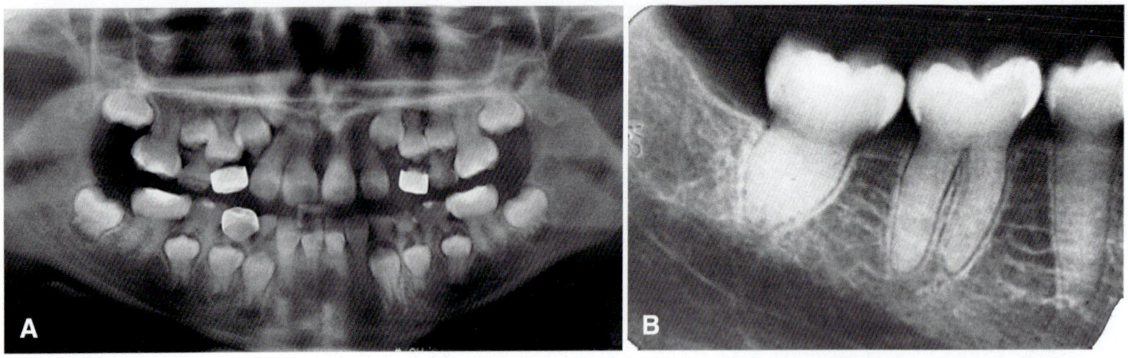

Fig. 19.34 Panoramic (A) and periapical (B) images of dentinogenesis imperfecta showing the characteristically bulbous crowns, constriction of tooth at the cementoenamel junction, short roots, and a reduced size of the pulp chamber and root canals.

condition, but mutations of the *DSPP* gene, the same gene that has been implicated in dentinogenesis imperfecta types II and III, have also been implicated in type II dentin dysplasia. Mutations in the *DSPP* gene can interfere with the normal mineralization of dentin, leading to the dental problems associated with dentin dysplasia. However, not all cases of dentin dysplasia are associated with mutations in the *DSPP* gene, implying that other unknown factors (possibly including other genes) may also contribute to this disorder. Recently, three other mutant genes have been detected with different genetic modes of inheritance: *SMOC2,* an inhibitor of mineralization; *VPS4B,* a gene involved in intracellular protein trafficking; and *SSUH2,* a gene involved in odontogenesis.

Clinical features. Dentin dysplasia occurs less frequently than dentinogenesis imperfecta (1:100,000 vs. 1:8000). Clinically, teeth with type I radicular dentin dysplasia have mostly normal color and shape in the primary and adult dentitions. Occasionally, a slight bluish brown translucency is apparent. The teeth are often misaligned in the arch, and patients may describe drifting and spontaneous exfoliation with little or no trauma. In type II coronal dentin dysplasia, the crowns of the primary teeth appear to be of the same color, size, and contour as teeth with dentinogenesis imperfecta—an interesting coincidence in light of the purported close genetic linkage between the two dentin abnormalities. Although not universally accepted, reports exist that primary teeth rapidly abrade. The permanent teeth have clinically normal-appearing crowns.

Imaging features. In type I dentin dysplasia, the roots of both the primary and the permanent teeth are either short or abnormally shaped (Fig. 19.35). The molar roots have been described as having a shallow W shape. The roots of primary teeth may be only thin spicules. The pulp chambers and root canals become completely obliterated before eruption; however, this is variable. In addition, about 20% of teeth with type I dentin dysplasia are associated with rarefying osteitis—likely the result of microscopic communications between the residual pulp and the oral cavity. Association of periapical inflammatory disease with noncarious teeth is an important feature for recognition of this particular entity. In type II dentin dysplasia, obliteration of the pulp chamber (Fig. 19.36) and reduction in the calibers of the root canals occur after eruption (at least by 5 or 6 years), in contrast with type I dentin dysplasia. As the pulp chambers of the molars are narrowed by hypertrophic dentin, the pulp chambers may become flame or thistle shaped, and there may be multiple pulp stones. Occasionally, the anterior teeth and premolars develop a pulp chamber that is thistle tube in shape because of its extension into the root. The roots of the coronal variety are normal in shape and proportions.

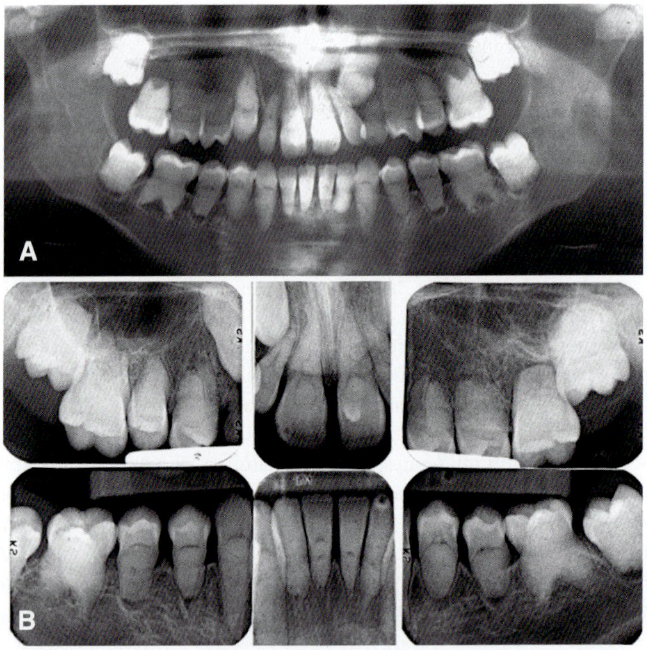

Fig. 19.35 Panoramic (A) and periapical (B) images of the same patient show the short, poorly developed roots; obliterated pulp chambers and root canals; and rarefying osteitis associated with type I (radicular) dentin dysplasia. Note the half-moon or "demilune" shape of the pulp chambers.

Differential interpretation. The differential interpretation for dentin dysplasia includes only dentinogenesis imperfecta because both abnormalities can appear clinically similar. Both entities can produce crowns with altered color and obliterated pulp chambers. The finding of a thistle tube–shaped pulp chamber in a single-rooted tooth strengthens the probability of dentin dysplasia. However, in type II dentin dysplasia, the pulp chambers become obliterated after eruption.

Sometimes crown size can help distinguish between the two. The teeth in dentinogenesis imperfecta typically have bulbous-shaped crowns with a constriction in the cervical region, whereas the crowns in dentin dysplasia are usually of normal shape, size, and proportion. If the roots are short and narrow, the condition is likely to be dentinogenesis imperfecta. Normal-appearing roots or practically no roots at all should suggest dentin dysplasia. Periapical rarefying osteitis in association with noncarious teeth is more commonly seen in dentin dysplasia.

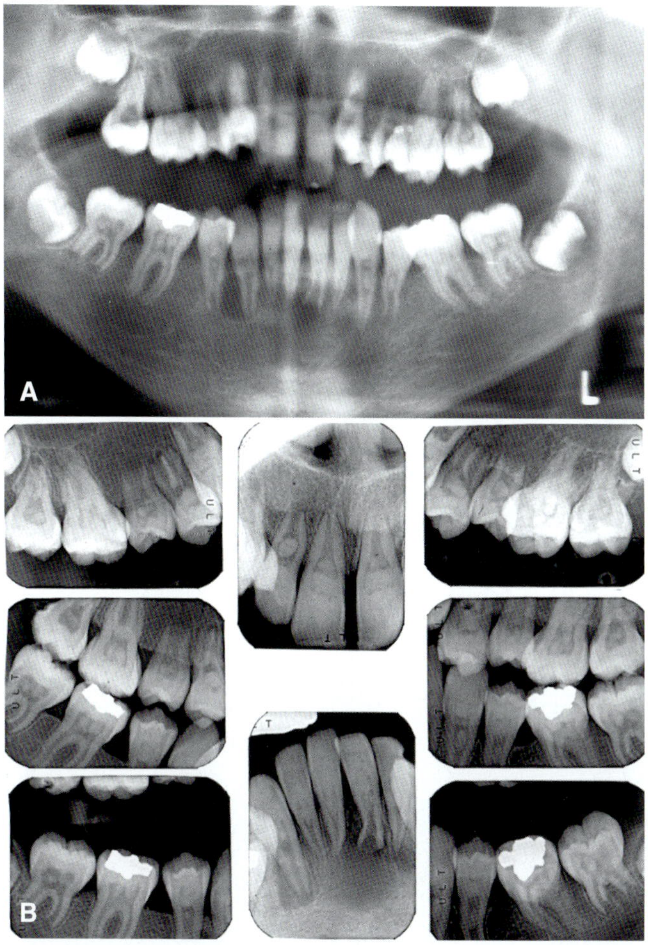

Fig. 19.36 Panoramic (A) and periapical (B) images of the same patient show obliteration of the pulp chamber, reduction in the caliber of root canals, and pulp stones obscuring the flame-shaped or thistle-shaped pulp chambers associated with type II (coronal) dentin dysplasia. Note the areas of rarefying osteitis associated with some of the mandibular anterior teeth.

Management. Teeth with type I dentin dysplasia have such poor bone support due to the short roots that prosthetic replacement is the only practical treatment. Teeth that are of normal shape, size, and support (type II) can have coronal coverage with fixed prosthodontic treatment, if they seem to be rapidly abrading. The esthetics of discolored anterior teeth can be improved by prosthetic treatment.

Regional Odontodysplasia

Disease mechanism. Regional odontodysplasia, or "ghost teeth," is a rare developmental disorder affecting dental tissues, which make both enamel and dentin hypoplastic and hypocalcified. The exact cause of this disorder is currently unknown. However, factors contributing to development of the disorder may include localized trauma, radiation, or a vascular issue. Some cases may suggest a possible genetic component, as it may occur more than once in a family, but in general, the etiology is unclear. The condition results in abnormal growth, calcification, and eruption of teeth. This localized arrest in tooth development typically affects only a few adjacent teeth in a quadrant—ergo the term "regional." These teeth may be either primary or permanent. If the primary teeth are affected, their successors are usually also involved.

Clinical features. Teeth affected with regional odontodysplasia are small and mottled brown as a result of staining of the hypocalcified and hypoplastic enamel. They are especially susceptible to caries, brittle, and subject to fracture and pulpal infection. Central incisors are most often affected, with lateral incisors and canines also occasionally exhibiting the defect (most often in the maxilla). Eruption of the defective teeth is often delayed, and in severe cases they may not erupt.

Imaging features. Because these teeth are very poorly mineralized, the images of teeth with regional odontodysplasia have been described as having a "ghost-like" appearance. The pulp chambers are large and the root canals are wide because the hypoplastic dentin is thin, serving just to outline the image of the root (Fig. 19.37). Also, the poorly outlined roots are short. The enamel likewise is thin and less dense than usual—sometimes so thin and poorly mineralized that it may not be evident on the image. The tooth is little more than a thin shell of hypoplastic enamel and dentin. Teeth that do not erupt are so hypomineralized and hypoplastic that they appear to be resorbing.

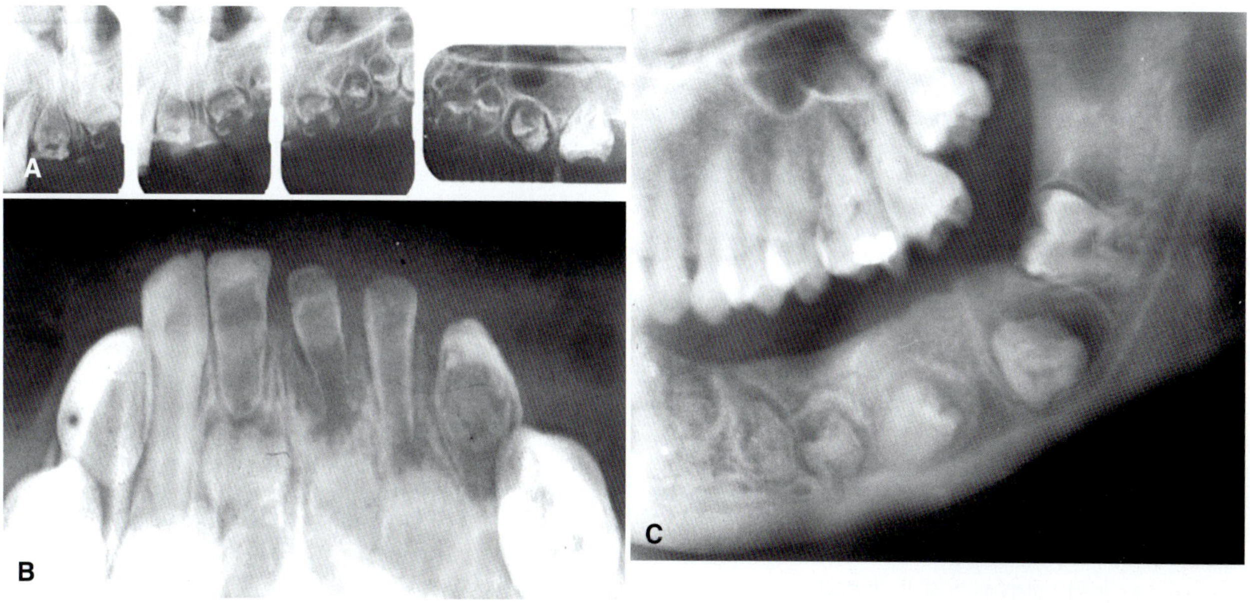

Fig. 19.37 Periapical (A), anterior occlusal (B), and cropped panoramic (C) images show the regional nature of tooth involvement in regional odontodysplasia. Note the lack of eruption and hypoplasia of enamel and dentin expressed mainly as short roots.

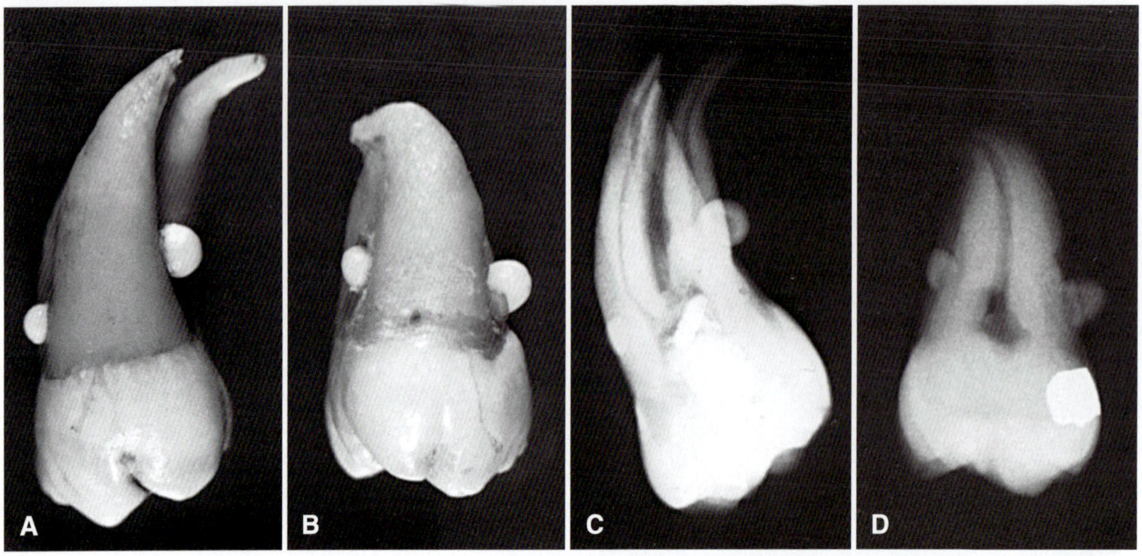

Fig. 19.38 Extracted teeth (A and B) and planar images (C and D) of enamel pearls. (Courtesy Dr. R. Kienholz, Dallas, TX.)

Differential interpretation. The malformed teeth occasionally seen in one of the expressions of dentinogenesis imperfecta occasionally may be confused with teeth in regional odontodysplasia. Only a few teeth of either dentition in an isolated segment of the arch are affected in regional odontodysplasia, whereas dentinogenesis imperfecta that resembles regional odontodysplasia is generalized. In addition, the enamel in regional odontodysplasia is hypoplastic, which is not the case in dentinogenesis imperfecta. Finally, the fact that the dentinogenesis imperfecta trait usually carries a history of familial involvement, in contrast to regional odontodysplasia (which is not hereditary), is another important distinguishing feature.

Management. With the advent of newer restorative materials, it is recommended to retain and restore the affected teeth as much as possible. Unerupted teeth should be retained during the period of skeletal growth. Severely damaged permanent teeth with pulpal involvement may require extraction and replacement.

Enamel Pearl

Disease mechanism. The enamel pearl or enameloma is a small formation of enamel 1–3 mm in diameter that can be found on the roots of deciduous and permanent teeth in or near the furcation areas of molar teeth, particularly the maxillary second or third molars (Fig. 19.38). Enamel pearls can be identified in approximately 3% of the population, probably formed by cells in the Hertwig epithelial root sheath before the epithelium loses its enamel-forming potential. Usually only one pearl develops, but occasionally more may develop. Enamel pearls may have a core of dentin and rarely a pulp horn extending from the chamber of the host tooth.

Clinical features. Most enamel pearls form apical to the gingival crest and are not detected during a clinical examination. They typically develop in or near the furcal areas of molar teeth, often lying at or just apical to the cementoenamel junction. Enamel pearls that form on the maxillary molars are usually in the mesial or distal furca, and pearls that develop in mandibular molars are located in the buccal or lingual furca. Usually no clinical symptoms are associated with their presence, although there may be a predisposition to the formation of a periodontal pocket.

Imaging features. The enamel pearl appears smooth, round, and comparable in degree of radiopacity to the enamel covering the crown (Figs. 19.39 and 19.40). Occasionally the dentin casts a small, round, radiolucent image in the center of the radiopaque sphere of enamel. If projected over the crown, it may be obscured.

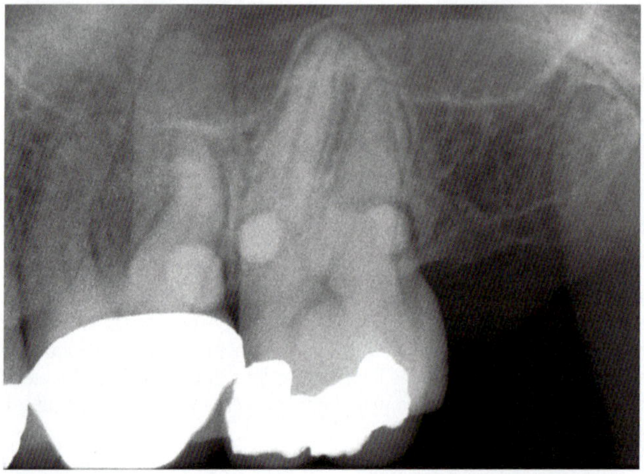

Fig. 19.39 Three enamel pearls (one attached to the first molar and two on the second molar) are apparent in this periapical image.

Differential interpretation. It is possible to mistake an enamel pearl for an isolated piece of calculus or a pulp stone. The differentiation between a pulp stone and an enamel pearl can be made by increasing the vertical angle of projection to move the image of the enamel pearl away from the pulp chamber. If the radiopacity is calculus, it is usually clinically detectable. Occasionally, oblique views of maxillary or mandibular molars may cause superimposition of a portion of the roots in the region of the furcation, producing a density that appears similar to that of an enamel pearl. In this case, producing another image at a slightly different horizontal angle eliminates this radiopaque region.

Management. As a rule, the recognition that a radiopaque mass superimposed on the tooth is an enamel pearl precludes the necessity for treatment. The clinician can remove the mass if its location at the cementoenamel junction predisposes to periodontal disease. The possibility must always be considered that it may contain a pulp horn.

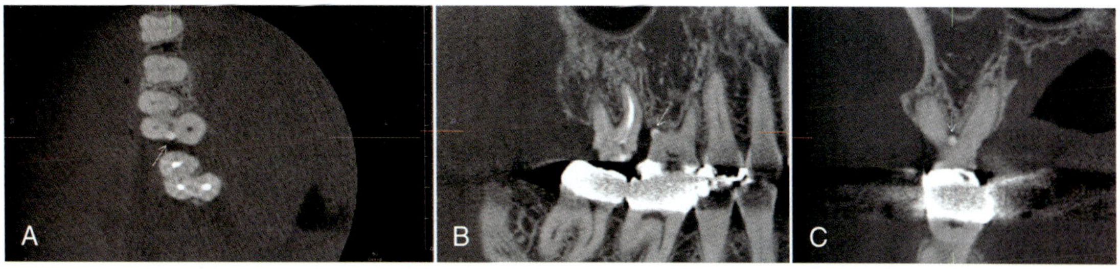

Fig. 19.40 Axial (A), corrected sagittal (B), and corrected coronal (C) cone beam computed tomographic images of an enamel pearl in the distal furcation of the maxillary right first molar resulting in furcation involvement (*arrows*).

Talon Cusp

Disease mechanism. The talon cusp is an anomalous hyperplasia of the cingulum of a maxillary or mandibular incisor, and the result is the formation of a supernumerary cusp. Normal enamel covers the cusp and fuses with the lingual aspect of the tooth. Any developmental grooves that are present may become caries-susceptible areas. The cusp may or may not contain an extension (horn) of the pulp. No apparent ethnic predilection exists.

Clinical features. The talon cusp is infrequently encountered. It may be found in either sex, and on both primary and permanent incisors. It varies in size from that of a prominent cingulum to a cusp-like structure extending to the level of the incisal edge. When viewed from its incisal edge, an incisor bearing the cusp is T shaped with the top of the incisal edge. Although it usually occurs as an isolated entity, its incidence has been reported to be increased in teeth related to cleft palate syndromes and in association with other anomalies.

Imaging features. The radiopaque image of a talon cusp is superimposed on that of the crown of the involved incisor (Fig. 19.41). The cuspal outline is smooth, and a layer of normal-appearing enamel is generally distinguishable. The image may not reveal a pulp horn. The cusp is often apparent before eruption and may simulate the presence of a supernumerary tooth.

Differential interpretation. The appearance of a talon cusp is quite distinctive. Although it may not be distinguishable from a supernumerary tooth with a single image, a second image with either the parallax or the buccal object technique can demonstrate continuity with the tooth.

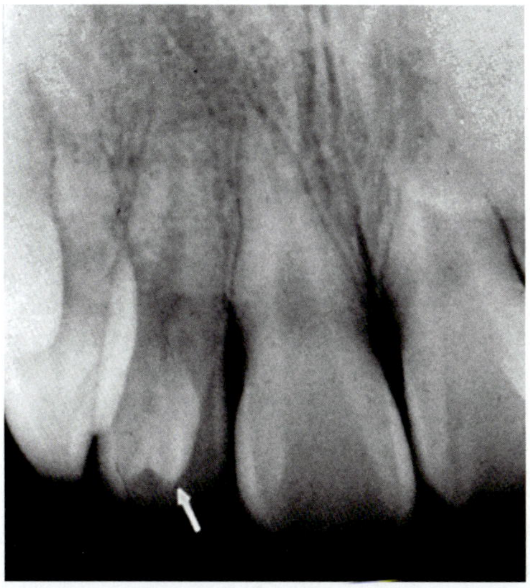

Fig. 19.41 Maxillary right lateral incisor bearing a talon cusp *(arrow)*. The tooth also has two enamel invaginations, one near the incisal edge and a second in the cingulum area. (Courtesy Dr. R. A. Cederberg, Dallas, TX.)

Management. If developmental grooves are present where the cusp fuses with the lingual surface of the incisor, treatment may be required to prevent the development of caries. If the cusp is large, it may pose an esthetic or occlusal problem. Slowly removing the cusp over a long period may stimulate the formation of secondary dentin and prevent exposure of a pulp horn.

Turner Hypoplasia

Disease mechanism. Turner hypoplasia, or Turner tooth, is a term used to describe a permanent tooth with a localized hypoplastic enamel defect. This defect may have been caused by the extension of periapical inflammatory disease from its deciduous predecessor, by mechanical trauma transmitted through the deciduous tooth or a protracted systemic illness affecting tooth mineralization. If the insult occurs while the crown is forming, it may adversely affect the ameloblasts of the developing tooth, and result in some degree of enamel hypoplasia or hypomineralization.

Clinical features. Turner hypoplasia most often affects the mandibular premolars, generally because of the relative susceptibility of the deciduous molars to caries, their proximity to the developing premolars, and their relative time of mineralization. The severity of the defect depends on the severity of the infection or mechanical trauma and on the stage of development of the permanent tooth. It may disturb matrix formation or calcification, in which case the result varies from a hypoplastic defect to a region of hypomineralization in the enamel. The hypomineralized area may become stained, and the tooth usually shows a brownish spot on the crown. If the insult is severe enough to cause hypoplasia, the crown may show pitting or a more pronounced defect.

Imaging features. The enamel irregularities associated with Turner hypoplasia alter the normal contours of the affected tooth and are often apparent on an image (Fig. 19.42). The involved region of the crown may appear as an ill-defined radiolucent region. A stained hypomineralized spot may not be apparent because of an insufficient difference in the degree of radiopacity between the spot and the crown of the tooth. Also, the hypomineralized areas may become remineralized by continued contact with saliva.

Differential interpretation. Other conditions that result in deformation of the tooth crown, such as the delivery of high-dose therapeutic radiation during tooth development should be considered, although usually several adjacent teeth are involved. Small defects may simulate the appearance of carious lesions but can be easily differentiated by clinical inspection.

Management. If an image of a tooth affected by Turner hypoplasia shows that the tooth has good root support, the esthetics and function of the deformed crown can be restored.

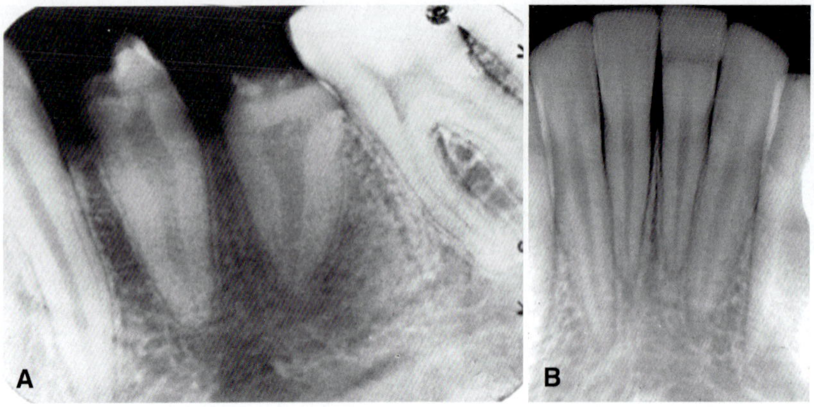

Fig. 19.42 Turner hypoplasia. Periapical images of the mandibular left premolar teeth (A) showing extensive malformation and hypomineralization of the crowns of the premolars. Periapical images of the mandibular incisors (B) shows a broad band of hypoplasia extending across the crown of the mandibular left central incisor.

Congenital Syphilis

Disease mechanism. Congenital syphilis is an infectious disease caused by *Treponema pallidum* transmitted by an infected mother to her baby during pregnancy or at birth. Late congenital syphilis is recognized within 2 or more years after birth. One of the main features is observed with the triad of Hutchinson, characterized by the presence of interstitial keratitis, eighth nerve deafness, and Hutchinson teeth. Approximately 30% of individuals with congenital syphilis have dental hypoplasia that involves the permanent incisors and first molars. Development of primary teeth is seldom disturbed. The affected incisors are called Hutchinson incisors and the molars are called "mulberry molars." The findings characteristic of the condition seem to result from degenerative changes in the enamel epithelium induced by the *T. pallidum* spirochete, leading to the complete destruction of the ameloblasts during odontogenesis. As a result, formation of abortive enamel and also cessation of enamel production occur. Premature loss of primary teeth associated with congenital syphilis has also been reported.

Clinical features. The affected incisor has a characteristic pointed or screwdriver-shaped crown, with the mesial and distal surfaces tapering from the middle of the crown to the incisal edge (Fig. 19.43). The effect is that the crown may be no wider mesiodistally than the cervical area of the tooth. The incisal edge is also frequently notched. Although maxillary central incisors usually demonstrate these syphilitic changes, the maxillary lateral and mandibular central incisors may also be involved.

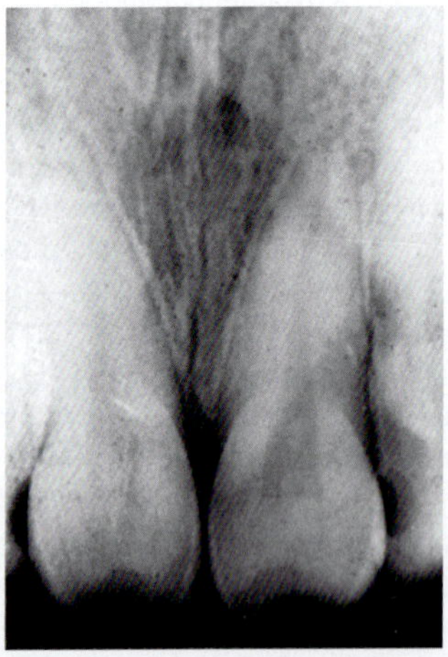

Fig. 19.43 Congenital syphilis may induce a developmental malformation of the maxillary central incisors referred to as "Hutchinson incisors." The abnormal morphology is characterized by tapering of the mesial and distal surfaces toward the incisal edge with notching of the incisal edge.

As with incisor crowns, the crowns of affected first molars are quite characteristic, usually smaller than normal, and may be even smaller than second molar crowns. The most distinctive feature is the constricted occlusal third of the crown, with the occlusal surface no wider than the cervical portion of the tooth. The cusps of these molars are also reduced in size and poorly formed. The enamel over the occlusal surface is hypoplastic, unevenly formed in irregular globules, similar to the surface of a mulberry, a small berry having an appearance similar to a blackberry.

Imaging features. The characteristic shapes of the affected incisor and molar crowns can be identified in the image. Because the crowns of these teeth form at about 1 year of age, images may reveal the dental features of congenital syphilis 4–5 years before the teeth erupt.

Management. Hutchinson teeth and mulberry molars often do not require dental treatment, although esthetic restorations may be used to correct the hypoplastic defects as indicated clinically.

ACQUIRED ABNORMALITIES

Acquired changes of the dentition—that is, changes that are initiated after development of the tooth—range in severity from changes that have no clinical significance to changes that cause tooth loss. In the latter case, early detection and treatment are required to preserve the tooth.

Attrition

Disease Mechanism

Attrition is physiologic wearing of the dentition resulting from occlusal contacts between the maxillary and mandibular teeth, and it can occur on the incisal, occlusal, and interproximal surfaces of the teeth. Interproximal wear causes the contact points to become broad and flat. Attrition occurs in more than 90% of young adults and is generally more severe in men than women. The extent of attrition depends on the abrasiveness of the diet, salivary factors, mineralization of the teeth, and stress. Physiologic attrition is also a component of the aging process. When the loss of dental tissue becomes excessive such as from bruxism, the attrition becomes pathologic.

Clinical Features

The tooth wear patterns from attrition are characteristic. Wear facets first appear on cusps, and marginal, oblique, and transverse ridges. The incisal edges of the maxillary and mandibular incisors show evidence of broadening. The wear facets on the occlusal surfaces of molars become more pronounced, with the lingual cusps of maxillary teeth and the buccal cusps of mandibular posterior teeth showing the most wear. When the dentin is exposed, it usually becomes stained, and the color contrast between stained dentin and enamel highlights the areas of attrition. The incisal edges of mandibular incisors tend to become pitted or "dished out" because the dentin wears more rapidly than its surrounding enamel. In the case of pathologic attrition, the patterns of wear are generally not as uniformly progressive as the patterns described for physiologic attrition. The wear facets develop at a faster rate. Moreover, attrition can be related to different cultural customs (dietary and otherwise) of a population.

Imaging Features

The imaging appearance of attrition results in a change in the normal outline of the tooth structure, altering the normal curved surfaces into flat planes. The crown is shortened in length and is bereft of the incisal or occlusal surface enamel (Fig. 19.44). Often many adjacent teeth in each arch show this wear pattern. Reduction in the size of the pulp chambers and canals may occur because attrition stimulates the deposition of secondary dentin. This secondary dentin may result in complete obliteration of the pulp chamber and canals. A simultaneous widening of the periodontal ligament space frequently occurs if the tooth is mobile. Occasionally, evidence of hypercementosis is present.

Differential Interpretation

Recognition of physiologic attrition is usually not difficult given the characteristic history, location, and extent of wear. The general pattern is predictable and familiar.

Management

Physiologic attrition does not generally require treatment unless the teeth become symptomatic or there is some cosmetic concern.

Abrasion

Abrasion is the nonphysiologic wearing of teeth as a result of increased friction produced when the tooth is in contact with a foreign material. A history or clinical examination usually reveals the cause. Although many causes exist, two occur with moderate frequency and can usually be eliminated: toothbrush and dental floss injury. In addition, a common magnifier of this effect is the abrasiveness associated with toothpaste ingredients. The particle size of the ingredients used in manufacturing toothpaste can lead to abrasion of the teeth. This, in combination with the hard bristles of a toothbrush, can cause more harm to the teeth than good. Other causes include pipe smoking, opening hairpins with the teeth, improper use of toothpicks, denture clasps, and cutting thread with the teeth.

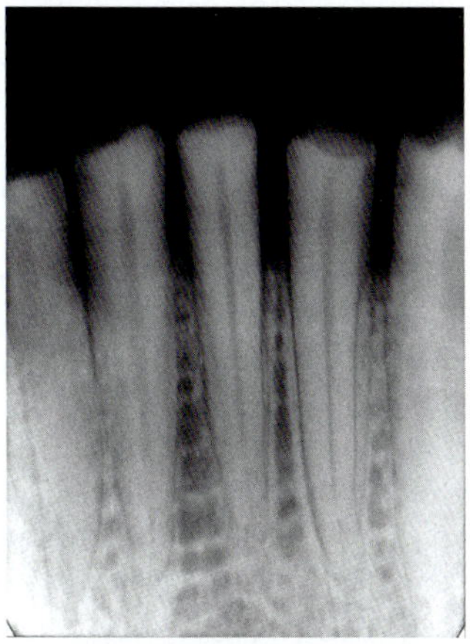

Fig. 19.44 Physiologic wear or attrition is demonstrated on this periapical image of the mandibular incisors.

Toothbrush Injury

Clinical features. Toothbrush abrasion is probably the most frequently observed type of injury to the dental hard tissues. The use of toothbrushes with hard bristles, or the improper horizontal "back-and-forth" movements of the toothbrush with heavy force can cause the bristles to create a V-shaped wedge defect into the cervical area of the tooth, usually involving enamel and the softer cementum.

Abraded teeth may become sensitive as the dentin is exposed. The abraded areas are usually most severe at the cementoenamel junction on the vestibular and labial surfaces of maxillary premolars, canines, and incisors, in approximately that order. The enamel generally limits the coronal extension of abrasion. The lesions are also more common and more pronounced on the left side for a right-handed person, and vice versa. The deposition of secondary dentin opposite the abraded areas usually keeps pace with the destruction at the surface, so pulpal exposure is rarely a complication.

Imaging features. The imaging appearance of toothbrush abrasion involves radiolucent defects at the cervical level of teeth. These defects have well-defined semicircular or semilunar shapes with borders of increasing radiopacity. The pulp chambers of the more seriously involved teeth are frequently partially or completely obliterated. The most common location of this injury is the premolar areas, usually in the upper arch.

Dental Floss Injury

Clinical features. Excessive and improper use of dental floss, particularly in conjunction with toothpaste, may result in abrasion of the dentition that presents as unusual irreversible notch-like lesions that often go undiagnosed (Fig. 19.45). The most frequent site is the cervical portion of the proximal surfaces, just above the gingiva.

Imaging features. The imaging appearance of dental floss abrasion is narrow semilunar radiolucency in the interproximal surfaces of the cervical area. Most often the radiolucent grooves on the distal surfaces of the teeth are deeper than the grooves on the mesial surfaces, probably

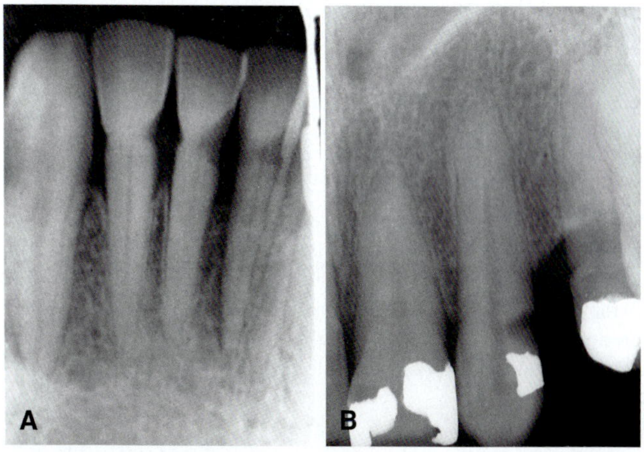

Fig. 19.45 (A) Abrasion of the cervical areas of these incisor teeth is evident from excessive (and improper) use of dental floss. Note the obliteration of the pulp chambers and reduction in size of the root canals. (B) Abrasion on the distal aspect of the maxillary canine from a denture clasp.

because it is easier to exert more pressure in a forward direction by pulling than by pushing the floss backward into the mouth.

Differential interpretation. Dental floss abrasion is readily identified by its clinical and imaging appearances. Its location provides some evidence regarding the nature of the cause. This can be verified by the patient history. Occasionally, the radiolucencies simulate carious lesions located at the cervical region of the tooth. The diagnosis can be confirmed by clinical inspection.

Management. The primary treatment recommended for abrasion is elimination of the causative agents or habits. Extensively abraded areas can be restored.

Erosion

Disease Mechanism

Erosion of teeth results from a chemical action not involving bacteria. Although in many cases the cause is not apparent, in others it is obviously the contact of acid with teeth. The source of the chemical may be acid from chronic vomiting or acid reflux from gastrointestinal disorders, eating disorders, or from a diet rich in acidic foods (e.g., citrus fruits, carbonated beverages). Eating disorders are associated with an increased risk of developing erosive lesions. In cases of bulimia, tooth erosion was 10 times more likely compared to healthy individuals. Regurgitated acids demineralize lingual or palatal tooth surfaces, and dietary acids primarily demineralize labial surfaces. Some occupations involve contact with acids that can induce dental erosion. The location of the erosion, the pattern of eroded areas, and the appearance of the lesion usually provide clues regarding the origin of the decalcifying agent. Additionally, it has been noted that in cases of xerostomia or hyposalivation the risk of dental erosion is also accentuated.

Clinical Features

Dental erosion usually affects incisors, often involving multiple teeth. The lesions are generally smooth, glistening depressions in the enamel surface, frequently near the gingiva. Erosion may result in so much loss of enamel that a pink spot shows through the remaining enamel.

Imaging Features

Areas of erosion appear as radiolucent defects on the crown. Their margins may be either well defined or diffuse. A clinical examination usually resolves any questionable lesions.

Differential Interpretation

The diagnosis of erosion is based on the clinical recognition of dished-out or V-shaped defects in the buccal and labial enamel and the dentinal surfaces. The margins of a restoration may project above the remaining tooth surface. The edges of lesions caused by erosion are usually more rounded off compared with lesions caused by abrasion.

Management

As with abrasion, erosion is managed with identification and removal of the causative agent. If the cause is chronic vomiting from an eating disorder, a daily fluoride rinse should be prescribed during counseling therapy. If the cause is unknown, management depends solely on restoration of the defect. Restoration prevents additional damage, possible pulp exposure, and objectionable esthetic appearance.

Resorption

Resorption is the removal of tooth structure by osteoclast-like cells, referred to as odontoclasts when they resorb tooth structure. Resorption is classified as internal or external on the basis of the surface of the tooth being resorbed. External resorption affects the outer surface of the tooth, and internal resorption affects the pulp chamber and root canal walls. These two types differ in their imaging appearance and treatment. The resorption discussed here is not that associated with the normal physiologic process that affects deciduous teeth. Although the etiology of most resorptive lesions is unknown, at least presumptive evidence exists that some lesions are the sequelae of chronic inflammation, excessive pressure and function, or adjacent tumors and cysts.

Internal Resorption

Disease mechanism. Internal resorption occurs within the pulp chamber or root canal system, and involves focal resorption of the adjacent dentin wall. This form of resorption results in a localized enlargement to the size of the pulp space at the expense of tooth structure, and may be transient and self-limiting, or progressive. The etiology of the recruitment and activation of odontoclasts is unknown but may be related to inflammation within the pulp. Internal resorption has been reported to be influenced by several potential predisposing factors including traumatic dental injuries, direct and indirect pulp capping, pulpotomy, and enamel invagination.

Clinical features. Internal resorption may affect any tooth in either the primary or the secondary dentitions. It occurs most frequently in permanent teeth, usually in central incisors, and first and second molars. The resorptive process most commonly begins during the fourth and fifth decades, and is more common in men. When the lesion originates in the pulp chamber of the crown, a radiolucent area may appear within the crown. If the enlarging pulp perforates the dentin and the enamel becomes involved, the area may appear clinically as a pink spot. If the condition is not intercepted, it may perforate the crown, with hemorrhagic tissue projecting from the perforation, and lead to pulpitis. When the lesion occurs in the root of a tooth, it is, for the most part, clinically silent. If resorption is extensive, it may weaken the tooth and result in fracture. It is also possible that the pulp may expand into the periodontal ligament space, and communicate with a deep periodontal pocket or the gingival sulcus, leading to pulpal inflammation.

Imaging features. Images can reveal symptomless early lesions of internal resorption. The lesions are localized; radiolucent; and round, oval, or elongated within the root or crown and are continuous with the image of the pulp chamber or root canal. These changes are now easily demonstrated using high resolution, limited, or small FOV CBCT. The outline is usually sharply defined and smooth or slightly scalloped. The result is an irregular widening of the pulp chamber or canal (Fig. 19.46). It is characteristically homogeneously radiolucent, without bony trabeculation or pulp stones. However, the internal structure may seem to be apparent if the surface of the resorbed tooth structure is very irregular and has a scalloped texture. In some cases, virtually the entire pulp chamber or root canal space may become involved, although more commonly the lesion remains localized (Fig. 19.47).

Differential interpretation. The most common lesions that can be confused with internal root resorption are dental caries on the buccal or lingual surface of a tooth and external root resorption. Carious lesions have more diffuse borders than lesions caused by internal root resorption. Clinical inspection quickly reveals caries on the buccal or lingual surface of a tooth. In addition, the mesial and distal surfaces of the pulp chamber and canal can usually be separated from the borders of the carious lesion. However, with internal root resorption, the image of the resorption cannot be separated from the pulp chamber or canal by altering the horizontal angulation of the x-ray beam.

Management. The management of internal resorption depends on the condition of the tooth. Prompt identification and management is important and is supported by annual clinical (pulp testing, etc.) and radiographic (periapical radiographs and/or CBCT) monitoring to

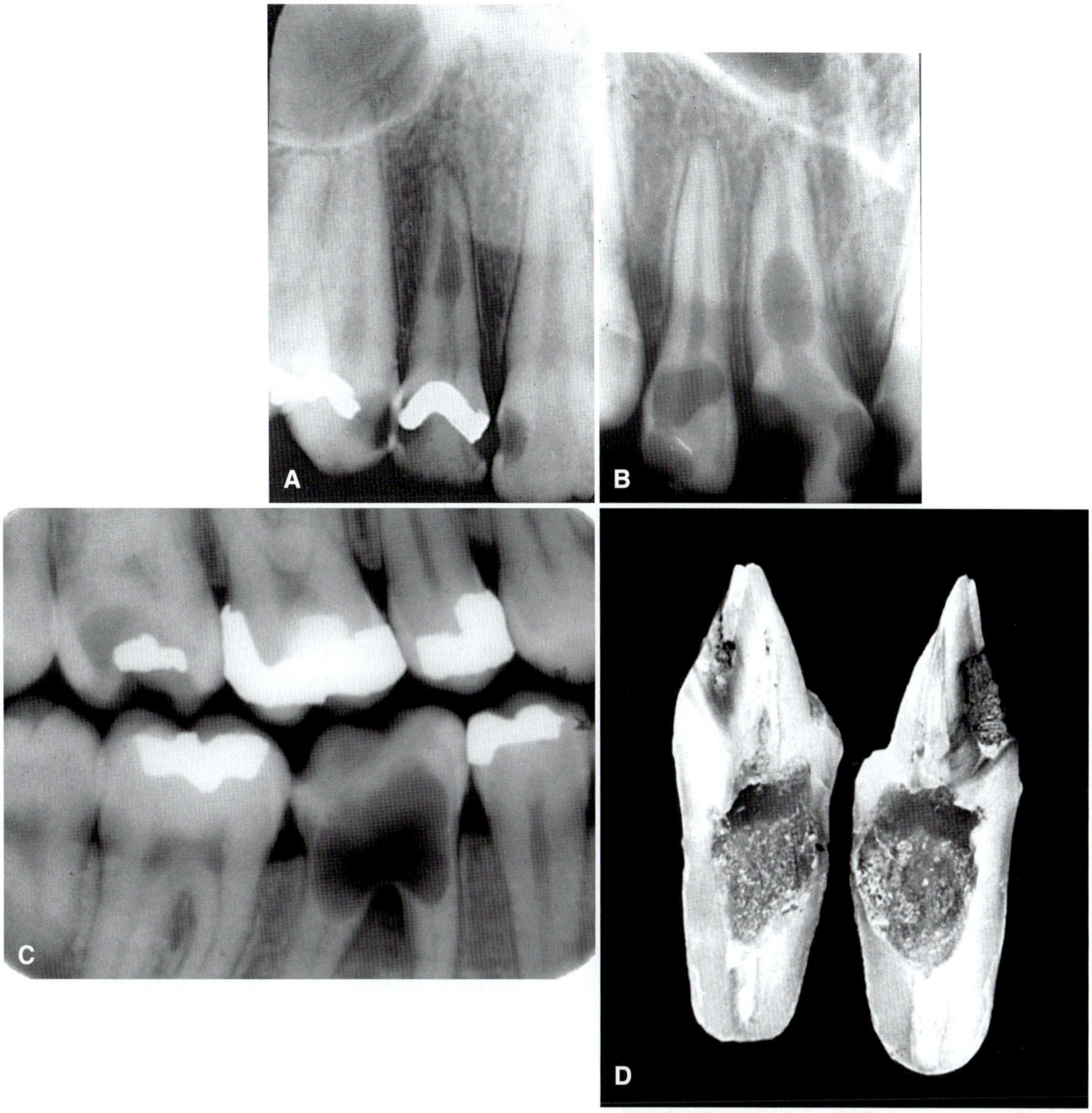

Fig. 19.46 Periapical (A and B) and bitewing images show internal resorption centered in the root canal system. Sectioned gross specimens (C and D) show internal resorption affecting both the crown and the roots in an incisor after crown reduction.

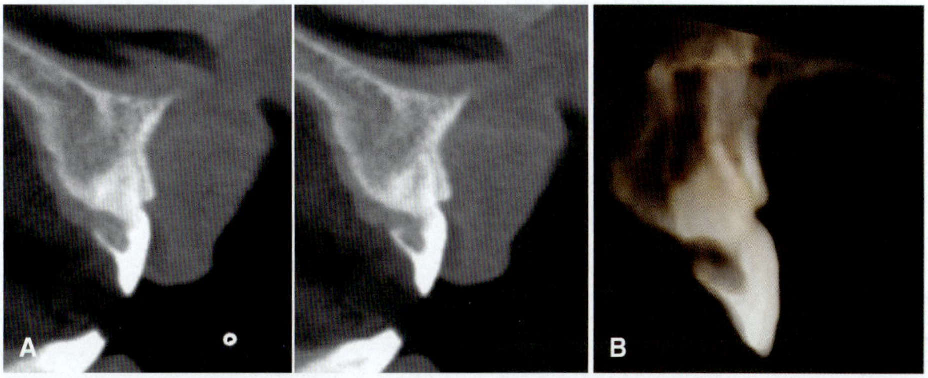

Fig. 19.47 (A) Cone beam computed tomographic cross-sectional images demonstrate an area of external resorption (invasive cervical resorption) affecting the palatal surface of the crown of a maxillary central incisor at the cementoenamel junction and proceeding internally into the tooth crown. (B) Three-dimensional surface rendering of the maxillary central incisor shows the resorptive defect on the palatal aspect of the tooth.

ensure early detection of possible complications. If the process has not led to a serious weakening defect in the structure, endodontic treatment halts the resorption. If the expanding pulp has not structurally compromised the tooth but a perforation of the root has occurred, the perforated surface may be surgically exposed and retrofilled. If the tooth has been badly resorbed and weakened by the resorption, extraction may be the only alternative. There is a lack of strong evidence for regenerative endodontic procedures for the management of internal root resorption.

External Resorption

Disease mechanism. In external resorption, odontoclasts resorb the outer surface of the tooth. This resorption most commonly involves the root surface but may also involve the cervical area of the tooth (invasive cervical resorption) or the crown of an unerupted tooth. The resorption may involve the dentin and cementum, and in some cases gradually extends to the pulp. Because the recruitment of odontoclasts requires an intact blood supply, only sections of the tooth with soft tissue coverage are susceptible to this resorption. This resorption may occur to a single tooth, multiple teeth, or in rare cases, all of the dentition. In many cases, the etiology is unknown, but many cases could very well be influenced by pressure exerted by trauma (luxation injuries), reimplanted teeth, orthodontic treatment, excessive occlusal forces, adjacent impacted teeth, a cyst, or a tumor.

Clinical features. External resorption is usually not recognized because often no characteristic signs or symptoms exist. Even when considerable loss of tooth structure occurs, the tooth in question is frequently firm and immobile in the dental arch. In advanced resorption, some nonspecific pain or fracture of the resorbed root occurs.

External resorption may appear at the apex of the tooth or on the lateral root surface, although it most commonly occurs in the apical and cervical regions. It is slightly more prevalent in mandibular teeth than in maxillary teeth and involves primarily the central incisors, canines, and premolars. External root resorption is common. One study of men and women 18–25 years old found that all patients exhibited some degree of external root resorption in four or more teeth.

Imaging features. Prior to potential management, a limited or small FOV CBCT is desirable to assess the nature of resorption as well as possible root canal perforation which could be easily missed by planar imaging. Common sites for external root resorption are the apical and cervical regions. When the resorptive event begins at the apex, it generally causes a smooth loss of tooth structure, resulting in blunting of the root apex (Fig. 19.48). Almost always, the bone and lamina dura follow the resorbing root and exhibit a normal appearance around this shortened structure—that is, the lamina dura and periodontal ligament space are preserved. When external root resorption occurs as the result of a periapical inflammatory disease, the lamina dura and periodontal ligament space are lost around the apex. After normal apexification (constriction of the walls of the pulp canal at the apex) of the pulp canal, it is very difficult or impossible to see the canal exit at the apex of the tooth. However, if resorption of the apical region has occurred, the pulp canal is visible and is abnormally wide at the apex.

Occasionally, external root resorption can involve the lateral surfaces of roots (Fig. 19.49). Such lesions tend to be irregular, may involve one side more than the other, and occur in any tooth.

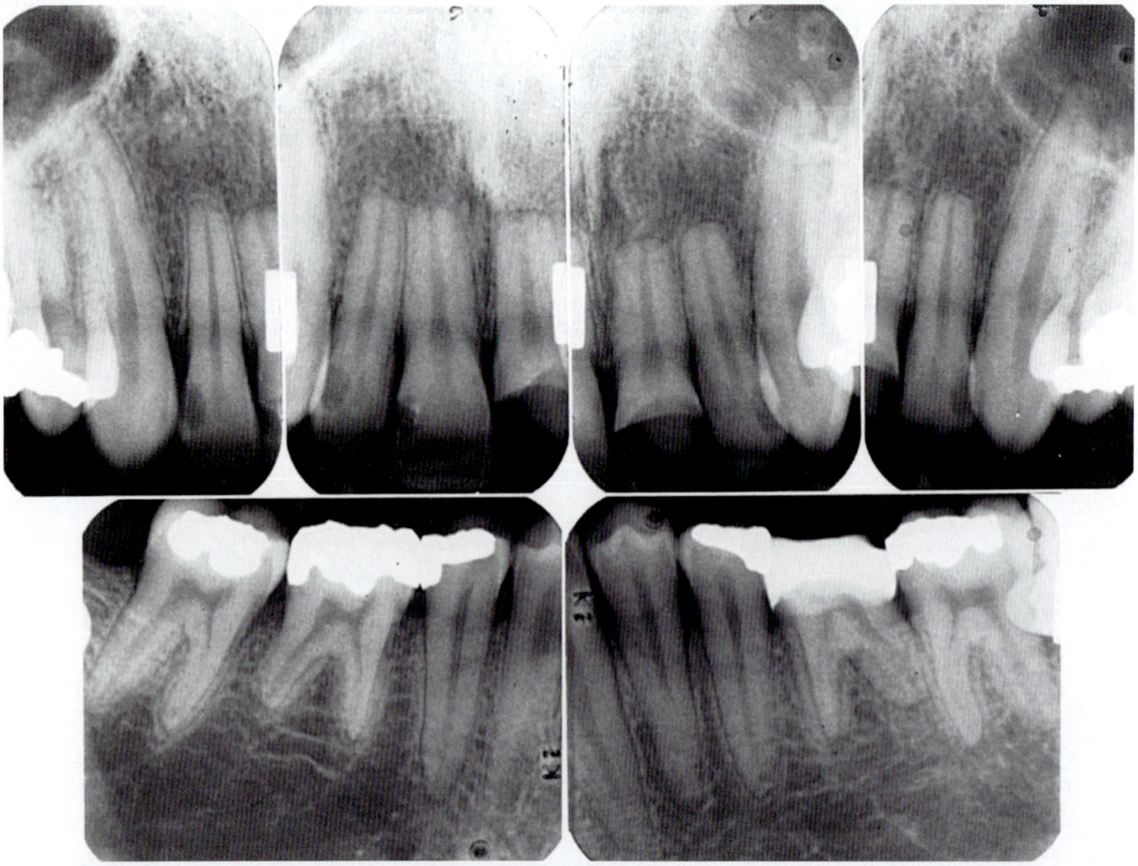

Fig. 19.48 External root resorption results in a loss of tooth structure from the apex. Note the blunted root apices, the widened pulp root canals, and the intact lamina dura.

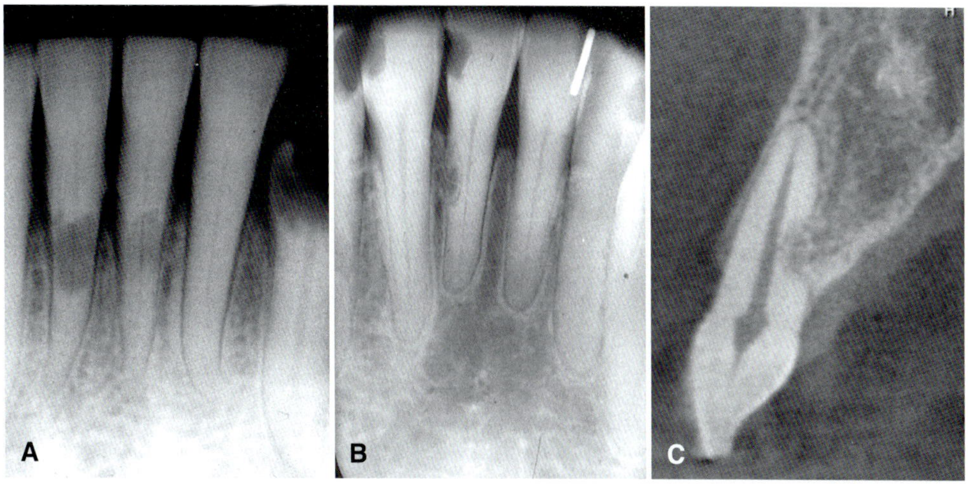

Fig. 19.49 External root resorption depicted as sharply defined radiolucencies confined to the root surfaces of the mandibular central incisors (A and B). In (B), the root has been replaced by an ingrowth of bone. This is sometimes referred to as inostosis. Corrected sagittal cone beam computed tomographic image (C) showing inostosis involving the palatal root surface of a maxillary incisor.

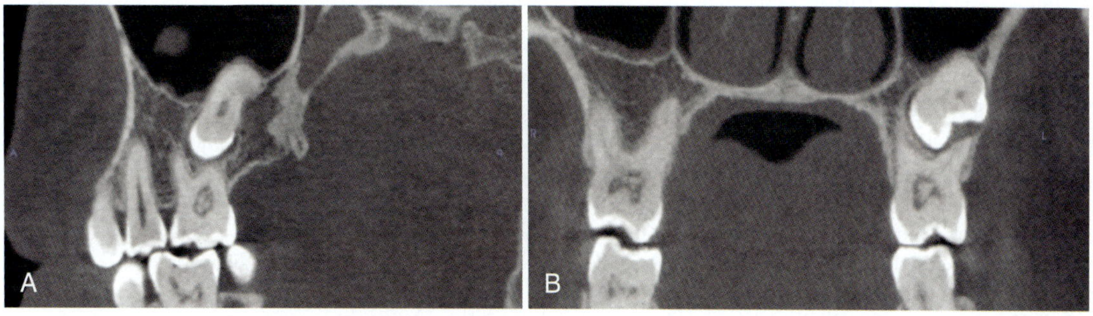

Fig. 19.50 Corrected sagittal (A) and coronal (B) cone beam computed tomographic images of external resorption involving the distobuccal root of a maxillary left first molar.

A common cause of external resorption on the side of a root is the presence of an unerupted adjacent tooth. Examples of external root resorption include resorption of the distal surfaces of the roots of a maxillary second molar by the crown of the adjacent third molar, and resorption of the root of a permanent central or lateral incisor, or both, by an unerupted maxillary canine (Fig. 19.50). External resorption of an entire tooth can occur when the tooth is unerupted and completely embedded in bone (Fig. 19.51), usually involving the maxillary canine or third molar. In such instances, the entire tooth, including the root and crown, may undergo resorption. Mandibular molar tooth roots can also become externally resorbed in the presence of an adjacent dense bone island; however, the resorption is self-limiting.

Differential interpretation. External root resorption on the apex or lateral surface of a root is easily visualized with imaging. When the lesion lies on the buccal or lingual surface of a root, and coronal to the adjacent bone, the differential interpretation includes caries and internal resorption. Internal resorption characteristically appears as a focal enlargement of the pulp chamber or root canal. In the case of external resorption, the image of the normal intact pulp chamber or canal may be traced through the radiolucent area of external resorption. Also, images made at different angles can be compared. The location of the radiolucency caused by external root resorption moves with respect to the pulp chamber, whereas the image of internal resorption remains fixed to the canal.

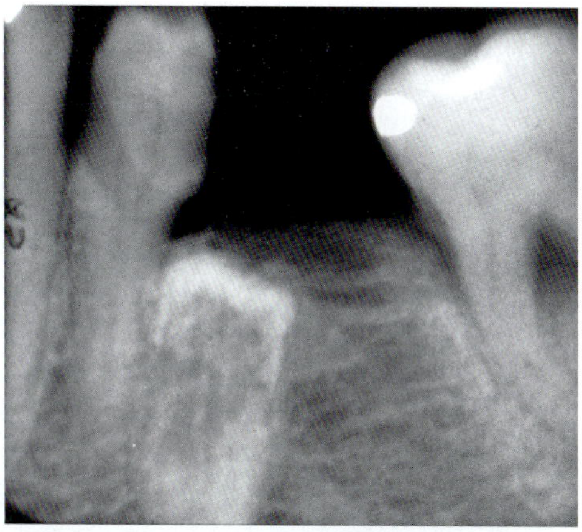

Fig. 19.51 External resorption of an impacted second premolar. Although both enamel and dentin have been resorbed, the residual enamel of the crown can still be seen, as well as a hint of a pulp chamber.

Management. When the cause of external root resorption is known, the treatment is usually to remove the etiologic factors. Treatment may involve cessation of excessive mechanical forces, surgical management of an adjacent impacted tooth, cyst, tumor, or source of inflammation. If the area of resorption is broad and on an accessible surface of the root (e.g., in a cervical location), curettage of the defect and the placement of a restoration usually stops the process.

Secondary Dentin

Mechanism

Secondary dentin is dentin deposited in the pulp chamber after the formation of primary dentin has been completed. Secondary dentin deposition may be part of physiologic aging, or it may result from more innocuous stimuli as chewing or minor trauma. Secondary dentin can also develop after long-term trauma from pathologic conditions such as moderately progressive caries, trauma, erosion, attrition, abrasion, or a dental restorative procedure. This specific stimulus promotes a more rapid and localized coronal response than that seen during normal aging. The term tertiary dentin has been suggested to identify dentin specifically initiated by nonphysiologic stimuli—that is, stimuli other than the normal aging response or normal biologic function.

Clinical Features

The response of odontoblasts in producing secondary dentin reduces the sensitivity of teeth to stimuli from the external environment. In elderly individuals with extensive secondary dentin formation, this reduced sensitivity may be especially pronounced. Similarly, the formation of an additional layer of dentin between the pulp and a region of insult reduces the sensitivity often felt by individuals with recent dental restorations or coronal fractures.

Imaging Features

Secondary dentin is indistinguishable from primary dentin on imaging. Its presence is manifested as a reduction in size of the normal pulp chamber and root canal (Fig. 19.52). When secondary dentin arises from the normal aging process, the result is a generalized reduction in pulp chamber area or volume and root canal caliber, maintaining a relatively normal shape. Often there remains only a thin, narrow pulp chamber and canal. The pulp horns usually disappear relatively early, followed by a reduction in size of the pulp chamber and narrowing of the canals. When more specific stimuli initiate secondary dentin formation, it begins in the region adjacent to the source of stimuli and alters the normal shape of the pulp chamber. Although formation of secondary dentin may continue until the pulp appears to be completely obliterated, histologic studies show that even in these extreme cases, a small thread of viable pulp tissue remains.

Differential Interpretation

Secondary dentin is recognized indirectly by the reduction in size of the pulp chamber. This appearance differs from that of the pulp stone. The pulp stone (see the following description) simply occupies some pulp chamber or canal space, but it has a round-to-oval shape (conforming to the chamber).

Management

Secondary dentin deposition per se does not require treatment. The precipitating cause is removed if possible, and the tooth is restored when appropriate.

Pulp Stones

Mechanism

Pulp stones are foci of calcification in the dental pulp. They are probably apparent microscopically in more than half of teeth of young people, and in almost all teeth of those older than 50 years. Although most are microscopic, they vary in size, with some 2 or 3 mm in diameter, almost filling the pulp chamber. Only larger pulp stones can be visualized on imaging. Although the larger stones represent only 15%–25% of pulpal calcification, they are a common imaging finding and may appear in a single tooth or several teeth. Their cause is unknown, and no firm evidence exists that they are associated with any systemic or pulpal disturbance. However, a significant association of orthodontic treatment with changes in pulp cavity volume and increased incidence of pulp stones was observed.

Clinical Features

Pulp stones are not clinically discernible.

Imaging Features

The imaging appearance of pulp stones is quite variable. They may be seen as radiopaque structures within pulp chambers or root canals, or they may extend from the pulp chamber into the root canals (Fig. 19.53). No uniform shape or number exists. They may occur as a single dense mass or as several small radiopacities. They may be round

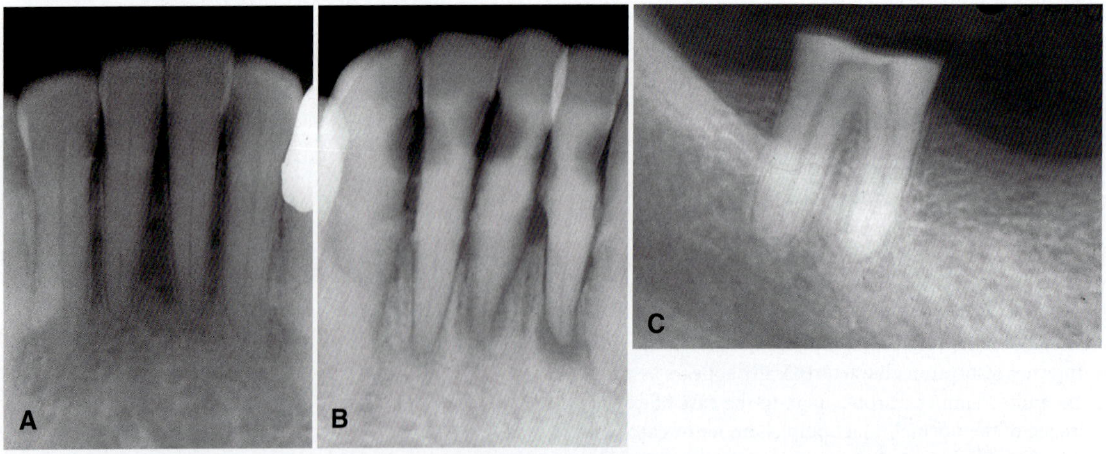

Fig. 19.52 Periapical images show normal formation of secondary dentin, causing recession of the pulp chamber and narrowing of the root canals of the mandibular incisor teeth (A). Secondary dentin has obliterated the pulp chambers and narrowed the root canals (B). This is likely a result of the carious lesions. Secondary dentin formation has obliterated the pulp chamber stimulated by the severe attrition of the coronal aspect of this molar (C).

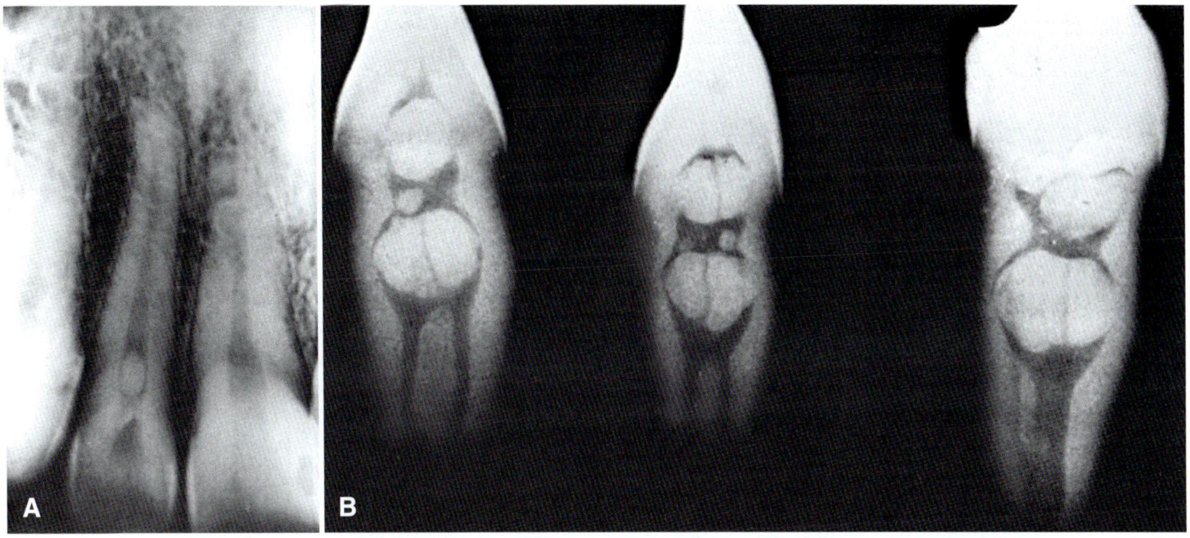

Fig. 19.53 Periapical image of pulp stones seen as isolated calcifications in the pulp. (A) Periapical radiograph shows a pulp stone in the coronal third of the root canal of the lateral incisor. (B) Planar images of extracted teeth show large pulp stones causing deformation of the pulp chamber and root canals.

or oval, and some pulp stones that potentially occupy most of the pulp chamber conform to its shape. Their outline likewise varies from sharply defined to a more diffuse margin. They occur in all tooth types but are most common in molars. In rare instances, the canal remodels and increases its girth to accommodate a large stone.

Differential Interpretation

Although pulp stones are variable in size and form, their recognition is usually not difficult. However, in some cases, differentiation from pulpal sclerosis is difficult.

Management

Pulp stones do not require treatment; however, when endodontic treatment is being considered for a tooth with pulp stones, careful planning to understand the location and extent is important for successful endodontic therapy. Small FOV CBCT is being used increasingly to preoperatively evaluate teeth with pulp stones undergoing endodontic treatment.

Pulpal Sclerosis

Mechanism

Pulpal sclerosis is another form of calcification in the pulp chamber and canals of teeth. In contrast to pulp stones, pulpal sclerosis is a diffuse process. Its specific cause is unknown, although its appearance correlates strongly with age. About 66% of all teeth in individuals 10–20 years old and 90% of all teeth in individuals 50–70 years old show histologic evidence of pulpal sclerosis. Histologically, the pattern of calcification is amorphous and unorganized, being evident as linear strands or columns of calcified material paralleling blood vessels and nerves in the pulp.

Clinical Features

Pulpal sclerosis is a clinically silent process without clinical manifestations.

Imaging Features

Early pulpal sclerosis, a degenerative process, is not demonstrable on imaging. Diffuse pulpal sclerosis produces a generalized, ill-defined collection of fine radiopacities throughout large areas of the pulp chamber and pulp canals (Fig. 19.54).

Differential Interpretation

The differential diagnosis includes small pulp stones, but this differentiation is academic because neither pulpal sclerosis nor pulp stones require treatment.

Management

Pulpal sclerosis does not require treatment. Pulp stones and pulpal sclerosis become important when endodontic therapy is indicated for other reasons.

Hypercementosis

Disease Mechanism

Hypercementosis is a complex and not yet well-defined condition, and generally refers to the excessive deposition of cementum on a tooth root. In most cases, its cause is unknown. Some forms of hypercementosis may be specific to a given etiology. Occasionally, hypercementosis can appear on a supraerupted tooth after the loss of an opposing tooth or as a response to inflammation. In this context, cementum is deposited on the root surface adjacent to the apex and a focus or rarefying osteitis. Hypercementosis occasionally has been associated with teeth that are in hyperocclusion or that have been fractured. Finally, hypercementosis occurs in patients with Paget disease of bone (see Chapter 23) and with hyperpituitarism (gigantism and acromegaly).

Clinical Features

Hypercementosis does not cause any clinical signs or symptoms.

Imaging Features

Hypercementosis is evident on images as an excessive accumulation of cementum around all or part of a root (Fig. 19.55). The root outline is usually smooth but occasionally may be seen as an irregular but bulbous enlargement of the root. It is most evident in the apical thirds of tooth roots, and is usually seen as a mildly irregular accumulation of cementum. This cementum is slightly more radiolucent than dentin. Of importance is the fact that the lamina dura and periodontal ligament space encompass the enlarged root. In the case of Paget disease of bone, the hypercementosis is more generalized, and usually very exuberant and irregular in outline.

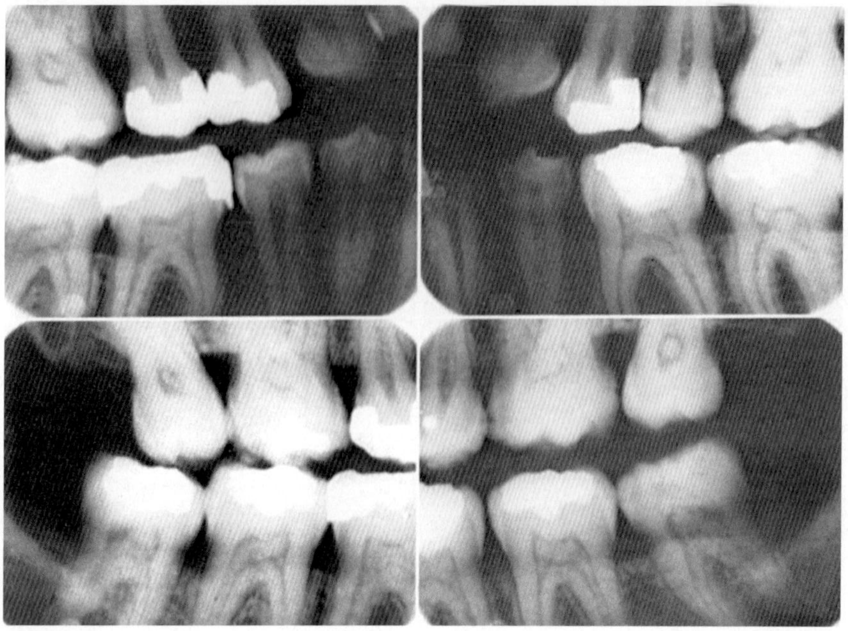

Fig. 19.54 Periapical images showing pulpal sclerosis as diffuse calcification of the pulp chamber and canals.

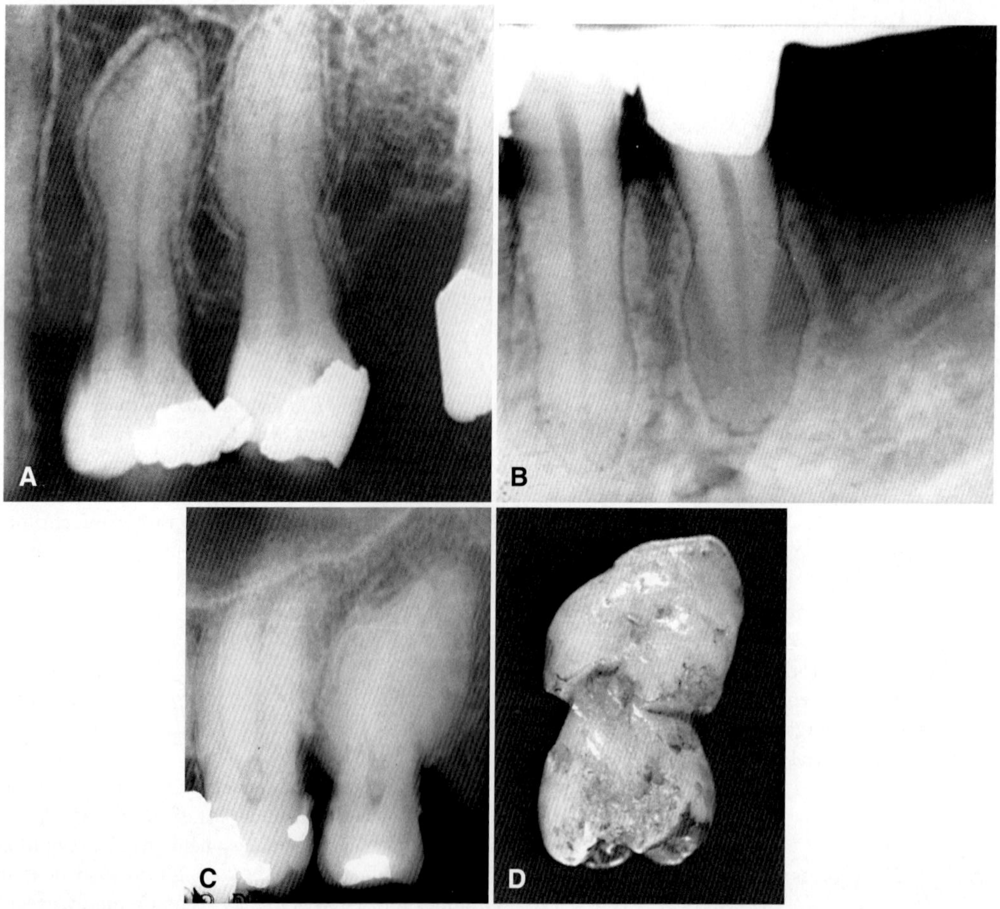

Fig. 19.55 Periapical images showing hypercementosis of the roots (A–C). In all cases, note the continuity of the lamina dura and the periodontal ligament space that encompasses the extra cementum. (D) An extracted molar exhibits extensive hypercementosis. (Courtesy Dr. R. Kienholz, Dallas, TX.)

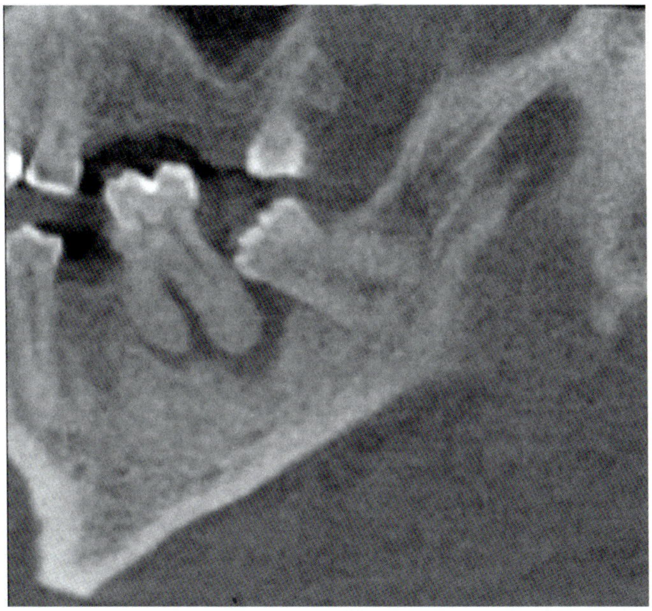

Fig. 19.56 Corrected sagittal cone beam computed tomographic image of hypercementosis involving the fully erupted mandibular left molar and associated bone loss.

Differential Interpretation

The differential interpretation may include any radiopaque structure that is seen within the vicinity of the root, such as a dense bone island or mature periapical osseous dysplasia. The differentiating characteristic is the presence of the periodontal ligament space around the hypercementosis. There may be a resemblance to a small cementoblastoma. Occasionally, a severely dilacerated root may have the appearance of hypercementosis.

Management

Hypercementosis requires no treatment. If a related condition, such as a periapical inflammatory disease, exists, treatment is necessary (Fig. 19.56). The primary significance of hypercementosis may relate to the difficulty that the root configuration can pose if extraction is indicated.

BIBLIOGRAPHY

Supernumerary Teeth

Ata-Ali F, Ata-Ali J, Peñarrocha-Oltra D, et al. Prevalence, etiology, diagnosis, treatment and complications of supernumerary teeth. *J Clin Exp Dent.* 2014;6:e414-e418. doi:10.4317/jced.51499.

Cammarata-Scalisi F, Avendaño A, Callea M. Main genetic entities associated with supernumerary teeth. *Arch Argent Pediatr.* 2018;116(6):437-444. doi:10.5546/aap.2018.eng.437.

Grahnen H, Lindahl B. Supernumerary teeth in the permanent dentition: a frequency study. *Odontol Revy.* 1961;12:290-294.

Grimanis GA, Kyriakides AT, Spyropoulos ND. A survey on supernumerary molars. *Quintessence Int.* 1991;22:989-995.

Lu X, Yu F, Liu J, et al. The epidemiology of supernumerary teeth and the associated molecular mechanism. *Organogenesis.* 2017;13:71-82. doi:10.1080/15476278.2017.1332554.

Rao SR. Supernumerary teeth. In: Bergsma D, eds. *Birth Defects Compendium.* 2nd ed. Alan R Liss; 1979.

Yusof WZ. Non-syndrome multiple supernumerary teeth: literature review. *J Can Dent Assoc.* 1990;56:147-149.

Developmentally Missing Teeth

Al-Ani AH, Antoun JS, Thomson WM, et al. Hypodontia: an update on its etiology, classification, and clinical management. *Biomed Res Int.* 2017;2017:9378325. doi:10.1155/2017/9378325.

Al-Emran S. Prevalence of hypodontia and developmental malformation of permanent teeth in Saudi Arabian school children. *Br J Orthod.* 1990; 17:115-118.

Baccetti T. A controlled study of associated dental anomalies. *Angle Orthod.* 1998;68(3):267-274. doi:10.1043/0003-3219(1998)068<0267:ACSOAD>2.3.CO;2.

Chung LK, Hobson RS, Nunn JH, Gordon PH, Carter NE. An analysis of the skeletal relationships in a group of young people with hypodontia. *J Orthod.* 2000;27(4):315-318. doi:10.1093/ortho/27.4.315.

Nieminen P. Genetic basis of tooth agenesis. *J Exp Zool B Mol Dev Evol.* 2009;312B(4):320-342. doi:10.1002/jez.b.21277.

O'Dowling IB, McNamara TG. Congenital absence of permanent teeth among Irish school-children. *J Ir Dent Assoc.* 1990;36:136-138.

Ogaard B, Krogstad O. Craniofacial structure and soft tissue profile in patients with severe hypodontia. *Am J Orthod Dentofacial Orthop.* 1995;108(5): 472-477. doi:10.1016/s0889-5406(95)70047-1.

Peck S, Peck L, Kataja M. Concomitant occurrence of canine malposition and tooth agenesis: evidence of orofacial genetic fields. *Am J Orthod Dentofacial Orthop.* 2002;122(6):657-660. doi:10.1067/mod.2002.129915.

Visioni AF, Lisboa-Costa TN, Pagnan NAB, et al. Ectodermal dysplasias: clinical and molecular review. *Am J Med Genet.* 2009;149A:1980-2002.

Macrodontia

Garn SM, Lewis AB, Kerewsky BS. The magnitude and implications of the relationship between tooth size and body size. *Arch Oral Biol.* 1968;13:129-131.

Koszowski R, Waśkowska J, Kucharski G, Śmieszek-Wilczewska J. Double teeth: evaluation of 10-years of clinical material. *Open Med.* 2014;9:254-263.

Mamdani S, Pathak D, Harrison M, Bhujel N. Macrodontia and double teeth: a review and case series. *Br Dent J.* 2023;234(5):315-321. doi:10.1038/s41415-023-5571-9.

Microdontia

Chen Y, Zhou F, Peng Y, et al. Non-syndromic occurrence of true generalized microdontia with hypodontia: a case report. *Medicine (Baltimore).* 2019;98(26):e16283. doi:10.1097/MD.0000000000016283.

Thomas C, Vaysse F, Courset T, et al. From child to adulthood, a multidisciplinary approach of multiple microdontia associated with hypodontia: case report relating a 15 year-long management and follow-up. *Healthcare (Basel).* 2021;9(9):1180. doi:10.3390/healthcare9091180.

Transposition

Schacter H. A treated case of transposed upper canine. *Dent Rec (London).* 1951;71:105-108.

Peck L, Peck S, Attia Y. Maxillary canine-first premolar transposition, associated dental anomalies and genetic basis. *Angle Orthod.* 1993;63(2):99-109. doi:10.1043/0003-3219(1993)063<0099:MCFPTA>2.0.CO;2.

Fusion

Hagman FT. Anomalies of form and number, fused primary teeth, a correlation of the dentitions. *ASDC J Dent Child.* 1988;55:359-361.

Sperber GH. Genetic mechanisms and anomalies in odontogenesis. *J Can Dent Assoc (Tor).* 1967;33:433-442.

Concrescence

Syed AZ, Alluri LC, Mallela D, et al. Concrescence: cone-Beam Computed Tomography Imaging Perspective. *Case Rep Dent.* 2016;2016:8597872. doi:10.1155/2016/8597872.

Gemination

Ferrazzano GF, Festa P, Cantile T, et al. Multidisciplinary approach to the treatment of double bilateral upper permanent incisors in a young boy. *Eur J Paediatr Dent.* 2017;18(2):94-98. doi:10.23804/ejpd.2017.18.02.02.

Grammatopoulos E. Gemination or fusion? *Br Dent J.* 2007;203:119-120. https://doi.org/10.1038/bdj.2007.699.

Tannenbaum KA, Alling EE. Anomalous tooth development: case report of gemination and twinning. *Oral Surg Oral Med Oral Pathol.* 1963;16:883-887.

Taurodontism

Haskova JE, Gill DS, Figueiredo JA, et al. Taurodontism-a review. *Dent Update.* 2009;36(4):235-236, 239-240, 243. doi:10.12968/denu.2009.36.4.235.

Pach J, Regulski PA, Tomczyk J, et al. Clinical implications of a diagnosis of taurodontism: a literature review. *Adv Clin Exp Med.* 2022;31(12): 1385-1389. doi:10.17219/acem/152120.

Dens in Dente

Oehlers FA. The radicular variety of dens invaginatus. *Oral Surg Oral Med Oral Pathol.* 1958;11:1251-1260.

Rushton MA. A collection of dilated composite odontomes. *Br Dent J.* 1937;63:65-86.

Soames JV, Kuyebi TA. A radicular dens invaginatus. *Br Dent J.* 1982;152:308-309.

Siqueira JF Jr, Rôças IN, Hernández SR, et al. Dens invaginatus: clinical implications and antimicrobial endodontic treatment considerations. *J Endod.* 2022;48(2):161-170. doi:10.1016/j.joen.2021.11.014.

Dens Invaginatus

Oehlers FA, Lee KW, Lee EC. Dens invaginatus (invaginated odontome): its structure and responses to external stimuli. *Dent Pract Dent Rec.* 1967;17:239-244.

Sykaras SN. Occlusal anomalous tubercle on premolars of a Greek girl. *Oral Surg Oral Med Oral Pathol.* 1974;38:88-91.

Yip WK. The prevalence of dens invaginatus. *Oral Surg Oral Med Oral Pathol.* 1974;38:80-87.

Gallacher A, Ali R, Bhakta S. Dens invaginatus: diagnosis and management strategies. *Br Dent J.* 2016;221:383-387. doi:10.1038/sj.bdj.2016.724.

Dens Evaginatus

Ponnambalam Y, Love RM. Dens evaginatus: case reports and review of the literature. *N Z Dent J.* 2006;102(2):30-34.

Molar-Incisor Malformation

Brusevold IJ, Bie TMG, Baumgartner CS, et al. Molar incisor malformation in six cases: description and diagnostic protocol. *Oral Surg Oral Med Oral Pathol Oral Radiol.* 2017;124(1):52-61. doi:10.1016/j.oooo.2017.03.050.

Kim JE, Hong JK, Yi WJ, et al. Clinico-radiologic features of molar-incisor malformation in a case series of 38 patients: a retrospective observational study. *Medicine (Baltimore).* 2019;98(40):e17356. doi:10.1097/MD.0000000000017356.

Lee HS, Kim SH, et al. A new type of dental anomaly: molar-incisor malformation (MIM). *Oral Surg Oral Med Oral Pathol Oral Radiol.* 2014;118(1): 101-109.e3. doi:10.1016/j.oooo.2014.03.014.

McCreedy C, Robbins H, Newell A, et al. Molar-incisor malformation: two cases of a newly described dental anomaly. *J Dent Child (Chic).* 2016;83:33-37.

Amelogenesis Imperfecta

Bailleul-Forestier I, Molla M, Verloes A, et al. The genetic basis of inherited anomalies of the teeth. Part 1: clinical and molecular aspects of non-syndromic dental disorders. *Eur J Med Genet.* 2008;51:273-291.

Crawford PJ, Aldred M, Bloch-Zupan A. Amelogenesis imperfecta. *Orphanet J Rare Dis.* 2007;2:17. doi:10.1186/1750-1172-2-17.

Gadhia K, McDonald S, Arkutu N, et al. Amelogenesis imperfecta: an introduction. *Br Dent J.* 2012;212(8):377-379. doi:10.1038/sj.bdj.2012.314.

Gasse B, Prasad M, Delgado S, et al. Evolutionary analysis predicts sensitive positions of MMP20 and validates newly- and previously-identified *MMP20* mutations causing amelogenesis imperfecta. *Front Physiol.* 2017;8:398. doi:10.3389/fphys.2017.00398.

Seymen F, Kim YJ, Lee YJ, et al. Recessive mutations in ACPT, encoding testicular acid phosphatase, cause hypoplastic amelogenesis imperfecta. *Am J Hum Genet.* 2016;99(5):1199-1205. doi:10.1016/j.ajhg.2016.09.018.

Witkop CJ Jr. Amelogenesis imperfecta, dentinogenesis imperfecta and dentin dysplasia revisited: problems with classification. *J Oral Pathol.* 1989;17: 547-553.

Wright JT. The molecular etiologies and associated phenotypes of amelogenesis imperfecta. *Am J Med Genet A.* 2006;140:2547-2555.

Dentinogenesis Imperfecta and Dentin Dysplasia

Chen D, Li X, Lu F, Wang Y, Xiong F, Li Q. Dentin dysplasia type I A dental disease with genetic heterogeneity. *Oral Dis.* 2019;25(2):439-446. doi:10.1111/odi.12861.

Kim JW, Simmer JP. Hereditary dentin defects. *J Dent Res.* 2007;86:292-299.

MacDougall M, Dong J, Acevedo AC. Molecular basis of human dentin diseases. *Am J Med Genet A.* 2006;140:2536-2546.

O Carroll MK, Duncan WK, Perkins TM. Dentin dysplasia: review of the literature and a proposed subclassification based on imaging findings. *Oral Surg Oral Med Oral Pathol.* 1991;72:119-125.

Regional Odontodysplasia

Crawford PJ, Aldred MJ. Regional odontodysplasia: a bibliography. *J Oral Pathol Med.* 1989;18:251-263.

Nijakowski K, Woś P, Surdacka A. Regional odontodysplasia: a systematic review of case reports. *Int J Environ Res Public Health.* 2022;19(3):1683. doi:10.3390/ijerph19031683.

Enamel Pearl

Meskin LH, Gorlin RJ. Agenesis and peg-shaped permanent lateral incisors. *J Dent Res.* 1963;42:1476-1479.

Moskow BS, Canut PM. Studies on root enamel, II: enamel pearls: a review of their morphology, localization, nomenclature, occurrence, classification, histogenesis, and incidence. *J Clin Periodontol.* 1990;17:275-281.

Natkin E, Pitts DL, Worthington P. A case of talon cusp associated with other odontogenic abnormalities. *J Endod.* 1983;9:491-495.

Rathva V. Ectopic enamel pearl. *Clin Pract.* 2012;2(2):e46. doi:10.4081/cp.2012.e46.

Turner Hypoplasia

Via WF Jr. Enamel defects induced by trauma during tooth formation. *Oral Surg Oral Med Oral Pathol.* 1968;25:49-54.

Congenital Syphilis

Bradlaw RV. The dental stigmata of prenatal syphilis. *Oral Surg Oral Med Oral Pathol.* 1953;6:147-158.

Pessoa L, Galvão V. Clinical aspects of congenital syphilis with Hutchinson's triad. *BMJ Case Rep.* 2011;2011:bcr1120115130. doi:10.1136/bcr.11.2011.5130.

Putkonen T. Dental changes in congenital syphilis: relationship to other syphilitic stigmata. *Acta Derm Venereol.* 1962;42:44-62.

Sarnat BG, Shaw NG. Dental development in congenital syphilis. *Am J Orthod.* 1943;29:270.

Acquired Abnormalities

Baden E. Environmental pathology of the teeth. In: Gorlin RJ, Goodman HM, eds. *Thoma's Oral Pathology.* Vol. 1. 6th ed. Mosby; 1970.

Mitchell DF, Standish SM, Fast TB. *Oral Diagnosis/Oral Medicine.* Lea & Febiger; 1978.

Pindborg JJ. *Pathology of the Dental Hard Tissues.* Saunders; 1970.

Shafer WG, Hine MK, Levy BM. *Oral Pathology.* 4th ed. Saunders; 1983.

Attrition

Johnson GK, Sivers JE. Attrition, abrasion, and erosion: diagnosis and therapy. *Clin Prev Dent.* 1987;9:12-16.

Murphy TR. Reduction of the dental arch by approximal attrition: quantitative assessment. *Br Dent J.* 1964;116:483-488.

Russell MD. The distinction between physiological and pathological attrition: a review. *J Ir Dent Assoc.* 1987;33:23-31.

Seligman DA, Pullinger AG, Solberg WK. The prevalence of dental attrition and its association with factors of age, gender, occlusion, and TMJ symptomatology. *J Dent Res.* 1988;67:1323-1333.

Abrasion

Bull WH, Callender RM, Pugh BR, et al. The abrasion and cleaning properties of dentifrices. *Br Dent J.* 1968;125:331.

Corica A, Caprioglio A. Meta-analysis of the prevalence of tooth wear in primary dentition. *Eur J Paediatr Dent.* 2014;15(4):385-388.

Erwin JC, Buchner CM. Prevalence of tooth wear in primary dentition. *Eur J Paediatr Dent.* 2014;15(4):385-388.

Priyam S, Sankeshwari R, Jalihal S, et al. Comparative evaluation of abrasiveness among three dentifrices: an in vitro study. *Int J Clin Pediatr Dent.* 2023;16(2):264-269. doi:10.5005/jp-journals-10005-2576.

Dental Floss Injury

Hunt I, Ryatt S. Aggressive flossing. *Br Dent J.* 2013;214(11):539. doi:10.1038/sj.bdj.2013.536.

Salas ML, McClellan AC, MacNeill SR, et al. Interproximal cervical lesions caused by incorrect flossing technique. *Int J Dent Hyg.* 2012;10(2):83-85. doi:10.1111/j.1601-5037.2011.00524.x.

Erosion

Bruggen Cate HJ. Dental erosion in industry. *Br J Ind Med.* 1968;25:249.

Carvalho TS, Colon P, Ganss C, et al. Consensus Report of the European Federation of Conservative Dentistry: erosive tooth wear diagnosis and management. *Swiss Dent J.* 2016;126(4):342-346.

Kisely S, Sawyer E, Siskind D, et al. The oral health of people with anxiety and depressive disorders - a systematic review and meta-analysis. *J Affect Disord.* 2016;200:119-132. doi:10.1016/j.jad.2016.04.040.

Kitasako Y, Tanabe T, Koeda M, et al. Patients with gastroesophageal reflux disease (both reflux oesophagitis and non-erosive reflux disease): prevalence and severity of erosive tooth wear and saliva properties. *J Oral Rehabil.* 2024;51(2):305-312. doi:10.1111/joor.13595.

Müller F, Chebib N, Maniewicz S, et al. The impact of xerostomia on food choices-A review with clinical recommendations. *J Clin Med.* 2023;12(14): 4592. doi:10.3390/jcm12144592.

Nijakowski K, Jankowski J, Gruszczyński D, et al. Eating disorders and dental erosion: a systematic review. *J Clin Med.* 2023;12(19):6161. doi:10.3390/jcm12196161.

Stafne EC, Lovestedt SA. Dissolution of tooth substance by lemon juice, acid beverages, and acid from some other sources. *J Am Dent Assoc.* 1947; 34:586-592.

Resorption

Bakland LK. Root resorption. *Dent Clin North Am.* 1992;36:91-507.

Bennett CG, Poleway SA. Internal resorption, postpulpotomy type. *Oral Surg Oral Med Oral Pathol.* 1964;17:228-234.

Goldman HM. Spontaneous intermittent resorption of teeth. *J Am Dent Assoc.* 1954;49:522-532.

Massler M, Perreault JG. Root resorption in the permanent teeth of young adults. *J Dent Child.* 1954;21:158-164.

Patel S, Krastl G, Weiger R, et al. ESE position statement on root resorption. *Int Endod J.* 2023;56(7):792-801. doi:10.1111/iej.13916.

Phillips JR. Apical root resorption under orthodontic therapy. *Angle Orthod.* 1955;20:1-22.

Simpson HE. Internal resorption. *J Can Dent Assoc.* 1964;30:355.

Solomon CS, Notaro PJ, Kellert M. External root resorption: fact or fancy. *J Endod.* 1989;15(5):219-223.

Tronstad L. Root resorption: etiology, terminology, and clinical manifestations. *Endod Dent Traumatol.* 1988;4:241-252.

Wang J, Feng JQ. Signaling pathways critical for tooth root formation. *J Dent Res.* 2017;96:1221-1228. doi:10.1177/0022034517717478.

Secondary Dentin

Kuttler Y. Classification of dentin into primary, secondary and tertiary. *Oral Surg Oral Med Oral Pathol.* 1959;12:966-969.

Pulp Stones

Moss-Salentijn L, Hendricks-Klyvert M. Calcified structures in human dental pulps. *J Endod.* 1988;14:184-189.

Da Silva EJNL, Prado MC, Queiroz PM, et al. Assessing pulp stones by cone-beam computed tomography. *Clin Oral Investig.* 2017;21(7):2327-2333. doi:10.1007/s00784-016-2027-5.

Farias Z, Sousa J, Faria C, et al. Pulpal calcifications in orthodontically moved teeth: scoping review. *J Clin Exp Dent.* 2023;15(9):e773-e780. doi:10.4317/jced.60777.

Hypercementosis

Massé L, Garot E, Maureille B, et al. Insights into the aetiologies of hypercementosis: a systematic review and a scoring system. *Arch Oral Biol.* 2023;146:105599. doi:10.1016/j.archoralbio.2022.105599.

Masood F, Benavides E. Alterations in tooth structure and associated systemic conditions. *Radiol Clin North Am.* 2018;56(1):125-140. doi:10.1016/j.rcl.2017.08.009.

20

Inflammatory Conditions of the Jaws

Ernest W.N. Lam

Inflammation is the most common pathologic condition arising in the jaws. Unlike the other bones in the skeleton, the jaws are unique in that the teeth create a direct pathway for agents or processes, be they pathogenic oral microorganisms, or chemical or physical agents, to enter bone. The subsequent inflammatory response that is mounted by the body attempts to isolate or eliminate the pathogen so that an environment can be established for the repair of the damaged tissue.

Under normal conditions, bone metabolism is a very complex balance of osteoblastic bone production and osteoclastic bone resorption. The pathogenicity of bacterial microorganisms, the host immune response, tissue vascularity, and time all play a role in tipping this balance in favor of either bone production or resorption. For the purposes of this chapter, all inflammatory conditions of bone, regardless of their specific etiology, are considered part of a spectrum of conditions with different clinical presentations and radiologic appearances.

Clinically, the four cardinal signs of inflammation (redness, swelling, heat, and pain) may be observed to varying degrees in the jaws. Acute processes tend to have a typically rapid onset and produce fever with pronounced swelling and pain. In contrast, chronic processes have a more prolonged course with generally less intense pain, and may be accompanied by intermittent, low-grade fever and the gradual development of a swelling of the tissues.

When the stimulus of the inflammatory response is bacterial, chemical, or physical trauma to the tooth pulp, the bone change is commonly restricted to the tooth root apex. This condition is referred to as periapical inflammatory disease. When bacterial dissemination occurs through the gingival tissues, the inflammatory response is referred to as periodontal disease if there is involvement of the supporting structures of the teeth. And when the response involves the crown of a partially erupted tooth, this is referred to as pericoronitis. Wider dissemination of the inflammatory response beyond the tooth may occur through the bone into adjacent tissue spaces via the Haversian and Volkmann systems of canals. This more widespread dissemination of inflammation is called osteomyelitis, and with this, there may be necrosis or death of bone.

PERIAPICAL INFLAMMATORY DISEASE

Terminology

Apical periodontitis, as well as radicular or periapical abscess, granuloma, and cyst are some of the many terms that have been used synonymously to refer to periapical inflammatory disease. The term apical periodontitis is used in endodontics to describe a clinical process of pulpal origin that results in inflammation of the apical periodontium; a change that may not always be apparent by viewing an image. Other terms such as abscess, granuloma, and cyst refer to processes that can only be identified and differentiated by an oral and maxillofacial pathologist under a microscope; these entities cannot be differentiated macroscopically by radiologic imaging.

"Rarefying osteitis" is the radiologic diagnosis for an inflammatory process occurring in bone associated with bone resorption at the root apex of a tooth, and typically, the pulpal tissues have become necrotic. In this context, the term "rarefying", which is derived from the word "rarefaction", refers to a loss of bone mineralization, while the term "osteitis" references inflammation of bone. The net result of this process is the appearance of a localized focus of increased radiolucency. In contrast, the term "sclerosing osteitis" references an inflammatory response of bone associated with bone deposition around the root of a tooth with a necrotic pulp. "Sclerosis" in this context refers to a "hardening" of the bone and radiologically, this appears as an increase in the radiopacity of bone. Commonly, sclerosing osteitis occurs at the periphery of an area of rarefying osteitis.

In the past, the terms "focal sclerosing osteitis" and "condensing osteitis" have both been used synonymously to refer to sclerosing osteitis on radiologic images, but their use should be discouraged. While the sclerotic response of bone can be focal, in inflammation, this response is almost always more diffuse and widespread. In radiologic imaging, "sclerosis" is used widely across all disciplines of radiology, including medical radiology, to refer to an increase in bone matrix density on an image. It is, therefore, the preferred contemporary term in radiologic diagnosis and one we will use in this text.

Disease Mechanism

The local response of the bone around a tooth root as a consequence of pulpal necrosis is the most common cause of periapical inflammatory disease. Necrosis of the pulp can occur because of bacterial, chemical, or physical trauma to the dental pulp, most commonly through dental caries. Metabolites derived from the necrotic pulp exit the tooth root apex, inciting an inflammatory response in the periodontal ligament space and surrounding bone (Fig. 20.1). This reaction is characterized histopathologically by an inflammatory infiltrate consisting of multinucleated cells such as neutrophils in the more acute stages, and monocytes/macrophages and lymphocytes in the more chronic stages.

Depending on the severity of the host response, tissue may necrose and pus may form, resulting in an abscess. This series of events is often thought of as being the acute inflammatory response. A granuloma is formed when the body attempts to isolate and eliminate the inflammatory response from the normal adjacent tissues with a cell infiltrate comprised predominantly of lymphocytes, plasma cells, and histiocytes (macrophages). Entrapped epithelium from the epithelial cell rests of Malassez may be stimulated to proliferate under these conditions, developing a lining within the area of apical bone resorption forming a cyst. Should the adjacent

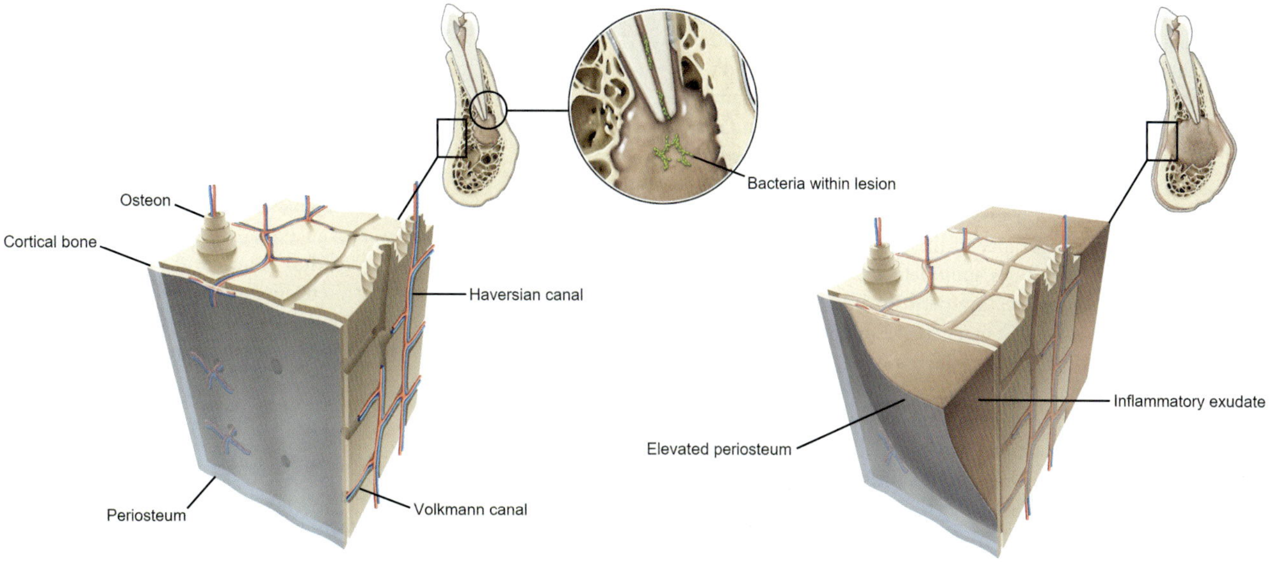

Fig. 20.1 Development and progression of periapical inflammatory disease located at the tooth root apex. The inflammatory response spreads through the bone via the Haversian and Volkmann canal systems. As the response reaches the bone surface through Volkmann canals, the exudate lifts and distends the surface periosteum.

surrounding bone and bone marrow become more involved, a compensatory response of the bone may be to isolate the inflammatory response by depositing bone at the periphery of the resorption; this is the process of sclerosis. Furthermore, should the inflammatory reaction become more widely disseminated, bacterial microorganisms and inflammatory mediators may reach the bone surface and the overlying periosteum.

The periosteum is a dense and irregularly thick layer of soft tissue that lines the floors of air cavities and covers the surfaces of the bones. Extensions of collagen from the bone called Sharpey fibers anchor the periosteum to the bone surface. The periosteum consists of two discrete cell layers: an inner osteogenic layer that harbors mesenchymal stem cells and an outer connective tissue layer that contains fibroblasts and collagen. When stimulated, the stem cells within the osteogenic layer can differentiate into osteoblasts, and these cells can produce bone. As the inflammatory response travels through the Haversian and Volkmann canal systems to the bone surface, the response may elevate and broadly distend the adherent periosteum (Fig. 20.1), and at the same time simulate mesenchymal stem cells in the osteogenic layer of the periosteum to differentiate into osteoblasts. As a result, new bone is deposited in a response called periosteal new bone formation (Fig. 20.2). However, as Sharpey fibers attach the periosteum to the bone surface, the amount of distension may be limited.

Internally within the bone, should bone deposition on the native trabeculae become extensive (i.e., sclerosis), marrow spaces containing small vascular channels may become smaller, effectively preventing the delivery of blood and nutrients. Should the local blood supply become compromised, the bone may undergo necrosis, giving rise to dying or dead bone called a sequestrum (singular) or sequestra (plural).

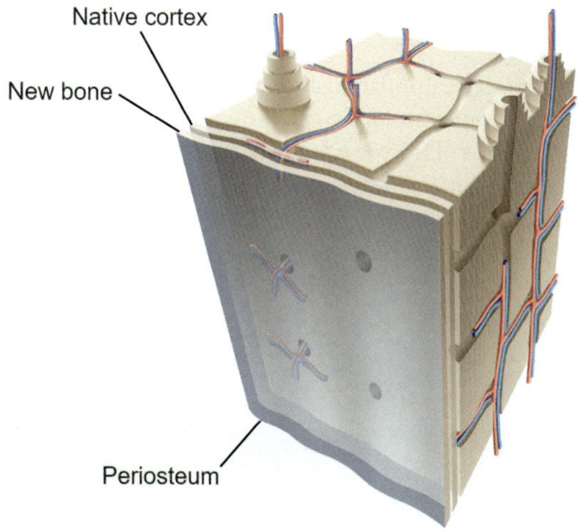

Fig. 20.2 Periosteal new bone formation, with the deposition of a single, new layer of bone at the bone surface.

Clinical Features

It is important for the dentist to recognize that the clinical presentation of periapical inflammatory disease may not necessarily correlate with the imaging findings. In the more acute stages of disease, inflammation can be associated with severe pain and swelling, including pain of the overlying tissues to palpation. As well, a tooth may become mobile and tender to percussion, and sometimes elevated in the tooth socket. Spontaneous drainage of pus into the oral cavity through a fistula or parulis may relieve pain. The acute lesion may evolve into one that becomes chronic and potentially asymptomatic, except for intermittent episodes of tooth pain which may be acute exacerbations of the chronic inflammatory response. In the more chronic phase of disease, the associated tooth may continue to be mobile and tender to percussion, or it may become asymptomatic. More often, however, periapical inflammation may arise in a chronic form de novo, and in this case, it may be completely asymptomatic.

Imaging Examination

An initial imaging examination consisting of one or more intraoral periapical images may identify the tooth involved. Occlusal and panoramic images may supplement this examination to characterize the extent of the lesion should the changes be more extensive and extend beyond the borders of the periapical image. While more extensive changes may be visible on panoramic imaging, occlusal images can be useful for identifying periosteal new bone formation at the bone surface. Depending on the exuberance of the bone response, cone beam computed tomography (CBCT) or multidetector computed tomography (MDCT) are useful for detecting periosteal new bone formation and bone sequestra. Additionally, magnetic resonance imaging (MRI) may be useful to visualize changes to the bone marrow, and a nuclear medicine examination with technetium (^{99m}Tc) and gallium (^{67}Ga) may confirm the diagnosis. With inflammatory lesions, a positive ^{99m}Tc result depicting increased bone metabolic activity and a positive ^{67}Ga scan in the same location reflecting an inflammatory cell infiltrate can confirm the MDCT, CBCT, or MRI results.

Imaging Features

The imaging features of periapical inflammatory disease may vary depending on the stage of the disease. Very early lesions may show little or no changes to the periapical tissues on images, and diagnosis may rely solely on tooth pulp vitality tests and the patient's clinical signs and symptoms (Fig. 20.3). More longstanding lesions may show a radiolucent region at the root apex of a tooth and a more diffuse, surrounding area of radiopacity.

Location

In most cases, periapical inflammatory disease develops around the tooth root apex or adjacent to the apical one-third of the tooth root, and within these areas of the periodontal ligament space. The epicenter of a periapical inflammatory lesion is located apical or subjacent to the apex of the involved tooth root (Fig. 20.4). However, as the lesion enlarges, the epicenter migrates in a more apical direction away from the tooth root apex. Less commonly, these lesions may be located adjacent to the surface of the tooth root at the exit of an accessory root canal, at the site of a perforation of the root surface from erroneous root canal instrumentation, or at the site of root fracture (Fig. 20.5).

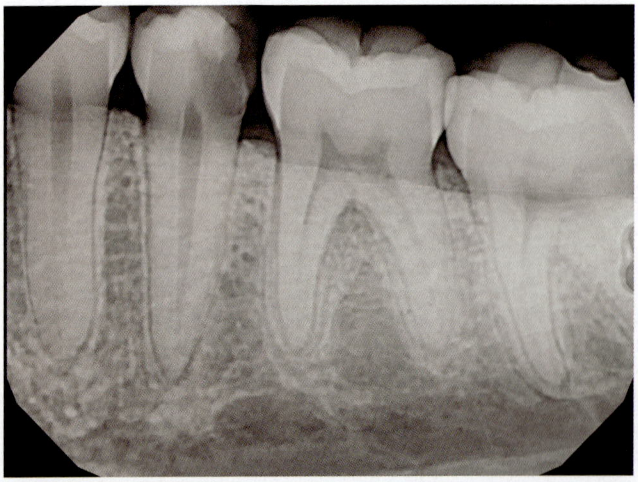

Fig. 20.3 An increase in the width of the periodontal ligament space in a very early lesion of rarefying osteitis involving the mandibular left second premolar. Note the large coronal caries. The lamina dura has been lost along the distal surface of the root near the root apex and an adjacent focus of sclerosing osteitis has also developed.

Periphery

The periphery of periapical inflammatory disease is typically poorly to moderately well defined, and the border can have a smooth, hydraulic contour, like the surface of a balloon. Beyond the border of the radiolucent area, the appearance of the bone may transition from something more radiopaque to an appearance that is more normal. The width of this transition (i.e., the "transition zone") will be determined by the amount of sclerosis present; a reflection of the chronicity of the inflammatory response (Fig. 20.6). Rarely is the periphery well defined and corticated, with a narrow zone of bone transition between the lesion and normal bone.

Internal Structure

Early periapical inflammatory disease may show no apparent change to the normal bone pattern at the apex of a tooth root. The inability to perceive a change may be due, in large part, to the amount of overlying cortical bone resorption necessary to visualize the change. Identifying early changes in demineralization may be a particular challenge in the mandibular premolar and molar areas because of this, and in the maxilla, the superimposition of adjacent anatomical structures may also mask early changes.

The earliest radiologic change to bone structure at the apex of a tooth root involves focal widening of the apical periodontal ligament space, and this may be accompanied by a loss of definition of the adjacent lamina dura (see Figs. 20.3 and 20.4A). As the radiolucent lesion enlarges, the epicenter of bone resorption is usually at, or just apical to the apex of the tooth root. This radiolucent region should not contain any areas of discrete internal mineralization. With time, there may be focal thickening of the apical lamina dura; an early indication of developing sclerosis.

Effects on Surrounding Structures

In the early stages of periapical inflammatory disease when the lesion is still small, there may be little or no effects on the adjacent bone. As the disease evolves, and the radiolucent portion of the lesion enlarges and extends to a bone border (e.g., the floor of an airspace such as the maxillary sinus, the cortex of the mandible or maxilla), the inflammatory response may perforate the bone surface through a cloaca.

Bone deposition may also be seen at the periphery of the focus of rarefaction, altering the normal morphology of the trabecular bone pattern and marrow spaces (see Figs. 20.6 and 20.7). The sclerotic bone reaction may include thicker than normal trabeculae, as well as an increase in the number of trabeculae per unit area. With time, the bone may become very dense, obscuring individual trabeculae and reducing the sizes of the marrow spaces. Depending on the aggressiveness of the pathogenic microorganisms, the exuberance of the host immune response, tissue vascularity and chronicity, the sclerotic response may extend to adjacent teeth, nontooth-bearing areas, or to a bone border. Occasionally, a lesion of periapical inflammatory disease may appear to be composed entirely of sclerotic bone (sclerosing osteitis), but usually some evidence exists of apical periodontal ligament space widening (Fig. 20.6A).

Should the inflammatory response arrive at a bone surface bordered by periosteum, periosteal new bone may form. The result of these processes is the deposition of paired layers of new bone and connective tissue oriented either mildly convex or nearly parallel to the bone surface. When this process occurs around the root apex adjacent to the floor of an airspace such as the maxillary sinus, the appearance is referred to as a "halo" pattern (Fig. 20.8). When the process occurs

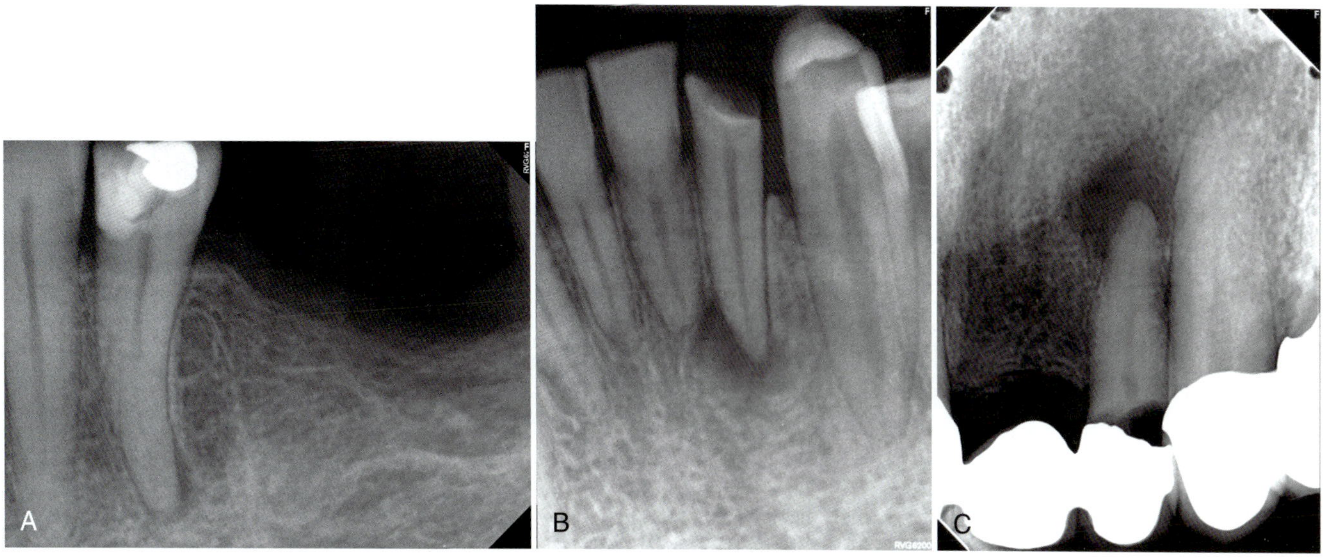

Fig. 20.4 Rarefying osteitis associated with a mandibular left first premolar (A), a mandibular left lateral incisor (B), and a maxillary left lateral incisor (C). Note the loss of definition of the lamina dura at the root apices and the migration of the epicenters away from the root surface as the lesions enlarge.

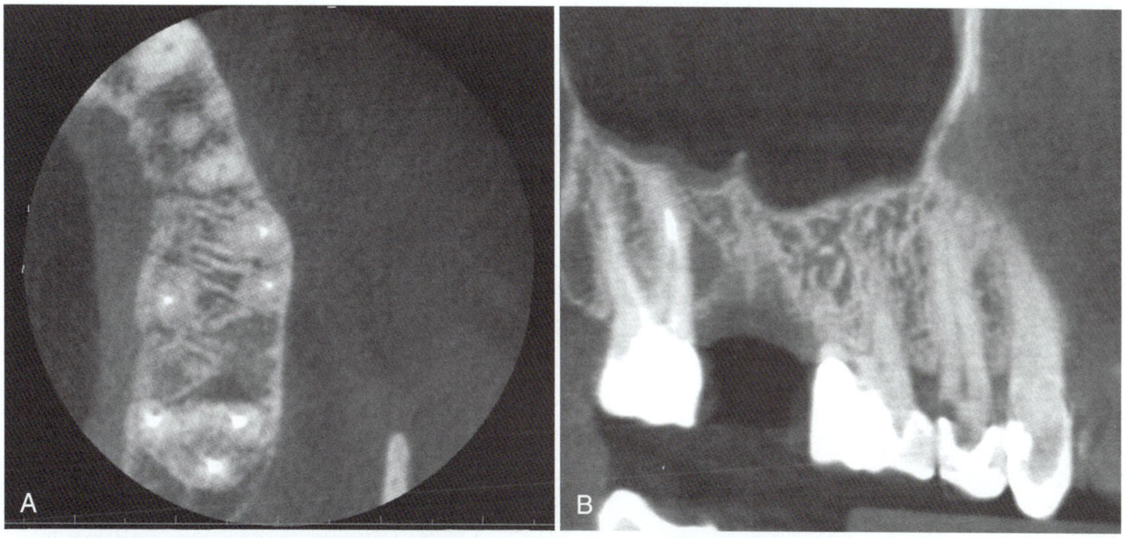

Fig. 20.5 Axial (A) and corrected sagittal (B) cone beam computed tomographic images of rarefying osteitis developing along the mesial surface of the mesiobuccal root of the maxillary right third molar at the midroot level. Rarefying osteitis in this location suggests the presence of a horizontal fracture of the mesiobuccal root.

at the bone surface, it is referred to as an "onion skin" pattern (Figs. 20.2 and 20.9).

Should periapical inflammatory disease involve the floor of the nasal fossa or maxillary sinus, inflammatory mediators may also stimulate the adjacent mucosal lining of the air cavity producing a localized thickening of the mucosa within the adjacent floor of the airspace called mucositis (Fig. 20.10).

Effects on Adjacent Teeth

In many regards, the response of the tooth to inflammation closely mirrors the response of the bone. Akin to bone rarefaction, tooth roots can undergo external resorption, and this may be seen on an image as a change in the normally smooth, tapering surface contour of the root. Alternatively (akin to bone sclerosis), tooth roots may undergo hypercementosis, and this may produce bulbous-shaped roots. The response of the tooth root, whether resorption or hypercementosis, may be asymmetric and nonuniform around the circumference of the root. When rarefying osteitis involves deciduous teeth, eruption of the underlying permanent dentition may be disrupted as these teeth may become displaced (Fig. 20.11).

Differential Interpretation

The two lesions that most commonly must be differentiated from periapical inflammatory disease are periapical cemento-osseous dysplasia (PCOD) and a dense bone island (DBI). In the early radiolucent phase of PCOD, the imaging characteristics cannot be used to reliably differentiate this lesion from periapical inflammatory disease (Fig. 20.12). The diagnosis may rely solely on the clinical examination; the pulpal

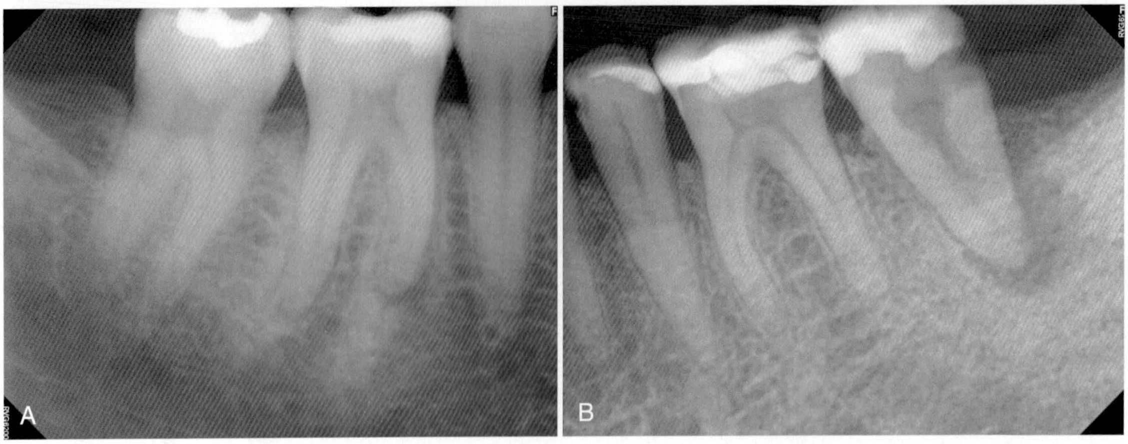

Fig. 20.6 Examples of both rarefying and sclerosing osteitis affecting a mandibular right first molar (A) and a mandibular left second molar (B). Note the similarity of the pattern with the radiolucent regions at the apices of the teeth and the diffuse radiopaque sclerotic bone reaction extending away from the areas of rarefaction into the adjacent bone.

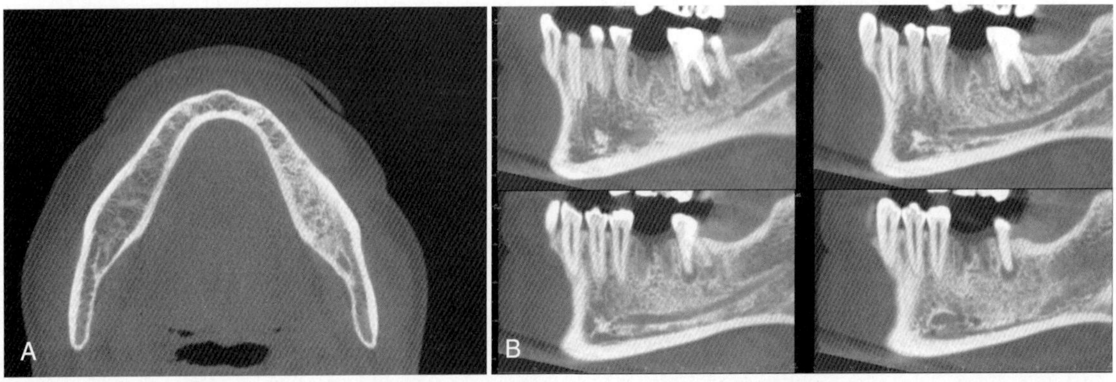

Fig. 20.7 Axial (A) and corrected sagittal (B) cone beam computed tomographic images of rarefying and sclerosing osteitis affecting the roots of a mandibular left second molar. Note the normal trabecular bone pattern of the mandible on the right side (A). The sclerotic response on the left side extends to the inferior cortex of the mandible (B). This change gives a particular prominence to the inferior alveolar canal.

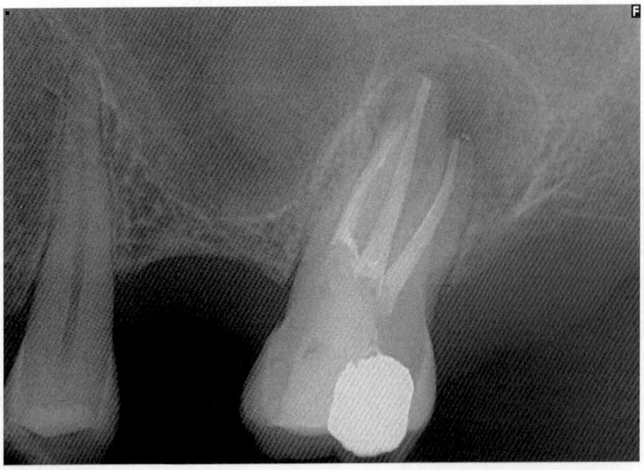

Fig. 20.8 Periosteal new bone formation emanating from the floor of the maxillary sinus as a result of an area of rarefying osteitis.

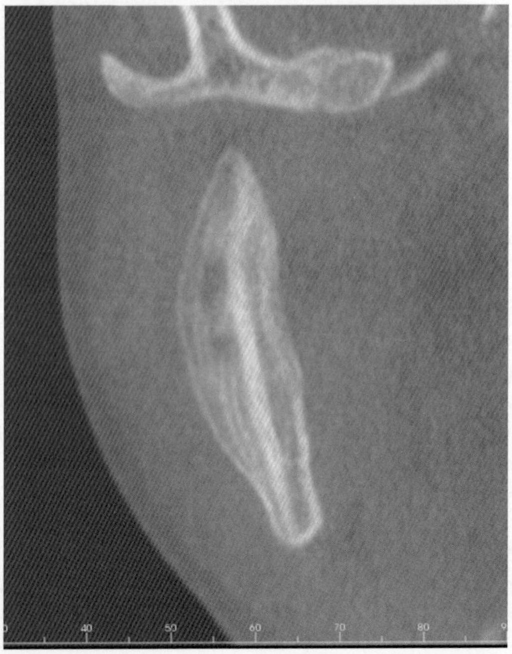

Fig. 20.9 Coronal cone beam computed tomographic image demonstrating prominent multilayered periosteal new bone formation along the lateral surface of the right mandibular ramus.

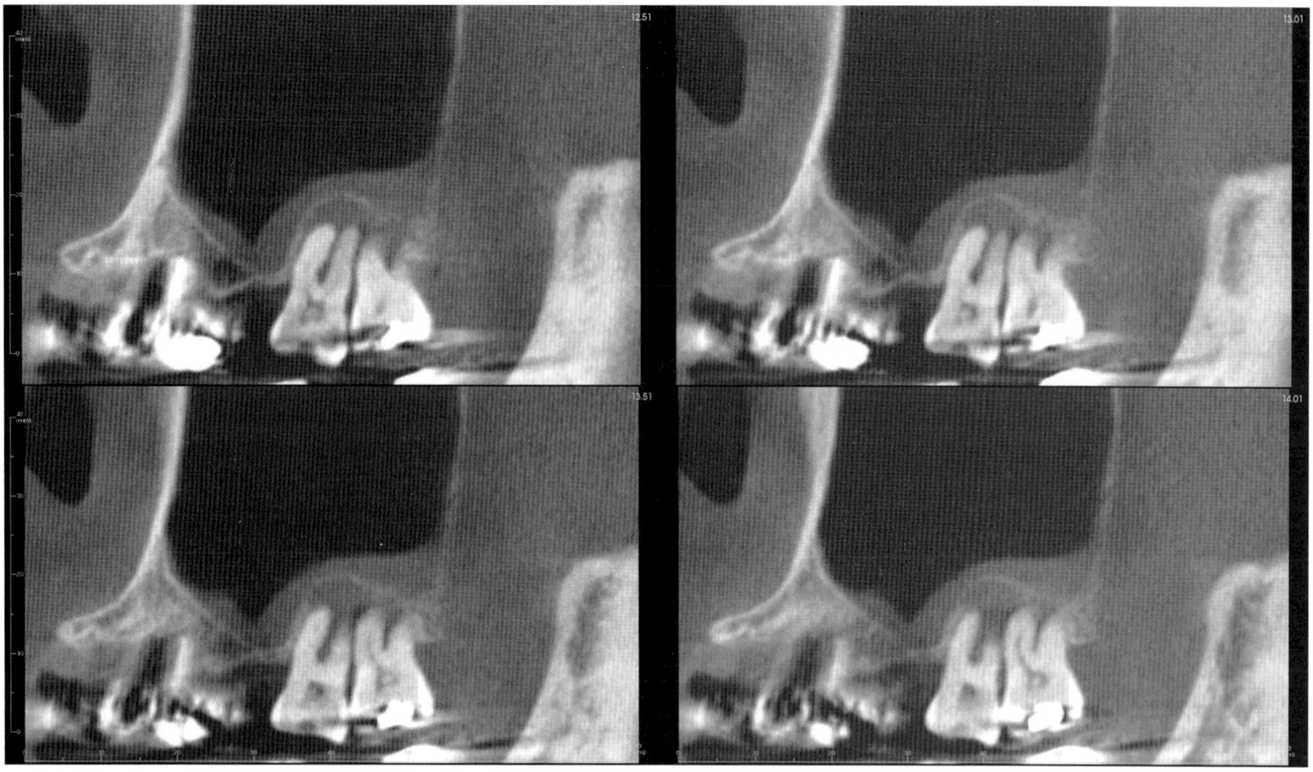

Fig. 20.10 Elevation of the maxillary sinus floor and sinus mucosal thickening (mucositis) adjacent to an area of rarefying osteitis. Mucositis is characterized by a radiopaque band of tissue adjacent to the elevated floor.

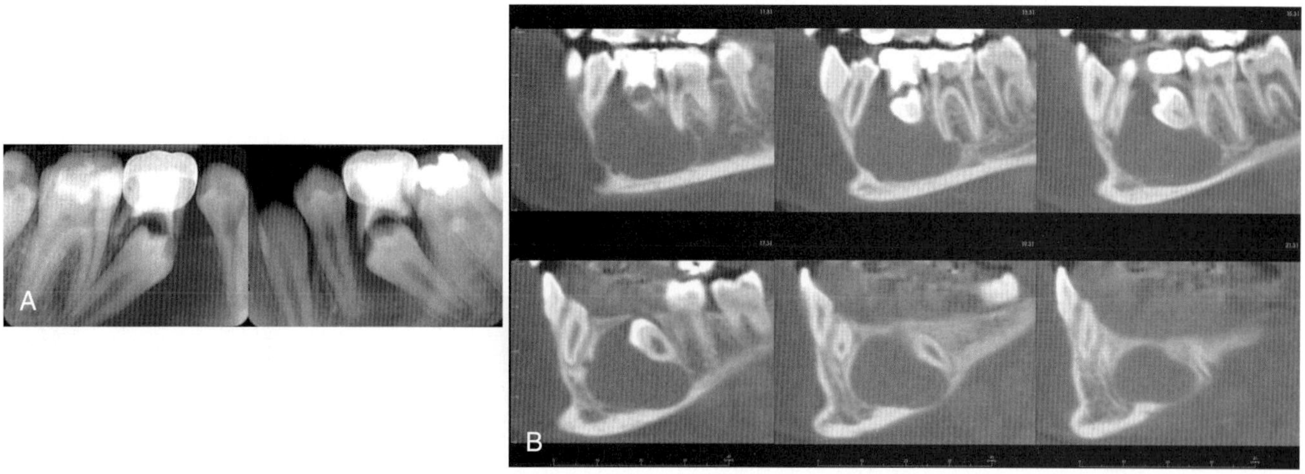

Fig. 20.11 (A) Periapical images of two areas of rarefying osteitis associated with the mandibular right and left second deciduous molars that have undergone pulpectomy procedures. Corrected sagittal (B) cone beam computed tomographic images of the area of rarefying osteitis associated with the mandibular left second deciduous molar. Note the curved, hydraulic characteristics of the border contours.

status of a tooth adjacent to a focus of PCOD will yield a vital test result, while the tooth adjacent to a lesion of periapical inflammatory disease will test nonvital. Depending on the age of the patient and the chronicity of the periapical inflammatory disease, the pulp chamber of the tooth with periapical inflammatory disease may also appear larger than the adjacent teeth with a vital pulp. More mature PCOD lesions may demonstrate a radiopaque focus centrally within the radiolucent area which helps in the differential interpretation since the radiopacity seen with periapical inflammatory disease occurs at the periphery of the radiolucent focus. External root resorption is also more commonly identified in inflammation than in PCOD where the change is typically one of hypercementosis.

When a DBI is centered on a tooth root apex, it may mimic a focus of sclerosing osteitis. In these instances, the DBI does not alter the width of the periodontal ligament space around the apex of the tooth (Fig. 20.13). Some DBIs, particularly when they develop adjacent to mandibular molar root apices, may cause external resorption of the tooth root. Although the amount of resorption is self-limiting, the root

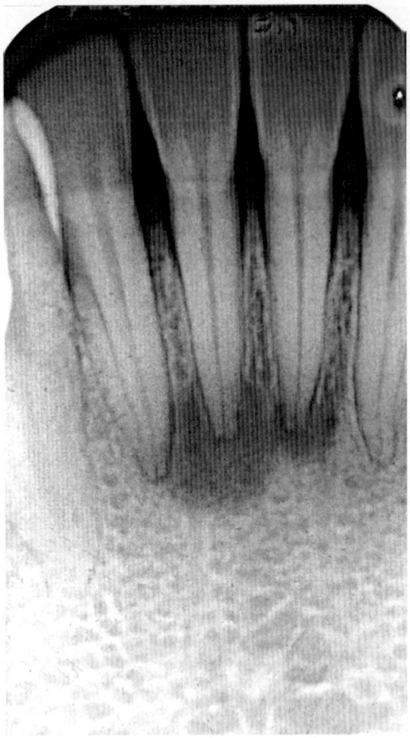

Fig. 20.12 Two early lesions of periapical cemento-osseous dysplasia located at the root apices of the mandibular central incisors. Note the similarities to rarefying osteitis.

apex of such a tooth may be blunted and nontapering. However, even in such instances, a retained, thin periodontal ligament space can be visualized between the resorbed root apex and the DBI, and the pulp of this tooth should test vital. Moreover, the zone of transition between the DBI and the normal adjacent bone is narrow, unlike in sclerosing osteitis.

In rare cases, metastatic lesions and blood-borne malignancies such as leukemia may develop within the apical periodontal ligament space. Close inspection of the surrounding bone may reveal other bone changes, which may include multiple, variably sized regions of cancellous bone destruction.

Persistent Periapical Inflammatory Disease

Persistent or recurrent periapical inflammatory disease may occur after orthograde endodontic treatment. In such instances, the persistence or reappearance of a radiolucent focus at the root apex of a tooth with a hydraulic periphery may be a clue that inflammation has persisted or recurred. Possible etiologies can include inadequate orthograde endodontic treatment, unusual root canal morphology, the presence of an untreated canal, perforation of a root surface, or root fracture (Fig. 20.14). Limited field-of-view CBCT may be useful in determining the etiology of persistent or recurrent disease (Fig. 20.14C). In the absence of a root fracture, orthograde endodontic retreatment or periapical endodontic surgery may be considered. However, if a root fracture is detected, management can involve extraction.

OSTEOMYELITIS

As the root "myel" in osteomyelitis references bone marrow, the term osteomyelitis is used to describe inflammation that involves the bone marrow. It is worth noting, however, that rarefying osteitis can also involve the bone marrow and extend through the bone producing sclerosis as well as surface periosteal new bone formation. Experienced clinicians see osteomyelitis as being a more extreme point along the inflammatory disease continuum that involves wider dissemination of the inflammatory response, and one that is more severe. Moreover, the diagnosis of osteomyelitis is also informed by the patient's clinical signs and symptoms.

For the novice clinician, the diagnosis of osteomyelitis can be among the most challenging to make. If, however, this diagnosis is not made in a timely manner and effectively managed, the infectious agent may persist and continue to spread in some patients, particularly those with preexisting chronic systemic conditions (e.g., sickle cell disease), immunosuppressive states (HIV/AIDS), and disorders of decreased vascularity (e.g., osteopetrosis).

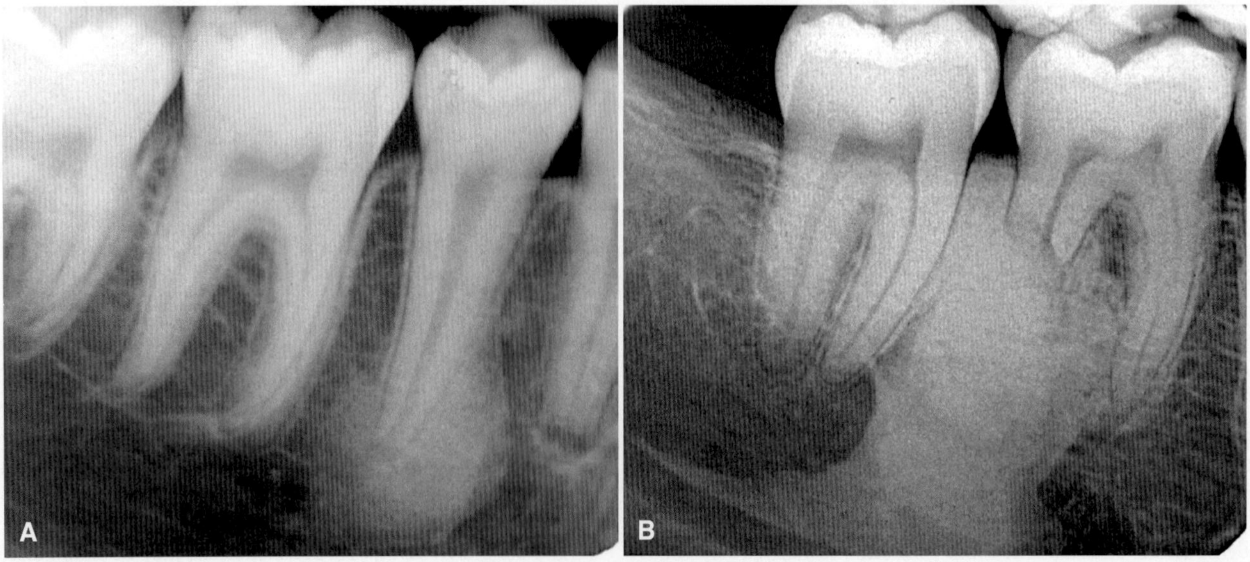

Fig. 20.13 Dense bone islands associated with mandibular right premolar (A) and molar (B) teeth. In comparison to sclerosing osteitis, the periodontal ligament space is unaffected and remains uniform in width.

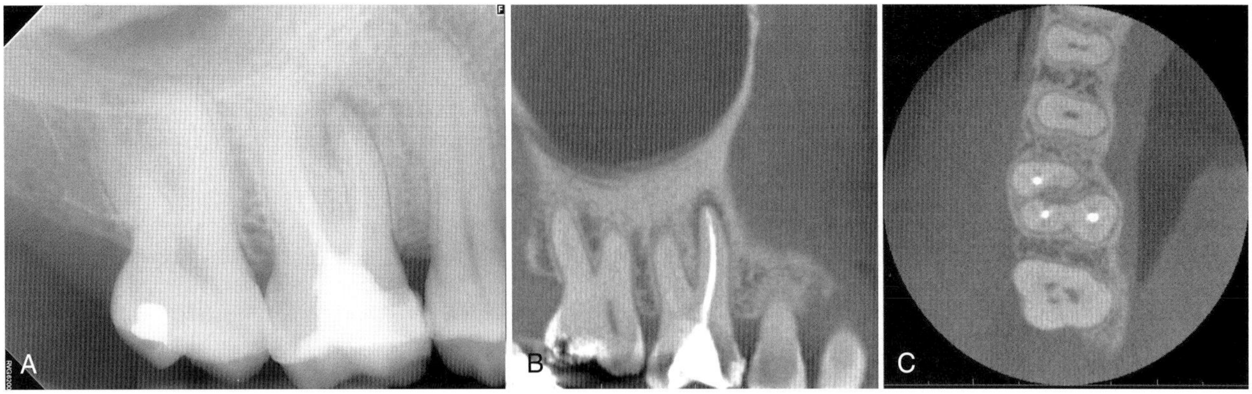

Fig. 20.14 (A) Periapical image of a maxillary right first molar showing periapical inflammatory disease following orthograde endodontic treatment 5 years prior. Corrected sagittal (B) and axial (C) cone beam computed tomographic images of the same patient showing extensive sclerosis extending to the floor of the maxillary sinus and mucositis along the sinus floor. The axial image (C) shows endodontic filling material located eccentrically in the mesiobuccal root of the tooth suggesting the presence of an untreated, more palatally positioned canal in the root.

Terminology

Numerous descriptors and eponyms have been used with the term osteomyelitis, and this has created a great deal of confusion about this disease process. In some instances, clinical progression is used as a descriptor (e.g., acute, chronic), while others make reference to an infectious agent (e.g., pyogenic), a clinical finding (e.g., suppurative), or a radiologic feature (e.g., proliferative periostitis, diffuse sclerosing). And some forms make use of multiple descriptors (Garrè chronic nonsuppurative sclerosing). For the sake of simplicity and to minimize confusion, we have chosen to categorize osteomyelitis and its associated imaging features with respect to its disease duration (e.g., acute, chronic), which we see as progression of the disease process along a continuum of severity, where one important variable is time.

Disease Mechanism

The acute phase of osteomyelitis is caused by spread of periapical inflammatory disease from a tooth with a nonvital pulp through the bone to more distant sites as dictated by bacterial pathogenicity and the host immune response. In this phase of the disease, the inflammatory cellular infiltrate within the medullary spaces consists predominantly of neutrophils and, to a lesser extent, mononuclear cells. Infection may also develop because of local spread from the gingiva or by hematogenous spread from a distant site through the bone to the bone surface and periosteum.

Clinical Features

The acute phase of osteomyelitis can affect people of all ages, and it has a strong male predilection. It is much more common in the mandible than in the maxillae, possibly a consequence of a more limited vascular network in the mandible. The typical signs and symptoms of acute osteomyelitis are rapid onset, pain, swelling of the adjacent soft tissues, fever, lymphadenopathy, and leukocytosis. The involved teeth may become mobile and sensitive to percussion, and purulent drainage also may be present. Paresthesia of the lower lip in the third division of the trigeminal nerve distribution has also been reported.

Chronic osteomyelitis may be a sequela of inadequately treated acute osteomyelitis, or it may arise very gradually de novo. Histopathologically, sparse involvement of the medullary spaces may be seen, together with marrow fibrosis and a chronic inflammatory cell infiltrate. In contrast to acute osteomyelitis, the signs and symptoms of chronic osteomyelitis may involve a more prolonged duration, but with intermittent recurrent episodes of swelling, fever, and lymphadenopathy. As with acute osteomyelitis, paresthesia and drainage with fistula formation also may occur. In some chronic cases, the patient may have little or no pain, or the pain may be limited to only times of disease exacerbation. If left untreated, the disease can continue to spread throughout the jaw. In the mandible, this can include the temporomandibular joint and can cause septic arthritis. Ear infections and infection of the mastoid air cells may also develop. Interestingly, in chronic osteomyelitis, bacterial culture results are usually negative, and pathogenic microorganisms are rarely found.

Imaging Examination

The goal of imaging is to identify one or more specific radiologic features of osteomyelitis. As we saw with rarefying osteitis, these features can include sclerosis of the bone, the development of a cloaca and periosteal new bone formation. In the case of osteomyelitis, the sclerotic reaction often extends beyond the tooth-bearing areas of the jaws. A hallmark diagnostic feature in osteomyelitis is the appearance of necrotic bone or sequestra, bone that has lost or is losing its blood supply.

An initial imaging examination consisting of intraoral periapical and occlusal, and panoramic images may be useful to characterize the extent of the disease process and the teeth involved. While rarefaction and sclerosis may be visible on panoramic imaging, occlusal images can be useful for depicting any periosteal new bone formation. CBCT or MDCT should be used for definitively identify periosteal new bone formation and sequestra, as these techniques are more sensitive to these findings.

MRI may be useful to visualize changes to the bone marrow and a nuclear medicine examination with technetium (^{99m}Tc) and gallium (^{67}Ga) may help to confirm the diagnosis. With acute inflammatory lesions, a positive ^{99m}Tc result depicting increased bone metabolic activity and a positive ^{67}Ga scan in the same location reflecting an inflammatory cell infiltrate can confirm the MDCT, CBCT, or MRI results during the acute phase. As the disease progresses into the chronic phase, a ^{67}Ga examination is not particularly useful because there may be no inflammatory cell population to detect.

Imaging Features

The imaging features of osteomyelitis may vary depending on the progression of the disease, and while inflammatory cells and exudate may be found in the bone, no changes may be apparent on the diagnostic images in the early acute phase of the disease.

Location

In general terms, the posterior body of the mandible is the most common site of disease, and this is, purportedly, a consequence of the relatively poor blood supply to the bone in this region. Osteomyelitis involving the maxilla is rare.

Periphery

Adjacent to normal bone, the acute phase of osteomyelitis most often demonstrates a poorly defined, noncorticated periphery. With time and increasing chronicity, the periphery may become better defined as the peripheral sclerotic response becomes more dense, and as the zone of transition between the normal cancellous bone and diseased bone widens.

As with rarefying osteitis, acute osteomyelitis may cause bone resorption or formation at the bone surface. Portions of cortical bone may be resorbed, and there may be new bone formation at the surface because of periosteal stimulation (Fig. 20.15). In some instances, however, the development of the "onion skin" pattern of periosteal new bone formation at the bone surface may be very faint depending on its degree of mineralization. As the inflammatory response may cycle through multiple rounds of activity and quiescence, multiple "onion skin" layers may develop. Eventually, a massive amount of new bone may be formed adjacent to the native bone surface (Fig. 20.16). This condition, also referred to as proliferative periostitis, is seen more often in children who have thicker and more loosely attached periosteum than adults, with higher osteogenic potential.

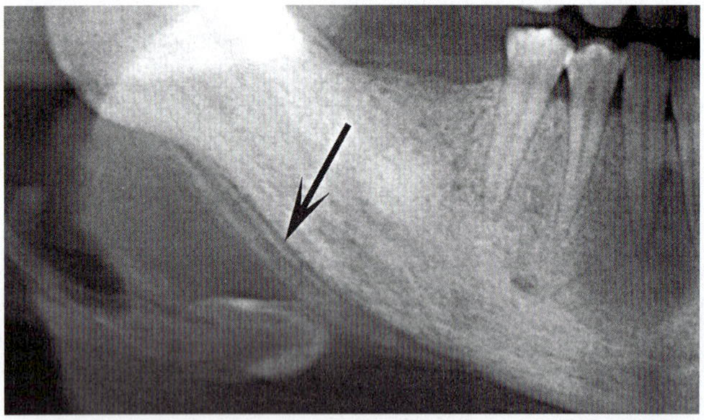

Fig. 20.15 Periosteal reaction involving the inferior cortex of the mandible. Note the radiolucent line *(arrow)* between the inferior cortex of the mandible and the first layer of periosteal new bone. A second radiolucent line separates the second layer of new bone from the first layer.

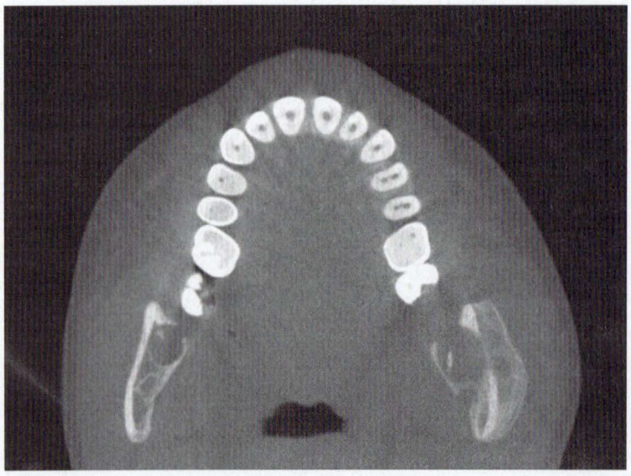

Fig. 20.16 Axial cone beam computed tomographic image shows exuberant multilayered periosteal new bone formation along the lateral surface of the left mandibular ramus.

Internal Structure

In the acute phase of osteomyelitis, there may be a slight decrease in the density of the involved bone, with a loss of definition of the existing trabeculae. As the disease process begins to spread, bone resorption becomes more profound with time, resulting in an area of radiolucency in one or more focal areas scattered regions throughout the bone. With increasing chronicity, sclerotic regions of bone begin to appear, and internal bone density may increase to the point where the cancellous bone is uniformly radiopaque with a density similar to cortical bone. Sequestra may begin to appear, and these can be identified by one or more fragments of radiopaque bone surrounded on all sides by a radiolucent periphery (Fig. 20.17). These islands of bone may vary in size from a small dot (smaller sequestra are usually seen in young patients) to larger islands of radiopaque bone separated from the surrounding bone (Fig. 20.18). CBCT or MDCT is superior to planar imaging for revealing the internal structure of the abnormal bone, and sequestra, especially in cases where the bone is very densely sclerotic or granular, obscuring individual bone trabeculae (Figs. 20.19 and 20.20).

Effects on Surrounding Structures

With time and disease chronicity, new bone may form at the bone surface within the more radiolucent connective tissue layer of the elevated

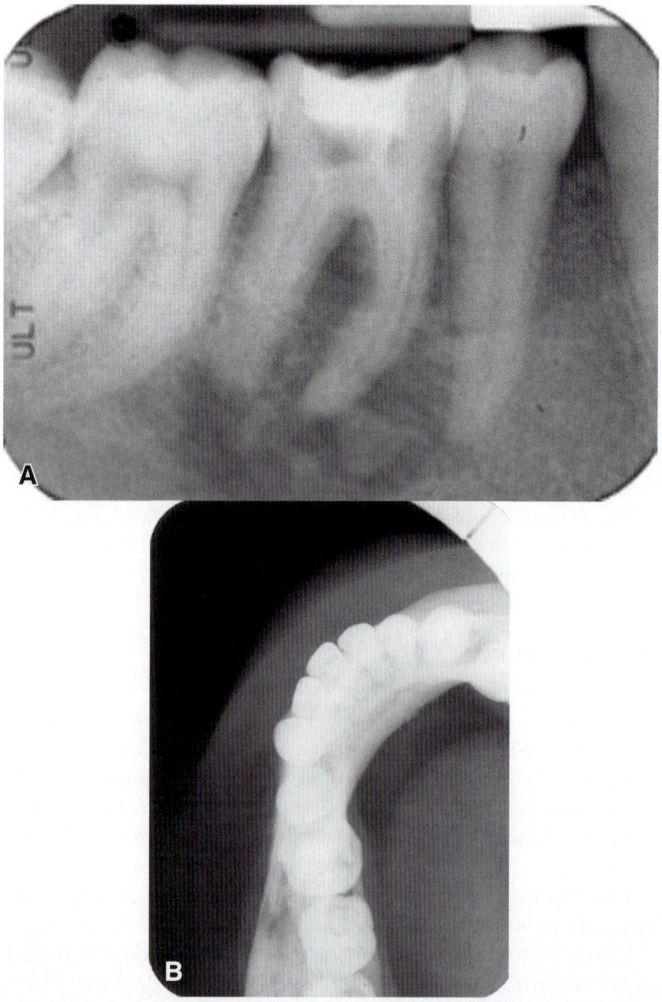

Fig. 20.17 Periapical image (A) showing a mixed radiolucent and radiopaque pattern around the roots of a mandibular right first molar. The cross-sectional occlusal image shows periosteal new bone formation on the buccal and lingual surfaces of the mandible (B).

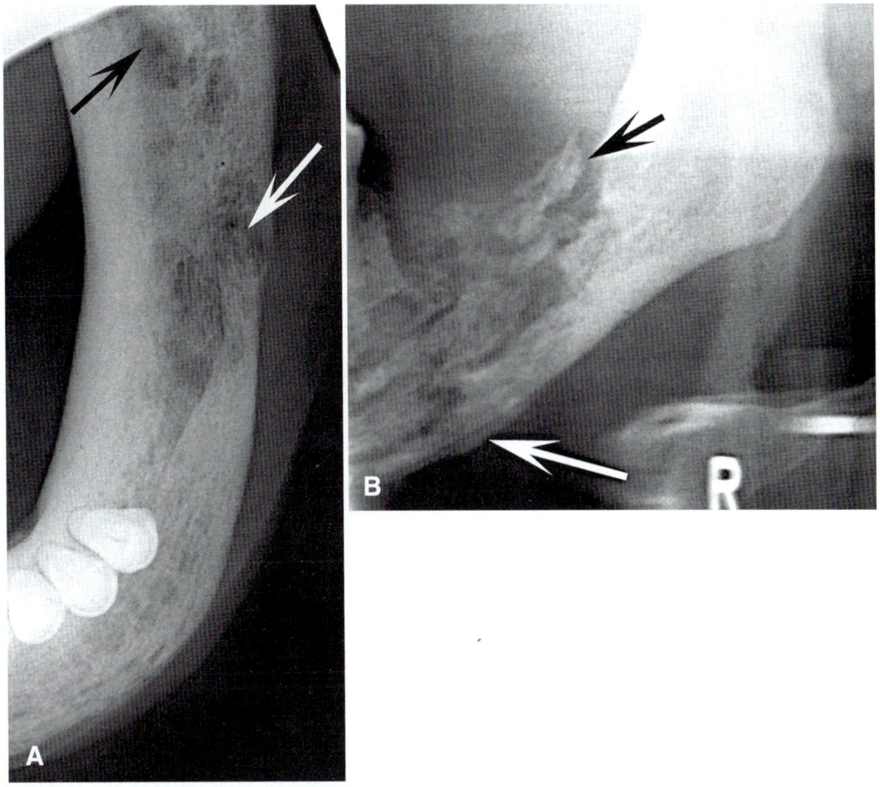

Fig. 20.18 Examples of sequestra. Cross-sectional occlusal image (A) demonstrates small sequestra as radiopaque islands of bone on a radiolucent background in osteomyelitis *(arrows)*. Cropped panoramic image (B) reveals a large sequestrum *(black arrow)* and a periosteal reaction at the inferior border of the mandible in osteomyelitis *(white arrow)*.

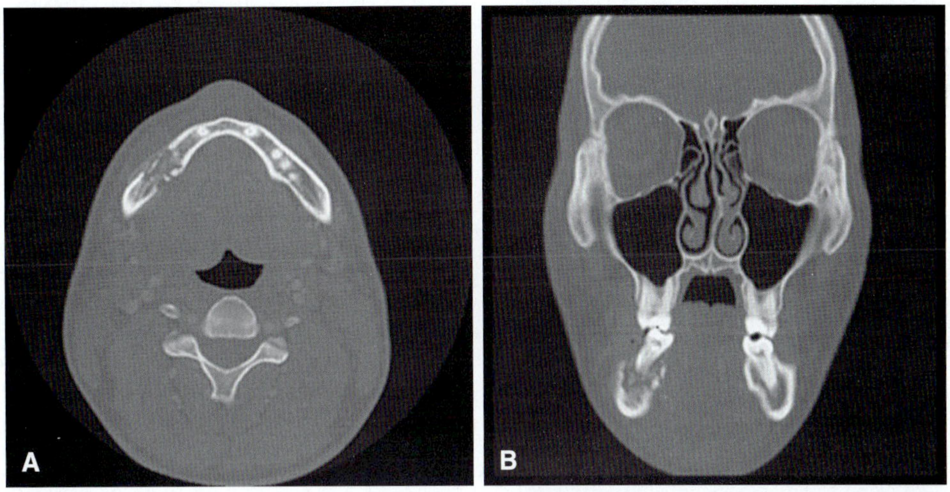

Fig. 20.19 Axial (A) and coronal (B) bone window multidetector computed tomographic images of the same patient shown in Fig. 20.17 shows sequestration of the lingual cortex.

periosteum as it begins to fill in with a granular or sclerotic bone pattern as intervening bone arcades increase in thickness and radiopacity (Fig. 20.21). When this occurs, it may be impossible to identify the original cortex or the individual layers of periosteal new bone, thus making it difficult to determine whether the new bone is derived from the periosteum. After a considerable amount of time, a bony hard asymmetry may be seen clinically on the affected side with an altered surface contour and morphology (Fig. 20.22). Should the disease not be adequately controlled, a cloaca, which may appear as a well-defined break in the outer cortex or in the periosteal new bone may form. Furthermore, the disease may slowly spread to the mandibular condyle and the temporomandibular joint resulting in septic arthritis. More distant spread may also involve the inner ear and mastoid air cells.

Effects on adjacent teeth. The effects on the teeth and lamina dura may be the same as the effects described for periapical inflammatory disease in the acute phase of osteomyelitis. The roots of teeth may undergo external resorption or hypercementosis, and the lamina dura may become less apparent with increasing sclerosis. If the tooth pulp is

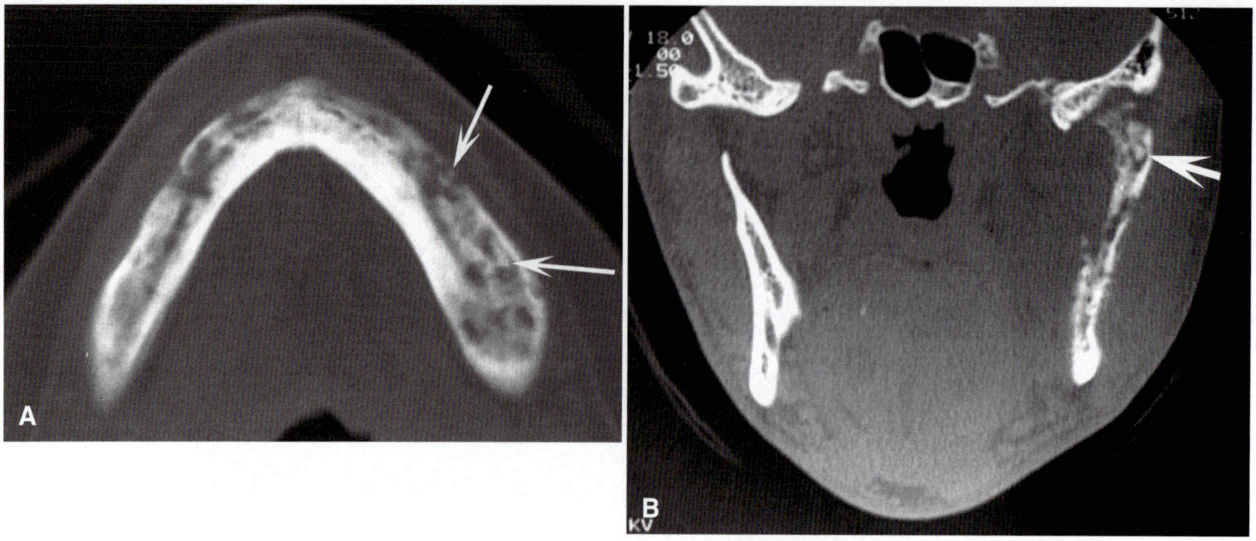

Fig. 20.20 Multidetector computed tomographic images showing multiple sequestra *(arrows)* within the body of the mandible (A) and in the condylar head (B).

nonvital, the widened periodontal ligament space at the root apex will be enlarged and appear prominent against the highly sclerotic bone.

DIAGNOSTIC IMAGING OF SOFT TISSUE INVOLVEMENT IN OSTEOMYELITIS

Diagnostic imaging may be used to confirm the presence and extent of soft tissue involvement. MDCT and MRI may be used to differentiate soft tissue neoplasia from inflammatory lesions that extend to the bone surface and into the adjacent soft tissues. If MDCT is acquired with an intravenous contrast agent, the imaging may demonstrate the soft tissue extension of the inflammatory response. This can appear as an increase in the attenuation (or radiopacity) of the normally low-attenuation (i.e., radiolucent) fat that underlies the skin. In these cases, one may observe a series of fine high-attenuation lines extending through the low-attenuation fat to the skin, with the lines being oriented perpendicular to the overlying skin surface. This is referred to as "fat streaking" (Fig. 20.23). In addition, one may see enlargement of the adjacent muscle and skin thickening and abnormal collections of gas in the soft tissue. Over time, the contrast between soft tissue planes may disappear, and the presence of an abscess may become evident as a well-defined region of low attenuation surrounded by a wide border of contrast-enhanced (i.e., more highly attenuated or radiopaque) tissue. T_1- or T_2-weighted MRI can be used with gadolinium enhancement and fat suppression to detect the presence of adjacent soft tissue involvement, including edema. Lymphadenopathy arising from infections also may be visualized on MDCT and MR images within the fascial spaces of the head and neck (Fig. 20.24).

Differential Interpretation

Clinically, the differential interpretation of a unilateral facial or jaw swelling may include osteomyelitis, fibrous dysplasia in children and adolescents, and malignancy in an adult. The clinical signs of acute inflammation may be helpful in guiding the imaging examination, and in the identification of key radiologic features that may allow the dentist to differentiate these different disease processes. On imaging, the presence of sequestra is a hallmark diagnostic feature of osteomyelitis.

In the acute phase of osteomyelitis in children and adolescents, the appearance of a unilateral jaw swelling may require an inflammatory

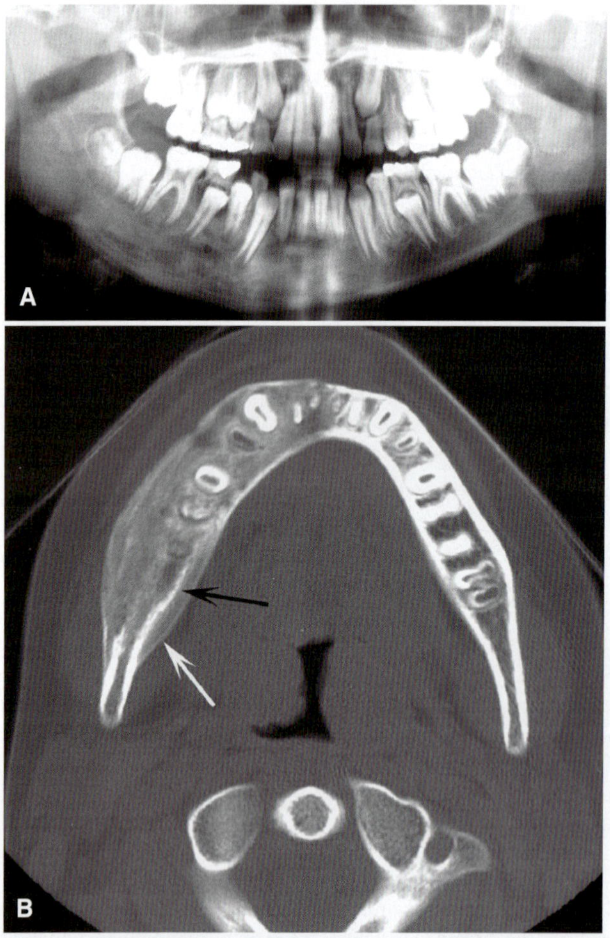

Fig. 20.21 Chronic osteomyelitis. The panoramic image (A) shows an increase in the height of the right mandibular body. The axial multidetector computed tomographic image (B) of the same patient shows periosteal new bone *(white arrow)* and evidence of the original cortex *(black arrow)*. There has been a general increase in bone density (sclerosis) on the right side and a loss of definition of the more low-attenuation (radiolucent) component of the response as the disease process has become more chronic.

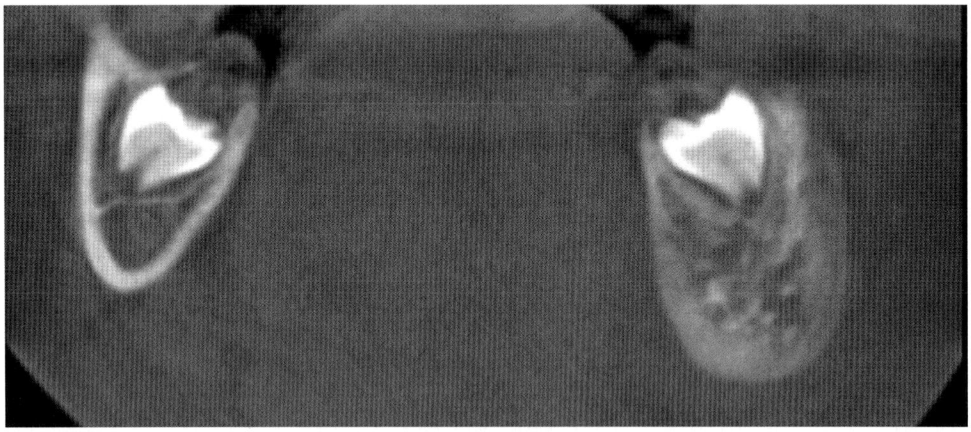

Fig. 20.22 Coronal cone beam computed tomographic image showing infilling of the periosteal new bone layers in chronic osteomyelitis involving the left mandibular body. Note the asymmetry of the mandibular body between the affected left side and the unaffected right side.

lesion to be differentiated from fibrous dysplasia. A useful radiographic feature in this instance may be the way in which the bone enlarges in response to the two diseases. In fibrous dysplasia, the new bone is manufactured from within. The outer cortex may be thinned by the changes, but the surface cortex remains intact as the bone enlarges. Also, bone sequestration is not seen in fibrous dysplasia. In contrast, the new bone that enlarges the jaws in osteomyelitis is deposited by periosteal new bone formation superficial to the native bone cortex. In the chronic phase of osteomyelitis, the native bone cortex may be indistinct or difficult to see. In such instances, inspection of the most peripheral surface of the bone may reveal subtle evidence of periosteal new bone formation that has not yet fully mineralized. These points of differentiation are important because the histopathologic appearance of a biopsy specimen of new periosteal bone in osteomyelitis may be similar to that of fibrous dysplasia, and the condition may be reported erroneously should a radiologic image not be made available to the oral and maxillofacial pathologist.

Malignant neoplasia, whether invading the jawbones from an adjacent soft tissue space or growing from within the bone may, at times, be difficult to differentiate from the acute phase of osteomyelitis. In particular, if the malignant neoplasm has become secondarily infected via an oral ulcer, it may be difficult to differentiate inflammatory radiologic features from those that are malignant. For example, Langerhans cell histiocytosis results in poorly defined, noncorticated, radiolucent regions of bone destruction, but the lesion rarely stimulates the sclerotic bone reaction seen in osteomyelitis. It is notable that some malignant neoplasms like Ewing sarcoma can also stimulate periosteum and create the "onion skin" type of appearance seen radiologically in osteomyelitis. Should there be destruction of adjacent structures or of the surface of the bone itself, the possibility of a malignant neoplasm should be more strongly considered. As well, Ewing sarcoma will be accompanied by an often rapidly growing and exuberant soft tissue mass, but these lesions usually also produce characteristic bone destruction. Malignant neoplasms such as osteosarcoma and chondrosarcoma have the capability of creating new bone within the lesion itself, but this may be accompanied by adjacent areas of bone destruction. Intralesional mineralization may have a wide range of appearances depending on the maturation of the cells, with some foci appearing more sporadic and irregular and others appearing more dense and granular. Paget disease of bone may affect the mandible bilaterally, which is rare in osteomyelitis. Periosteal new bone formation and sequestra are also not seen in Paget disease.

Chronic osteomyelitis is similar to the bone lesions described in chronic recurrent multifocal osteomyelitis (CRMO) and SAPHO syndrome; synovitis (inflammatory arthritis), acne (pustulosa), pustulosis (psoriasis, palmoplantar pustulosis), hyperostosis (acquired), and osteitis (osteomyelitis) with respect to the imaging findings, negative microbiologic cultures, and clinical features such as intermittent recurrent pain and swelling of the involved bone. These forms of osteomyelitis arise *de novo* without going through an acute phase of osteomyelitis where a pathogenic microorganism can be identified. Some authors have used the term "primary chronic osteomyelitis" to describe this group of diseases and "secondary chronic osteomyelitis" to describe the entity that evolves from the acute phase of osteomyelitis where a pathogenic microorganism can be identified. A similar appearance can be seen in cases of SAPHO syndrome (Fig. 20.25).

CRMO is a condition that often occurs symmetrically in the long bones in children and is characterized by pain of the affected bone without or with swelling. CRMO has been described as a nonpurulent osteomyelitis with negative microbiologic cultures. The imaging features are identical to chronic osteomyelitis, which have been described here. Treatment consists of systemic steroids, nonsteroidal antiinflammatory drugs (NSAIDs), and bisphosphonates because antibiotic and surgical therapy have not been effective treatments. Chronic osteomyelitis of the jaw in children not having a clear etiology may be a unifocal variant of CRMO.

Management

As with all inflammatory lesions of the jaws, removal of the source of inflammation (e.g., removal of a tooth, root canal treatment) is the primary goal of therapy. Antimicrobial treatment is the mainstay of treatment of acute osteomyelitis, along with surgical incision and drainage.

Chronic osteomyelitis may be more difficult to manage than the acute form. In cases involving an extreme osteoblastic response where the bone may become very sclerotic, the subsequent decrease of blood supply into the bone may work against healing. Hyperbaric oxygen therapy and creative modes of long-term antibiotic delivery have been used with limited success. Surgical intervention, which may include sequestrectomy, decortication, or resection, often is necessary. The probability of successful treatment, especially when using long-term antibiotic therapy with decortication is greater in the first and second decades of life. If microbiological cultures are negative, antibiotic therapy is not effective. It may be that the inflammatory response has become the main disease process, and antiinflammatory agents, such as steroids and NSAIDs, may be more effective. More recently, the use of bisphosphonate therapy has provided some therapeutic success.

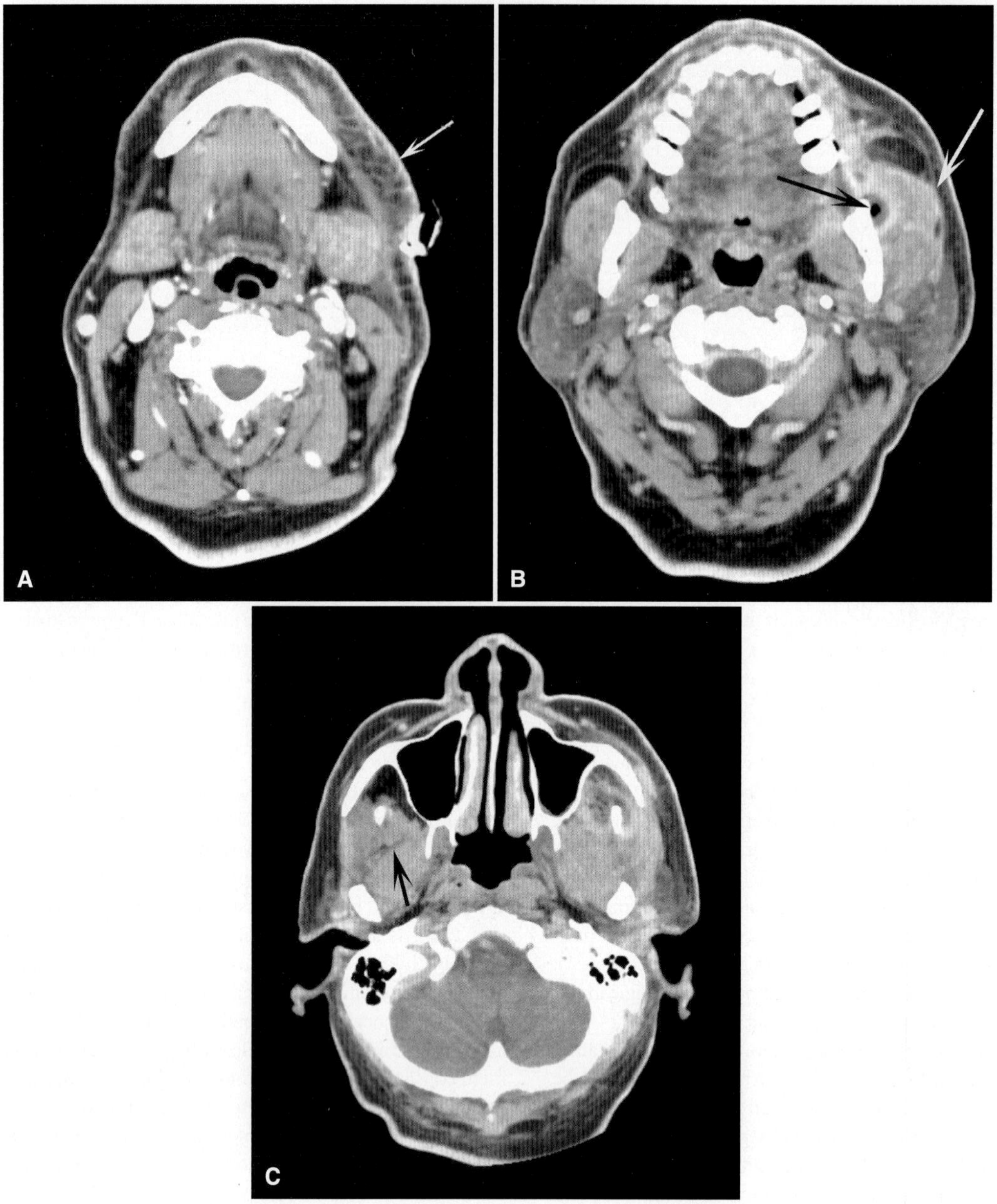

Fig. 20.23 Three axial multidetector computed tomographic soft tissue window images with contrast showing an infection involving the soft tissues overlying the left mandibular ramus. There is streaking or reticulation of the fat underlying the adjacent skin as well as thickening of the skin *(arrow)* compared with the unaffected contralateral side. Also, there is thickening of the masseter muscle *(white arrow)* and a radiolucent pocket of gas *(black arrow)* adjacent to the bone (B). Furthermore, there is a loss of distinctive fat tissue planes between the soft tissues (C). Note that the individual muscles defined by fat planes (the lateral border of the normal lateral pterygoid muscle *[arrow]* is not apparent on the opposite affected side). (Courtesy Stuart White, DDS, Los Angeles, CA.).

RADIATION-INDUCED CHANGES TO THE JAWS

Disease Mechanism

Many of the imaging features identified in osteomyelitis may also be seen with changes to bone following physical or chemical trauma. However, without a clinical history, it may be difficult, if not impossible, to differentiate the imaging features of these diseases from one another.

Therapeutic radiation is an example of physical trauma, prescribed for the treatment of a malignancy in the head and neck. Radiation damages the cellular elements of bone and periosteum as well as those structures contained within the bone. At the macromolecular level, this damage may involve DNA, protein, or lipid molecules, and these changes could impair DNA replication, enzyme function, or cell membrane permeability. Moreover, such changes could result in the misrepair of radiation-induced DNA damage, arrested cell division, or cell death. The stage of differentiation of cells as well as the dose, dose rate, and fractionation of radiation are all factors that affect how the bone will respond to this injury.

At very low radiation doses in the order of 1–4 Gy, radiation has been reported to have a stimulatory effect on osteoblasts, and this may

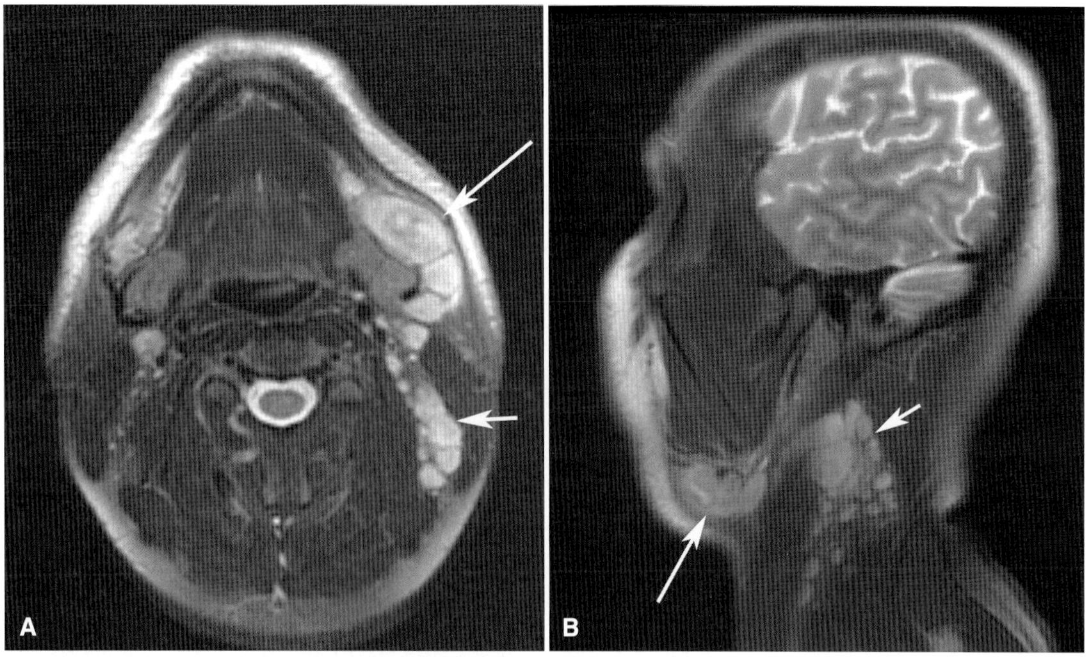

Fig. 20.24 Axial (A) and sagittal (B) T2-weighted magnetic resonance images of a patient with tuberculosis. Note the significant lymphadenopathy involving the submandibular lymph nodes *(long arrows)* and level II nodes *(short arrows)*.

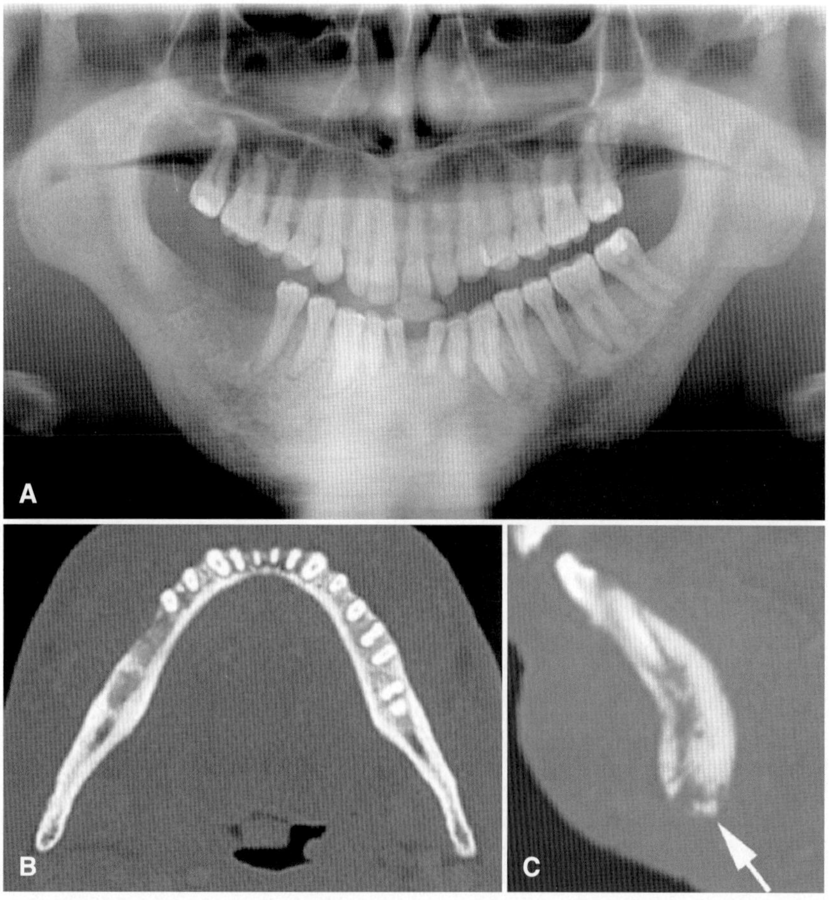

Fig. 20.25 A case of SAPHO in which both the wrist and the mandible were involved. The panoramic image (A) shows a diffuse, generalized sclerotic bone reaction, bone resorption of the inferior border of the mandibular body, and widening of the periodontal ligament spaces around many teeth. The axial multidetector computed tomographic image (B) shows the mostly sclerotic bone reaction with some regions of bone resorption, while the sagittal image of the anterior mandible (C) shows resorption of the inferior cortex and a sequestrum *(arrow)*.

be seen radiographically as sclerosis. Above this dose range, however, therapeutic doses of 10 Gy can result in chondroblast and osteoblast cell death. At even higher doses of 20 Gy, the long bones in a young child can sustain irrevervsible growth retardation resulting in short stature. In contrast, mature bone is much more radiation resistant, with damage occurring with higher doses ranging from 60 to 70 Gy.

It is important to recognize that bone contains a number of other tissues that may also be affected by radiation. One such tissue system is the vasculature. Indeed, many of the late effects of radiation injury involving bone may arise because of damage to the vasculature. Although vascular endothelial cells in large vessels are generally radioresistant, the thinner walls of smaller vessels may be more sensitive. Damage to this population of cells lining the walls of small vessels may compromise their ability to proliferate, and the bone may become hypocellular and hypovascular as a result. The lack of sufficient vascularity results in a hypoxic environment in which healing of bone is compromised. Should the dose, dose rate, or fractionation scheme of radiation delivery exceed the tolerance of the bone to repair, the bone may undergo death or necrosis, and this is referred to as osteoradionecrosis. Therapeutic radiation exposure can cause bone damage and changes without necrosis, although it is possible that such changes may make the bone more susceptible to necrosis, especially after surgical intervention.

Radiation-induced necrosis or osteoradionecrosis is characterized by the presence of exposed bone after the delivery of radiation therapy. The exposed bone may become a sequestrum, often leading to the involvement of more bone. Although bone located anywhere within the jaws is susceptible, the posterior mandible is affected more often than other areas because it is frequently in the radiation field, particularly when lymph nodes are included in the treatment field for a head and neck malignancy. Intense pain may occur with intermittent swelling and drainage extraorally. However, many patients feel no pain with bone exposure. The loss of normal structure may compromise the integrity of the bone, and in some cases, the bone can fracture.

Histopathologically, bone necrosis is defined by the absence of osteocytes within lacunae. The overlying mucosal covering can be lost, and the necrotic bone becomes exposed to the oral environment where it can become secondarily infected. It is also possible that irradiated bone becomes more susceptible to necrosis from an odontogenic infection, dental extraction, or denture trauma. And finally, depending on the extensiveness of the necrosis, the bone may become susceptible to fracture.

Imaging Examination

An initial imaging examination consisting of panoramic, as well as intraoral periapical and occlusal images may be useful to image the teeth and periodontal structures. Also, as many of the imaging features overlap with the features seen in osteomyelitis, a CBCT or MDCT examination should be obtained for the identification of sequestra.

Imaging Features

Immediately following radiation therapy, there may be no visible changes on imaging. The earliest changes may be seen in the posterior mandible because this region of the jaws is generally less well vascularized. An early change seen in the outer cortical plate of the mandible is a sharply defined region of bone resorption, and within the bone, there may be irregular, poorly defined, noncorticated areas of bone resorption and sclerosis. In the maxilla, parts of the cortical borders of the sinus, for example, may be lost (Fig. 20.26). Should the normal architecture of the bone be sufficiently disrupted, jaw fractures may also be seen.

In the alveolar processes of the jaws, the most frequent change is an irregular but uniform widening of the periodontal ligament space

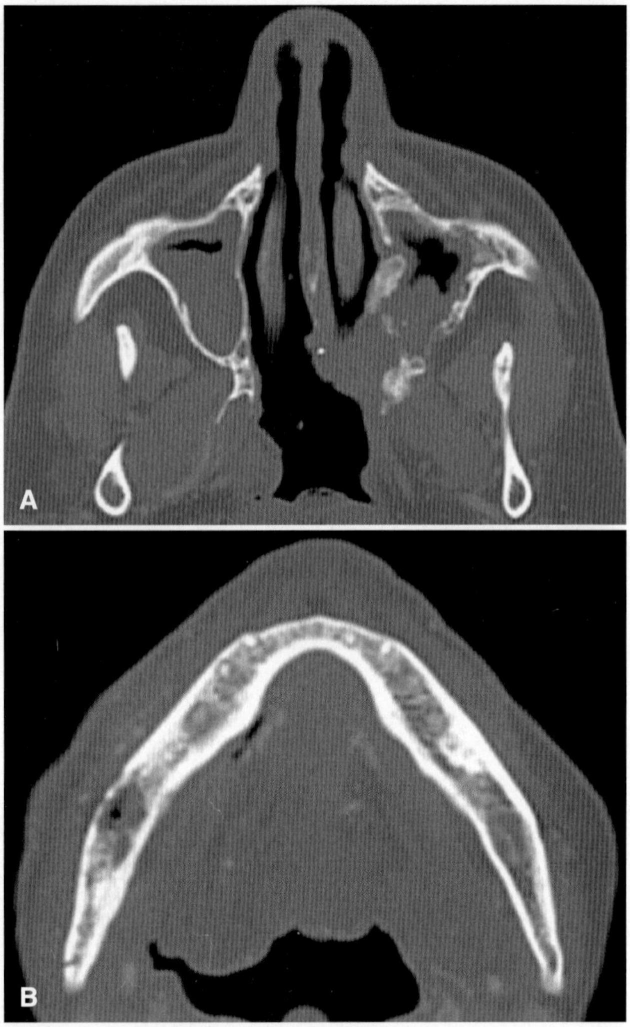

Fig. 20.26 Multidetector computed tomographic images show radiation changes with significant resorption of the left maxilla (A) and resorption and sclerosis in the posterior right mandible (B).

encircling the teeth. Furthermore, the widening that is seen lacks a discrete epicenter (Fig. 20.27) and there is no bone loss, differentiating these changes from periapical inflammatory disease (Fig. 20.4). A recent study has shown the cumulative incidence of periodontal ligament space widening ranges from 12% in the first 12 months following radiation therapy to 34% in the second year, and finally, to 55% in the third year with widening becoming more significant with cumulative mandibular doses greater than 45 Gy. Other changes that may also be seen include periodontal disease like bone loss and sclerosis.

The radiologic interpretation of osteoradionecrosis relies on the identification of sequestra in addition to the patient history (Fig. 20.28). Although fractures of the bone can develop (Fig. 20.29), the appearance of a fracture is not necessarily diagnostic. Bone sequestra are seen more commonly in the mandible, and often the sequestra are fragments of detached cortical bone. The presence of osteoradionecrosis cannot always be diagnosed from the diagnostic image, and often clinically obvious signs of exposed necrotic bone may not have significant changes in the panoramic image. In these cases, CBCT or MDCT imaging is required.

Of note is the dampened periosteal response in osteoradionecrosis. Likely, this is due to the radiation-induced death of the relatively

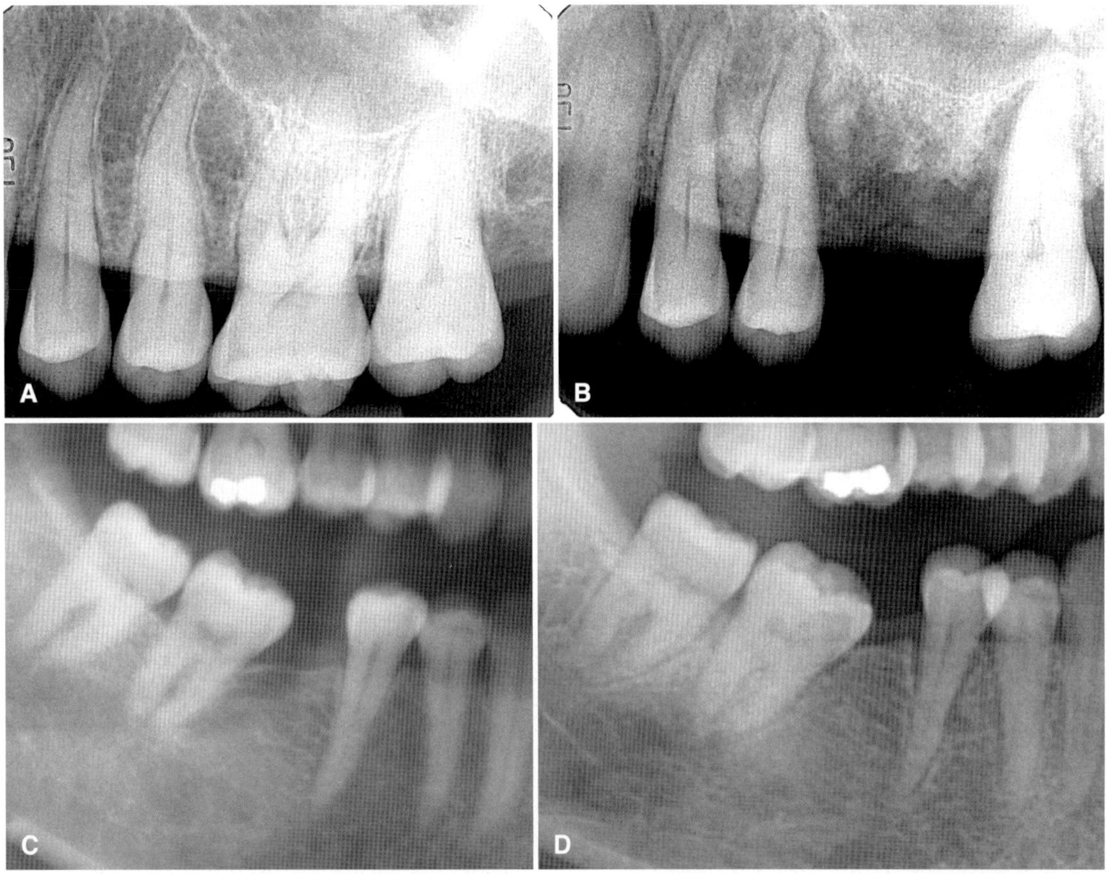

Fig. 20.27 Changes to the periodontal ligament spaces after therapeutic radiation. Periapical (A) and cropped panoramic (C) images were made prior to radiation therapy, and images (B) and (C) were made of the same patients following radiation. Note the combination of bone destruction and sclerosis, and the nonconcentric widening of the periodontal ligament space.

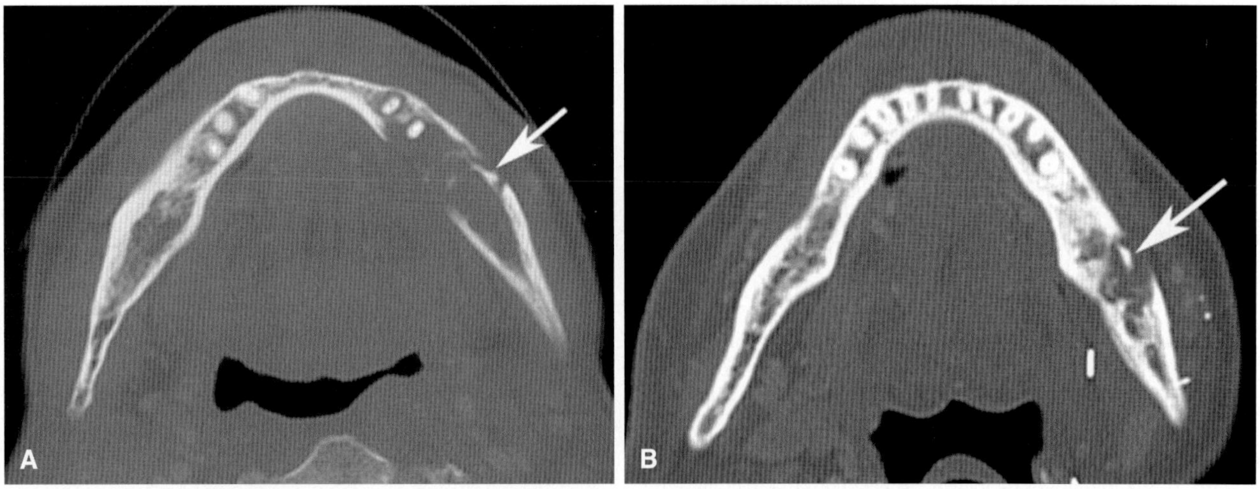

Fig. 20.28 Examples of radiation-induced necrosis (osteoradionecrosis). Axial multidetector computed tomographic images show extensive bone resorption and sequestra *(arrow)* (A). The sclerotic response is more prominent in (B).

radiosensitive mesenchymal stem cell population in the inner osteogenic layer of the periosteum.

Differential Interpretation

Radiation-induced widening of the periodontal ligament space must be distinguished from periapical inflammatory disease to avoid unnecessary endodontic treatment or tooth extraction. In periapical inflammatory disease, a circular or "hydraulic" enlargement of the periodontal ligament space is seen at the apex of the tooth root, and an epicenter is visible apical to the root apex. In periodontal disease, the change in the width of the periodontal ligament space is seen at the alveolar crest. Vitality testing of the tooth pulp and a thorough patient history and

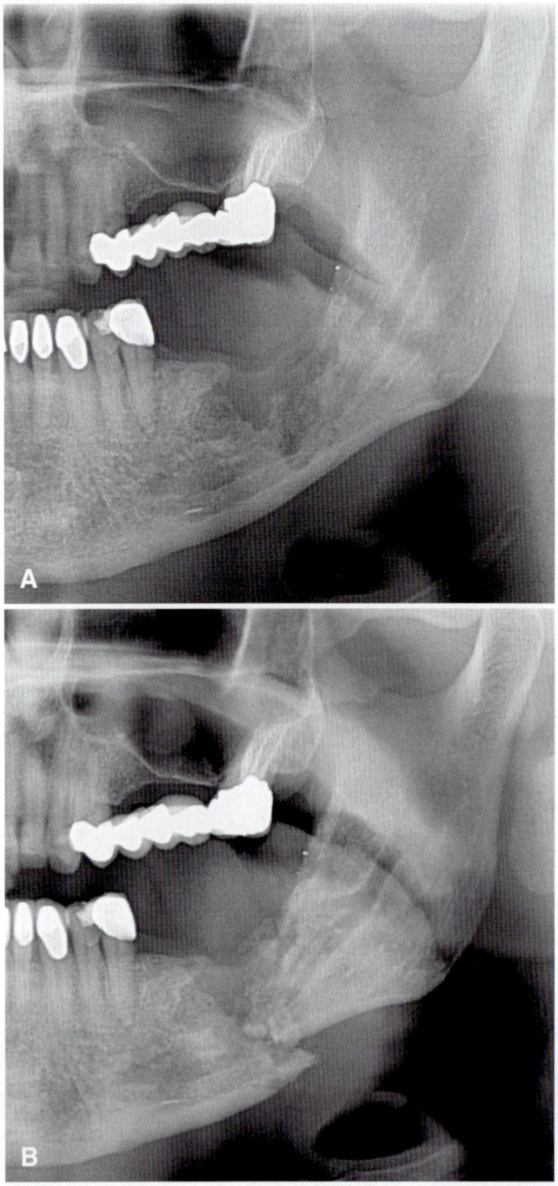

Fig. 20.29 Cropped panoramic images of a patient with bone resorption secondary to therapeutic radiation (A) and the development of a fracture secondary to the loss of bone integrity in the same patient 3 months later (B).

clinical examination are important to avoid unnecessary endodontic treatment or extraction. Radiation-induced periodontal bone-like loss is difficult to differentiate from conventional periodontal disease as the regions of bone resorption and sclerosis may be very similar.

Bone resorption secondary to radiation therapy may simulate bone destruction from a malignant neoplasm, especially in the maxilla. For this reason, the detection of a recurrence of the malignant neoplasm in the presence of osteoradionecrosis may be very difficult. If the recurrence of a malignancy is suspected, MDCT or MRI may be used to detect an associated soft tissue mass. Differentiating radiation-induced changes from osteomyelitis is less difficult because of the history of radiation therapy.

Management

Treatment of radiation-induced necrosis at the present time is unsatisfactory. Decortication with sequestrectomy and hyperbaric oxygen with antibiotics have been used with limited success because of poor healing following surgery. More conservative approaches, which aim to maintain the integrity of the mandible by keeping the site free of infection and the patient free of pain, may prove more successful in the long term. The incidence of osteoradionecrosis has declined because of the use of intensity-modulated radiotherapy (IMRT) and preventive therapies that can include the removal of teeth with a poor periodontal or pulpal prognosis before radiation treatment. Excellent oral and denture hygiene continue to remain the mainstays of preventive regimens.

MEDICATION-RELATED OSTEONECROSIS OF THE JAWS

Some medications can cause chemical trauma to bone, altering the balance of osteoblast and osteoclast activities, creating a disease state. As with therapeutic radiation, many of the imaging features identified in medication-related osteonecrosis of the jaws overlap with osteomyelitis.

Disease Mechanism

Bisphosphonates and receptor activator of nuclear factor kappa-B ligand (RANK-L) inhibitors are drugs that act to inhibit osteoclast function and therefore, bone resorption. Although these drugs have become important treatment modalities of the bone lesions of multiple myeloma, hypercalcemia of malignancy, metastatic disease, and osteoporosis, the intraoral exposure of necrotic bone in patients undertaking this pharmacologic treatment is now a well-known complication. The bone exposure occurs more commonly in patients receiving intravenous injections of the drug, and with the more potent aminobisphosphonates after an invasive procedure, such as tooth extraction, periodontal or endodontic surgery, or implant placement. More recently, this has become a more common finding in patients who use oral bisphosphonates.

Clinical Features

Clinically, patients typically develop an area of exposed bone after an invasive dental surgical procedure, although cases related to denture trauma and spontaneous cases have also occurred (Fig. 20.30). Ulceration of palatal tori, for example, resulting in bone exposure, is most likely the result of trauma. The most common areas affected

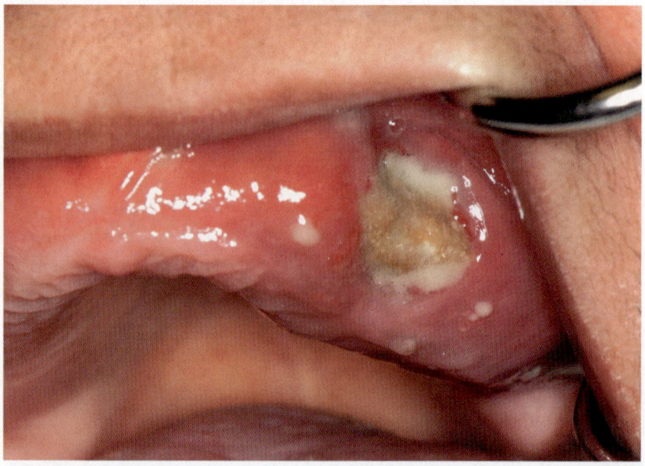

Fig. 20.30 A clinical image showing exposed bone along the vestibular surface of the edentulous maxillary premolar region in a patient with a history of bisphosphonate use.

are the posterior mandible (60%) and the maxilla (40%), although both jaws (9%) may be affected. The incidence of bone exposure is difficult to determine, but more recent studies suggest that approximately 3% of patients receiving these drugs have exposed bone. The patients may be asymptomatic or may present with pain and swelling.

Imaging Features

A spectrum of radiographic findings may or may not correlate well with the clinical symptoms. Often, there are no specific imaging findings with the clinically exposed bone; however, imaging may demonstrate the detachment. These changes can appear quickly, and they may be dramatic (Fig. 20.31). In some cases, the radiographic changes may be indistinguishable from osteomyelitis (Fig. 20.32). Other reported findings include widening of the periodontal membrane space seen with radiation and thickening of the lamina dura (Fig. 20.33).

Management

Treatment of medication-related bone exposure is unsatisfactory as surgical intervention and hyperbaric oxygen therapy have not been consistently successful. The mainstay of therapy is preventive in nature. Patients who are scheduled to be administered the drugs intravenously should have a dental examination to remove potential and existing sources of infection to obviate the need for invasive dental procedures in the future. The situation is further complicated by the fact that the half-life of some of these drugs in bone can be as long as 12 years. Once bone is exposed, management is aimed at controlling the symptoms of pain and infection with antibiotic mouth rinses and systemic antibiotic therapy.

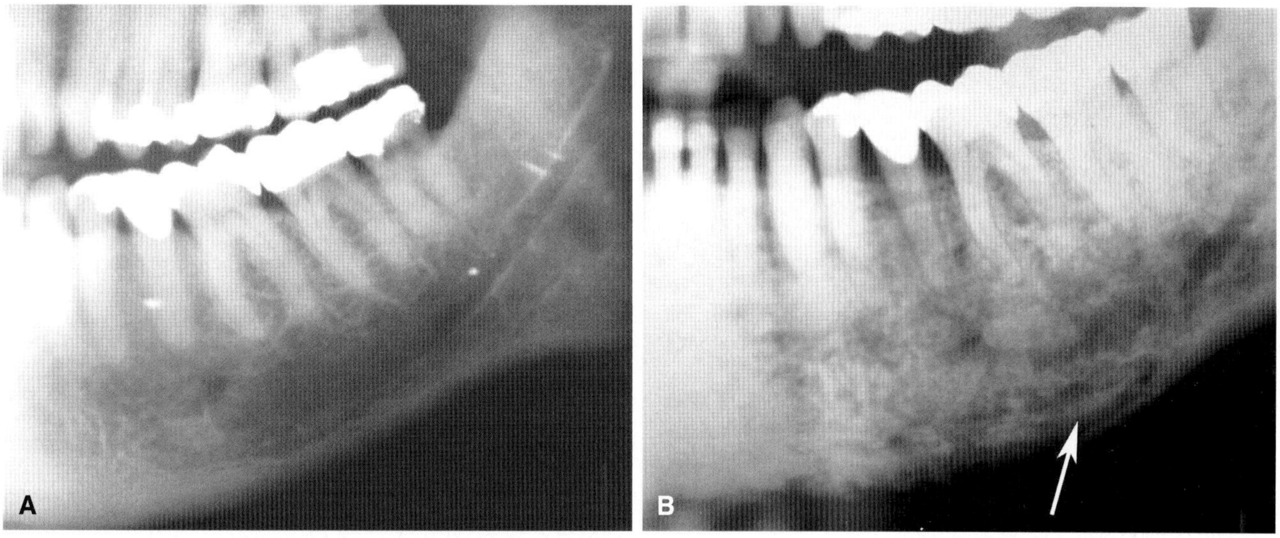

Fig. 20.31 Two cropped panoramic images (A and B) of the same patient taken 1 year apart show the dramatic changes to the normal bone pattern following bisphosphonate therapy. Note the developing sclerotic bone pattern and the sequestrum *(arrow)* of the inferior cortex.

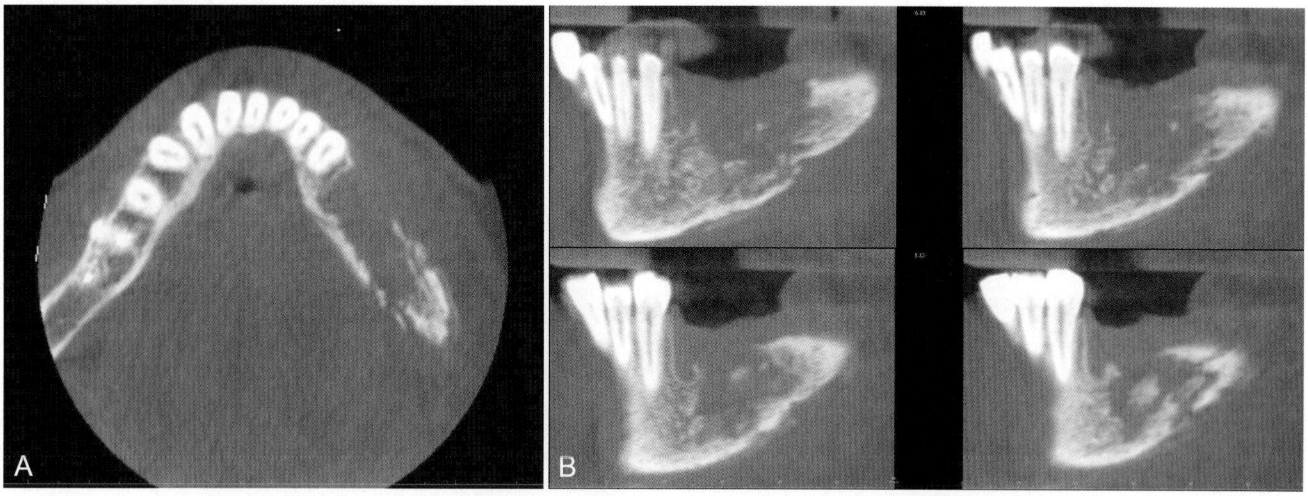

Fig. 20.32 Axial (A) and corrected sagittal (B) cone beam computed tomographic images of a patient receiving intravenous bisphosphonate therapy showing bone destruction in the left posterior mandible with periosteal new bone formation on the buccal and lingual surfaces of the bone (A) and sequestra.

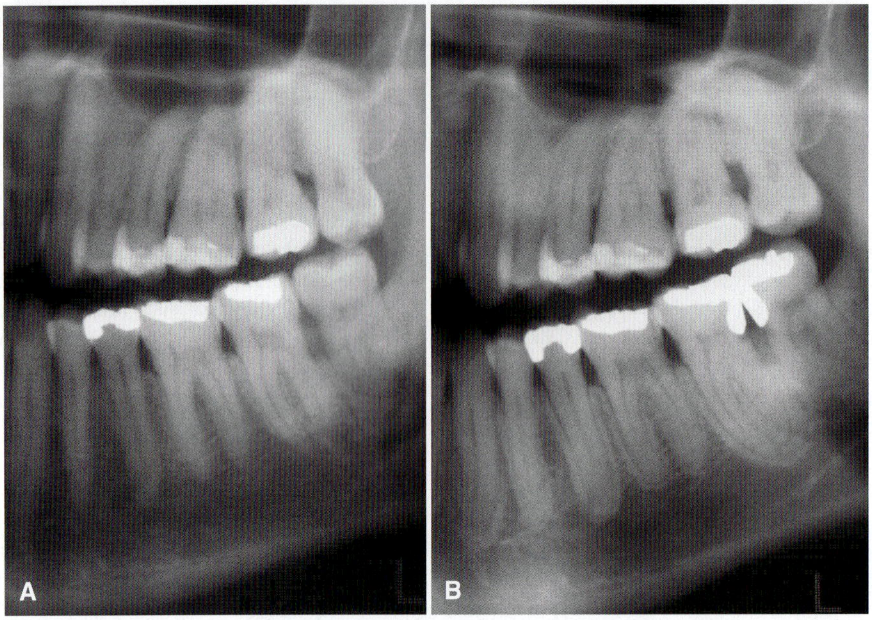

Fig. 20.33 Two cropped panoramic images (A and B) of a patient receiving bisphosphonate therapy made 7 years apart, reveal thickening of the lamina dura around the teeth.

PERICORONITIS

Disease Mechanism

Pericoronitis is a clinical diagnosis that refers to inflammation of the soft tissue operculum surrounding the crown of a partially erupted tooth. This condition, also referred to as operculitis, is seen most often in association with mandibular third molars in young adults. The gingiva surrounding the erupted portion of the crown becomes inflamed when food or microbial debris become trapped under the soft tissue. The gingiva subsequently becomes swollen and may become secondarily traumatized by the opposing occlusion. This inflammation may also extend into the bone surrounding the crown of the tooth.

Clinical Features

Pericoronitis can affect patients of any age or sex, but it is most commonly seen during the time of eruption of the third molars in young adults. Patients with pericoronitis typically complain of pain and swelling, with trismus being a common presentation. When the partially erupted tooth is a mandibular third molar, pain is often felt on occlusion with an ulcerated operculum usually the source of the pain.

Imaging Features

The imaging features of pericoronitis can range from no changes when the inflammatory lesion is confined to the soft tissues to localized rarefaction around the tooth crown and root to sclerosis of the adjacent bone. Should the inflammatory response become more exuberant, the changes can extend to the bone surface, resulting in the development of osteomyelitis in the most severe cases.

Location

The mandibular third molar region is the most common location, and the bone change is on the follicular space or the portion of the crown still embedded in bone or in close proximity to bone.

Periphery

The periphery of the bone change is poorly defined with a wide zone of transition between the normal trabecular pattern and the sclerotic bone.

Internal Structure

The internal structure of bone adjacent to the area of pericoronitis is most often sclerotic with thickened trabeculae (Fig. 20.34). An area of bone loss or radiolucency immediately adjacent to the crown that enlarges the follicular space may be seen. If this lesion spreads considerably, the internal pattern appears identical to the imaging features of osteomyelitis.

Effects on Surrounding Structures

As with periapical inflammatory disease, pericoronitis may cause rarefaction and/or sclerosis of the surrounding bone. With more extensive involvement, evidence of periosteal new bone formation may be seen along an adjacent bone surface (Fig. 20.35), and this may extend superiorly as high as the sigmoid notch of the mandible.

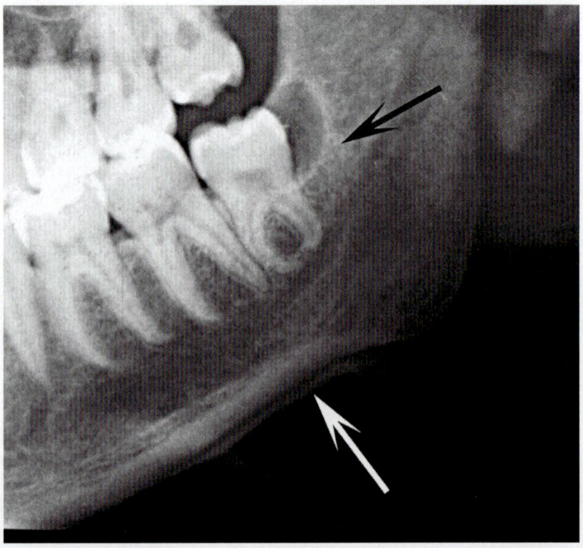

Fig. 20.34 Cropped panoramic image of a case of pericoronitis related to the partially erupted mandibular left third molar. Note the sclerotic bone reaction adjacent to the follicular cortex *(black arrow)* and the periosteal reaction *(white arrow)*.

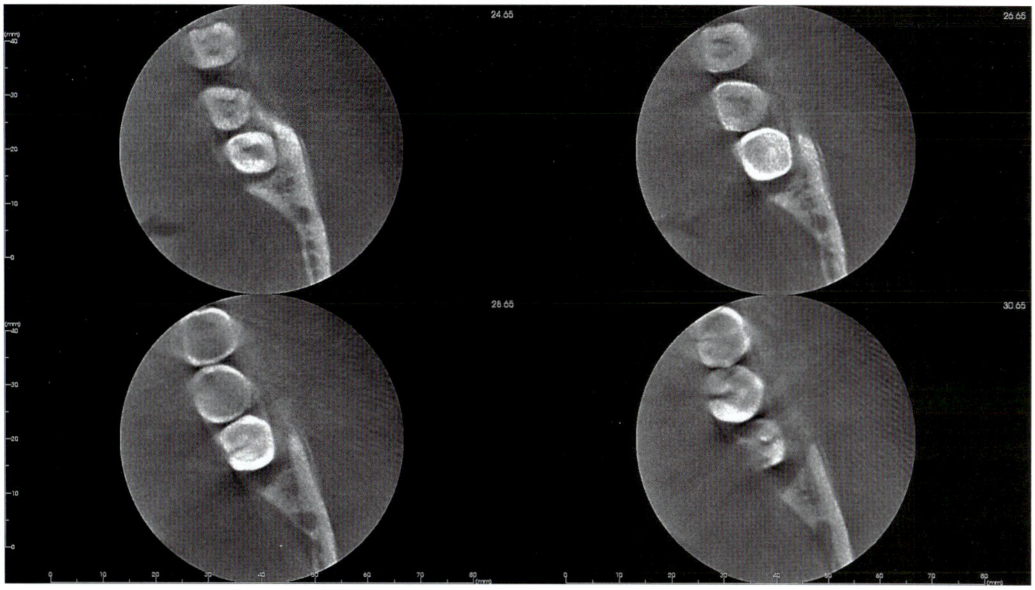

Fig. 20.35 Axial cone beam computed tomographic images showing periosteal new bone formation adjacent to the lateral surface of the ramus in a patient with pericoronitis.

Differential Interpretation

Although the diagnosis of pericoronitis is made clinically rather than radiographically, the differential interpretation can include other mixed radiolucent and radiopaque, or sclerotic, entities that can exist adjacent to the crown of a partially erupted third molar. These may include a DBI and fibrous dysplasia. The clinical symptoms, which are indicative of inflammation, usually exclude these intraosseous conditions. Neoplasms to be considered include squamous cell carcinoma (in older patients) and the sclerotic form of osteosarcoma. The occurrence of squamous cell carcinoma developing within a preexisting inflammatory lesion may be difficult to identify. Features characteristic of malignant neoplasia, such as profound cortical bone destruction and invasion, may assist with the diagnosis.

Management

The treatment aim of pericoronitis is removal of the partially erupted tooth. However, in the acute phase, when trismus may prevent adequate access, antibiotic therapy should relieve symptoms until definitive treatment can be provided.

BIBLIOGRAPHY

Periapical Inflammatory Lesions

Jalali P, Tahmasbi M, Augsburger RA, et al. Dynamics of bone loss in cases with acute or chronic apical abscess. *J Endod.* 2019;45:1114-1118.

Lam EWN, Law AS, Nguyen RHN, et al. Interexaminer agreement in the radiologic identification of apical periodontitis/rarefying osteitis in the National Dental Practice-Based Research Network PREDICT Endodontic Study. *J Endod.* 2021;47:1575-1582.

Pericoronitis

Blakey GH, White RP Jr, Offenbacher S, et al. Clinical/biological outcomes of treatment for pericoronitis. *J Oral Maxillofac Surg.* 1996;54:1150-1160.

Osteomyelitis

Baba A, Kurokawa R, Kurokawa M, et al. Advanced imaging of head and neck infections. *J Neuroimaging.* 2023;33:477-492.

Mardini S, Gohel A. Imaging of odontogenic infections. *Radiol Clin North Am.* 2018;56:31-44.

Orpe EC, Lee L, Pharoah MJ. A radiological analysis of chronic sclerosing osteomyelitis of the mandible. *Dentomaxillofac Radiol.* 1996;25:125-129.

Petrikowski CG, Pharoah MJ, Lee L, et al. Radiographic differentiation of osteogenic sarcoma, osteomyelitis, and fibrous dysplasia of the jaws. *Oral Surg Oral Med Oral Pathol Oral Radiol Endod.* 1995;80:744-750.

Tiwari P, Bera RN, Kanojia S, et al. Assessing the optimal imaging modality in the diagnosis of jaw osteomyelitis. A meta-analysis. *Br J Oral Maxillofac Surg.* 2021;59:982-992.

Radiation-Induced Changes to Bone

McBride WH, Schaue D. Radiation-induced tissue damage and response. *J Pathol.* 2020;250:647-655.

Williams HJ, Davies AM. The effect of x-rays on bone: a pictorial review. *Eur Radiol.* 2006;16:619-633.

Osteoradionecrosis

Chan KC, Perschbacher SE, Lam EW, et al. Mandibular changes on panoramic imaging after head and neck radiotherapy. *Oral Surg Oral Med Oral Pathol Oral Radiol.* 2016;121:666-672.

Lajolo C, Rupe C, Gioco G, et al. Osteoradionecrosis of the jaws due to teeth extractions during and after radiotherapy: a systematic review. *Cancers (Basel).* 2021;13:5798.

Topkan E, Kucuk A, Somay E, Yilmaz B, Pehlivan B, Selek U. Review of osteoradionecrosis of the jaw: radiotherapy modality, technique and dose as risk factors. *J Clin Med.* 2023;12:325.

Medication-Related Osteonecrosis

Goker F, Grecchi E, Grecchi F, et al. Treatment of medication-related osteonecrosis of the jaw (MRONJ). A systematic review. *Eur Rev Med Pharmacol Sci.* 2021;25:2662-2673.

Jadu F, Lee L, Pharoah M, et al. A retrospective study assessing the incidence, risk factors and comorbidities of pamidronate-related necrosis of the jaws in multiple myeloma patients. *Ann Oncol.* 2007;18:2015-2019.

Nicholatou-Galitis O, Schiødt M, Mendes RA, et al. Medication-related osteonecrosis of the jaw: definition and best practice for prevention, diagnosis, and treatment. *Oral Surg Oral Med Oral Pathol Oral Radiol.* 2019;127:117-135.

21

Cysts

Ernest W.N. Lam

A true cyst is an epithelially lined pathologic cavity within bone that may contain a small amount of fluid drawn from adjacent cells and tissues. The epithelial cells may be derived from odontogenic or nonodontogenic sources. Odontogenic sources include the dental lamina, the reduced enamel epithelium, and the epithelial rests of Malassez, quiescent remnants of Hertwig epithelial root sheath. Nonodontogenic sources of cyst linings may include respiratory epithelium or remnant epithelial cells found within areas of tissue fusion. A thin connective tissue layer underlies the epithelium and separates the epithelial basal cell layer from the adjacent bone. Pseudocysts are a group of cysts that may lack an epithelial lining, or they may not be cavities in the bone at all. Rather, pseudocysts are grouped in this category because they may have some but not all of the radiologic features of a true cyst.

DISEASE MECHANISM

The proliferation of remnant epithelial cells within the bone is the initiating event in the pathogenesis of a true cyst. Epithelial proliferation may be the result of a genetic mutation or the release of a signaling molecule or mediator from an adjacent cell or tissue that stimulates proliferation. As the cells proliferate, osteoclasts are recruited to accommodate this growing population and space is made available for their increasing numbers. Debris from the proliferating cells accumulates at the center of the developing cavity, and the increasing osmotic gradient that develops draws fluid into the cavity from adjacent cells and tissues. With time, the developing cavity increases in size as more debris accumulates centrally and as more fluid is drawn in. In addition, a thin connective tissue layer develops beneath the basal epithelial cells. The end result is a cavity within the bone that expands much as a balloon would expand as it is filled with water (Fig. 21.1).

CLINICAL FEATURES

The most common clinical feature is a firm to bony-hard swelling that may be accompanied by pain if the cyst is related to a tooth with a nonvital pulp, or if the cyst has become secondarily infected.

IMAGING EXAMINATION

Diagnostic imaging has many important roles in the diagnosis and management of a cyst. First, imaging may reveal characteristic features that may lead to the diagnosis of a particular cyst. And second, imaging may reveal the extent of both intra- and extraosseous involvement, and assist in determining the best site for biopsy.

Intraoral images may reveal subtle changes around the teeth, including the effects of the cyst on the periodontal ligament space and lamina dura. Panoramic imaging can provide additional information about the extensiveness of bone involvement and reveal other relevant changes such as alterations to the borders of the maxillary sinus. However, from the standpoint of being able to visualize fine detail, intraoral imaging is more optimal. Both cone beam computed tomography (CBCT) and multidetector computed tomography (MDCT) may be useful to demonstrate the three-dimensional involvement of bone, as well as effects on structures not apparent on 2D planar imaging. Should the cyst grow large enough to involve adjacent soft tissues, MDCT and magnetic resonance imaging (MRI) may show the extent of such involvement.

IMAGING FEATURES

Location

Cysts may occur anywhere centrally within the maxillae or mandible but are rare in the condylar and coronoid processes of the mandible. Odontogenic cysts are typically found in the tooth-bearing areas of the jaws; in the mandible, they develop superior to the inferior alveolar canal. Some nonodontogenic cysts can originate within the antrum, whereas others can develop in the soft tissues around the face and neck.

Periphery

True cysts that arise centrally from within bone have a well-defined periphery and a cortex characterized by a fairly uniform, thin, radiopaque line. When a cyst becomes secondarily infected, which may happen if the cyst develops a communication with oral microorganisms, the cortex may become thicker and sclerotic, demonstrating a less radiopaque appearance. In addition, some cysts may insinuate themselves around the roots of teeth or against a bone cortex, creating a series of contiguous arcs; this is referred to as *scalloping*.

Shape

Cysts have smooth, curved borders that may give them a contour similar to the surface of a fluid-filled balloon. This contour is often described using the word "hydraulic," and the pattern of enlargement is described as a "hydraulic pattern of growth" within the bone.

Internal Structure

Cysts are most often uniformly radiolucent; however, long-standing cysts may contain cellular debris, including cholesterol granules or dystrophic calcification, both of which can impart sparse, particulate radiopacities against the more radiolucent background. In some cysts, different regions of the epithelium can proliferate at different rates, with some areas showing slower or faster regions of proliferation. This type of differential proliferation may give the cyst a multilocular

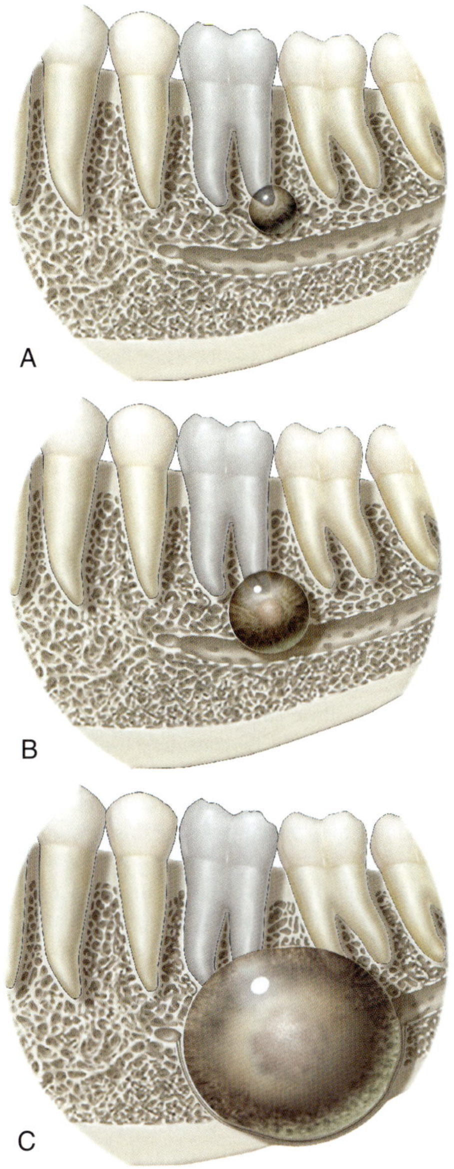

Fig. 21.1 The balloon-like "hydraulic" development and enlargement of a cyst in the jaws, and displacement of the adjacent teeth and compression of the inferior alveolar canal as it increases in size.

appearance and result in the development of bony walls or septa between the loculations. Occasionally scalloping of the cyst border against the endosteal or inner surface of the bone cortex may give the false impression of septation, particularly on planar imaging.

Effects on Surrounding Structures

Cysts develop and increase in size slowly, and when the periphery encounters an adjacent bone border, the bone border thins where it engages the cyst periphery. With time, the bone will expand to accommodate the cyst, and the pattern of expansion produces a smooth, curved surface. Cysts may displace the inferior alveolar nerve canal in an inferior or lingual direction, or displace the floor of the maxillary sinus in a superior direction, maintaining a thin layer of bone separating the cyst cavity from the airspace.

Effects on Adjacent Teeth

The slowly growing nature of a cyst can cause displacement of adjacent teeth as well as external resorption of tooth roots producing an often sharp, curved edge that mirrors the curvature of the cyst border. This is referred to as directional external resorption. As well, the lamina dura and the periodontal ligament space may be lost.

ODONTOGENIC CYSTS

Radicular Cyst

The radicular cyst is discussed in Chapter 20 in the context of periapical inflammatory disease. As the radiologic features of a radicular cyst cannot be reliably differentiated from those of a radicular abscess or granuloma, the "umbrella term" *rarefying osteitis* is used in oral and maxillofacial radiology as a radiologic diagnosis to describe a localized inflammatory condition arising from a tooth with a necrotic pulp. It is only after a focus of rarefying osteitis has undergone biopsy that the oral and maxillofacial pathologist can determine the presence of an epithelial lining, and diagnose a radicular cyst. The lining of a radicular cyst is derived from the epithelial cell rests of Malassez, and these cells are stimulated to proliferate by inflammatory mediators and signals derived from a tooth with a nonvital pulp.

Dentigerous Cyst

Disease Mechanism

The dentigerous or follicular cyst develops from the proliferation of the reduced enamel epithelium. Consequently, the cyst is associated with the crown of an impacted tooth or supernumerary tooth. The eruption cyst is the soft tissue counterpart of a dentigerous cyst.

Clinical Features

Dentigerous cysts are the second most common type of cyst in the jaws. Clinical examination may reveal a missing tooth or teeth and possibly a hard swelling that can manifest as a facial asymmetry.

Imaging Features

Location. The epicenter of a dentigerous cyst is located coronal to the crown of the involved tooth, most commonly a third molar or a maxillary canine (Fig. 21.2). An important diagnostic point is that the periphery of the cyst engages the tooth at its cementoenamel junction. A dentigerous cyst developing in association with a maxillary third molar tooth will enlarge into the maxilla and displace the tooth superiorly as well as the floor of the maxillary sinus as it enlarges. Cysts developing in association with a mandibular third molar may displace the tooth distally, sometimes a considerable distance into the base of the ramus.

Periphery. Dentigerous cysts have a well-defined and corticated periphery. If the periphery of the cyst perforates an adjacent bone surface, a portion of the cortex may be lost (Fig. 21.3). This loss of bone surface integrity may facilitate the entry of oral microorganisms into the cyst cavity. Secondary infection of the cyst in this way may affect the visibility of the periphery and the cortex.

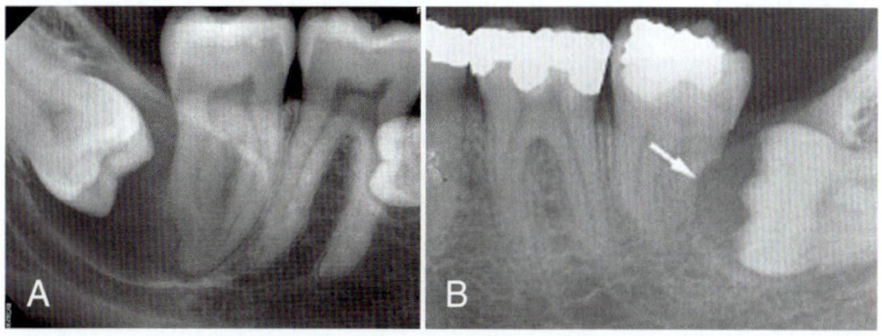

Fig. 21.2 A dentigerous cyst surrounds the crown of the mandibular right (A) and left (B) third molar. Note the associations of the cysts with the cementoenamel junctions. In (B), the cyst has caused external resorption of the distal root of the mandibular left second molar *(arrow)*.

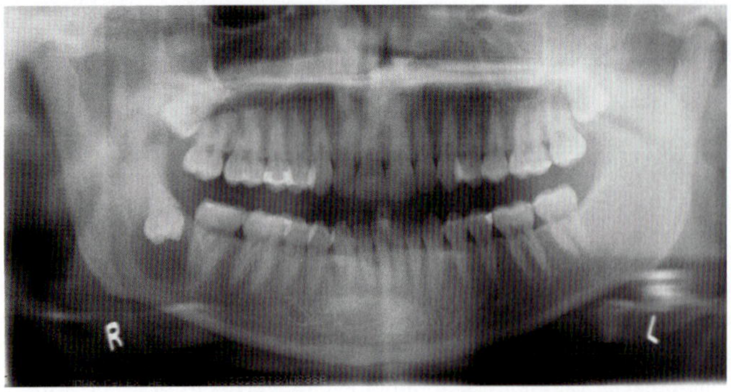

Fig. 21.3 A panoramic image shows a dentigerous cyst associated with the mandibular right third molar. The alveolar crest distal to the mandibular right second molar has been lost and the cortical boundary is no longer continuous around the entire cyst. As well, the third molar has been displaced into the mandibular ramus and the inferior alveolar canal has been displaced inferiorly around the cyst.

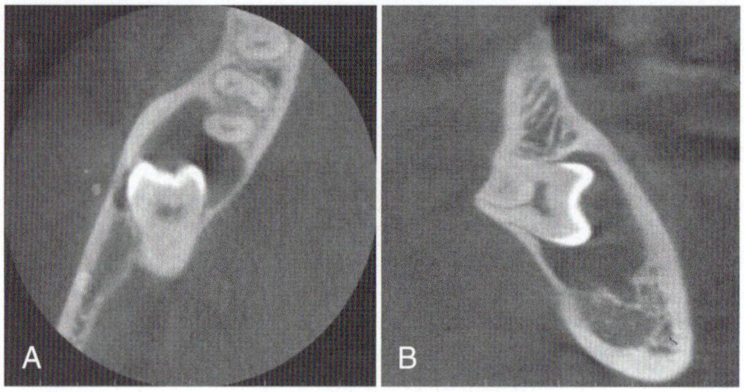

Fig. 21.5 Axial (A) and corrected sagittal (B) cone beam computed tomographic images of a dentigerous cyst associated with a mandibular right third molar. Note the displacement into the lingual cortex of the mandible, which has remodeled itself to accommodate the displaced tooth (A). The association with the cementoenamel junction is clearly visible (B).

Internal structure. Internally, a dentigerous cyst is completely radiolucent except for the crown of the involved tooth.

Effects on surrounding structures. As dentigerous cysts are slow growing, adjacent bone borders—whether the floor of the maxillary sinus or an adjacent cortex of bone—may become displaced as the cyst enlarges. Furthermore, adjacent anatomic structures such as the inferior alveolar canal can be displaced apically, away from the cyst (Fig. 21.3). In cases where the border of the dentigerous cyst has perforated the crest of the alveolar process, the intraluminal osmotic pressure will have been relieved, and the cyst may be in a state of decompression. In these instances, the hydraulic contour may become less evident, and the cyst may be less capable of expanding or affecting adjacent structures.

Effects on adjacent teeth. A dentigerous cyst has a propensity to displace and resorb adjacent teeth (see Fig. 21.2B). In addition, a dentigerous cyst can displace the associated tooth in an apical direction, away from the cyst epicenter, and this may be considerable. For instance, maxillary third molars (Fig. 21.4) or canine teeth may be displaced superiorly toward the floor of the orbit, and mandibular third molars may be displaced distally or superiorly into the ramus, condylar or coronoid processes, or lingually or inferiorly in the mandible (Figs. 21.5 and 21.6).

Differential Interpretation

The histopathologic appearance of the reduced enamel epithelium lining a dentigerous cyst is not specific. Therefore, the diagnosis relies on both the radiographic interpretation and surgical observation of the attachment of the cyst to the cementoenamel junction. However, histopathologic examination should be performed to eliminate other similar-appearing lesions.

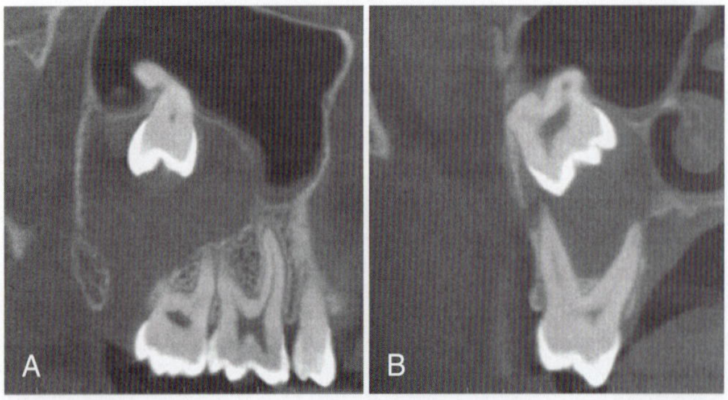

Fig. 21.4 Corrected sagittal (A) and coronal (B) cone beam computed tomographic images of a dentigerous cyst associated with the maxillary right third molar. Note the displaced floor of the adjacent maxillary sinus and the displacement of the tooth in a superior direction.

One of the most difficult differential interpretations to make is between a hyperplastic follicle developing around a tooth crown and a dentigerous cyst. A cyst should be considered with any evidence of tooth displacement or expansion of the bone, or if the follicle is enlarging asymmetrically. If uncertainty remains, the region should be reexamined in 4–6 months to detect any change in shape or influence on surrounding structures.

The differential interpretation of a dentigerous cyst may also include an odontogenic keratocyst (OKC), an ameloblastic fibroma, a developing odontome, and a unicystic or other pattern of ameloblastoma. An OKC does not expand the bone in a buccal-lingual direction to the same degree as a dentigerous cyst, is less likely to resorb teeth, and may attach further apically on the root surface or coronally on the tooth crown instead of at the cementoenamel junction. The tooth associated with a dentigerous cyst may display complete tooth root development, and this feature may potentially be used to differentiate it from an OKC or unicystic ameloblastoma. It may be impossible to differentiate a small ameloblastic fibroma, developing odontome, or some patterns of ameloblastoma from a dentigerous cyst if there is no internal structure. Other less common lesions that may have a pericoronal relationship to an impacted tooth include the adenomatoid odontogenic tumor, the calcifying epithelial odontogenic tumor, and calcifying odontogenic cyst (COC), but the incidence of these entities is generally more rare, and there may be evidence of radiopaque foci in these lesions. Occasionally rarefying osteitis developing at the apex of a primary tooth may appear to envelop the crown of the developing permanent tooth positioned apical to it, giving the false impression of a dentigerous cyst associated with the permanent tooth. This most often occurs with mandibular deciduous molars and the developing premolar teeth. In these cases, the clinician should look for extensive caries or large restorations in the primary tooth (an etiology that would support an interpretation of rarefying osteitis), or angular displacement of the permanent tooth, as opposed to apical displacement.

Management

Dentigerous cysts are managed by surgical removal, which usually includes the tooth as well. Large cysts may be treated by marsupialization before removal. The cyst lining should be submitted for histopathologic

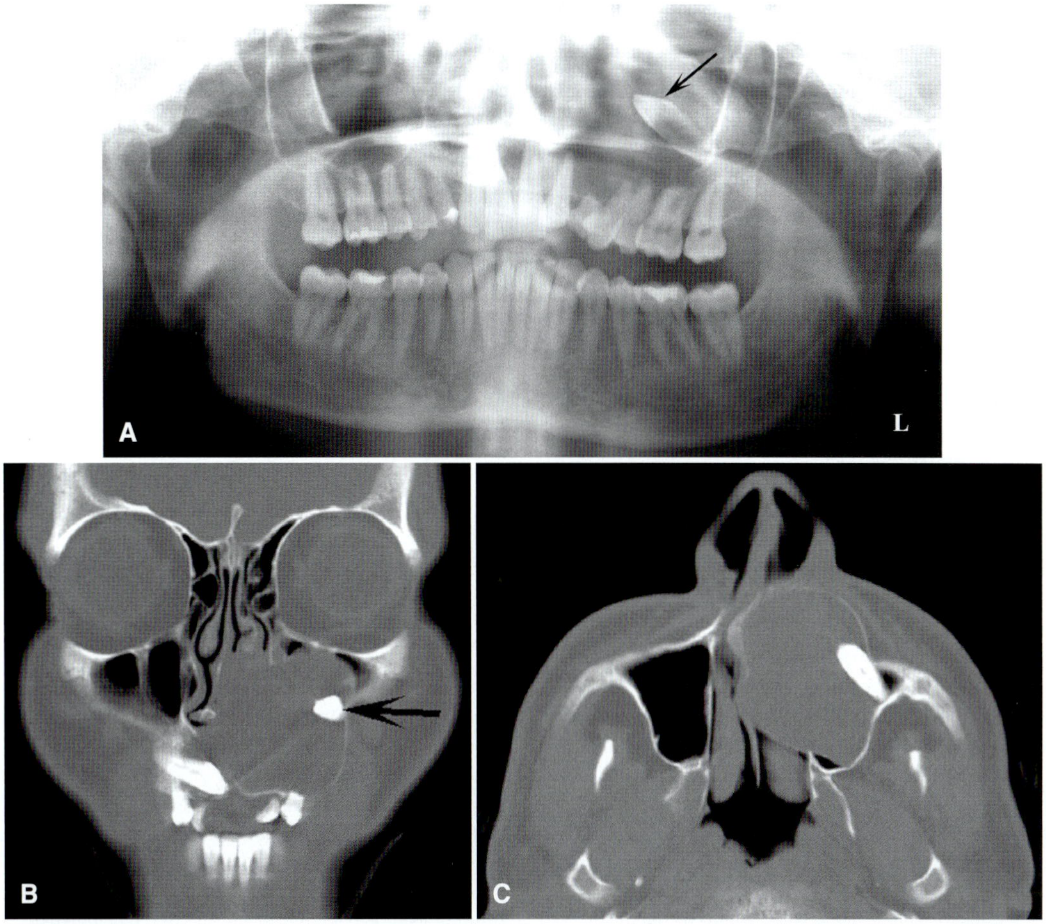

Fig. 21.6 (A) A panoramic image revealing the presence of a large dentigerous cyst associated with the left maxillary canine *(arrow)*, which has been displaced. Note the displacement and resorption of other teeth in the left maxilla. Coronal (B) and axial (C) multidetector computed tomographic images of the same case show superolateral displacement of the canine, expansion of the anterior wall of the maxilla, and expansion of the floor of the nasal fossa.

examination because other lesions have been reported to arise, albeit rarely, from the epithelial lining of a dentigerous cyst; namely ameloblastoma, squamous cell carcinoma, and mucoepidermoid carcinoma.

Odontogenic Keratocyst

Disease Mechanism

The epithelial lining of the OKC is derived from the dental lamina and is distinctive for its thin, keratinized epithelium of four to eight epithelial cell layers thick under light microscopy. When the keratin sloughs from the surface of the epithelium, a collection of viscous or "cheesy" material can be found in the cyst lumen. In contrast to most cysts which are thought to enlarge solely by intraluminal osmotic pressure, the epithelium in the OKC appears to have some innate growth potential due to a mutation of the human homolog of the *Drosophila PTCH* gene, a gene that controls cell proliferation and specialization. Occasionally bud-like proliferations of cells from the basal layer of the epithelium may develop and grow into the underlying connective tissue. These islands of epithelial cells may give rise to satellite microcysts, which can enlarge independently. The differences in these mechanisms of growth can give the OKC a different radiographic appearance from other cysts, and contribute to its sometimes unique behavior.

Clinical Features

OKCs can develop as solitary entities or in association with an unerupted tooth. Although they usually cause no symptoms, mild swelling may occur, and patients may report pain if the cyst becomes secondarily infected by oral microorganisms. Aspiration of the cavity may reveal keratin deposits in the form of thick, yellow, cheesy material. In contrast to other odontogenic cysts, OKCs have a great propensity for recurrence, possibly because of small satellite microcysts or fragments of epithelium left behind during surgical removal.

Imaging Features

Location. As the epithelial lining of OKCs is derived from the dental lamina which is ubiquitous in the tooth-bearing areas of the jaws, OKCs can develop almost anywhere. Most commonly, they may be found in the posterior body of the mandible and ramus. The epicenter is located superior to the inferior alveolar canal. OKCs may also develop as solitary entities in or around the teeth.

Periphery. OKCs have a well-defined and corticated periphery. The periphery is smooth, but its border may scallop an adjacent thick bone cortex (Fig. 21.7).

Internal structure. The internal structure is most commonly radiolucent. Should there be foci of sloughed keratin, radiopaque foci may

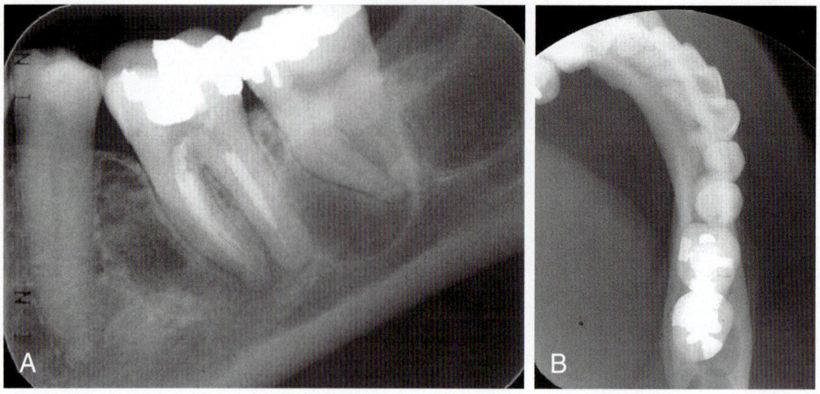

Fig. 21.7 Periapical image (A) shows the corticated and smooth, "hydraulic" periphery of an OKC in the left posterior body of the mandible. The cross-sectional occlusal image (B) shows little, if any buccal/lingual expansion of the bone.

be seen. In some cases, curved internal septa may be present, giving the lesion a multilocular appearance.

Effects on surrounding structures. An important characteristic of the OKC in the mandible is its propensity to grow longitudinally through the bone without significant bone expansion (Figs. 21.8 and 21.9). This "tunneling" type of growth pattern with minimal expansion is an important feature in the mandible but may potentially contribute to late detection. In the ramus, more prominent expansion may be seen due to the very thin medial-lateral dimension of the bone. The tunneling effect can also be seen within the alveolar process of the maxilla (Fig. 21.10). Adjacent to an airspace such as the nasal fossa or maxillary sinus, OKC enlargement is more concentric and balloon-like (see Fig. 21.10C), which is more classic for a cyst. In these locations, as the cyst enlarges, the volume of the adjacent airspace may be reduced. Occasionally the bone expansion created by a large lesion may exceed the capacity of the bone to remodel and contain the OKC. In such instances, the cyst epithelium may contact soft tissue adjacent to the outer surface of the bone through surface perforations. As well, the inferior alveolar nerve canal may be displaced inferiorly.

Effects on adjacent teeth. Occasionally, they may also have an association with the crown of an unerupted or impacted tooth, making them difficult to distinguish from a dentigerous cyst. A change to the contour of the follicle coronal to the cementoenamel junction (Fig. 21.8A) or asymmetry of the follicle are features of an OKC which may allow the clinician to distinguish it from a dentigerous cyst. OKCs occasionally displace teeth and resorb tooth roots, but to a lesser degree than dentigerous cysts.

Differential Interpretation

When an OKC develops in a pericoronal position, it may be indistinguishable from a dentigerous cyst. The lesion is likely to be an OKC if the cyst periphery is associated with the tooth at a point apical or coronal to the cementoenamel junction, or if tooth root development is incomplete. In the mandible, OKCs will produce little or no expansion of the bone. The scalloped margin or a multilocular appearance of an OKC may resemble an ameloblastoma, but the latter has a far greater propensity to expand bone. Occasionally a large lateral periodontal cyst, especially in the maxilla, has a growth pattern similar to that of an OKC, with minimal bone expansion. The mild expansion and multilocular appearance of the odontogenic myxoma may make it indistinguishable from an OKC, particularly if little or no internal structure is seen. A simple bone cavity (SBC) often has a scalloped border and minimal bone expansion, like an OKC; however, the cortex of the SBC is more delicate and often more difficult to detect, particularly on a panoramic image. As well, an SBC has little or no effect on adjacent teeth, lamina dura, or a tooth follicle.

Management

If an OKC is suspected, referral to an oral and maxillofacial radiologist for a complete radiologic examination is advisable. If, on planar imaging,

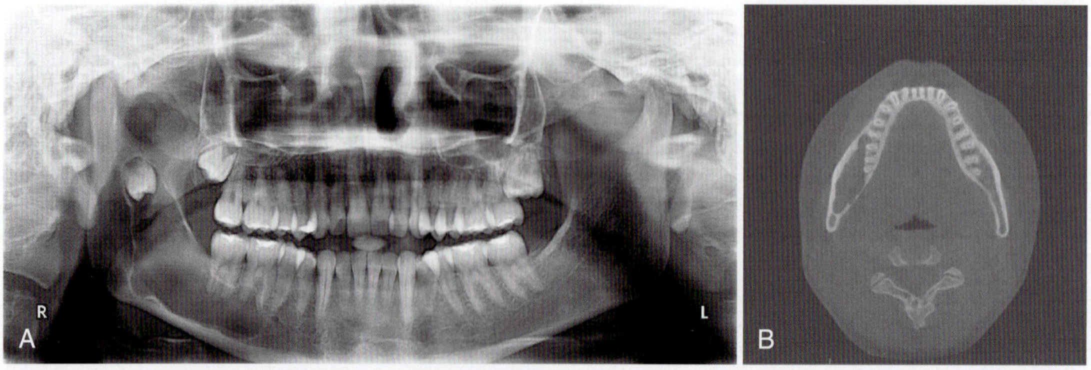

Fig. 21.8 A large odontogenic keratocyst is associated with the follicle of the displaced mandibular right third molar. Note the change to the contour of the third molar follicle located coronal to the cementoenamel junction of the third molar (A). Despite the large size of the cyst, the buccal and lingual surfaces of the mandible have been expanded only slightly (B).

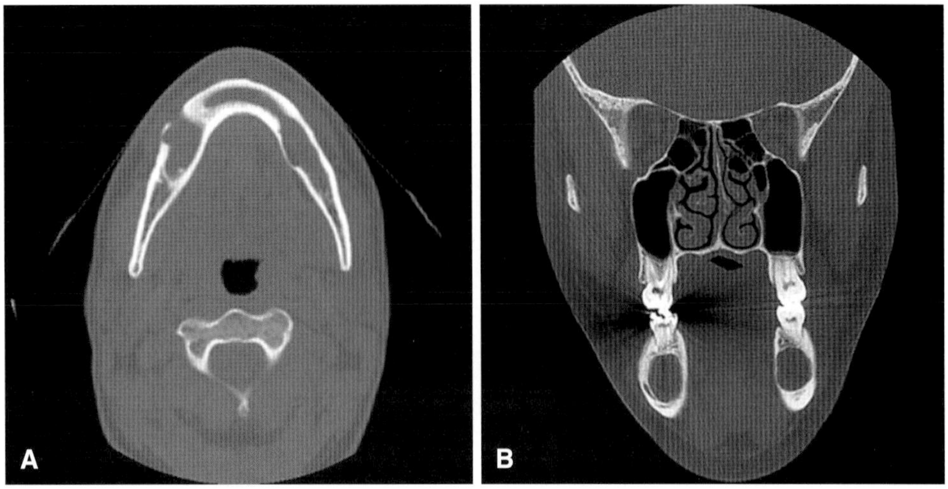

Fig. 21.9 (A) A large odontogenic keratocyst tunneling through the body of the mandible and crossing the midline to involve both the right and left sides. (B) Despite the cyst's very large size, there has been little, if any, buccal or lingual expansion of the bone.

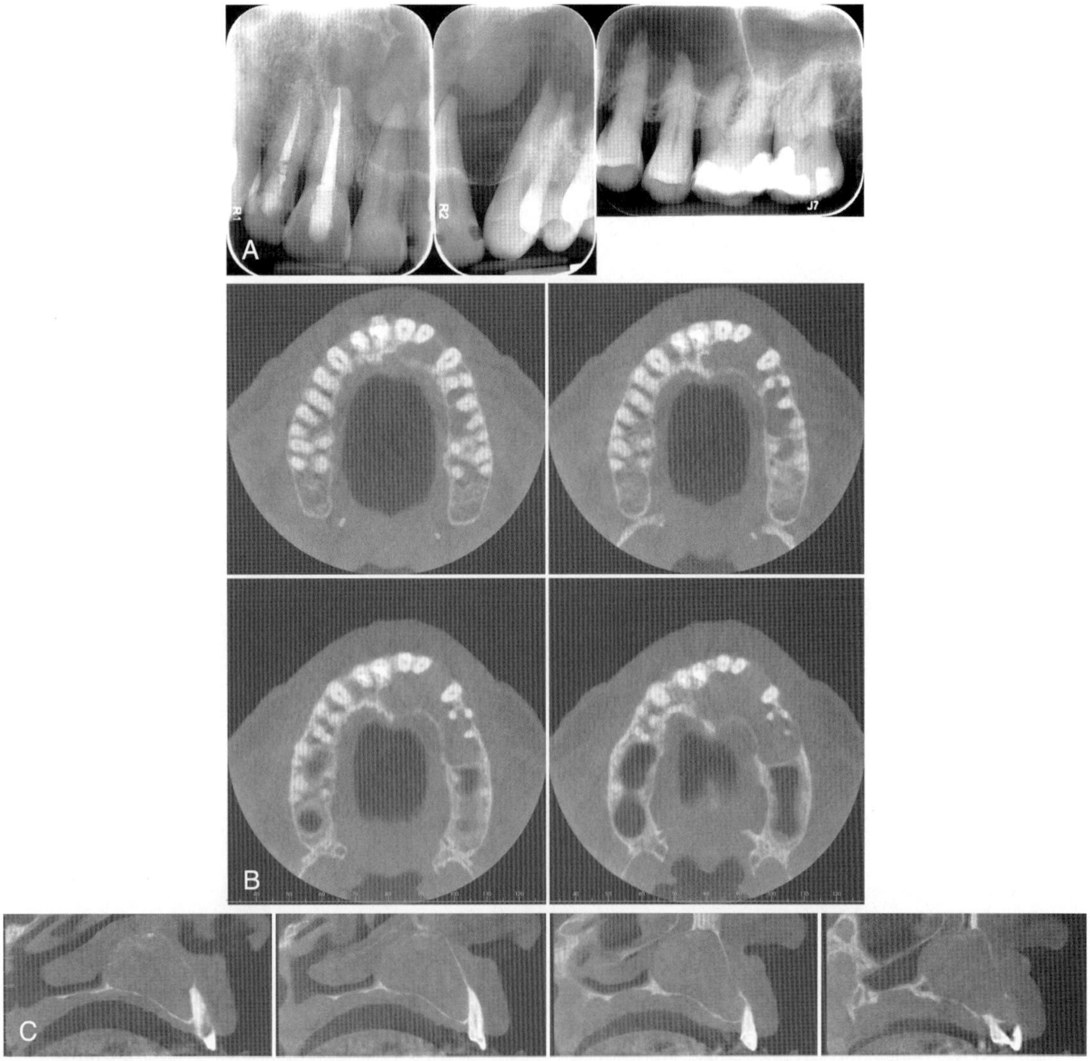

Fig. 21.10 Periapical (A), axial (B), and cross-sectional (C) cone beam computed tomographic images of a maxillary odontogenic keratocyst. Note that the OKC is generally confined to the borders of the bone in the axial (B) and cross-sectional (C) images, except superiorly, where there has been hydraulic expansion of the nasal floor.

cortical perforation is detected, MDCT should be used to investigate the possibility of soft tissue extension. Otherwise CBCT can be ordered. Because this entity has a propensity to recur, an accurate determination of the extent and location of any cortical perforations with soft tissue extension is best achieved with MDCT. In the case shown in Fig. 21.9A, the MDCT identified a perforation of the buccal cortex in the mandibular right premolar area, and this was a site of recurrence some 15 years later (Fig. 21.11).

Surgical treatment may vary and can include resection, curettage, or marsupialization to reduce the size of large lesions before surgical excision. More attention is usually devoted to the bony walls adjacent to the cyst to reduce the chance of recurrence. Following surgical treatment, it is important to reexamine the patient at regular intervals to detect any recurrence. Recurrent lesions usually develop within the first 5 years but may occur as many as 10 years later or more.

Nevoid Basal Cell Carcinoma Syndrome

Disease Mechanism

Nevoid basal cell carcinoma or Gorlin–Goltz syndrome, is an autosomal-dominant disorder related to a mutation of the human homolog of the *Drosophila PTCH* gene.

The expressivity of the phenotypes is variable, although they may include multiple basal cell carcinomas of the skin, palmar and plantar pitting, skeletal abnormalities such as bifid ribs, vertebral fusion, polydactyly, shortening of the metacarpals, temporal and temporoparietal bossing, minor hypertelorism, mild prognathism, calcification

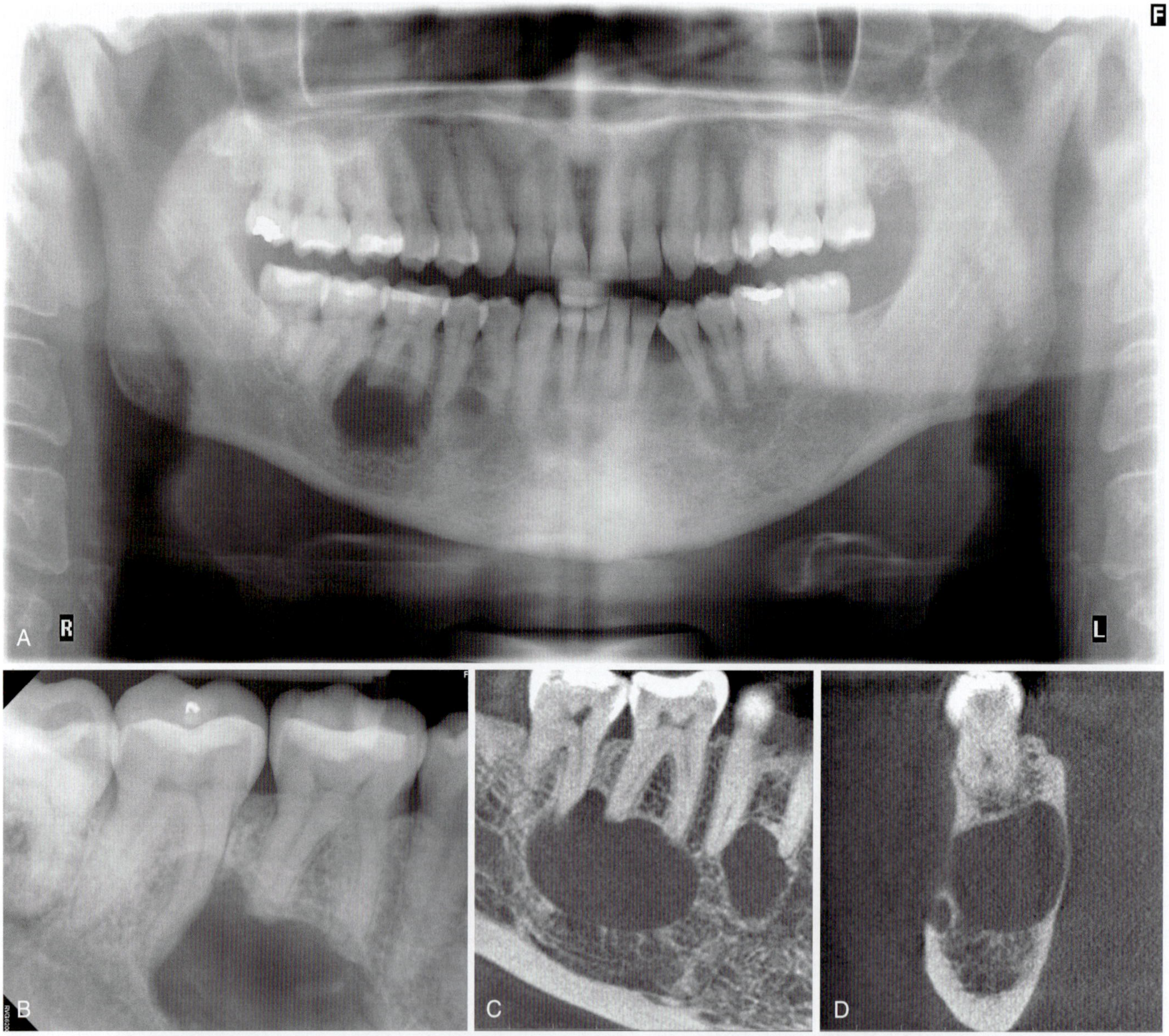

Fig. 21.11 Recurrence of the OKC from Fig. 21.9, 15 years later. The patient was treated by marsupialization of the OKC. Panoramic (A) and periapical (B) images show the multifocal recurrence in the right posterior mandible. Corrected sagittal (C) and coronal (D) cone beam computed tomographic images show the molar area recurrence. Note the scalloping of the OKC around the molar root apices, the external resorption of the mandibular right first molar distal root and the lack of significant buccal/lingual expansion (D). The granular bone pattern in the left mandible (A) is consistent with healing.

of the falx cerebri and other parts of the dura, medulloblastoma, and multiple OKCs.

Clinical Features

Nevoid basal cell carcinoma syndrome may be detected early in life, usually in the second or third decade, with the development of OKCs within the jaws and/or skin basal cell carcinomas. Although genetic testing of relatives is a useful diagnostic tool, approximately 20% of new diagnoses represent spontaneous mutations of the *PTCH* gene. Typically, multiple OKCs develop in multiple quadrants earlier in life (Fig. 21.12). A thorough radiologic examination that includes CBCT or MDCT is required to detect all the cysts, and regular follow-up of patients is important to identify new and recurrent OKCs early, particularly because the recurrence rate of OKCs associated with the syndrome is higher than that of solitary OKCs.

Imaging Features

The imaging features of OKCs that arise in nevoid basal cell carcinoma syndrome are identical to those associated with solitary OKCs.

Differential Interpretation

The presence of a corticated periphery and the hydraulic features of the OKCs differentiates nevoid basal cell carcinoma syndrome from other abnormalities characterized by multiple radiolucencies, including multiple myeloma. Cherubism presents with bilateral multilocular, radiolucent lesions with internal septations, but these usually develop with epicenters in the mandibular rami and produce significant jaw expansion, features that are not characteristic of OKCs. In addition, the lesions of cherubism displace teeth anteriorly, which is a distinctive characteristic. Although it is conceivable that patients may present with multiple dentigerous cysts, in such instances, the dentigerous cysts should develop a more expansile pattern of enlargement.

Management

OKCs in nevoid basal cell carcinoma syndrome are treated more aggressively than solitary OKCs because they appear to have an even greater propensity for recurrence. It is reasonable to examine the patient annually for new and recurrent cysts with panoramic and intraoral imaging. Should these images reveal areas that are suspicious for new or recurrent OKCs, CBCT or MDCT should be ordered. A referral to a medical geneticist should also be made.

Buccal Bifurcation Cyst

Disease Mechanism

The epithelial lining of the buccal bifurcation cyst (BBC) is probably derived from the epithelial cell rests of Malassez in the bifurcation of multirooted teeth. As the histopathologic characteristics of the epithelial lining are not distinctive and overlap with other odontogenic cysts, both histopathologic and radiologic findings are necessary for diagnosis. The etiology of the BBC is not known. One hypothesis identifies inflammation as the stimulus for epithelial proliferation, but inflammation is not always present.

It is possible that the paradental cyst of the third molar and the BBC are the same entity. An associated enamel extension into the furcation of third molars with paradental cysts has not been documented with molars with BBC. In addition, the inflammatory component associated with paradental cysts is not always present with BBCs.

Clinical Features

Commonly the BBC is associated with mandibular permanent molars. Rarely, the BBC may develop in association with a maxillary molar. On clinical examination, the molar may be unerupted, or partially erupted with its lingual cusp tips abnormally protruding through the mucosa, more occlusally than the position of the buccal cusps. The first molar is involved more frequently than the second molar, and the pulps of these teeth are vital.

A hard swelling may be palpable buccal to the involved molar, and if the cyst has been secondarily infected, the patient may complain of pain. The age of detection is younger, within the first two decades of life rather than in the third decade, which is more common for a paradental cyst of the third molar.

Imaging Features

Location. The BBC is most commonly associated with the mandibular first permanent molar followed by the second molar (Fig. 21.13). Occasionally BBCs can occur bilaterally (Fig. 21.14). The epicenter of the cyst is always located buccal to the furcation of the affected molar. On panoramic or periapical images, the lesion may appear to be centered slightly distal to the furcation of the involved tooth because of x-ray beam obliquity.

Periphery. In some cases, the periphery is not always readily apparent, and the lesion may have a very subtle radiolucent appearance superimposed over the roots of the molar. In other cases, the lesion may have a well-defined and corticated border.

Internal structure. The internal structure is radiolucent.

Effects on surrounding structures. As the cyst enlarges and engages the buccal surface of the bone, expansion of the surface is seen. Owing to its very slow growth rate, the surface of the bone will remodel to accommodate the cyst. With the expansion of the bone surface, the cortex remains intact but is often significantly thinned. If the cyst is secondarily infected, periosteal new bone formation may be seen adjacent to the involved tooth (Fig. 21.15).

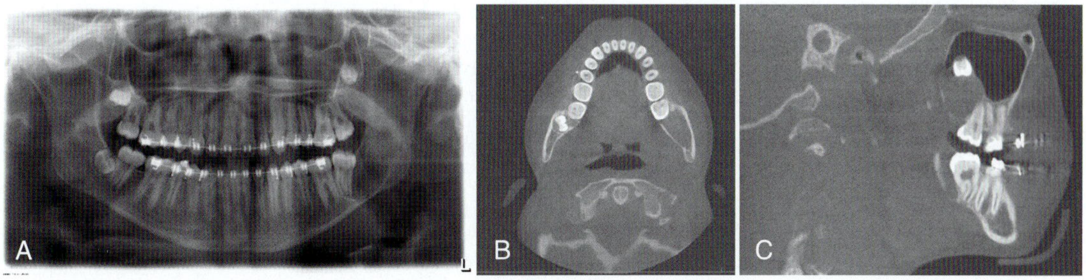

Fig. 21.12 Panoramic (A), axial (B), and sagittal (C) cone beam computed tomographic images of a case of nevoid basal cell carcinoma syndrome. Note the large OKCs developing in the left mandibular ramus displacing the roots of the mandibular second molar mesially, and in the left maxilla, displacing the developing maxillary left third molar superiorly. Another small OKC, not visible on the panoramic image (A), can be identified between the mandibular right second molar and the developing mandibular left third molar (B).

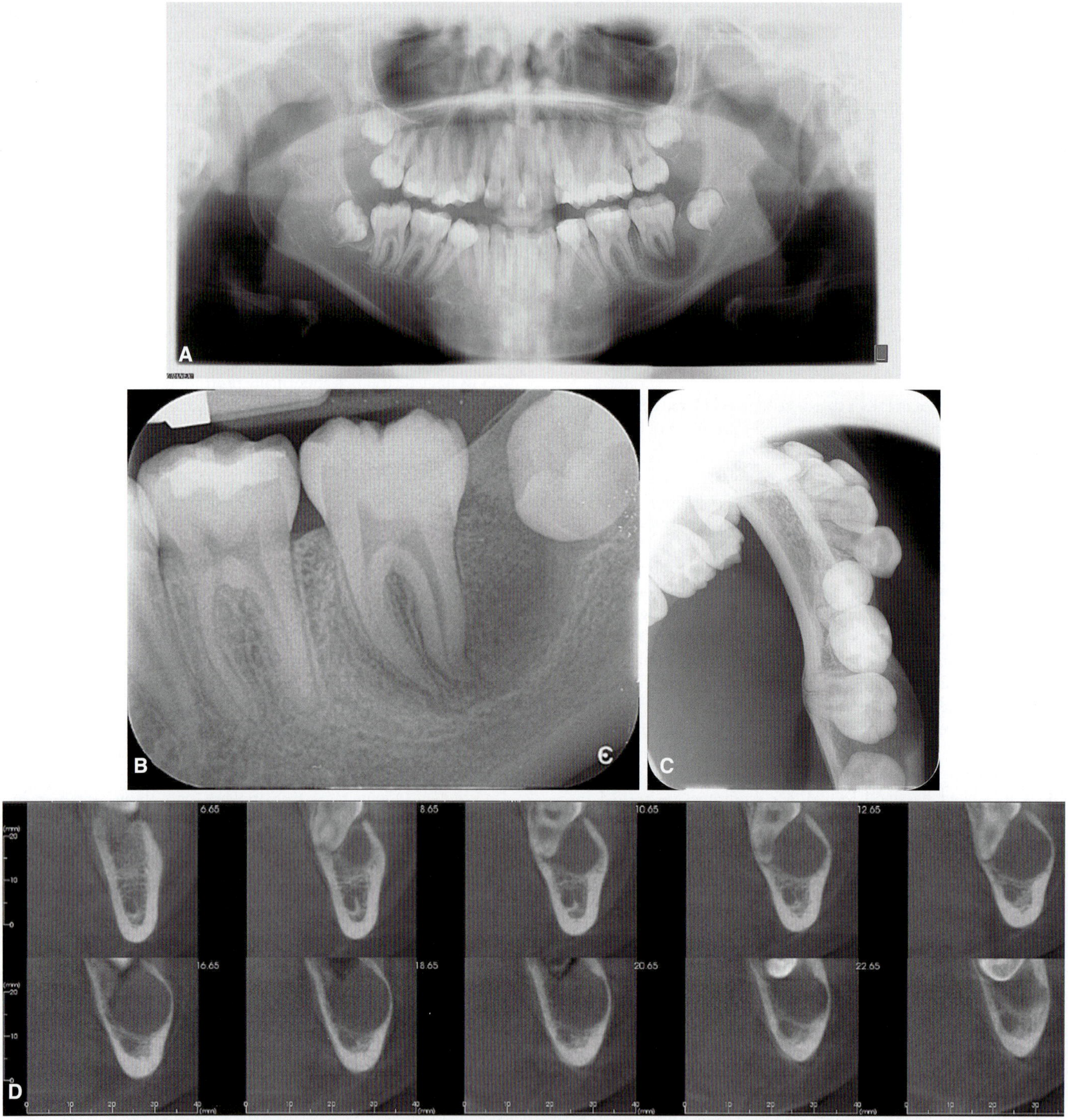

Fig. 21.13 Panoramic (A), periapical (B), and cross-sectional occlusal (C) images of the left posterior mandible show a buccal bifurcation cyst associated with a tipped mandibular left second molar. Note the tipping of the tooth crown in (A) and the displacement of the roots of the second molar into the lingual cortex of the mandible (C). The buccal epicenter of the cyst is seen in the buccal lingual cross-sectional cone beam computed tomographic images, as is the compression of the inferior alveolar canal (D).

Effects on adjacent teeth. The most striking diagnostic characteristic of the BBC is the tipping of the roots of the involved molar into the lingual cortex of the mandible and concomitant tipping of the tooth's occlusal surface in a buccal direction (see Figs. 21.13C and D, and 21.14B and C). This accounts for the lingual cusp tips being positioned higher than the buccal tips on a periapical or panoramic image. The best diagnostic image is the cross-sectional mandibular occlusal image, which demonstrates the abnormal position of the tooth roots adjacent to or within the lingual cortex.

Differential Interpretation

The differential interpretation of the BBC includes rarefying osteitis, OKC, and dentigerous cyst. Rarefying osteitis can easily be excluded because the lesion epicenter is located apical to the root apex of the

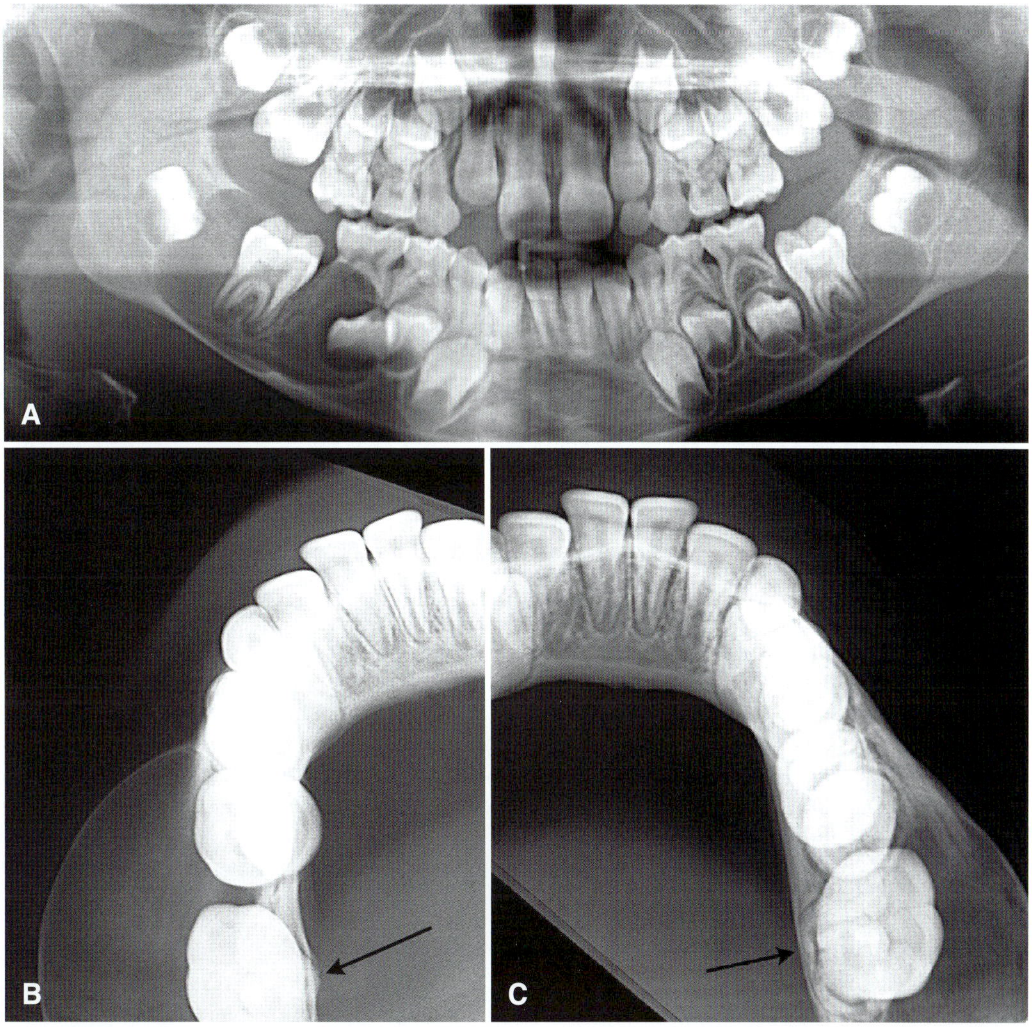

Fig. 21.14 Bilateral buccal bifurcation cysts. A panoramic image (A) shows cysts related to the mandibular first molars. The occlusal surface of each tooth has been tipped in relation to the other teeth, and adjacent teeth have been displaced. Occlusal images of the same case (B and C). Note the smooth curved expansion of the buccal surface and the displacement of the roots of the first molars into the lingual cortex *(arrows)*.

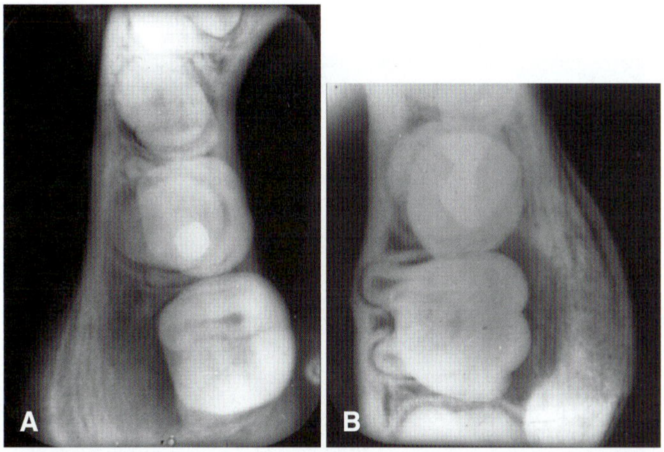

Fig. 21.15 Occlusal views (A and B) of buccal bifurcation cysts that have been secondarily infected. Note the laminated periosteal new bone formation on the buccal aspect of the first molars and the abnormal position of the roots of the first molar in (B). (Courtesy Dr. Doug Stoneman, University of Toronto.)

involved tooth, whereas the epicenter of the BBC is located buccally, at the level of the furcation. Although obliquity of the x-ray beam may superimpose the BBC near the crown of an unerupted or partially erupted developing molar, the occlusal image will readily show the focal expansile nature of the bone adjacent to the molar furcation which may help differentiate BBC from OKC. Should the BBC become secondarily infected and periosteal new bone formation or sclerosis can be visualized, the cyst could be confused with a periodontal abscess or Langerhans cell histiocytosis. The fact that only a BBC tilts the molar as described helps to differentiate it from other lesions.

Management

A BBC is managed by conservative curettage, although some cases have resolved without intervention. The involved molar tooth does not require removal, and BBC does not recur.

Residual Cyst

Disease Mechanism

A residual cyst is an entity that develops after incomplete removal of the epithelial cell layer associated with a previous cyst. The most common sources of this epithelium include a radicular cyst (i.e., rarefying osteitis) and a dentigerous cyst.

Clinical Features

A residual cyst is usually asymptomatic and is often identified in an edentulous site in a radiologic examination. If not identified, the cyst can enlarge, resulting in a painless swelling of the jaw. If it is secondarily infected, the presence of a residual cyst may be identified by the pain it elicits.

Imaging Features

Location. Residual cysts can occur in both jaws, although they are found slightly more often in the mandible than the maxilla. The epicenter of a residual cyst is located in an area formerly occupied by a tooth, and in the mandible, it is always superior to the inferior alveolar canal (Fig. 21.16).

Periphery. A residual cyst has a well-defined and corticated border unless it has become secondarily infected.

Internal structure. Internally, the residual cyst typically is radiolucent, although dystrophic calcifications may develop in long-standing cysts.

Effects on surrounding structures. Residual cysts may cause expansion of an adjacent bone surface and thinning of the overlying cortex. A residual cyst may displace the floor of the maxillary sinus, or course of the inferior alveolar canal.

Effects on adjacent teeth. Residual cysts can displace teeth or resorb tooth roots.

Differential Interpretation

Without a patient history and/or previous images, clinicians may have difficulty determining whether a solitary cyst in the jaws is a residual cyst. Other examples of common solitary cysts include the OKC, however, a residual cyst has greater potential for expansion of bone than an OKC. The mandibular lingual bone depression or Stafne defect has an epicenter that is usually inferior to the inferior alveolar canal; however, the cortex of the depression is usually very thick.

Management

The treatment of residual cysts is surgical removal, marsupialization, or both if the cyst is large.

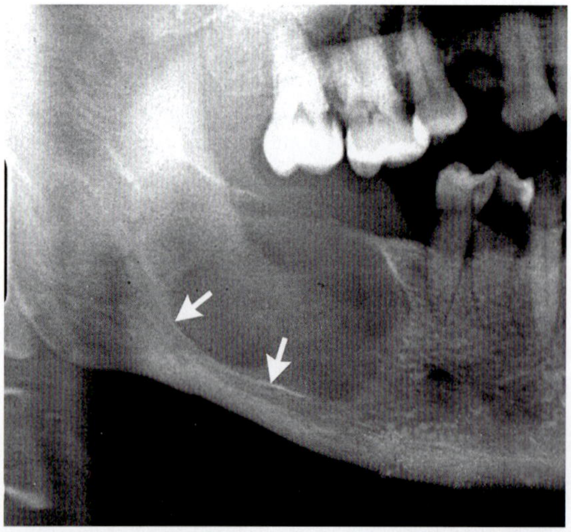

Fig. 21.16 The epicenter of this residual cyst is located superior to the inferior alveolar canal; it has displaced the canal in an inferior direction *(arrows)*. The cortical boundary is not continuous around the entire cyst.

Lateral Periodontal Cyst

Disease Mechanism

The lateral periodontal cyst is thought to arise from remnants of the epithelial cell rests of Malassez in the periodontal ligament space adjacent to the surface of the tooth root. This lesion is usually unicystic, however, in some cases, it may appear as a cluster of small cystic cavities. Although this variant has been termed a "botryoid odontogenic cyst" radiologically, the term is related more to its histopathologic appearance. It has been postulated that a lateral periodontal cyst is the intrabony counterpart of the gingival cyst in an adult.

Clinical Features

The lateral periodontal cyst is often small and usually asymptomatic (Fig. 21.17). If these cysts become secondarily infected, they can mimic a lateral periodontal abscess.

Imaging Features

Location. The lateral periodontal cyst usually develops in the incisor and premolar areas of the mandible. In the maxilla, it usually develops in the lateral incisor and the canine areas.

Periphery. A lateral periodontal cyst has a well-defined and corticated border. Although it is most often round to oval in shape, a larger cyst can take on a more irregular appearance.

Internal structure. Internally, the lateral periodontal cyst is radiolucent.

Effects on surrounding structures. Occasionally, a large lateral periodontal cyst may have a growth pattern similar to that of an OKC with minimal expansion of the bone (see Fig. 21.18).

Effects on adjacent teeth. The lateral periodontal cyst may efface the lamina dura of the adjacent root, and larger cysts can displace adjacent teeth.

Differential Interpretation

The lateral periodontal cyst is sometimes said to be an interpretation of exclusion. Because the radiographic appearance of a lateral periodontal cyst is similar to that of many other solitary cysts, the following lesions should be included in the differential interpretation: a small OKC, SBC, ameloblastoma, and a focus of rarefying osteitis located at the foramen of a lateral (accessory) root canal. If the lateral periodontal cyst has a botryoid appearance radiologically, it may also resemble a small ameloblastoma.

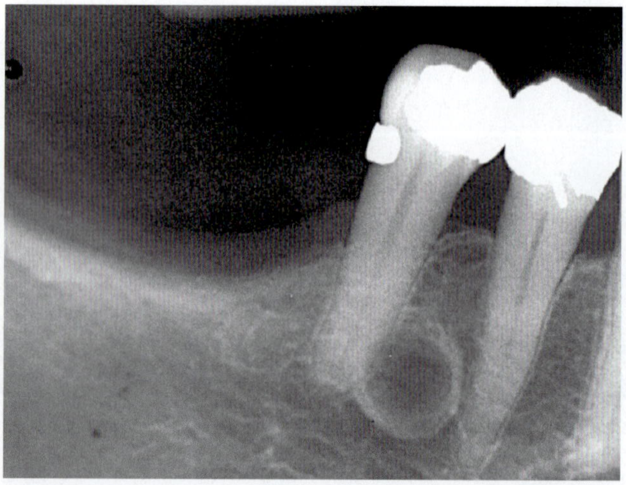

Fig. 21.17 A lateral periodontal cyst in the mandibular premolar region. Note the classic well-defined cortical border and the "hydraulic" shape.

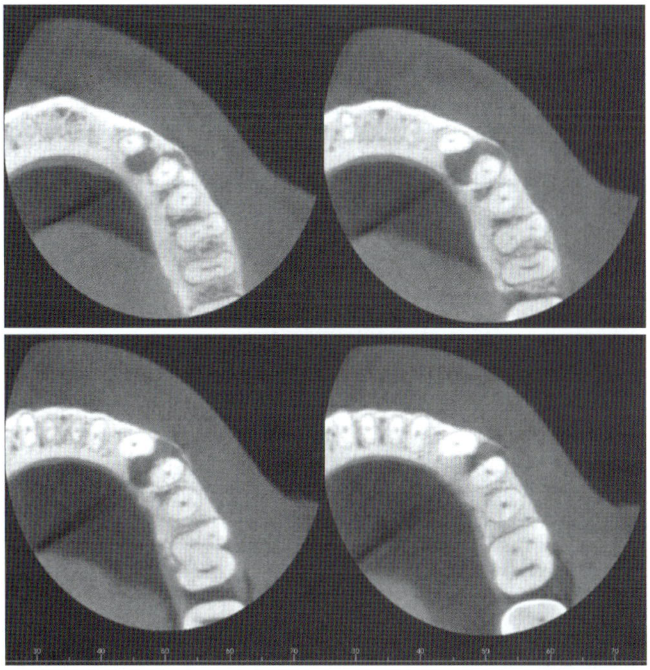

Fig. 21.18 Axial cone beam computed tomographic images of a lateral periodontal cyst developing between the roots of a mandibular left canine and first premolar tooth showing minimal buccal/lingual expansion of the bone.

Management

Lateral periodontal cysts usually do not require sophisticated imaging beyond intraoral or panoramic images because of their small size. Excisional biopsy or simple enucleation is the treatment of choice because these cysts do not tend to recur.

Glandular Odontogenic Cyst

Disease Mechanism

The glandular or sialo-odontogenic cyst is a rare cyst derived from odontogenic epithelium with a spectrum of microscopic characteristics including salivary gland features such as mucous-producing cells. Some authors hypothesize a relationship to the central mucoepidermoid carcinoma.

Clinical Features

There is a slight female predilection with a mean age in the fifth decade of life. This cyst shows aggressive behavior and a tendency to recur after surgery.

Imaging Features

Location. The glandular odontogenic cyst occurs more commonly in the mandible and most often in the anterior mandible and the maxilla.

Periphery. There is usually a cortical border that may be smooth or scalloped.

Internal structure. The glandular odontogenic cyst may be radiolucent, although multilocular lesions have been reported (Fig. 21.19).

Effects on surrounding structures. Expansion of an adjacent bone border has been reported, with perforation through the cortex.

Effects on adjacent teeth. Displacement of adjacent teeth has been reported.

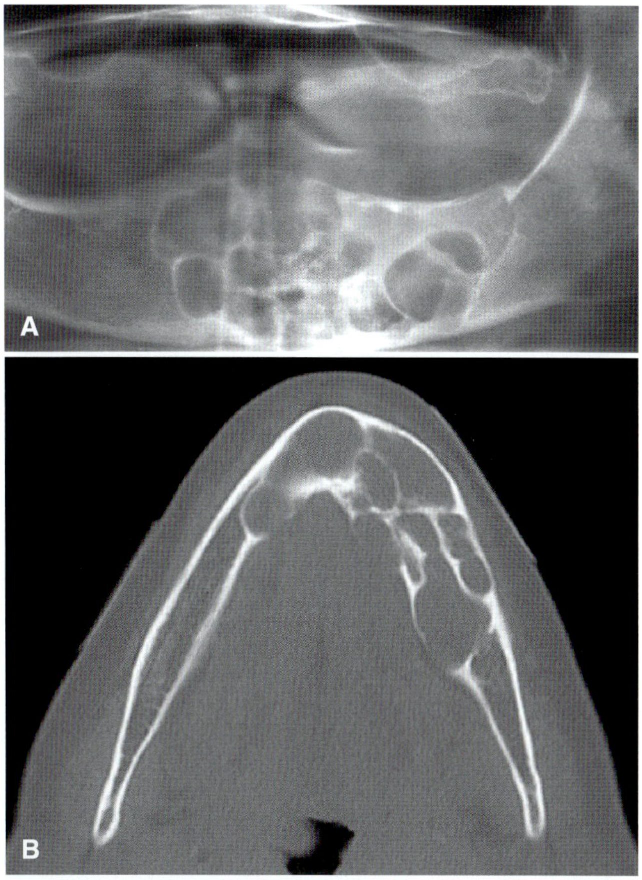

Fig. 21.19 A cropped panoramic image (A) of a glandular odontogenic cyst with a multilocular appearance very similar to an ameloblastoma. Axial multidetector computed tomographic image (B) detailing the multilocular internal cystic structure.

Differential Interpretation

This cyst can appear similar to any unilocular or multilocular radiolucent entity, including OKC, ameloblastoma, and central mucoepidermoid carcinoma.

Treatment

Because of the high rate of recurrence with conservative treatments such as enucleation, more aggressive management, including resection, may be considered. Treated cases should be followed with periodic radiographic examinations to assess for recurrence.

Calcifying Odontogenic Cyst

Disease Mechanism

The COC is known by several other names, including calcifying epithelial odontogenic cyst, dentinogenic ghost cell tumor, and Gorlin cyst. COCs are uncommon, slow growing, benign lesions. They have a spectrum of appearances with the characteristics of a cyst, but in some instances, the characteristics of a solid neoplasm. The cells within this lesion can produce a calcified matrix identified as dysplastic dentin; in some instances, the lesion is associated with an odontome. This lesion also sometimes contains a more solid component that gives it an appearance resembling that of an ameloblastoma, although it does not behave like one.

Clinical Features

The COC has a wide age distribution. Clinically the lesion usually presents as a slow growing, painless swelling in the jaw. Occasionally

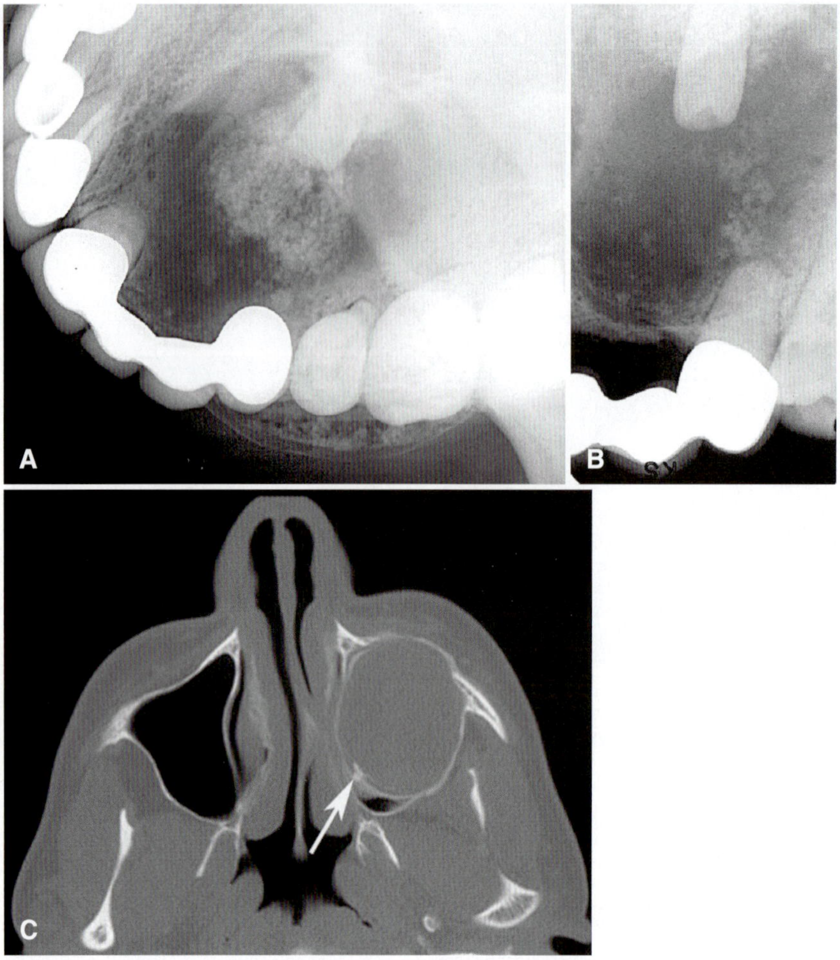

Fig. 21.20 Calcifying odontogenic cyst (COC) developing adjacent to a maxillary lateral incisor (A and B). Note the well-defined corticated border, internal calcifications, and resorption of part of the root of the central incisor. Axial multidetector computed tomographic image (C) of a large COC invaginating and effacing the maxillary sinus. Note the small calcifications along the posterior border *(arrow)*.

the patient may complain of pain. Aspiration often yields a viscous granular yellow fluid.

Imaging Features

Location. Most COCs occur centrally in bone, with a nearly equal distribution between the jaws. Most (approximately 75%) occur mesial to the first molar, especially in the incisor and canine areas, where the tumor can sometimes manifest as a pericoronal radiolucency.

Periphery. The periphery can vary from being well defined and corticated with a curved, hydraulic periphery to being poorly defined and irregular.

Internal structure. The internal structure can vary. The lesion may be completely radiolucent or may show evidence of small foci of calcified material that appear as white flecks or small smooth pebbles, an appearance associated with more long-standing cysts. Also, larger, more solid amorphous radiopaque masses can be seen (Fig. 21.20). In rare cases, the lesion may appear multilocular.

Effects on surrounding structures. The lesion may expand the bone and perforate an adjacent cortex when it is large enough to extend to the bone surface.

Effects on adjacent teeth. In 20%–50% of cases, the COC is associated with an unerupted or impacted tooth (most commonly a canine) that impedes its eruption. Displacement of adjacent teeth and resorption of roots may also occur.

Differential Interpretation

When there is no evidence of internal calcifications, the COC may be radiologically indistinguishable from a dentigerous cyst or an OKC. Other lesions to be considered that have internal calcifications include an adenomatoid odontogenic tumor, developing odontome, and calcifying epithelial odontogenic tumor. It is not, however, common for the COC to occur in locations where these latter two entities commonly arise.

Management

The COC is treated with enucleation and curettage. Because clinicians generally have little experience with the more solid neoplastic variants, it is wise to follow treatment with periodic imaging examinations for recurrence.

NONODONTOGENIC CYSTS

Nasopalatine Duct Cyst

Disease Mechanism

The nasopalatine duct or incisive canal usually contains remnants of the nasopalatine duct, a primitive organ of smell, as well as the nasopalatine vessels and nerves. The nasopalatine duct cyst forms in the nasopalatine canal when the embryonic epithelial remnants within the canal undergo proliferation.

Clinical Features

The nasopalatine duct cyst accounts for approximately 10% of jaw cysts, and while the age distribution is broad, most cases are discovered in the fourth through sixth decades with the incidence being three times higher in males than females.

Most nasopalatine duct cysts are asymptomatic; however, as they increase in size, the most frequent chief complaint is a swelling just posterior to the palatine papilla. This swelling is usually fluctuant, and the mucosa may take on a blue hue if the cyst is near the surface. A less superficial nasopalatine cyst is covered by normal-appearing mucosa unless it is ulcerated from masticatory trauma. As the cyst enlarges, it may penetrate the labial cortex and produce a swelling below the maxillary labial frenulum or to one side of it. The lesion may also expand superiorly toward the floor of the nasal cavity and distort the nasal septum. Pressure from the cyst on the adjacent nasopalatine nerves that occupy the same canal may cause a burning sensation or change in sensation over the palatal mucosa. In some cases, cystic fluid may drain into the oral cavity through a sinus tract or a remnant of the nasopalatine duct, and the patient may report a salty taste.

Imaging Features

Location. Most nasopalatine duct cysts are centered in the maxillary midline in the area of the nasopalatine foramen or canal. This cyst can also expand asymmetrically, extending posteriorly into the hard palate or laterally into the lateral incisor area.

Periphery. The nasopalatine duct cyst has a well-defined and corticated periphery, and it is round or oval in shape (Fig. 21.21). On a planar image, the image of the anterior nasal spine may become superimposed over the cyst, giving it a heart shape.

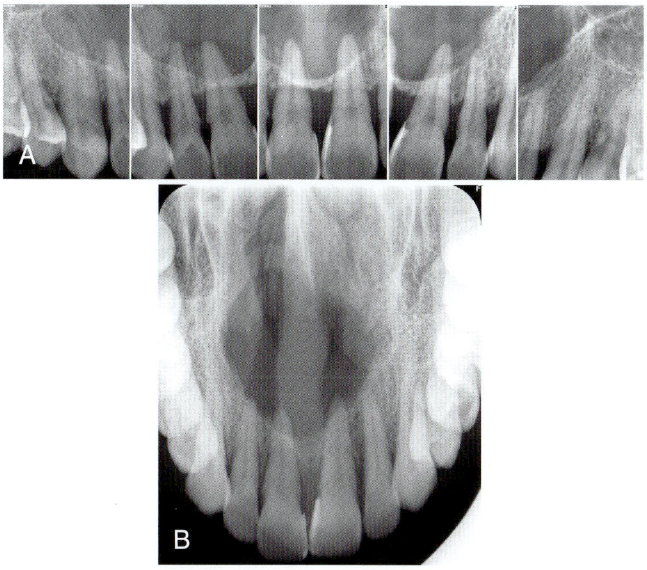

Fig. 21.21 Periapical (A) and anterior occlusal (B) images of a nasopalatine duct cyst. Note the uniform periodontal ligament space around all the apices of the adjacent tooth roots.

Internal structure. Most nasopalatine duct cysts are radiolucent. Rarely, nasopalatine cysts may develop internal dystrophic calcifications; these may appear as ill-defined, amorphous, scattered radiopacities.

Effects on surrounding structures. Seen from a lateral perspective, the nasopalatine duct cyst may expand the labial or palatal cortices of the maxilla. If the cyst is large enough, the floor of the nasal fossa may be displaced in a superior direction. It should also be noted that the canal can expand asymmetrically, resulting in an asymmetric nasopalatine duct cyst (Fig. 21.22).

Effects on adjacent teeth. The nasopalatine duct cyst can affect the teeth, depending on the location of the cyst epicenter. Larger cysts can abut the palatal surfaces of the maxillary incisors, and displace the roots of the central incisors so they diverge, and occasionally cause root resorption.

Differential Interpretation

The normal horizontal diameter of the incisive canal can range up to 10 mm, so the most common differential interpretation is a large incisive foramen. As an internal reference, the horizontal dimension of the canal can be compared with the mesial/distal width of the permanent maxillary central incisor crown, approximately 8 mm.

Clinical examination should reveal the expansile features characteristic of a cyst and other changes that occur with a space-occupying lesion, such as tooth displacement. Two periapical images made at different horizontal angulations may show the cyst to be located palatal to the adjacent teeth. An anterior occlusal image or a limited field-of-view CBCT examination centered in the maxillary midline may demonstrate the size change and expansion in the palatal direction. Rarefying osteitis associated with a central incisor can appear similar to an asymmetric nasopalatine cyst; however, the absence of the lamina dura with enlargement of the apical periodontal ligament space can differentiate rarefying osteitis from a nasopalatine duct cyst. As well, vitality testing of the central incisor tooth pulp may also be useful.

Management

The management of a nasopalatine cyst is enucleation, preferably from the palate to avoid the nasopalatine nerve. If the cyst is large and there is danger of devitalizing the tooth or creating a naso-oral or oroantral fistula, the surgeon may elect to perform marsupialization.

PSEUDOCYSTS

Simple Bone Cavity

Disease Mechanism

The simple bone cyst is not a true cyst because it lacks an epithelial lining, although it is a cavity within the bone. Many names have been given to this entity. Some of these have been descriptive (e.g., simple, solitary,

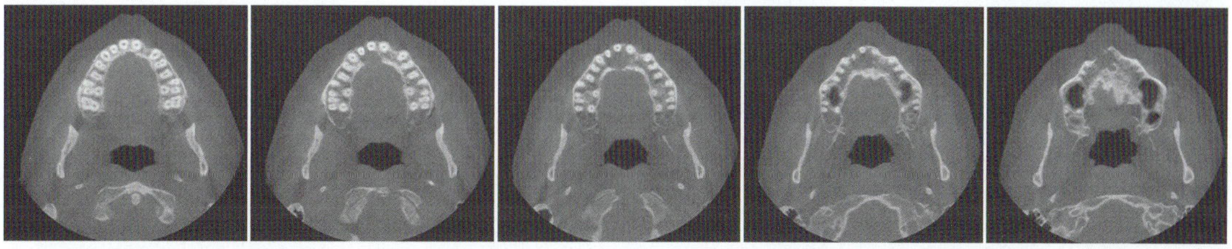

Fig. 21.22 Axial cone beam computed tomographic images of an asymmetric incisive canal cyst. Note the continuity of the cyst cavity with the midline incisive canal.

unicameral, cavity), while others are related to a presumptive etiopathogenesis (e.g., hemorrhagic, idiopathic, traumatic, cyst). Given the confusion that has developed because of these many different names, we have elected to refer to this entity as a "simple bone cavity" (SBC). Lining this cavity may be a thin layer of connective tissue layer, although it may also contain a small amount of blood or serosanguinous fluid.

The etiology of the SBC is not known, although there are several hypotheses. The one that makes the most biologic sense is that the SBC arises from a local disturbance between normal osteoblast differentiation during bone growth and development, and osteoclastic coordination. The dysregulation of these processes is believed to give rise to the empty bone cavity. There is no evidence to support a traumatic etiology for the SBC.

Clinical Features

A solitary SBC is very common, with most occurring in the first 2 decades of life; the mean age is approximately 18 years. One or more SBCs can develop in association with bone dysplasias; however, when this occurs with the cemento-osseous dysplasias, the mean age of occurrence is in the fifth decade of life with a striking female preponderance of 4:1.

The SBC is asymptomatic in most cases, but occasionally pain or tenderness may be present, especially if the cyst has become secondarily infected in association with a cemento-osseous dysplasia. Expansion of the mandible is also possible; however, tooth movement is unusual. If teeth are involved, the pulps of these teeth remain vital.

Most SBCs are found incidentally during imaging examinations made for other purposes, particularly in adolescents. Although SBCs can become quite large, there is no evidence that they cause fractures of the jaws unlike SBCs in the appendicular skeleton.

Imaging Features

Location. Almost all SBCs are found in the mandible; they rarely develop in the maxilla. The lesion can occur anywhere in the mandible but is more commonly found in the posterior mandible during the second decade of life, and in older patients when it is associated with a bone dysplasia.

Periphery. SBCs have well-defined, delicately corticated borders. In some instances, the border may be so delicate that it is difficult to see, particularly on a panoramic image. On intraoral images, the thickness of the cortex may be similar to the thickness of a normal trabecula. The boundary is usually better seen in the alveolar process around the teeth than in the body of the mandible. When the SBC encounters a tooth root, the periphery scallops around the roots of the teeth with a gentle, smooth curve (Fig. 21.23A).

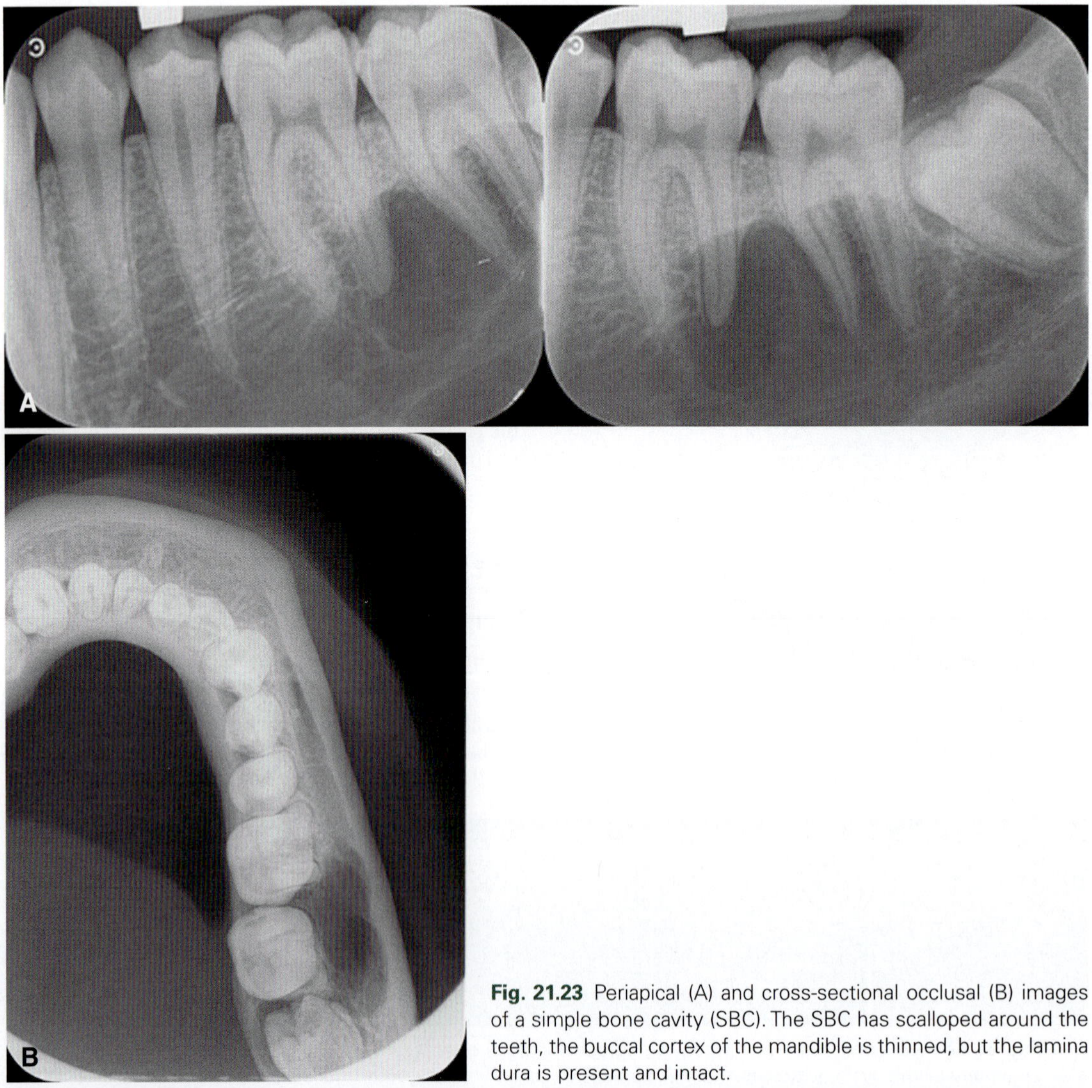

Fig. 21.23 Periapical (A) and cross-sectional occlusal (B) images of a simple bone cavity (SBC). The SBC has scalloped around the teeth, the buccal cortex of the mandible is thinned, but the lamina dura is present and intact.

Internal structure. The internal structure is totally radiolucent, although occasionally a larger SBC may appear to display delicate internal septation. These septa, often referred to as pseudosepta, are the result of pronounced scalloping of the SBC border into the endosteal surface of either the buccal or lingual cortex of the mandible (see Fig. 21.23B). The ridging of the internal surface of the bone cortex produced by two adjacent endosteal bone scallops gives rise to the appearance of septa on panoramic or periapical images.

Effects on surrounding structures. Although some SBCs may expand the bone surface (see Fig. 21.24), they have a general propensity to scallop the endosteal surface of a bone cortex. Larger SBCs can, however, cause expansion (Fig. 21.25).

Effects on adjacent teeth. In most cases, SBCs have no effect on adjacent teeth, although rare cases of tooth displacement and resorption have been documented. SBCs may cause minimal disruption to the lamina dura, although most commonly, there is no disruption (Fig. 21.21A). Similarly, the lesion spares the cortical boundary of the follicle around a developing tooth (Fig. 21.25); this is a highly characteristic feature and can be used to differentiate the SBC from other cystic or cyst-like entities.

Differential Interpretation

SBCs may have an appearance like that of a central giant cell lesion; however, the giant cell lesion has a greater propensity to displace teeth, cause external root resorption, and develop areas of internal mineralization. Because smaller SBCs may grow through the bone and scallop bone borders, they may appear like OKCs. However, OKCs usually have a more definitive cortex, resorb and displace teeth, and displace or disrupt the integrity and shape of tooth follicles. As the SBC may displace bone from around teeth without affecting the teeth themselves, there may be a tendency to include a malignant lesion in the differential interpretation. However, the maintenance of some lamina dura, and the lack of an invasive periphery and bone destruction should be enough to remove this category of disease from consideration. The diagnosis of the SBC relies primarily on radiographic interpretation, and less so on the surgical finding of no epithelial lining.

SBCs can heal spontaneously, and when they do, the formation of the new, immature bone may be detected internally (Fig. 21.26). In these cases, the bone pattern may appear reminiscent of a bone dysplasia such as fibrous dysplasia or a benign tumor like a cemento-ossifying fibroma. Should there be biopsy of such a site, it is important for the oral and maxillofacial pathologist to consult the imaging.

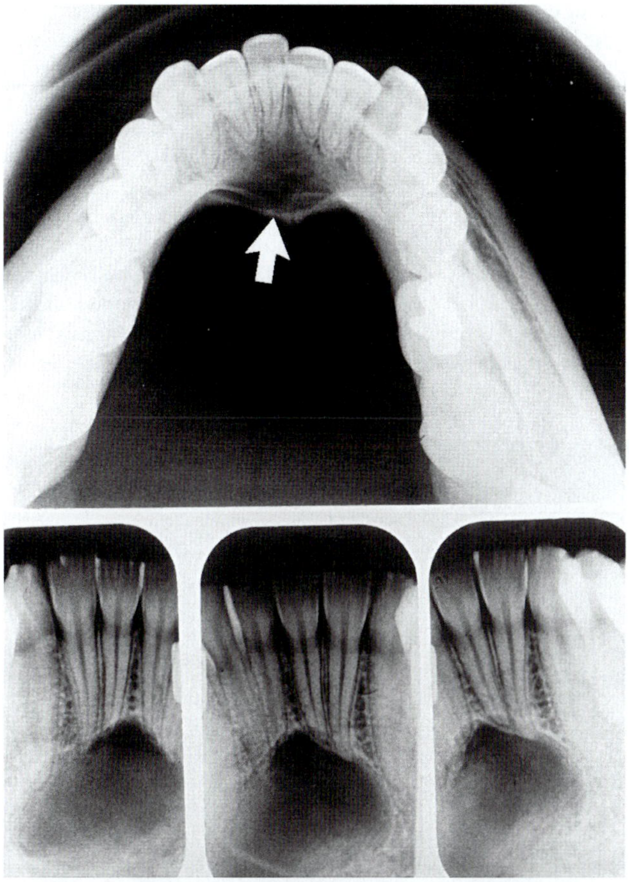

Fig. 21.24 Simple bone cavity *(arrow)* positioned in the anterior of the mandible. The superior aspect of the peripheral cortex is better defined than the inferior border, and there is evidence of some expansion of the lingual surface of the mandible, which may be due in part to muscle attachment at the genial tubercles.

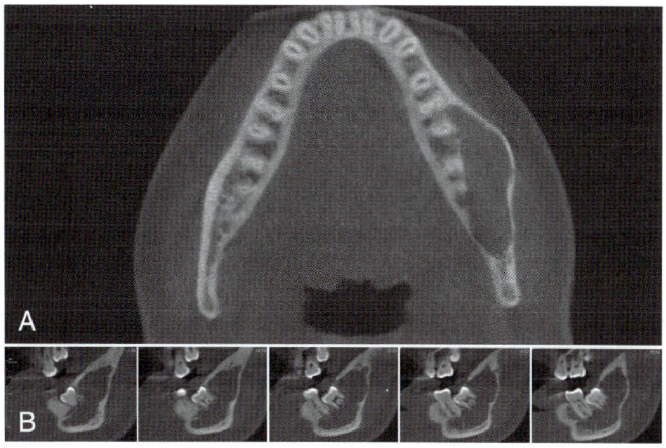

Fig. 21.25 Axial (A) cone beam computed tomographic image shows buccal expansion of the left mandibular body and ramus by a simple bone cavity. Despite its size, the apical root sheath structures are intact and unaffected (B).

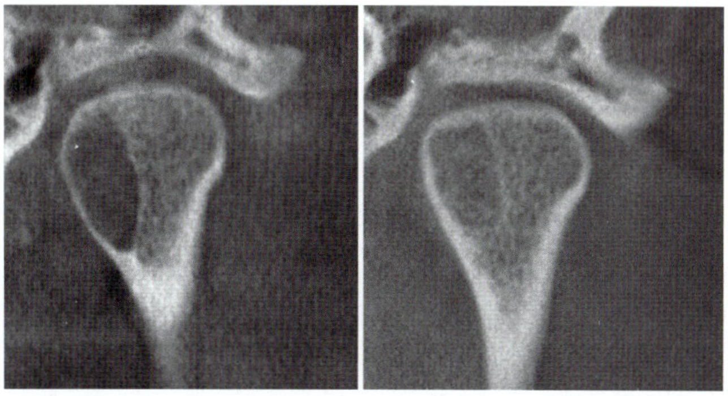

Fig. 21.26 A simple bone cavity developing in the medial pole of the left condylar head shows the process of healing after 8 years of periodic monitoring. Note the fine internal granular bone and very slight expansion of the ramus.

Management

The management of SBCs may be observation with follow-up imaging, or a puncture of the cavity wall to elicit healing by secondary intention. Spontaneous healing has also been reported for SBCs. Solitary SBCs do not recur, although those associated with a cemento-osseous dysplasia may.

Mandibular Lingual Bone Depression

Disease Mechanism

The mandibular lingual bone depression or Stafne defect is not a true cyst because it is neither a cavity in the bone nor is it lined by epithelium. Rather, it is a depression or defect within the lingual surface of the mandible. It is classified as a pseudocyst because of its shape; the often round or oval appearance of the depression simulates the radiologic features of a cyst.

First described by Stafne in the posterior mandible in a small cohort of adult patients, the depressions were found to develop in adulthood, and are not congenitally or related to the development of the adjacent submandibular salivary gland. Although the pathogenesis of the depression is not known, surgical exploration and imaging studies of the depressions have revealed the presence of several different tissues within the defect, including muscle, fat, lymph node, and salivary gland tissue, to name a few.

Clinical Features

The depression has a peak incidence in the fourth and fifth decades of life. Although rare, the lingual bone depression in the posterior mandible has an incidence of between 0.10% and 0.48%, although many likely go unseen. In the premolar area of the mandible, the incidence is much lower, at 0.009%. The defect may increase in size over time, but the ultimate size of the defect can vary.

Imaging Features

Location. All lingual bone depressions are found in the mandible. The more posterior variant of the depression has an epicenter located inferior to the inferior alveolar canal and anterior to the antegonial notch. In the premolar area of the mandible, the depression is located in the periapical region of the mandibular premolars, superior to the mylohyoid ridge.

Periphery. The mandibular lingual bone depression has a well-defined periphery and appears corticated radiologically. The inferior cortex of the mandible is often continuous with the periphery of the depression, although the thickness of the cortex can vary depending on the depth of the depression. More shallow depressions may have a very thick cortex (Fig. 21.27), while deeper depressions may display a thinner cortex, one that may mimic the cortex of an odontogenic cyst (Fig. 21.28).

Internal Structure. The internal structure is totally radiolucent.

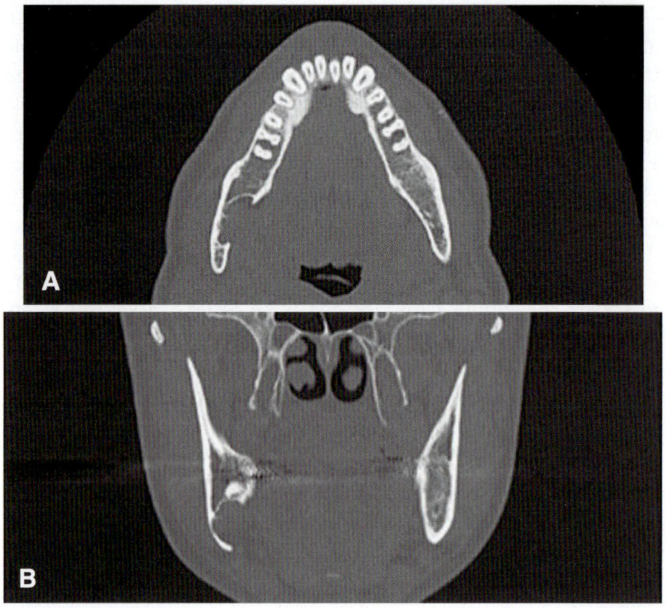

Fig. 21.28 Axial (A) and coronal (B) multidetector computed tomographic images showing a large mandibular lingual bone depression in the right posterior mandible. There has been substantial thinning of the mediolateral dimensions of the ramus.

Effects on surrounding structures. In addition to the change in the contour of the lingual surface of the mandible, there may be thinning of the lingual mandibular cortex within the depression depending on the depth of the depression. When the depression is substantial, the lingual cortex may abut the endosteal surface of the buccal cortex.

Effects on adjacent teeth. There are no effects on the teeth.

Differential Interpretation

When the cortex of the depression is thick, it should not be confused with any other lesion occurring centrally within the bone. If the depression increases in depth and overlaps the inferior alveolar canal or develops a thinner cortex, benign odontogenic and nonodontogenic entities should be considered. These may include a central giant cell lesion if the cortex is thin and the epicenter is located further away

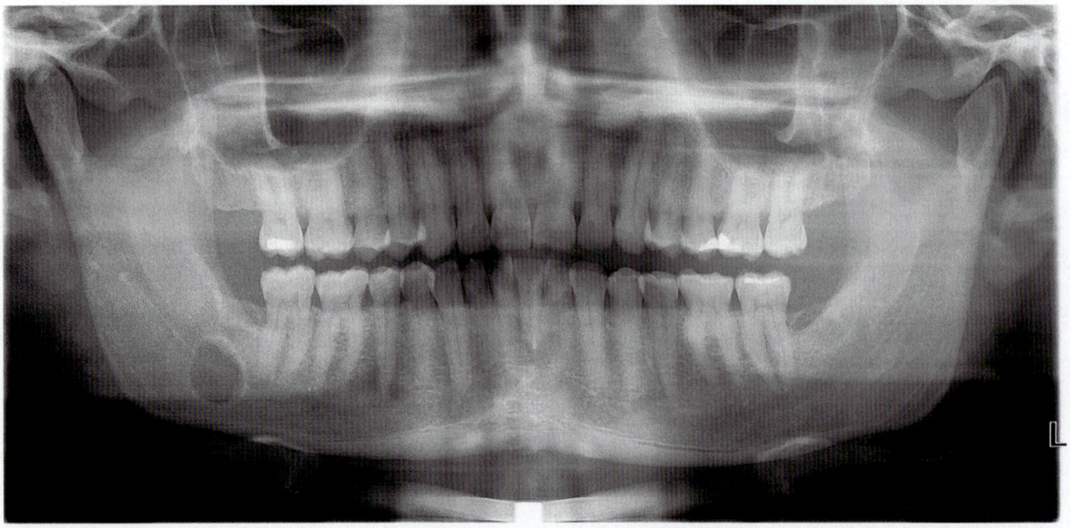

Fig. 21.27 Panoramic image of a mandibular lingual bone depression (Stafne defect) in the right posterior mandible. Note the thickness of the cortex.

from a tooth-bearing area of the jaws, or an OKC if the epicenter is closer.

Management

Recognition of the depression should preclude the need for surgical intervention or advanced imaging.

CYSTS ORIGINATING IN SOFT TISSUES

Nasolabial Cyst

Disease Mechanism

The origin of the nasolabial or nasoalveolar cyst is not known. The epithelial component of these cysts may arise from remnant epithelial rests during the merging of the embryonic nasal and maxillary processes. Alternatively, the source of the epithelium may be the embryonic nasolacrimal duct, which initially lies on the bone surface.

Clinical Features

The nasolabial cyst is rare. The age of detection ranges from 12 to 75 years with a mean age of 44 years, and approximately 75% of these lesions occur in females. When the lesion is small, it may produce a very subtle, unilateral swelling of the nasolabial fold and may elicit discomfort or pain. When large, it may distend the overlying soft tissues, flaring the nasal alae, distorting the nostrils, and creating fullness of the philtrum and upper lip. In addition, the floor of the nasal cavity may become displaced, causing some obstruction. If infected, the cyst may drain into the nasal cavity. Although the nasolabial cyst is usually unilateral, some bilateral lesions have been reported.

Imaging Features

Location. Nasolabial cysts are primarily soft tissue lesions located adjacent to the alveolar process, superior to the roots of the incisor teeth. Because this is a soft tissue lesion and planar imaging may not show any detectable changes, the investigation could include either MDCT or MRI (Fig. 21.29).

Periphery. Soft tissue window MDCT images with contrast enhancement will reveal a circular or oval lesion with slight soft tissue enhancement of the periphery.

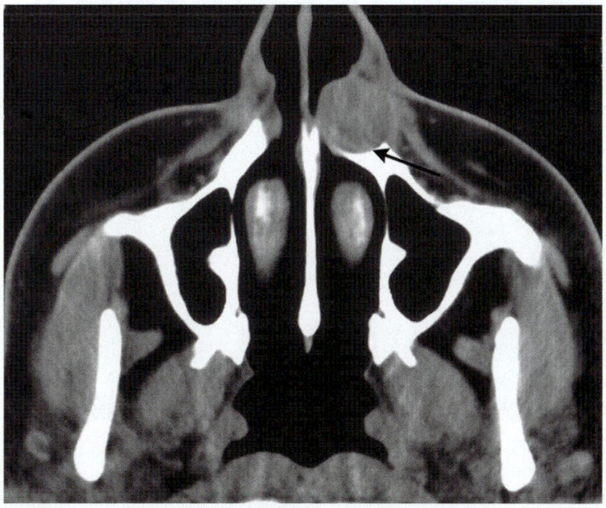

Fig. 21.29 Nasolabial cyst shown in an axial multidetector computed tomographic image with a soft tissue algorithm. Note the well-defined periphery and the erosion of the labial aspect of the alveolar process *(arrow)*.

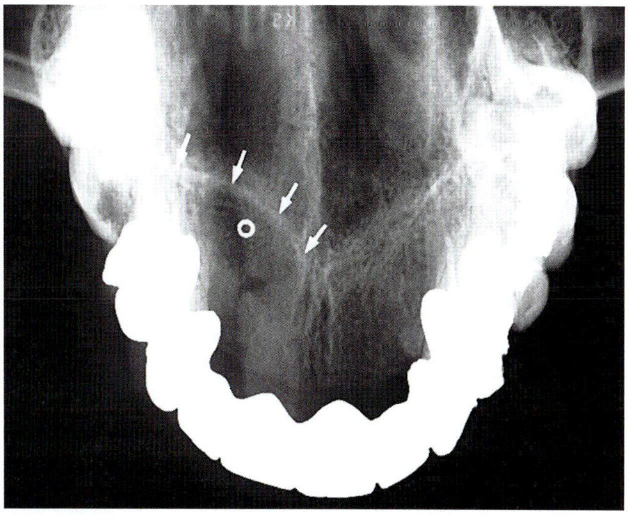

Fig. 21.30 Occlusal image of a nasolabial cyst. The image shows erosion of the alveolar bone *(o)* and elevation of the floor of the nasal fossa *(arrows)*. (From Chinellato LE, Damante JH. Contribution of radiographs to the diagnosis of naso-alveolar cyst. *Oral Surg Oral Med Oral Pathol.* 1984;58:729–735.)

Internal structure. In enhanced MDCT images, the cavity of the cyst will appear homogeneously low attenuation (radiolucent) with respect to the surrounding soft tissues.

Effects on surrounding structures. Occasionally a cyst may resorb the adjacent bone (Fig. 21.30), producing a "saucer-like" depression of the surface. This can result in an increased radiolucency of the alveolar process underlying the cyst and apical to the incisor teeth. Also, the outline of the floor of the nasal fossa may become distorted, resulting in a posterior bowing of this surface.

Differential interpretation. The swelling caused by an infected nasolabial cyst may simulate periapical inflammatory disease, therefore it is important to establish the vitality of the adjacent tooth pulps. This cyst may also resemble a nasal furuncle if it pushes upward into the floor of the nasal cavity. A large minor salivary gland mucocele or a cystic salivary adenoma should also be considered in the differential diagnosis of an uninfected nasolabial cyst.

Management. The nasolabial cyst requires excision, but cysts do not tend to recur.

Thyroglossal Duct Cyst

Disease Mechanism

The thyroglossal duct cyst develops from epithelial remnants of the embryonic thyroglossal duct, which extends from the foramen cecum in the midline of the dorsal surface of the tongue to the isthmus of the thyroid gland. This cyst is the most common congenital cyst and midline soft tissue mass in the head and neck.

Clinical Features

The cyst manifests as a slow-growing, painless mass, unless it is secondarily infected; it is found in the midline of the neck, and most are detected in the first and second decades of life. Such cysts may occur along any portion of the former track of the duct and extend from below the hyoid bone to the tongue.

Imaging Features

Many thyroglossal duct cysts have a close proximal relationship with the hyoid bone. The periphery of the cyst is usually well defined, and the hydraulic periphery is characteristic of a cyst. The shape of the cyst may be influenced by the impingement of the surrounding structures. The internal structure on MDCT images is homogeneous and of low attenuation, equivalent to fluid (Fig. 21.31A).

Branchial Cleft Cyst

Disease Mechanism

The etiology of the branchial cleft cyst is controversial but seems to be related to remnants of epithelium from one of the four embryonic branchial arches. The cyst wall usually has a lining of stratified squamous cells with some lymphoid tissue elements.

Clinical Features

The branchial cleft cyst arises in the lateral aspect of the neck, anterior to the sternocleidomastoid muscle, in the second and third decades of life. If the cyst is related to the first branchial arch, it may be located in an area extending from the angle of the mandible to the parotid and preauricular regions. This cyst usually manifests as a slow-growing, painless, fluctuant swelling unless it is secondarily infected.

Imaging Features

The imaging appearance of the branchial cleft cyst is very similar to that of the thyroglossal duct cyst in terms of both shape and internal image density (see Fig. 21.31B). The lateral position of the branchial

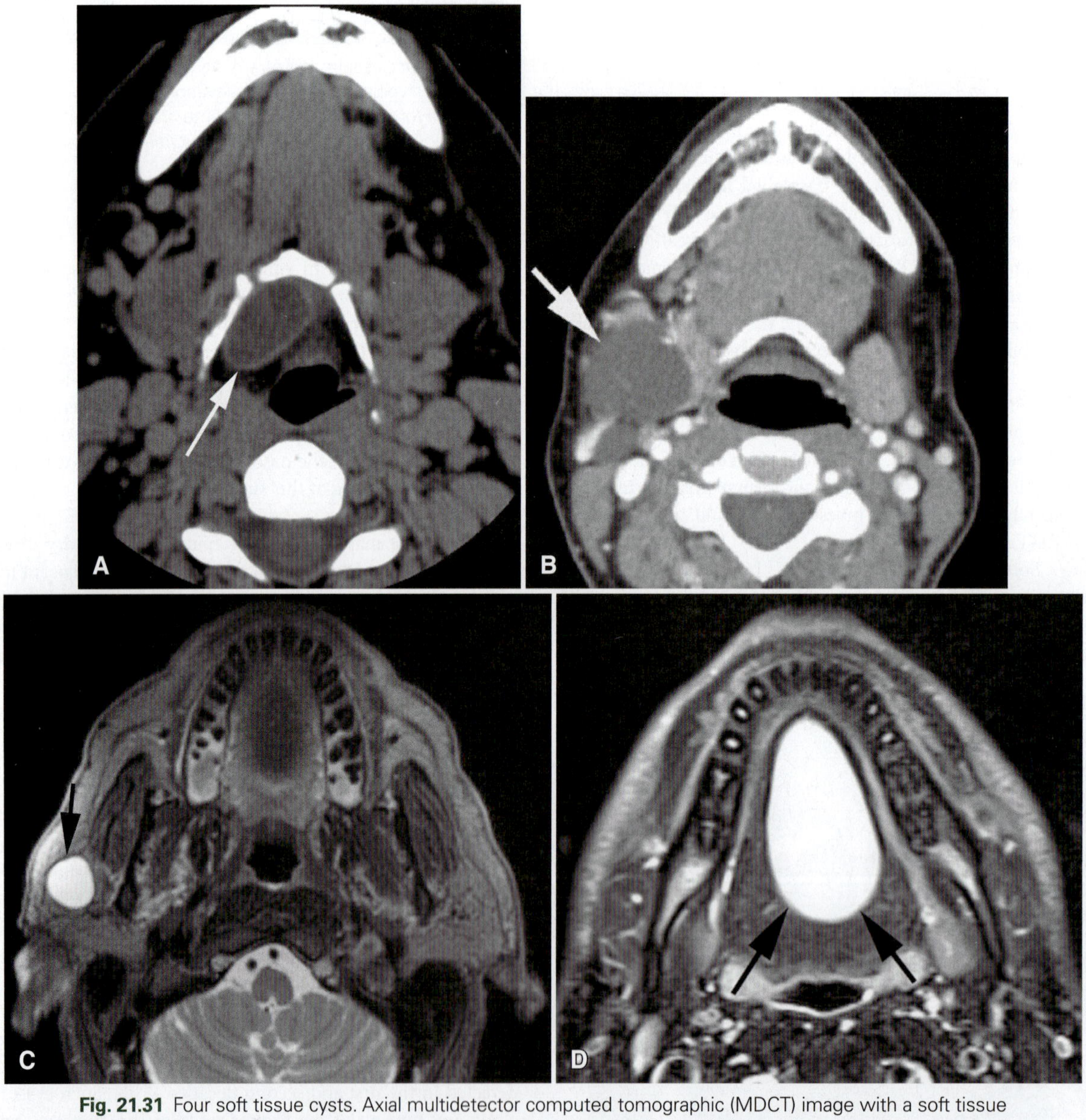

Fig. 21.31 Four soft tissue cysts. Axial multidetector computed tomographic (MDCT) image with a soft tissue algorithm of a thyroglossal duct cyst *(arrow)* positioned adjacent to the hyoid bone. Note the cystic shape and homogeneous low attenuation of the internal structure (A). Axial MDCT scan using soft tissue algorithm of a branchial cleft cyst *(arrow)* positioned just inferior the angle of the mandible and displacing the submandibular salivary gland medially (B). Axial T2-weighted magnetic resonance image of a lymphoepithelial cyst *(arrow)* positioned in the right parotid gland (C). Note the homogeneous high-signal *(white)* internal structure, indicating fluid. Axial T2-weighted magnetic resonance image of a dermoid cyst *(arrows)* in the floor of the mouth (D).

cleft cyst in the neck differentiates it from a thyroglossal duct cyst. When it is associated with the parotid gland, it may be difficult to differentiate from a lymphoepithelial cyst.

Lymphoepithelial Cyst of the Parotid Gland

Disease Mechanism

The lymphoepithelial parotid cyst, once also known as a branchial cyst, is commonly located within the parotid gland and its histopathologic features are very similar to that of a branchial cleft cyst.

Clinical Features

The mean age of the appearance of this cyst is the fifth decade with a slight female predominance. Usually manifesting as a slow-growing enlargement in the parotid gland, such a cyst may be associated with human immunodeficiency virus infections.

Imaging Features

Most commonly this cyst is located within the parenchyma of the parotid gland, and they are spherical or circular in shape with internal densities in advanced imaging examinations that are reminiscent of fluid (see Fig. 21.31C).

Dermoid Cyst

Disease Mechanism

The dermoid cyst is a cystic form of the teratoma, thought to develop from entrapped pluripotent embryonic cells. The cyst is lined with epidermis and cutaneous appendages, and is filled with keratin or sebaceous material. In rare cases, it may contain bone, teeth, muscle, or hair, in which case they are properly called teratomas.

Clinical Features

The dermoid cyst usually becomes clinically apparent between ages 12 and 25 years, and manifests as slow, painless swelling. Although few (up to 10%) arise in the head and neck with the orbital regions being the most common, only 1%–2% develop in the oral cavity. Of these, approximately 25% occur in the floor of the mouth and on the tongue. When located in the neck or floor of the mouth, these cysts may interfere with breathing, speaking, and eating. On palpation, the cyst may be fluctuant or doughy soft, according to their contents.

Imaging Features

The dermoid cysts have a well-defined periphery and a cystic shape. Internally, the cyst may have the density of fluid, or it may have a soft tissue multilocular appearance (see Fig. 21.31D). If teeth or bone form in the cyst, these densities may become apparent on planar imaging.

Differential Interpretation

Lesions that are clinically similar to the dermoid cyst includes the ranula in the floor of the mouth, the thyroglossal duct cyst, the cystic hygroma, and the branchial cleft cyst.

BIBLIOGRAPHY

Johnson NR, Gannon OM, Savage NW, et al. Frequency of odontogenic cysts and tumors: a systematic review. *J Investig Clin Dent.* 2014;5:9-14.

Rajendra Santosh AB. Odontogenic cysts. *Dent Clin North Am.* 2020;64:105-119.

Soluk-Tekkesin M, Wright JM. The World Health Organization classification of odontogenic lesions: a summary of the changes of the 2022 (5th) edition. *Turk Patoloji Derg.* 2022;38:168-184.

Odontogenic Cysts–Buccal Bifurcation Cyst

Packota GV, Hall JM, Lanigan DT, et al. Paradental cysts on mandibular first molars in children: report of five cases. *Dentomaxillofac Radiol.* 1990;19:126-132.

Pompura JR, Sandor GK, Stoneman DW. The buccal bifurcation cyst: a prospective study of treatment outcomes in 44 sites. *Oral Surg Oral Med Oral Pathol Oral Radiol Endod.* 1997;83:215-221.

Ruddocks LA, Fitzpatrick SG, Bhattacharyya I, et al. Buccal bifurcation cyst: A case series and review of the literature. *J Am Dent Assoc.* 2022;153:421-428.

Odontogenic Cysts–Calcifying Odontogenic Cyst

de Arruda JAA, Schuch LF, Abreu LG, et al. A multicentre study of 268 cases of calcifying odontogenic cysts and a literature review. *Oral Dis.* 2018;27:1282-1293.

Yoshiura K, Tabata O, Miwa K, et al. Computed tomographic features of calcifying odontogenic cysts. *Dentomaxillofac Radiol.* 1998;27:12-16.

Odontogenic Cysts–Dentigerous Cyst

Nahajowski M, Hnitecka S, Antoszewska-Smith J, et al. Factors influencing an eruption of teeth associated with a dentigerous cyst: a systematic review and meta analysis. *BMC Oral Health.* 2021;21:180.

Xu GZ, Jiang Q, Yu CQ, et al. Clinicopathologic features of dentigerous cysts in the maxillary sinus. *J Craniofac Surg.* 2012;23:e226-e231.

Odontogenic Cysts–Glandular Odontogenic Cyst

MacDonald-Jankowski DS. Glandular odontogenic cyst: systematic review. *Dentomaxillofac Radiol.* 2010;39:127-139.

Noffke C, Raubenheimer EJ. The glandular odontogenic cyst: clinical and radiologic features: review of the literature and report of nine cases. *Dentomaxillofac Radiol.* 2002;31:333-338.

Odontogenic Cysts–Lateral Periodontal Cyst

Weathers DR, Waldron CA. Unusual multilocular cysts of the jaws (botryoid odontogenic cysts). *Oral Surg Oral Med Oral Pathol.* 1973;36:235-241.

Wysocki GP, Brannon RB, Gardner DG, et al. Histogenesis of the lateral periodontal cyst and the gingival cyst of the adult. *Oral Surg Oral Med Oral Pathol.* 1980;50:327-334.

Odontogenic Cysts–Odontogenic Keratocyst

Borghesi A, Nardi C, Giannitto C, et al. Odontogenic keratocyst: imaging features of a benign lesion with an aggressive behaviour. *Insights Imaging.* 2018;9:883-897.

Stoelinga PJW. The odontogenic keratocyst revisited. *Int J Oral Maxillofac Surg.* 2022;51:1420-1430.

Odontogenic Cysts–Nevoid Basal Cell Carcinoma Syndrome

Kalogirou EM, Thermos G, Zogopoulos V, et al. The immunohistochemical profile of basal cell nevus syndrome-associated and sporadic odontogenic keratocysts: a systemic review and meta-analysis. *Clin Oral Investig.* 2021;25:3371-3367.

Lam EWN, Lee L, Perschbacher SE, et al. The occurrence of keratocystic odontogenic tumours in nevoid basal cell carcinoma syndrome. *Dentomaxillofac Radiol.* 2009;38:475-479.

Titinchi F. Novel recurrence risk stratification of odontogenic keratocysts: a systematic review. *Oral Dis.* 2022;28:1749-1759.

Odontogenic Cysts–Residual Cyst

Titinchi F, Morkel J. Residual cyst of the jaws: a clinic-pathologic study of this seemingly inconspicuous lesion. *PLoS One.* 2020;15:e0244250.

Nonodontogenic Cysts–Nasolabial Cyst

Sheikh AB, Chin OY, Fang CH, et al. Nasolabial cysts: a systematic review of 311 cases. *Laryngoscope.* 2016;126:60-66.

Yuen H, Julian CY, Samuel CL. Nasolabial cysts: clinical features, diagnosis and treatment. *Br J Oral Maxillofac Surg.* 2007;45:293-297.

Nonodontogenic Cysts–Nasopalatine Cyst

Mraiwa RJ, Jacobs R, Van Cleynenbreugel J, et al. The nasopalatine duct cyst revisited using 2D and 3D CT imaging. *Dentomaxillofac Radiol.* 2004;33:396-402.

Swanson KS, Kaugars GE, Gunsolley JC. Nasopalatine duct cyst: an analysis of 334 cases. *J Oral Maxillofac Surg*. 1991;49:268-271.

Soft Tissue Cysts–Branchial Cleft Cyst

Fanous A, Morcrette G, Couloigner V, et al. Diagnostic approach to congenital cystic masses of the neck from a clinical and pathologic perspective. *Dermatopathology (Basil)*. 2021;8:342-358.

Soft Tissue Cysts–Dermoid Cyst

Pryor SG, Lewis JE, Weaver AL, et al. Pediatric dermoid cysts of the head and neck. *Otolaryngol Head Neck Surg*. 2005;132:938-942.

Seward GR. Dermoid cysts of the floor of the mouth. *Br J Oral Surg*. 1965;3:36-47.

Soft Tissue Cysts–Lymphoepithelial Cyst

Suto T, Kato H, Kawaguchi M, et al. MRI findings of sporadic/simple lymphoepithelial cyst of the parotid gland. *Neuroradiol J*. 2023;36(5): 541-547. https://doi.org/10.1177/19714009231163558.

Soft Tissue Cysts–Thyroglossal Duct Cyst

Tanitame K, Nonishi H. Thyroglossal duct cyst. *N Engl J Med*. 2019;380:2563.

Pseudocysts–Mandibular Lingual Bone Depression

Stafne EC. Bone cavities situated near the angle of the mandible. *J Am Dent Assoc*. 1942;29:1969-1972.

Pseudocysts–Simple Bone Cavity

Chadwick JW, Alsufyani NA, Lam EW. Clinical and radiographic features of solitary and cemento-osseous dysplasia-associated simple bone cysts. *Dentomaxillofac Radiol*. 2011;40:230-235.

Lima LB, de Freitas Filho SA, Barbosa de Paulo LF, et al. Simple bone cyst: description of 60 cases seen at a Brazilian School of Dentistry and review of international literature. *Med Oral Patol Oral Cir Bucal*. 2020; 25:e616-e625.

22

Benign Tumors and Neoplasms

Ernest W.N. Lam

DISEASE MECHANISM

A benign neoplasm is an abnormal mass of tissue that develops as a result of uncontrolled cell proliferation. Moreover, the potential for cell proliferation in a neoplasm is unlimited. Although the term tumor is often used synonymously for neoplasm, a tumor is a more generic term that refers to a tissue mass. So while all neoplasms are tumors, not all tumors are neoplasms.

The loss of growth control in neoplasia is often the result of an identifiable gene mutation that dysregulates normal cell turnover. The molecular abnormality is then propagated through cell division, which results in a population of cells, each of which contains the same genetic abnormality. This type of clonal proliferation or propagation is a hallmark of neoplasia. Unlike malignant neoplasms, benign neoplasms lack the ability to metastasize; that is, benign neoplastic cells do not have the ability to form satellite masses at distant sites.

Benign neoplasms tend to resemble the tissue of their origin histologically. For example, an ameloblastoma, a neoplasm that is derived from odontogenic epithelium, is composed of cells that resemble ameloblasts. Benign neoplasia should, however, be differentiated from hyperplasia, metaplasia, and hamartomatous proliferation. While these processes may produce a tissue mass, cell proliferation is limited. Hyperplasia is a proliferation of cells that develops in response to a stimulus. In metaplasia, a stimulus transforms one mature cell type into another mature cell type. For both hyperplasia and metaplasia, when the stimulus is removed, the altered cell types revert to their native cell types. A hamartoma is a mass of disorganized normal tissue with limited growth potential that would normally be found at the site of growth.

CLINICAL FEATURES

In general, odontogenic neoplasms are rare. They may be found incidentally on radiologic examinations made for other purposes, or they may be detected clinically by an enlargement of the jaws or movement of teeth. Sometimes the radiologic examination is performed to try to discover the reason for these changes. Benign neoplasms typically have an insidious onset and grow slowly. These neoplasms are painless, but they can be locally aggressive and extend into adjacent tissue spaces.

APPLIED DIAGNOSTIC IMAGING

If an abnormal enlargement of the jaw is suspected, a radiologic examination should be performed to document the extent of the enlargement, and the imaging characteristics of the abnormality. This examination often begins with a panoramic image to identify the site and extent of the abnormality, and intraoral periapical and/or occlusal images should be acquired to evaluate the effects of the abnormality on the teeth and the surrounding structures. For abnormalities developing centrally within the bone, the addition of cone beam computed tomography (CBCT) or multidetector computed tomography (MDCT) is essential for further refining radiologic feature identification and diagnosis. If clinically, or on panoramic or intraoral imaging, the abnormality appears to extend into the adjacent soft tissues, MDCT or magnetic resonance imaging (MRI) may be required to characterize soft tissue involvement.

A systematic, thorough imaging examination allows the dentist to characterize all the important key features of an abnormality, allowing them to differentiate the benign neoplasm from other processes. On the one hand, some imaging features may be so specific of an entity that a preliminary diagnosis of the type of benign neoplasm can be made. On the other hand, should the imaging features overlap with other similar appearing entities and a preliminary diagnosis cannot be made, other diagnostic tests must be ordered. A thorough imaging examination may also direct the clinician to the most favorable biopsy site, should biopsy be necessary. In all cases, however, the imaging examination should be performed prior to biopsy, as the biopsy procedure could alter the radiologic appearances of the tissues in such a way as to mask characteristic features.

IMAGING FEATURES

Location

Some benign neoplasms have a specific anatomic predilection because of their biology. For example, lesions that develop from odontogenic cell sources occur in the alveolar processes superior to the inferior alveolar nerve canal where odontogenic cells and teeth reside. Lesions of vascular and neural origin develop within or in close proximity to the inferior alveolar canal, and cartilaginous neoplasms occur in locations where chondrocytes may reside, such as around the mandibular condyle. Although some neoplasms can develop more commonly in a particular region of the jaws (i.e., the posterior body of the mandible) than another, this type of "common location" approach should be used sparingly as it can oversimplify the diagnostic process and result in error.

Periphery

Benign neoplasms grow generally slowly as their cell populations increase in number (Fig. 22.1). As a result, the borders of benign neoplasms are well defined. The amount of cortication at the lesion periphery can, however, vary. If the neoplasm exhibits a slower or more indolent growth rate, the cortex is often more apparent. In contrast, if the neoplasm grows more quickly or aggressively, the cortex will be less clearly seen or there may be discontinuities or breaks.

The clonal nature of cell proliferation in a benign neoplasm often results in what appears to be a concentric or near-spherical pattern of enlargement. However, unlike the smooth, hydraulic border of an

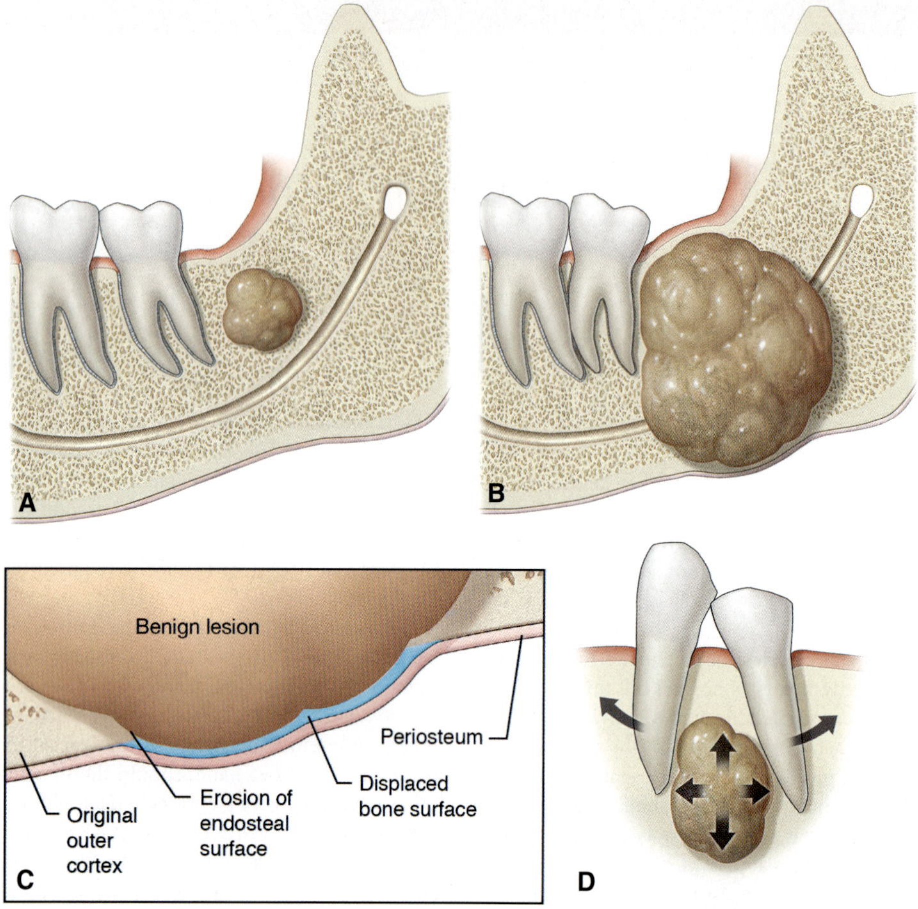

Fig. 22.1 Benign lesions grow concentrically in bone (A). They can be round to oval, or lobulated (B). As they grow, benign lesions can displace adjacent bone borders (C) and teeth (D), and externally resorb tooth roots.

enlarging cyst, the type of concentric growth of a benign neoplasm results in a border that is more irregular or even lobulated. As the neoplastic cells proliferate, different subpopulations within the mass may experience different microenvironments that support or slow local growth. For example, in areas where the vascular supply is richer, the cells may proliferate at a faster rate and this region of the neoplasm may enlarge more quickly than an adjacent area that may be less well vascularized. This type of differential growth may be appreciated radiologically as a lobulated periphery, where larger lobules reflect regions of faster growth and smaller lobules regions of slower growth.

Internal Structure

The internal structure may be completely radiolucent or radiopaque, or it may be a mixture of both radiolucent and radiopaque areas. Normal bone that is trapped between adjacent lobules of a benign neoplasm are called septa (or septum, if there is just one). These septa can be linear, curvilinear, or curved depending on the neoplasm, and vary in thickness. Curved septa are a characteristic feature of ameloblastoma. While the cells in an ameloblastoma do not produce bone, the trapped residual bone between the lobules of the neoplasm is remodeled into curvilinear or curved structures by internal changes to the mass during growth. Should the sizes of adjacent lobules be larger and the entrapped bone become more significantly compressed, the septum will appear thinner. In contrast, smaller adjacent lobules may result in a thicker septum. Although residual bone in the form of septa may give rise to a mixed radiolucent and radiopaque internal structure, some clinicians differentiate septa (residual bone) from mineralized matrices produced de novo by the tumor cells themselves.

Cells in some neoplasms have developed the capability to produce a mineralized matrix if the cells have reached an appropriate level of differentiation or specialization. These “true” mixed radiolucent and radiopaque lesions contain mineralized areas that can take the form of tooth material or bone. Because the most mature part of the neoplasm is located more centrally, mineralization often occurs in this location first, before it spreads to more peripheral areas within the neoplasm. A cemento-ossifying fibroma often has an internal granular radiopaque pattern produced by the abnormal or immature bone that is being manufactured by the neoplastic cells. The internal pattern can be highly characteristic for a specific type of neoplasm, and this may aid in the interpretation. A neoplasm with a totally radiolucent internal structure may not be as useful an aid to interpretation.

Effects on Surrounding Structures

The manner in which a benign neoplasm affects adjacent tissues may suggest biological behavior that is closer to the indolent or aggressive ends of the growth-rate spectrum. As the neoplasm enlarges, it may displace neighboring structures. If the growth pattern is indolent or slow, adjacent structures may respond by remodeling around the enlarging mass. For example, the surface of the bone may enlarge, and the cortex may thin as the bone is remodeled to accommodate the growing mass (Fig. 22.1B). This appearance is caused by simultaneous resorption of bone along the inner (endosteal) surface of the cortex and deposition of bone along the outer cortical surface by the

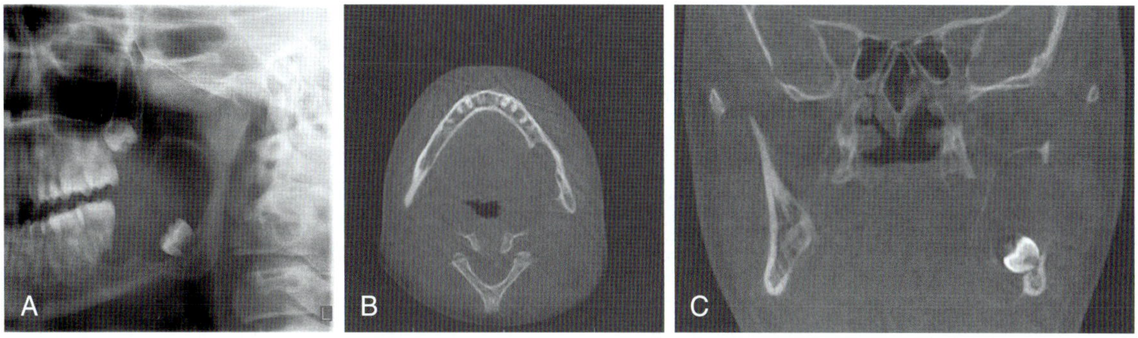

Fig. 22.2 Cropped panoramic (A), and axial (B) and coronal (C) cone beam computed tomographic images show a unicystic ameloblastoma developing in the left posterior mandible. There has been significant expansion of the mandibular body (B) and ramus (C) to the sigmoid notch, and inferior displacement of the mandibular left third molar and root resorption of the mandibular left second molar (A).

periosteum (Fig. 22.1C). Because the remodeling process is slow, the cortex maintains its integrity and resists perforation. In contrast, a faster, more aggressively growing neoplasm may exceed the capacity of the bone to remodel, resulting in perforation of the cortex. Internal structures such as the inferior alveolar canal or the floor of the maxillary sinus may also be displaced to accommodate a developing adjacent benign neoplasm.

Effects on Adjacent Teeth

Benign neoplasms may also cause tipping or bodily displacement of adjacent teeth (see Fig. 22.1D). Any orthodontist will tell you that tooth movement is a very slow process, and the movement of teeth by a benign neoplasm is no different. The roots of teeth may also be resorbed in a directional manner as the edge of the neoplasm encounters the root surface. Benign neoplasms tend to resorb the adjacent root surfaces in a smooth fashion.

ODONTOGENIC TUMORS AND NEOPLASMS

Disease Mechanism

Odontogenic neoplasms arise from odontogenic tissues in the jaws. According to the World Health Organization (WHO), these neoplasms can be classified on the basis of the cell or tissue of origin of each neoplasm: neoplasms composed of odontogenic epithelium; mixed neoplasms composed of both odontogenic epithelium and odontogenic ectomesenchyme (connective tissue); and neoplasms composed of primarily ectomesenchyme. Odontogenic neoplasms are relatively rare, accounting for only 1.3%–15% of all oral neoplasms.

Benign jaw neoplasms are presented in this chapter according to their tissues of origin. This format should assist the reader in learning to correlate the radiographic appearance of neoplasms with the underlying pathologic mechanism of the disease process.

ODONTOGENIC EPITHELIAL NEOPLASMS

Ameloblastoma

Disease Mechanism

Ameloblastoma is the most well-known of the odontogenic neoplasms. This neoplasm arises from odontogenic epithelium derived from remnants of the dental lamina and the enamel organ. Although several different subtypes have been described, all involve proliferation of these cell remnants. The unicystic ameloblastoma may develop as a single entity or from within the epithelial lining of a dentigerous cyst; this is also called a mural (i.e., within the wall) ameloblastoma (Fig. 22.2). More commonly, ameloblastomas are solid cell masses developing within the bone, or they may develop peripheral to the bone. For those ameloblastomas that develop within the bone, these neoplasms can develop cystic internal areas (cystic or multicystic) or induce the proliferation of fibrous connective tissue (desmoplastic).

Clinical Features

The age range for the diagnosis of ameloblastoma is very broad. While the unicystic ameloblastoma occurs more generally in younger people, the classic ameloblastoma has a wide age range, and has been identified in children as young as 3 years and in adults over 80 years. Most patients are, however, between 20 and 50 years of age, with the average age at discovery about 40 years.

Ameloblastomas grow slowly, and few, if any, symptoms occur in the early stages. When small, the neoplasm may be an incidental finding, discovered during a new patient or recall dental examination. As the neoplasm increases in size, the patient may experience tooth movement or a change in their occlusion. Eventually, they may notice a gradually increasing facial asymmetry. Swelling of the cheek, gingiva, or hard palate has been reported as the chief complaint in 95% of untreated maxillary ameloblastomas. The mucosa over the mass is normal, and in most cases, patients do not report pain or other sensory changes. As the neoplasm enlarges further, the surface may be bony hard to palpation, or there may be crepitus if the bone surface has thinned. If the overlying bone becomes perforated, the swelling may feel firm or fluctuant.

An untreated benign neoplasm may grow to a great size, and is typically more of a concern in the maxilla where it can impinge on vital structures as it approaches the skull base. Recurrence rates are higher in older patients and in patients with multilocular lesions. As seen with other jaw neoplasms, local recurrence, whether detected radiographically or histopathologically, may have a more aggressive character than the original neoplasm.

Imaging Features

Worth, in his 1963 book, describes four patterns of ameloblastoma: a unilocular radiolucent cavity (Fig. 22.3), a unilocular radiolucent cavity with partial division by coarse septa (Fig. 22.4), multilocular radiolucent cavities separated by curved septa of variable lengths (Fig. 22.5), and a honeycomb pattern consisting of many radiolucent compartments separated by small, curved septa (Figs. 22.6 and 22.7). It should be noted that although a unicystic ameloblastoma is a unilocular entity, a unilocular appearance is not necessarily reflective of a unicystic ameloblastoma.

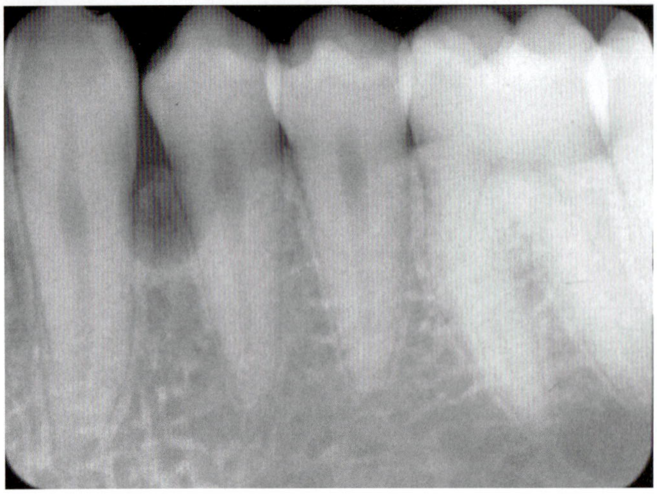

Fig. 22.3 A small unilocular ameloblastoma developing near the crest of the alveolar process of the mandible reducing definition of the crestal cortex.

Location. Although remnants of odontogenic epithelium may be located anywhere within the jaws, most ameloblastomas (80%) develop in the molar/ramus region of the mandible. In the maxilla, most ameloblastomas develop in the third molar area, subjacent to the floor of the maxillary sinus or more anteriorly, adjacent to the nasal floor (Fig. 22.8).

Periphery. The ameloblastoma has well-defined borders, although the thickness of the cortex as well as its continuity peripherally can vary depending on the relative aggressiveness of individual neoplasms. For example, a faster, more aggressively growing neoplasm may exhibit a less visible cortex. The borders are often curved, and for smaller lesions, an ameloblastoma may be indistinguishable from a cyst (see Fig. 22.3). The periphery of ameloblastoma in the maxilla is usually less well defined, and this may be due to the native cancellous bone pattern in the maxilla and relative aggressiveness of maxillary lesions.

Internal structure. The internal structure of ameloblastomas can vary from one that is unilocular and radiolucent (see Fig. 22.3) to one that has many small locules separated by radiopaque septa (see Fig. 22.6). Indeed, Worth notes that the presence of a septum within

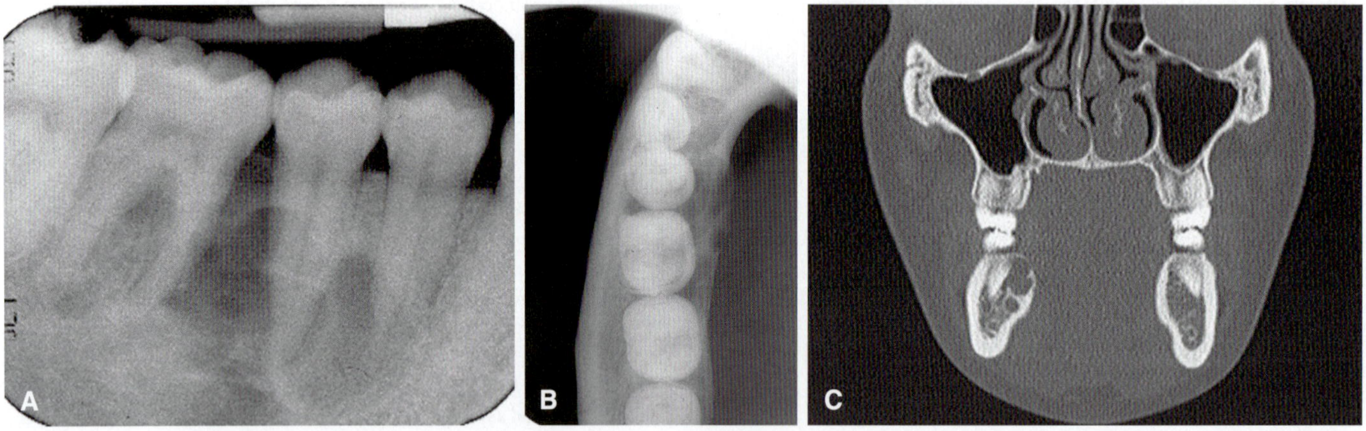

Fig. 22.4 Periapical (A) and cross-sectional occlusal (B) images showing short septa developing in an ameloblastoma. The partial loculations that result are seen in the coronal multidetector computed tomographic image (C).

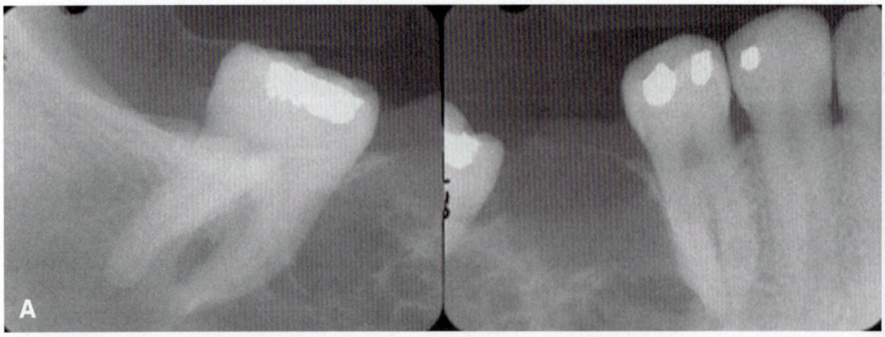

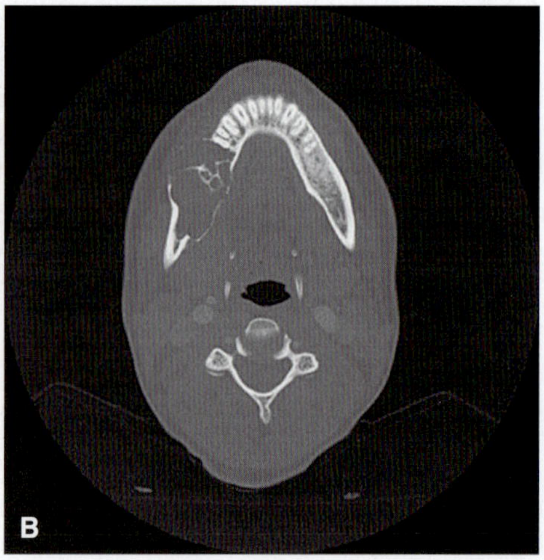

Fig. 22.5 A large multilocular ameloblastoma developing in the right posterior mandible. Note the coarse, curved septations dividing the larger cavity into smaller, more discrete regions on the periapical images (A). The multidetector computed tomographic image of the same patient (B) shows the variability in the sizes of these cavities.

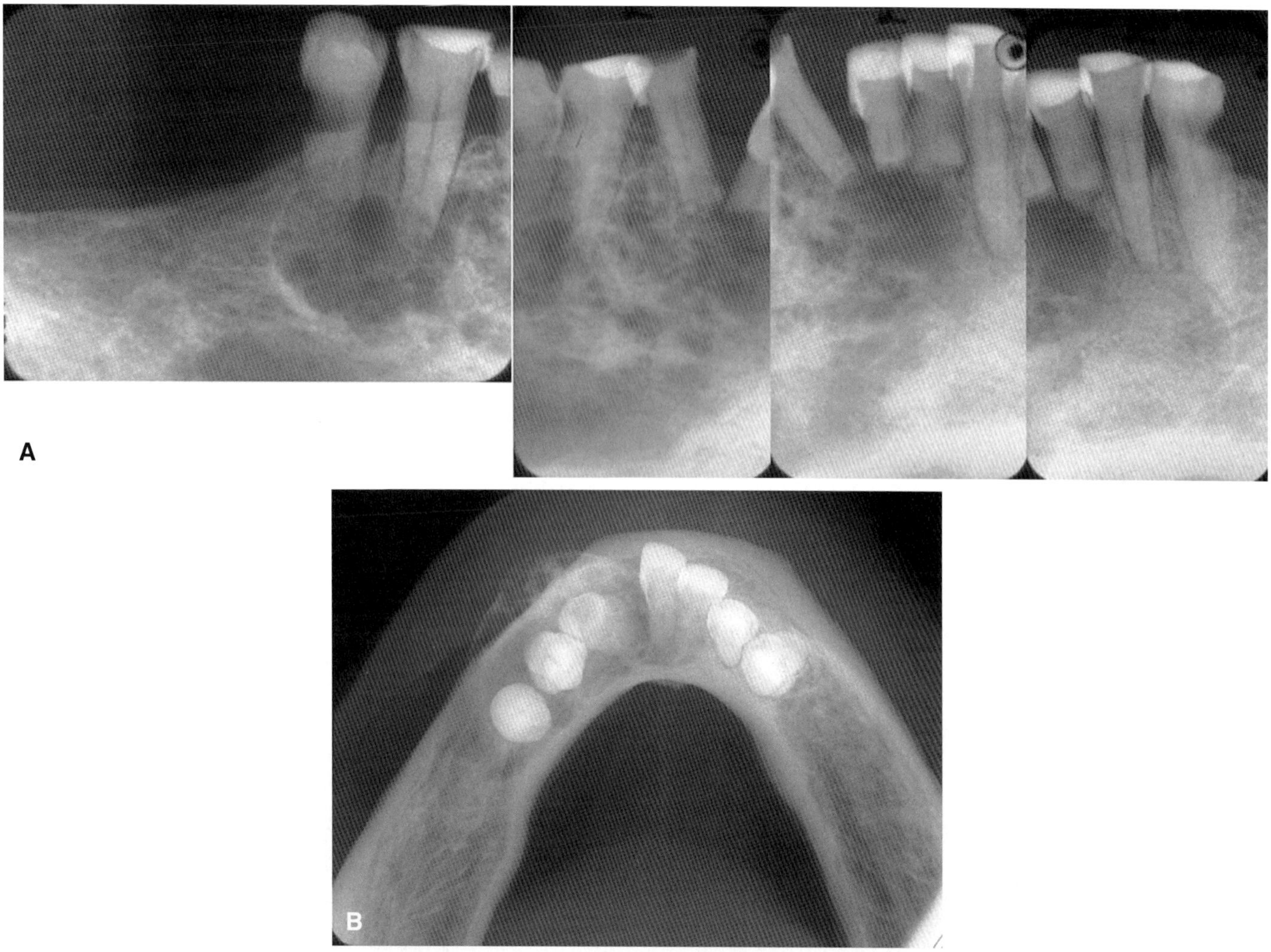

Fig. 22.6 Periapical (A) and cross-sectional occlusal (B) images showing the honeycomb appearance of an ameloblastoma. Note the short, curved septa and the small, closely spaced compartments of tumor reminiscent of honeycombs in a beehive.

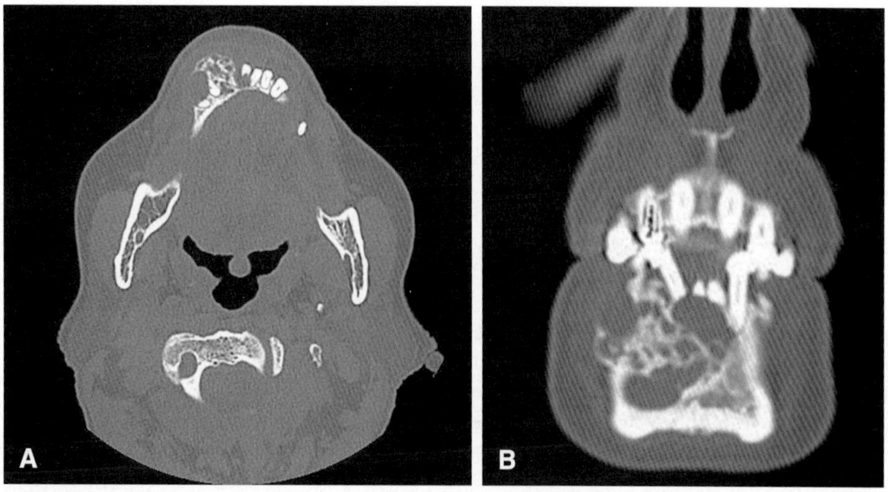

Fig. 22.7 Axial (A) and coronal (B) multidetector computed tomographic images of the same patient in Fig. 22.6 showing the short, curved septa and the small, closely spaced tumor compartments.

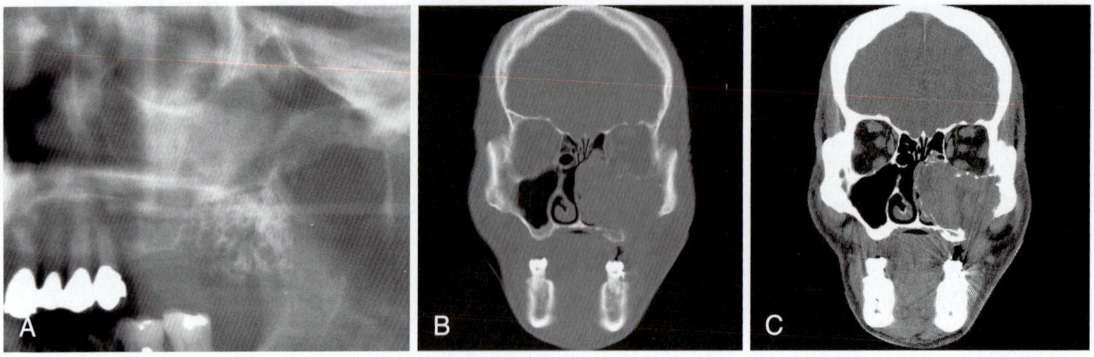

Fig. 22.8 Cropped panoramic image (A) of an ameloblastoma involving the left maxilla. Note the multilocular appearance in the tuberosity region. It is impossible to determine the extent of the lesion with the panoramic image, but the coronal multidetector computed tomographic images in bone (B) and soft tissue (C) windows show the extensions more clearly. Note the aggressive nature of the tumor as it has displaced both the sinus and nasal fossa floors, and perforated the lateral border of the maxilla.

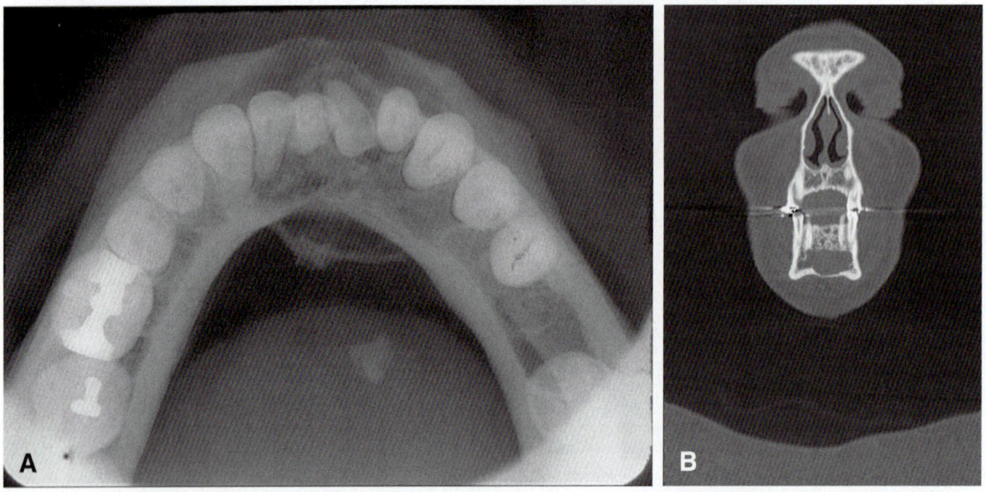

Fig. 22.9 Cross-sectional occlusal (A) and coronal multidetector computed tomographic (B) images showing the irregular sclerotic bone developing around the teeth in a desmoplastic ameloblastoma.

a larger cyst-like cavity or a septum that produces partial loculation within a cavity adds greatly to the possibility of ameloblastoma (see Figs. 22.4 and 22.5).

Most commonly, the septa in ameloblastomas are coarse and curved, partially dividing a unilocular cavity into multiple smaller, variably sized cavities (see Fig. 22.5C). Because this neoplasm frequently has internal cyst-like cavities, in some cases, the septa are remodeled into curves creating a soap bubble (compartments of variable size) or a honeycomb (numerous small compartments) pattern (see Fig. 22.6). Generally, the loculations are larger in the posterior mandible and smaller in the anterior mandible. In the desmoplastic variety, the internal structure can be composed of a very irregular bone pattern resembling a bone dysplasia or bone-forming neoplasm (Fig. 22.9).

Effects on surrounding structures. A cross-sectional occlusal image may demonstrate the concentric growth pattern with thinning of an adjacent cortex leaving a thin "eggshell" of remnant bone at the surface (see Fig. 22.5B). Where the crest of the alveolar process of the mandible in the retromolar area or the anterior border of the mandibular ramus has been perforated or lost, the probability of ameloblastoma is greatly increased. The unicystic ameloblastoma, for example, may cause extreme expansion of the mandibular ramus (Fig. 22.2). CT images often reveal regions of perforation of the displaced bone cortex owing to the inability of the production of periosteal new bone as the ameloblastoma expands (Fig. 22.2B).

Effects on adjacent teeth. There is a pronounced tendency for ameloblastomas to cause extensive root resorption (Fig. 22.6A). Tooth displacement is also common (Fig. 22.6B), and in some cases, this displacement can be apical.

Recurrent ameloblastoma. Ameloblastomas may recur when the initial surgical excision inadequately removes the entire neoplasm. A recurrent neoplasm has a characteristic appearance of multiple small cyst-like structures with very coarse, almost sclerotic borders (Fig. 22.10). Depending on how the neoplasm recurs, these small cyst-like areas may be separated by normal bone.

Additional imaging. If a preliminary interpretation of ameloblastoma is made based on planar imaging, MDCT is highly recommended. MDCT may also more accurately demonstrate the anatomic extent and effects on the adjacent bone borders and soft tissues (see Fig. 22.11). In this regard, MDCT imaging has an advantage over CBCT imaging because it can display the extension of the neoplasm's soft tissue outside of the bone and into adjacent spaces. If soft tissue extension is extensive, an MRI can provide superior images of the nature and extent of the extension. MDCT is also an essential tool in the postsurgical follow-up assessment of ameloblastoma.

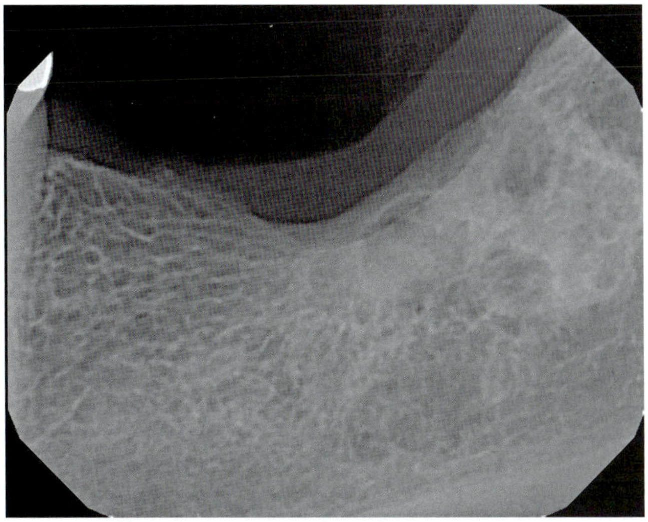

Fig. 22.10 Periapical image of a recurrent ameloblastoma in the left mandible. Note the thick, sclerotic borders of the small locules. (Courtesy Dr. T. Blight, Winnipeg, MB.)

Differential interpretation. A small unilocular ameloblastoma cannot be easily differentiated from an odontogenic keratocyst. If the ameloblastoma develops around the crown of an unerupted tooth, it often cannot be differentiated from a dentigerous cyst. Because the appearance of internal septa is important for the interpretation of ameloblastoma, other types of lesions that also have internal septa such as odontogenic keratocyst, mucoepidermoid carcinoma, and odontogenic myxoma, or those that produce internal linear mineralizations such as the central giant cell (CGC) lesion, may have a similar appearance.

An odontogenic keratocyst may contain curved septa, but in the mandible, the odontogenic keratocyst will grow along the bone without marked buccal/lingual bone expansion, a growth feature not characteristic of ameloblastoma. The mucoepidermoid carcinoma may have features that overlap a recurrent ameloblastoma, and these may be indistinguishable without a clinical history. Radiologically, the mucoepidermoid carcinoma may display similarly thick, almost sclerotic internal septa. Odontogenic myxomas may have similar-appearing septa; however, there are usually one or two thin sharp, straight septa, which is characteristic of the myxoma. The presence of straight septa oriented perpendicularly to one another greatly adds to the probability of myxoma. Also, myxomas are not as expansile as ameloblastomas, and like odontogenic keratocysts, they tend to grow along the bone. Giant cell lesions, in addition to occurring in a younger age group, have more granular or wispy ill-defined internal patterns as the mineralization is produced de novo by the cells within the lesion.

Management. The size of the ameloblastoma often dictates the aggressiveness of its management. The most common treatment is en bloc surgical resection. The surgical procedure should take into account the tendency of the neoplasm to perforate adjacent bone borders and extend into the adjacent soft tissues. The maxilla is usually treated more aggressively because of the tendency of ameloblastoma to encroach upon vital structures near or in the skull base.

Calcifying Epithelial Odontogenic Tumor

Disease Mechanism

The calcifying epithelial odontogenic tumor (CEOT) or Pindborg tumor is a very rare neoplasm, accounting for about 1% of odontogenic neoplasms. This neoplasm usually arises within bone, and its cells may produce a mineralized matrix as well as amyloid.

Clinical Features

A CEOT is a less aggressive neoplasm than an ameloblastoma, but is found in a similar age group: 8–92 years, with an average age of about 42 years. Rarely does this neoplasm have an extraosseous location. Jaw expansion is a regular feature and usually the only symptom. Palpation of the swelling reveals a hard mass.

Imaging Features

Location. Similar to ameloblastoma, the CEOT develops more commonly in the mandible than the maxilla, with a ratio of at least 2:1. Most develop in the premolar and molar areas, and approximately 52% have an association with an unerupted or impacted tooth. In about half of cases, images made early in the development of these neoplasms reveal a radiolucent area associated with the crown of a mature, unerupted tooth.

Periphery. The periphery has a well-defined and corticated border with a smooth, hydraulic periphery. In some neoplasms, however, the boundary may be irregular and poorly defined.

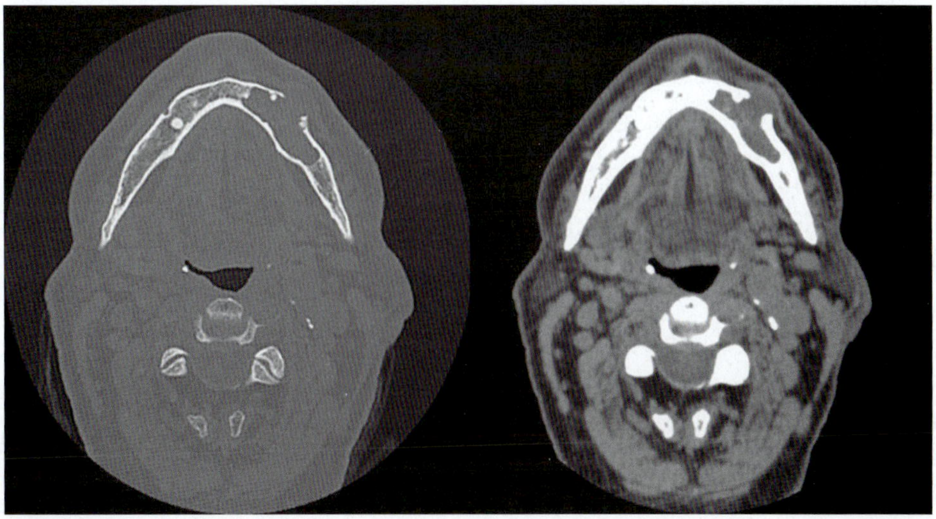

Fig. 22.11 Axial bone *(left)* and soft tissue *(right)* windowed multidetector computed tomographic images of an ameloblastoma in the mandible showing perforation of the buccal cortex of the bone, and outgrowth of the tumor into the adjacent soft tissues.

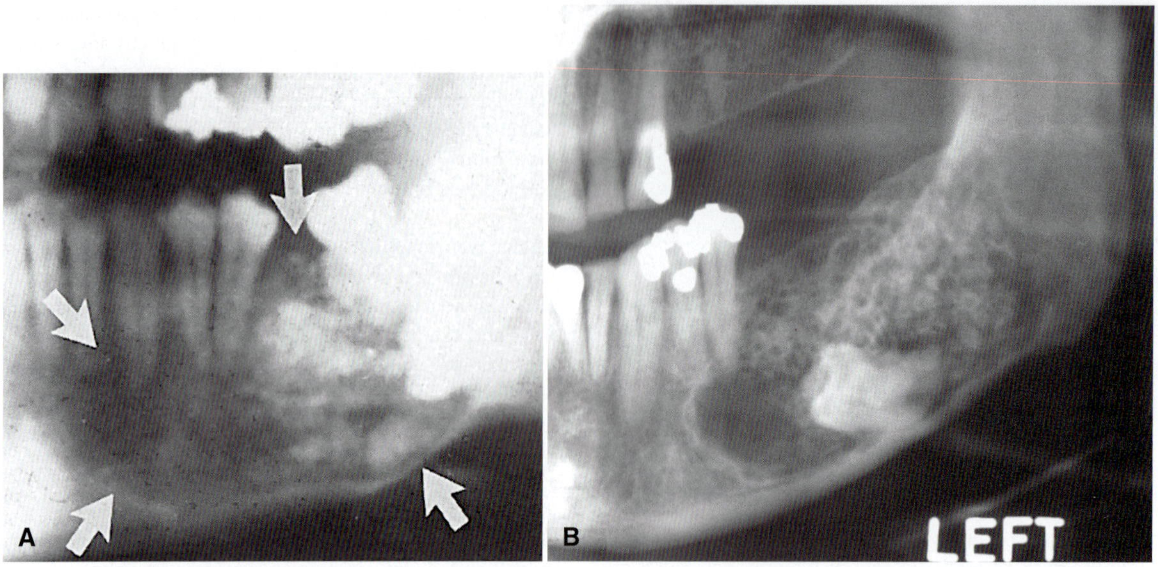

Fig. 22.12 Calcifying epithelial odontogenic tumor (A) *(arrows)*. The tumor appears as a mixed radiolucent and radiopaque lesion (B) associated with an unerupted tooth. (A, Courtesy Dr. M. Gornitsky, Montreal, QB. B, Courtesy Dr. D. Lanigan, Saskatoon, SK.)

Internal structure. Internally, the CEOT may appear unilocular or multilocular with numerous scattered radiopaque internal foci of variable sizes and densities. Some of these foci may have a crescent or a doughnut shape with a radiolucent center. The most characteristic finding is the appearance of the radiopacities close to the crown of the unerupted or impacted tooth (Fig. 22.12). In addition, small, thin, opaque trabeculae may cross the radiolucency in many directions.

Effects on surrounding structures. There may be expansion of the bone; however, the cortical boundary is often maintained.

Effects on surrounding teeth. CEOTs may displace a developing tooth or prevent its eruption because of its pericoronal epicenter.

Differential Interpretation

A CEOT with a completely radiolucent internal structure may resemble a dentigerous cyst or an odontogenic keratocyst. Lesions with radiopaque foci may resemble adenomatoid odontogenic tumor (AOT), a developing odontome and calcifying odontogenic cyst. However, the prominent location of the CEOT and the age of the patient help in the differential interpretation.

Management

The management of a CEOT is local resection, a more conservative approach than ameloblastoma.

MIXED EPITHELIAL AND MESENCHYMAL ODONTOGENIC TUMORS AND NEOPLASMS

Ameloblastic Fibroma

Disease Mechanism

The ameloblastic fibroma is a benign mixed neoplastic proliferation of odontogenic epithelium and primitive mesenchymal components resembling the dental papilla. These cells do not deposit a mineralized matrix on the tumor cell bed.

Clinical Features

The ameloblastic fibroma arises in the first and second decades of life during the period of tooth formation, with an average age of about 15 years. They usually produce a painless, slow-growing soft tissue mass overlying the bone, preventing teeth from erupting (Fig. 22.13). Although the most common signs are swelling, delayed eruption, or a missing tooth, this neoplasm may also be discovered incidentally on imaging made for another purpose.

Imaging Features

Location. Ameloblastic fibroma often develops in the posterior mandible, extending as far posteriorly as the mandibular ramus and as far mesially as the premolar and molar areas. A common location is coronal to an unerupted tooth and near the crest of the alveolar process (Fig. 22.14), or it may arise in an area where a tooth has failed to develop.

Periphery. The borders of an ameloblastic fibroma are well defined and often corticated in a manner like that of a cyst.

Internal structure. An ameloblastic fibroma is more commonly totally radiolucent and unilocular (see Figs. 22.13 and 22.14). Less commonly, these lesions may have a multilocular appearance with indistinct curved septa (Fig. 22.15).

Effects on surrounding structures. If the lesion is large, there may be expansion with an intact overlying cortex.

Effects on adjacent teeth. The associated tooth or teeth may be inhibited from normal eruption or may be displaced in an apical direction.

Differential Interpretation

It may not be possible to differentiate a small ameloblastic fibroma with a coronal relationship to an unerupted tooth from a hyperplastic follicle or a small dentigerous cyst on imaging as the radiologic features may overlap, lacking specificity.

Although the ameloblastic fibroma may have similar features to an ameloblastoma, the ameloblastic fibroma occurs at an earlier age, and the septa in an ameloblastoma are more well defined and coarse. In comparison, the septa in ameloblastic fibroma are infrequent and often very fine. CGC lesions may appear multilocular, but these neoplasms usually have an epicenter anterior to the mandibular first molar in young patients, and the internal radiopacities are characteristically more granular, wispy, and poorly defined. Odontogenic myxomas can

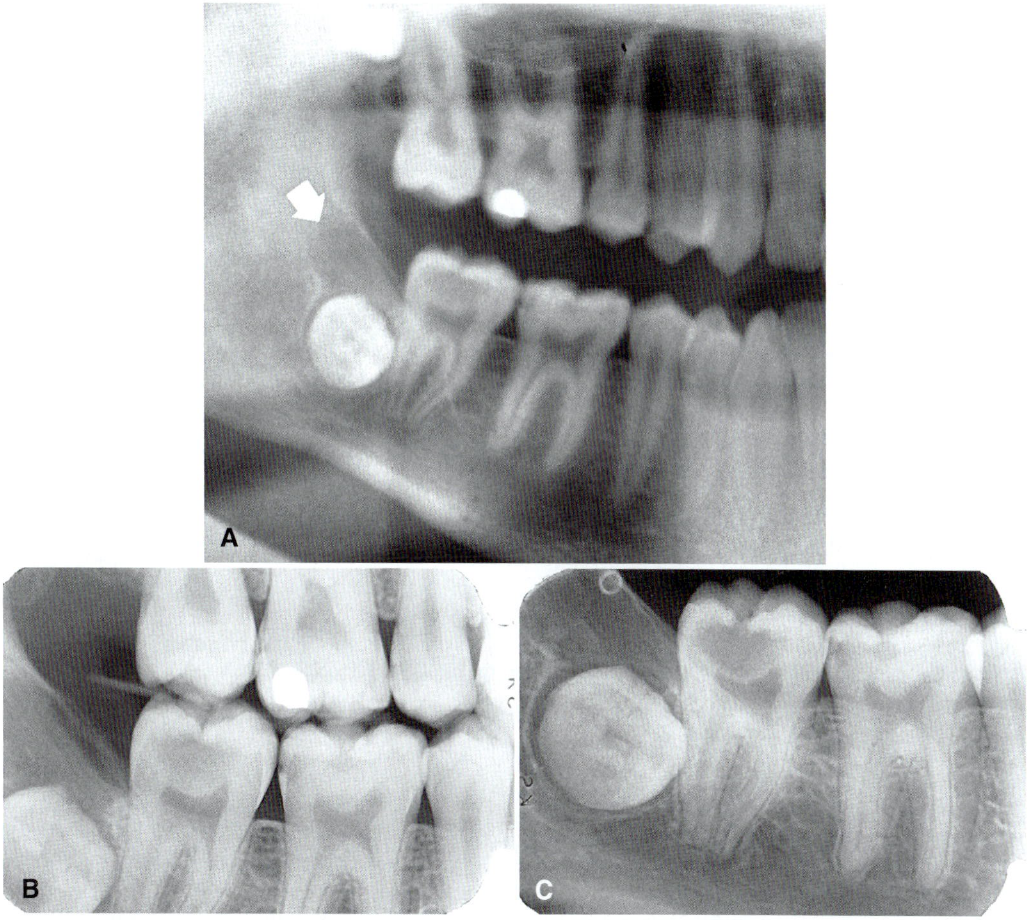

Fig. 22.13 (A) An ameloblastic fibroma is seen as a radiolucency coronal to the unerupted third molar *(arrow)*. Bite-wing (B) and periapical (C) images of the same lesion (B). (Courtesy Dr. G. Sanders, La Crosse, WI.)

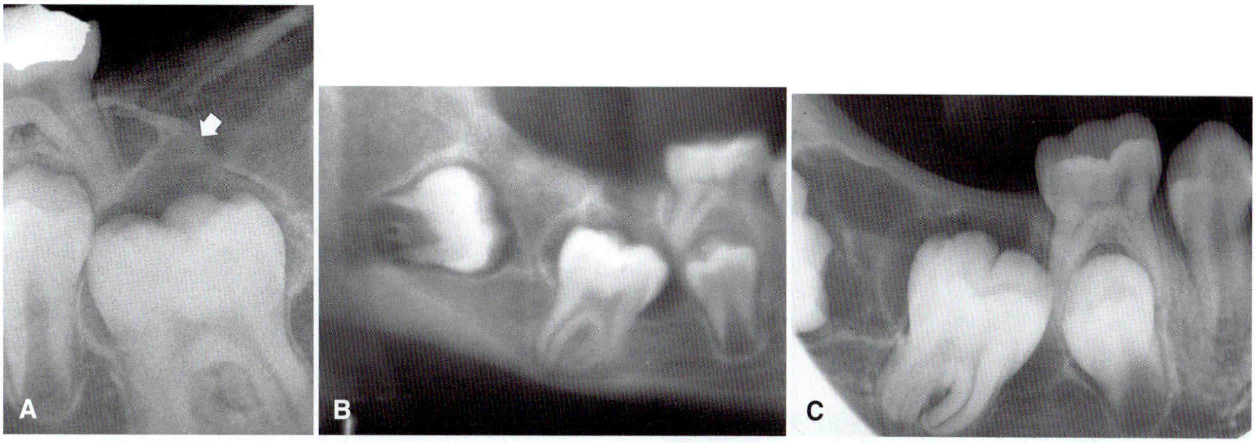

Fig. 22.14 Ameloblastic fibroma appearing as a unilocular outgrowth of the follicle of the unerupted first permanent molar (A). Periapical and cropped panoramic (B) images illustrating an ameloblastic fibroma associated with the crowns of the first and second molars.

appear multilocular, but usually a few sharp straight septa can be identified, which are not characteristic of ameloblastic fibromas. Moreover, myxomas usually occur in an older age group.

Management

The management of ameloblastic fibroma is conservative surgical enucleation and mechanical curettage of the surrounding bone. This approach is reported to be successful, and there is no recurrence.

Odontome

Disease Mechanism

Like supernumerary teeth, the odontome develops in a jaw that harbors an excess of dental lamina. Many now consider the entity formerly known as odontoma to be a hamartoma, characterized by the production of mature enamel, dentin, cementum, and pulp tissue, but without the capacity for continuous growth. As part of this

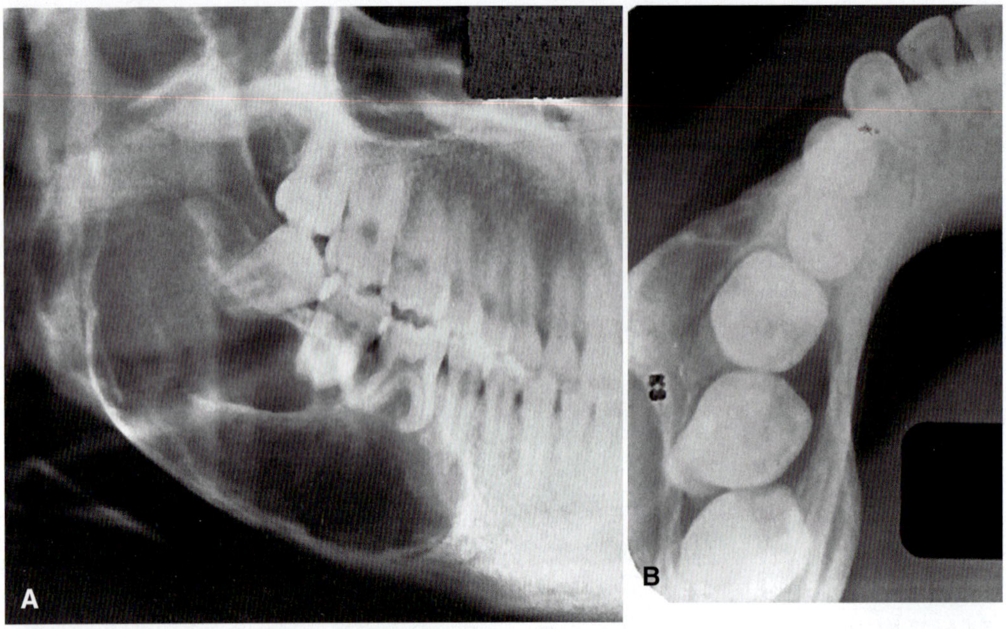

Fig. 22.15 Panoramic (A) and cross-sectional occlusal (B) images of an ameloblastic fibroma in the body and ramus of the right mandible. Note the expansion of the mandible on the occlusal image.

philosophical change, we have elected to refer to this entity as an odontome rather than odontoma, and what was previously known to as the "ameloblastic fibro-odontoma" as a "developing odontome." As hamartomas, the developing odontome and odontome demonstrate limited growth potential, although they can be locally disruptive.

The structure of the component tissues may vary from being a nondescript but heterogeneous mass of the dental hard tissues referred to as a complex odontome, to more discrete, multiple well-formed teeth (denticles) called a compound odontome. A third variety of odontome, the dilated odontome, is a single entity that may be a severe expression of a dens invaginatus or dens in dente.

Clinical Features

Odontomes are very common, and often, they may develop in an area of the jaws with a missing tooth or interfere with the eruption of a permanent tooth (Fig. 22.16). The odontome shows no sex predilection, and most form while the dentition is developing in the first or second decades of life. As with ameloblastic fibroma, an odontome may be found during the investigation of retained primary teeth or delayed eruption of permanent teeth. In rare cases, odontomes are associated with primary teeth.

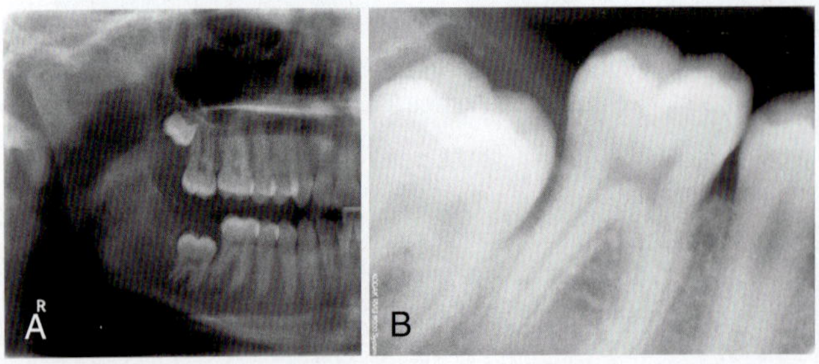

Fig. 22.16 A developing odontome located coronal to the mandibular right second molar preventing eruption of the mandibular right second molar (A). The mineralization can be faint and may only be appreciated on a periapical image (B). (Courtesy Dr. H. Grubisa, Oakville, ON.)

Compound odontomes are about twice as common as the complex type. Although the compound variety forms equally between men and women, 60% of complex odontomes occur in women. In very rare circumstances, a compound odontome may erupt into the mouth. Left unidentified or untreated, odontomes will not increase in size, but they may have an effect on the adjacent dentition or bone.

Imaging Features

Location. As odontomes develop from excess dental lamina, they may occur anywhere in the tooth-bearing areas of the jaws. The majority of compound odontomes (62%) occur in the anterior maxilla in association with the crown of an unerupted canine tooth. In contrast, 70% of complex odontomes are found in the mandibular first and second molar area.

Periphery. The border of odontomes is well defined, with a smooth but irregular periphery. These lesions have a cortical border.

Internal structure. The contents of these lesions are heterogeneously radiopaque with the degree of radiopacity determined by the density of the mineralization. In general, developing odontomes appear less radiopaque than their more mature compound, complex, or dilated brethren (Fig. 22.17). Complex odontomes contain an irregular but somewhat more homogeneous mass of calcified tissue (Fig. 22.18). The density of the mineralized matrix within these lesions may vary, reflecting differences in the amount and type of hard tissue that has been formed. In some cases, enamel, dentin, and pulp spaces can be visualized (Fig. 22.19), thereby contributing to the heterogeneous appearance. Compound odontomes have a number of variably sized toothlike structures or denticles that have the appearance of small, malformed teeth (Fig. 22.20). A dilated odontome is a single calcified structure with a more radiolucent central portion and has an overall form like a doughnut (see Fig. 22.21). The radiopaque component of odontomes is surrounded by a thin, radiolucent rim that has a similar appearance to the follicle surrounding a developing tooth crown.

Effects on surrounding structures. Large odontomes may cause expansion of bone, but with maintenance of the cortical boundary.

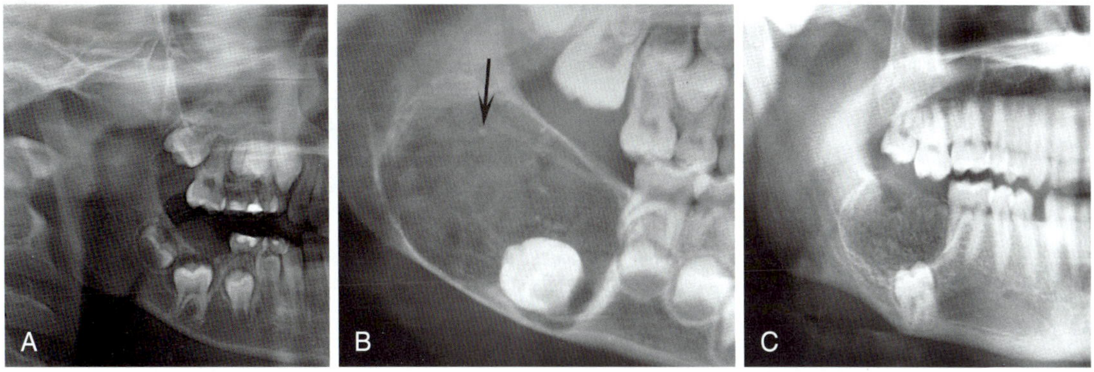

Fig. 22.17 Cropped panoramic image of a developing odontome located occlusal to the mandibular right first molar (A). Cropped panoramic images (B and C) of a mixed radiolucent and radiopaque entity with more diffuse mineralization and scattered radiopacities (B, *arrow*).

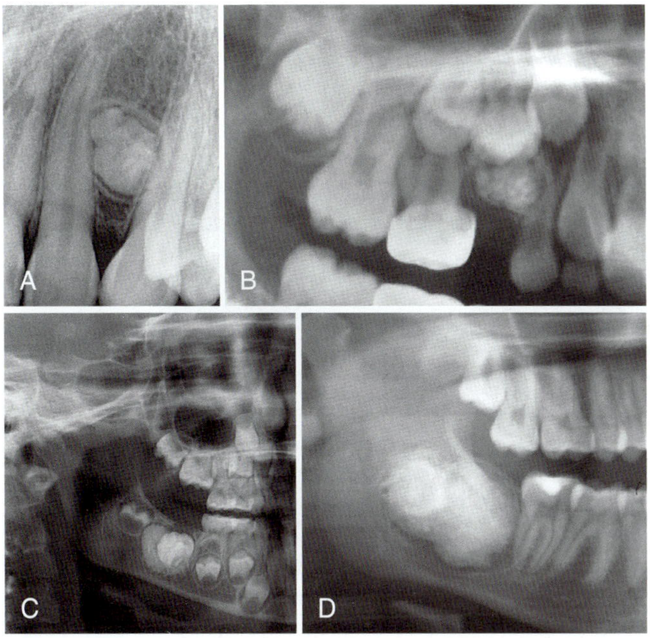

Fig. 22.18 Complex odontomes shown on periapical (A) and cropped panoramic images (B to D). Note the toothlike density of the radiopaque mass, the thin radiolucent rim surrounding the mineralized tissue, and disruptions to the normal eruption or position of the associated tooth.

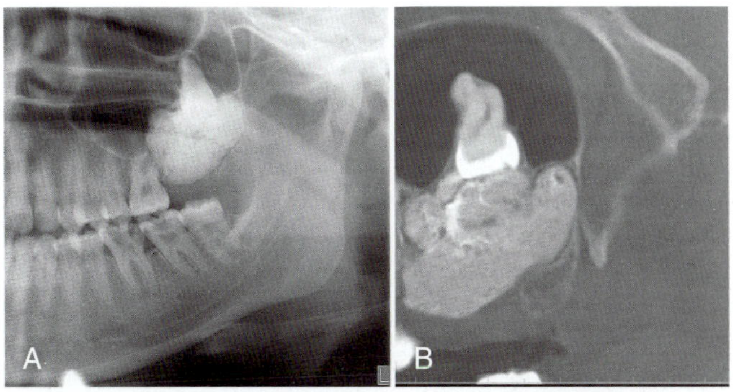

Fig. 22.19 Cropped panoramic (A) and corrected sagittal cone beam computed tomographic image (B) of a complex odontome in the posterior maxilla. Note the variation of densities within the mass and the thin, radiolucent line that surrounds it.

Effects on adjacent teeth. Odontomes can interfere with the normal eruption of teeth, and most (70%) are associated with impacted or malposed teeth, diastema, aplasia, malformation, or devitalization of adjacent teeth.

Differential Interpretation

The appearance of small, toothlike radiopaque structures within a well-defined entity leads to easy recognition of a compound odontome. A complex odontome can differ from a cemento-ossifying fibroma by its tendency to be associated with an unerupted tooth, and they are usually more radiopaque than a cemento-ossifying fibroma due to the presence of mature tooth material.

The fully mature stage of periapical cemento-osseous dysplasia may resemble a complex odontome but there may be multiple areas of cemento-osseous dysplasia with epicenters at the root apices. Furthermore, odontomes are more radiopaque than the dysplastic bone found in the cemento-osseous dysplasias. DBIs, while radiopaque, lack the radiolucent rim surrounding the radiopaque focus that odontomes do.

Management

Odontomes are removed by simple excision. They do not recur.

Adenomatoid Odontogenic Tumor

Disease Mechanism

AOT is an uncommon, nonaggressive neoplasm of odontogenic epithelium. Although the cells of origin of AOT may be from enamel organ epithelium, it is classified as a mixed tumor because it also contains connective tissue elements as well as calcifications that have been interpreted as dentin- or enamel-like material. AOT accounts for approximately 3% of all oral neoplasms, and they can occur both centrally within the bone and peripherally. Furthermore, the central AOT may be divided into a follicular type, associated with the crown of an unerupted or impacted tooth, and the extrafollicular type, not associated with a tooth. Approximately 73% of central lesions are the follicular type.

Clinical Features

The AOT occurs across a wide age range: 5–50 years. A majority develop in the second decade of life, with an average age of 16 years. In addition, the tumor has a 2:1 female predilection.

The follicular type is identified earlier than the extrafollicular type, probably because they may be associated with an unerupted tooth. The tumor is slow growing and manifests as a gradually enlarging, painless swelling or asymmetry.

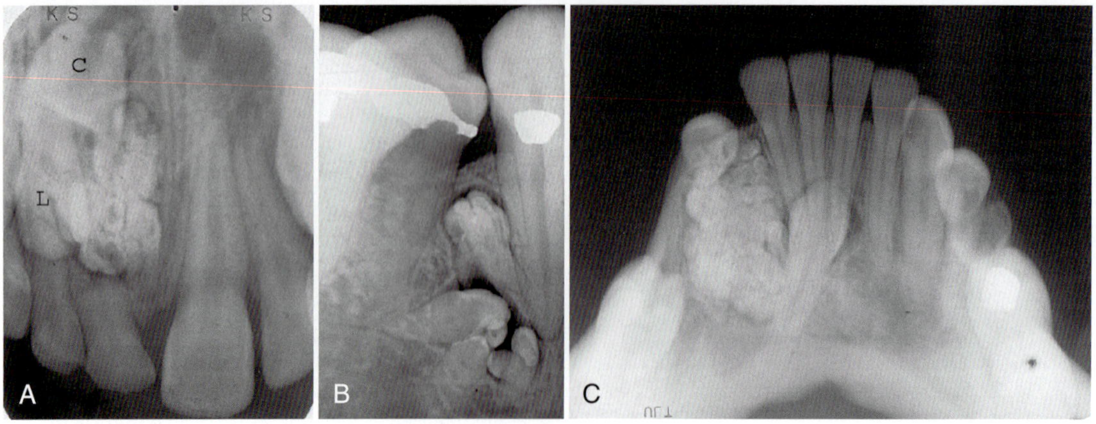

Fig. 22.20 Periapical (A and B) and anterior occlusal (C) images of compound odontomes. Note the numerous small toothlike entities (denticles) and the radiolucent periphery.

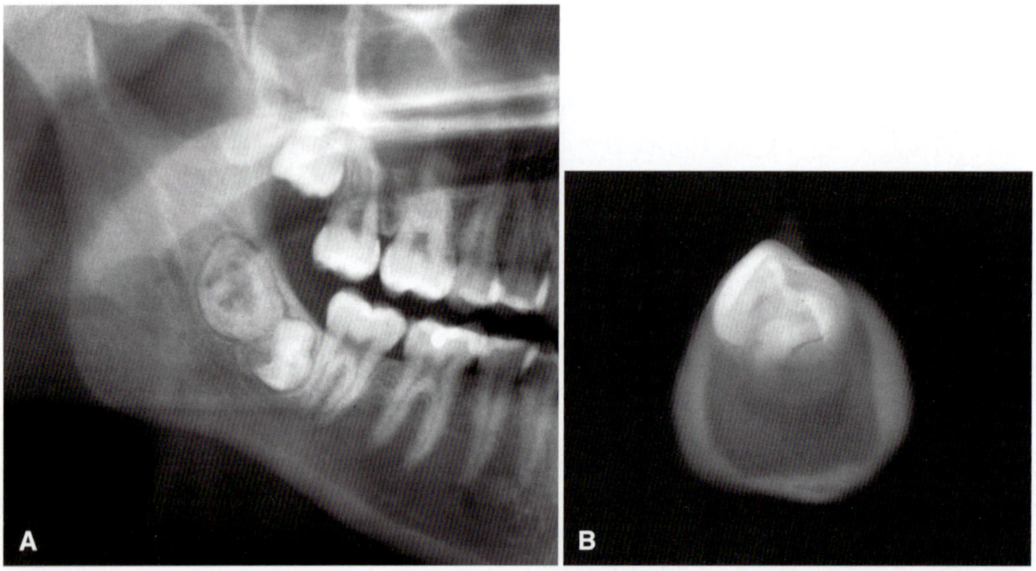

Fig. 22.21 A cropped panoramic image demonstrating a dilated odontome located distal to the unerupted third molar (A). The image of the excised specimen shows the crown-like morphology of the lesion (B).

Imaging Features

Location. At least 75% of AOTs occur in the anterior maxilla and mandible, with the canine region being the most common area in both jaws (Fig. 22.22). Although the follicular type may have a relationship with an impacted tooth (most often a canine), it may often not have an association with the cementoenamel junction; rather, it may surround a greater part of the tooth crown and root (Fig. 22.23).

Periphery. The periphery is well defined and corticated, although the cortex may show some variation in thickness.

Internal structure. The internal appearance may be radiolucent (see Fig. 22.23A), or mixed radiolucent and radiopaque (Fig. 22.23B); the mixed type may be seen in up to two-thirds of cases. The appearance of the mixed type may vary from an appearance of faint, delicate radiopaque foci to more dense clusters of ill-defined radiopacities. Occasionally, the calcifications may appear very well defined, like a cluster of small pebbles (see Fig. 22.22C). Intraoral imaging may be required to demonstrate these calcifications which may not be visible on other imaging due to lower spatial resolution. Histopathologic studies have verified that the size, number, and density of the small radiopacities may vary from case to case, although they seem to increase with age.

Effects on adjacent structures. As the neoplasm enlarges, some expansion of the jaw may occur; however, the outer cortex remains intact.

Effects on surrounding structures. AOT may cause the displacement of adjacent teeth; however, root resorption is rare. If the epicenter of the lesion is located coronal to a developing tooth, it may inhibit eruption of the tooth.

Differential Interpretation

When the AOT is completely radiolucent and has a follicular relationship with an impacted tooth, differentiation from a dentigerous cyst or an odontogenic keratocyst may be difficult. If the relationship of the radiolucent entity is located more apical to the cementoenamel junction, a dentigerous cyst can be discounted; however, this would not exclude an odontogenic keratocyst. If there are radiopaque foci within the tumor, other lesions with calcifications might be entertained in the differential interpretation. The maxillary and mandibular anterior regions are also common sites for the calcifying odontogenic cyst, and it may be difficult to differentiate this cyst from the extrafollicular type of AOT. A developing odontome and CEOT may be considered; however, they may develop more commonly in the posterior mandible.

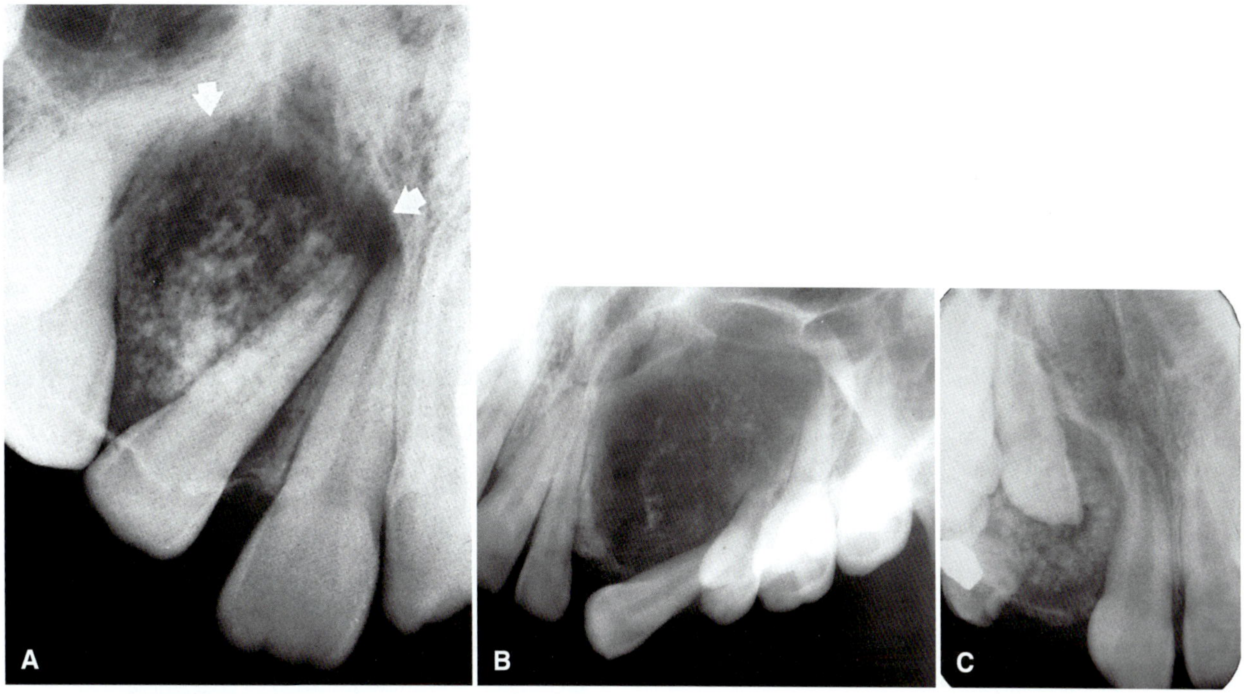

Fig. 22.22 Periapical images of extrafollicular adenomatoid odontogenic tumors with moderate (*arrows*, A) and faint mineralization (B) patterns within the maxilla. A periapical image of an intrafollicular AOT with pebble-like calcifications. (A, Courtesy Dr. R. Howell, Morgantown, WV.)

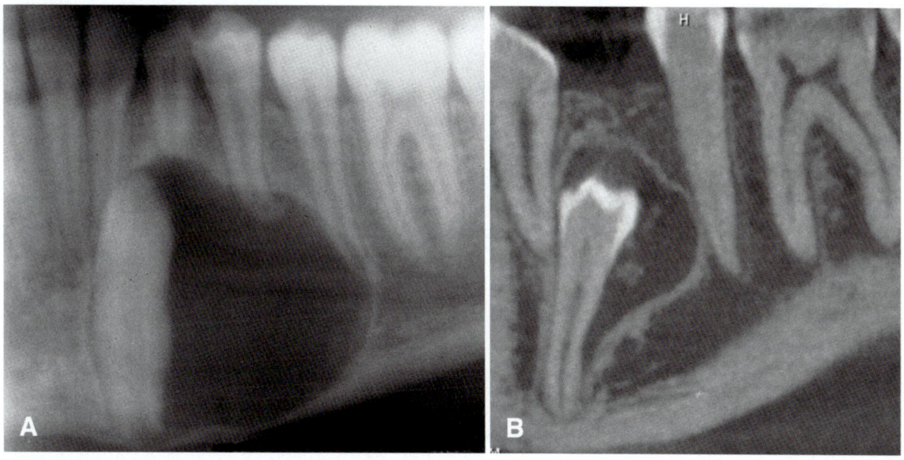

Fig. 22.23 Cropped panoramic image (A) shows no apparent internal calcifications in an adenomatoid odontogenic tumor. Cone beam computed tomographic image (B) of an adenomatoid odontogenic tumor related to the first premolar. Note the pebble-like calcifications distal to the premolar. (Courtesy Dr. M. Madhavji, Toronto, ON.)

Management

Conservative surgical excision is adequate because the tumor is not locally invasive, is well encapsulated, and is easily separable from the bone. The recurrence rate is very low at approximately 0.2%.

MESENCHYMAL ODONTOGENIC TUMORS

Odontogenic Myxoma

Disease Mechanism

The odontogenic myxoma resembles the mesenchymal portion of the dental papilla, which arises from odontogenic ectomesenchyme. This neoplasm is so named for its loose, gelatinous internal matrix of connective and mucoid tissues. Although nonodontogenic myxomas may arise in the other areas of the skeleton, the presence of odontogenic epithelium that can be identified microscopically is the rationale behind its inclusion as an odontogenic tumor.

Clinical Features

The odontogenic myxoma is uncommon, accounting for approximately 3%–6% of odontogenic tumors. They have a slight female predilection, and although the lesion can occur at any age, more than half are detected in individuals between 10 and 30 years; it rarely occurs before age 10 or after age 50. These neoplasms are slow growing,

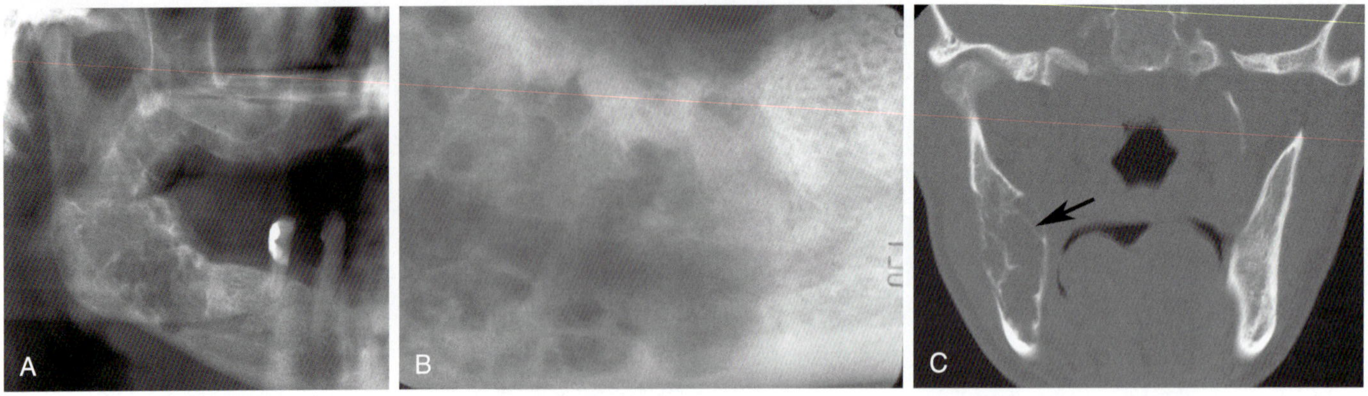

Fig. 22.24 Panoramic (A), periapical (B), and coronal multidetector computed tomographic (C) images of a myxoma in the body and ramus of the right mandible. Notice the presence of a straight, short septa (*arrow*, C) and the small loculations produced by these.

although they may be locally aggressive, particularly in the maxilla. Recurrence rates of 25% have been reported, and this high rate may be explained by the lack of encapsulation of the mass and the ability of the myxomatous matrix within the tumor to extend into marrow spaces where it may be difficult to detect and remove surgically.

Imaging Features

Location. Myxoma is more commonly found in the mandible by a margin of 3:1. In the mandible, these tumors occur in the premolar and molar areas, and only rarely in the ramus and condyle. Myxomas in the maxilla usually involve the alveolar process in the premolar and molar regions, and the zygomatic process.

Periphery. The lesion is usually well defined, and it may have a corticated margin (Fig. 22.24). In the maxilla, however, the periphery is most often poorly defined.

Internal structure. When it occurs in a pericoronal area, an odontogenic myxoma may appear cyst-like and radiolucent internally. Residual bone trapped within the tumor may impart a multilocular appearance to the tumor, and characteristically, these septa are straight, thin, and "etched" (Fig. 22.25). The sometimes-linear appearance of septa in the odontogenic myxoma has been described as the strings of a tennis racket or a stepladder, but these patterns are rarely seen. Most septa are curved and coarse, but the finding of one or two straight septa often helps in the interpretation of this neoplasm.

Effects on adjacent structures. In the mandible, the odontogenic myxoma tends to "tunnel" through the bone like an odontogenic keratocyst, without the same amount of expansion seen with other benign neoplasms (Fig. 22.25B and C); however, when they become very large, there may be considerable expansion.

Effects on adjacent teeth. When the odontogenic myxoma arises in a tooth-bearing area of the jaws, it displaces teeth, and they may become mobile. Myxomas rarely cause resorption of tooth roots. The lesion also frequently scallops between the roots of adjacent teeth like a simple bone cavity.

Additional Imaging

MDCT imaging and, in particular, MRI can help in establishing the intraosseous involvement of the tumor and guide the surgeon in planning the resection margins. The myxomatous matrix within the tumor produces a very characteristic high tissue signal on T_2-weighted magnetic resonance images, and this is particularly useful in establishing both extension of the tumor in bone and the presence of a recurrence (Fig. 22.26).

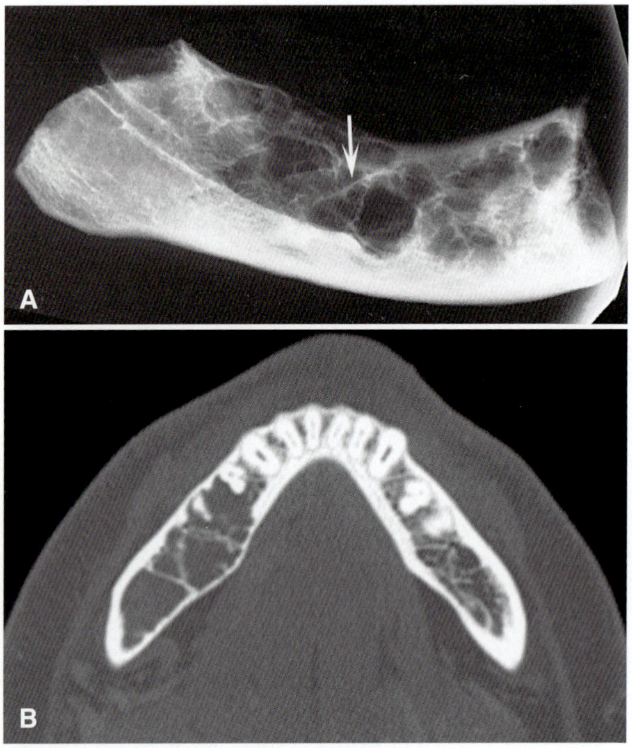

Fig. 22.25 Image of an excised surgical specimen of an odontogenic myxoma (A) and the tumor, in situ (B), on an axial multidetector computed tomographic image. Note the sharp, straight "etched" septum *(arrow)*.

Differential Interpretation

Because odontogenic myxoma most often has a multilocular internal pattern, the differential interpretation should include other multilocular lesions, such as ameloblastoma, mucoepidermoid carcinoma, odontogenic keratocyst, CGC lesion, and central hemangioma. The finding of characteristic thin, straight septa with less than expected bone expansion is very useful in the differential interpretation. Occasionally, a small area of expansion with straight septa may be projected over an intact outer bony cortex and give a spiculated appearance. Careful inspection of this area of expansion, however, reveals a thin but intact outer cortex. An odontogenic fibroma occasionally has many of the same radiographic characteristics and cannot be reliably differentiated from a myxoma.

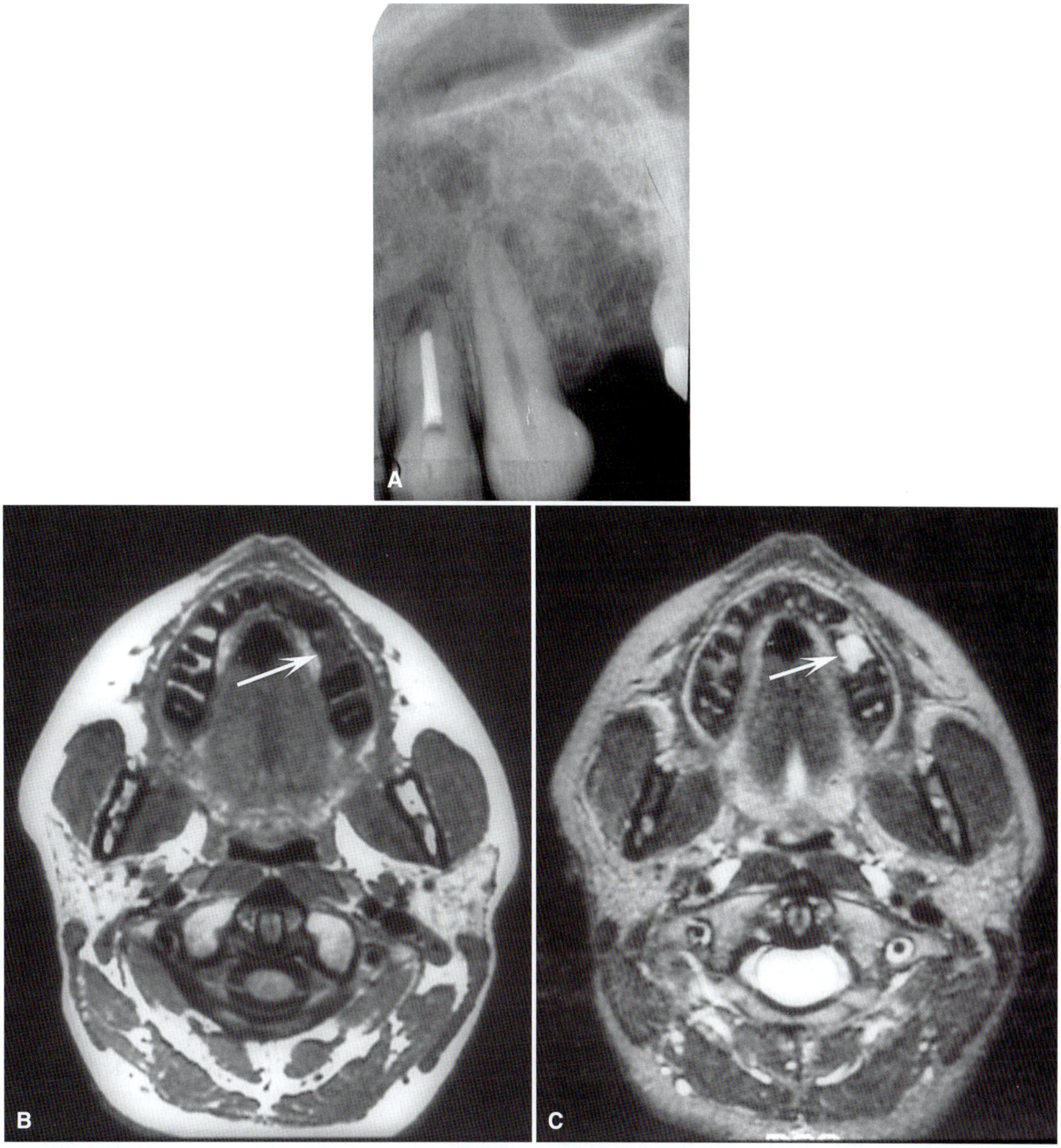

Fig. 22.26 Periapical image (A) obtained to investigate a possible recurrence of an odontogenic myxoma in the maxillary left premolar area after treatment by surgical curettage. (B) Axial T_1-weighted magnetic resonance image shows a low *(black)* signal from the segment of the alveolar process while the T_2-weighted image shows a high *(white)* signal (C), which is characteristic of an odontogenic myxoma, confirming the presence of a recurrence.

Management

Odontogenic myxomas are treated by resection with a generous amount of surrounding bone to ensure removal of the myxomatous material that may infiltrate the adjacent marrow spaces. With appropriate treatment, the prognosis is good.

Cementoblastoma

Disease Mechanism

The cementoblastoma is a slow-growing, mesenchymal neoplasm of cementoblasts. The neoplasm manifests as a bulbous growth of cementum that envelops the root and root apex of a tooth.

Clinical Features

Cementoblastomas are uncommon, although likely, they occur more often than published accounts indicate. The lesion is more common in males than females. The age range is from 12 to 65 years, although most patients are younger.

The neoplasm most often develops in association with a permanent tooth but in rare cases occurs with a primary tooth. The tumor is solitary and slow growing, but if large enough, it can displace adjacent teeth. The involved tooth pulp is vital, and if accompanied with pain, the pain is often reported to be relieved by nonsteroidal antiinflammatory drugs.

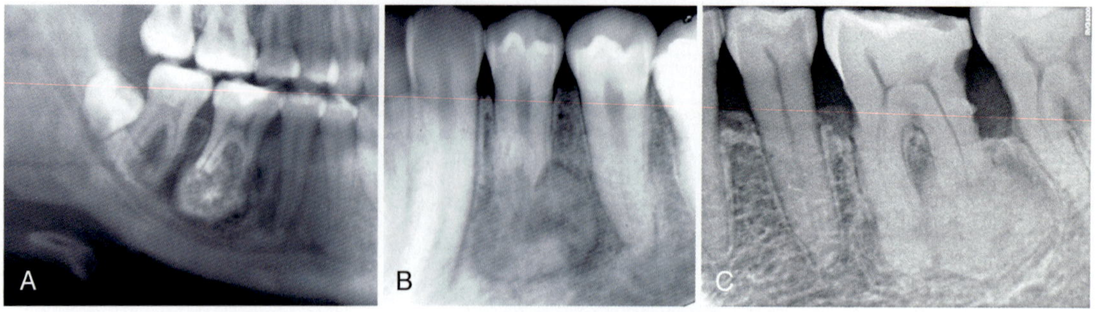

Fig. 22.27 Cropped panoramic image showing a large, bulbous, radiopaque mass obscuring the roots of the mandibular right first molar (A). A radiolucent rim can be seen surrounding the mass, and root resorption of the molar roots has occurred. Periapical images of a lesion associated with a premolar (B) and a molar (C). (A, Courtesy Dr. B. Pynn, Toronto, ON. B, Courtesy Dr. B. Pynn, Toronto, ON. C, Courtesy Dr. M. Huang, Toronto, ON.)

Imaging Features

Location. Cementoblastoma develops on the root surfaces of the mandibular dentition (78%), notably a premolar or first molar (90%).

Periphery. The lesion has a well-defined and corticated border.

Internal structure. The cementoblastoma is a mixed radiolucent and radiopaque neoplasm in which most of the internal structure is radiopaque (Fig. 22.27). The resulting pattern may be amorphous, or a wheel-spoke pattern may be seen with the radiopaque structures radiating from the center to the periphery of the mass. The density of the cemental mass usually obscures the outline of the enveloped root. This central radiopaque mass is surrounded by a radiolucent band indicating that the tumor is maturing from the center to the periphery.

Effects on adjacent structures. If large enough, this neoplasm can cause expansion of the bone, and in some cases, there is a perforation through the outer cortical plate without periosteal reaction.

Effects on adjacent teeth. If the root outline is apparent, in most cases, varying amounts of external resorption of the root can be seen.

Differential Interpretation

The most common lesion from which a cementoblastoma must be differentiated is a solitary lesion of periapical cemento-osseous dysplasia. The differential interpretation may be difficult in some cases. The presence or absence of symptoms, or observation of the lesion over a period of time may be required. Generally, the radiolucent internal periphery around the cementoblastoma is better defined and uniform than with cemento-osseous dysplasia. Also, owing to the pattern of concentric growth of the cementoblastoma, the overall shape is more uniform and spherical than the more irregular outline of the cemento-osseous dysplasia. Similarly, the epicenter of the cemento-osseous dysplasia is commonly located periapical to the root, whereas in cementoblastoma, the epicenter is located on the root. Other lesions that may be included in the differential interpretation are dense bone island and hypercementosis. Dense bone islands do not have a radiolucent internal periphery like cementoblastoma. Although a periodontal ligament space may be seen surrounding a region of hypercementosis, the tooth root does not increase in size concentrically like cementoblastoma. Finally, the width of the periodontal ligament space in hypercementosis is usually thinner than the internal radiolucent rim of the cementoblastoma, and root resorption or jaw expansion is not seen with hypercementosis.

Management

Cementoblastomas are managed with endodontic treatment and root amputation. In very large cases, excision and extraction of the associated tooth may be necessary.

Central Odontogenic Fibroma

Disease Mechanism

The central odontogenic fibroma is a very rare neoplasm that resembles the odontogenic myxoma. Indeed, some authors theorize that these entities represent two processes along a spectrum of connective tissue-type neoplasms. Two types of central odontogenic fibromas have been described according to histopathologic appearances, the simple type and the WHO type, although these cannot be differentiated radiologically.

Clinical Features

Most cases of central odontogenic fibroma occur between the ages of 11 and 39 years, and there is a definite female preponderance with a reported ratio of 2.2:1. An unusual, but rather distinctive feature of some maxillary cases is a cleft or depression in the palatal mucosa where expansion by the neoplasm would be expected (Fig. 22.28A).

Imaging Features

Location. Central odontogenic fibromas occur somewhat more often in the mandible. The most common site is the molar–premolar region in the mandible and anterior to the first molar in the maxilla.

Periphery. The periphery is usually well defined, and there may be a corticated border.

Internal structure. Some lesions are totally radiolucent, with smaller lesions being unilocular. Some display unorganized internal calcifications, and larger lesions have a multilocular pattern. The internal septa may be fine and straight, as in odontogenic myxomas, or may be granular, resembling the internal structure seen in CGC lesions.

Effects on adjacent structures. A central odontogenic fibroma may cause expansion with maintenance of a thin cortical boundary, or occasionally can grow along the bone with minimum expansion.

Effects on adjacent teeth. Tooth displacement is common, and root resorption has been reported. Some maxillary lesions have a distinctive behavior of resorbing the bone around teeth without tooth displacement or resorption (see Fig. 22.28B).

Differential Interpretation

The differential interpretation includes odontogenic keratocyst, odontongenic myxoma, and central desmoplastic fibroma. When the neoplasm exhibits tunneling enlargement in the bone, it may be difficult to differentiate central odontogenic fibroma from an odontogenic keratocyst or myxoma. Central desmoplastic fibroma is a more aggressive neoplasm, and tends to break through the bone cortex and extend into the adjacent soft tissue. The septa in desmoplastic fibroma are very

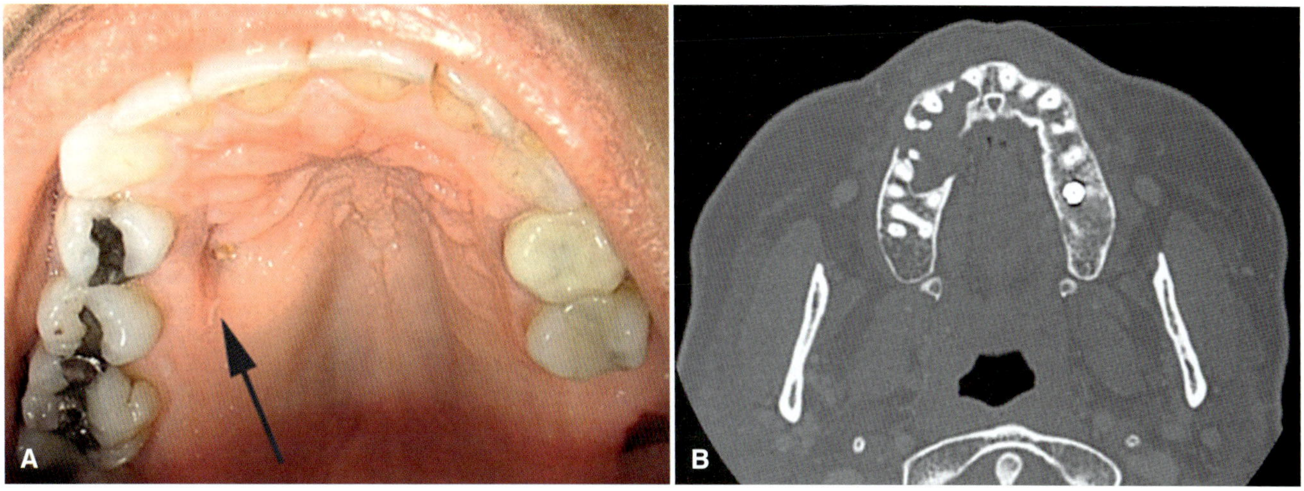

Fig. 22.28 Clinical photograph (A) of a central odontogenic fibroma of the maxilla demonstrating a cleft *(arrow)* in the palatal mucosa. Axial computed tomographic image (B) of the same case showing loss of both the buccal and the palatal cortical plates without extension into the surrounding tissues and resorption of bone around the roots of the maxillary teeth with displacement or root resorption.

thick, straight, and angular. If thin, straight septa are seen, it may be impossible to differentiate this neoplasm from an odontogenic myxoma on radiographic criteria alone. If fine, granular septa are present, the appearance may be identical to a CGC lesion.

Management

Central odontogenic fibromas are treated with simple excision. These lesions have a very low recurrence rate.

NONODONTOGENIC TUMORS AND NEOPLASMS

Neuroma

Disease Mechanism

Despite its name, the neuroma is not a neoplasm, but rather a reactive hyperplasia arising from the abnormal proliferation of scar tissue following trauma of a peripheral nerve. The proliferating nerve cells form a disorganized network of nerve fibers composed of varying proportions of axons, perineural connective tissue, Schwann cells, and scar tissue. Nerve trauma may be the result of mechanical or chemical injury caused by bone fracture, surgery, biopsy or excision of a cyst or neoplasm, extrusion of endodontic material, dental implant placement, or tooth extraction. Consequently, "traumatic neuroma" and "amputation neuroma" have been used synonymously for this entity.

Clinical Features

Neuromas seldom become large, rarely exceeding 1 cm in diameter, and the mandibule and sacrum are the most common site for these lesions. Neuromas may cause various symptoms, including severe pain resulting from pressure applied as the tangled mass develops within the bone, or as the result of external trauma. The patient may also develop a neuralgia, with pain referred to the eyes, face, and head.

Imaging Features

The imaging features of a neuroma relate to the extent and shape of the proliferating mass of neural tissue within the bone.

Location. The most common location for neuroma is the mental foramen. Less commonly, neuromas may be found in the anterior maxilla and the posterior mandible.

Periphery. The borders of the neuroma are well defined and corticated. Although it may occur in various shapes depending on the amount of resistance to expansion offered by the surrounding bone, when a neuroma arises in the mandibular canal, its periphery usually takes on the cortication of the canal borders.

Internal structure. The internal structure of a neuroma is totally radiolucent.

Effects on adjacent structures. If the neuroma extends to the mandibular foramen or the mental foramen, there can be enlargement of these foramina. The cortex of the canal is maintained.

Effects on adjacent teeth. There are no effects on the teeth.

Differential Interpretation

When small, it is impossible to differentiate a neuroma from a schwannoma or neurofibroma on imaging.

Management

The management of neuroma is excision. As neuromas can enlarge, they may also cause pain. Recurrence is uncommon after simple excision.

Schwannoma

The schwannoma or neurilemmoma is a true neoplasm of neuroectodermal origin arising solely from Schwann cells, the cells that produce the myelin sheath surrounding the axons of peripheral nerves.

Clinical Features

Schwannomas are slow growing, and they can occur at any age (but most commonly arise in the second and third decades) and occur with equal frequency in males and females. The mandible and sacrum are the most common sites.

Schwannomas cause few symptoms other than those related to the location and size of the neoplasm. The usual chief complaint is an unexplained swelling. Although pain is uncommon with schwannoma unless the neoplasm encroaches on adjacent nerves, paresthesia may arise, especially with lesions originating in the inferior alveolar canal. Pain, when present, usually develops at the site of the tumor. If paresthesia occurs, it is felt distal (i.e., more peripheral) to the neoplasm.

Imaging Features

The radiological appearances of neuroma and schwannoma may appear similar, making it impossible to differentiate one from the other on imaging.

The imaging features of a neuroma and schwannoma relate to the extent and shape of the proliferating mass of neural tissue within the bone.

Location. The schwannoma is most commonly located within an expanded inferior alveolar nerve canal between the mandibular foramen and the mental foramen (Fig. 22.29). Fewer than 1 in 10 cases of schwannoma occur in the maxilla.

Periphery. In keeping with their slow growth rate, the borders of the schwannoma are well defined and corticated. When a schwannoma arises in the mandibular canal, its periphery usually takes on the cortication of the canal. Small schwannomas may appear cyst-like, but more commonly the shape of the neoplasm expands the canal in a more fusiform manner.

Internal structure. The internal structure of the schwannoma is totally radiolucent. Larger schwannomas may develop a scalloping outline which may give a false impression of a multilocular pattern.

Effects on adjacent structures. If the soft tissue masses extend to the mandibular foramen or the mental foramen, there can be enlargement of these foramina. Fusiform expansion of the inferior alveolar canal in schwannoma is slow with an epicenter within the canal. The cortex of the canal is maintained.

Effects on adjacent teeth. If a schwannoma becomes large, it may extend superiorly to involve the tooth-bearing areas of the jaws and cause root resorption of adjacent teeth (Fig. 22.30).

Differential Interpretation

When small, it is impossible to differentiate a neuroma from a schwannoma on imaging. Should a schwannoma become large, a hemangioma or arteriovenous (A-V) malformation should also be considered. However, as schwannomas have a distinct epicenter within the canal, vascular lesions usually cause a more uniform widening of the entire length of the canal without an obvious epicenter. Furthermore, vascular lesions may alter the course of the canal, and it may take on a serpiginous or snakelike appearance. Invasion of the canal by a malignant lesion will produce irregular widening with destruction of the canal cortex.

Management

The management for a schwannoma is excision. A soft tissue capsule usually is present, facilitating surgical removal, although occasionally

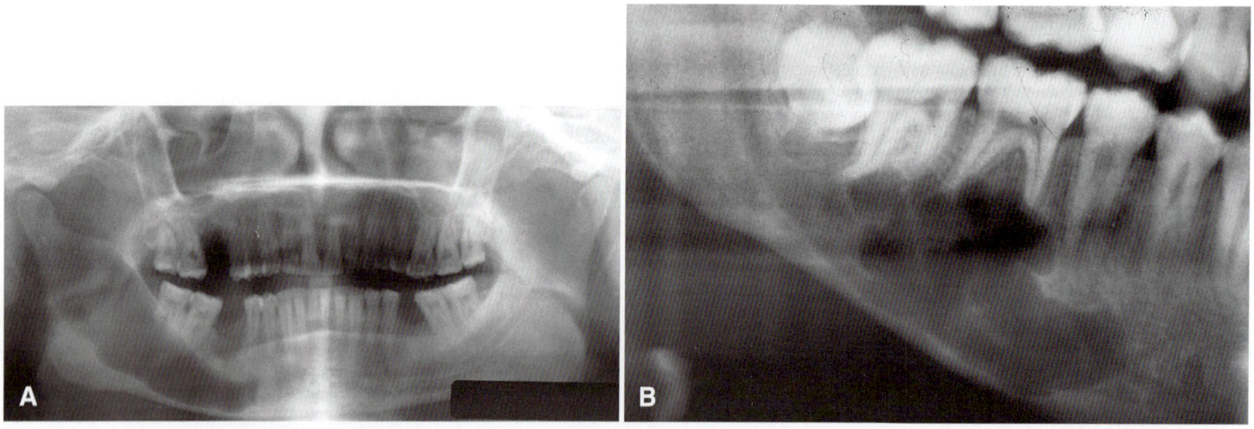

Fig. 22.29 Cropped panoramic images show a neurofibroma forming in the mandibular body along the path of the mandibular canal (A) producing external root resorption of the molar teeth. Note the fusiform shape of the canal as the tumor displaces its borders (B).

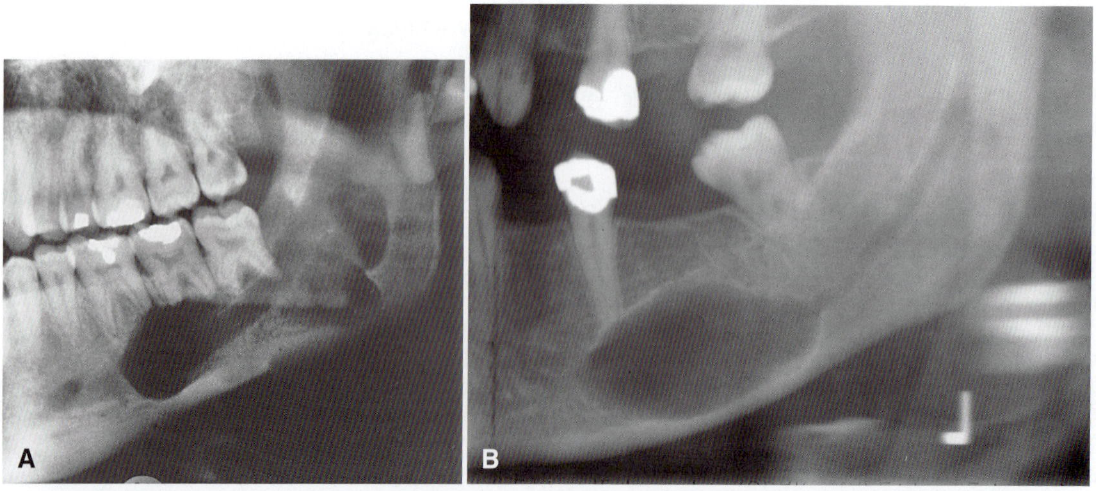

Fig. 22.30 Panoramic image of a large schwannoma expanding the entire length of the right mandibular canal from the mandibular to the mental foramen (A). Cropped panoramic image of a smaller tumor (B). Note the resorption of the molar root apices.

preservation of the nerve may not be possible. Periodic examination is indicated to check for recurrence.

Neurofibroma and Neurofibromatosis

Disease Mechanism

Neurofibromas are neoplasms of Schwann cells that also incorporate nerve fibers such as peripheral nerve axons and the connective tissue of the sheath of Schwann in a disorderly pattern. Neurofibromas can be solitary in nature and are typically intraosseous. Multiple neurofibromas, including multiple soft tissue neurofibromas, can develop in neurofibromatosis or von Recklinghausen disease.

Neurofibromatosis is a member of a family of diseases known as the phakomatoses, a group of multisystem diseases that may involve the central nervous system, the eyes, and the skin. Three disease processes have been defined: neurofibromatosis type 1 (NF1), neurofibromatosis type 2 (NF2), and schwannomatosis. The *NF1* gene encodes a protein called neurofibromin, which behaves as a tumor suppressor protein and is produced by peripheral Schwann cells. Mutations in *NF1* result in uncontrolled proliferation of Schwann cells and/or fibroblasts along peripheral nerves. In contrast, *NF2* encodes a protein called merlin or schwannomin, which also has tumor suppressor qualities, and controls cell shape, growth, and adhesion. Mutations of *NF2* result in unmediated control of cell cycle progression, enhancing cell division and proliferation. Little is currently known of schwannomatosis; however, mutations of two genes have been identified, *SMARCB1* and *LZTR1*, both of which function as tumor growth suppressor genes.

Clinical Features

Solitary intraosseous neurofibromas can occur at any age, but they are usually found in young patients. Those solitary lesions that develop in association with the inferior alveolar nerve may produce pain or paresthesia. They may also expand and perforate the bone cortex, and produce a swelling that is firm or hard to palpation.

Neurofibromatosis type 1 or von Recklinghausen disease is the form of neurofibromatosis that can commonly involve the oral and maxillofacial region. Furthermore, it is one of the most common genetic diseases, affecting approximately 1:3000 births. The most common manifestations are the development of cutaneous and subcutaneous neurofibromas, and larger plexiform neurofibromas. Skin pigmentation called *café au lait* spots can also be identified, with the spots becoming larger and more numerous with age. Most patients eventually have more than six spots larger than 1.5 cm in diameter. The expression of NF1 may also include abnormalities of the bones of the head and neck, including the ramus of the mandible, and the greater and lesser wings of the sphenoid bone.

Imaging Features

Solitary intraosseous neurofibromas can develop within the inferior alveolar canal, the cancellous bone, and underlying the periosteum. Intraosseous neurofibromas are well defined and may be corticated depending on the growth rate of the neurofibroma. The solitary neurofibroma is usually unilocular but occasionally, it may have a multilocular appearance. Within the inferior alveolar canal, a developing neurofibroma may cause fusiform enlargement of the inferior alveolar canal in much the same way as a schwannoma (Fig. 22.30). It is impossible to differentiate a solitary intraosseous neurofibroma from a neuroma or schwannoma.

The morphologic changes in the jaws with NF1 can be a characteristic. These changes are often unilateral and can include the following alterations in the shape of the mandible: enlargement of the coronoid notch in the horizontal and/or the vertical dimensions; the development of an obtuse mandibular angle; lengthening and deformity of the condylar head; and lateral bowing and thinning of the mandibular ramus (Fig. 22.31). Changes in mandibular morphology can continue to increase in severity through the second decade. Other radiographic changes include enlargement of the mental and mandibular foramina, the inferior alveolar canal, and an increased incidence of canal branching. Erosive changes to the outer contour of the mandible and interference with normal eruption of the molars also may occur. Changes to the sphenoid wing can result in an increase in the medial-lateral width of the superior orbital fissure and the appearance on an occipitomental (Waters) view as an "empty orbit." Abnormal accumulations of fatty tissue within deformities of the mandible and sphenoid bone have been observed in images produced by MDCT imaging (Fig. 22.31C).

Management

Solitary intraosseous neurofibromas that have been excised seldom recur. However, it is wise to reexamine the area periodically because these tumors are not encapsulated, and some undergo malignant change. In von Recklinghausen disease, small cutaneous and subcutaneous neurofibromas can be removed if they are painful, but large plexiform neurofibromas should be observed. Malignant conversion of these lesions has occurred in rare cases.

MESENCHYMAL TUMORS AND NEOPLASMS

Dense Bone Island

Disease Mechanism

The dense bone island (DBI), otherwise known as enostosis or idiopathic osteosclerosis, is the "internal" counterpart of exostosis. They represent localized hamartomatous growths of cortical bone into the cancellous bone space.

Clinical Features

DBIs are asymptomatic and are discovered incidentally on images made for other purposes.

Imaging Features

Location. DBIs are more common in the mandible than in the maxilla. They occur most often in the premolar and molar areas (Fig. 22.32), although their presence does not correlate with the presence or absence of teeth (Fig. 22.32A).

Periphery. DBIs directly abut adjacent normal cancellous bone. The periphery is usually well defined, and occasionally, the periphery blends with the trabeculae of the surrounding bone (Fig. 22.32).

Internal structure. The internal pattern of DBIs can vary from a ground glass-like pattern (Fig. 22.33) to one that is uniformly radiopaque (Fig. 22.32). In some cases, heterogeneous radiolucent areas may be visualized, depending on the thickness of the DBI. Three-dimensional imaging may show continuity of the dense bone island with an adjacent cortex of bone, which may explain the high internal density (Fig. 22.34).

Effects on adjacent structures. There are no effects on adjacent structures.

Effects on adjacent teeth. A DBI located periapical to a tooth root can cause external root resorption (see Fig. 22.33). The tooth most often involved is the mandibular first molar. In all circumstances, the tooth pulp is vital, and the root resorption appears to be self-limiting. A visible periodontal ligament space may be visible between the resorbed tooth root and the DBI. In very rare cases, DBIs can inhibit the eruption of a tooth and even displace a tooth.

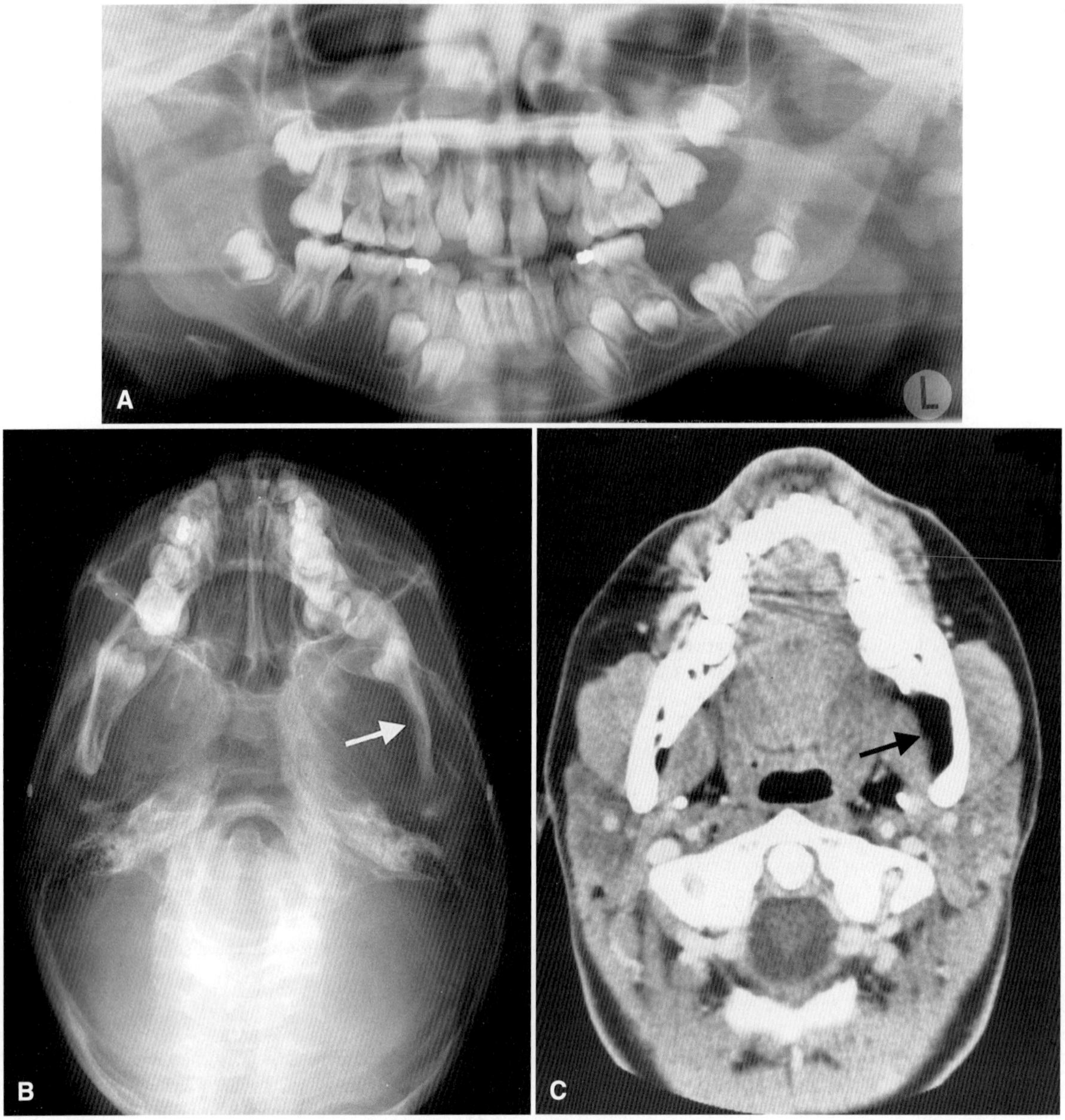

Fig. 22.31 Example of neurofibromatosis involving the mandible. Panoramic image (A) demonstrates enlargement of the left coronoid notch, enlargement of the mandibular foramen, and interference of the eruption of the first and second molars. Basal skull view (B) of the same case reveals thinning and bowing of the ramus in a lateral direction *(arrow)*. The axial multidetector soft tissue window computed tomographic image (C) shows fat to be located adjacent to the abnormal mandibular ramus *(arrow)*.

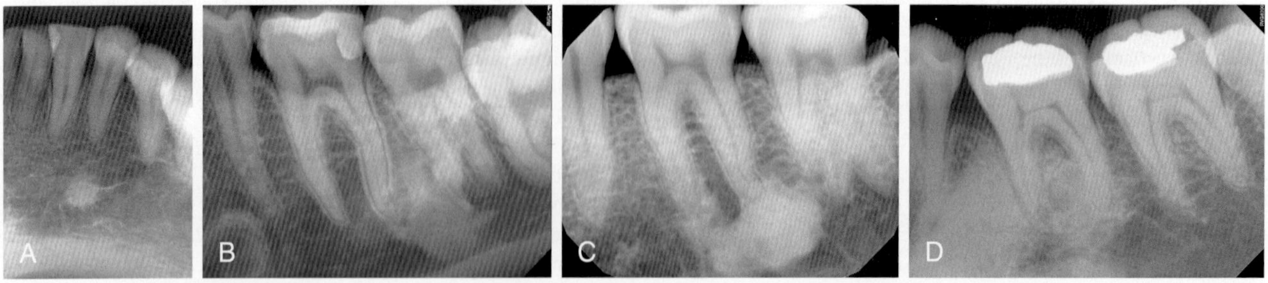

Fig. 22.32 Periapical images of dense bone islands (DBIs) in the mandible (A to D). Note the lack of a radiolucent rim surrounding these entities. Also, some of the surrounding trabeculae appear to merge into the periphery of the radiopacities (see A and D). Note the continuity of the DBIs with the lamina dura and the normal appearing periodontal ligament spaces.

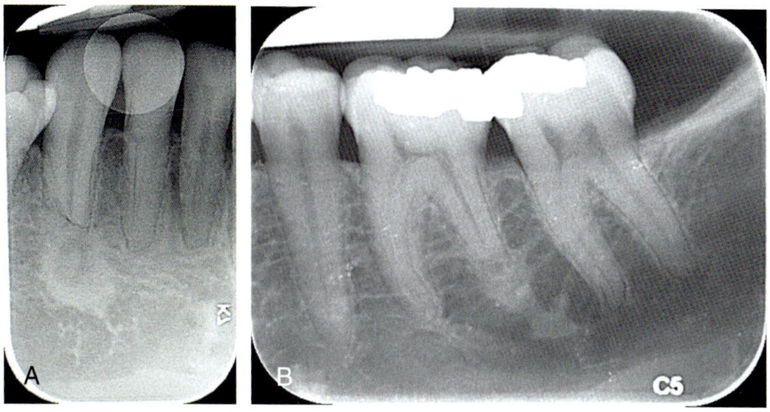

Fig. 22.33 Dense bone islands causing external resorption of the roots in a mandibular right canine (A) and a mandibular left first molar (B). Note the ground glass pattern within (A).

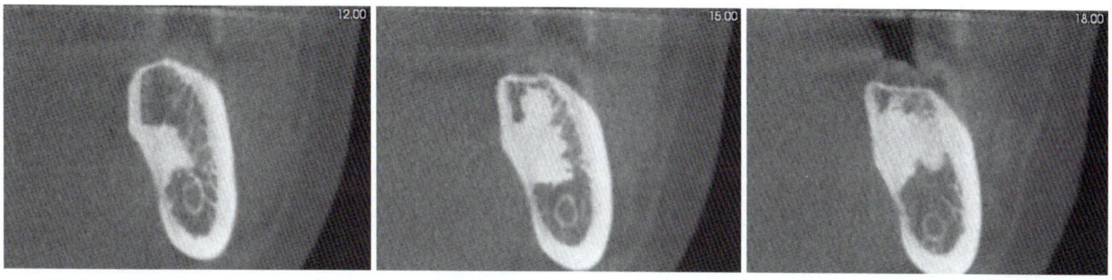

Fig. 22.34 Cross-sectional cone beam computed tomographic images of a dense bone island demonstrating its continuity with the lingual cortex of the mandible.

Differential Interpretation

Several radiopaque entities must be considered in forming a differential interpretation. When a DBI is located at a root apex, it may resemble sclerosing osteitis. However, in sclerosing osteitis, there is often an area of rarefying osteitis located adjacent to the tooth root apex, and the area of sclerosis is located more peripheral to this. Similarly, periapical inflammatory disease may have an apparent etiology, such as a large restoration or carious lesion.

Dense bone islands may also have similarities to periapical cemento-osseous dysplasia, hypercementosis, or cementoblastoma. In these cases, there should be a radiolucent periphery between the radiopaque center of these lesions and the adjacent normal bone.

DBIs are often static in size, but they may increase in size, especially when there is active growth of the jaws. If five or more DBIs are present, adenomatous polyposis coli should be considered.

Management

DBI does not require treatment. If multiple DBIs are present, the patient's family history should be reviewed for the presence of colonic polyps, and a referral should be made to their physician and a medical geneticist.

Exostoses of Bone

Disease Mechanism

Exostoses are exophytic, hamartomatous masses of mostly cortical bone, arising from the bone surface. Occasionally, they may incorporate a small amount of internal cancellous bone, particularly when they arise on the maxillary alveolar processes. Although the etiology of exostoses is unknown, it has been hypothesized that elevated masticatory forces may be a factor in their underlying formation.

Clinical Features

Exostoses may develop on the buccal surfaces of the maxillary alveolar processes, usually in the canine or molar area, and they may be solitary or multiple, flat prominences, nodular or pedunculated (Fig. 22.35). Occasionally, they may also occur on the palatal surface or crest, and less commonly on the mandibular alveolar process, where they may develop under the pontic of a fixed partial denture. Published studies suggest a male predominance and an increase in frequency with age.

A torus is a more location-specific exostosis arising in the midline of the hard palate or the lingual surface of the mandible (Figs. 22.36 and 22.37). The palatal torus (Fig. 22.38) occurs in about 20% of the population while the mandibular torus is less common, occurring in approximately 8% of the population. Interestingly, various studies have shown marked differences between the sexes and ethnic groups. For example, tori develop commonly in the Asian and Inuit populations, and about twice as often in women than men. Furthermore, in women, the occurrence of the mandibular torus correlates with occurrences of the palatal torus.

In the hard palate, the base of the torus extends along the roof of the hard palate, and the bulk extends downward into the oral cavity. These lesions have been described as flat, lobulated, nodular, or mushroom-like. In the mandible, single or multiple tori can develop, and they can be unilateral or bilateral, most often developing in the premolar region (see Fig. 22.37). Mandibular tori can also vary in size, ranging from an outgrowth that is barely palpable to one that contacts a torus on the opposite side. In contrast to palatal tori, mandibular tori develop later in life, in middle-aged adults. Although tori may be discovered at any age, they usually develop in young adults before 30 years of age, and they may continue to enlarge slowly during a lifetime.

Normal mucosa covers the exostoses or tori; however, the mucosa may be thin and appear pale. Consequently, if traumatized, the mucosa

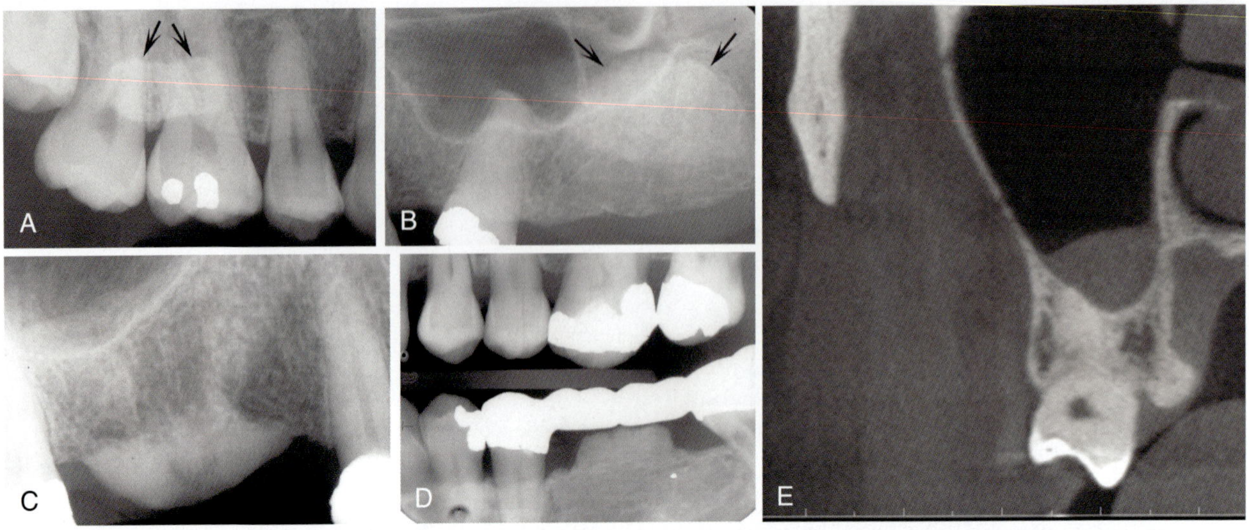

Fig. 22.35 Periapical images showing superimpositions of areas of exostosis overlying the roots (A) and alveolar process (B) in the maxilla. Periapical (C) and bite-wing (D) images of hyperostosis located at the crest of the alveolar process of the maxilla and underlying a fixed partial denture pontic in the mandible. Coronal cone beam computed tomographic image (E) of an exostosis located on the palatal surface of the maxillary right alveolar process.

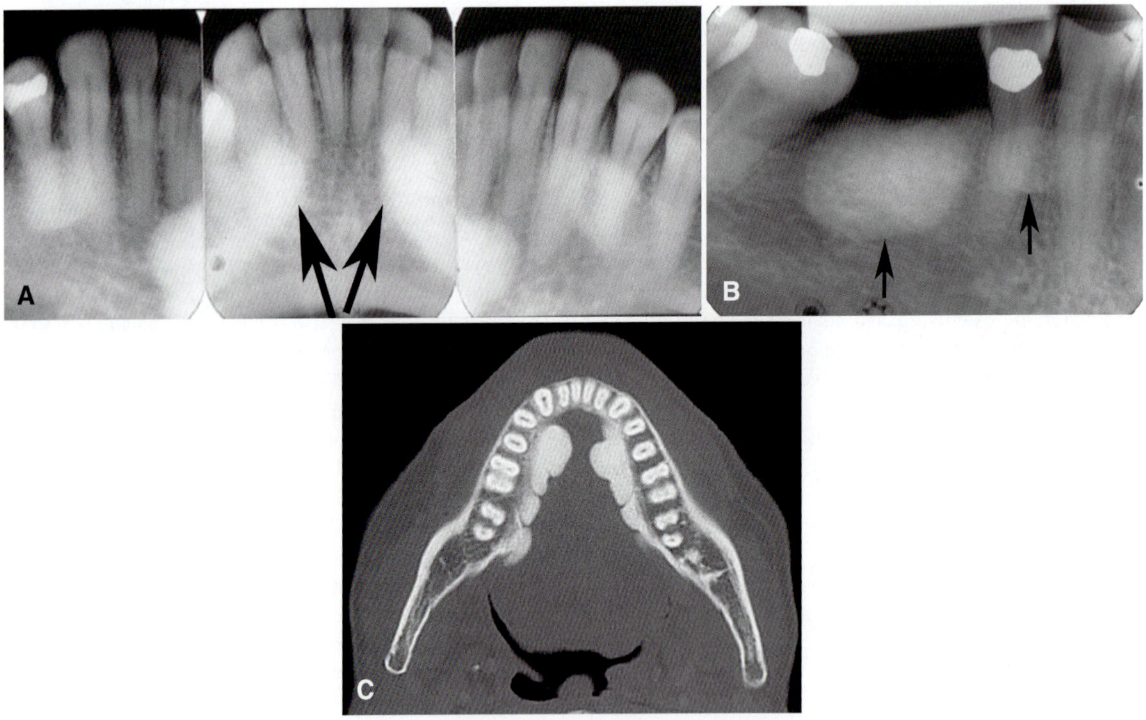

Fig. 22.36 Mandibular tori usually are seen as homogenously radiopaque entities on periapical images (A and B) superimposed over the roots of the teeth *(arrows)*. Axial multidetector computed tomographic image (C) shows a case with bilateral mandibular tori.

overlying a torus may easily ulcerate. Patients are often unaware of having tori, and sometimes, patients who do discover them may insist that they have arisen suddenly and have grown rapidly.

Imaging Features

Location. The maxillary alveolar process is the most common location for an exostosis, and the image of the exostosis is superimposed over the roots of the adjacent teeth (Fig. 22.35A). On a panoramic image, a palatal torus appears as a dense radiopaque structure superimposed over the crowns and/or roots of the maxillary premolar and molar dentition. The recognition of mandibular tori relies on their appearance and location. Their presence bilaterally reinforces this impression, although they can occur unilaterally. On mandibular periapical images, a mandibular torus appears as a radiopaque entity, usually superimposed on the roots of premolars and molars near the crest of the alveolar process, and occasionally over a canine or incisor (Fig. 22.36).

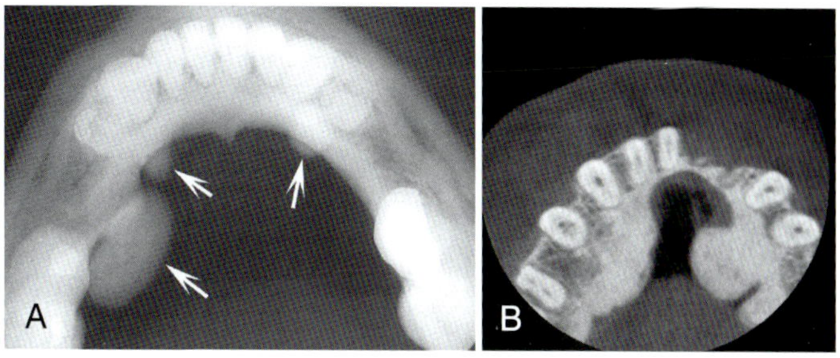

Fig. 22.37 Cross-sectional occlusal (A) and axial cone beam computed tomographic image (B) shows lobulated and asymmetric mandibular tori.

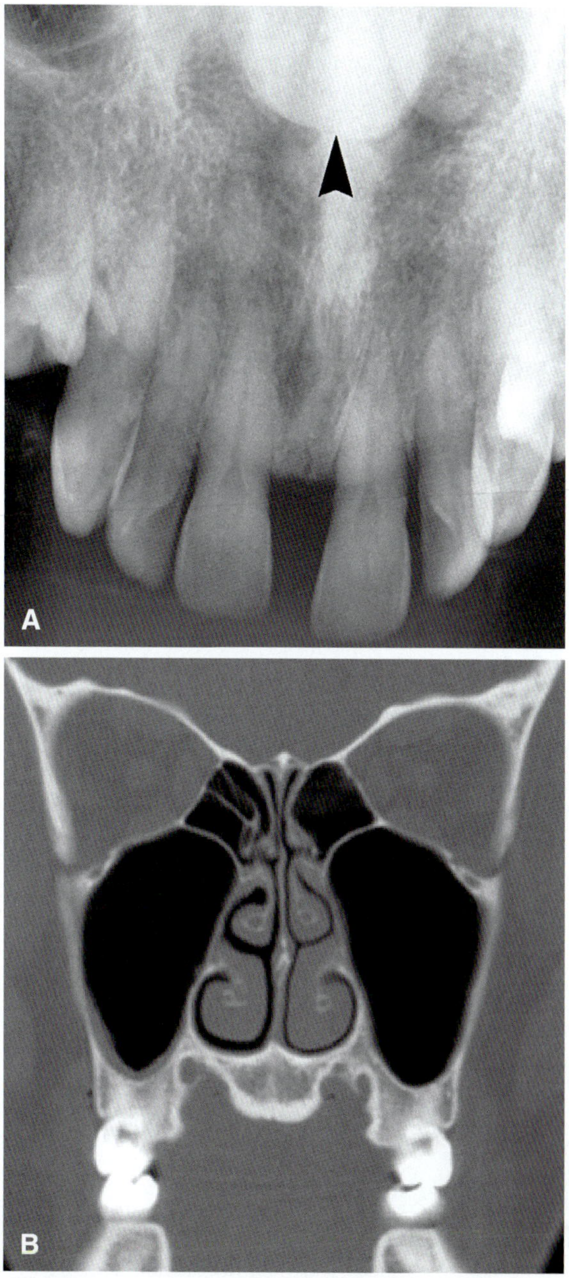

Fig. 22.38 Anterior occlusal image of the maxilla (A) shows a palatal torus *(arrowhead)*. Coronal multidetector computed tomographic image shows a midline palatal torus (B).

Periphery. The periphery of exostoses is usually well defined and smoothly contoured with a curved border (Fig. 22.37). However, some may have poorly defined borders that blend into the surrounding normal bone. Tori may also demonstrate a lobulated outline. Mandibular tori, in particular, can appear very sharply demarcated on intraoral images (Fig. 22.36).

Internal structure. The internal structure of a exostoses usually is homogeneous and radiopaque. Although maxillary alveolar process exostoses can have an internal cancellous bone pattern, they most often consist only of cortical bone (Fig. 22.35A, C, D).

Effects on adjacent structures. Exostoses are continuous with the bone surface, although the continuity may be difficult to appreciate with planar imaging. In the mandible, the continuity of tori may be visualized on cross-sectional occlusal images (Fig. 22.37A).

Effects on adjacent teeth. Exostoses have no effects on the teeth.

Management

Exostoses do not require treatment, although removal may be necessary to accommodate a partial or complete removable denture.

Osteoma

Disease Mechanism

The etiology of the slow-growing osteoma is obscure, and it is unclear whether osteomas are true neoplasms or another example of an exostosis. Consequently, the behavior and radiologic appearances overlap considerably with DBIs and exostoses. Osteomas develop from the periosteum and may occur either externally on a bone surface or within the paranasal sinuses from cartilage or embryonal periosteum.

Clinical Features

Osteomas can occur at any age but are most frequently found in individuals older than 40 years. One or more osteomas can develop simultaneously in a single bone or in multiple bones. Although most osteomas are small, some may become large enough to impact anatomy or function in the oral and maxillofacial region. Osteomas that arise within the frontal sinus and ethmoid air cells may do so without any clinical signs or symptoms. If they become large enough, they can block the outflow of mucus secretions from these air spaces creating the conditions for the formation of a mucocele.

Osteomas originate from the periosteum and may occur either externally on a bone surface or within the paranasal sinuses (Fig. 22.39).

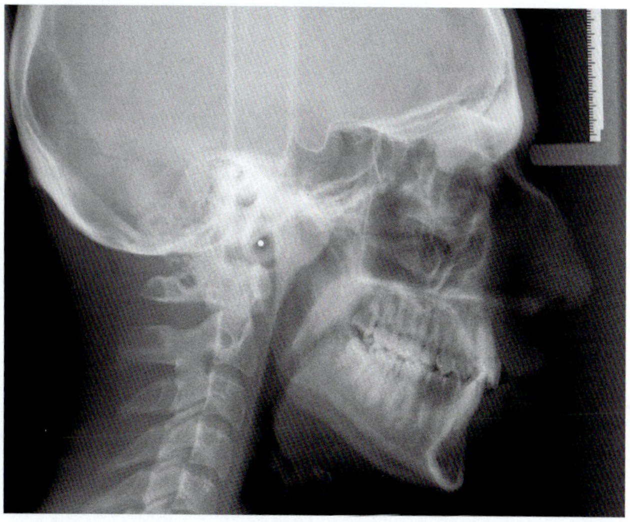

Fig. 22.39 A lateral cephalometric skull image shows an osteoma occupying the frontal bone, obscuring the frontal sinus.

When osteomas develop on the bone surface, a patient may perceive a hard swelling. The swelling is painless until its size or position interferes with function. The osteomas are attached to the cortex of the jaw by a pedicle or along a wide base. Structurally, osteomas can be divided into three types: lesions composed of cortical bone (also called ivory osteomas); lesions composed of cancellous bone; and lesions composed of a combination of both.

Imaging Features

Location. The mandible is more commonly involved than the maxilla. This entity is found most frequently on the inferior border of the mandible in the molar area (Fig. 22.40) or on the medial surface of the mandibular ramus (Fig. 22.41). The mandibular lesions are exophytic, and may be either pedunculated or sessile, extending into adjacent soft tissues. Osteomas also occur in the paranasal sinuses, especially the frontal sinus and ethmoid air cells.

Periphery. Osteomas have well-defined borders. Cortical osteomas lack a discernable cortex while osteomas with a cancellous bone core may have a corticated periphery.

Internal structure. Osteomas composed solely of cortical bone are uniformly radiopaque, whereas osteomas containing cancellous bone show evidence of internal trabecular structure.

Effects on surrounding structures. Large lesions can displace adjacent soft tissues, such as the muscles of mastication, and cause jaw dysfunction. In some cases, there is a sclerotic bone reaction within the cancellous portion of the parent bone and adjacent to the base of the osteomas. The appearance of this sclerotic bone reaction is identical to a DBI.

Differential Interpretation

The appearance of an osteoma is characteristic. A small osteoma may be similar in appearance to an exostosis. Osteomas involving the condylar head can be difficult to differentiate from osteochondromas, osteophytes, or condylar hyperplasia. Furthermore, osteomas involving the coronoid process may be similar to osteochondromas.

Management

Unless the osteoma interferes with normal function or presents a cosmetic problem, this lesion may not require treatment. In such cases, the osteoma should be kept under observation. Resection of osteomas is possible but may be difficult if the osteoma is of the cortical (ivory) type.

Familial Adenomatous Polyposis Syndrome

Disease Mechanism

Familial adenomatous polyposis is a genetic disorder caused by a mutation of the adenomatous polyposis coli *(APC)* gene. This mutation results in the development of multiple colonic polyps, and these can undergo malignant transformation at an average age of 39 in the classic form, or at an average age of 59 years in the attenuated form.

Gardner syndrome is a subtype of familial adenomatous polyposis syndrome. Multiple osteomas are a feature of Gardner syndrome, as are multiple dense bone islands, epidermoid cysts, and subcutaneous desmoid tumors, including desmoplastic fibroma. The associated osteomas appear during the second decade of life, and are most common in the frontal and sphenoid bones, the maxillae, and the mandible (Fig. 22.42). Because osteomas and DBIs often develop before intestinal polyps are

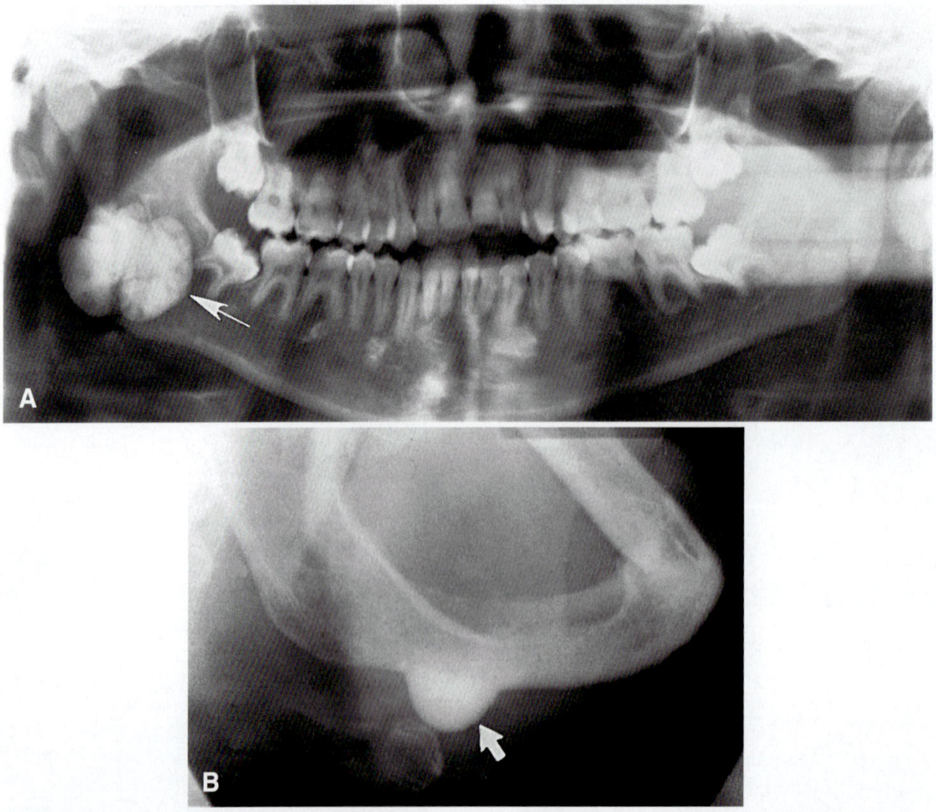

Fig. 22.40 Panoramic image (A) of an osteoma located near the right mandibular angle *(arrow)*. A lateral oblique image of the mandible (B) shows an osteoma as a sessile, exophytic, radiopaque mass attached to the inferior border of the mandible *(arrow)*. (A, From Matteson SR. *Dent Radiogr Photogr.* 1985;57(1–4):3–16, 53–59.)

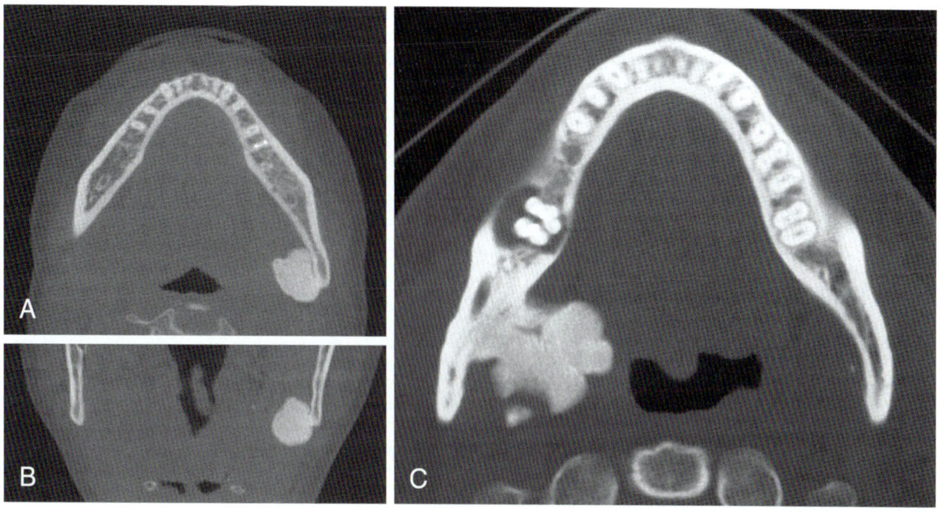

Fig. 22.41 Axial (A) and coronal (B) cone beam computed tomographic images of an osteoma attached to the base of the left mandibular ramus. Axial multidetector computed tomographic image (C) of a lobulated osteoma on the medial surface of the mandibular ramus (A).

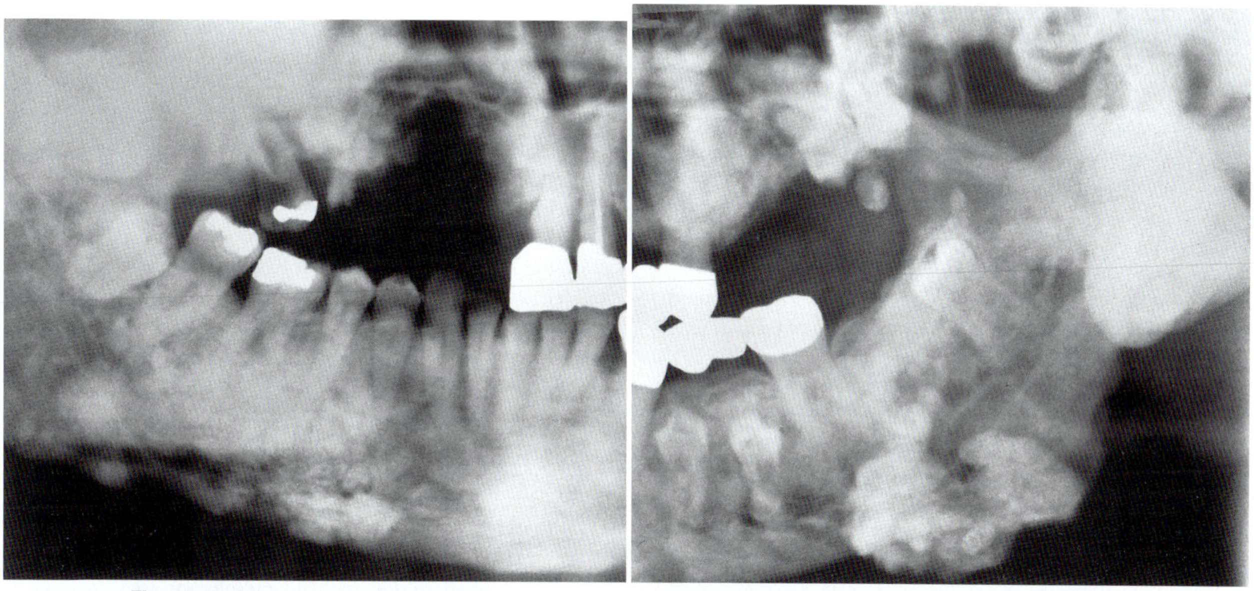

Fig. 22.42 Panoramic image shows multiple osteomas and dense bone islands throughout both jaws in a patient with familial adenomatous polyposis syndrome. Note the impacted mandibular left premolars.

identified, early recognition of the syndrome may be lifesaving for a patient. Occasionally, osteomas may not be present but the presence of five or more DBIs may indicate a familial multiple polyposis syndrome (Fig. 22.43). Also, dental abnormalities include an increased frequency of supernumerary and impacted teeth, and odontomes may also occur in Gardner syndrome.

Management

Generally, the removal of osteomas is unnecessary unless the tumors interfere with normal function or present a cosmetic concern. It is most important to recognize the relationship of multiple osteomas and multiple DBIs with familial adenomatous polyposis syndrome for early diagnosis. A family history of colorectal cancer may also help. These patients should be referred to their physician and to a medical geneticist for diagnosis and management.

Osteoblastoma

Disease Mechanism

An osteoblastoma is benign neoplasm of osteoblasts. These osteoblasts have the capacity to deposit osteoid and immature bone within the neoplasm.

Clinical Features

Osteoblastomas arise most commonly in the vertebrae of a young person and have a male-to-female ratio of 2:1. The average age of occurrence is 17 years, with most lesions occurring in the second and third decades of life. Clinically, patients often report pain and swelling of the affected region.

Imaging Features

Location. Osteoblastomas are found in the tooth-bearing regions and the temporomandibular joint (within the condylar or the temporal bone components).

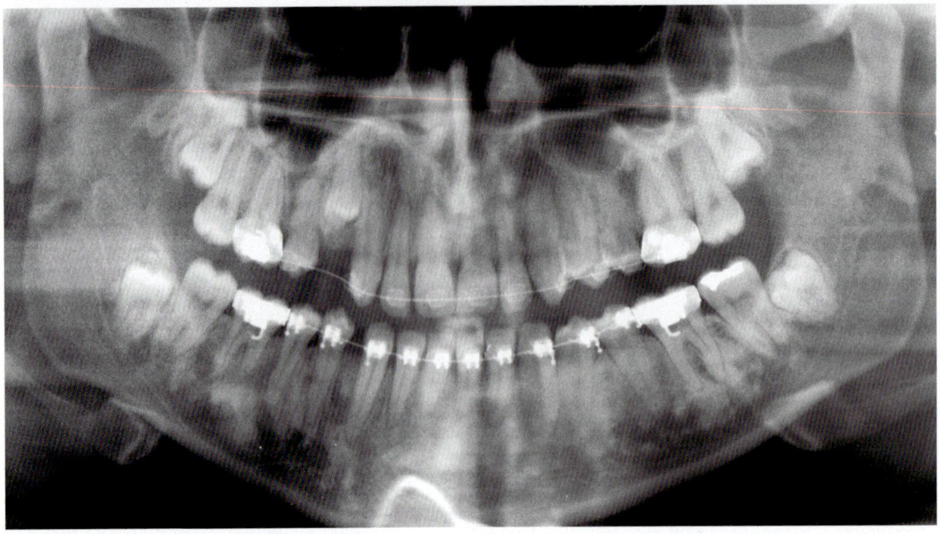

Fig. 22.43 Panoramic image multiple dense bone islands, one of which may have interfered with the eruption of the maxillary right first premolar, in a patient with familial adenomatous polyposis syndrome.

Periphery. The periphery may be diffuse or may show evidence of a cortex. Lesions often have an internal radiolucent border surrounding the more central areas of abnormal bone deposition (Fig. 22.44).

Internal structure. The internal structure may be entirely radiolucent in early developing tumors, or there may be areas of varying central mineralization. The internal calcification may take the form of fine granular bone trabeculae.

Effects on adjacent structures. Osteoblastomas can expand bone, but usually a thin outer cortex is maintained. This lesion may invaginate the maxillary sinus or the middle cranial fossa.

Effects on adjacent teeth. If osteoblastomas develop in a tooth-bearing area within the jaws, there may be movement of teeth or external root resorption.

Differential Interpretation

Osteoblastomas and osteoid osteomas have very similar, if not identical, appearances. The agreement that osteoblastomas and osteoid osteomas are different lesions is increasing; they differ only in size and in their morphologic histopathologic features. Osteoid osteomas are usually smaller and have an associated sclerotic bone reaction at the periphery. Sometimes the appearance of an osteoblastoma may be similar to a large focus of cemento-osseous dysplasia. Both may have internal radiolucent peripheries that surround central radiopaque foci, but the osteoblastoma behaves more aggressively like a neoplasm.

An important differential interpretation is osteosarcoma. This differentiation may rely on the identification of benign features of the osteoblastoma as revealed in diagnostic images. Osteoblastomas do not normally perforate cortical boundaries or invade adjacent soft tissue.

Management

Osteoblastomas are treated with curettage or local excision, and recurrences have been described.

Osteoid Osteoma

Disease Mechanism

The osteoid osteoma is a benign neoplasm of osteoblasts that bears a close resemblance to osteoblastoma. The core consists of osteoid and immature bone within highly vascularized, osteogenic connective tissue. The tumor usually develops within the outer bone cortex but may also form within the cancellous bone.

Clinical Features

Osteoid osteomas occur most often in young people between the ages of 10 and 25 years and have a 2:1 male-to-female predilection; they seldom occur before age 4 years or after age 40. Most of the lesions occur in the femur and tibia; the jaws are rarely involved. The osteoid osteoma has a small, oval or round, tumorlike core approximately 1 cm in diameter. Larger osteoid osteomas have been reported to reach approximately 5 or 6 cm. The osteoid trabeculae in an osteoid osteoma are generally smaller with more narrow trabecular spacing. In addition, the soft tissue over the involved bony area may be swollen and tender. Osteoid osteomas produce severe bone pain that can be characteristically relieved with nonsteroidal antiinflammatory drugs.

Imaging Features

Location. The lesion is most common in the cortex of the appendicular skeleton and spine. In the jaws, osteoid osteomas are more common in the body of the mandible.

Periphery. The borders are well defined by a rim of sclerotic bone (Fig. 22.45).

Internal structure. The internal structure of young lesions is composed of a small round or ovoid radiolucent area. In more mature lesions, the appearance may have a mixed radiolucent and radiopaque appearance, as abnormal bone is deposited.

Effects on adjacent structures. As previously mentioned, this tumor can stimulate a sclerotic bone reaction within the peripheral bone, and cause thickening of the cortex by stimulating periosteal new bone formation.

Differential Interpretation

The differential interpretation of osteoid osteoma, particularly because of the peripheral sclerotic bone reaction, should include sclerosing osteitis, cemento-ossifying fibroma, cementoblastoma, and cemento-osseous dysplasia. The presence of a central radiolucency usually eliminates dense bone island from the differential. Bone scintigraphy may assist in the interpretation by revealing considerable vascularity in the blood pool phase and a very high comparative bone metabolism.

Management

Spontaneous remission has been reported, although the data are insufficient for identifying such cases in advance. Complete excision

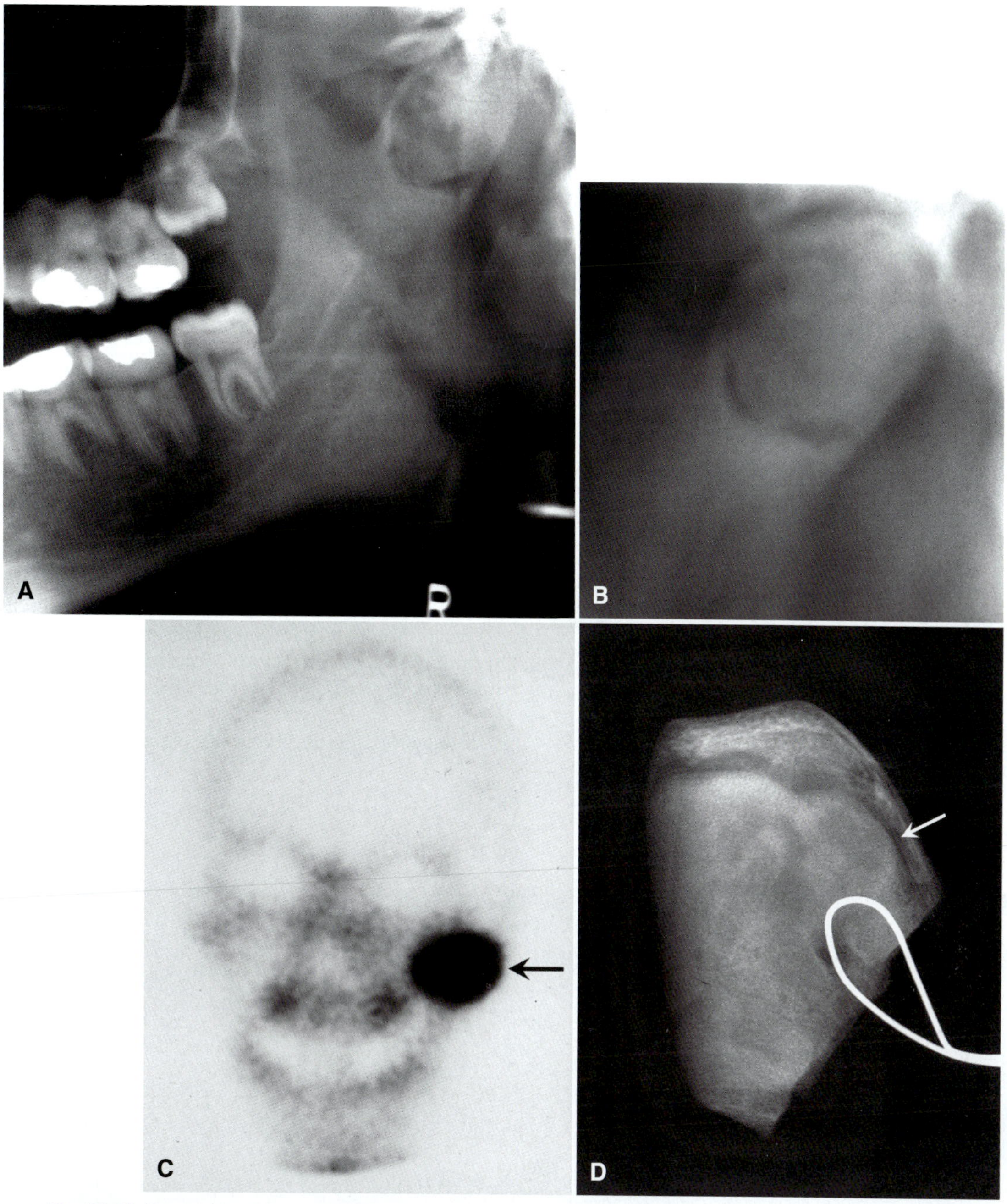

Fig. 22.44 Cropped panoramic image (A) of an osteoblastoma arising within the left mandibular condyle. Note the enlargement of the condyle and presence of the radiolucent rim that surrounds an internal structure of granular bone. Conventional tomograph (B) of the left condyle. ^{99m}Tc nuclear medicine image (C) demonstrates increased bone activity in the left condyle *(arrow)*. Image of the surgical specimen (D). Note the internal granular bone and the radiolucent rim *(arrow)*.

currently is the recommended treatment because it often relieves pain. A new, more conservative treatment involving radiofrequency thermoablation is obtaining success rates of 76%–100%.

Cemento-ossifying Fibroma

Disease Mechanism

The cemento-ossifying fibroma is a neoplasm that contains highly cellular, fibrous connective tissue with varying amounts of abnormal, immature bone, and cementum or cementum-like tissue. Other internal regions of this tumor can have irregular trabeculae of woven or lamellar bone.

Clinical Features

The clinical behavior of cemento-ossifying fibroma can vary from indolent to aggressive. Cemento-ossifying fibroma can occur at any age but usually is found in young adults. Females are more often affected than males. Juvenile ossifying fibroma is a very aggressive form of cemento-ossifying fibroma that occurs in the first two decades of life. Although the pathogenesis of this juvenile ossifying fibroma is controversial, the radiologic appearance has similarities to that of cemento-ossifying fibroma but may be much more expansile.

Cemento-ossifying fibroma is usually asymptomatic at the time of discovery. Occasionally, facial asymmetry develops. Displacement of

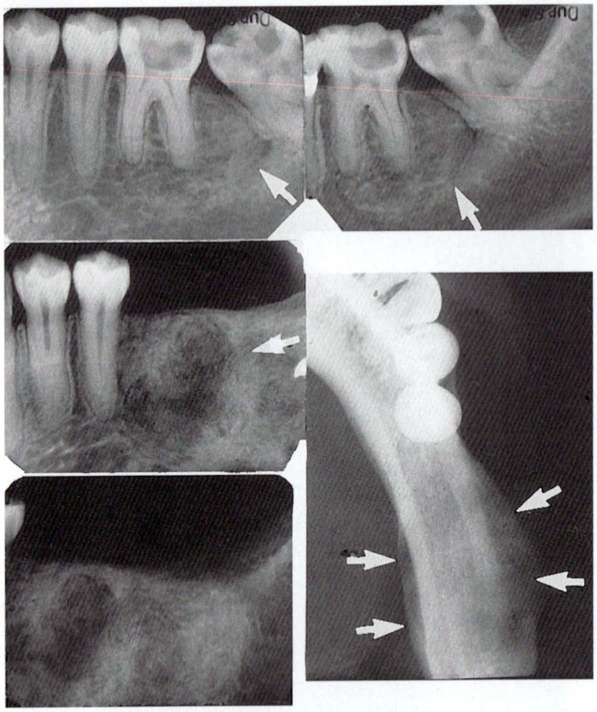

Fig. 22.45 Osteoid osteoma *(single arrow)* appears as a mixed radiolucent and radiopaque lesion in the molar region. The lesion has caused expansion of the buccal and lingual cortex of the mandible *(multiple arrows)*. (Courtesy Dr. A. Shawkat, Radcliff, KY.)

the teeth may be an early clinical feature, although most lesions are discovered during routine dental examinations. In cases of juvenile ossifying fibroma, rapid growth may occur in a young patient, resulting in deformity of the involved jaw.

Imaging Features

Location. Cemento-ossifying fibroma appears almost exclusively in the facial bones and most commonly in the mandible where it arises apical to the premolars and molars, and superior to the inferior alveolar canal. In the maxilla, cemento-ossifying fibroma occurs most often in the area of the canine fossa and in the region of the zygomatic process of the maxilla.

Periphery. The borders are usually well defined, and the cortex may appear thickened to the point of sclerosis.

Internal structure. The internal structure is mixed radiolucent and radiopaque with a pattern that depends on the amount and form of mineralization. In some instances, the internal structure may appear almost totally radiolucent with just a hint of calcified material. In the type that contains mainly abnormal trabeculae of bone, the pattern may appear like the ground glass pattern seen in fibrous dysplasia, or it may appear wispy (similar to stretched tufts of cotton) or flocculent (similar to clouds or large, heavy snowflakes) (Fig. 22.46). Lesions that produce more amorphous bone may contain solid, homogeneously radiopaque regions that do not have any intrinsic pattern. A thin, radiolucent line, representing connective tissue, separates the more centrally occurring radiopaque area from the normal surrounding bone (see Fig. 22.47).

Effects on adjacent structures. Cemento-ossifying fibroma can be distinguished from fibrous dysplasia by its pattern of growth.

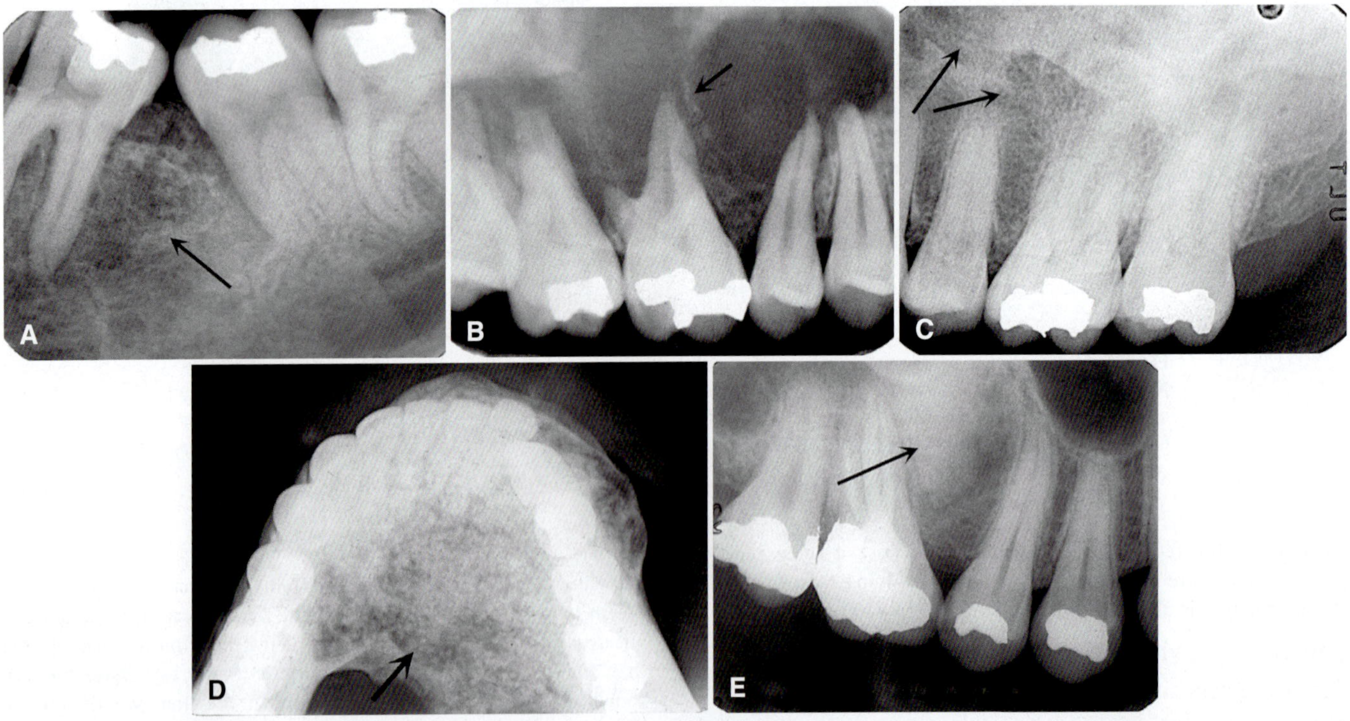

Fig. 22.46 Variations of the bone pattern seen in cemento-ossifying fibroma. These may range from wispy trabecular patterns (A) *(arrow)* and (B), to a granular pattern *(arrows)* (C) reminiscent of fibrous dysplasia. Also, there may be a flocculent pattern with larger tufts of bone formation *(arrow)* (D) and a more solid, radiopaque pattern *(arrow)* (E).

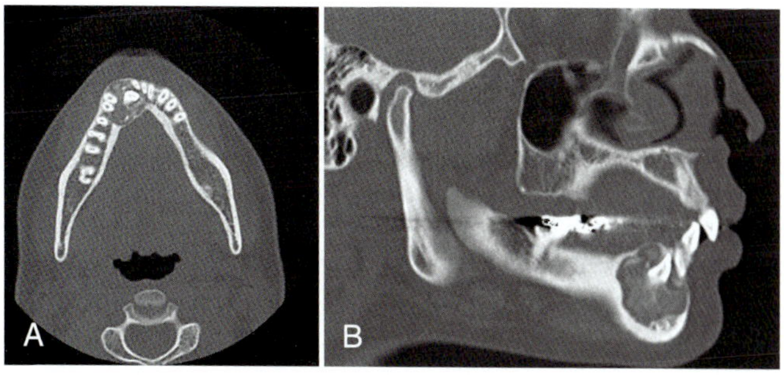

Fig. 22.47 Axial (A) and sagittal (B) cone beam computed tomographic images of a cemento-ossifying fibroma with a thin, low-attenuation (radiolucent) rim at the lesion's internal periphery.

Enlargement of the lesion is concentric within the medullary part of the bone, with outward, concentric growth. This can result in displacement of the inferior alveolar canal and expansion of the adjacent bone cortices. A significant point is that the outer cortices, although displaced and thinned, remain intact. Cemento-ossifying fibroma that develops in the maxilla can cause significant displacement of the borders of the maxillary sinus and almost completely efface the sinus (Fig. 22.48). There is, however, a bony partition that separates the air-filled space from the neoplasm.

Effects on adjacent teeth. Cemento-ossifying fibroma can displace teeth. In addition, the lamina dura of involved teeth usually is missing, and resorption of teeth may occur.

Differential Interpretation

The differential interpretation of cemento-ossifying fibroma includes lesions with a mixed radiolucent and radiopaque internal structure. The differentiation from fibrous dysplasia can be very difficult. The boundaries of cemento-ossifying fibroma usually are better defined, and these lesions occasionally have a cortex with an adjacent internal radiolucent rim, whereas thc periphery of fibrous dysplasia usually blends with surrounding bone. The internal structure of fibrous dysplasia lesions in the maxilla may be more homogeneous and show less pattern variation. Both types of lesions can displace teeth, but cemento-ossifying fibroma displaces from a specific point or epicenter. Fibrous dysplasia rarely resorbs teeth. The expansion of the jaws associated with cemento-ossifying fibroma is more concentric about a definitive epicenter than fibrous dysplasia, which enlarges the bone while distorting the overall shape with a fusiform type of growth pattern. In the maxilla, great difficulty may arise in differentiating cemento-ossifying fibroma from fibrous dysplasia when the lesion involves the maxillary antrum. Fibrous dysplasia usually displaces the lateral wall of the maxilla into the maxillary antrum; however, the pyramidal shape of the air cavity is maintained. The periphery of cemento-ossifying fibroma has a more convex shape, and therefore imparts a concavity to the floor of the air-filled antrum (see Fig. 22.48A). With respect to the teeth, fibrous dysplasia may alter the bone pattern around the teeth without displacing the teeth from an obvious epicenter of a concentrically growing benign tumor. The importance of this differentiation lies in the treatment, which is resection for a cemento-ossifying fibroma and observation for fibrous dysplasia.

The differential interpretation of the type of cemento-ossifying fibroma that produces a mainly homogeneous amorphous bone from periapical cemento-osseous dysplasia (PCOD) may be difficult, especially with large single lesions of PCOD. However, PCOD is often multifocal, whereas cemento-ossifying fibroma is not. Also, the presence of a simple bone cavity is a characteristic of either florid cemento-osseous dysplasia or PCOD but not cemento-ossifying fibroma. A wider sclerotic border is more characteristic of the slow-growing cemento-osseous dysplasia as well as a more undulating expansion.

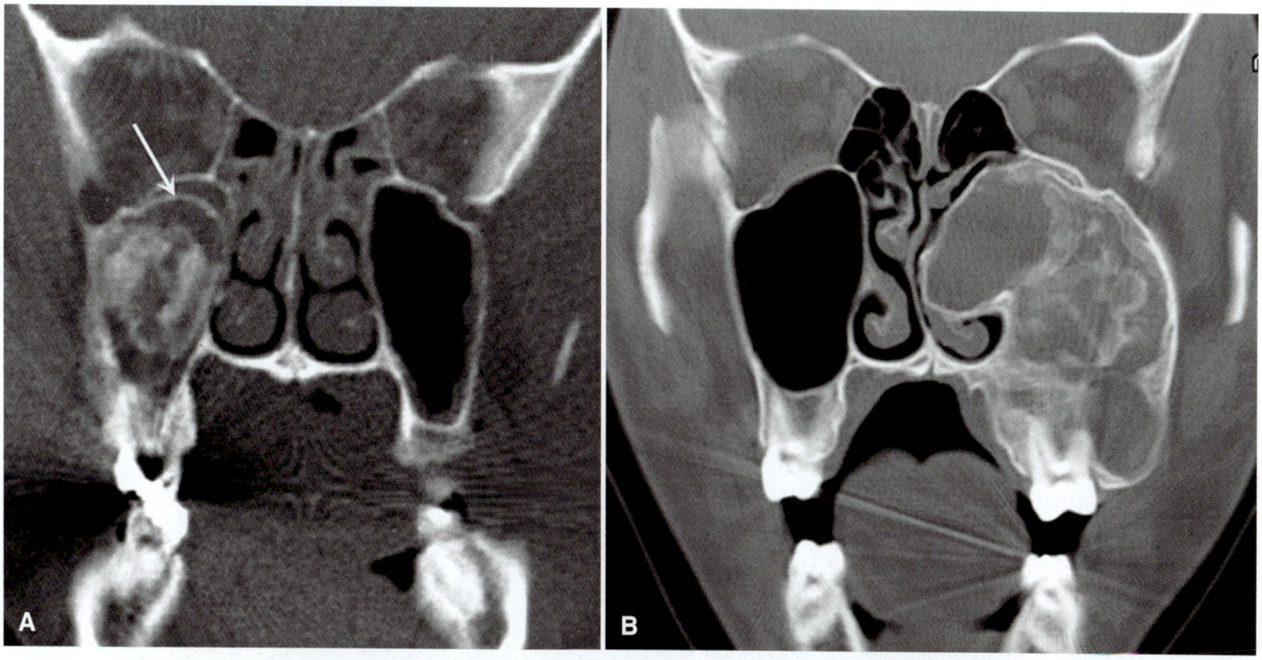

Fig. 22.48 Coronal multidetector computed tomographic images of a cemento-ossifying fibroma in the maxilla displacing the floor of the maxillary sinus. In contrast to fibrous dysplasia where the remnant contours of the maxillary sinus are preserved, the cemento-ossifying fibroma effaces the air cavity leaving only a crescent-shaped remnant of the airspace. Note the displacement of the medial wall of the maxilla in the nasal fossa (B).

Other lesions to be considered include those that have internal calcifications similar to the pattern seen in cemento-ossifying fibroma. These include giant cell lesions, calcifying odontogenic cysts, calcifying epithelial odontogenic (Pindborg) tumor, and AOT. Occasionally, the interpretation of osteogenic sarcoma is considered. However, characteristics suggesting a malignant lesion should be seen, such as cortical bone destruction and invasion into the surrounding soft tissues and along the periodontal ligament space.

Management

The prognosis of cemento-ossifying fibroma is favorable with surgical enucleation or resection. Large lesions require a detailed determination of the extent of the lesion, which can be obtained with CBCT or MDCT imaging. Even if the lesion has reached appreciable size, it usually can be separated from the surrounding tissue and completely removed. Recurrence after removal is unlikely.

Central Giant Cell Lesions

Disease Mechanism

As the origin of this entity remains controversial, we will refer to them as a CGC lesion rather than CGC granuloma or CGC tumor. Despite the name, CGC lesions consist primarily of fibroblasts, with numerous vascular channels; giant cells are a minority of the cell population in these lesions. Because the behavior and imaging characteristics of CGC lesions are similar in many respects to benign tumors, they are included in this chapter.

Clinical Features

CGC lesions affect mostly adolescents and young adults; at least 60% of cases occur in individuals younger than 20 years old. Many CGC lesions are asymptomatic; however, when on the surface of the bone, the most common presenting sign is a swelling. Palpation of the area may elicit tenderness, and in some cases, the patient may complain of pain. Because of the highly vascular nature of these lesions, the overlying mucosa may have a purple color. The rate of lesion growth is variable with faster growing lesions creating the suspicion of a malignancy.

Imaging Features

Location. CGC lesions develop in the mandible twice as frequently as in the maxilla. Within the first two decades of life, there is a tendency for the epicenter of the lesion to be located mesial to the first molar in the mandible, and mesial to the canine in the maxilla. In older individuals, CGC lesions can occur with greater frequency in the posterior regions of the jaws.

Periphery. Slower growing lesions have a well-defined periphery, but in most cases, the periphery shows no evidence of a cortex. They may have more poorly defined borders; an appearance that may appear more aggressive.

Internal structure. Some CGC lesions show no evidence of internal structure and may be radiolucent (Fig. 22.49). This is especially true of small lesions. Other lesions have a subtle granular pattern of calcification that may require a change in image brightness to perceive, and occasionally, this granular bone pattern is organized into wispy striations (Fig. 22.50). Unlike conventional septa, the striations seen in CGC lesions are manufactured by the cells within the lesion; they do not represent remnant normal bone. When present, these striations are characteristic of CGC lesions, especially if they emanate at right angles from the periphery of the lesion. This characteristic appearance is further brought to prominence if a small indentation of the expanded cortex is seen at the point where this right-angled striation originates (Fig. 22.51). In some instances, the striations are better defined, and these can divide the lesion into compartments, creating a multilocular appearance.

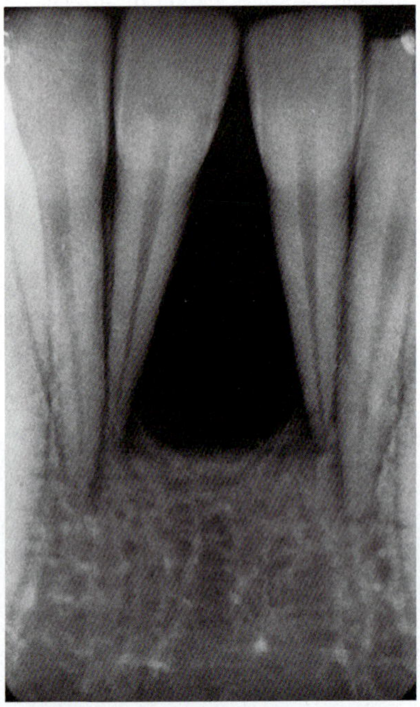

Fig. 22.49 Periapical image of a central giant cell lesion in the anterior mandible with no evidence of internal structure.

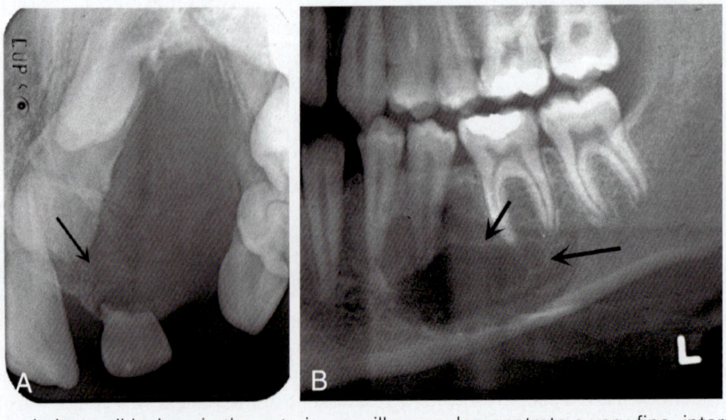

Fig. 22.50 Central giant cell lesions in the anterior maxilla may demonstrate a very fine, internal pattern (A). In the posterior mandible, the internal pattern may show wispy, granular linear patterns of mineralization (B).

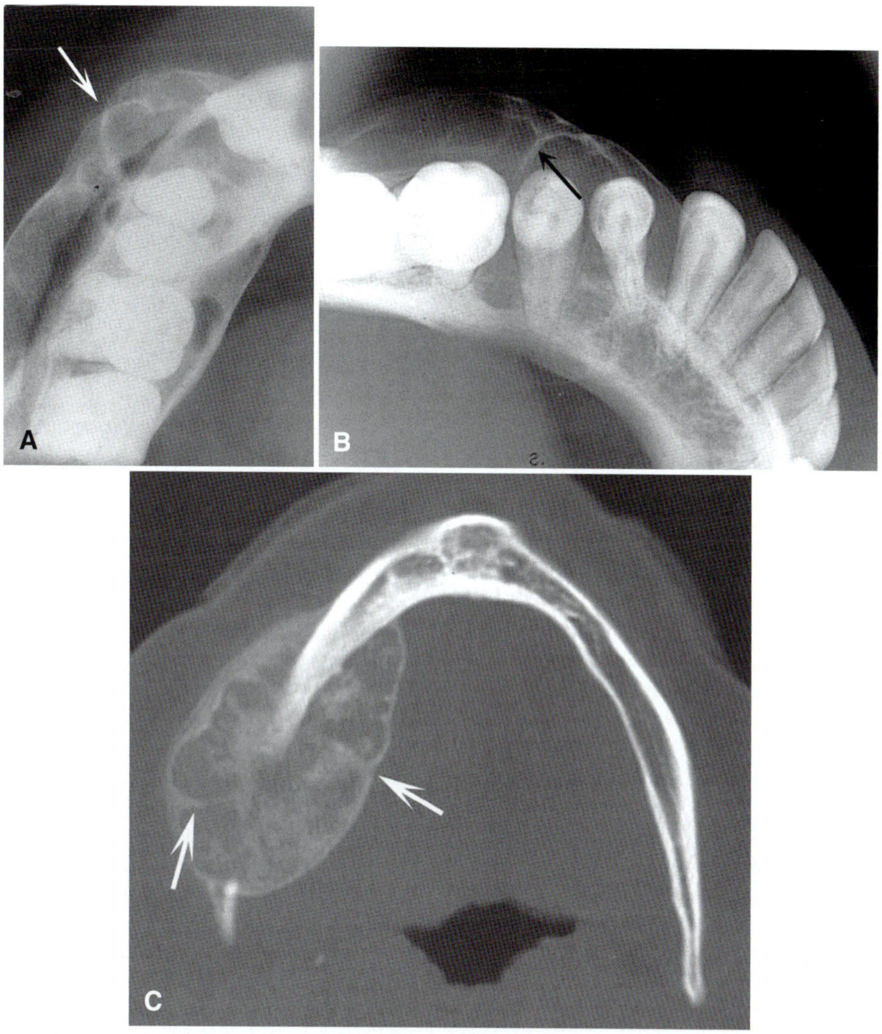

Fig. 22.51 Central giant cell lesions characteristically expand the bone, although the expansion may be uneven (*arrow*, A). Occlusal (B) and axial multidetector computed tomographic (C) images show surface indentations with a pattern of right-angle, linear mineralized striations.

Effects on adjacent structures. CGC lesions have a strong propensity to expand bone borders and displace anatomic structures. At the lesion's periphery, the periphery may overlap the native buccal cortex, a pattern of growth referred to as "flow-around" that may give the appearance of a double boundary (Fig. 22.52). The bone forming the border of the expanded mandible often has a more granular quality compared with cortical bone, sometimes making it difficult to visualize. In some instances, the bone cortex is destroyed and not expanded; this occurs more often in the maxilla, where the cortical bone destruction may give the lesion a more aggressive appearance. The inferior alveolar canal may be displaced in an inferior direction.

Effects on adjacent teeth. CGC lesions often displace and resorb tooth roots (see Fig. 22.50). Resorption of tooth roots is not, however, a consistent feature, but when it occurs, it may be profound and irregular in outline. The lamina dura of teeth within the lesion are usually lost.

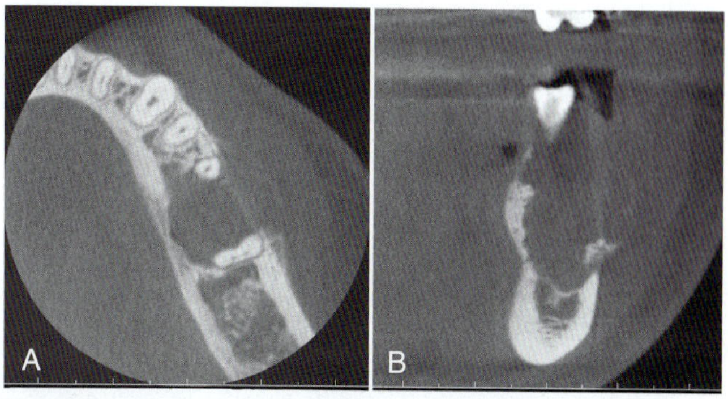

Fig. 22.52 Axial (A) and cross-sectional (B) cone beam computed tomographic images of a central giant cell lesion showing expansion of the buccal surface of the mandible and the so-called flow-around effect of the lesion's growth over the buccal surface of the bone at the lesion periphery.

Differential Interpretation

A small CGC lesion that is totally radiolucent may appear similar to a cyst, especially a simple bone cavity. Evidence of tooth displacement or root resorption of an adjacent tooth or expansion is more characteristic of neoplastic behavior.

If the internal structure of the CGC lesion contains radiopaque striations, the differential interpretation may include odontogenic myxoma, aneurysmal bone cyst (ABC), and ameloblastoma. If the internal structure appears less striated, cemento-ossifying fibroma may be considered. Useful characteristics for differentiating an ameloblastoma may include the thickness and curvature of the septa compared to what is seen with CGC lesions; they tend to be more coarse, curved, and well defined, whereas CGC lesion striations are more delicate, granular, and wispy, some of which are oriented at a right angle to the periphery. Odontogenic myxomas occur in an older age group, may have sharper and straighter septa, and do not have the same propensity to expand bone as CGC lesions. ABCs can appear identical to CGC lesions, radiologically, especially the appearance of the internal striations. ABCs are, however, comparatively rare lesions that occur more often in the posterior aspect of the jaws, and usually cause profound expansion.

The radiologic appearance of a brown tumor of hyperparathyroidism is identical to a CGC lesion. Also, the appearance of the CGC lesion may also be identical to the bilateral lesions seen in cherubism. The lesions in cherubism are, however, multiple and have epicenters that are located in the mandibular body and ramus, and posterior maxillae.

Management

CBCT may be useful to identify the presence of internal structure, particularly, the radiopaque striations of immature bone within the lesion. MDCT may not be able to discern the delicate striations as effectively as a small field-of-view CBCT system with a smaller voxel size. MDCT imaging is required for large lesions to determine whether the lesion has extended through the cortex to involve the overlying soft tissue. Occasionally, CGC lesions can behave very aggressively. If a CGC lesion occurs after the second decade of life, hyperparathyroidism should be considered, and serum testing for elevated parathyroid hormone should be ordered.

Treatment may include intralesional delivery of corticosteroids and/or calcitonin if the lesion is large, followed by enucleation and curettage. Some lesions are also resected. The patient should be followed carefully to rule out recurrence, especially if a more conservative management strategy is used. Although recurrences are rare, they tend to be more common in the maxilla.

Cherubism

Disease Mechanism

Cherubism is a rare, inherited disease caused by a germline mutation of the *SH3BP2* gene that has a role in immune response signaling. It is, however, likely that other mutations are also involved. The lesions that develop are identical to CGC lesions histopathologically and radiologically.

Clinical Features

Cherubism develops in early childhood, between the ages of 2 and 6 years. The most common presenting sign is a firm, painless, bilateral swelling of the cheeks due to the expansile nature of the lesions. Enlargement of the submandibular lymph nodes may also occur, but no systemic abnormalities are involved. Because children's faces are often chubby, mild cases may go undetected for some time. Profound swelling of the maxilla may result in stretching of the skin of the cheeks, which depresses the lower eyelids, exposing a thin line of sclera and causing the appearance of upturned eyes, "raised to heaven". Cherubism is, however, a time-limited disease, and the lesions involute and regress without treatment around the time of skeletal maturity.

Imaging Features

Location. The lesions of cherubism are bilateral, and both jaws can be affected. When present in only one jaw, the mandible is the most common location. The epicenters of these lesions are always in the posterior body and ramus of the mandible, or in the tuberosity of the maxilla (Fig. 22.53). The lesions grow concentrically, and in severe cases can extend to the midline.

Periphery. The periphery is well defined and corticated.

Internal structure. The internal appearance is similar to the appearance within CGC lesions. That is, there may be fine, granular bone oriented in wispy striations, imparting a multilocular pattern to the lesions.

Effects on adjacent structures. Expansion of the surfaces of the maxilla and mandible by cherubism can result in severe enlargement of the jaws. Maxillary lesions can displace the maxillary sinus floors, and in the mandible, there may be substantial displacement of the medial and lateral surfaces of the ramus. Of particular concern is that the extensive medial displacement of the soft tissues adjacent to the mandible can compromise the airway.

Effects on adjacent teeth. Because the epicenters of these lesions are in the posterior mandible and maxilla, the teeth are displaced toward the midline. The degree of displacement can be severe, and developing tooth buds may be aggressively disrupted with some lesions.

Differential Interpretation

Although the radiologic appearances of the lesions in cherubism are similar to solitary CGC lesions, the lesions in cherubism are bilateral with epicenters in the posterior mandible and maxillae. Differentiating cherubism from fibrous dysplasia should not present any difficulties

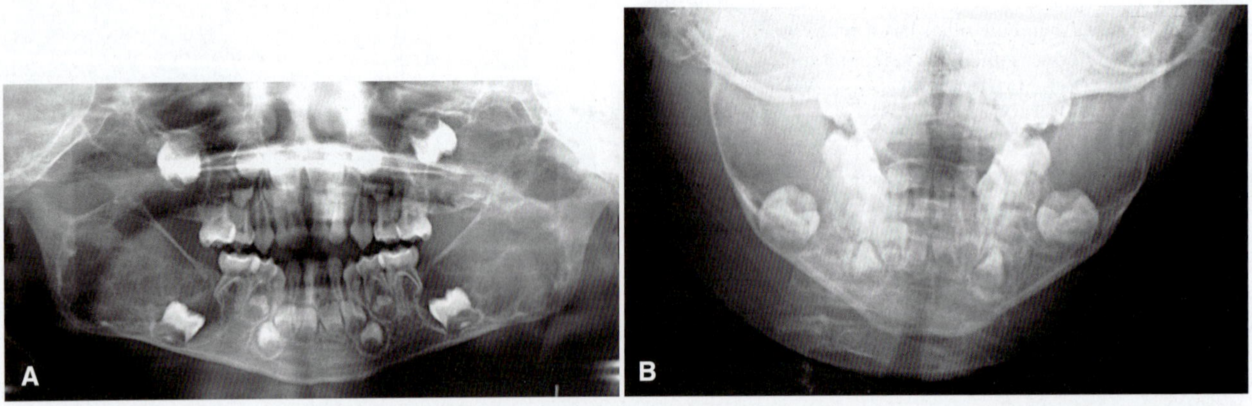

Fig. 22.53 Panoramic image (A) shows four lesions in the maxillae and mandible in a patient with cherubism. The epicenters of the lesions are in the maxillary tuberosity and mandibular ramus. Note the mesial displacement of the unerupted maxillary first molars. Internally, the mandibular lesions contain a faint, linear mineralization pattern. A posterior–anterior planar image of the mandible (B) shows the expanded mandible.

because fibrous dysplasia is a unilateral abnormality. Furthermore, the sometimes multilocular appearance of the lesions in cherubism, and the aggressive bodily displacement of tooth follicles and erupted teeth are more characteristic of cherubism. Cherubism may also have some similarities to odontogenic keratocysts in nevoid basal cell carcinoma syndrome. The bilateral symmetry of cherubism, anterior displacement of teeth, and multilocular appearances of the lesions are characteristics that can help with the differential interpretation.

Management

Significant enlargement of the posterior mandible may affect the patency of the airway in exuberant cases. Treatment can be delayed because the lesions may cease their growth, and infill granular bone during adolescence and at skeletal maturity. After skeletal growth has stopped, conservative surgical procedures, if required, may be done for cosmetic problems. Surgery also may be required to uncover displaced teeth, and orthodontic treatment may be needed.

Aneurysmal Bone Cyst

Disease Mechanism

The ABC has long been considered to be a reactive lesion of bone, although recently, a chromosomal aberration of the *USP6* gene has given some credence to a neoplastic etiology. As this lesion has both clinical and radiologic features that can mimic a benign albeit aggressive neoplasm, we have included the ABC in this chapter. The ABC represents a proliferation of fibroblasts and small vessels; osteoclast-like cells; and reactive, poorly calcified woven bone.

Clinical Features

More than 90% of ABCs that arise within the jaws occur in individuals younger than 30 years old, and the condition appears to have a predilection for females. An ABC in the jaw usually manifests as a rapidly growing bony swelling. Pain is an occasional complaint, and the involved area may be tender on palpation. ABCs occasionally develop in association with other primary lesions, such as fibrous dysplasia, central hemangioma, CGC lesions, and osteosarcoma.

Imaging Features

Location. The mandible is involved more often than the maxilla by a ratio of 3:2. Furthermore, the molar and ramus regions are more often involved than the anterior regions of the jaws (Fig. 22.54).

Periphery. The periphery of ABCs is well defined, and it may be partially corticated, depending on the aggressiveness of its growth. The shape is usually circular and the periphery "hydraulic," resembling the classical shape of a cyst.

Internal structure. Small initial lesions may show no evidence of an internal structure. Larger lesions, however, develop internal areas of mineralization that bear a striking resemblance to the wispy, sometimes granular-appearing striations present in CGC lesions. This can give the ABC a multilocular appearance (Fig. 22.54). Striations positioned at right angles to the outer expanded border are another similar finding. In MDCT soft tissue algorithm images, the low-attenuation or radiolucent areas may have a somewhat circular shape and represent large vascular spaces within the lesion (Fig. 22.55).

Effects on adjacent structures. When an ABC becomes large, there can be extreme expansion of the bone surface with displacement and thinning of the bone cortices (see Fig. 22.54). This characteristic is highly dramatic in ABCs, more so than in almost any other lesion.

Effects on adjacent teeth. ABCs can displace and resorb tooth roots.

Differential Interpretation

The radiologic appearances of ABC and CGC lesions may be identical. ABCs may expand the bone to a far greater degree, and they are more common in the posterior regions of the mandible than the anterior. ABCs may also show a similarity to the lesions in cherubism; however, cherubism is a bilateral disease. Ameloblastoma may be considered, but generally, ameloblastomas occur in an older age group. The diagnosis is based on biopsy results. A hemorrhagic aspirate favors the diagnosis of ABC.

Management

MDCT or MRI are recommended to determine the extent of the lesion better, and to characterize the very vascular nature of these lesions. Surgical curettage and partial resection are the primary means of treatment. The recurrence rate ranges from 19% to about 50% after curettage, and approximately 11% after resection. Careful follow-up is needed.

Desmoplastic Fibroma

Disease Mechanism

A desmoplastic fibroma arising in bone is an aggressive, infiltrative neoplasm that produces abundant collagen fibers.

Clinical Features

Patients usually complain of facial swelling, pain (in rare cases), and sometimes dysfunction, especially when the neoplasm is located close to the temporomandibular joint. The lesion has a slight female predilection and most cases of the neoplasm are found in individuals under the age of 30. Although it originates in bone, the tumor may invade the surrounding soft tissue extensively. One or more desmoplastic fibromas may also occur as part of familial adenomatous polyposis (Gardner syndrome).

Imaging Features

Location. Desmoplastic fibromas of bone may occur in the mandible or maxilla, but the most common site is the posterior mandible and ramus.

Periphery. The periphery most often is poorly defined, and has an invasive characteristic commonly seen in malignant tumors.

Internal structure. Internally, the desmoplastic fibroma may be totally radiolucent, especially when the lesion is small. Larger lesions appear to be multilocular with very coarse, thick septa. These wide septa may be straight or may have an irregular shape (Fig. 22.56).

Effects on surrounding structures. Desmoplastic fibromas of bone can expand bone and often break through the outer cortex, extending into the adjacent soft tissue. Usually, MDCT or MRI is required to determine the soft tissue extent of the lesion.

Differential Interpretation

Distinguishing desmoplastic fibroma from fibrosarcoma may be difficult both radiologically and histopathologically. However, the presence of coarse, irregular, and sometimes straight septa may help support the correct diagnosis. The appearance of these septa also helps differentiate the lesion from other multilocular tumors. Very small lesions may resemble simple bone cavities.

Management

Resection of this neoplasm with adequate margins is recommended because of its high recurrence rate. Patients who have been treated for the condition should be followed closely with frequent radiologic examinations.

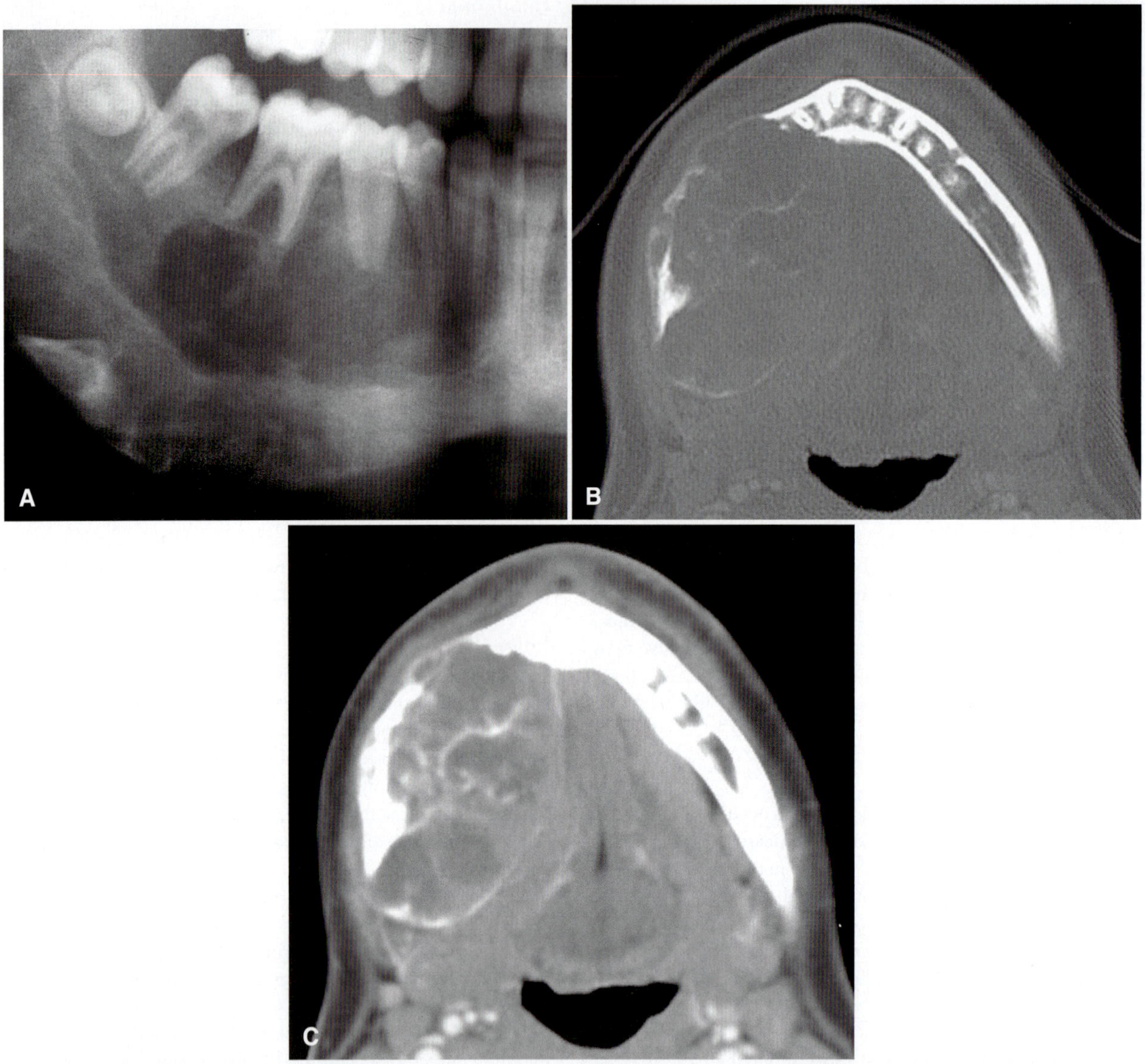

Fig. 22.54 Cropped panoramic image (A) of an aneurysmal bone cyst occupying the right mandibular body. Axial bone (B) and soft tissue (C) window multidetector computed tomographic images show the exuberant expansion of the bone, and faint, wispy mineralized striations within the lesion. Also note the low-attenuation *(dark)* areas on the soft tissue window image that demonstrate a fluidlike density.

Central Hemangioma

Disease Mechanism

A hemangioma is a proliferation of blood vessels creating a mass that resembles a neoplasm, although in many cases it is actually a hamartoma. The etiology of hemangiomas may be developmental or traumatic in origin. Hemangiomas can occur anywhere in the body but are most frequently noticed on the skin and subcutaneous tissues. The central (intraosseous) type most often is found in the vertebrae and skull, and rarely in the jaws.

Clinical Features

Hemangiomas occur most commonly in the first decade of life, although they may also occur later in life, and with a strong 2:1 female prevalence. Enlargement of the bone is slow, producing a nontender expansion of the jaw that occurs over several months or years. Pain, if present, is of the throbbing type. Some tumors may be compressible or pulsate should they involve adjacent soft tissues, and a bruit may be detected on auscultation. Anesthesia of the skin can also occur should the lesion compress an adjacent peripheral nerve. Bleeding may occur from the gingiva around affected teeth, and teeth may be loosened or displaced. Some teeth may demonstrate rebound mobility; that is, when depressed into their sockets, they return to their original position within several minutes because of pressure from the vascular network around the tooth roots. Aspiration with a syringe produces arterial blood that may be under considerable pressure.

Imaging Features

Location. Hemangiomas affect the mandible about twice as often as the maxilla. In the mandible, the most common site is the posterior body and ramus, and within the inferior alveolar canal.

Periphery. The range of appearances of intraosseous hemangiomas may be quite variable. In some instances, the periphery is well defined and corticated; however, some lesions may exhibit a poorly defined periphery, simulating the appearance of a malignant neoplasm.

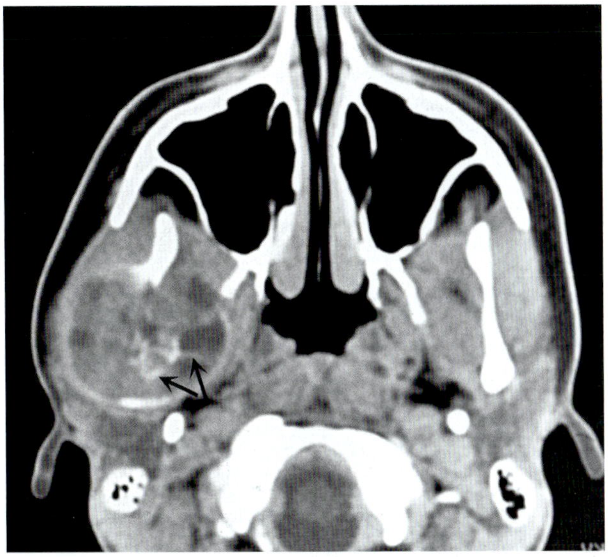

Fig. 22.55 Axial soft tissue window multidetector computed tomographic image of an aneurysmal bone cyst in the left mandibular condylar head. Note the very significant expansion of the bone and the wispy linear striations *(arrows)*.

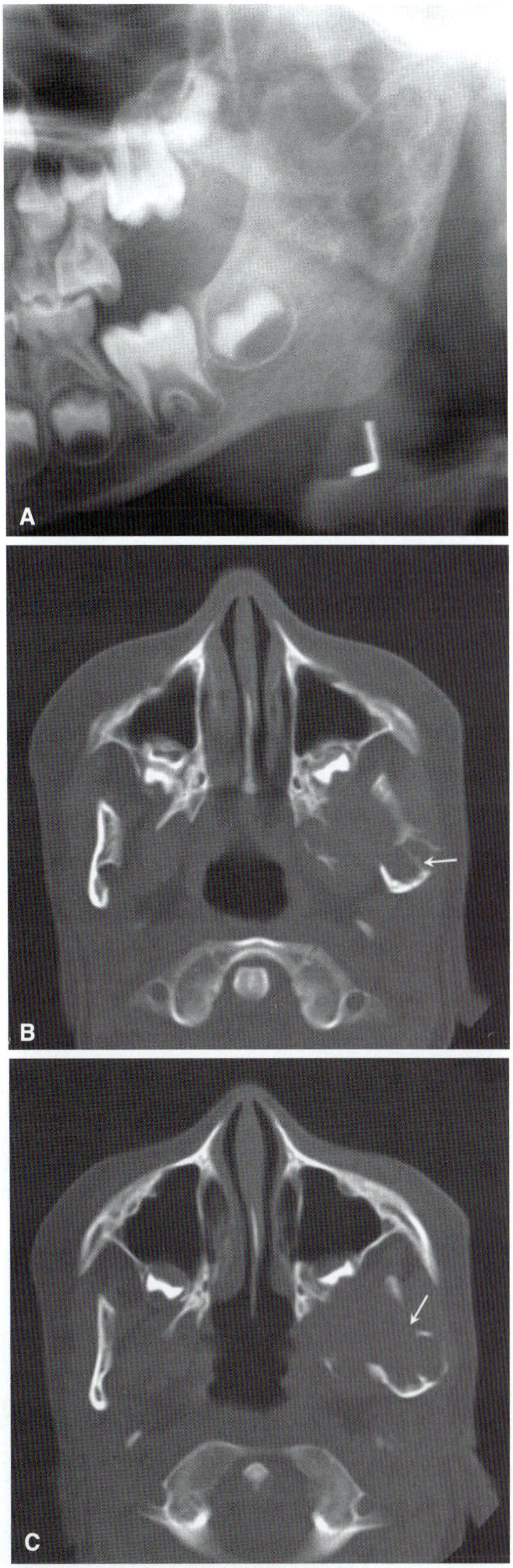

Fig. 22.56 Cropped panoramic image of a central desmoplastic fibroma centered within the left condyle and ramus (A). Axial bone window multidetector computed tomographic image (B) reveals thick straight septa *(arrows)*. More superiorly, (C) computed tomographic images reveal that the tumor has perforated the anterior cortex of the condylar head.

Internal structure. Intraosseous hemangiomas may be totally radiolucent; however, when there is residual bone trapped around the proliferating blood vessels, hemangiomas can take on a multilocular appearance. Small radiolucent locules may resemble enlarged marrow spaces surrounded by coarse, dense, and well-defined trabeculae (Fig. 22.57). These internal trabeculae may produce a honeycomb pattern composed of small circular radiolucent spaces that represent blood vessels that are oriented along the path of the incident x-ray beam.

Effects on adjacent structures. When the inferior alveolar canal is involved, the entire canal may appear enlarged, and often the normal path of the canal may develop a serpiginous or snakelike course (Fig. 22.58). The mandibular and mental foramen may also be enlarged. In addition, the involved bone may be enlarged and have coarse, internal trabeculae. When an intraosseous hemangioma extends beyond the bone surface, distending and displacing the periosteum, linear spicules of bone can be seen emanating from bone surface in a sunray-like pattern (Fig. 22.59).

When a hemangioma involves soft tissue, focal, circular areas of mineralization can be seen on imaging called phleboliths (Fig. 22.60). As discussed in Chapter 29, phleboliths are calcified thrombi which develop in vessels as a result of stagnant flow, and are composed of crystals of calcium carbonate-fluorohydroxyapatite.

Effects on adjacent teeth. The roots of teeth are often resorbed or displaced by an adjacent vascular lesion. Also, developing teeth may be larger and erupt earlier when in an intimate relationship with a hemangioma (Fig. 22.61).

Differential Interpretation

Contrast-enhanced MDCT, conventional MR, and MR angiography are useful modalities for aiding the differential interpretation of any vascular lesion and other neoplasms of the jaws. Conventional angiography is a radiologic procedure performed by injecting a radiopaque contrast agent into an artery. The distribution of the contrast in the vascular neoplasm can be seen in real time, and provide important information about both size and extent, as well as the vessels involved in feeding the hemangioma. MR angiography is now being used routinely for the same purposes without the necessity of an intraarterial

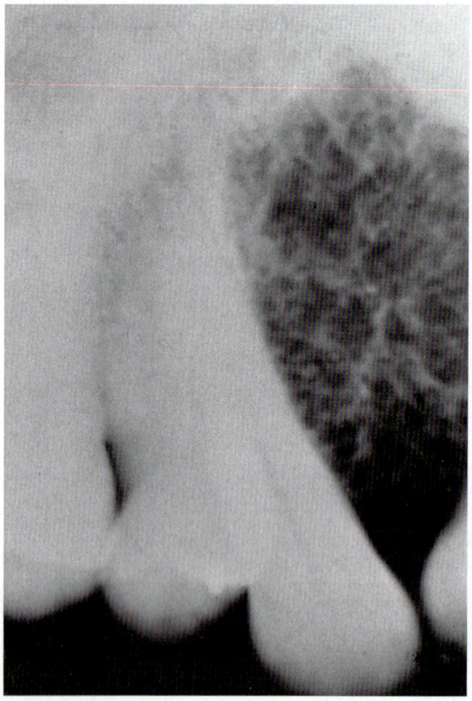

Fig. 22.57 Hemangioma in the anterior maxilla shows a coarse trabecular pattern. (Courtesy Dr. E. J. Burkes, Chapel Hill, NC.)

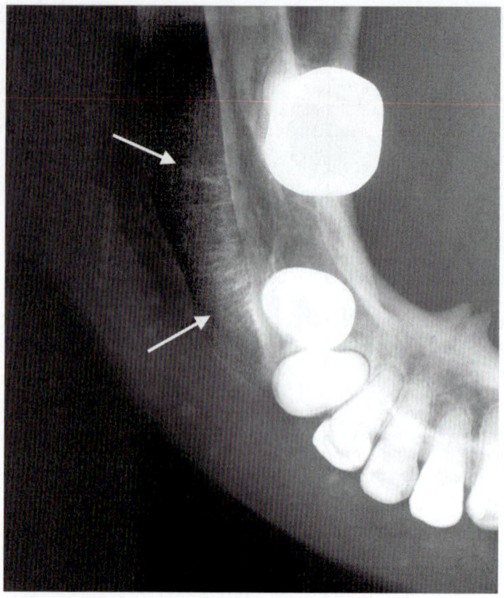

Fig. 22.59 Occlusal image of a central hemangioma of the mandible with adjacent spiculation (arrows). This pattern has a very similar appearance to the spiculation seen in osteosarcoma.

injection of contrast. When a hemangioma produces a sunray, spiculated bone pattern at its periphery, the appearance may be difficult to differentiate from a bone-forming malignancy.

Management

Central hemangiomas should be treated without delay because trauma that disrupts the integrity of the affected jaw may result in lethal exsanguination. Specifically, embolization (introduction of inert materials into the lesion through the vasculature), surgery (en bloc resection with ligation of the feeder vessel), and sclerosing techniques have been used to manage hemangiomas.

Arteriovenous Malformation

Disease Mechanism

The arteriovenous malformation (A-V) is not a neoplasm. Rather, it represents a direct communication between an artery and a vein that bypasses the intervening capillary system. The A-V malformation is included in this chapter because its pattern of enlargement has similarities to the way in which a neoplasm enlarges.

An A-V malformation can occur anywhere in the body, and it usually develops as a result of trauma, but in rare instances it may be a developmental anomaly. The head and neck are the most common sites, and A-V malformations can arise centrally in the jaw and the adjacent soft tissues.

Clinical Features

The clinical appearance of a central A-V malformation can vary considerably, depending on the extent of bone or soft tissue involvement. The lesion may expand bone, and a mass may be present in the overlying soft tissue. The soft tissue swelling may have a purple discoloration, and palpation or auscultation of the swelling may reveal a pulse. Furthermore, aspiration produces blood. Recognition of the hemorrhagic nature of these lesions is of utmost importance because extraction of an associated tooth may be immediately followed by life-threatening bleeding.

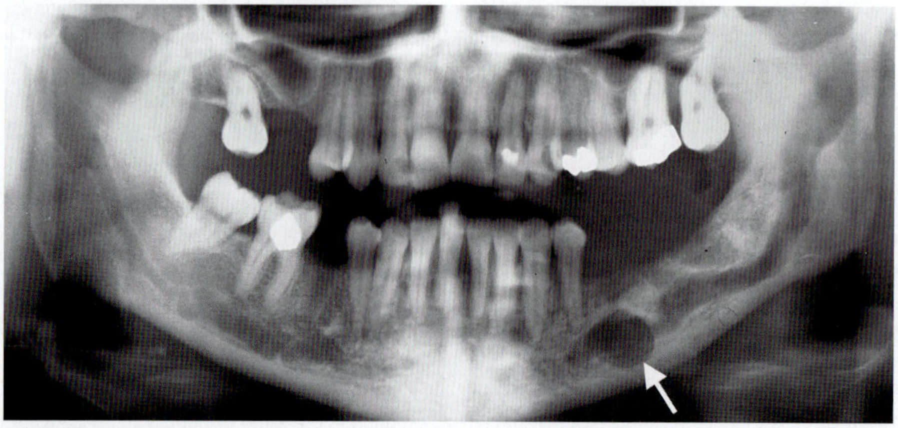

Fig. 22.58 Panoramic image of a vascular lesion within the left mandibular canal. The canal is enlarged and has an irregular, serpiginous path, and the mental foramen is enlarged *(arrow)*.

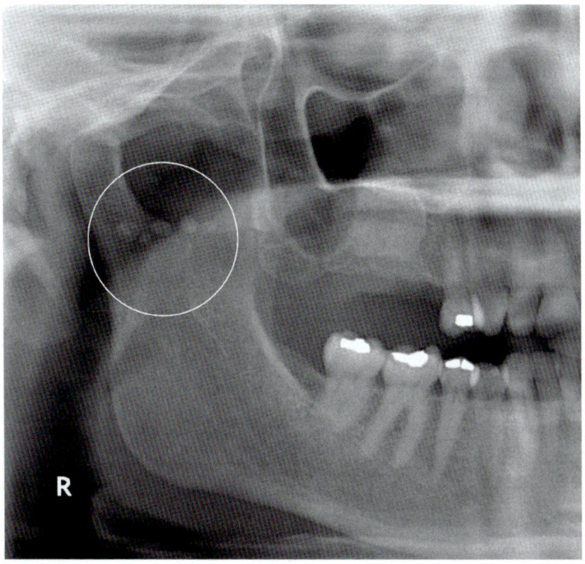

Fig. 22.60 A cropped panoramic image shows multiple phleboliths superimposed over the right mandibular condylar neck and sigmoid notch area of the mandible *(circle)*.

Imaging Features

Location. These lesions most commonly develop in the retromolar area of the mandible and ramus, and involve the mandibular canal.

Periphery. The borders are usually well defined and corticated.

Internal structure. The A-V malformation is radiolucent, although the tortuous path of an enlarged vessel in bone may give it a multilocular appearance (Fig. 22.62).

Effects on surrounding structures. Both central lesions and lesions in adjacent soft tissue can resorb bone. The inferior alveolar canal may take on a serpiginous appearance in a manner similar to hemangioma.

Effects on adjacent teeth. The roots of teeth may be resorbed or displaced by an adjacent vascular lesion.

Differential Interpretation

As with hemangiomas, contrast-enhanced MDCT, conventional MR, and MR angiography are useful modalities for aiding the differential interpretation of A-V malformations as well as the identification of a feeder vessel (Fig. 22.63). The differential interpretation is similar to hemangiomas and includes multilocular lesions.

Management

An A-V malformation is treated surgically.

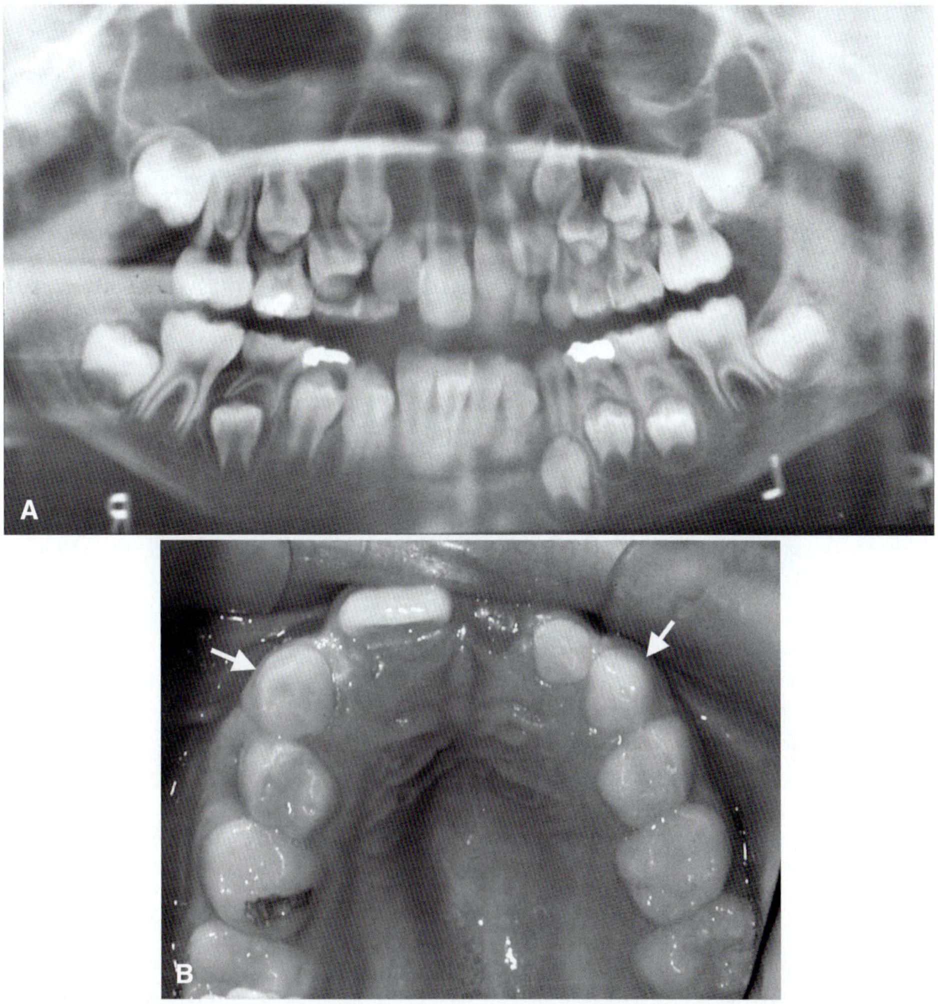

Fig. 22.61 A panoramic image (A) demonstrates the effect of an adjacent soft tissue hemangioma on the developing dentition. The root development and eruption of the maxillary right canine and premolar teeth are significantly advanced compared with the left side. A clinical photograph (B) from the same case shows the size asymmetry of the maxillary deciduous canine teeth.

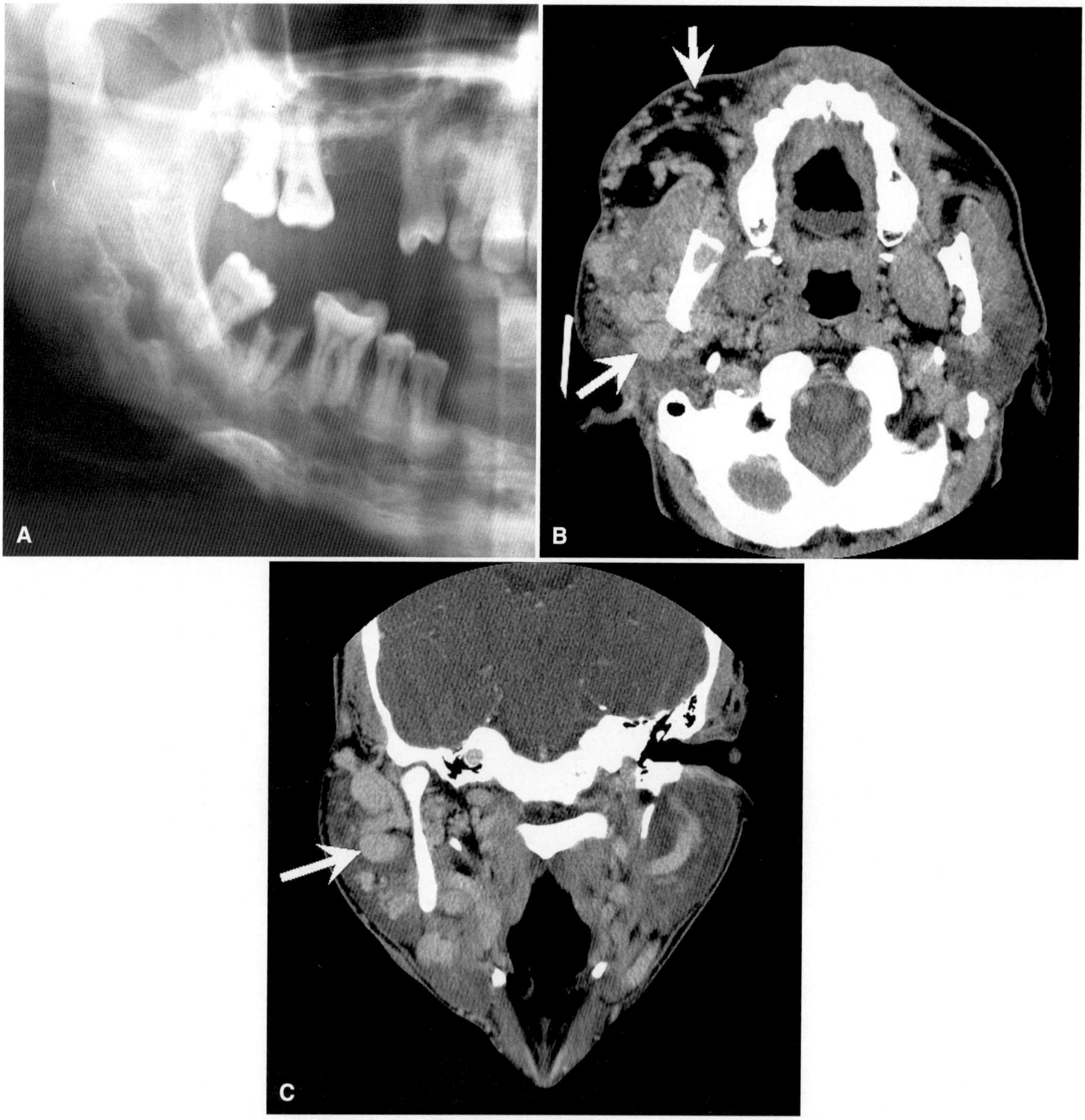

Fig. 22.62 Panoramic image of a patient with an A-V malformation. Note the enlarged, serpiginous inferior alveolar canal (A). Axial (B) and coronal (C) soft tissue multidetector computed tomographic images obtained after administration of intravascular contrast medium fills the feeder vessels of the malformation, and causes the blood vessels to be more radiopaque *(arrows)*.

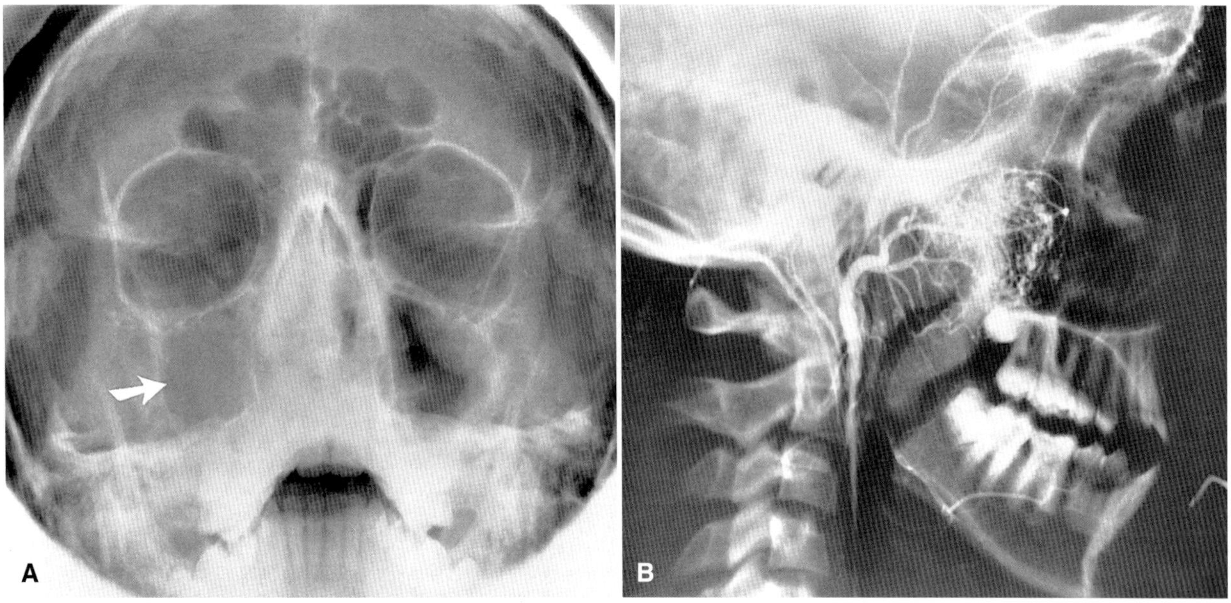

Fig. 22.63 Waters image radiograph shows a radiopacified right maxillary sinus *(arrow)* due to the presence of an A-V malformation (A). The lateral skull view (B) was made following the injection of radiopaque contrast material as part of an angiographic examination. The contrast agent serves to enhance visualization. (Courtesy Dr. G. Himadi, Chapel Hill, NC.)

BIBLIOGRAPHY

Gomes IP, Bastos VC, Guimarães LM. The molecular basis of odontogenic cysts and tumours. *J Oral Pathol Med.* 2023;52:351-356.

Nosé V, Lazar AJ. Update from the 5th edition of the World Health Organization classification of head and neck tumors: familiar tumor syndromes. *Head Neck Pathol.* 2022;16:143-157.

Soluk-Tekkesin M, Wright JM. The World Health Organization classification of odontogenic lesions: a summary of the changes of the 2022 (5th) edition. *Turk Patoloji Derg.* 2022;38:168-184.

Adenomatoid Odontogenic Tumor

Bansal SP, Shaikh S, Arvandekar AS, et al. Analysis of 55 cases of adenomatoid odontogenic tumor in an Indian population and review of the literature. *Med Oral Patol Oral Cir Bucal.* 2022;27:e85-e92.

Reichart PA, Philipsen HP, Khongkhunthian P, et al. Immunoprofile of the adenomatoid odontogenic tumor. *Oral Dis.* 2017;23(6):731-736. doi:10.1111/odi.12572.

Ameloblastic Fibroma

Atarbashi-Moghadam S, Ghomayshi M, Sijanivandi S. Unusual microscopic changes of ameloblastic fibroma and ameloblastic fibro-odontoma: a systematic review. *J Clin Exp Dent.* 2019;11:e476-e481.

Buchner A, Vered M. Ameloblastic fibroma: a stage in the development of a hamartomatous odontoma or a true neoplasm? Critical analysis of 162 previously reported cases plus 10 new cases. *Oral Surg Oral Med Oral Pathol Oral Radiol.* 2013;116:598-606.

Ameloblastoma

da Silva LAM, Filho SRC, Saraiva MJD, et al. Clinical radiographic and histopathologic analysis of craniopharyngeomas and ameloblastomas: a systematic review. *Head Neck Pathol.* 2022;16:1195-1222.

Kim S, Jang HS. Ameloblastoma: a clinical, radiographic, and histopathologic analysis of 71 cases. *Oral Surg Oral Med Oral Pathol Oral Radiol Endod.* 2001;91:649-653.

Aneurysmal Bone Cyst

Buraczewski J, Dabska P. Pathogenesis of aneurysmal bone cyst: relationship between the aneurysmal bone cyst and fibrous dysplasia of bone. *Cancer.* 1971;28:597-604.

Restrepo R, Zahrah D, Pelaez L, et al. Update on aneurysmal bone cyst: pathophysiology, histology, imaging and treatment. *Pediatr Radiol.* 2022;52:1601-1614.

Triantafillidou K, Venetis G, Karakinaris G, et al. Variable histopathological features of 6 cases of aneurysmal bone cysts developed in the jaws: review of the literature. *J Craniomaxillofac Surg.* 2012;40:33-38.

Calcifying Epithelial Odontogenic Tumor

Ruddocks LA, Fitzpatrick SG, Bhattacharyya I, et al. Calcifying epithelial odontogenic tumor: a case series spanning 25 years and review of the literature. *Oral Surg Oral Med Oral Pathol Oral Radiol.* 2021;131:684-693.

Kaplan I, Buckner A, Caleron S, et al. Radiological and clinical features of calcifying epithelial odontogenic tumor. *Dentomaxillofac Radiol.* 2001; 30:22-28.

Cementoblastoma

Ide F, Sakamoto S, Miyazaki Y. The true history of cementoblastoma. *Head Neck Pathol.* 2023;17:528-533.

Van Hoe S, Shaheen E, de Faria Vasconcelos K, et al. Contribution of three-dimensional images in the planning of cementoblastoma resection. *BJR Case Rep.* 2021;7:20200156.

Central Central Giant Cell Lesions

Carlos R, Sedano HO. Intralesional corticosteroids as an alternative treatment for central giant cell granuloma. *Oral Surg Oral Med Oral Pathol Oral Radiol Endod.* 2002;93:161-166.

de Lang J, van den Akker HP, Veldhujzen van Zanten GO, et al. Calcitonin therapy in central giant cell granuloma of the jaw: a randomized double-blind placebo-controlled study. *Int J Oral Maxillofac Surg.* 2006;35: 791-795.

Tahmasbi-Arashlow M, Patel PB, Nair MK, et al. Cone-beam computed tomographic imaging of central giant cell granuloma. A comprehensive review. *Imaging Sci Dent.* 2022;52:123-131.

Central Odontogenic Fibroma

Handlers JP, Abrams AM, Melrose RJ, et al. Central odontogenic fibroma: clinicopathologic features of 19 cases and review of the literature. *J Oral Maxillofac Surg.* 1991;49:46-54.

Correa Pontes FS, Lacerda de Souza L, Paula de Paula L, et al. Central odontogenic fibroma: an updated systematic review of cases reported in the literature with emphasis on recurrence influencing factors. *J Craniomaxillofac Surg*. 2018;46:1753-1757.

Cherubism

Bianchi SD, Boccardi A, Mela F, et al. The computed tomographic appearances of cherubism. *Skeletal Radiol*. 1987;16:6-10.

Schreuder WH, van der Wal JE, de Lange J, et al. Multiple versus solitary giant cell lesions of the jaw: similar or distinct entities. *Bone*. 2021; 149:115935.

Dense Bone Island

McDonnel D. Dense bone island: a review of 107 patients. *Oral Surg Oral Med Oral Pathol*. 1993;76:124-128.

Petrikowski GC, Peters E. Longitudinal radiographic assessment of dense bone islands of the jaws. *Oral Surg Oral Med Oral Pathol Oral Radiol Endod*. 1997;83:627-634.

Desmoplastic Fibroma

Kahraman D, Karakoyunlu B, Karagrece U, et al. Desmoplastic fibroma of the jaw bones: a series of twenty-two cases. *J Bone Oncol*. 2020;26:100333.

Hemangioma

Lund BA, Dahlin DC. Hemangiomas of the mandible and maxilla. *J Oral Surg*. 1964;22:234-242.

Zlotogorski A, Buchner A, Kaffe I, et al. Radiological features of central haemangioma of the jaws. *Dentomaxillofac Radiol*. 2005;34:292-296.

Hyperostosis

Jainkittivong A, Langlais RP. Buccal and palatal exostosis: prevalence and concurrence with tori. *Oral Surg Oral Med Oral Pathol Oral Radiol Endod*. 2000;90:48-53.

Odontogenic Myxoma

Chrcanovic BR, Gomez RS. Odontogenic myxoma: an updated analysis of 1,692 cases reported in the literature. *Oral Dis*. 2019;75:676-683.

Dotta JH, Miotto LN, Spin-Neto R, et al. Odontogenic myxoma: systematic review and bias analysis. *Eur J Clin Invest*. 2020;50:e13214.

Neurofibromatosis

Ahlawat S, Blakeley JO, Langmead S, et al. Current status and recommendations for imaging in neurofibromatosis type 1, neurofibromatosis type 2, and schwannomatosis. *Skeletal Radiol*. 2020;49:199-219.

Lee L, Yan YH, Pharoah MJ. Radiographic features of the mandible in neurofibromatosis: a report of 10 cases and review of the literature. *Oral Surg Oral Med Oral Pathol Oral Radiol Endod*. 1996;81:361-367.

Tamura R. Current understanding of neurofibromatosis Type 1, 2 and schwannomatosis. *Int J Mol Sci*. 2021;22:5850.

Odontoma

Kaugars GE, Miller ME, Abbey LM. Odontomas. *Oral Surg Oral Med Oral Pathol*. 1989;67:172-176.

Pippi R. Odontomas and supernumerary teeth: is there a common origin? *Int J Med Sci*. 2014;11:1282-1297.

Soluk Tekkesin M, Pehlivan S, Olgac V, et al. Clinical and histopathological investigation of odontomas: review of the literature and presentation of 160 cases. *J Oral Maxillofac Surg*. 2012;70:1358-1361.

Osteoblastoma

Alvares Capelozza AL, Gião Dezotti MS, Casati Alvares L, et al. Osteoblastoma of the mandible: systematic review of the literature and report of a case. *Dentomaxillofac Radiol*. 2005;34:1-8.

Jones AC, Prihoda TJ, Kacher JE, et al. Osteoblastoma of the maxilla and mandible: a report of 24 cases, review of the literature, and discussion of its relationship to osteoid osteoma of the jaws. *Oral Surg Oral Med Oral Pathol Oral Radiol Endod*. 2006;102:639-650.

Osteoma

Dinarvand P, Davaro EP, Doan JV, et al. Familial adenomatous polyposis syndrome: an update and review of extraintestinal manifestations. *Arch Pathol Lab Med*. 2019;143:1382-1398.

Earwaker J. Paranasal osteomas: a review of 46 cases. *Skeletal Radiol*. 1993; 22:417-423.

Thakker NS, Evans DG, Horner K, et al. Florid oral manifestations in an atypical familial adenomatous polyposis family with late presentation of colorectal polyps. *J Oral Pathol Med*. 1996;25:459-462.

Schwannoma

Minowa K, Sakakibara N, Yoshikawa K, et al. CT and MRI findings of intraosseous schwannoma of the mandible: a case report. *Dentomaxillofac Radiol*. 2007;36:113-116.

Torus

Eggen S, Natvig B. Concurrence of torus mandibularis and torus palatinus. *Scand J Dent Res*. 1994;102:60-63.

Eggan S, Natvig B, Gåsemyr J. Variation in torus palatinus prevalence in Norway. *Scand J Dent Res*. 1994;102:54-59.

23

Diseases Affecting the Structure of Bone

Ernest W.N. Lam

DISEASE MECHANISM

Coordination of the activities of bone-forming (i.e., osteoblasts), bone-maintaining (i.e., osteocytes), and bone-removing (i.e., osteoclasts) cells regulates the normal structure of bone. Indeed, it has been estimated that between 5% and 10% of total bone volume in the adult skeleton is replaced each year. Some disease processes may produce abnormalities in the bone through disturbances in the balance of serum concentrations of calcium and phosphate, and these may dysregulate osteoblasts, osteocytes, and osteoclasts (Fig. 23.1). A disease that alters the balance of calcium and phosphate levels can result in the abnormal formation of bone and teeth.

Bone dysplasias form another group of abnormalities, characterized by a dysregulation of the normally coordinated activities of osteoblasts and osteoclasts; however, here the normal bone is replaced with a proliferation of fibrous connective tissue and immature or poorly formed bone. These entities, often referred to by the histopathologic term "fibro-osseous lesions," encompass a broad group of disease processes ranging from conditions of bone cell dysregulation to neoplasms. In oral and maxillofacial radiology, we prefer the more macroscopic term of "bone dysplasia" to describe the uncoordinated activity of bone cells.

DIAGNOSTIC IMAGING

Diagnostic imaging has many important roles in the assessment and follow-up of diseases and conditions that affect bone and bone turnover. Imaging may be useful in describing the extent of disease and determining if one or more bones are involved. Furthermore, imaging, particularly intraoral imaging, may be useful in characterizing changes in the bone pattern of the jaws.

Various imaging modalities may be used to aid in these diagnoses. Intraoral images are often the first step in an investigation as they provide the best spatial resolution and reveal subtle changes to the intraosseous architecture of the jaws, as well as involvement of the periodontal ligament (PDL) space and lamina dura. Panoramic imaging and skull imaging can help delineate the extent of bone involvement, and cone beam computed tomography (CBCT) and multidetector computed tomography (MDCT) can demonstrate the involvement of areas of bone that cannot be resolved on planar images. Imaging in the form of nuclear medicine may provide useful information as to the metabolic activity of the bone.

Because some of the diseases affecting bone may involve the skeleton more broadly, the changes manifested in the appearance of the jaws in diagnostic images are usually generalized and often nonspecific, making it difficult to identify the diseases based on imaging characteristics alone (Table 23.1). The general changes that can be seen in the jaws may include the following:

1. Change in size and shape of the bone
2. Change in the number, size, and orientation of trabeculae
3. Change in the number and size of marrow spaces
4. Altered thickness and density of cortical borders
5. Increase or decrease in overall bone density

Changes to the bone cortex or trabeculae can result in a decrease or increase in bone density. Because many of the technical parameters used to produce diagnostic images influence the density of the image (i.e., exposure time, kVp, and mA), it may be difficult to detect genuine changes in the density of bone caused by systemic disease. Systemic conditions that decrease bone density do not affect mature teeth; however, the normal density of the teeth may appear more prominent than normal against the generally more radiolucent-appearing jawbone. In severe cases, the teeth may appear to lose bone support. As well, cortical structures can appear thin, become less defined, and occasionally may not be visualized. A true increase in bone density may be detected by a loss of contrast between the inferior cortex of the mandible and the cancellous bone as the radiopacity of the cancellous bone approaches that of cortical bone. Often the radiolucent outline of the inferior alveolar nerve canal appears more distinct in contrast to the surrounding radiopaque dense bone.

Some systemic diseases that occur during tooth formation may result in dental alterations. Lamina dura is part of the bone structure of the alveolar process, but because it is usually examined in conjunction with the PDL space and roots of teeth, it is included with the description of the dental structures (Table 23.2). Changes to teeth and associated structures include the following:

1. Accelerated or delayed eruption
2. Tooth hypoplasia
3. Tooth hypocalcification
4. Loss of a distinct lamina dura

The teeth and their supporting structures often exhibit no detectable changes associated with systemic diseases. However, the first symptoms of a disease may occasionally manifest as a dental problem.

METABOLIC BONE ABNORMALITIES

Osteopenia

Disease Mechanism

Osteopenia is a radiologic appearance that reflects an imbalance that favors resorption. This change is reflected as a generalized loss of normal cancellous bone architecture as well as cortical density and a generalized increase in the radiolucency of the bone. Bone mass normally increases from infancy to about 30 years of age; however, after this age, there is a gradual and progressive decline, occurring at a rate of about 8% per decade in females and 3% per decade in males. The onset of osteopenia is barely perceptible, but it may become more prominent as patients age. To some degree, it can be considered a variation of normal.

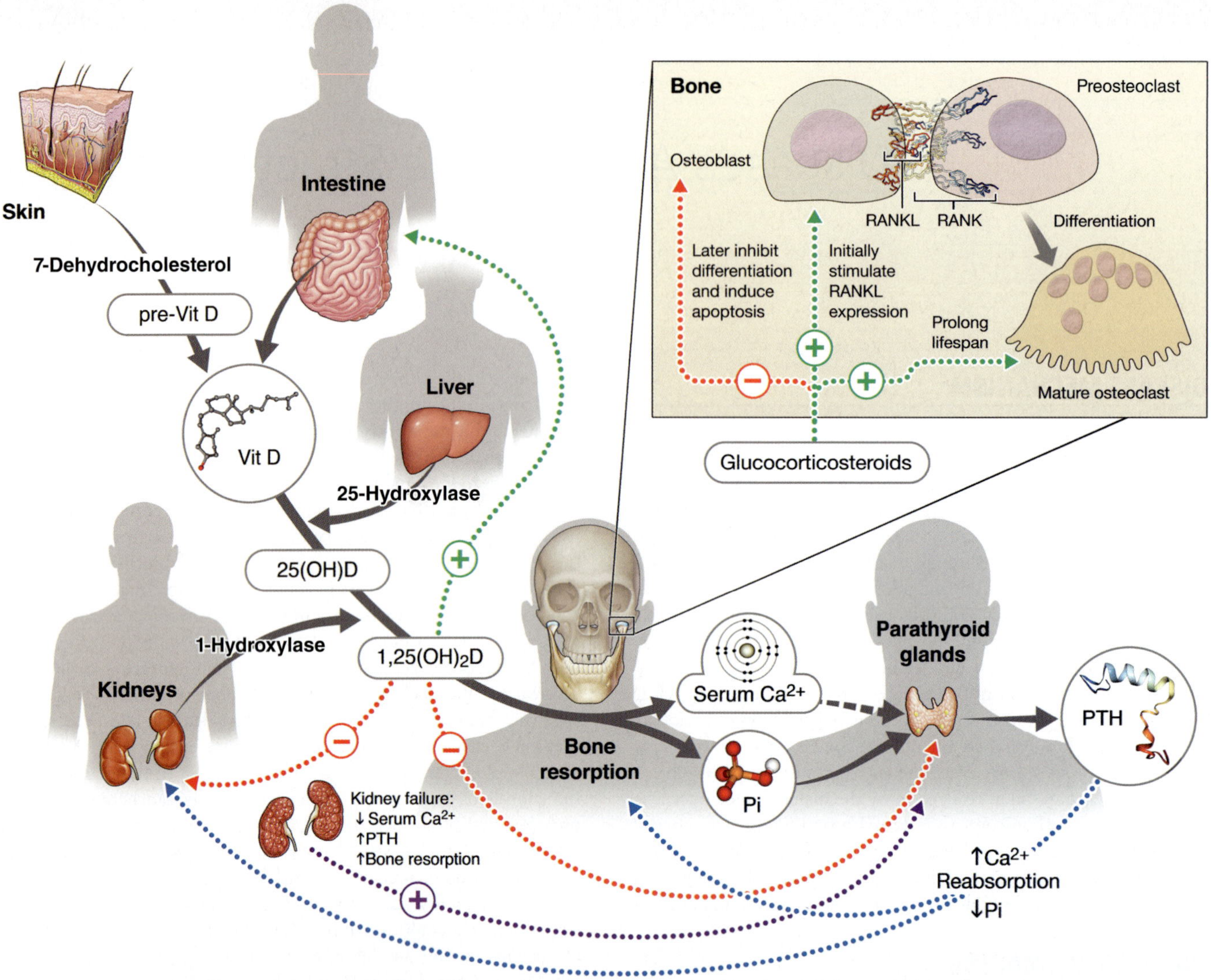

Fig. 23.1 This figure shows the activity of vitamin D, parathyroid hormone *(PTH)*, and glucocorticosteroids in bone and other tissues and outlines their roles in maintaining normal serum levels of calcium *(Ca^{2+})* and inorganic phosphate *(Pi)* in bone metabolism. Bone metabolism is a balance of osteoblastic bone formation and osteoclastic bone resorption. A plus *(+)* sign indicates a promotion effect, and a minus *(−)* sign indicates an inhibitory effect. Vitamin D, either ingested or produced in the skin, undergoes a series of hydroxylation reactions, first in the liver and then in the kidneys, to the active form of 1,23-dihydroxy vitamin D *(1,23$(OH)_2$D)* *(solid dark gray arrows)*. 1,23$(OH)_2$D promotes Ca^{2+} and Pi absorption in the intestine *(dotted green line)* and tips the balance of bone metabolism in favor of resorption, releasing Ca^{2+} and Pi from the bone to the serum. Bone resorption is accomplished through the expression of receptor activator of nuclear factor kappa-B ligand *(RANKL)* by osteoblasts, which interacts with a receptor activator of nuclear factor kappa-B *(RANK)* receptor on preosteoclasts. This induces differentiation of these cells into active osteoclasts that can resorb the bone *(upper right inset box)*. 1,23$(OH)_2$D can also inhibit the last hydroxylation of its precursor (23(OH)D) within the kidneys *(dashed red arrow)* and inhibit the parathyroid glands from producing PTH *(dashed red arrow)*. PTH can increase serum Ca^{2+} by directly increasing bone resorption through promoting the expression of RANKL and the differentiation of osteoclasts *(dashed blue arrow)*. PTH also increases serum Ca^{2+} by increasing reabsorption of Ca^{2+} in the kidneys and promoting the hydroxylation of vitamin D to its active form in the kidneys *(dashed blue arrow)*. However, elevated serum Ca^{2+} can reduce production of PTH by the parathyroid glands *(dashed dark gray arrow)*. In the event of kidney failure, PTH may be upregulated to increase serum calcium *(dashed purple arrow)*. Glucocorticosteroids initially increase bone resorption through increased osteoblastic expression of RANKL, thus increasing osteoclast differentiation; thus, they can prolong the lifespan of the osteoclast. Later, glucocorticosteroids reduce bone formation by limiting differentiation and inducing apoptosis of osteoblasts.

TABLE 23.1 Changes in Bone Observed in Systemic Disease[a]

	BONES				
			TRABECULAE		
Systemic Disease	Density	Size of Jaws	Increase	Decrease	Granular
Hyperparathyroidism	Decrease	No	Yes	Yes	Yes
Hypoparathyroidism	Rare increase	No	No	No	No
Hyperpituitarism	No	Large	No	No	No
Hypopituitarism	No	Small	No	No	No
Hyperthyroidism	Decrease	No	No	No	No
Hypothyroidism	No	Small	No	No	No
Cushing syndrome	Decrease	No	No	Yes	Yes
Osteoporosis	Decrease	No	No	Yes	No
Rickets	Decrease	No	No	Yes	No
Osteomalacia	Rare decrease	No	No	Rare decrease	No
Hypophosphatasia	Decrease	No	No	Yes	No
Renal osteodystrophy	Decrease; rare increase	Large	Rare	Yes	Yes
Hypophosphatemia	Decrease	No	No	Yes	Yes
Osteopetrosis	Increase	Large			
Sickle cell anemia	Decrease	Large maxilla			
Thalassemia	Decrease	Large maxilla			

[a]This table summarizes the major imaging changes to bone with endocrine and metabolic bone diseases. It does not include all the possible variable appearances.

TABLE 23.2 Effects on Teeth and Associated Structures[a]

Systemic Disease	Hypocalcification	Hypoplasia	Large Pulp Chamber	Loss of Lamina Dura	Loss of Teeth	Eruption
Hyperparathyroidism	No	No	No	Yes	Rare	No
Hypoparathyroidism	No	Yes	No	No	No	Delayed
Hyperpituitarism	No	No	No	No	No	Supraeruption
Hypopituitarism	No	No	No	No	No	Delayed
Hyperthyroidism	No	No	No	Thin	Yes	Early
Hypothyroidism	No	No	No	No	Yes	Delayed
Cushing syndrome	No	No	No	Partial	No	Premature
Osteoporosis	No	No	No	Thin	No	No
Rickets	Yes, enamel	Yes, enamel	No	Thin	No	Delayed
Osteomalacia	No	No	No	Thin	No	No
Hypophosphatasia	Yes	Yes	Yes	Yes	Yes	Delayed
Renal osteodystrophy	Yes	Yes	No	Yes	No	No
Hypophosphatemia	Yes	Yes	Yes	Yes	Yes	No
Osteopetrosis	Yes	Rare	No	Thick	Yes	Delayed

[a]This table summarizes the major imaging changes that can occur to teeth and associated structures with endocrine and metabolic bone diseases. It does not include all the possible variable appearances.

Clinical Features

When osteopenia becomes pronounced, patients may undergo a diagnostic test known as dual-energy x-ray photon absorptiometry (DEXA), and they may be diagnosed with osteoporosis. Postmenopausal women are most at risk. The most important clinical concern of osteoporosis is fracture, which may involve the distal radius, proximal femur, ribs, and vertebrae. Patients may also develop bone pain. Planar imaging techniques used in dentistry such as a panoramic image cannot be used to reliably diagnose osteoporosis.

Imaging Features

Effects on the teeth and jaws. Osteopenia is seen as a generalized reduction in bone density, and this change can be observed by comparing the bone to the adjacent teeth. In a patient with osteopenia, the teeth tend to appear relatively more radiopaque and stand out against the relatively more radiolucent-appearing bone. The trabeculae may appear shorter and more delicate in nature, although any reduction in the number of trabeculae may be less evident in the alveolar processes, possibly because of loading forces applied to bone by teeth. There may also be a loss of cortical homogeneity and thickness, and these changes can commonly affect the inferior cortex of the mandible (Fig. 23.2). Occasionally the lamina dura may also appear thinner.

Attempts have been made to use commonly acquired periapical and panoramic images to determine the risk of osteoporosis; however, this has proven unreliable. Novel techniques to analyze the trabecular pattern in intraoral images are, however, being developed.

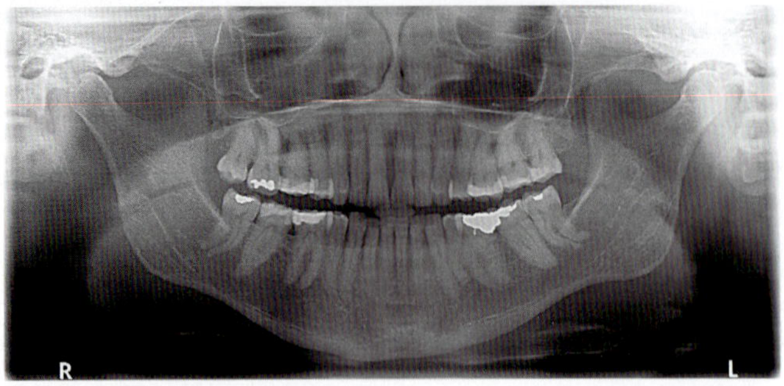

Fig. 23.2 Generalized osteopenia is evident as a change to the normal trabecular bone pattern, an increase in cortical heterogeneity, and thinning of the inferior cortex of the mandible. Note the prominence of the dentition on the background of the demineralized bone.

Management

Should the osteopenic appearance be subsequently diagnosed as osteoporosis, weight-bearing exercise programs, the administration of estrogen, calcium, vitamin D, and in more severe cases, pharmacologic inhibitors of osteoclastic bone resorption (i.e., bisphosphonates) and receptor activator of nuclear factor kappa-B ligand (RANKL) may help reduce the rate of bone mineral loss.

Rickets and Osteomalacia

Disease Mechanism

The term *rickets* is given to a group of disorders that result in the development of soft, fragile bones in growing children. Nutritional rickets is caused by inadequate ingestion of vitamin D (calciferol), or calcium and phosphorus, while hypophosphatemic rickets (formerly vitamin D–resistant rickets) results from a dysregulation of phosphate excretion by the kidneys. In contrast, the term *osteomalacia* is used when the nutritional deficiency affects the adult skeleton.

Calcitriol is the active form of vitamin D, and humans ingest an inactive precursor, calciferol, in our diets. Humans also synthesize calciferol in skin during exposure to the ultraviolet B radiation in sunlight. Calcitriol is synthesized in subsequent chemical reactions in the liver and kidney, although more recent studies suggest that this reaction can occur in other organ systems as well. Rickets and osteomalacia may therefore develop from a lack of sun exposure, inadequate ingestion of vitamin D or calcium in the diet, an inability to synthesize calcitriol in the liver and kidney, or malabsorption of vitamin D in the gastrointestinal tract. In contrast, hypophosphatemic rickets is a group of inherited X-linked disorders in which there is a decrease in serum phosphate levels due to malabsorption of phosphorus in the distal renal tubules of the kidneys.

Normal calcification of the osseous structures requires the correct amounts and ratio of serum calcium and phosphate. Low serum levels can cause low-density bone development, which can result in the abnormal formation of trabeculae. The trabeculae may be short and irregular, and the bone can develop a granular pattern (Fig. 23.3A). Low serum phosphate can also interfere with the normal calcification of dentin, resulting in larger than normal pulp chambers and root canals.

Clinical Features

Rickets. In the first 6 months of life, sharp flexion of the wrist (tetany) or convulsions are the most common clinical signs of rickets. Later in infancy, the skeletal effects of the disease may be more clinically prominent. Craniotabes, a regional softening of the parietal bones, may be the initial sign of the disease. Children with rickets usually have short stature and deformity of the extremities including bowing of the legs, and there may be swelling of the wrists and ankles. Eruption and development of the dentition is delayed, and the enamel and dentin may be hypocalcified.

Osteomalacia. Most patients with osteomalacia have some degree of bone pain as well as muscle weakness of varying severity. Other clinical features include a peculiar waddling or "penguin gait," and tetany.

Imaging Features

Effects on the teeth and jaws. Rickets in infancy or early childhood may result in hypoplasia of the developing teeth with thin enamel and large pulp chambers and root canals (Figs. 23.3B and C and 23.4). This early manifestation of rickets can be seen in diagnostic images and involve both unerupted and erupted teeth. Diagnostic images may also document delayed tooth eruption in early rickets. The cortical borders of tooth follicles may be thin or absent, and the lamina dura of erupted teeth may be thin and sparse. If the disease occurs before the age of 3 years, enamel hypoplasia is fairly common. Rarefying osteitis may occur frequently without an apparent etiology as defects in the dentin and the large pulp chambers may promote ingress of oral microorganisms resulting in pulp necrosis. If the disease is severe, the patient will have premature loss of the teeth.

Effects on the skeleton. The earliest and most prominent feature of rickets is widening of the epiphyses of the long bones. This is a manifestation of the wide uncalcified osteoid seams that are seen histologically. The abnormal biomechanics that result lead to cupping and fraying of the metaphases of the long bones, and the soft weight-bearing bones such as the femur and tibia undergo a characteristic bowing.

In children, incomplete or "greenstick" fractures can occur in bones, while in adults, thin bone cortices can induce pseudofractures, which are poorly calcified, ribbon-like zones extending into bone at approximate right angles to the margin of the bone. These can be seen in the ribs, pelvis, and weight-bearing long bones.

Management

Treatment consists of administering vitamin D supplements, phosphates, and anticalciurics. Serum calcium concentrations must be closely monitored to prevent hypercalcemia and its complications. Nephrocalcinosis is a long-term complication that may arise from treatment.

Hypophosphatasia

Disease Mechanism

Hypophosphatasia is a rare inherited disorder caused by a reduction in the activity of the tissue nonspecific alkaline phosphatase, one of a family of enzymes produced by osteoblasts and odontoblasts that is required for the normal mineralization of osteoid and teeth. When deficient, the enzyme fails to cleave phosphate-containing substances such as inorganic pyrophosphate, which results in the extracellular accumulation of inorganic pyrophosphate—a known inhibitor of hydroxyapatite formation.

Six clinical forms of the disease are recognized, depending on the age at diagnosis: two perinatal forms, one that is nonlethal (benign) and one that is lethal; infantile, childhood, and adult forms; and odontohypophosphatasia. The disease in individuals with homozygous involvement has an early onset in utero and is usually severe, leading to death within the first year. The less severe forms of the condition have an autosomal recessive mode of transmission, and the milder forms have variable patterns of inheritance.

Clinical Features

Infants demonstrate bowed limbs and a marked deficiency of skull ossification. Individuals with the milder forms of the disease show poor growth and deformities similar to rickets. There may be a history of

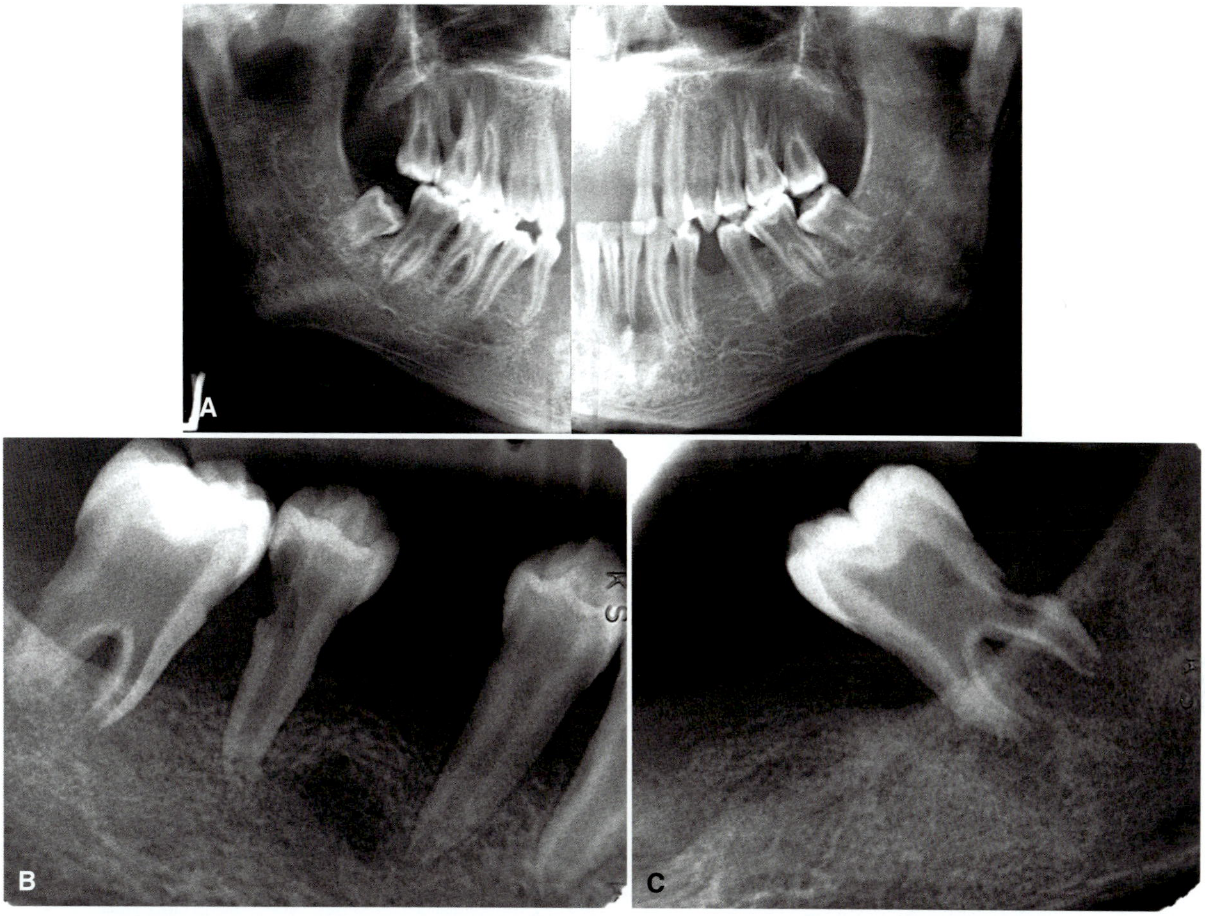

Fig. 23.3 Panoramic image (A) of a patient with hypophosphatemic rickets. Note the generalized osteopenic appearance of the jaws, the lack of bone density, and the large pulp chambers. Periapical images (B and C) of a different patient demonstrate apparent bone loss around the teeth, a granular bone pattern, large pulp chambers, and the open root apices.

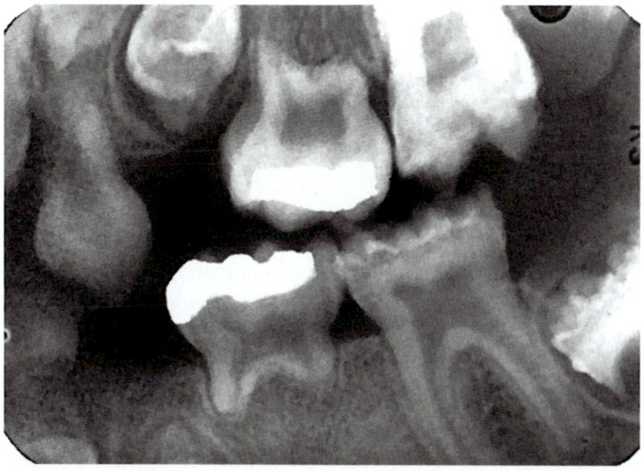

Fig. 23.4 The bite-wing image shows thinning (hypoplasia) and decreased mineralization (hypocalcification) of the enamel in a child with rickets. (Courtesy Dr. H. G. Poyton, Toronto, ON.)

fractures, delayed walking, or bone pain. Approximately 85% of these children show premature loss of the primary teeth, particularly the incisors, and delayed eruption of the permanent dentition. Dental findings are often the first clinical sign of hypophosphatasia and the only sign of odontohypophosphatasia.

Imaging Features

Effects on the teeth and jaws. Both primary and permanent teeth have a thin enamel layer and large pulp chambers and root canals (Fig. 23.5). The teeth may also appear hypoplastic, and they may be lost prematurely. In the jaws, there is a generalized osteopenic appearance to the bones. The cortical bone and lamina dura are thin, and the alveolar processes are poorly calcified and may appear deficient.

Effects on the skeleton. In young children with hypophosphatasia, the long bones show irregular defects in the epiphyses and the skull is poorly calcified. In older children, premature closure of the skull sutures results in gyral impressions on the inner table of the skull that resemble hammered metal (i.e., "beaten copper"). The skull may assume a brachycephalic shape. In adults, there may be generalized osteopenia.

Management

There is no curative treatment for hypophosphatasia; however, enzyme replacement therapy is currently being investigated and has demonstrated efficacy in children with life-threatening hypophosphatasia.

Osteopetrosis

Disease Mechanism

Osteopetrosis, also known as marble bone disease or Albers-Schönberg disease, is an inherited disease that affects the differentiation and function of osteoclasts. The disease is inherited in either an autosomal

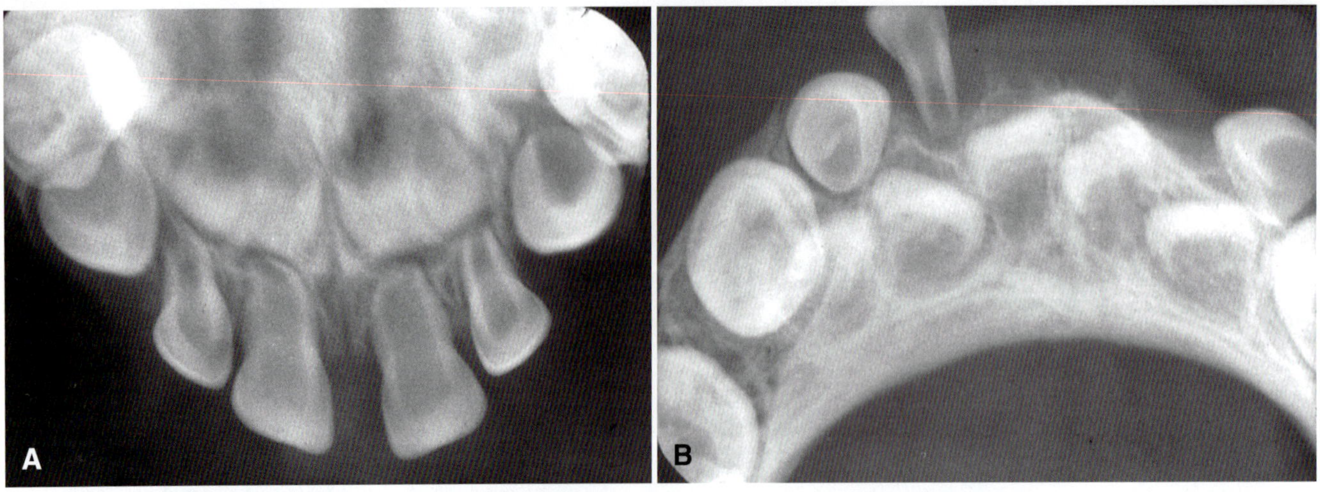

Fig. 23.5 Note the very large pulp chambers in the deciduous dentition in a patient with hypophosphatasia (A) and premature loss of the mandibular incisors (B) on these anterior occlusal images. (Courtesy Dr. H. G. Poyton, Toronto, ON.)

recessive (osteopetrosis congenita) or autosomal dominant (osteopetrosis tarda) manner and results in abnormally functioning osteoclasts that affect the formation of the primary skeleton and abnormal bone turnover thereafter. The failure of bone to remodel normally causes the bones to become densely mineralized, susceptible to infection, and perhaps counterintuitively, fragile and susceptible to fracture.

Clinical Features

The more severe, recessive form of osteopetrosis affects infants and young children; it is invariably fatal early in life. There is progressive deposition of bone, resulting in narrowing of bony canals and foramina. These changes create morphologic defects from hydrocephalus, as well as sensorineural and sensorimotor deficits, including blindness, deafness, vestibular nerve dysfunction, and facial nerve paralysis. The benign, dominant form appears in adults and may be entirely asymptomatic or accompanied by mild signs and symptoms. It may be discovered at any time from childhood to adulthood as an incidental finding, or it may manifest as a bone fracture. The loss of marrow spaces secondary to the deposition of bone in patients with osteopetrosis may also affect the development of red and white blood cells and platelets, resulting in anemia, leukopenia, and thrombocytopenia. Consequently, patients may develop lethargy, be prone to infection, and have longer than normal bleeding times.

In some more chronic cases, bone pain and cranial nerve palsies caused by neural compression may be clinical problems. The increased bone density and relatively poor vascularity result in an increased susceptibility to osteomyelitis, usually from odontogenic inflammatory lesions. This problem is more common in the mandible, where periapical and periodontal inflammatory conditions are common.

Imaging Features

Effects on the teeth and jaws. Effects on teeth may include early tooth loss, missing teeth, malformed roots and crowns, and teeth that are poorly calcified and prone to caries. The normal eruption pattern of the primary and secondary dentitions may be delayed because of the increased bone density or ankylosis. The lamina dura and bone cortices may appear thicker than normal.

The increased radiopacity of the jaws may be so great that the diagnostic image may fail to reveal detail of the bone or the roots of the teeth. The normal interface between cortical and cancellous bone may be lost, and in the mandible, the inferior alveolar canal may appear very prominent. On planar imaging, the bone may appear underexposed due to failure of the incident x-ray beam to penetrate it.

Effects on the skeleton. Bones may become mildly enlarged and show greatly increased radiopacity. Because this condition is systemic, the changes affect all bones bilaterally (Fig. 23.6). The bones can become so radiopaque that the trabecular pattern may not be visible. The homogeneous radiopacity of the cancellous bone also reduces the contrast with the bone cortex.

Management

Treatment of osteopetrosis consists of bone marrow transplantation in an attempt to stimulate the formation of functional osteoclasts. The hematologic complications are managed with systemic steroids. When osteomyelitis develops (Fig. 23.7), it is difficult to treat, and a combination of antibiotics and hyperbaric oxygen therapy is used. It is therefore imperative that odontogenic inflammatory disease not develop in these individuals.

Endocrine Disturbances

Diagnostic Imaging Features

Endocrine disturbances affect the entire body, and the changes manifested in the appearances of the teeth and jaws in diagnostic images are usually generalized and often nonspecific. Therefore, it may be difficult to identify the diseases based on imaging characteristics alone (see Table 23.1).

When systemic diseases manifest during tooth development, the teeth may appear hypoplastic or hypocalcified, and their eruption may be accelerated or delayed. Because the lamina dura is often examined in conjunction with the PDL space and the roots of teeth, it may become less distinct or lost. If the teeth have developed, no detectable changes may be visible. However, the first symptoms of a disease may occasionally manifest as a dental problem.

The general changes that can be seen in the jaws can include thickening of the trabeculae and bone cortices and changes to the sizes and shapes of the bones. Because both technical and patient factors can determine the appearance of bone on a diagnostic image, it may be difficult to detect and quantify genuine changes in bone density when they arise. For example, systemic conditions that may decrease bone

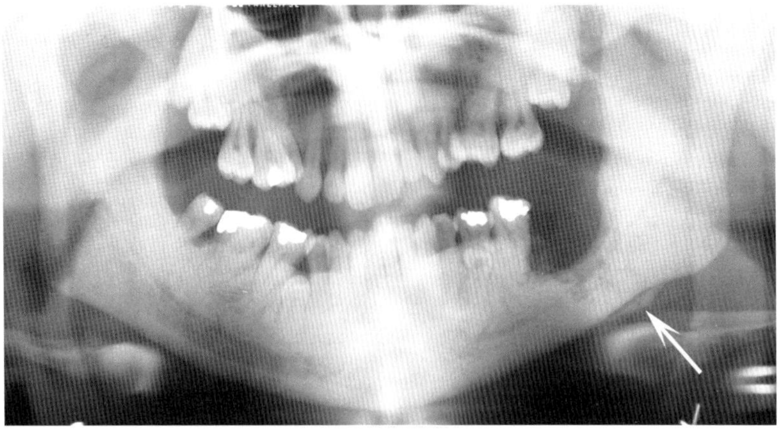

Fig. 23.6 A significant and generalized increase in the radiopacity of the bones is seen on this panoramic image of a patient with osteopetrosis. The inferior alveolar canals are prominently seen and narrowed. Also, there is osteomyelitis in the body of the left mandible with periosteal new bone formation *(arrow)*.

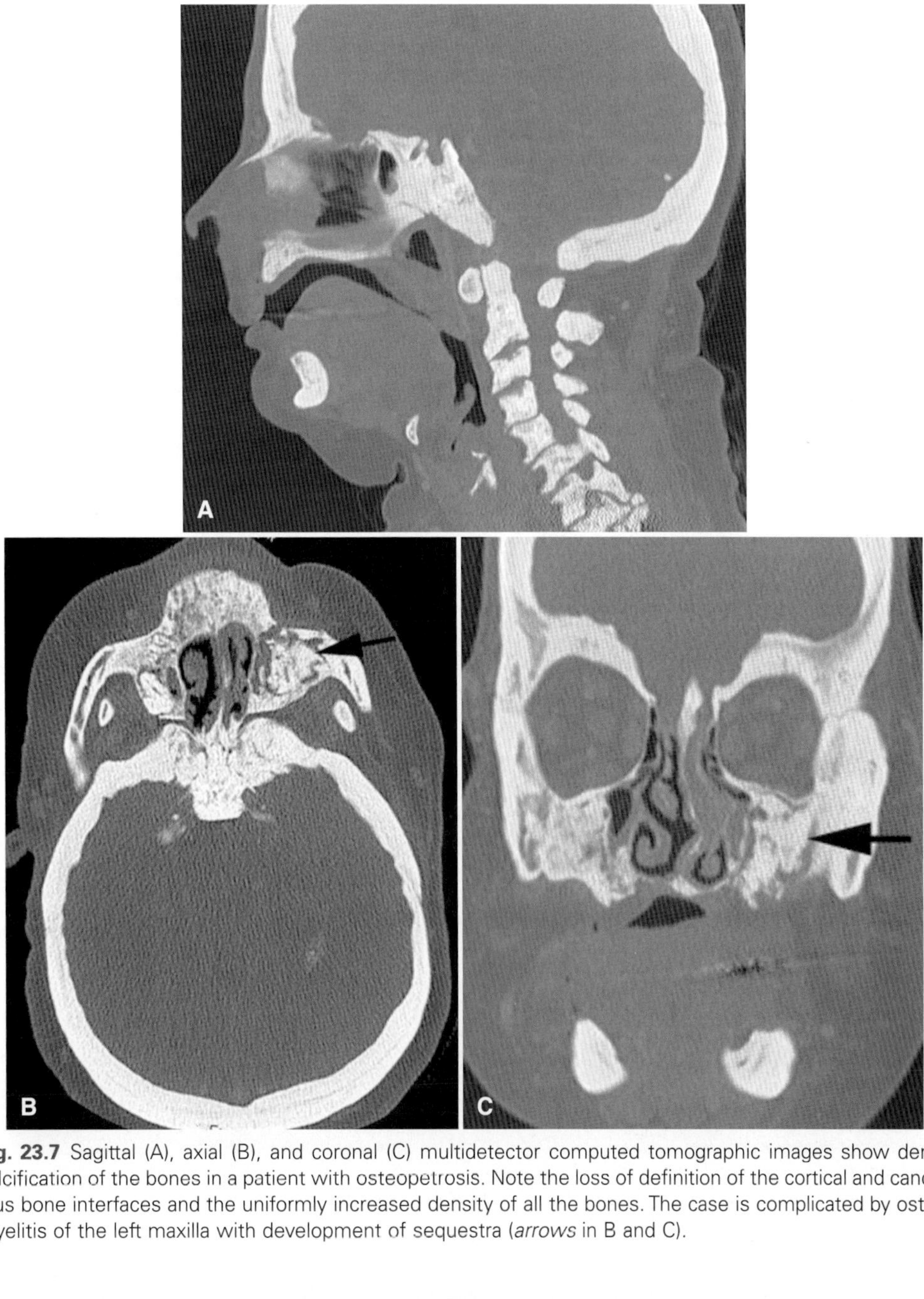

Fig. 23.7 Sagittal (A), axial (B), and coronal (C) multidetector computed tomographic images show dense calcification of the bones in a patient with osteopetrosis. Note the loss of definition of the cortical and cancellous bone interfaces and the uniformly increased density of all the bones. The case is complicated by osteomyelitis of the left maxilla with development of sequestra (*arrows* in B and C).

density generally do not affect mature teeth, and the images of the teeth may appear more prominent against a generally more osteopenic bone pattern in the jaws. In severe cases, the normal supporting structures around the teeth may not be visible. Also, cortical structures may appear thin and less well defined; occasionally they may even disappear. In contrast, an increase in bone density may be seen as a loss of contrast of the cortical/cancellous bone interface as the radiopacity of the cancellous bone approaches that of the cortical bone. Moreover, the radiolucent outline of the inferior alveolar nerve canal may appear more prominent in contrast to the surrounding radiopacity of the more dense bone.

Hyperparathyroidism

Disease Mechanism

Hyperparathyroidism is an endocrine abnormality in which there is an excess of circulating parathyroid hormone (PTH). This excess favors osteoclastic resorption of bone, which mobilizes calcium from the skeleton. The change can alter the normal morphology of bone trabeculae by increasing the renal tubular reabsorption of calcium and increasing calcitriol production. The net result of these changes is an increase in serum calcium levels (Fig. 23.8).

In 80% to 85% of cases, primary hyperparathyroidism is the result of PTH overproduction from an adenoma arising from one of the four parathyroid glands. The incidence of primary hyperparathyroidism is about 0.1%, and the condition can be sporadic or part of a hereditary syndrome, such as hyperparathyroidism–jaw tumor syndrome, which involves tumors of parathyroid glands, jaws, and kidneys. Less frequently, in 10% to 15% of cases, patients may have hyperplastic parathyroid glands that secrete excess PTH.

Secondary hyperparathyroidism develops as a compensatory response in response to hypocalcemia. The underlying hypocalcemia may result from inadequate dietary intake, poor intestinal absorption of vitamin D, or deficient metabolism of vitamin D in the liver or kidneys (renal osteodystrophy). Chronic renal failure produces bone changes by interfering with calcitriol synthesis in the kidneys. The various biologic functions of calcitriol outlined in Fig. 23.1 are hindered, especially the absorption of calcium from the intestines. The result is a state of hypocalcemia and hyperphosphatemia that prevents the normal calcification of bone and teeth, stimulating the parathyroid gland to secrete PTH so that more calcium can be liberated into the blood.

Clinical Features

Primary hyperparathyroidism affects females two to three times more commonly than males, typically in adults 30 to 60 years of age. The clinical manifestations of the disease are related to hypercalcemia, and they cover a broad range of signs and symptoms often summarized as the triad of "stones, bones, and groans": renal calculi; bone complications including osteoporosis, arthritis, and fracture; and gastrointestinal symptoms including peptic ulcers. The combination of hypercalcemia and an elevated serum level of PTH is diagnostic of primary hyperparathyroidism. Serum alkaline phosphatase level, a reliable indicator of bone turnover, may also be elevated in hyperparathyroidism.

The clinical features of secondary hyperparathyroidism are the same as those seen in chronic renal failure. In children, growth retardation and frequent bone fractures may occur. Adults may have a gradual softening and bowing of the bones.

Imaging Features

Effects on the teeth and jaws. In children, there may be hypoplasia and hypocalcification of the teeth which may make enamel difficult to discern on diagnostic images. One of the earliest manifestations of hyperparathyroidism is loss of lamina dura on intraoral images, which occurs in approximately 10% of patients. The extensiveness of this change will depend on the duration and severity of the disease. The loss of lamina dura may also give the root a more tapered appearance because of the loss of image contrast between the tooth and the bone. However, as PTH mobilizes minerals from the skeleton, teeth that are already fully formed are unaffected.

Only about one in five patients with hyperparathyroidism has observable bone changes. In the jaws, there may be demineralization and thinning of bone cortices including the inferior border of the mandible, the cortical borders of the inferior alveolar canal, and the cortical borders of the maxillary sinuses. The density of the jawbones is decreased, resulting in an osteopenic appearance that contrasts with the normal, unaltered density of the teeth (see Fig. 23.8). The elevated rate of bone remodeling can result in an abnormal bone pattern, and the normal trabeculae are replaced by numerous small, more randomly

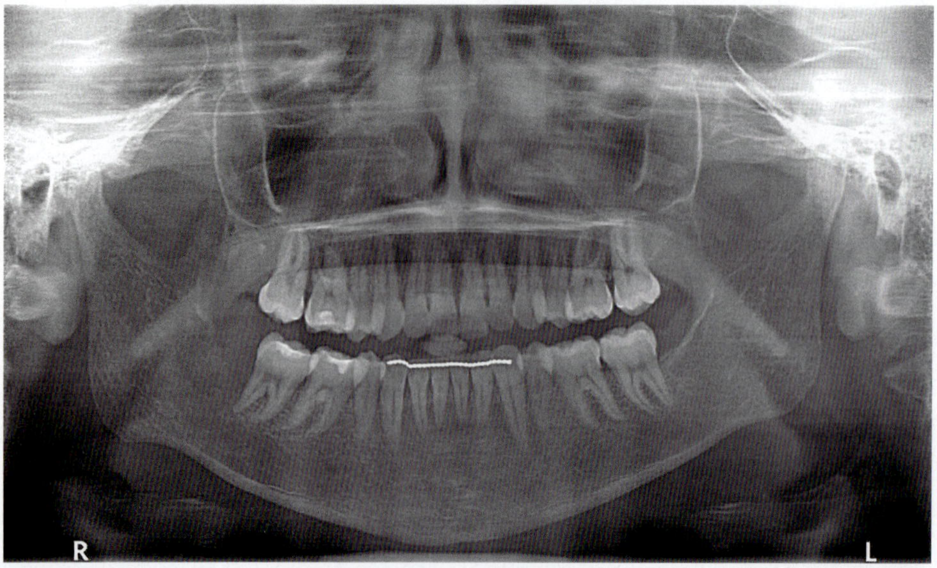

Fig. 23.8 This panoramic image shows generalized osteopenia in a 20-year-old patient with primary hyperparathyroidism. Note how the teeth stand out in contrast to the osteopenic bone.

oriented trabeculae, creating a ground-glass appearance in the diagnostic image (Figs. 23.9 and 23.10). In the skull, the calvarium may take on a granular appearance that is classically known as the "salt and pepper" skull—an appearance caused by loss of the central (diploic) trabeculae and thinning of the cortical tables (Fig. 23.11).

Brown tumors of hyperparathyroidism, which are central giant cell lesions, may also appear in bone, and these are frequently found in the facial bones and jaws, particularly in cases of long-standing disease (Figs. 23.12 and 23.13). The lesions are called brown tumors because of their brown or reddish-brown appearances on gross examination. Brown tumors may be solitary or multiple within a single bone. If a giant cell lesion occurs later than the second decade of life, the patient should be screened for increases in serum calcium, PTH, and alkaline phosphatase.

Effects on the skeleton. One of the earliest and most reliable changes with hyperparathyroidism is subtle erosions of bone from the subperiosteal surfaces of the phalanges of the hands. Demineralization of the skeleton may result in generalized osteopenia; the bone appears "gray" and somewhat "bland." In advanced cases, there may be localized regions of bone loss produced by osteoclastic activity; this is known as osteitis fibrosa cystica. And finally, the increased levels of serum calcium may precipitate in the soft tissues, forming punctate or nodular calcifications in the joints and kidneys.

The features of secondary hyperparathyroidism can be highly variable, with some changes resembling those seen in rickets, and other

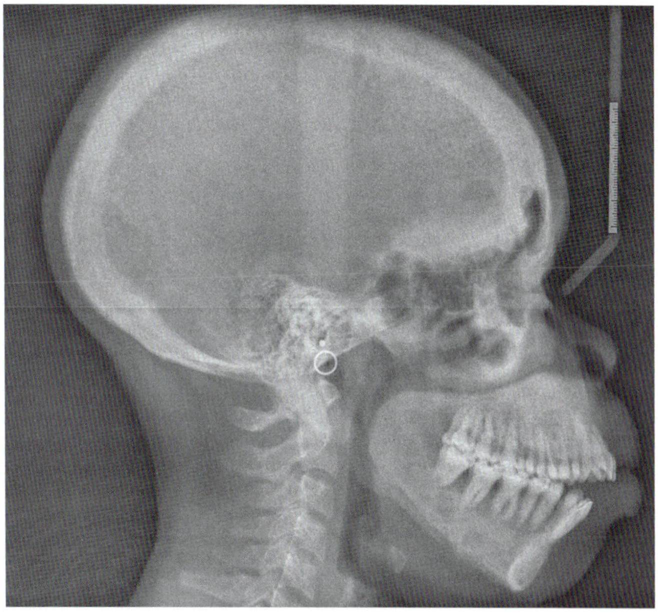

Fig. 23.10 Lateral cephalometric skull image of a patient with renal osteodystrophy reveals a generalized granular bone pattern. Note the loss of a clear interface between the cancellous bone and the cortical bone. (Courtesy Dr. G. Packota, Saskatoon, SK.)

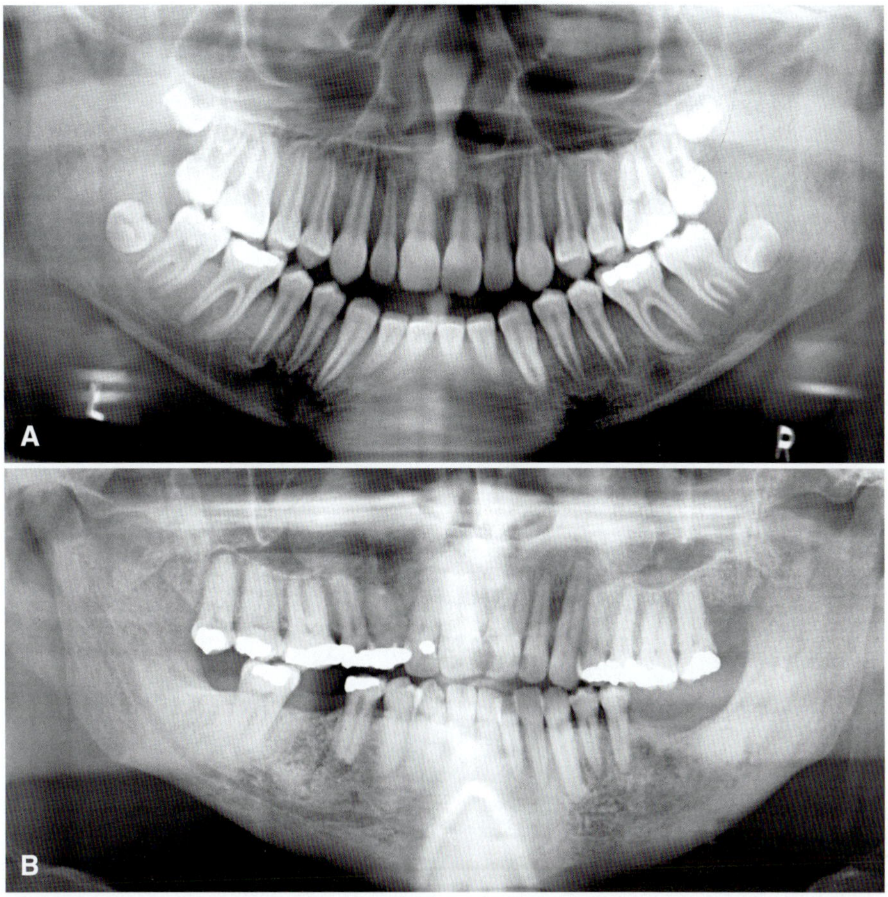

Fig. 23.9 Two cases of renal osteodystrophy. Panoramic image (A) shows radiolucent areas of bone loss, loss of distinct lamina dura and a sclerotic bone pattern around the teeth. Panoramic image (B) shows a generalized sclerotic bone pattern and a loss of a clear interface between the cancellous bone pattern and the cortical bone.

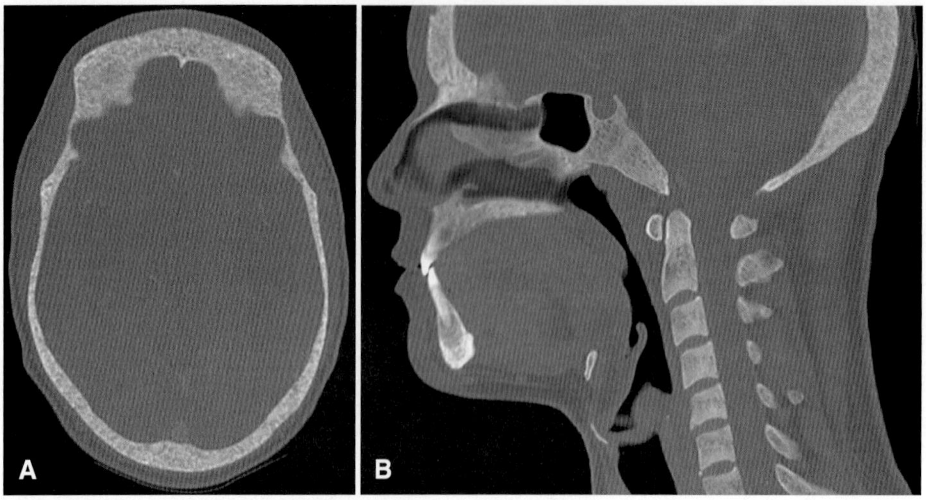

Fig. 23.11 Axial (A) and sagittal (B) multidetector computed tomographic images in a patient with secondary hyperparathyroidism. Note the generalized thinning and loss of definition of the cortical bone and the internal granular pattern of the bone.

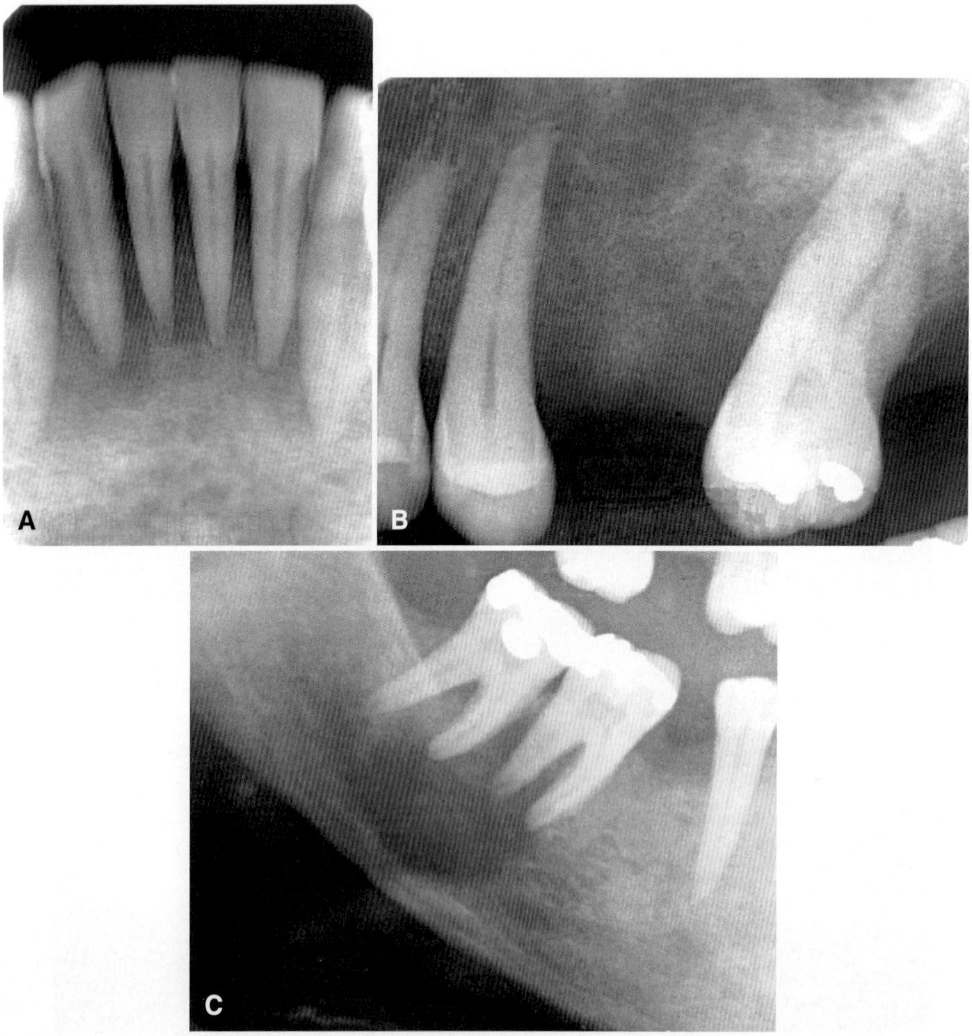

Fig. 23.12 Periapical images (A and B) show loss of lamina dura around the teeth in a patient with hyperparathyroidism. Also, note the loss of definition of the floor of the maxillary antrum (B). The cropped panoramic image (C) of the same patient reveals a central giant cell lesion (brown tumor) developing apical to the mandibular molars.

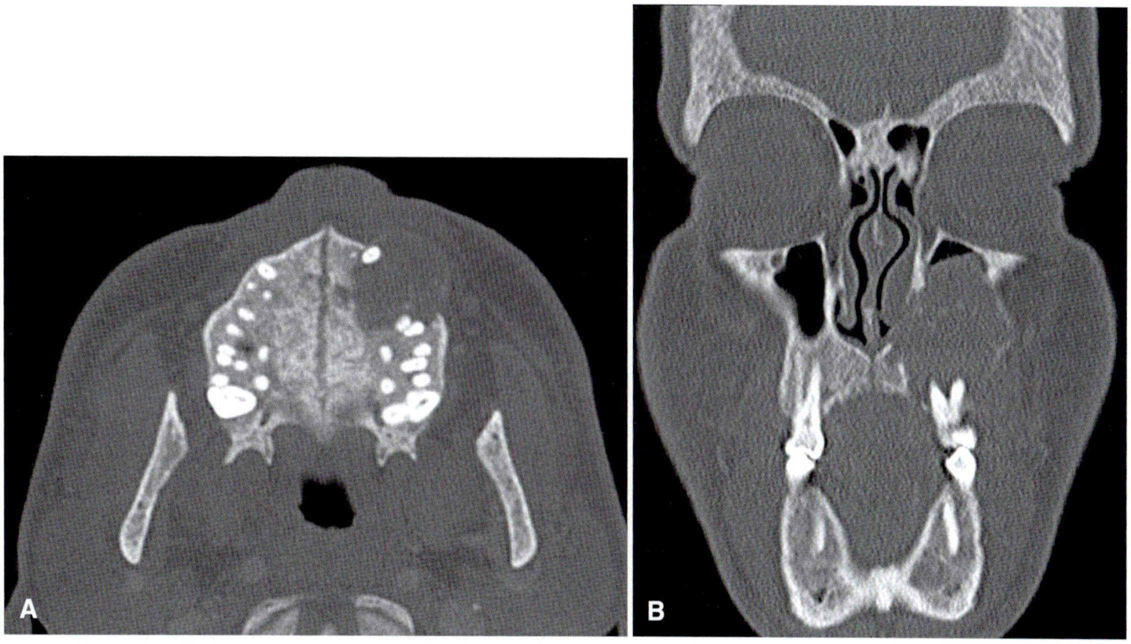

Fig. 23.13 Axial (A) and coronal (B) multidetector computed tomographic images in a patient with secondary hyperparathyroidism and a central giant cell lesion (brown tumor) involving the left maxilla.

changes consistent with primary hyperparathyroidism. Interestingly, one may also see an increase in bone density in some patients. There may also be brown tumors, but these are less frequently seen compared to primary hyperparathyroidism.

Management

After successful surgical removal of the causative parathyroid adenoma, almost all changes revert to normal. The only exception may be the site of a brown tumor, which often heals with bone that is more sclerotic than normal. In secondary hyperparathyroidism, patients with renal osteodystrophy are given vitamin D supplements and phosphate binders. The imaging features of secondary hyperparathyroidism may persist even after a successful renal transplant because of hyperplasia of the parathyroid glands secondary to the previous chronic low serum levels of calcium.

Hypoparathyroidism and Pseudohypoparathyroidism

Disease Mechanism

Hypoparathyroidism is an uncommon condition in which insufficient secretion of PTH occurs. Several causes exist, but the most common is unintended damage or removal of the parathyroid glands during thyroid surgery. In pseudohypoparathyroidism, there is a defect in the response of the target tissue cells to normal levels of PTH. In both cases, the result is low serum levels of calcium.

Clinical Features

There is a variety of clinical manifestations, although some patients may show no changes. Patients with pseudohypoparathyroidism often have early closure of certain bony epiphyses and manifest short stature or disproportionate extremities. Some patients experience sensorineural abnormalities, and these may include paresthesia of the hands or feet, or the area around the mouth. There may also be neurologic changes that may include anxiety and depression, epilepsy, parkinsonism, chorea, tetany of the wrist, and carpopedal spasm. Chronic forms may produce a reduction in intellectual capacity.

Imaging Features

Effects on the teeth and jaws. Imaging of the jaws may reveal enamel hypoplasia, external root resorption, delayed eruption, or root dilaceration (Fig. 23.14).

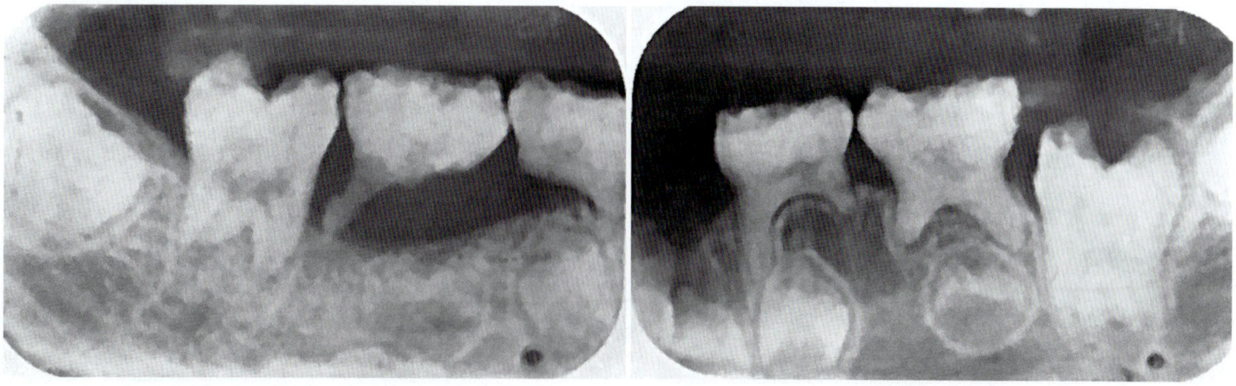

Fig. 23.14 Anomalies of tooth development in a patient with pseudohypoparathyroidism. (Courtesy Dr. S. Bricker, San Antonio, TX.)

Effects on the skeleton. On skull images, ectopic soft tissue calcifications within the brain may result in the appearance of flocculent, bilateral calcifications within the cerebral hemispheres on posteroanterior skull images. Centrally there is calcification of the basal ganglia.

Management

These conditions are managed with orally administered supplemental calcium and vitamin D.

Hyperpituitarism

Disease Mechanism

Hyperpituitarism in the form of gigantism and acromegaly results from hyperfunction of the anterior lobe of the pituitary gland, with the usual cause being a benign secretory tumor of growth hormone-secreting cells (somatotrophs). In skeletally immature children, the condition is known as gigantism, and in skeletally mature adults, the condition is known as acromegaly. An excess of growth hormone causes overgrowth of all tissues in the body, including bone, which is still capable of growth.

Clinical Features

In children, there is generalized overgrowth of most hard and soft tissues. Active growth occurs in bones in which the epiphyses have not fused with the bone shaft. During adolescence, generalized skeletal growth is excessive and may be prolonged, and affected individuals may ultimately attain heights of 7 to 8 feet (2.1 to 2.4 m) or more but with remarkably normal proportions. The eyes and other parts of the central nervous system do not enlarge except in rare cases in which the condition manifests in infancy.

In adults, acromegaly has an insidious clinical course, quite different from what is seen in children. In adults, the clinical effects develop quite slowly because many tissues have already lost the capacity for growth, including much of the skeleton. Interestingly, an excess of growth hormone can stimulate enlargement of the mandible, as well as the phalanges of the hand and the supraorbital ridges, and the underlying frontal sinus may also enlarge. Excess growth hormone in adults also results in hypertrophy of some soft tissues including the lips, tongue, nose, and soft tissues of the hands and feet, sometimes to a striking degree.

Imaging Features

Effects on the teeth and jaws. The tooth crowns are unaffected, but the roots of premolar and molar teeth often develop hypercementosis. This condition may be the result of altered functional and structural demands on teeth rather than an effect of the increased hormone level. Supraeruption of the posterior teeth may occur, which compensates for the growth of the mandible.

Hyperpituitarism causes enlargement of the jaws, most notably the mandible (Fig. 23.15). Mandibular condylar growth may be very prominent, and patients can develop a prominent skeletal class III appearance with a strongly prognathic mandible. The thickness and height of the alveolar processes may also increase, as well as the length of the dental arch resulting in increased spacing of the teeth. The mandibular angle may also become more obtuse. This change, in combination with the flaring of the anterior teeth caused by enlargement of the tongue (macroglossia), may result in the development of an anterior open bite. The sign of incisor flaring is a helpful point of differentiation between acromegalic prognathism and inherited prognathism.

Effects on the skeleton. Although functional adenomas of the pituitary gland may not enlarge the sella turcica at all, in some cases there is enlargement or "ballooning" of the sella (see Fig. 23.15B). Skull images characteristically reveal enlargement of the paranasal sinuses (especially the frontal sinus). The sinuses are more prominent in acromegaly than in pituitary gigantism because bone pneumatization in gigantism tends to be more in step with the generalized enlargement of the facial bones. Acromegaly also produces diffuse thickening of the outer cortex of the skull.

Management

Surgical removal of the pituitary gland is the first line of treatment. If surgery fails or is not possible, medications may be used to reduce growth hormone levels. Radiation therapy may also be considered, but this usually takes several years to show an effect.

Hypopituitarism

Disease Mechanism

Hypopituitarism is the result of decreased secretion of pituitary hormones, the most common of which is growth hormone.

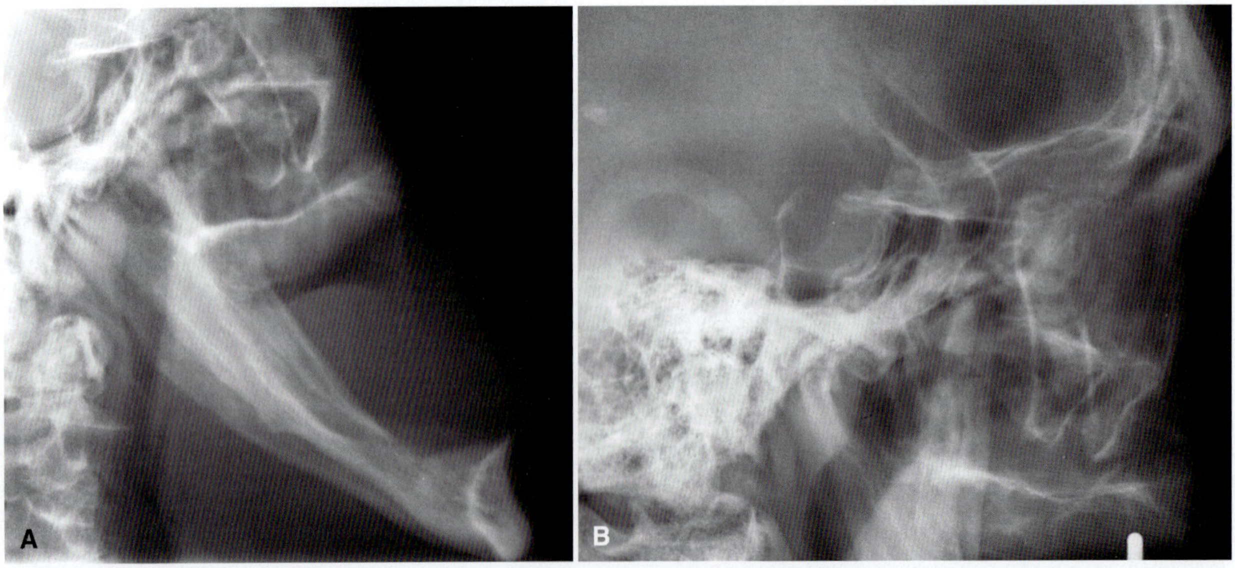

Fig. 23.15 (A) A patient with acromegaly manifesting in growth of the mandible and the development of a class III skeletal relationship of the jaws. (B) A portion of a lateral skull image of the same patient demonstrates enlargement of the sella turcica.

Clinical Features

Individuals with this condition exhibit dwarfism but have relatively well-proportioned bodies. One study reported a marked failure of development of the maxilla and mandible, and the dimensions of these bones in adults with this disorder were approximately the same as those in normal children 5 to 7 years of age.

Imaging Features

Effects on the teeth and jaws. Eruption of the primary dentition occurs at the normal time, but exfoliation is delayed by several years. The crowns of the permanent teeth also develop normally, but their eruption is delayed several years. The third molar buds may be completely absent.

Effects on the skeleton. In hypopituitarism, the jaws, especially the mandible, are small, which results in crowding of the teeth and malocclusion.

Management

Treatment is usually directed toward removal of the cause or replacement of the pituitary hormones or hormones of its target gland. The response of the dentition to treatment with growth hormone is variable but seems to parallel the skeletal response.

Hyperthyroidism

Disease Mechanism

Hyperthyroidism is a disease process that involves excessive production of thyroxine in the thyroid gland. The most common forms of hyperthyroidism are diffuse toxic goiter (Graves disease), toxic nodular goiter (Plummer disease), and toxic adenoma, a benign tumor of the thyroid gland. Each of these conditions results in increased levels of circulating thyroxine.

Clinical Features

Excessive thyroxine causes a generalized increase in the metabolic rate of all body tissues, resulting in tachycardia, increased blood pressure, sensitivity to heat, and irritability. Hyperthyroidism is more common in females.

Imaging Features

Effects on the teeth and jaws. Hyperthyroidism results in an accelerated rate of dental development and early eruption, with premature loss of the primary teeth.

Effects on the skeleton. Hyperthyroidism results in an increased rate of bone turnover that is imbalanced in favor of excessive bone resorption. This resorption is manifest in adults as a generalized loss of bone density or bone volume in edentulous areas.

Management. Radioactive iodine (^{131}I) is the most common treatment for hyperthyroidism followed by antithyroid medications and surgical removal of the thyroid gland.

Hypothyroidism

Disease Mechanism

Hypothyroidism or cretinism results from insufficient secretion of thyroxine by the thyroid glands despite the levels of circulating thyroid-stimulating hormone.

Clinical Features

In children, hypothyroidism may result in retarded mental and physical development. The base of the skull shows delayed ossification, and the paranasal sinuses show only partial development. Dental development is delayed, and the primary teeth are slow to exfoliate.

Hypothyroidism in adults results in myxedematous swelling but not the dental or skeletal changes seen in children. Adult symptoms may range from lethargy, poor memory, inability to concentrate, constipation, and cold intolerance to the more florid clinical picture of a dull and expressionless face, periorbital edema, large tongue, sparse hair, and skin that feels "doughy" to the touch.

Imaging Features

Effects on the teeth and jaws. There may be delayed eruption of teeth, teeth with short roots, and thinning of the lamina dura. There may also be external root resorption and premature tooth loss. Patients with adult hypothyroidism may develop periodontal disease and diastemas of the teeth as a result of enlargement of the tongue. The maxilla and mandible may be relatively small.

Effects on the skeleton. Features in children include delayed closure of the epiphyses. In the calvarium, skull sutures may exhibit wormian bone formation—that is, the formation of one or more islands of bone within a suture.

Management

Patients with hypothyroidism are managed with hormone replacement and careful monitoring to prevent the development of iatrogenic hyperthyroidism.

Hypercortisolism

Disease Mechanism

Hypercortisolism arises from prolonged exposure to elevated levels of either exogenous or endogenous glucocorticoids. Hypersecretion of endogenous glucocorticoids may be the result of adrenal hyperplasia, adenoma, or adenocarcinoma, or it may be due to a pituitary adenoma secreting adrenocorticotrophic hormone (Cushing disease). The increased concentration of glucocorticoid results in a loss of bone mass from reduced osteoblastic function and either directly or indirectly increased osteoclastic function.

Clinical Features

This condition affects females three to five times as frequently as males, and onset may occur at any age but is usually seen in the third or fourth decades of life. Patients with hypercortisolism often exhibit fat accumulation that spares the extremities but is more pronounced in the face ("moon facies") and upper back ("buffalo hump"). These patients also demonstrate violaceous striae and muscle weakness and may have hypertension and concurrent diabetes.

Imaging Features

Effects on the teeth and jaws. The teeth may erupt prematurely, and partial loss of the lamina dura may occur (Fig. 23.16).

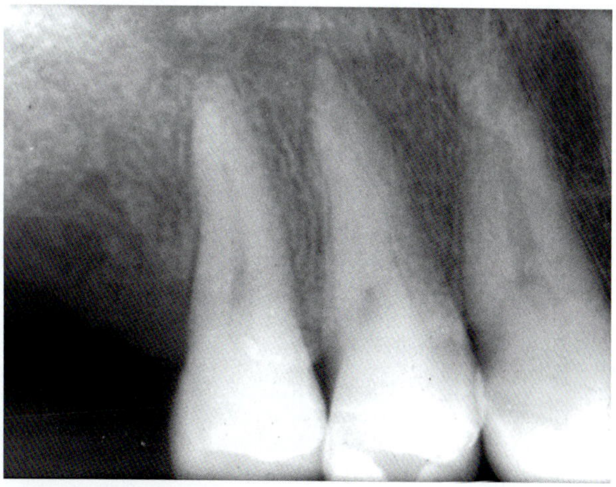

Fig. 23.16 Cushing disease manifested in the jaws as thinning or loss of the lamina dura around the teeth and generalized osteopenia. (Courtesy Dr. H. G. Poyton, Toronto, ON.)

Effects on the skeleton. Altered osteoblastic and osteoclastic activity can result in thinning of the skull, which may be accompanied by a mottled appearance of the bone. There may be generalized osteopenia secondary to reduced osteoblastic and increased osteoclastic activity, and the bone may also exhibit a granular pattern because of the abnormal formation of numerous short and randomly oriented trabeculae. Skeletal osteopenia may also result in fractures.

Systemic Sclerosis

Disease Mechanism

Systemic sclerosis or scleroderma is a connective tissue disease that causes excessive collagen deposition resulting in hardening (sclerosis) of the skin and other tissues. Involvement of the gastrointestinal tract, heart, lungs, and kidneys usually results in more serious complications. The cause of the disease is unknown.

Clinical Features

Systemic sclerosis is a disease of middle age with the greatest incidence between 30 and 50 years of age; it is rarely seen in adolescents and elderly adults. Females are affected about three times as often as males.

The condition may be localized or generalized with the localized form only affecting the skin and adjacent teeth with no major organ involvement. In contrast, the generalized systemic form can also involve other organ systems. In most patients with moderate to severe systemic sclerosis, the involved skin has a thickened, leathery quality that drapes the underlying tissues tightly. Involvement of the facial region may restrict normal mandibular opening. Patients may also present with xerostomia, as well as an increased number of decayed, missing, or filled teeth. Also, patients are more likely to have periodontal involvement. Patients with cardiac and pulmonary involvement may have varying degrees of heart failure and respiratory insufficiency. Renal involvement usually leads to some degree of uremia with or without hypertension.

Imaging Features

Effects on the teeth and jaws. The most common manifestation of systemic sclerosis in images of the jaws is nonconcentric PDL space widening around the teeth. Approximately two-thirds of patients can exhibit this feature, and the change can be localized (Fig. 23.17) or generalized (Fig. 23.18). In such instances, PDL width can be at least twice as wide as normal. The lamina dura remains normal. Despite the

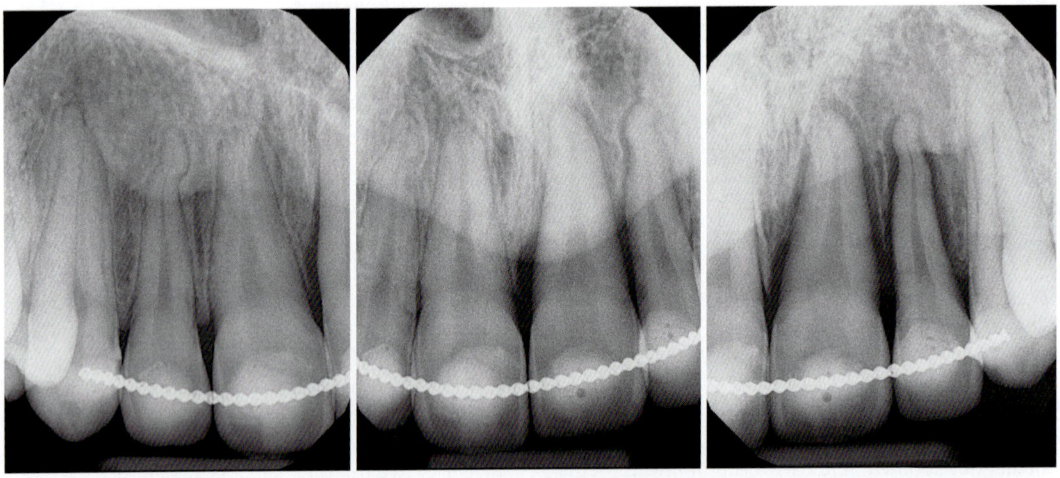

Fig. 23.17 Periapical images showing local widening of the periodontal ligament spaces around the maxillary left incisor teeth in the localized form of systemic sclerosis. (Courtesy Dr. P. Chauvin, Montreal, QC.)

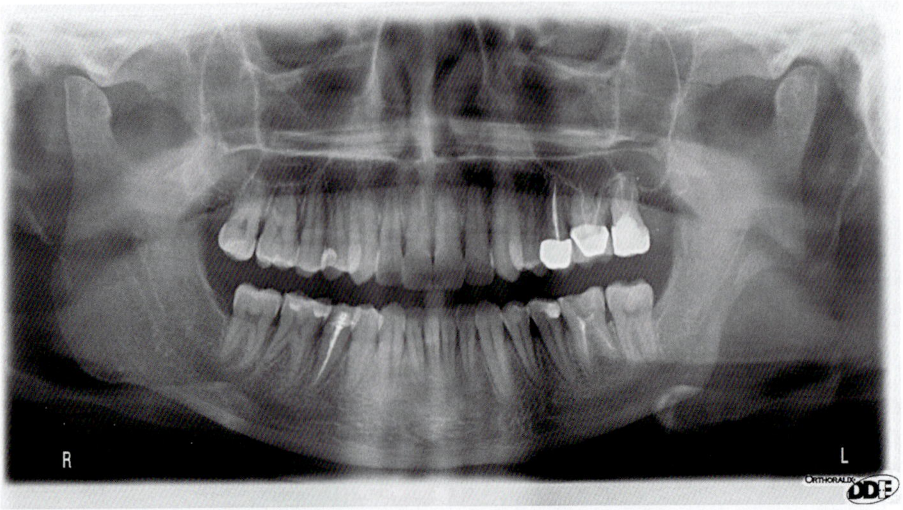

Fig. 23.18 Generalized widening of the periodontal ligament spaces throughout the dentition in a patient with systemic sclerosis. (Courtesy Dr. B. Friedland, Boston, MA.)

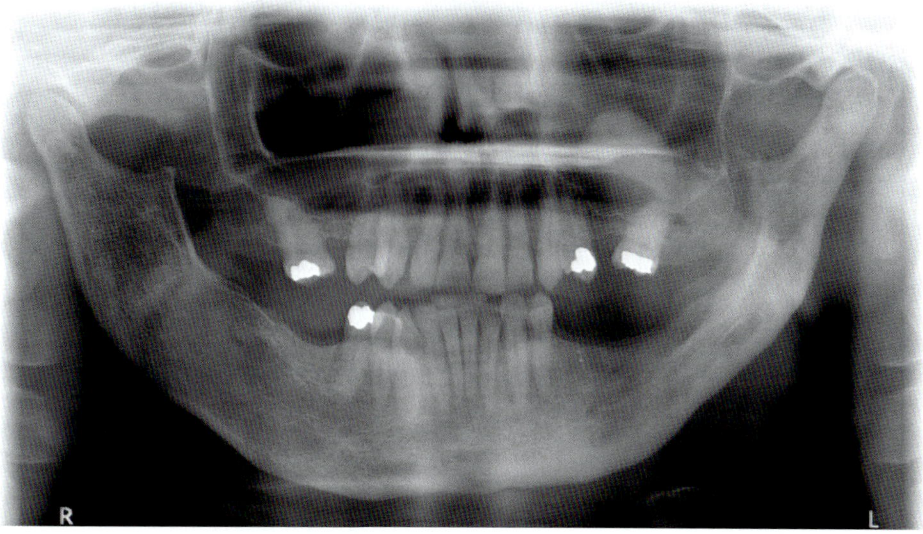

Fig. 23.19 Resorption of the mandibular angles, the insertion sites of the masseter and medial pterygoid muscles in a patient with systemic sclerosis. (Courtesy Dr. H. Grubisa, Oakville, ON.)

widening of the PDL spaces, the clinician finds that the involved teeth are often not mobile, and their gingival attachments are usually intact.

Another characteristic feature in some cases of systemic sclerosis is an alteration to the morphology of the mandible at the tendinous attachments of the masticatory muscles. These sites include the angles of the mandible, the coronoid processes, the lingual surface of the anterior mandible, and the condylar heads (Fig. 23.19). The alteration is typically bilateral and symmetric. Most of these erosive borders are smooth and sharply defined, and the changes may progress with the disease.

Differential Interpretation

Other causes of PDL space widening include "traumatic occlusion," orthodontic tooth movement, intermaxillary fixation with arch bars, and invasion of the PDL by malignant neoplasms. Widening of the PDL space with malignant neoplasia is more localized than generalized, asymmetric, and accompanied by destruction of the lamina dura.

Management

The progressive loss of bone in the region of the mandibular angle is more serious because of potential fracture. It is reasonable to obtain initial and periodic panoramic images in all patients with systemic sclerosis to assess mandibular integrity.

DYSPLASIAS OF BONE

Disease Mechanism

Bone dysplasias are a group of conditions in which normal bone is replaced with abnormal immature bone and a rich fibrous connective tissue matrix (Fig. 23.20). Although the mechanism is not well understood, it has been hypothesized that osteoblast and osteoclast functions become dysregulated, favoring the activity of one cell type over the other.

For both the clinician and the patient, it is important to understand that in the context of bone, the term "dysplasia" does not imply that the process is premalignant. This is in contrast to the use of the term in the context of epithelium where epithelial dysplasia is premalignant. Furthermore, bone dysplasias are not neoplasms and therefore should not be managed as such.

Cemento-osseous Dysplasia

Disease Mechanism

The cemento-osseous dysplasias are conditions in which one or more areas of normal bone metabolism are altered, and cancellous bone is replaced by a mixture of fibrous connective tissue containing varying amounts of immature, abnormal bone. Periapical cemento-osseous dysplasia (PCOD) is the more localized form, affecting one sextant of the jaws, while florid cemento-osseous dysplasia (FCOD) is a more widespread form affecting two or more sextants. In some cases, a familial trend can be seen in FCOD. As the entities mature and more abnormal bone is deposited, the vascular supply can be compromised—a condition that likely contributes to its increased susceptibility to infection.

Foci of cemento-osseous dysplasia occur in the periapical areas of the teeth, which may be erupted or unerupted, or impacted. The replacement of normal bone undergoes three stages. In the first, the normal bone is resorbed, and in the second and third stages, immature, new bone is deposited in increasing amounts, centrally within the resorptive area.

Clinical Features

PCOD typically arises during the fourth and fifth decades of life. The condition occurs more often in women than men, and commonly affects non-Caucasian populations. PCOD is usually found incidentally on images made for other purposes. In some patients, the foci can become quite large, causing a notable expansion of the alveolar process and thinning of adjacent cortices. As well, these areas may continue to expand slowly. The pulps of the adjacent teeth are vital, and the patient usually has no history of pain or tooth sensitivity, although occasionally, patients may note the development of a swelling or an area of low-grade, intermittent, poorly localized pain, especially when a simple bone cavity has developed within the abnormality.

Should foci of FCOD become secondarily infected because of exposure to oral microorganisms, osteomyelitis may develop, and there may be mucosal ulceration and fistulous tracts with suppuration and pain. The development of osteomyelitis is of particular concern when the abnormalities are in their most mature, radiopaque states. If

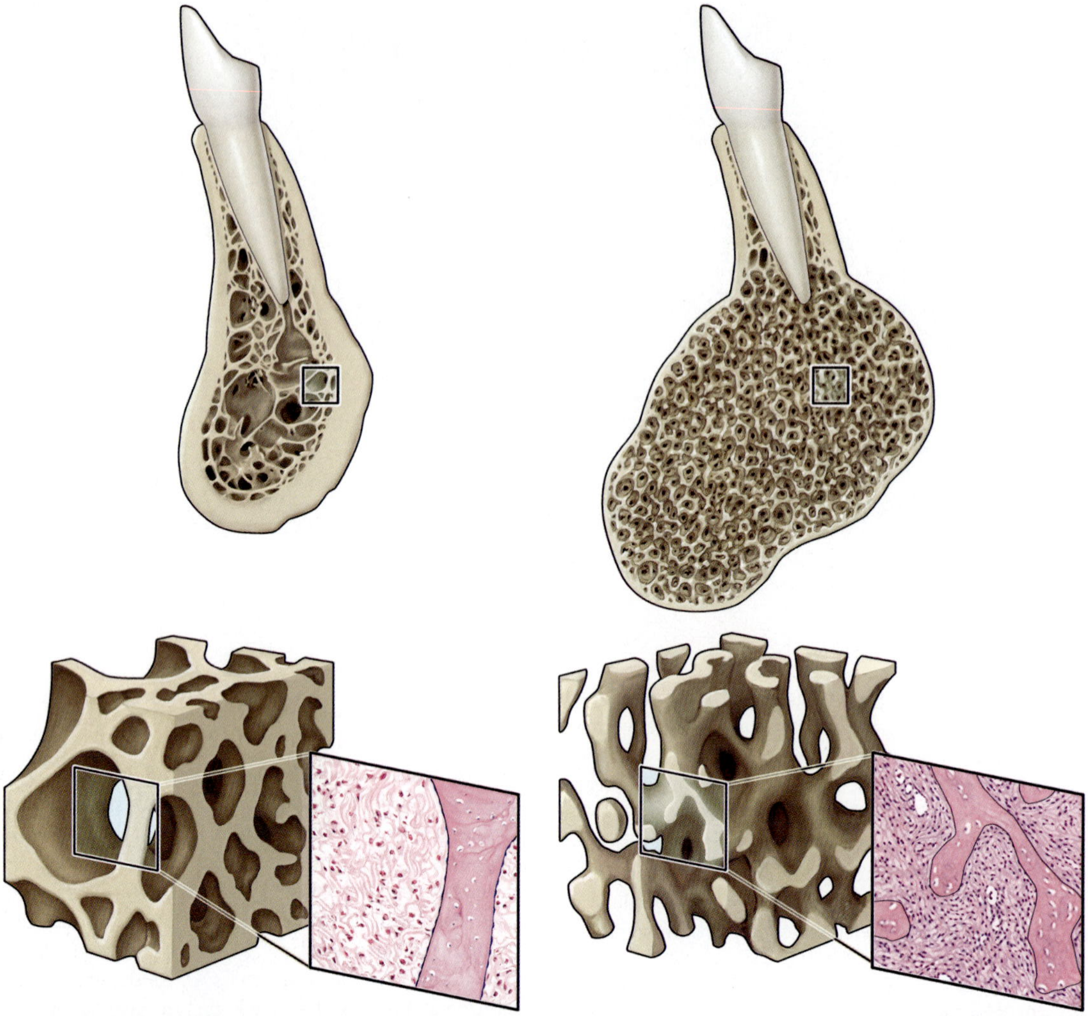

Fig. 23.20 Dysplastic lesions of bone alter the normal bone architecture. Normal bone *(left)* is replaced by irregularly shaped, short trabeculae and a dense fibrous connective tissue matrix *(right)*.

osteomyelitis is suspected, CBCT or MDCT should be ordered to determine the extent of involvement.

Imaging Features

Location. The epicenter of cemento-osseous dysplasia is located in the periapical areas of the teeth, within the alveolar processes of the jaws (Fig. 23.21). In rare cases, the epicenter is located slightly more coronally and may be nearer to the apical third of the root. In the mandible, the epicenters are located superior to the inferior alveolar canal.

There may be one or more foci of abnormal bone within the same sextant in PCOD. FCOD is diagnosed when two or more sextants are involved, and these abnormal foci may be found in both jaws (Fig. 23.22). However, when they are present in only one jaw, the mandible is the more common location. If the involved tooth has been extracted, a focus can still develop, but the periapical location may be less clear (Fig. 23.23).

Periphery. PCOD may be irregularly shaped or have a round or oval shape. In most cases, the periphery of a PCOD is well defined, and the cortex can vary in width to the point of appearing thickened. Internally there may be a variably wide radiolucent rim surrounding the radiopaque center, which sometimes can be difficult to visualize in very mature cases (Fig. 23.24). As the focus matures, a band of more variably thick bone can appear at the external periphery.

Internal structure. The internal appearance of PCOD can vary, depending on the degree of maturity. In the early stage, normal bone is resorbed and replaced with fibrous connective tissue that is usually continuous with the PDL space (causing loss of the lamina dura). This appears as a radiolucency at the apex of the involved tooth (see Fig. 23.21A and B).

In the second and more mature stage, a radiopaque focus appears within the center of the radiolucent zone, and this can vary in appearance from a small oval or circular region of mineralization with a cotton-wool appearance to a larger, irregular, amorphous area of calcification. The radiopaque pattern can resemble the granular or "ground-glass" pattern seen in fibrous dysplasia (Figs. 23.25A and 23.26A and B). Alternatively, the dysplastic bone can form a swirling pattern (Figs. 23.25D and 23.26C and D). The internal density of larger FCOD foci can vary from a mixture of radiolucent and radiopaque regions (Fig. 23.26E) to almost complete radiopacity (Figs. 23.25E and 23.26F). In some cases, prominent radiolucent regions may develop, which usually represent a simple bone cavity (Fig. 23.27). These cavities may enlarge with time even beyond the boundary of the abnormality into the surrounding normal bone and later fill in with abnormal dysplastic bone.

In the third and most mature stage, the internal pattern may be completely radiopaque without any obvious pattern. A variably wide but thin radiolucent internal border can usually be seen at the periphery of the

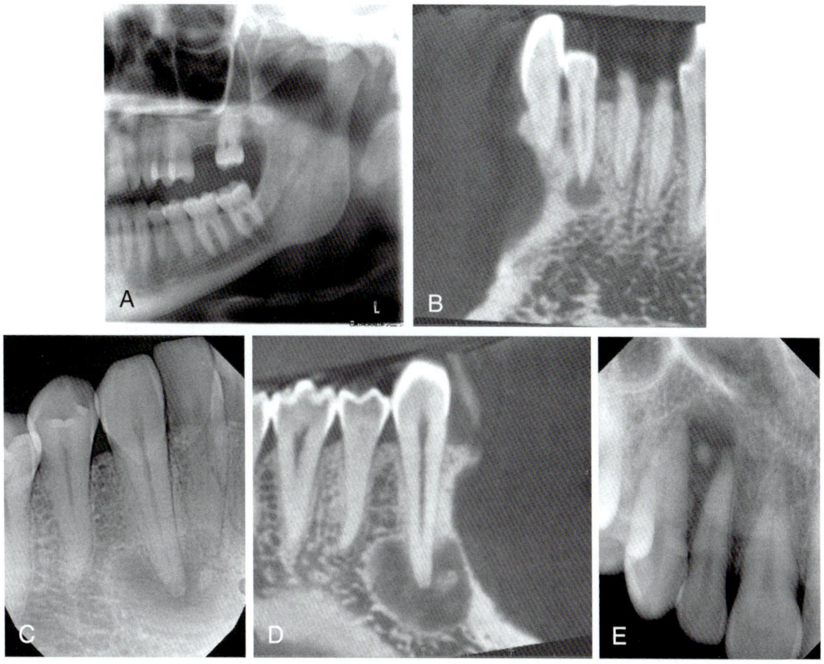

Fig. 23.21 Cropped panoramic (A), buccal/lingual cross-sectional cone beam computed tomographic (B and D), and periapical (C and E) images of early periapical cemento-osseous dysplasia. The images show loss of the periodontal ligament spaces around the root apices of the involved teeth and retention of the periodontal ligament space in (C). Note the small foci of dysplastic bone developing adjacent to the tooth roots in images (C), (D), and (E).

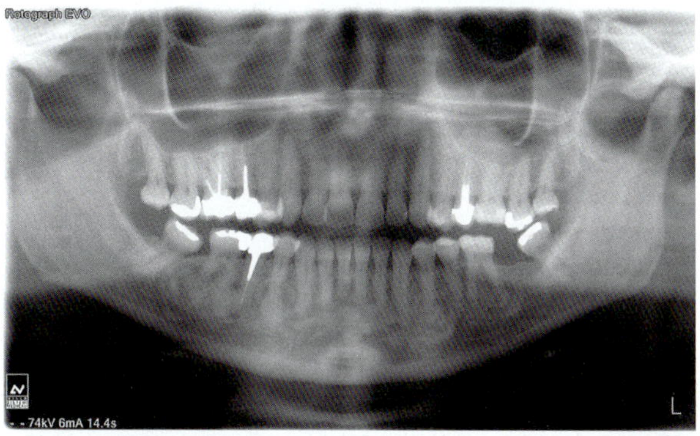

Fig. 23.22 Panoramic image showing multiquadrant involvement of mature florid cemento-osseous dysplasia. Note the appearance of the peripheral radiolucent border encircling the dysplastic bone and the hypercementosis of the teeth.

radiopacity because the focus mineralizes from the center (Fig. 23.28). Occasionally an internal radiolucent border is not apparent, which makes the differential interpretation more difficult. The internal structure may appear dramatically radiolucent if a simple bone cavity (Fig. 23.29) develops in association with cemento-osseous dysplasia.

Effects on adjacent structures. Some foci of PCOD may stimulate a peripheral reaction from the surrounding bone. Smaller foci do not expand the jawbone; however, larger ones can cause expansion (Fig. 23.25E). In such cases, a thin intact outer cortex can be visualized like that seen in fibrous dysplasia. The surface of the bone does not usually expand in a fusiform manner like fibrous dysplasia, but rather the border may exhibit irregular undulations. In the maxilla, cemento-osseous dysplasia can displace the floor of the maxillary sinus superiorly. In the mandible, they can displace the inferior alveolar canal inferiorly and cause enlargement of the alveolar bone by displacement of the buccal and lingual cortical plates.

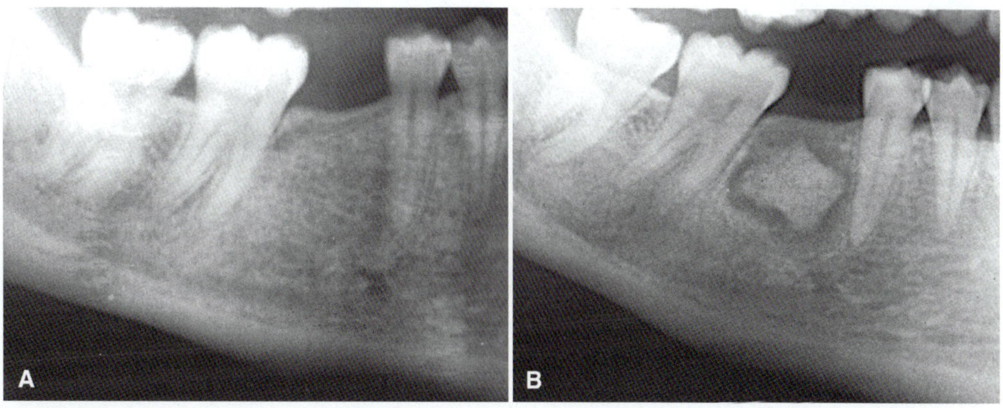

Fig. 23.23 Cropped panoramic images showing interval development of a solitary focus of PCOD in the edentulous first molar area. The images (A and B) were made at two time points, 3 years apart.

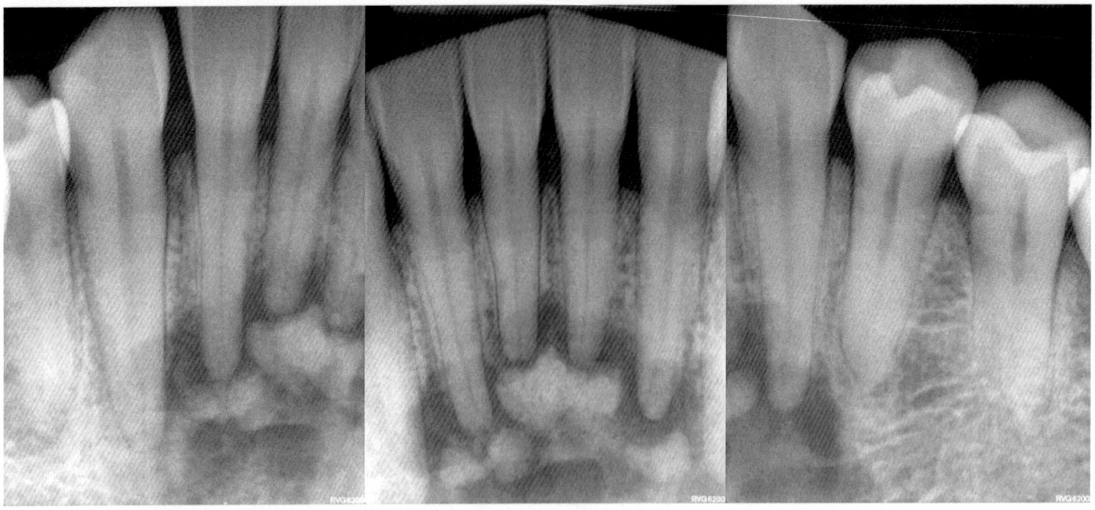

Fig. 23.24 The mixed radiolucent and radiopaque appearance of a more mature stage of periapical cemento-osseous dysplasia. Note the radiolucent rim encircling the radiopaque foci of dysplastic bone.

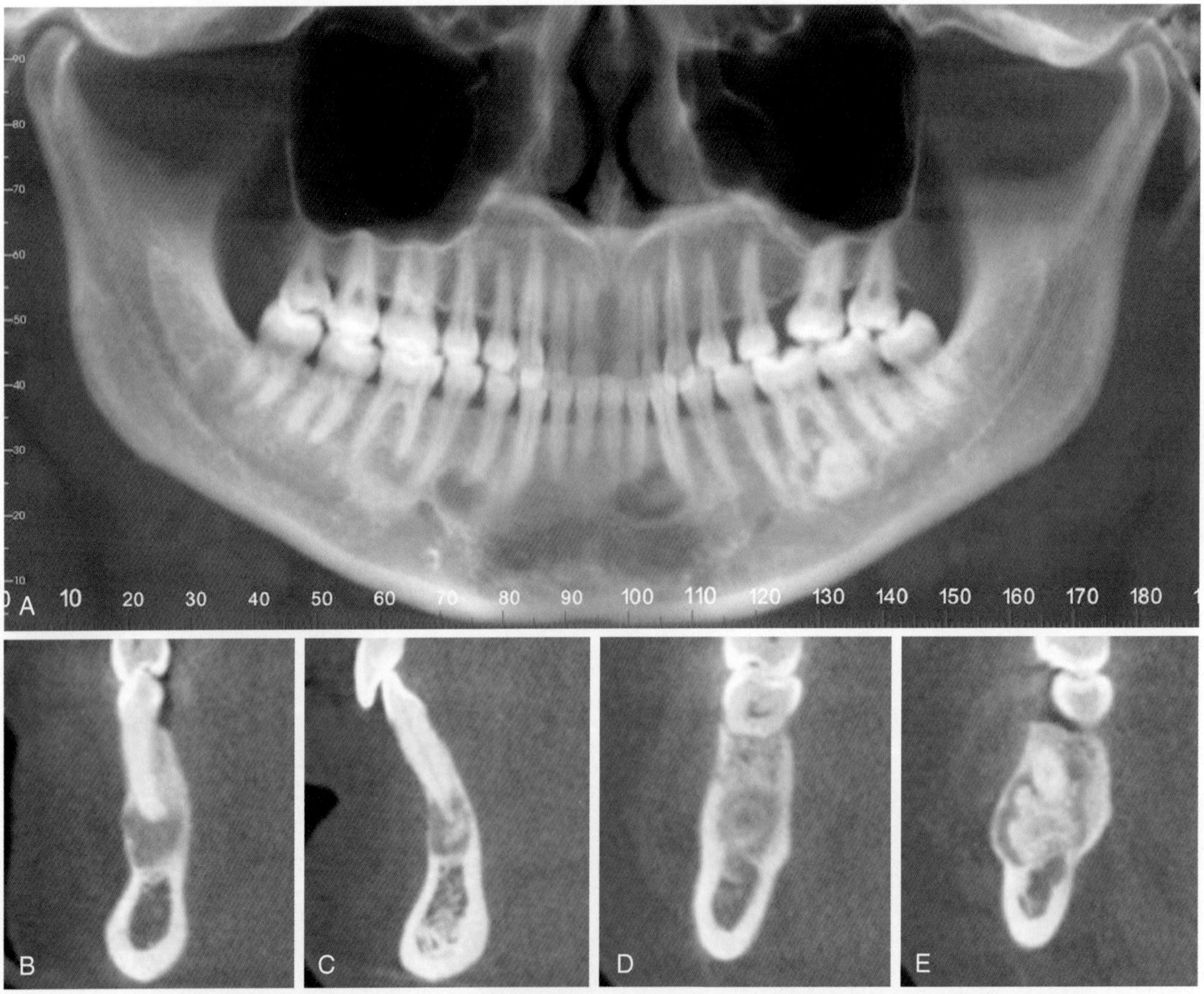

Fig. 23.25 A reconstructed panoramic image (A) from a cone beam computed tomographic examination of the jaws shows multiple foci of cemento-osseous dysplasia. Buccal/lingual reconstructions of the cone beam computed tomographic volume shows a ground-glass internal pattern (B), early central deposition of dysplastic bone (C), and a swirling pattern of dysplastic bone deposition (D). The radiopaque component is the dominant pattern in image (E) with a thin radiolucent periphery. Note the thinning of the buccal cortex and the expansion of the bone surface.

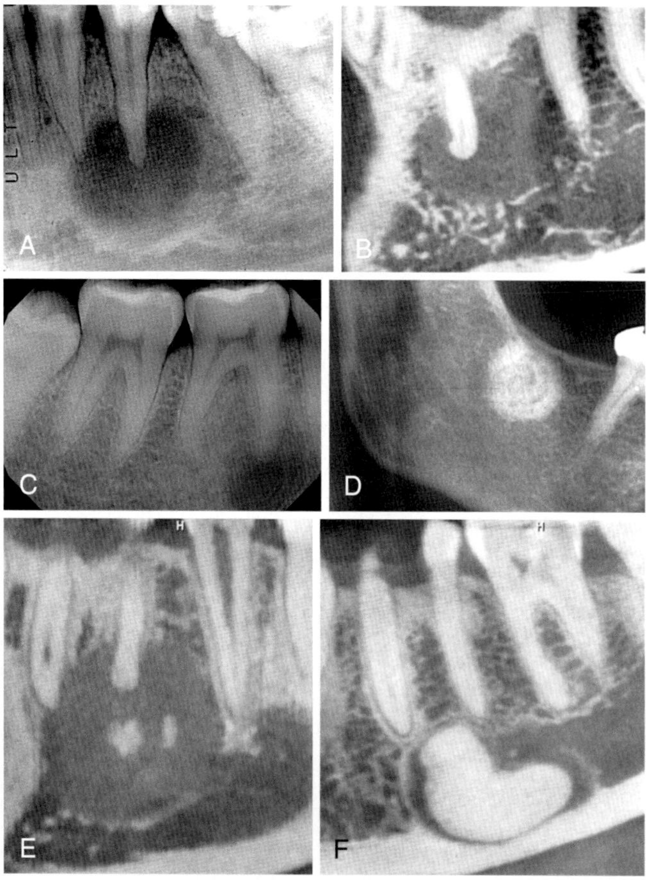

Fig. 23.26 Several unique internal patterns can be seen in the cemento-osseous dysplasias ranging from those that are more ground-glass–like (A and B) to ones that have a swirl pattern (C and D). Internal foci of amorphous bone can also be seen (E) and in extreme cases, the dystrophic bone can appear dense and uniform (F). (C, Courtesy Dr. G. Krishnamoorthy, Toronto, ON.)

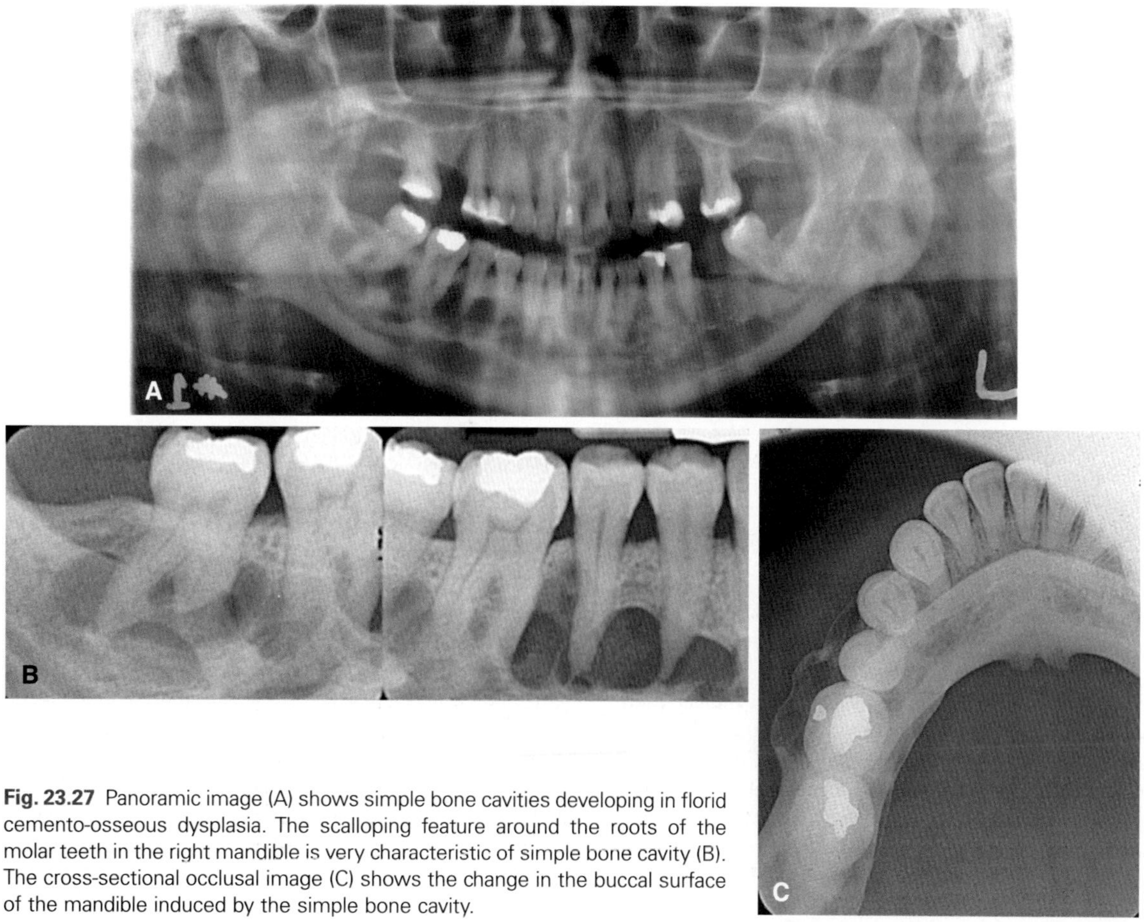

Fig. 23.27 Panoramic image (A) shows simple bone cavities developing in florid cemento-osseous dysplasia. The scalloping feature around the roots of the molar teeth in the right mandible is very characteristic of simple bone cavity (B). The cross-sectional occlusal image (C) shows the change in the buccal surface of the mandible induced by the simple bone cavity.

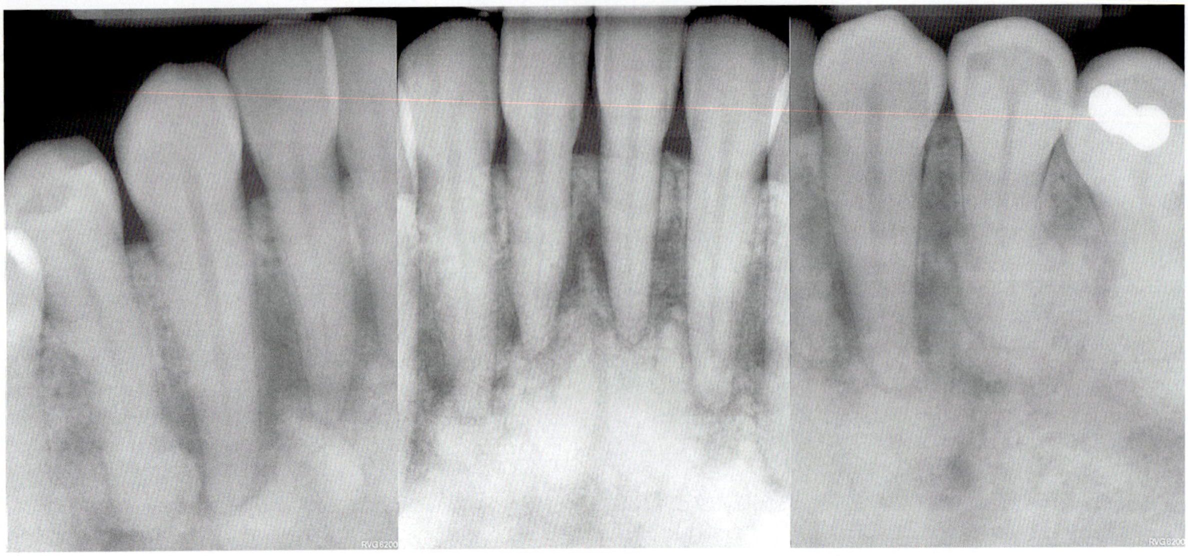

Fig. 23.28 Very mature lesions of periapical cemento-osseous dysplasia. The radiopaque component dominates the images and the radiolucent periphery is very thin.

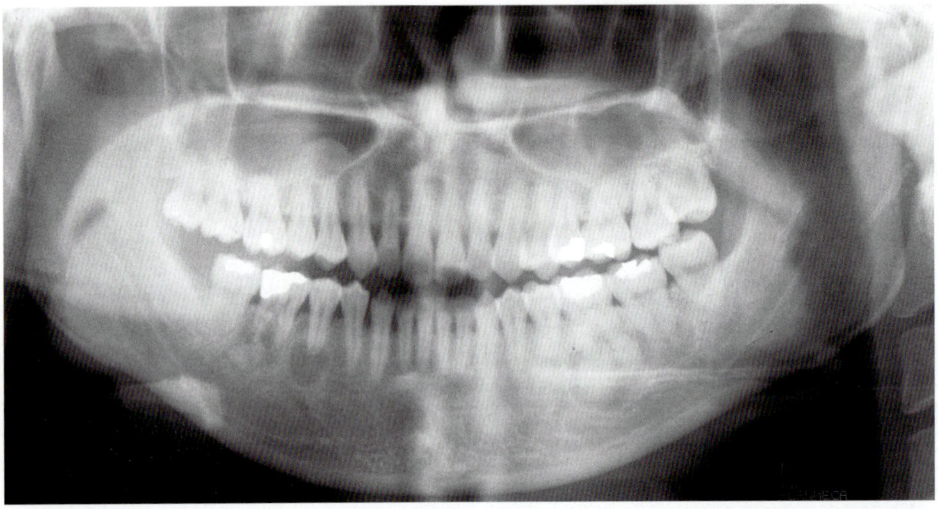

Fig. 23.29 Panoramic image showing multiple stages of maturation of florid cemento-osseous dysplasia. A simple bone cavity is developing at the apex of the mandibular right second premolar. (Courtesy Dr. C. Poon-Woo, Toronto, ON.)

Effects on adjacent teeth. The lamina dura around the involved tooth root apices can be lost, making the PDL space either less apparent or apparently wider (Fig. 23.21). The tooth structure is usually not affected, although roots may develop hypercementosis, particularly in FCOD, making extraction difficult.

Differential Interpretation

Early foci of PCOD are radiolucent, and the most important differential interpretation is rarefying osteitis. Occasionally PCOD cannot be distinguished from rarefying osteitis by radiologic characteristics alone. In such instances, the final diagnosis must rely on clinical information, such as pulp vitality testing of the adjacent tooth.

In the case of a solitary, mature focus of PCOD, the differential interpretation may include a cementoblastoma, especially when the focus is located more coronally and in close proximity to a tooth root. As cementoblastoma is attached to the surface of the root, the root may be partially resorbed. Also, the peripheral radiolucency may be better defined in cementoblastoma, and there may be a unique pattern to the internal structure, such as a spoke or radiating pattern. Expansion of the bone in cementoblastoma is more concentric without the surface undulation seen in PCOD. The presence or absence of clinical symptoms may also help to distinguish PCOD from cementoblastoma. Another entity to consider is an odontome. Although odontomes often arise occlusal to a tooth and prevent its eruption, some odontomes may have a more periapical position. The appearance of tooth-like structures and the identification of enamel (which is very radiopaque) can help in the differential interpretation. Also, the peripheral cortex of an odontome is often more well defined, and the internal radiolucent periphery is more uniform in width. Mature PCOD lesions may also resemble a dense bone island. The appearance of a radiolucent periphery in PCOD, even if very slight, points to PCOD. Solitary entities, particularly those that expand the bone, may be difficult to differentiate from cemento-ossifying fibroma.

The fact that PCOD and FCOD may be multifocal and centered in the alveolar processes helps in differentiating the cemento-osseous dysplasias from other entities. Paget disease of bone may also display cotton-wool radiopaque regions with associated hypercementosis. However, Paget disease affects the bone of the entire mandible more generally. Furthermore, Paget disease of bone is often polyostotic, involving other bones as well as the jaws. The better defined border of FCOD with its radiolucent internal periphery and surrounding sclerotic border are also useful in making the differential diagnosis. Another disease that may resemble FCOD is osteomyelitis, particularly if large areas of sclerosis develop. The radiopaque foci in FCOD may appear similar to the sequestra seen in osteomyelitis. This should not, however, be confused with a situation where FCOD has become secondarily infected, resulting in osteomyelitis. The foci of an amorphous bone that has become secondarily infected have a wider and more profound radiolucent border (Fig. 23.30). CBCT or MDCT imaging is essential if osteomyelitis is suspected, to determine the extent of involvement.

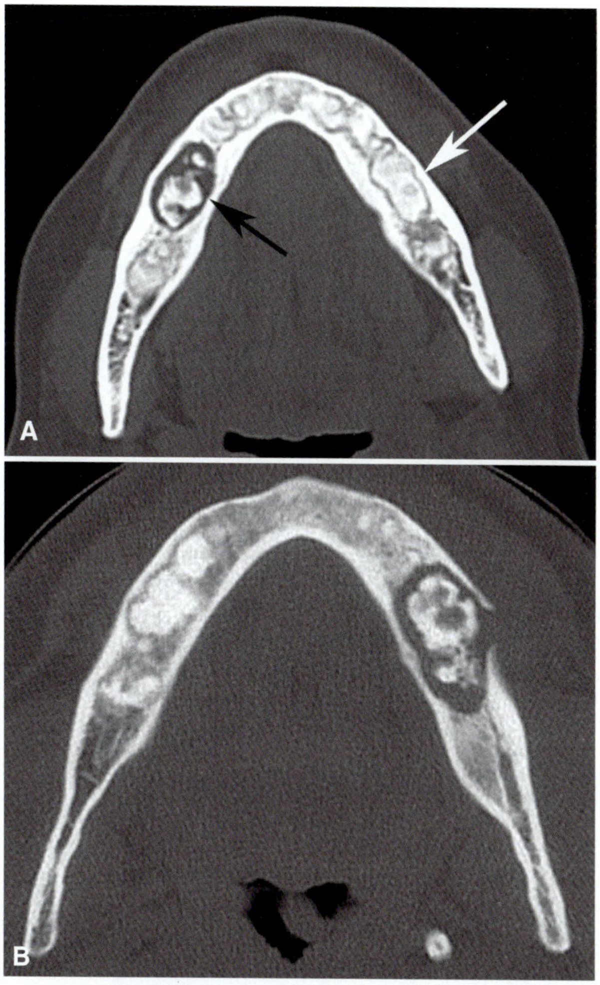

Fig. 23.30 Axial multidetector computed tomographic images of florid cemento-osseous dysplasia. Note the radiolucent rim *(white arrow)* on the patient's left side around a mature focus of dysplastic bone and the focus on the right side with a more pronounced radiolucent border (A). The more pronounced and irregular border suggests that the focus is secondarily infected *(black arrow)*. A different case (B) of osteomyelitis caused by a secondarily infected focus of cemento-osseous dysplasia. Note the discontinuity of buccal cortex where the lesion is draining into the adjacent soft tissues.

Management

The cemento-osseous dysplasias do not require treatment, although there is value in obtaining a panoramic image to establish the extent of involvement. Because of the propensity for the most mature lesions to become secondarily infected, the patient should be encouraged to maintain an effective oral hygiene program to avoid odontogenic infections and bone loss due to periodontal disease. However, if the teeth have been removed and if considerable atrophy of the alveolar ridge has occurred, the foci of dysplastic bone may reach the mucosal surface, much in the same way stones become exposed in old, worn concrete. These foci of abnormal bone can perforate the mucosa, particularly when located under a denture, and can become secondarily infected. If osteomyelitis occurs, the avascular foci of amorphous bone will become large sequestra, and the inflammatory response may spread slowly throughout the jaw from one region of FCOD to another. Biopsy of cemento-osseous dysplasia is not required, as a possible complication of doing this is secondary infection.

Fibrous Dysplasia

Disease Mechanism

Fibrous dysplasia is another bone dysplasia where the cancellous bone is replaced by a mixture of fibrous connective tissue containing varying amounts of immature, abnormal bone. Fibrous dysplasia develops as a postzygotic mutation of the *GNAS1* gene—a regulator of bone formation and remodeling. Mutations of this gene have been detected in 93% of cases. At the histopathologic level, the result is the appearance of numerous short, irregularly shaped trabeculae of woven bone. Unlike normal bone, where trabeculae are oriented in response to stresses and strains placed on the bone, trabeculae in fibrous dysplasia are oriented randomly. And compared to normal bone, there are more trabeculae per unit volume within the cancellous component of the involved bone.

Clinical Features

Fibrous dysplasia commonly affects the skeleton unilaterally and can affect one or more bones in the body depending on the timing of the mutation. Should the mutation occur soon after zygote formation, there will be more involvement of the skeleton, including systemic manifestations. A mutation developing later will result in fewer manifestations.

The most common sites of bone involvement include the ribs, femur, tibia, maxilla, and mandible. The solitary or monostotic form of fibrous dysplasia accounts for approximately 70% of all cases and is the most commonly identified type in the jaws. *Polyostotic fibrous dysplasia* is the term used when multiple bones are affected. When polyostotic fibrous dysplasia is accompanied by cutaneous light brown pigmentation (café au lait spots), the abnormality is referred to as *Jaffe or Jaffe–Lichtenstein syndrome*. And when polyostotic involvement is accompanied by café au lait spots and endocrine hyperfunction abnormalities, this is termed *McCune–Albright syndrome*.

Polyostotic fibrous dysplasia is usually identified in children younger than 10 years of age, whereas monostotic disease is typically discovered in a slightly older age group. The lesions usually become static when skeletal growth ceases but bone changes may continue, particularly in the polyostotic form. Furthermore, lesions may become active during pregnancy or with the use of oral contraceptives. Studies of the sex distribution of fibrous dysplasia show no sexual predilection except for McCune–Albright syndrome, which affects females almost exclusively.

Symptoms of fibrous dysplasia may be absent or mild, depending on the degree of involvement. Monostotic fibrous dysplasia is often discovered as an incidental finding in images made for other purposes. Patients with jaw involvement may first experience a unilateral facial swelling or an enlarging deformity of the alveolar process. Pain and pathologic fractures are rare. If craniofacial lesions involve the skull base, the bone changes may impinge on neural foramina and peripheral sensorineural deficits may arise.

Imaging Features

Location. Fibrous dysplasia affects the maxilla almost twice as often as the mandible and is more frequently seen in the more posterior regions of the jaw (Fig. 23.31). Involvement of the axial skeleton is more commonly unilateral, but when fibrous dysplasia affects a single midline bone such as the mandible, or the frontal or sphenoid bones, the changes can cross the midline.

Periphery. The periphery of fibrous dysplasia lesions is most commonly poorly defined, with a gradual and broad zone of transition between normal and dysplastic bone. Some refer to the broadness of the transition zone as "blending" of the dysplastic bone into the normal trabecular pattern. Occasionally the boundary between the dysplastic and normal bone can appear better defined and even corticated, especially in early lesions (Fig. 23.32).

Internal structure. The density and internal pattern of fibrous dysplasia can vary considerably, with the variation being more pronounced in the mandible than in the maxilla. The internal density of the dysplastic bone may be radiolucent, radiopaque, or a mixture of both compared to normal bone. Early lesions may be more radiolucent (Fig. 23.33) than mature ones. In the maxilla and skull base, where the bone changes tend to be more homogeneous, the bone may appear more radiopaque. In the mandible, where the lesion may be more heterogeneous, one may appreciate granular internal septa, giving a multilocular appearance to the abnormal bone.

The abnormal trabeculae in fibrous dysplasia are usually shorter, thinner, and more irregularly shaped and oriented. In addition, the trabeculae may be more numerous than in normal bone. These changes create a series of classical radiologic patterns that can include an appearance referred to as granular or ground glass, resembling the appearance of sandblasted or etched glass (Figs. 23.32 and 23.33). Another common pattern is one that resembles the surface texture of an orange or a lemon (Fig. 23.34). This is termed *peau d'orange*—(French for "orange skin"). A distinctive characteristic is the organization of the abnormal trabeculae into a swirling pattern similar to a fingerprint (Fig. 23.35A). And one final pattern has a wispy arrangement that resembles loose to dense cotton (Fig. 23.35B). Occasionally radiolucent regions may occur in mature lesions of fibrous dysplasia; these are simple bone cavities.

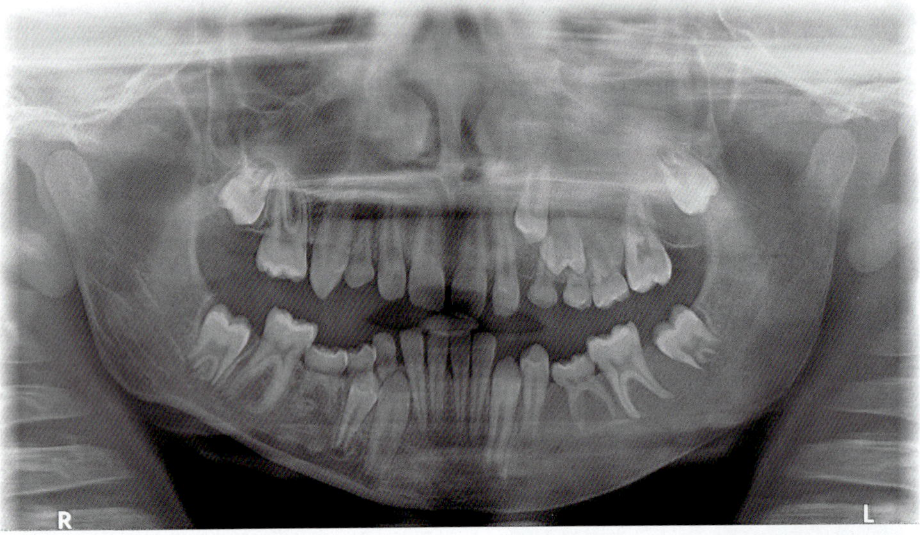

Fig. 23.31 Fibrous dysplasia involving the left maxilla and mandible. Note the ground-glass bone pattern in both bones as well as the enlargement of the left maxillary tuberosity and the inferior surface of the mandible. (Courtesy Dr. H. Grubisa, Oakville, ON.)

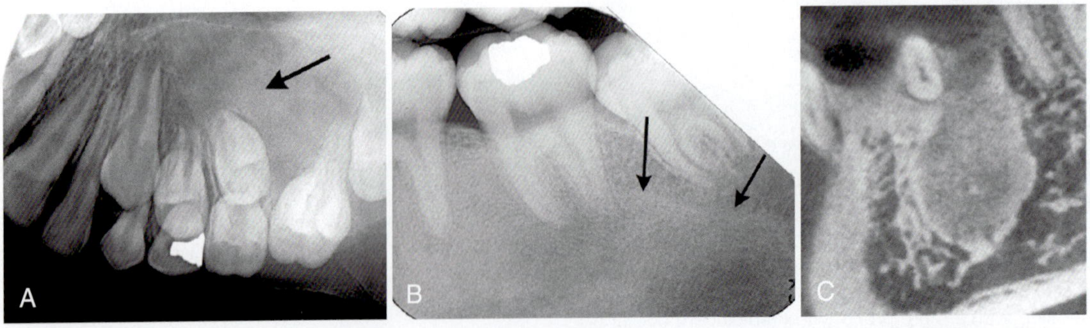

Fig. 23.32 The periapical image shows the granular bone pattern *(arrow)* of fibrous dysplasia blending into the adjacent normal bone in the region of the unerupted maxillary left canine tooth (A). In (B), the border in this case of fibrous dysplasia has a better defined, almost corticated border *(arrows)*. The corrected sagittal cone beam computed tomographic image (C) shows a border that is definitively corticated, although irregular in width.

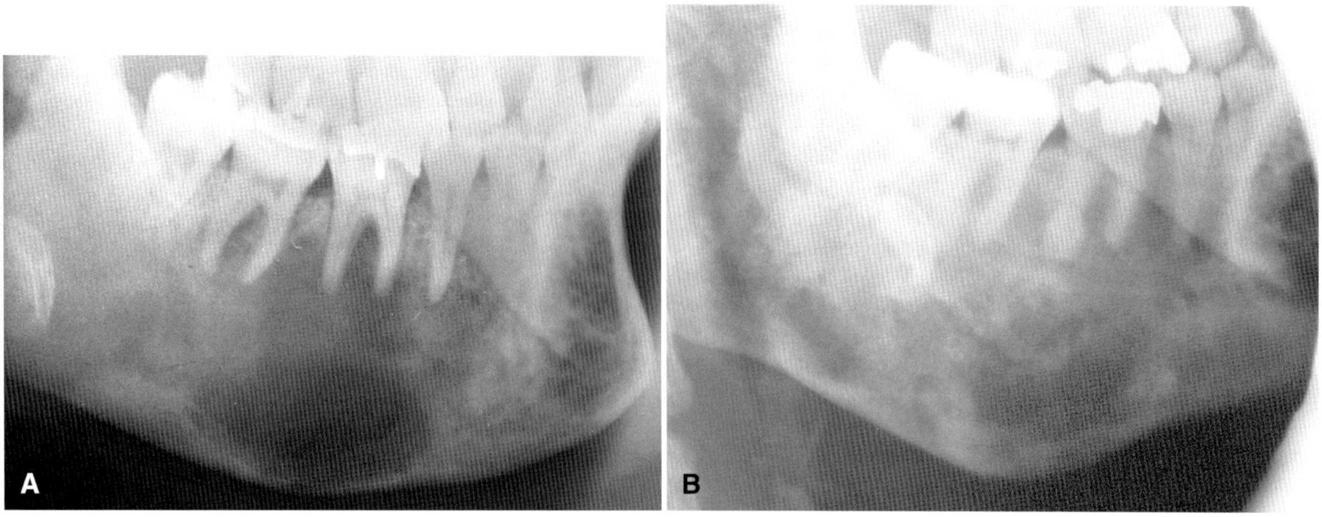

Fig. 23.33 Cropped panoramic images showing an earlier, more radiolucent stage of fibrous dysplasia (A) and, after 18 years, a more radiopaque appearance (B).

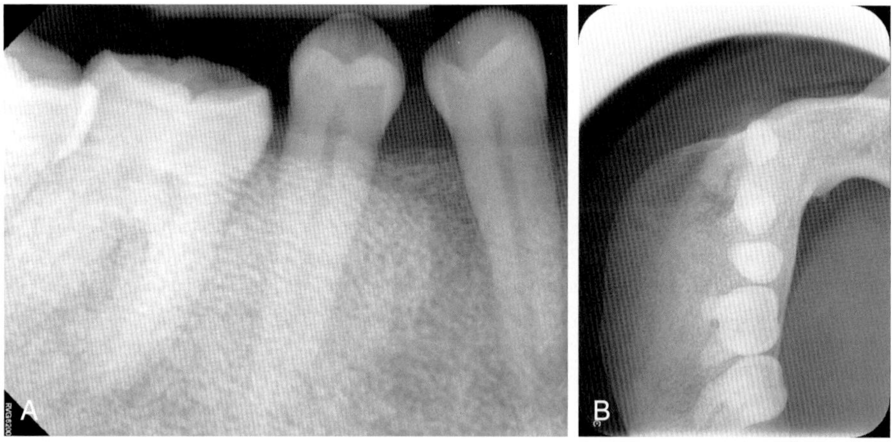

Fig. 23.34 Periapical (A) and right cross-sectional occlusal (B) images show the stippled orange-peel pattern of fibrous dysplasia. Note the significant enlargement of the right mandibular body in (B). (Courtesy Dr. T. Thang, Toronto, ON.)

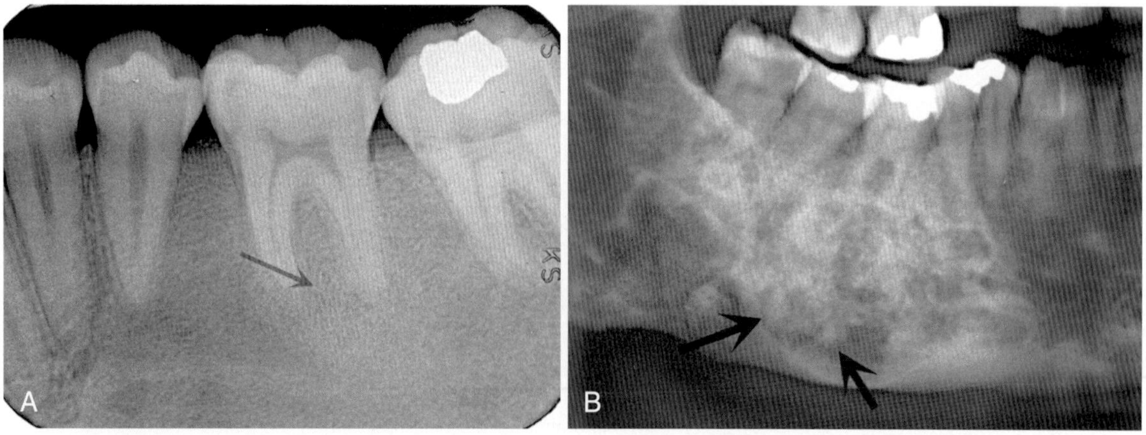

Fig. 23.35 A periapical image (A) shows the fingerprint pattern of fibrous dysplasia around the roots of the mandibular left first molar *(arrow)*. The cropped panoramic image (B) shows a more heterogeneous cotton-wool pattern that includes both radiolucent and radiopaque foci *(arrows)*.

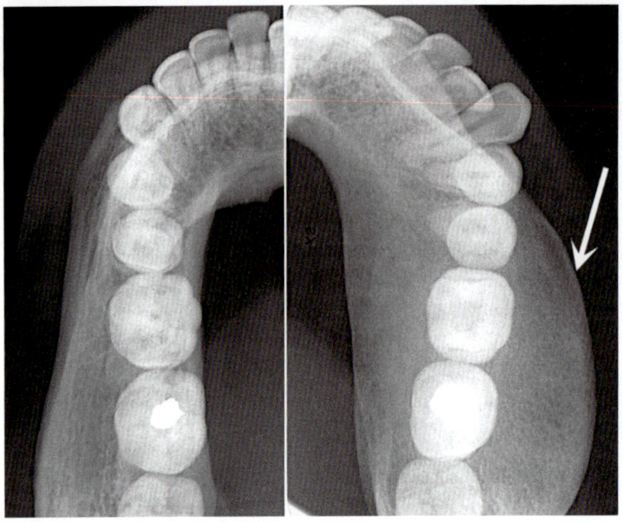

Fig. 23.36 Cross-sectional occlusal images of the right and left mandibular bodies in the same patient show the noted enlargement of the left mandibular body by fibrous dysplasia. The buccal cortex has been significantly thinned, but it is intact *(arrow)*.

Effects on adjacent structures. When a focus of fibrous dysplasia is small, it may have no effect on surrounding structures, and this is referred to as subclinical fibrous dysplasia. As the focus increases in size, there will be bone enlargement, with maintenance of a thinned cortex (Fig. 23.36). In the mandible, the pattern of gentle enlargement can affect the bone more evenly along its length; this is referred to as fusiform enlargement. This pattern of enlargement should be contrasted with the more concentric type of expansion seen with benign neoplasms.

Fibrous dysplasia arising in the maxilla can displace the cortical borders of the maxillary sinus, reducing the size of the air cavity. The lateral wall of the maxillary sinus is often the first to be impacted, and the last region of the sinus to be involved is usually the most posterosuperior border. A characteristic of involvement of the maxilla and maxillary sinus, in particular, is a miniaturized airspace that approximates the normal anatomic shape of the antrum (Fig. 23.37A).

Cortical boundaries, such as the floor of the antrum, may also become less distinct when the dysplastic bone involves the bone cortex. And when the growth epicenter of fibrous dysplasia occurs inferior to the inferior alveolar canal, it may displace the canal in a superior direction (see Fig. 23.37B).

Effects on adjacent teeth. Often the bone surrounding the teeth is altered without affecting the dentition. In such instances, the lamina dura becomes much less distinct as the dysplastic bone blends with this structure (see Fig. 23.34). If there is an increase in bone density, the PDL space may appear to have been narrowed. Fibrous dysplasia can displace teeth or interfere with normal eruption, complicating orthodontic therapy. In very rare instances, some root resorption or hypercementosis may occur.

Differential Interpretation

Other processes can produce the ground-glass pattern of fibrous dysplasia. This pattern is often seen where there has been healing of bone by secondary intention, when immature new bone grows into the connective tissue matrix of granulation tissue. Commonly, this may be seen following tooth extraction or orthograde endodontic treatment of rarefying osteitis. Occasionally PCOD may show a similar bone pattern, but these lesions are often multifocal, with an epicenter in the periapical area of the tooth. As well, PCOD occurs in an older age group. Healing of a simple bone cavity may also create a similar pattern; indeed, both the histopathologic and radiologic appearances of the healed bone may mimic what is seen in fibrous dysplasia.

Metabolic bone diseases such as primary hyperparathyroidism may produce a ground-glass pattern in the bone; however, these changes are often more generalized, bilateral, and polyostotic. Unlike fibrous dysplasia, there is no bone enlargement in hyperparathyroidism. Paget

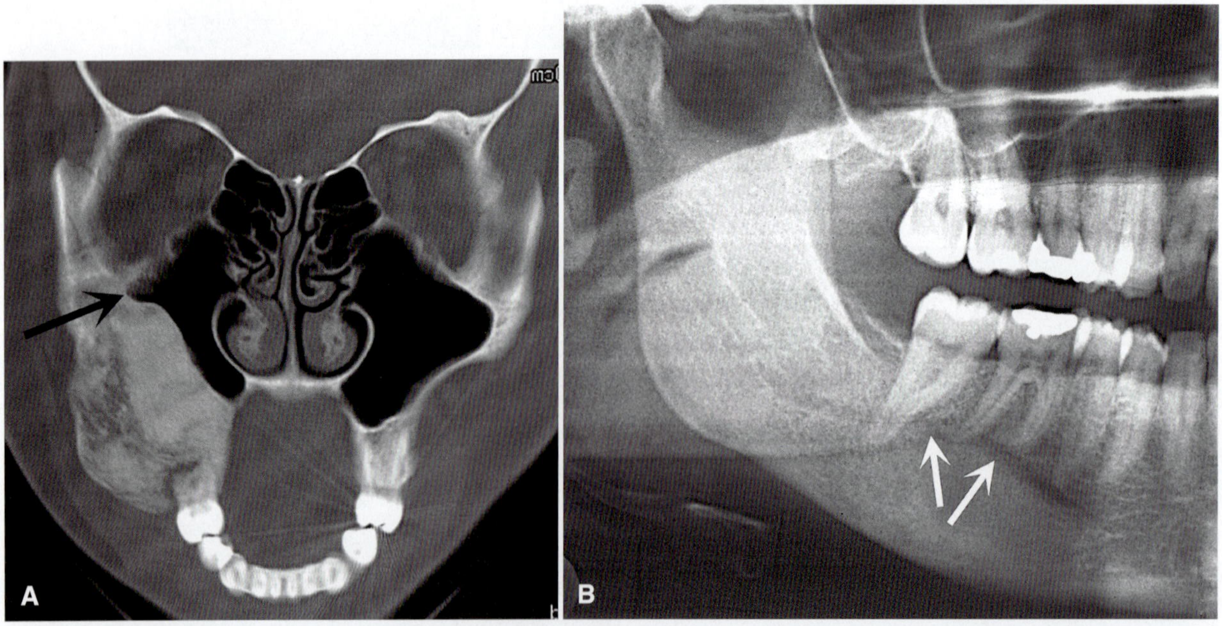

Fig. 23.37 Coronal multidetector computed tomographic image of a region of fibrous dysplasia in the right maxilla (A) shows nonconcentric expansion of the lateral surface of the maxilla and the altered airspace of the maxillary sinus. Note that the right maxillary sinus appears as a smaller version of the unaffected left maxillary sinus and the retained right zygomatic recess *(arrow)*. The cropped panoramic image (B) shows superior displacement of the inferior alveolar nerve canal by a focus of fibrous dysplasia *(arrows)*.

disease of bone may produce a cotton-wool type of pattern, and there may be expansion with bilateral bone involvement.

Of paramount importance is the differentiation of osteomyelitis, cemento-ossifying fibroma, and osteosarcoma from fibrous dysplasia. Although these entities can have very similar histopathologic and radiologic appearances, their management is dramatically different. Therefore, a careful analysis of the imaging features is paramount. Whereas osteomyelitis may cause a bone to increase in size, the additional bone is generated at the bone surface by the periosteum. The new bone that is laid down on the surface of the outer cortex in osteomyelitis may reveal evidence of the original cortex and lamellar periosteal new bone formation. In contrast, fibrous dysplasia enlarges the bone from within, displacing and thinning the outer cortex as the bone grows so that the remaining cortex maintains its position at the outer surface of the bone. The identification of sequestra aids in the differentiation of osteomyelitis from fibrous dysplasia. Osteosarcoma may produce a similar internal pattern depending on the degree of differentiation of the malignant osteoblasts, but it should show other malignant and more aggressive radiologic features (see Chapter 24). Some difficulty may arise in differentiating cemento-ossifying fibroma of the maxilla, especially the juvenile type. Cemento-ossifying fibroma grows in a more concentric manner. If the bone pattern is altered around the teeth and the teeth are displaced from a specific epicenter, the lesion is more likely cemento-ossifying fibroma rather than fibrous dysplasia. In the maxilla, the shape of the enlarged bone of fibrous dysplasia adjacent to the antrum maintains the contour of the antral wall, which is different from the more convex pattern of expansion of a neoplasm.

Management

In most cases, the clinical and radiologic features of fibrous dysplasia are sufficient to allow the practitioner to make a diagnosis without a biopsy. However, consultation with an oral and maxillofacial radiologist is advisable. The radiologist may supplement a conventional imaging examination with CBCT or MDCT, so that features not seen on planar imaging may become more apparent. Such an examination may also serve as a baseline for future comparisons.

It is reasonable to continue occasional monitoring of the involved bone or ask the patient to report any changes. With many lesions, bone enlargement slows at skeletal maturation; orthodontic treatment and cosmetic surgery may be delayed until after this time. Sarcomatous changes are unusual and exceptionally rare but have been reported, especially if radiation therapy has been administered.

Paget Disease of Bone

Disease Mechanism

Paget disease of bone, or osteitis deformans, is a polyostotic skeletal disorder that may involve a paramyxovirus infection and subsequent changes to the host cell genome. Mutations have been identified in three genes involved in bone remodeling: *SQSTM1, TNFRSF11A,* and *TNFRSF11B*. Of these, the most commonly identified mutation involves the *SQSTM1* gene. Abnormal osteoclasts produce an intense wave of bone resorption. After a period of time, this is followed by vigorous osteoblastic activity, forming poor-quality woven bone. The condition may involve many bones simultaneously, but it is not a generalized skeletal abnormality.

Clinical Features

Paget disease of bone is seen most frequently in the United Kingdom and Australia and less often in North America. It has an incidence of approximately 3.5% of individuals above 40 years of age, and at age 65, the incidence in men is approximately twice that in women. Of note is that the worldwide incidence of Paget disease of bone is declining, and this may be related to the increased uptake of vaccinations against airborne viruses.

The affected bone is enlarged and commonly deformed because of the poor quality of the bone that is formed. This can result in bowing of the legs, curvature of the spine, and enlargement of the skull. Also, there may be enlargement of the jaws which can cause tooth movement, diastema, and malocclusion. Removable dentures may become tight or fit poorly in patients.

Bone pain is an inconsistent symptom and is most often directed toward the weight-bearing bones; facial or jaw pain is uncommon. Patients with Paget disease of bone may also have ill-defined sensorineural pain due to the impingement neural foramina and canals. They also often have severely elevated levels of serum alkaline phosphatase (greater than with any other disorder) during osteoblastic phases of the disease. These patients also often have high levels of hydroxyproline in the urine—a marker of collagen degradation.

Imaging Features

Location. Paget disease of bone occurs most often in the pelvis, femur, skull (Figs. 23.38 and 23.39), and vertebrae. Whenever the jaws are involved, which is generally infrequently, the maxilla is affected approximately twice as often as the mandible. Although bone involvement is generally bilateral, occasionally only one maxilla is involved or the involvement may be significantly greater on one side. In the mandible, the entire bone is usually involved.

Internal structure. The internal appearance of the bone is variable and depends on the developmental stage of the disease. Classically, Paget disease of bone has three radiologic stages, although these may often overlap. In the early stage of primarily osteoclastic activity, the bone appears radiolucent. In the intermediate stage of the disease, granular or ground-glass–patterned bone appears within the radiolucent areas. Finally, in the most mature stage, the bone becomes dense and radiopaque with a pattern that has been described as "cotton-wool."

In the jaws, the trabeculae are altered in number and shape. In the early stage, trabeculae numbers are decreased. During the intermediate and late stages, the trabeculae may become elongated and align themselves in a linear pattern—an appearance that is more common in the mandible. Trabeculae may be short, with random orientations, and may have a granular pattern similar to that which is seen in fibrous dysplasia. A third pattern occurs when the trabeculae are organized into rounded, radiopaque patches of abnormal bone, creating a cotton-wool appearance (Fig. 23.39).

Effects on adjacent structures. Paget disease of bone always enlarges an affected bone to some extent, even in the early stage. Often the bone

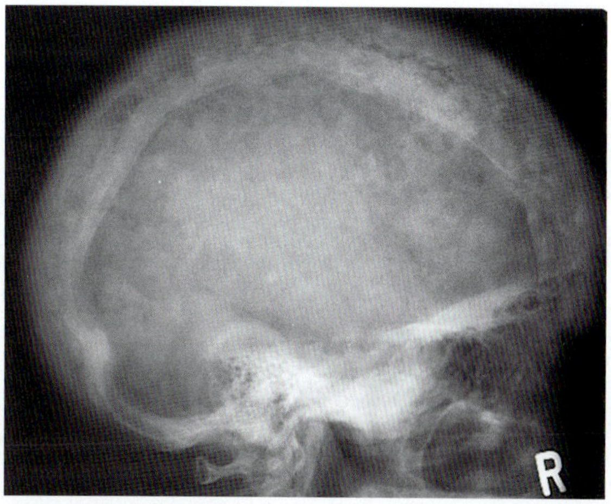

Fig. 23.38 A lateral image of the calvarium showing the flocculent cotton-wool appearance of the bone and substantial thickening of the skull bones. (Courtesy Dr. K. Dolan, Iowa City, IA.)

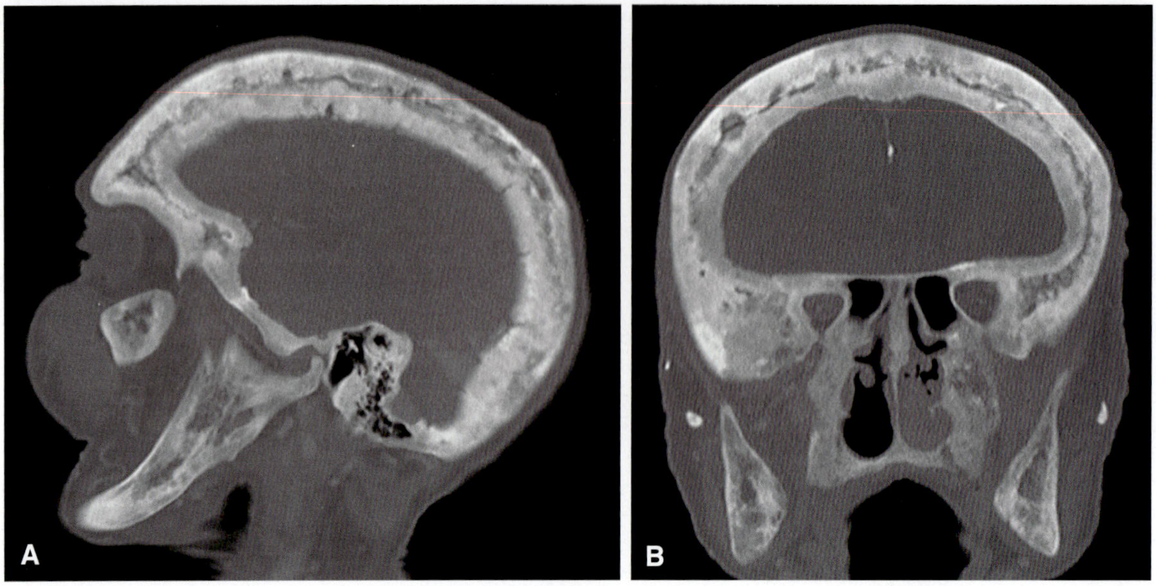

Fig. 23.39 Sagittal (A) and coronal (B) multidetector computed tomographic images in a patient with Paget disease of bone. Note the increase in thickness of the bones and the bone density.

enlargement is impressive. The thickness of the bones of the calvarium may increase three or four times their normal thickness. In enlarged jaws, the cortex may be thinned but remains intact, and it may have a laminated appearance in occlusal images (see Fig. 23.40). When the maxilla is involved, the disease invariably involves the sinus floor. However, the airspace is usually not diminished to a great extent. The sinus floor may appear more granular and less apparent as sharp boundaries.

Effects on adjacent teeth. The lamina dura may become less evident and may be altered into the abnormal bone pattern. Hypercementosis often develops, and this may be exuberant and irregular, which is characteristic of Paget disease (Fig. 23.41).

Differential Interpretation

Paget disease of bone may appear similar to fibrous dysplasia; however, the disease occurs in an older age group and is almost always bilateral. In the maxilla, fibrous dysplasia has a tendency to encroach on the sinus airspace, whereas Paget disease does not. The linear trabeculae and cotton-wool appearance of Paget disease are distinctive. Lesions of cemento-osseous dysplasia are more focal and less generalized than Paget disease of bone, and there are areas of normal intervening bone between the foci of cemento-osseous dysplasia. Although the cemento-osseous dysplasias may also have an internal cotton-wool pattern, these abnormalities have an epicenter that is located superior to the inferior

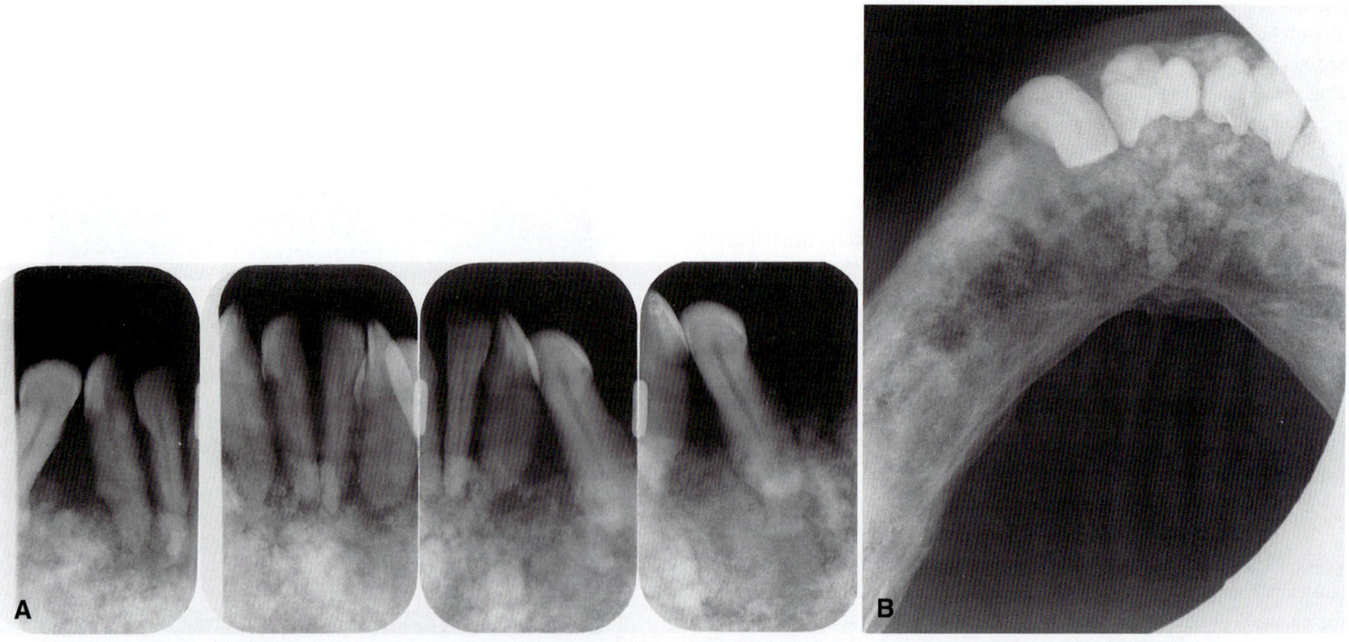

Fig. 23.40 Periapical and occlusal images of Paget disease of bone with a cotton-wool appearance (A) and mandibular enlargement (B). Note the maintenance of the thin cortices on the occlusal image and the laminated appearance of the lingual cortex.

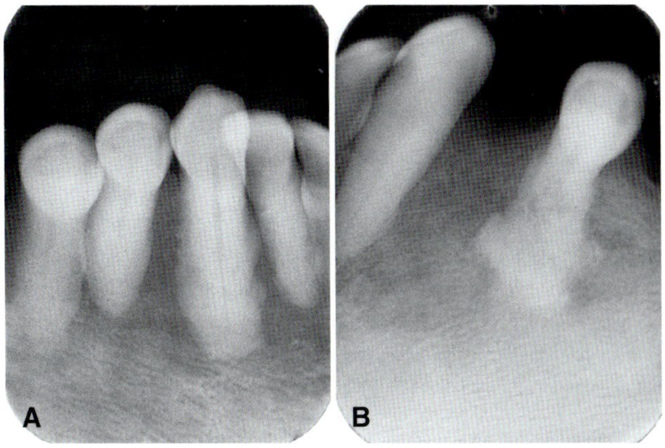

Fig. 23.41 Two periapical images (A and B) of Paget disease of bone showing exuberant hypercementosis of the roots.

alveolar nerve canal, and an internal radiolucent border may be appreciated. The bone pattern in Paget disease of bone may show some similarities to the bone pattern in metabolic bone diseases, and both conditions may be bilateral. However, Paget disease enlarges bone and metabolic diseases tend not to. The specific bone pattern changes, the late age of onset, the enlargement of the involved bone, and the extreme elevation of serum alkaline phosphatase aid in the differential diagnosis.

Management

Paget disease of bone is usually managed medically, using calcitonin or, more recently, bisphosphonates. The medication relieves pain and reduces the serum alkaline phosphatase levels and osteoclastic activity. Surgery may be required to correct deformities of the long bones and treat fractures.

There are complications of this disease that are of concern. Extraction sites heal slowly, and the incidence of osteomyelitis is higher. Approximately 10% of cases with polyostotic disease develop osteosarcoma.

INTRAOSSEOUS HEALING

Disease Mechanism

After the extraction of a tooth or successful orthograde endodontic treatment, or following the successful excision of an intraosseous lesion, the defect fills with bone as healing occurs by secondary intention. The potential for the defect to infill with bone and "heal" is dictated by the availability of nearby bone-forming cells that migrate into the defect, the size of the defect, and time. Should the bone defect be large, the contribution of adjacent bone cells from the surface or periosteum to healing may be insufficient, particularly if the lesion extends to both adjacent bone cortices. Time is also an important variable, as complete healing can take many months to upwards of a year, making early signs of healing difficult to visualize radiologically. Moreover, should the patient be older and osteopenic, there may be fewer available bone cells to infill the defect.

Osseous infilling begins at the periphery of the defect, as osteoblasts grow inward from the internal surface of the defect. Early healing may be difficult to visualize due to the poor mineralization of the new bone, and the radiolucent appearance may persist for some time. If the radiologic interpretation is uncertain, the patient's treatment history, as well as the clinical signs and symptoms, may inform the interpretation. Histopathologically, the new bone that is formed may appear similar to that seen in a bone dysplasia.

Clinical Features

The patient will be asymptomatic. It is important, however, to correlate a finding of potential healing with a history of endodontic treatment or surgery. If prior imaging is available, this may also help inform the interpretation and diagnosis.

Imaging Features

Periphery

As osseous healing begins at the periphery, any cortex previously visible on the image will slowly be lost as new bone begins to grow inward. The periphery may become less well defined depending on bone cell availability and maturation. Should the endpoint of the healing process be a fibrous scar, the internal surface of the healing defect can appear corticated.

Shape

The area of healing may appear irregular. When an entity heals in the maxilla that has also displaced the floor of the maxillary sinus superiorly, the healed contour of the sinus floor can take on the appearance of a deflated balloon as the defect fills with bone (Fig. 23.42). This is referred to as a lesion that has "collapsed" (e.g., collapsed cyst).

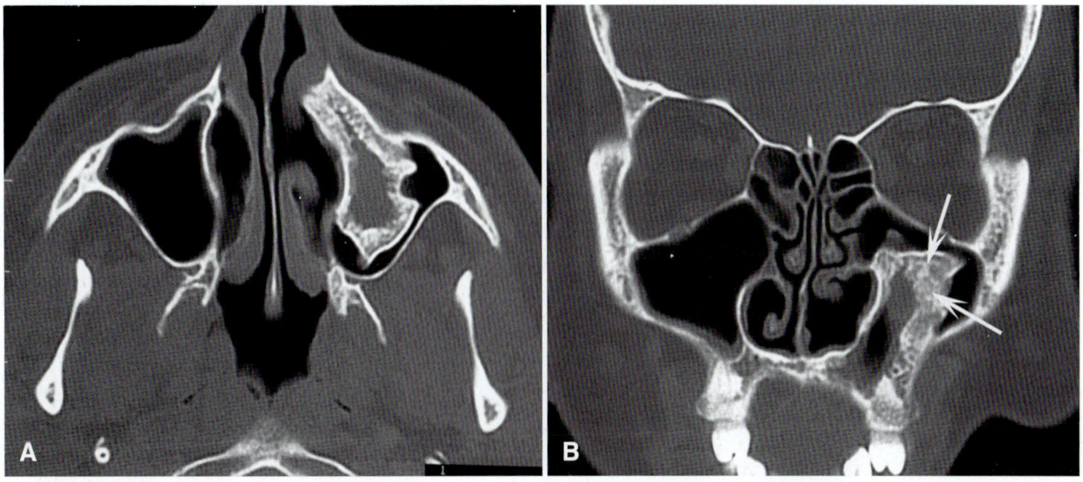

Fig. 23.42 Axial (A) and coronal (B) bone window multidetector computed tomographic images of a collapsed cystic lesion in the left maxilla. Note the irregular shape and contour to the collapsing lesion and the new bone that is being deposited from the periphery. (Courtesy Drs. S. Ahing and T. Blight, Winnipeg, MB.)

Internal Structure

New bone may first be visible around the periphery of the radiolucent defect, adjacent to the normal cancellous bone. The periphery of the radiolucent area may display a granular type of bone pattern consisting of short trabeculae and small, punctate radiolucent spaces (Fig. 23.43). With time, the central radiolucent focus decreases in size as new bone grows inward toward the center. As the bone matures, there may be a series of radiating trabeculae extending from the border of the normal adjacent bone inward toward the center of the defect. This pattern at the periphery is sometimes described as having a rolled border, or a doughnut pattern. Such entities have been described as sites of "incomplete osseous healing," a "fibrous scar," or "healing with an altered bone pattern" (Fig. 23.44).

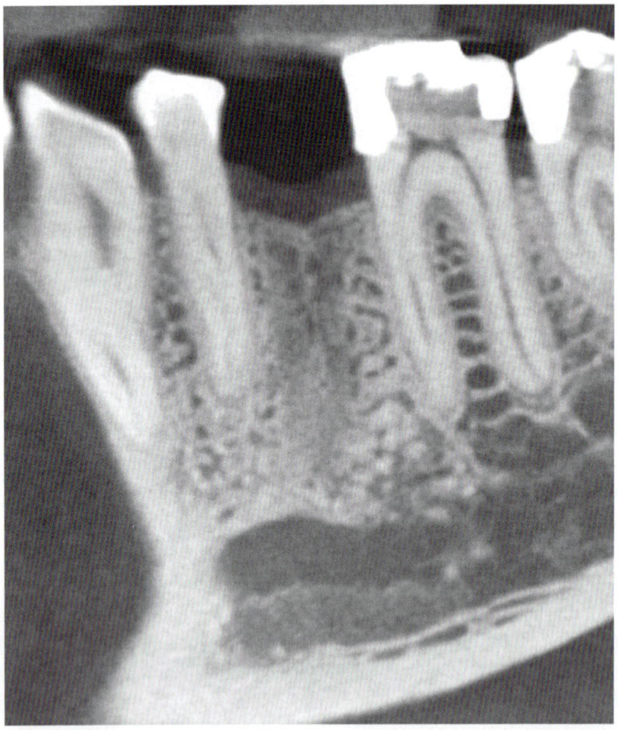

Fig. 23.43 Corrected sagittal cone beam computed tomographic image showing a ground-glass pattern of bone healing following extraction of the mandibular left second premolar.

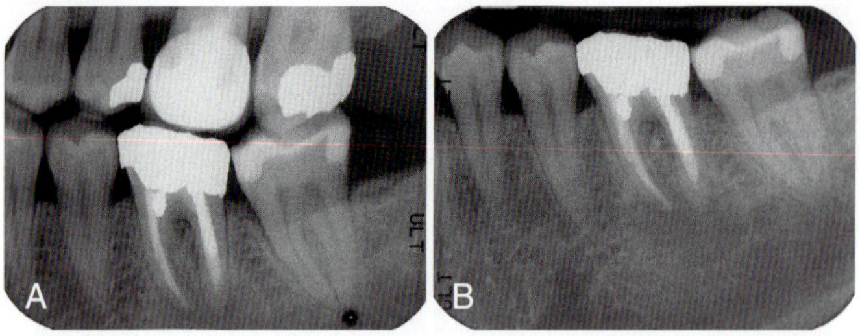

Fig. 23.45 Bitewing (A) and periapical (B) images showing a ground-glass pattern of bone healing following successful orthograde endodontic treatment. Note the uniform periodontal ligament spaces located at the root apices of the mandibular left first molar.

Effects on Surrounding Structures

There may be no effects on the adjacent structures. In a young person with a great deal of healing potential, the new bone that develops can appear as if the defect had never been present, with normal trabeculae and cortical borders being completely reestablished.

Effects on Adjacent Teeth

The PDL space should be reestablished around the teeth in the event of healing as well as the lamina dura (Fig. 23.45).

HEMOGLOBINOPATHIES

Disease Mechanism

Sickle cell anemia and thalassemia are both hereditary hemoglobinopathies that arise as a result of errors in hemoglobin molecule synthesis. In sickle cell anemia, a mutation of the *HBB* gene that encodes the beta globulin subunit of the hemoglobin molecule results in a morphological alteration to the red blood cell leading to the sickle shape that is seen under light microscopy. The sickled cells prevent the normal delivery of oxygen to tissues. In contrast, thalassemia can affect either the *HBB* gene or one of the *HBA* genes, the *HBA* gene being the one that encodes one of the two alpha globulin subunits of hemoglobin. In thalassemia, an inadequate amount of hemoglobin is synthesized, and this results in lower red blood cell numbers and lower oxygen levels in tissues. In response to the hemoglobinopathies, the hematopoietic system attempts to increase the production of red blood cells, inducing a compensatory hyperplasia of the bone

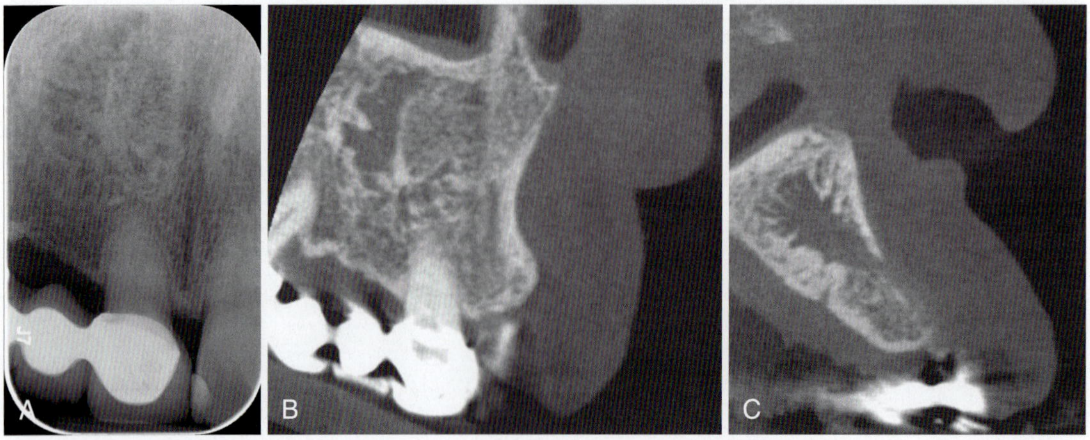

Fig. 23.44 Periapical (A), and corrected sagittal (B) and buccal/lingual cross-sectional (C) cone beam computed tomographic images of a fibrous scar in the anterior right maxilla. Note the radiating pattern of the bone toward the center of the defect and the absence of mineralization at the center.

marrow in regions of the skeleton that once had the ability to produce red blood cells.

Clinical Features

The most severe form of sickle cell anemia, the homozygous recessive form, affects approximately 1 in every 400 individuals of African descent. Although the heterozygous genotype is present in about 6% to 8% of this population, these individuals do not show related clinical findings. In contrast, thalassemia affects individuals from Mediterranean countries.

The signs and symptoms of sickle cell anemia vary considerably, and most patients with the disease normally manifest mild, chronic features. Prolonged episodes of hemolytic quiescence occur, occasionally punctuated by exacerbations known as sickle cell crises. During the crisis state, patients often have severe abdominal, muscle and joint pain and a high temperature; they may also experience circulatory collapse. During milder periods, a patient may complain of fatigue, weakness, shortness of breath, and muscle and joint pain. As in other chronic anemias, the heart is usually enlarged and a murmur may be present. The disease occurs mostly in children and adolescents, and affected individuals may experience a life expectancy that is 20 years less than those unaffected. Patients with thalassemia can often present with the milder symptoms of fatigue and weakness. Their skin may be pale, and their face develops prominent cheekbones and a protrusive premaxilla, resulting in a "rodent-like" face.

Imaging Features

The hyperplasia of the bone marrow at the expense of cancellous bone is the primary reason for the abnormal manifestations of the hemoglobinopathies seen in diagnostic images.

Effects on the Teeth and Jaws

The jaws appear osteopenic with thinning of the cortical borders and enlargement of the marrow spaces as these spaces are recruited to produce more red blood cells. The trabeculae are elongated and coarse as the marrow spaces enlarge. Severe bone marrow hyperplasia prevents development of the paranasal sinuses, especially the maxillary sinus, and causes an expansion of the maxilla resulting in malocclusion.

Effects on the Skeleton

The effects of the hemoglobinopathies on the skeleton generally result from reactivation and hyperplasia of the quiescent bone marrow (Fig. 23.46). The thinning of individual cancellous trabeculae and cortices is most common in the vertebral bodies, long bones, skull,

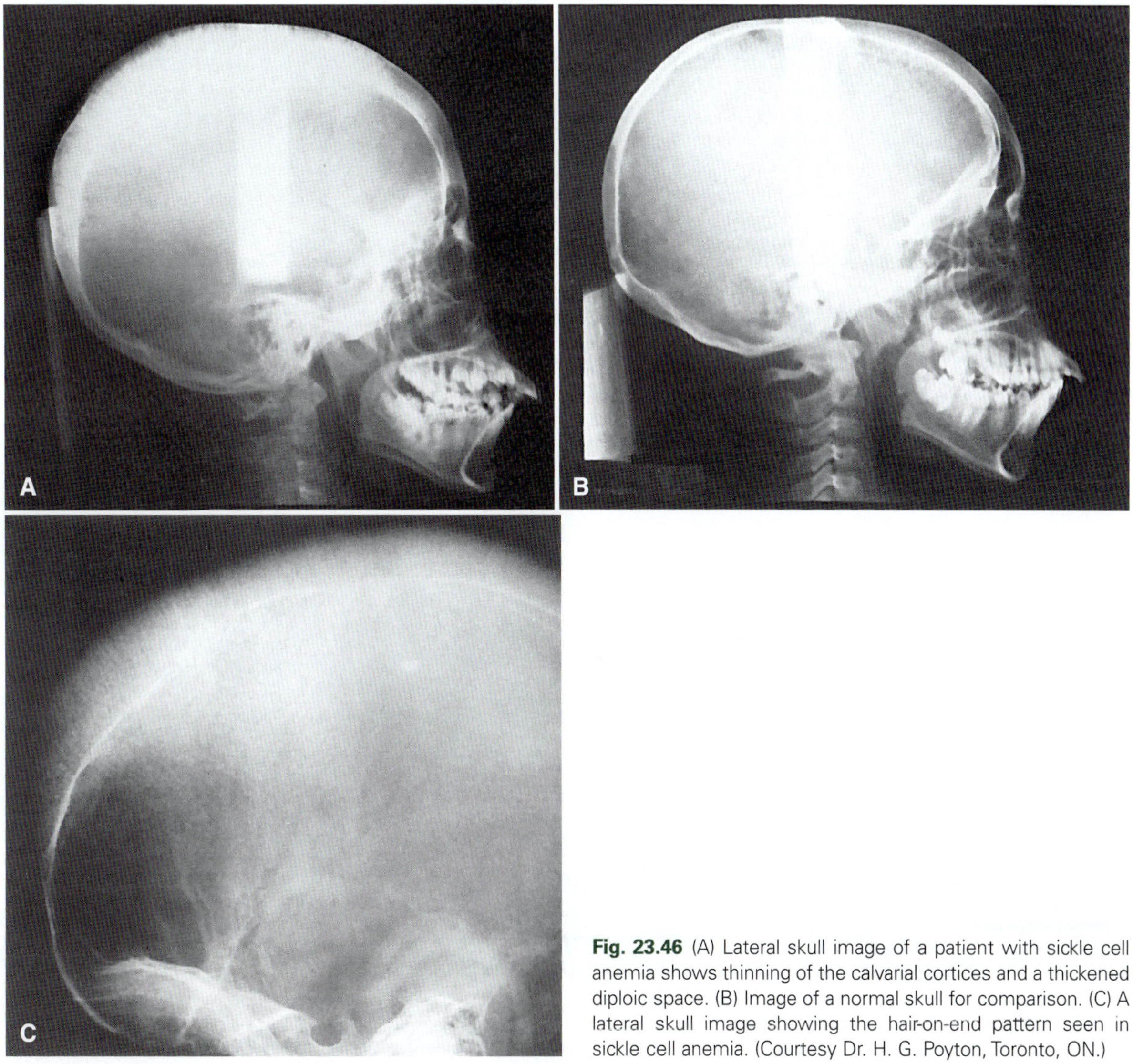

Fig. 23.46 (A) Lateral skull image of a patient with sickle cell anemia shows thinning of the calvarial cortices and a thickened diploic space. (B) Image of a normal skull for comparison. (C) A lateral skull image showing the hair-on-end pattern seen in sickle cell anemia. (Courtesy Dr. H. G. Poyton, Toronto, ON.)

and jaws. The skull may show widening of the diploic space and thinning of the inner and outer cortices (Figs. 23.47 and 23.48). In extreme cases (5%), the surface cortex of the skull cannot be visualized, and a hair-on-end appearance may develop as an exuberant reaction in an attempt to increase the volume of marrow space for the production of new red blood cells. Small areas of infarction may be present within bones if there has been blockage of the microvasculature; these are seen as areas of localized bone sclerosis. Osteomyelitis may complicate the hemoglobinopathies if infection begins in one of these areas of pronounced hypovascularity.

Management

Management of patients with sickle cell anemia is supportive and aims to control the symptoms and prevent the complications of this multisystem disease. Bone marrow transplantation is a curative option, but its applicability is limited because of the associated risks. Patients with thalassemia minor require no treatment except for iron supplementation when iron deficiency is confirmed. Patients with thalassemia major require regular hypertransfusion to maintain their hemoglobin levels and iron chelation therapy to prevent iron overload.

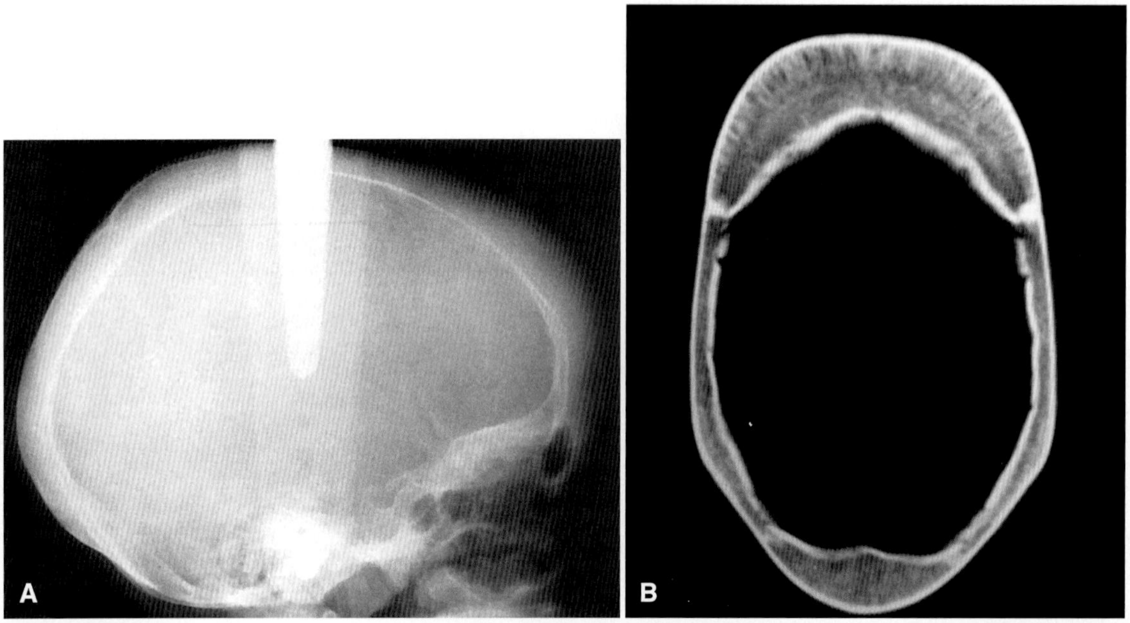

Fig. 23.47 Lateral skull (A) and axial multidetector computed tomographic (B) images of a patient with thalassemia. Note the granular appearance of the skull and thickening of the diploic space. The computed tomographic image shows the hair-on-end appearance in the frontal bone. (A, Courtesy Dr. H. G. Poyton, Toronto, ON.)

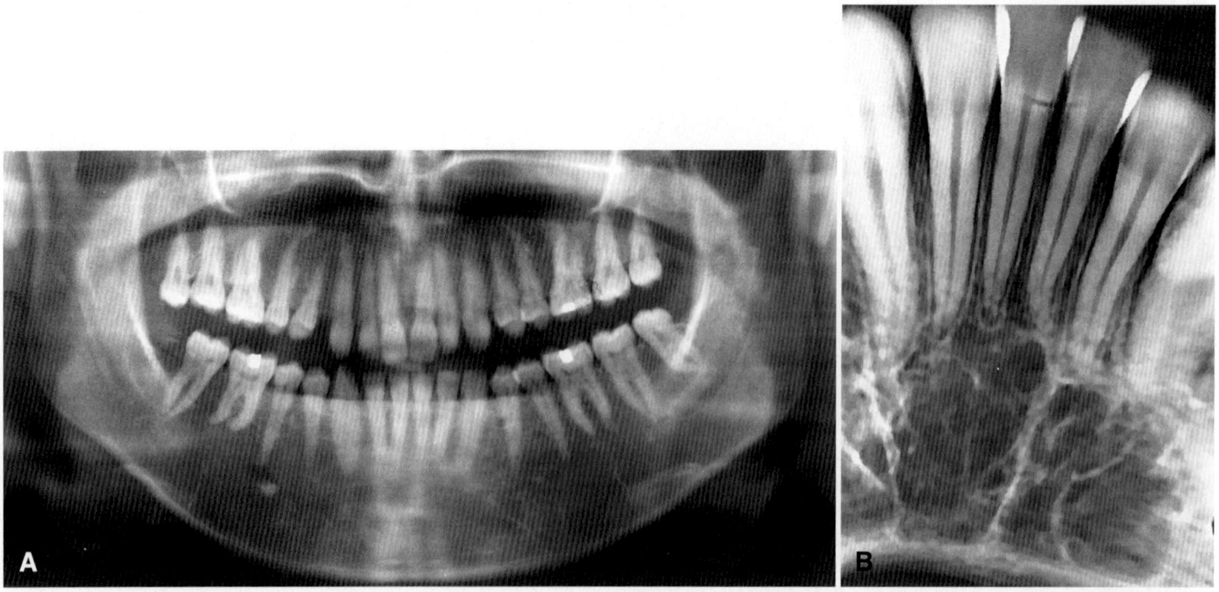

Fig. 23.48 Panoramic image (A) of a patient with thalassemia. Note the thickened body of the mandible, the sparse trabeculae, and absent maxillary sinuses. In the periapical image (B) of a different patient, note the thick trabeculae and large bone marrow spaces. (Courtesy Dr. H. G. Poyton, Toronto, ON.)

BIBLIOGRAPHY

Fibrous Dysplasia

Davidova LA, Bhattacharyya I, Islam MN, et al. An analysis of clinical and histopathologic features of fibrous dysplasia of the jaws: a series of 40 cases and review of the literature. *Head Neck Pathol.* 2020;14:353-361.

Kushchayeva YS, Kushchayev SV, Glushko TY, et al. Fibrous dysplasia for radiologists: beyond ground glass bone matrix. *Insights Imaging.* 2018;9: 1035-1056.

Petrikowski CG, Pharoah MJ, Lee L, et al. Radiographic differentiation of osteogenic sarcoma, osteomyelitis and fibrous dysplasia of the jaws. *Oral Surg Oral Med Oral Pathol Oral Radiol Endod.* 1977;50:1-7.

Van de Voorde N, Mortier GR, Vanhoenacker FM. Fibrous dysplasia, Paget's disease of bone, and other uncommon sclerotic bone lesions of the craniofacial bones. *Semin Musculoskelet Radiol.* 2020;24:570-578.

Hypercortisolism

Barbot M, Zilio M, Scaroni C. Cushing's syndrome: overview of clinical presentation, diagnostic tools and complications. *Best Pract Res Clin Endocrinol Metab.* 2020;34:101380.

Hyperthyroidism

Aytekin Z, Yilmaz SG. Evaluation of osseous changes in dental panoramic radiography using radiomorphometric indices in patients with hyperthyroidism. *Oral Surg Oral Med Oral Pathol Oral Radiol.* 2022;133:492-499.

Hyperparathyroidism

Guimarães LM, Valeriano AT, Rebelo Pontes HA, et al. Manifestations of hyperparathyroidism in the jaws: concepts, mechanisms, and clinical aspects. *Oral Surg Oral Med Oral Pathol Oral Radiol.* 2022;133:547-555.

Minisola S, Arnold A, Belaya Z, et al. Epidemiology, pathophysiology, and genetics of primary hyperparathyroidism. *J Bone Miner Res.* 2022;37: 2315-2329.

Torresan F, Iacobone M. Clinical features, treatment, and surveillance of hyperparathyroidism-jaw tumor syndrome: an up-to-date and review of the literature. *Int J Endocrinol.* 2019;2019:1761030.

Hypoparathyroidism

Bilezikian JP. Hypoparathyroidism. *J Clin Endocrinol Metab.* 2020; 105:1722-1736.

Frensilli J, Stoner R, Hinrichs E. Dental changes of idiopathic-hypoparathyroidism: report of three cases. *J Oral Surg.* 1971;29:727-731.

Hypophosphatasia

Jedrychowski JR, Duperon D. Childhood hypophosphatasia with oral manifestations. *J Oral Med.* 1979;34:18-22.

Macfarlane JD, Swart JGN. Dental aspects of hypophosphatasia: a case report, family study, and literature review. *Oral Surg Oral Med Oral Pathol.* 1989;67:521-526.

Whyte MP. Hypophosphatasia – aetiology, nosology, pathogenesis, diagnosis and treatment. *Nat Rev Endocrinol.* 2016;12:233-246.

Hypopituitarism

Conley H, Steflik DE, Singh B, et al. Clinical and histologic findings of the dentition in a hypopituitary patient: report of case. *ASDC J Dent Child.* 1990;57:376-379.

Okawa R, Kokomoto K, Nakano K. Dental effects of enzyme replacement therapy in case of childhood-type hypophosphatasia. *BMC Oral Health.* 2021;21:323.

Cemento-Osseous Dysplasias

Alsufyani NA, Lam EW. Cemento-osseous dysplasia of the jaw bones: key radiographic features. *Dentomaxillofac Radiol.* 2011;40:141-146.

Chadwick JW, Alsufyani NA, Lam EW. Clinical and radiographic features of solitary and cemento-osseous dysplasia-associated simple bone cysts. *Dentomaxillofac Radiol.* 2011;40:230-235.

Kato CNAO, de Arruda JAA, Mendes PA, et al. Infected cemento-osseous dysplasia: analysis of 66 cases and literature review. *Head Neck Pathol.* 2020;14:173-182.

MacDonald-Jankowski DS. Florid cemento-osseous dysplasia: a systematic review. *Dentomaxillofac Radiol.* 2003;32:141-149.

Osteoporosis

Mupparapu M, Akintoye SO. Application of panoramic radiography in the detection of osteopenia and osteoporosis-current state of the art. *Curr Osteoporos Rep.* 2023;21(4):354-359.

White SC. Oral radiographic predictors of osteoporosis. *Dentomaxillofac Radiol.* 2002;31:84-92.

Osteopetrosis

Calder AD, Arulkumaran S, D'Arco F. Imaging in osteopetrosis. *Bone.* 2022;165:16560.

Nilesh K. Extensive maxillary osteomyelitis following tooth extraction in a patient with osteopetrosis. *BMJ Case Rep.* 2020;13:e235091.

Ruprecht A, Wagner H, Engel H. Osteopetrosis: report of a case and discussion of the differential diagnosis. *Oral Surg Oral Med Oral Pathol.* 1988;66:674-679.

Younai F, Eisenbud L, Sciubba JJ. Osteopetrosis: a case report including gross and microscopic findings in the mandible at autopsy. *Oral Surg Oral Med Oral Pathol.* 1988;65:214-221.

Paget Disease of Bone

Amaya N, Itoiz ME, Paparella ML. Paget's disease of the jaws: histological features of a series of 31 cases. *Acta Odontol Latinoam.* 2021;34:237-262.

Gennari L, Rendina D, Merlotti D, et al. Update on the pathogenesis and genetics of Paget's disease of bone. *Front Cell Dev Biol.* 2022;10:932065.

Lombardi AF, Aihara AY, Fernandes ADRC, et al. Imaging of Paget's disease of bone. *Radiol Clin North Am.* 2022;60:561-573.

Rao V, Karasick D. Hypercementosis: an important clue to Paget disease of the maxilla. *Skeletal Radiol.* 1982;9:126-128.

Systemic Sclerosis

Alexandridis C, White SC. Periodontal ligament changes in patients with progressive systemic sclerosis. *Oral Surg Oral Med Oral Pathol.* 1984;58: 113-118.

Burchfield C, Vorrasi J. Maxillofacial implications of scleroderma and systemic sclerosis: a case report and literature review. *J Oral Maxillofac Surg.* 2019;77: 1203-1208.

Rickets

Harris R, Sullivan HR. Dental sequelae in deciduous dentition in vitamin-D resistant rickets: case report. *Aust Dent J.* 1960;5:200-203.

Marks SC, Lindahl RL, Bawden JW. Dental and cephalometric findings in vitamin D resistant rickets. *J Dent Child.* 1965;32:239.

Opsahl VS, Gaucher C, Bardet C, et al. Tooth dentin defects reflect genetic disorders affecting bone mineralization. *Bone.* 2012;50:989-997.

Sickle Cell Anemia

Costa SA, Ribeiro CCC, Thomaz EBAF, et al. Mechanisms underlying the adaptive pulp and jaw bone trabecular changes in sickle cell anemia. *Oral Dis.* 2023;29:786-795.

White SC, Cohen JM, Mourshed FA. Digital analysis of trabecular pattern in jaws of patients with sickle cell anemia. *Dentomaxillofac Radiol.* 2000;29: 119-124.

Thalassemia

Bayrak S, Göller Bulut D, Orhan K, et al. Evaluation of osseous changes in dental panoramic radiography of thalassemia patients using mandibular indexes and fractal size analysis. *Oral Radiol.* 2020;36:18-24.

Movahhedian N, Akbarizadeh F, Khojastepour L, et al. Assessment of mandibular characteristics in patients affected with b-thalassemia major: a retrospective case control study. *Int Orthod.* 2020;18:776-783.

24

Malignant Neoplasms

Ernest W.N. Lam

DISEASE MECHANISM

Malignant neoplasms are abnormal growths of tissue that develop as a result of uncontrolled cell proliferation. In contrast to benign neoplasms, malignant neoplasms generally show more aggressive growth patterns, invade adjacent normal tissues, and have the ability to metastasize to regional lymph nodes or distant sites through the lymphatic or vascular systems, or by perineural spread. Malignant neoplasms that arise de novo are referred to as primary neoplasms, and a lesion that originates from a distant primary malignant neoplasm is termed a metastasis. The term "cancer," synonymous with malignant neoplasia, references the crab-like infiltration of malignant cell populations into adjacent tissue spaces seen under a microscope.

The loss of control of cell proliferation in malignant neoplasia is the result of now often identifiable gene mutations. Such mutations can be caused by viruses (e.g., Epstein–Barr virus), high-dose radiation exposure, or exposure to carcinogenic agents (e.g., tobacco). As with benign neoplasia, the molecular abnormality in a malignant cell is propagated through cell division, resulting in a clonal population of abnormal cells.

The most practical method of classification of malignant neoplasms is based on the cell of origin. In this chapter, malignancies that commonly involve the jaws have been divided into four categories: lesions of epithelial origin or carcinomas; lesions of mesenchymal origin or sarcomas; lesions of hematopoietic origin; and metastatic lesions. Of these, carcinomas are by far the most common malignant neoplasm in the head and neck.

The prognosis for the patient is related to early detection. Often, malignant neoplasms are not recognized early enough, are misdiagnosed as other disease processes such as inflammation, and are, thus, mismanaged. Discussions of unusual malignant neoplasms have been omitted from this chapter to concentrate on more common lesions that a general practitioner may encounter.

CLINICAL FEATURES

The clinical signs and symptoms that suggest a lesion may be malignant can include a rapidly growing mass, ulceration of the mass and hemorrhage, and the presence of a firm (indurated) or rolled tissue border. The mass may develop without any overt dental cause, and teeth may become mobile as the bone supporting the teeth is lost. Moreover, the mass may develop a foul smell if it has been colonized by oral microorganisms, and the patient may have difficulty swallowing (dysphagia), speaking (dysphonia), and tasting (dysgeusia). There may also be rapid weight loss, sensorineural or sensorimotor deficits, and lymphadenopathy.

Dentists should vigilantly watch for signs of malignant disease in their patients, particularly those who may engage in high-risk behaviors or have a genetic predisposition. Because the incidence of oral malignancies (primarily carcinomas) can vary widely around the world, some general dentists may rarely or never see a patient with a malignant neoplasm. This scarcity may make a dentist less likely to recognize a malignancy when it is present. The failure to identify a malignancy in its early stages may result in delayed diagnosis and treatment and an increased need for aggressive treatment with added morbidity, and, in the worst case, premature death. Indeed, it has been said that *it is always better to suspect a malignancy and to be wrong than to not suspect one at all and to be proven wrong.*

APPLIED DIAGNOSTIC IMAGING

Diagnostic imaging has many important roles in the diagnosis and management of a patient with a malignant neoplasm. Oral and maxillofacial imaging may help establish an initial diagnosis. Intraoral and panoramic imaging can demonstrate involvement of the tooth bearing areas of the jaw as well as adjacent structures such as the maxillary sinus. Small field of view, small voxel cone-beam computed tomography (CBCT) may also be useful in demonstrating early bone involvement, while multidetector computed tomography (MDCT) and magnetic resonance imaging (MRI) may show the extent of the neoplasm and the involvement of adjacent soft tissue structures. MRI has been found to be particularly useful for demonstrating perineural spread of disease and lymph node involvement. Positron emission tomographic imaging, a technique capable of detecting abnormal cellular metabolic activity associated with malignant neoplasms, has been used with MDCT and MRI to describe the extent of disease; specifically, local and lymph node involvement and more distant sites of spread. Radiologic investigations may also help stage and grade the neoplasm for management and prognosis. Biopsy is always required in cases of malignancy for a definitive diagnosis, but this should only be done following imaging. A thorough diagnostic imaging examination is also part of the postoperative treatment plan of a patient who has survived cancer, who is often rendered xerostomic, neutropenic, and susceptible to dental caries, periodontal disease, and systemic infection.

IMAGING FEATURES

Malignant neoplasms grow quickly and aggressively, leaving little if any time for the normal tissues around them to respond. Consequently, the imaging features of malignancy are, by and large, destructive in nature.

Location

Malignant neoplasia may occur anywhere in the oral and maxillofacial region. Squamous cell carcinoma, the most common primary malignant neoplasm of the head and neck, may arise from any epithelial surface within the oral and perioral areas and the aerodigestive tract (e.g., the floor of the mouth, the tongue, the retromolar area in the mandible, the oropharyngeal tonsillar area, the soft palate, the lip, and the gingiva). Malignant neoplasms arising from any of these sites may involve the jawbones by direct extension. Sarcomas, arising from cells with a mesenchymal lineage, are more common in the mandible and in the posterior regions of both jaws, while metastatic disease is most common in the posterior mandible and maxilla. Rarely, do metastases develop at the apices of teeth or in the follicles of developing teeth (Fig. 24.1D).

Periphery

The borders of a malignant neoplasm are commonly irregular, and their peripheries can vary from those that are more well defined to those that are very poorly defined. This variation often reflects the aggressiveness of the neoplasm's growth characteristics. Malignant neoplasms also lack the border cortication associated with slower growing, benign masses that allow bone the opportunity to remodel as the mass enlarges. For example, some oral squamous cell carcinomas invading the mandible may have more well-defined borders, particularly if the invading neoplasm has a very broad surface. Other malignancies may create more irregular, poorly defined borders, as smaller populations of malignant cells invade the bone in a more piecemeal manner; this is referred to as an infiltrative pattern of destruction (see Fig. 24.1A). Evidence of destruction of a cortical border with an adjacent soft tissue mass is highly suggestive of malignancy (see Fig. 24.1B).

Internal Structure

Most malignancies that develop in or around the jaws do not produce bone or stimulate the formation of reactive bone. Consequently, such neoplasms are internally radiolucent. Occasionally, residual islands of bone may be visualized, resulting in a pattern of patchy destruction at the lesion periphery. Primary sarcomas of bone as well as metastases, particularly from the breast or the prostate, can stimulate abnormal bone production, giving the appearance of a somewhat irregular or disorganized, patchy, radiopaque pattern internally.

Effects on Adjacent Structures

Malignant neoplasia is a destructive process, and the effects on surrounding structures mirror this behavior. These changes can destroy the normal trabecular bone pattern, external bone cortices, the floor of the maxillary sinus (see Fig. 24.1B), the cortex of the inferior alveolar canal, and the follicular cortices of developing tooth crowns. Malignant neoplasms may also invade the periodontal ligament space resulting in nonconcentric widening with destruction of the lamina dura (see Fig. 24.1C). This type of widening has been termed "Garrington sign."

Usually, no periosteal reaction occurs where the neoplasm has destroyed the outer cortex of bone; however, some malignant neoplasms may grow so quickly that when they reach the bone surface, they can lift the periosteum and stimulate surface and mesenchymal progenitor cells in the periosteum to deposit osteoid along Sharpey fibers and blood vessels. This can give rise to a pattern of alternating linear radiolucent and radiopaque lines emanating at 90 degrees from the bone surface (see Fig. 24.1E). These patterns have been referred to as "hair-on-end" or "sunburst" patterns depending on the exuberance of the mineralization pattern.

Effects on Adjacent Teeth

Rapidly growing malignant neoplasms typically destroy the supporting bone and associated structures around the teeth so that the teeth may appear to be "floating in space" (see Fig. 24.1F). Teeth are rarely affected by a malignant neoplasm, except in a small number of cases where root resorption can occur, a finding that is more common with some hematogenous malignancies and sarcomas.

CARCINOMAS

Squamous Cell Carcinoma Arising in Soft Tissue

Disease Mechanism

Squamous cell carcinoma is the most common primary malignancy in the head and neck, accounting for over 95% of malignancies. These neoplasms arise from the surface epithelium lining the oral and perioral structures, and the upper aerodigestive tract. The disease etiology is multifactorial, with chronic tobacco and alcohol use implicated as risk factors. Although a number of different gene mutations have been identified in both human and animal cell models of oral cancer, none have been definitively linked to disease pathogenesis. Prior human papillomavirus and Epstein–Barr virus infections have, however, been implicated in the development of some tonsillar, tongue, and laryngeal carcinomas.

Histopathologically, squamous cell carcinoma is characterized initially by invasion of malignant epithelial cells through the basement membrane into the underlying connective tissue with subsequent spread into adjacent tissue spaces.

Clinical Features

Squamous cell carcinoma appears initially as a white and/or red surface mucosal lesion. With time, these lesions may exhibit central necrosis and ulceration and develop a rolled or indurated border— a sign of malignant cell infiltration into adjacent normal tissues. There may also be palpable infiltration into other adjacent tissues, including muscle. Regional nonpainful lymph nodes may develop in the neck, and these may or may not be fixed to underlying structures. Other clinical features may include the presence of a visible soft tissue mass, altered sensation, foul smell, trismus, tooth mobility, or hemorrhage. Large lesions can obstruct the airway, the opening of the Eustachian tube orifice (leading to diminished hearing) or the nasopharynx. Patients often report significant weight loss and feel unwell, and the condition is fatal if untreated.

Imaging Features

Location. Squamous cell carcinoma commonly involves the floor of the mouth, the retromolar trigone area of the mandible, the tonsillar pillars, and the dorsum of the tongue. A common site of bone invasion is the lingual surface of the mandible adjacent to these involved areas. Lesions involving the attached gingiva may cause bone loss that mimics periodontal disease.

Periphery. Squamous cell carcinoma may invade into the underlying bone from any direction, producing a radiolucency that may appear more broadly based at the bone surface. This has been described as a "cookie bite" pattern of bone destruction. Invasion is characterized most commonly by a noncorticated border that is usually poorly defined (Fig. 24.2). Lesions that have a broader surface may have a more well-defined border, with a narrower transition zone between abnormal and normal bone. Other lesions have an irregular and poorly defined border with a wider transition zone with finger-like destruction of the surrounding bone. Should the bone become structurally compromised by the invading mass, fracture can occur, and the borders will show sharpened thinned bone ends with displacement of segments. Sclerosis may also develop in the bone adjacent to the neoplasm if there has been infiltration of the neoplasm by oral microorganisms.

Internal structure. The internal structure of the invaded bone is radiolucent where the original bone structure has been lost. Occasionally, small islands of residual normal trabecular bone may remain visible within this area of bone destruction.

Effects on adjacent structures. Destruction of adjacent bone border (Fig. 24.2) or internal cortical boundaries, such as the floor of the

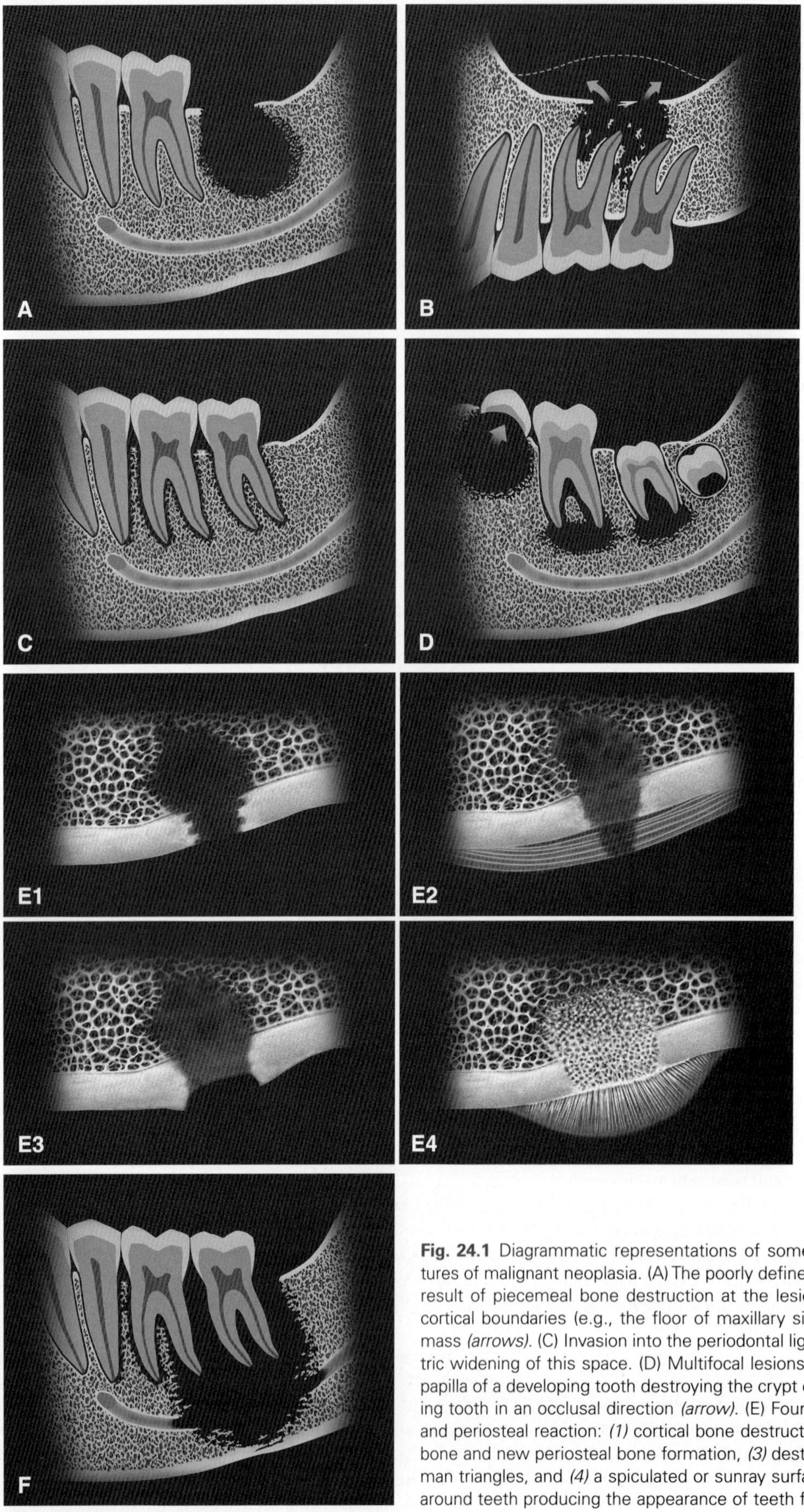

Fig. 24.1 Diagrammatic representations of some of the important radiologic features of malignant neoplasia. (A) The poorly defined borders of a malignancy are the result of piecemeal bone destruction at the lesion's periphery. (B) Destruction of cortical boundaries (e.g., the floor of maxillary sinus) with an adjacent soft tissue mass *(arrows)*. (C) Invasion into the periodontal ligament space causing nonconcentric widening of this space. (D) Multifocal lesions located at root apices and in the papilla of a developing tooth destroying the crypt cortex and displacing the developing tooth in an occlusal direction *(arrow)*. (E) Four types of effects on cortical bone and periosteal reaction: *(1)* cortical bone destruction, *(2)* destruction of the cortical bone and new periosteal bone formation, *(3)* destruction of cortical bone with Codman triangles, and *(4)* a spiculated or sunray surface reaction. (F) Bone destruction around teeth producing the appearance of teeth floating in space.

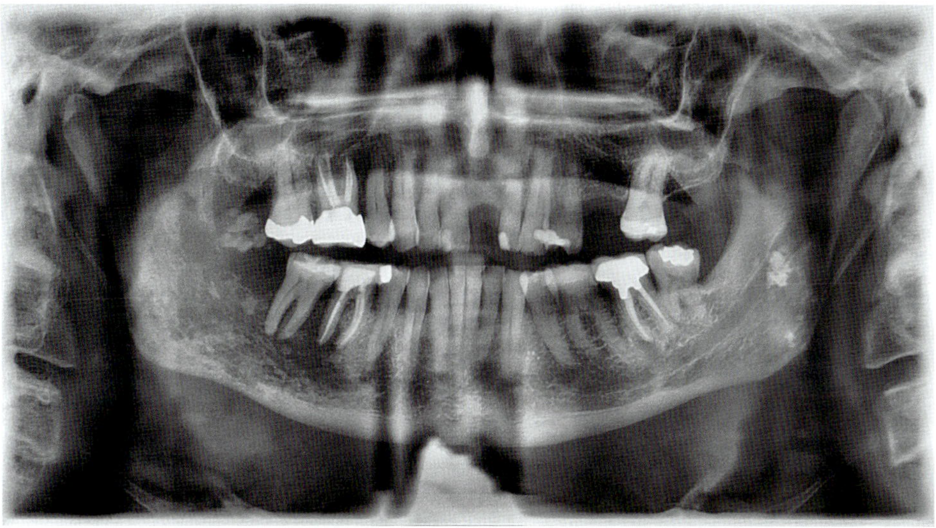

Fig. 24.2 Panoramic image of a squamous cell carcinoma invading the right posterior mandibular body, alveolar process and ramus. (Courtesy Dr. C. Fenton, Peterborough, ON.)

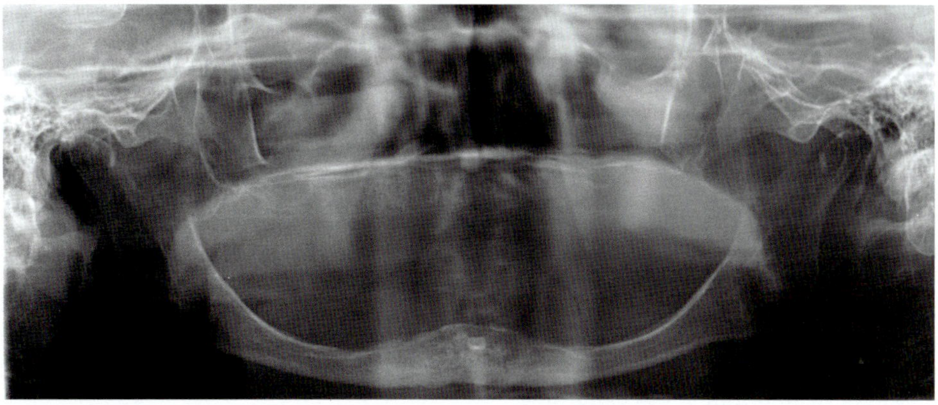

Fig. 24.3 Panoramic image of a squamous cell carcinoma destroying the floor of the right maxillary sinus and the adjacent alveolar process of the maxilla. (Courtesy Dr. P. Chauvin, Montreal, QC.)

nose and maxillary sinus, can occur (Fig. 24.3), and bone cortices may be thinned or lost resulting in fracture (Fig. 24.4).

Effects on adjacent teeth. Evidence of bone involvement adjacent to the teeth may first appear as widening of the periodontal ligament space with loss of the adjacent lamina dura. Teeth may appear to "float in space," bereft of any bone support but are otherwise unaffected (Fig. 24.5). In a very rapidly growing neoplasm, the soft tissue mass may carry the teeth from their normal positions resulting in gross displacement.

Differential Interpretation

The bone loss from squamous cell carcinoma originating in the soft tissues of the alveolar process may appear very similar to periodontal disease (see Fig. 24.6A and B). Enlargement of a recent extraction socket without evidence of healing can indicate the presence of squamous cell carcinoma (see Fig. 24.5B).

Involvement of the mandibular canal by squamous cell carcinoma can occur through a neurovascular foramen, enlarging the caliber of the canal. In contrast to a benign entity, such as a vascular malformation involving the canal, malignant invasion would destroy the canal's cortex (Fig. 24.6C). As well, a direct extension of a surface malignancy can cause destruction of the superior cortex (Fig. 24.6D).

Destruction of bone may also occur in inflammation (i.e., osteomyelitis), as well as a result of chemical (e.g., medication-related osteonecrosis of the jaws) or physical (e.g., radiation) trauma. Occasionally, it may be difficult to differentiate osteomyelitis from squamous cell carcinoma, especially when oral microorganisms have gained entry to the bone surrounding the neoplasm. All of these processes can be destructive, leaving remnant islands of bone. Loss of normal anatomical structures together with evidence of profound bone destruction can help differentiate malignancy from these other processes that result in perhaps relatively milder forms of bone destruction. But even this may sometimes be problematic. Osteomyelitis and medication-related osteonecrosis of the jaws may produce a periosteal reaction, whereas radiation damage and squamous cell carcinoma do not. If bone destruction is present, patient history, biopsy, and advanced imaging prove vital to the diagnosis.

Management

Head and neck squamous cell carcinoma is commonly managed by radiation therapy and surgery. The choice of which modality is used, and in what sequence, depends on the protocol of the treatment facility and the location and severity of the neoplasm. Generally, chemotherapy is not a common treatment modality.

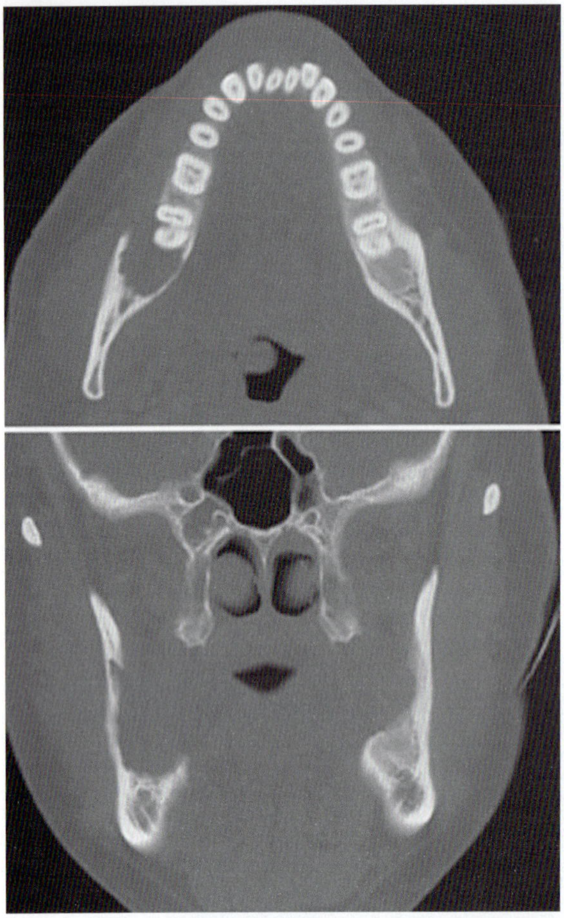

Fig. 24.4 Axial (top) and coronal (bottom) multidetector computed tomographic images of bone destruction in the mandibular retromolar area by a squamous cell carcinoma.

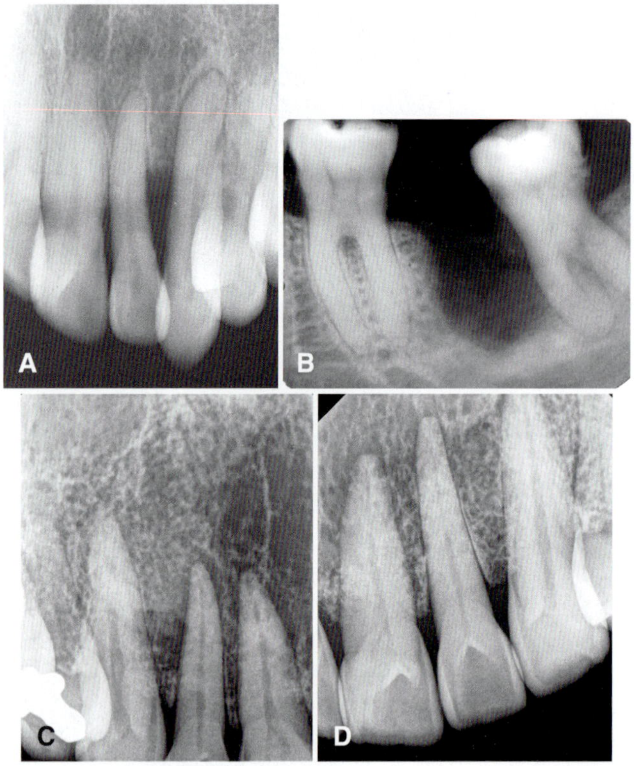

Fig. 24.5 Periapical image reveals bone destruction similar to periodontal disease around the lateral incisor from a squamous cell carcinoma originating in the soft tissues of the alveolar process (A). Note the lack of a sclerotic bone reaction at the periphery. The tooth socket from an extracted second molar has enlarged in size and has not healed because of the presence of a squamous cell carcinoma (B). Periapical images (C and D) of a squamous cell carcinoma invading the alveolar process from the nasal cavity. In (C), note the wide transition zone from the bone destruction near the midline to the more normal bone pattern distal to the maxillary right canine tooth.

Squamous Cell Carcinoma Originating in the Maxillary Sinus

Disease Mechanism

Risk factors for developing squamous cell carcinoma in the mucosal lining of the maxillary sinus include chronic sinusitis, inhaled organic chemicals used in manufacturing, wood dust, and metals such as nickel and chromium.

Clinical Features

Maxillary sinus squamous cell carcinoma occurs most commonly in patients of African and Asian heritage, with men affected more commonly than women. The initial signs may be very similar to inflammatory disease and may include recurrent sinusitis, nasal obstruction, epistaxis, sinus pain, and facial paresthesia.

Imaging Features

Squamous cell carcinoma arising in the mucosal lining of the maxillary sinus may manifest as soft tissue opacification of the maxillary sinus and destruction of the sinus cortical border and the adjacent maxillary alveolar process (Fig. 24.3). An associated noncorticated soft tissue mass may also project into the oral cavity.

Squamous Cell Carcinoma Originating in Bone

Disease Mechanism

Primary squamous cell carcinoma arising centrally within the jawbones with no connection with the surface epithelium is exceptionally rare. In such instances, surface squamous cell carcinoma or metastases must be excluded. Typically, the surface epithelium is invariably normal in appearance. Such primary carcinomas are presumed to arise from intraosseous remnants of odontogenic epithelium, such as the dental lamina or the lining of an odontogenic cyst.

Clinical Features

These neoplasms may remain clinically silent until they have reached a fairly large size. Pain or other sensorineural changes such as lip paresthesia, jaw fracture, and lymphadenopathy may accompany the neoplasm. This primary neoplasm is more common in men and in patients in their fourth to eighth decade of life.

Imaging Features

Location. As intraosseous squamous cell carcinoma arises from remnants of the dental lamina, they only originate in the tooth-bearing areas of the jaw. These neoplasms have a predilection for the mandibular molar region and are less frequently seen in the anterior parts of the jaws (Fig. 24.7A).

Periphery. The periphery of most lesions is poorly defined. They are most often round or irregular in shape, with an irregular border that reflects destruction and invasion into bone. The degree of irregularity may reflect the aggressiveness of the lesion. If sufficient in size, bone cortices may be thinned or destroyed, and jaw fracture can occur.

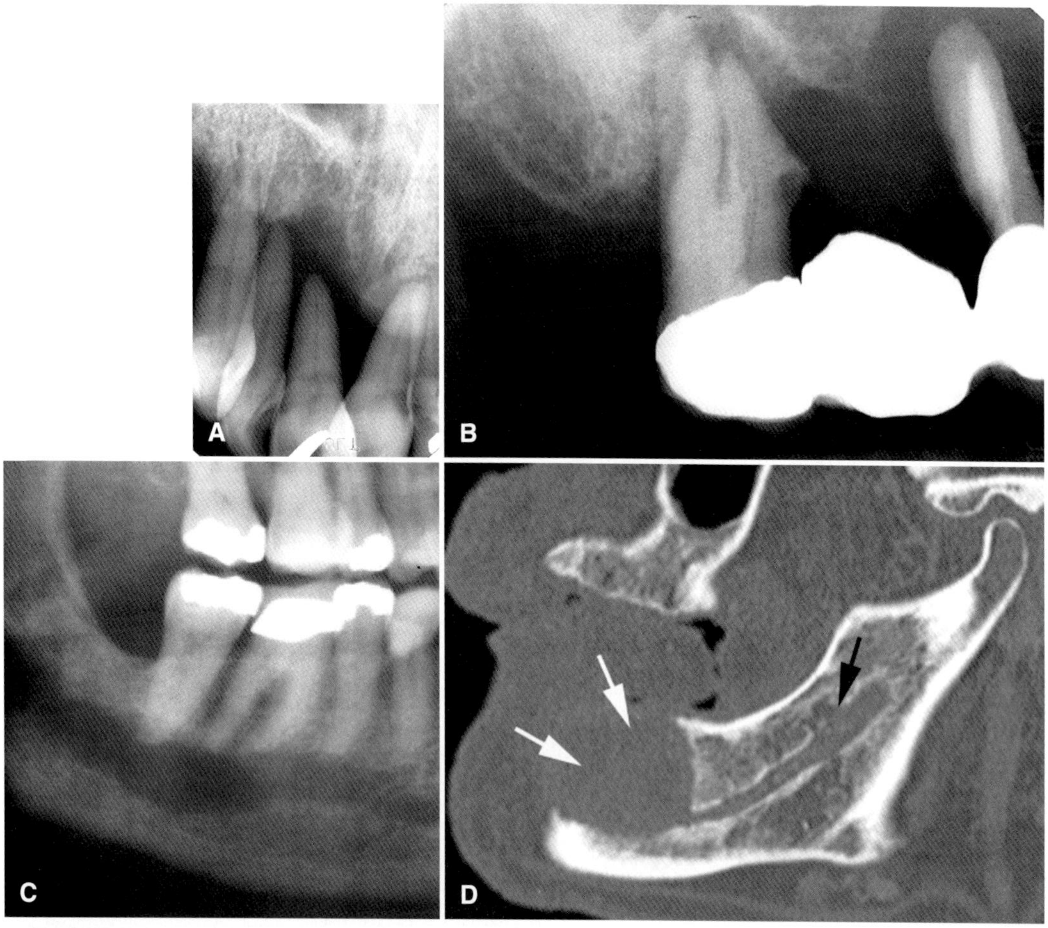

Fig. 24.6 Periapical images (A and B) of two cases of squamous cell carcinoma involving the maxillary alveolar processes. Bone destruction around the tooth roots leaves the teeth bereft of any bone support. Cropped panoramic image of a squamous cell carcinoma involving the mandibular canal (C). Note the irregular width of the canal and destruction of its cortical borders. Sagittal multidetector computed tomographic image of another case of a squamous cell carcinoma destroying the mandible in the region of the mental foramen *(white arrows)*, extending to the canal. Again, note the destruction of the cortices of the canal *(black arrow)* (D).

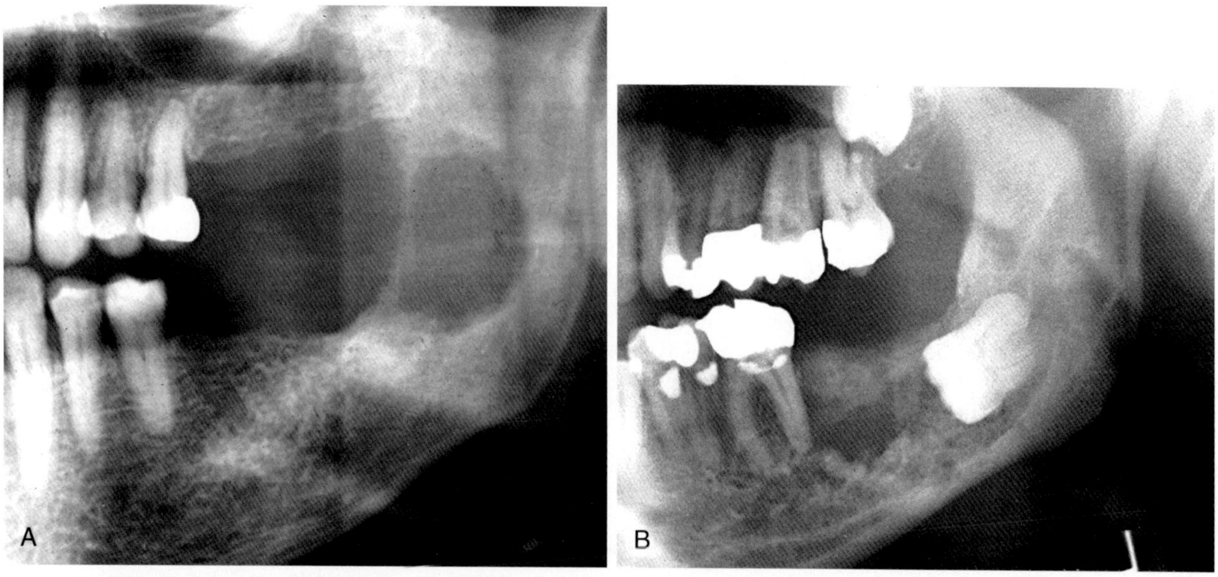

Fig. 24.7 Rare cases of primary intraosseous carcinoma developing in the left mandibular ramus (A) and within a dentigerous cyst (B) associated with the mandibular left third molar. In (B), note the absence of the cyst cortex, the invasion into adjacent bone, and the poorly defined borders.

Internal structure. The internal structure within the bone is radiolucent with no evidence of bone production, and very little residual bone is left within the center of the lesion. If the lesion is located in the mandible and it is small, the adjacent bone cortices may mask the internal bone change.

Effects on adjacent structures. These lesions are capable of causing extensive destruction of the nasal and antral borders, the cortex of the inferior alveolar canal, and the lamina dura.

Effects on adjacent structures. Carcinoma arising in an odontogenic cyst can thin and destroy the lamina dura of adjacent teeth.

Effects on adjacent teeth. Teeth that lose bone support appear to be "floating in space." Lamina dura is lost, but root resorption is unusual.

Differential Interpretation

If the lesions are less aggressive and have a smooth border, the radiolucent area may be mistaken for rarefying osteitis. Alternatively, if lesions are not centered about the root apex, occasionally it may be difficult to differentiate this condition from an odontogenic cyst or benign odoontogenic neoplasm. If the border is infiltrative with extensive bone destruction, a solitary plasmacytoma or a metastatic lesion must be excluded. Examination of the oral cavity and especially the surface epithelium assists in differentiating this condition from surface squamous cell carcinoma.

Management

Such lesions are managed in much the same way as squamous cell carcinoma arising from the oral soft tissues.

Squamous Cell Carcinoma Originating in a Cyst

Disease Mechanism

Squamous cell carcinoma may develop from the epithelial cell lining of an odontogenic cyst.

Clinical Features

The development of squamous cell carcinoma from the lining of an odontogenic cyst is such an exceptionally rare occurrence. This malignancy must be differentiated from primary intraosseous carcinoma, metastasis, or invasion from a surface carcinoma. The most common presenting sign or symptom is pain. The pain may be characterized as dull and of several months' duration. Swelling is occasionally reported. Jaw fracture, fistula formation, and regional lymphadenopathy may occur. If the maxilla is involved, sinus pain, epistaxis, or swelling may be present.

Imaging Features

Location. This neoplasm may occur anywhere that odontogenic epithelium may be present, including the lining of an odontogenic cyst. Most cases occur in the mandible (see Fig. 24.7B), with a few cases reported in the anterior maxilla.

Periphery. The appearance of squamous cell carcinoma arising within a cyst wall may not be visible until the abnormality attains a size that is large enough to impact adjacent bone. As the malignant cells progressively replace the cyst lining, the smooth, well-defined, and corticated border is lost or it becomes poorly defined. In more advanced stages, the shape and contour of the cyst become less "hydraulic" and the border takes on a poorly defined, infiltrative quality.

Internal structure. This lesion is radiolucent, perhaps more so than invasive surface carcinoma, owing to loss of bone during cyst development.

Effects on adjacent teeth. There is destruction of adjacent bone surfaces including the inferior border of the mandible or floor of the nose or maxillary sinus. It can also produce complete destruction of the alveolar process.

Differential Interpretation

If an odontogenic cyst has become secondarily infected by oral microorganisms, it may lose its cortex and appear ragged and identical to a malignant lesion arising in a preexisting cyst. However, with inflammation, there will be a peripheral sclerotic response in the bone. This sclerosis is not normally present in a cyst that has undergone malignant transformation. Nevertheless, the two may be difficult to differentiate radiologically, and the epithelium from an excised cyst must be submitted for histopathologic examination. A solitary plasmacytoma may be difficult to distinguish, especially if it has a well-defined periphery and a cyst-like shape. Metastatic disease may be similar, although it is commonly multifocal.

Management

The treatment of squamous cell carcinoma originating in a cyst is identical to the treatment described for squamous cell carcinoma arising in soft tissue.

Central Mucoepidermoid Carcinoma

Disease Mechanism

Central mucoepidermoid carcinoma is an epithelially derived malignant salivary gland neoplasm arising in bone and is histologically indistinguishable from its soft tissue counterpart. The malignant cells are believed to arise from malignant transformation of mucus secreting cells in odontogenic epithelium or those cells that have been entrapped in bone. The clinician must exclude the possibility of an invasive overlying mucoepidermoid carcinoma or odontogenic neoplasm.

Clinical Features

Depending on the histopathologic grade, a low-grade central mucoepidermoid carcinoma can mimic a benign neoplasm in terms of its growth rate, whereas a high-grade lesion can have more aggressive growth characteristics. The most common patient complaint is a swelling that may have been present for months or years, which has caused a facial asymmetry. Occasionally, patients may feel as if teeth have been displaced or a denture no longer fits. Paresthesia involving the distribution of the inferior alveolar nerve and spreading of the lesion to regional lymph nodes have also been reported. In contrast to other oral malignancies, central mucoepidermoid neoplasm is more common in females than males.

Imaging Features

Location. Mucoepidermoid carcinoma is three to four times more common in the mandible than the maxilla and usually develops in the premolar and molar regions. The lesion most commonly has an epicenter superior to the mandibular canal in the tooth-bearing areas of the jaws, similar to benign cysts and neoplasms of odontogenic origin.

Periphery. Mucoepidermoid carcinoma manifests as a unilocular or multilocular expansile mass (Fig. 24.8). The border is most often well defined and corticated with a scalloped or undulating periphery, which is similar to the appearance of a benign neoplasm of odontogenic origin. The peripheral cortication may be impressively thick and almost sclerotic, which belies its malignant nature.

Internal structure. The internal structure can have features similar to a benign neoplasm such as a recurrent ameloblastoma. Lesions are often described as being multilocular or having a round, radiolucent, "soap bubble" or honeycomb-like internal structure. Also, there may be regions of adjacent sclerotic bone, although this bone is not produced by the neoplasm; it is merely remodeled residual bone.

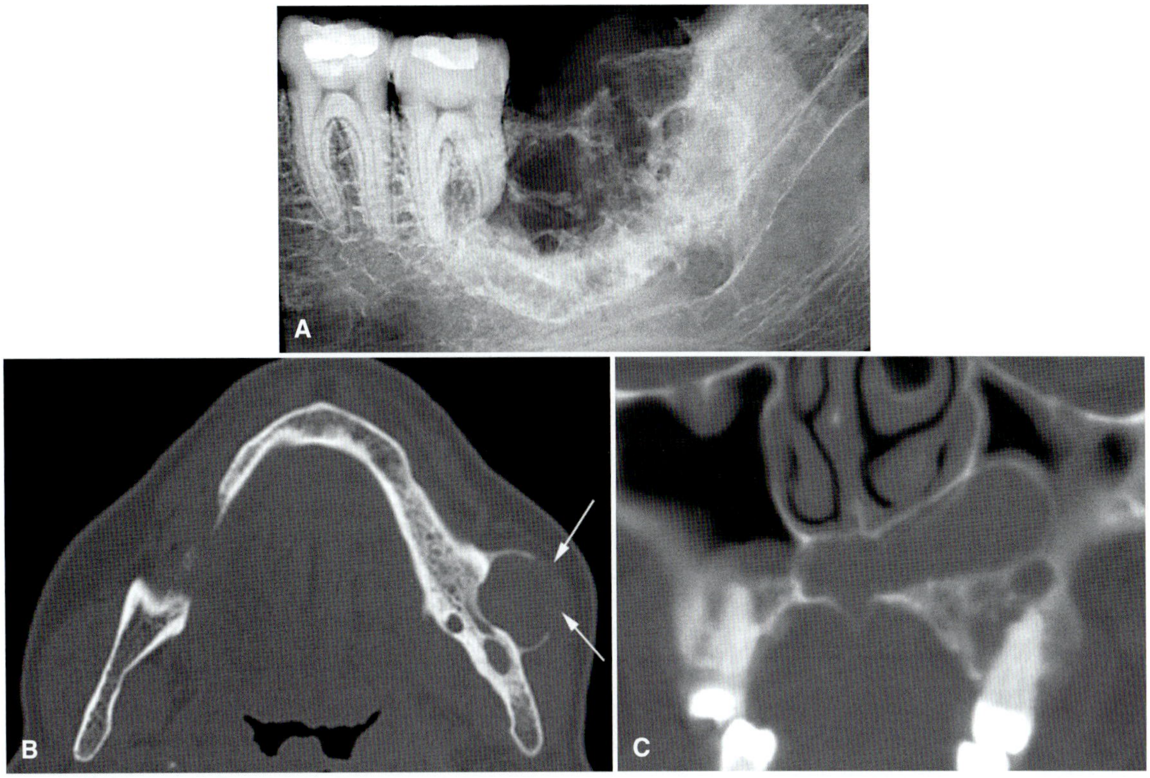

Fig. 24.8 Multilocular radiolucency is characteristic of central mucoepidermoid carcinoma (A). This lesion has destroyed the crest of the alveolar process and the bone distal to the second molar and has displaced the mandibular canal inferiorly. Axial multidetector computed tomographic image (B) reveals multiple cyst-like epicenters, some surrounded by sclerotic bone and expansion of the mandible with extension into the surrounding soft tissue *(arrows)*. Coronal multidetector computed tomographic image (C) of a central mucoepidermoid carcinoma in the maxilla with a multilocular internal structure.

Effects on adjacent structures. Central mucoepidermoid carcinoma can cause bone expansion and displacement of adjacent cortices, often with perforation and sometimes extension into the surrounding soft tissues. Similar to a benign neoplasm of odontogenic origin, the mandibular canal may be displaced.

Effects on adjacent teeth. Teeth remain largely unaffected by this disease, although adjacent lamina dura may be lost.

Differential Interpretation

Some imaging characteristics of this neoplasm may appear similar to a benign neoplasm of odontogenic origin. Its malignant nature is revealed if there is expansion with cortical perforation with extension of the neoplasm into the surrounding soft tissues. The primary differential interpretation is ameloblastoma (both primary and recurrent forms), with which it shares similarities in its peripheral and internal features; it may be impossible to differentiate the two. Biopsy is required to make a definitive diagnosis.

Management

Central mucoepidermoid carcinoma is treated surgically with en bloc resection encompassing a margin of adjacent normal bone. Neck dissection and postoperative radiation therapy may be required to control the spread to the lymph nodes.

"Malignant Ameloblastoma" and Ameloblastic Carcinoma

Disease Mechanism

Although counterintuitive, "malignant ameloblastoma" is defined as being an ameloblastoma with typical benign histopathologic features but is deemed malignant because of its ability to metastasize. Ameloblastic carcinoma is an ameloblastoma exhibiting the histopathologic features of a malignant neoplasm, such as increased and abnormal mitosis and hyperchromatic, large, pleomorphic nuclei. Both the "malignant ameloblastoma" and the ameloblastic carcinoma are exceptionally rare.

Clinical Features

Clinically and radiologically, these lesions may be impossible to differentiate from the classic ameloblastoma. They present as hard expansile masses with displaced and perhaps loosened teeth and normal overlying mucosa. Tenderness of the overlying soft tissue has been reported. Metastatic spread may be to the cervical lymph nodes, lung, or other viscera, and the skeleton—especially the spine. Local extension may occur into adjacent bones, connective tissue, or salivary glands. These neoplasms occur most commonly between the first and sixth decades of life and are more common in males than in females.

Imaging Features

Location. These lesions occur more common in the mandible than in the maxilla. Most occur in the premolar and molar regions where classic ameloblastoma is typically found.

Periphery. These lesions may appear similar to classic ameloblastoma with a well-defined and corticated border and scalloping of the adjacent bone cortex. "Malignant ameloblastoma" may show more aggressive behavior commonly seen in malignant neoplasm, that is, loss of and perforation of a cortical boundary and invasion into the adjacent soft tissue.

Internal structure. The lesions are either unilocular or more commonly multilocular, giving the appearance of the same honeycomb or soap-bubble pattern that is seen in classic ameloblastoma. Most of the septa are robust and thick.

Effects on adjacent structures. The bone borders may be perforated or lost, and as with classic ameloblastoma, the lesions may displace adjacent anatomy. The inferior alveolar canal may also be displaced or the cortices lost.

Effects on adjacent teeth. Teeth may be moved bodily by the neoplasm and may exhibit root resorption similar to a benign neoplasm.

Differential Interpretation

The differential interpretation of these lesions should include classic ameloblastoma, odontogenic keratocyst, odontogenic myxoma, and central mucoepidermoid carcinoma, from which it may not be distinguishable radiologically. If the lesion is locally invasive and this is apparent radiologically, the interpretation of carcinoma arising from within the bone or from an odontogenic cyst should be considered. If the patient is young and the location of the lesion is anterior to the second permanent molar, a central giant cell lesion may mimic some of its radiologic features. Biopsy is required for a definitive diagnosis.

Management

These lesions are most often treated with en bloc surgical resection. However, many may not be identified as being malignant until the time of biopsy. Because the histopathologic appearance of these lesions may reveal classic ameloblastoma, the initial treatment may be inadequate. In addition, the metastatic lesions may not appear for many months or years after treatment of the primary neoplasm, adding another reason for treatment failure.

METASTATIC DISEASE

Disease Mechanism

Metastasis is the process whereby new foci of a malignant neoplasm are established at a distant site. For patients, metastasis is often the terminal event in the clinical course of cancer. Metastatic disease that involves the jaws usually occurs when the primary lesion is located anatomically inferior to the clavicles. In most instances, the primary malignant neoplasm has already been identified, although occasionally the presence of a metastasis may reveal the presence of a silent primary malignancy.

Less than 0.1% of cells within a primary malignant neoplasm develop the phenotypic ability to successfully metastasize, and most often, this process involves the vascular system. Although the process is complex, two broad sets of events occur. The first arises within the primary tissue or organ (the proximal metastatic event), and the second occurs within the distant tissue or organ (the distal metastatic event). During the proximal event, the neoplastic cell loses its adhesion to adjacent cells within the mass and migrates through the basement membrane (if present) into the underlying connective tissue where it may encounter a blood vessel. The malignant cell then passes through the basement membrane and endothelial cell layers of the vessel wall and enters the circulation. Once in the circulation, the malignant cell must evade the body's immune system, travelling through the vessel until it adheres to a distant endothelial cell, where the distal metastatic event occurs. The metastasizing cell then repeats the same events but in the reverse order; that is, the cell moves across the endothelial cell and its basement into the adjacent connective tissue. Should the microenvironment in this location be favorable, the malignant cell is able to proliferate, and a metastatic focus develops. It should also be noted that the spread of malignant disease through the lymphatic system and along nerve axons may also contribute to disease dissemination.

Metastatic disease involving the jaws accounts for less than 1% of metastatic malignancies found in bone, with most affecting the bones of the vertebrae, pelvis, skull, ribs, and humerus. Most metastases arise from carcinomas, the most common being from breast, lung, and prostate, with colorectal, kidney, thyroid, gastrointestinal, melanoma, testicular, bladder, ovarian, and cervical cancers rounding out the list. In children, metastatic disease may arise from neuroblastoma, retinoblastoma, and Wilms tumor.

Clinical Features

Metastatic disease is the most common malignancy that develops in bone. Women develop almost twice the number of metastatic neoplasms as men. Metastatic disease is more common in patients in their fifth to seventh decades of life, and breast metastases outnumber all other types. Patients may complain of dental pain, develop unexplained paresthesia or anesthesia involving the third branch of the trigeminal nerve, or hemorrhage from the tumor site. Patients may also experience a change to their occlusion should the neoplasm grow large enough for teeth to lose their bone support or from jaw fracture.

Imaging Features

Location

The posterior mandible is most commonly affected (Fig. 24.9) given the rich vascular supply to this area of the bone. The maxilla and maxillary sinus are the next most common sites, followed by the anterior hard palate and mandibular condyle. Frequently, metastatic lesions of the mandible are seen bilaterally (see Fig. 24.9B and C). Also, occasionally, lesions may develop in the periodontal ligament space (sometimes at the root apex), mimicking periapical inflammatory disease or periodontal disease, or in the papilla of a developing tooth.

Periphery

Metastatic lesions may have moderately well-defined to poorly defined peripheries, without any cortex (see Fig. 24.9A). The lesions typically exhibit a lobular or polymorphous shape owing to the microenvironment of the bone. In general, areas with a more supportive microenvironment may see a greater proliferation of metastatic neoplastic cells, while areas with a less supportive microenvironment may see less proliferation—thus, the contours of adjacent regions within the same neoplasm may appear lobular and heterogeneous.

Internal Structure

Most metastatic lesions are generally radiolucent relative to bone, although foci of residual normal trabecular bone may be appreciated in association with the more osteolytic areas. Some metastatic lesions from prostate and breast lesions may also stimulate osteoblasts within the bone to produce an osteoblastic response that produces sclerosis.

The metastatic focus may begin as a few smaller areas of bone destruction separated by normal bone. As the metastatic cell populations begin to proliferate and coalesce, smaller regions may develop into a larger, poorly defined region over time, and the jaw may become enlarged. If osteoblastic metastases are present, the normally poorly defined radiolucent focus may develop areas of patchy sclerosis as the result of new bone formation (Fig. 24.10). If the neoplasm is seeded into multiple regions of the bone, the result may be multiple variably sized radiolucent lesions with normal bone between the metastatic foci.

Effects on Adjacent Structures

The cortical borders of adjacent structures, including neurovascular canals and airspaces, may be destroyed. Occasionally, the metastatic

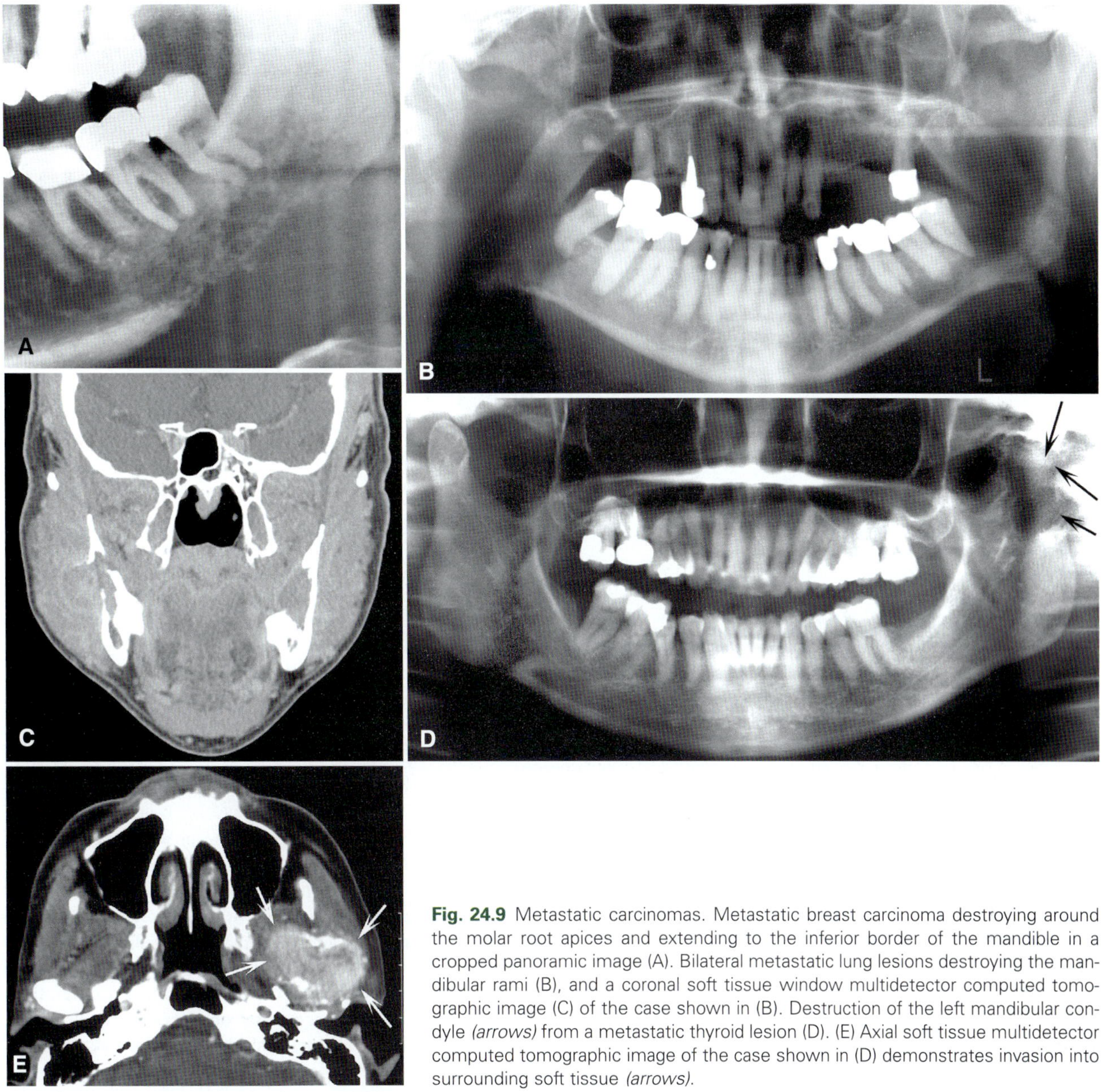

Fig. 24.9 Metastatic carcinomas. Metastatic breast carcinoma destroying around the molar root apices and extending to the inferior border of the mandible in a cropped panoramic image (A). Bilateral metastatic lung lesions destroying the mandibular rami (B), and a coronal soft tissue window multidetector computed tomographic image (C) of the case shown in (B). Destruction of the left mandibular condyle *(arrows)* from a metastatic thyroid lesion (D). (E) Axial soft tissue multidetector computed tomographic image of the case shown in (D) demonstrates invasion into surrounding soft tissue *(arrows)*.

lesion may breach the outer cortex of the jaws and extend into surrounding soft tissues, manifesting as an intraoral mass.

Some metastatic carcinomas, namely from the prostate and breast, may stimulate intraosseous new bone deposition (see Fig. 24.10). When a metastatic focus reaches the bone surface and cortex, the neoplasm may lift the periosteum from the bone surface, stimulating surface and progenitor osteoblasts within the periosteum to deposit a mineralized matrix along Sharpey fibers and vascular channels, both of which are oriented perpendicular to the bone surface.

Effects on Adjacent Teeth

Typical of malignancy, a metastasis can invade the lamina dura and irregularly widen the periodontal ligament space. Teeth may seem to be floating in a soft tissue mass, and their position may be altered because of a loss of bony support. Extraction sockets may fail to heal and may increase in size. Resorption of teeth, a feature commonly seen with benign neoplasms, is generally rare, although this is sometimes seen with multiple myeloma, chondrosarcoma, and osteosarcoma.

Differential Interpretation

In most cases, if a known primary malignancy has been identified, the diagnosis of metastasis is straightforward. Hematogenous malignancies including multiple myeloma may be confused with metastatic disease; however, the border of multiple myeloma is usually better defined than a metastatic focus. When a lesion originates within the periodontal ligament space of a tooth, the appearance may be identical to that of periapical inflammatory disease. A point of differentiation is that the periodontal ligament space widening from inflammation occurs in a more concentric manner at the tooth root apex with loss of the adjacent lamina dura. In contrast, metastatic disease usually causes irregular periodontal ligament space widening, which may extend longitudinally along the side of the root. Odontogenic cysts, if secondarily infected, may have a poorly defined border giving a similar appearance to a metastatic lesion; however, if multiple lesions are seen, the possibility of a metastasis is more likely. Invasion of the jaws by head and neck squamous cell carcinoma may be difficult to distinguish from metastatic disease. In general, the epicenter of

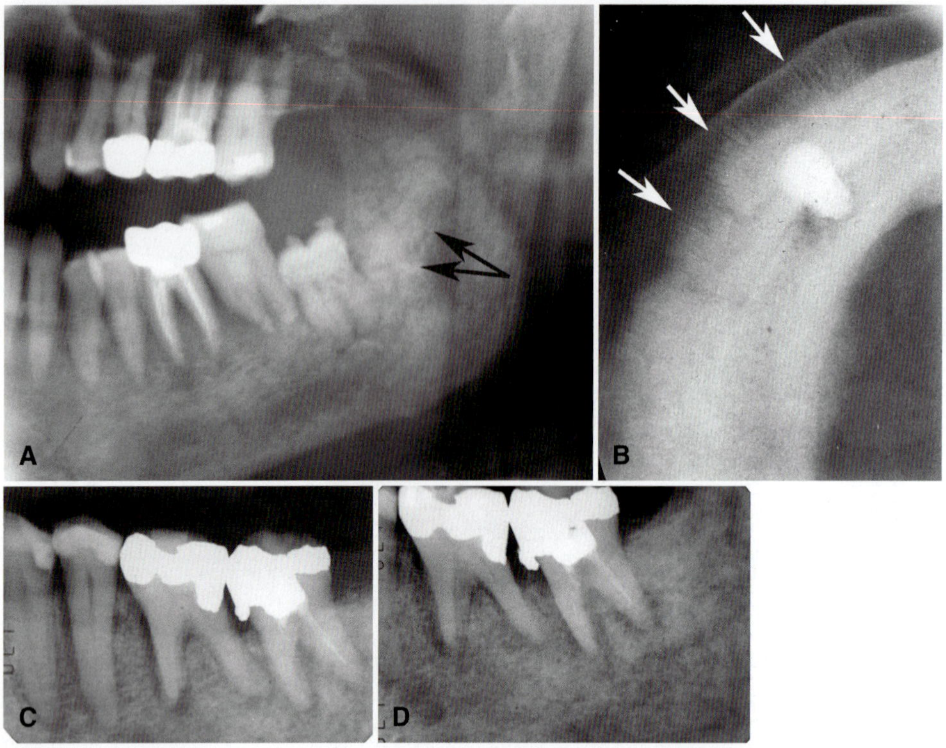

Fig. 24.10 Cropped panoramic image of metastatic prostate lesions involving the body and ramus of the body (A). Note the osteoblastic (sclerotic) bone reaction *(arrows)*. Occlusal image (B) of a metastatic prostate lesion producing sclerosis and a spiculated surface sunray reaction *(arrows)*. Two periapical images of a metastatic breast lesion (C and D) showing the sclerotic bone reaction around the molar roots as well as the nonconcentric widening of the periodontal ligament spaces.

squamous cell carcinoma will be nearer the surface of the bone, and a "cookie bite" defect of the bone surface may be appreciated. In contrast, a metastasis should have an epicenter within the bone, and the shape of the lesion would be more circular or oval.

Management

The identification of metastasis in the jaws is the harbinger of a poor prognosis. If the appearance in the images is suspicious, an opinion from an oral and maxillofacial radiologist should be sought, and the tissue biopsied and submitted for histopathology. Radiologic examination of the body with planar imaging or nuclear medicine may be useful to detect other metastatic lesions. On the rare occasion that the jaw is the first diagnosed site of metastasis, it is imperative that the patient be referred quickly to their physician of record for prompt management.

SARCOMAS

Osteosarcoma

Disease Mechanism

Osteosarcoma is a malignant neoplasm of osteoblasts in which osteoid is produced directly by the malignant cells. As with all malignancies, the development of osteosarcoma is due to the loss of control of cell proliferation, which is the result of a gene mutation. In osteosarcoma, it is interesting to note that these neoplasms can arise within Paget disease of bone and fibrous dysplasia after radiation therapy.

Clinical Features

Osteosarcoma of the jaws is very rare and accounts for approximately 7% of all osteosarcomas. The lesion occurs in males twice as frequently as females, and jaw lesions typically occur with a peak in the fourth decade, about 10 years later, on average, than long bone osteosarcomas.

The dentist may be the first health professional to identify an osteosarcoma developing in the jaws, with the most commonly reported sign or symptom being a rapidly enlarging swelling that may be present 6 months before diagnosis. Other signs and symptoms may include pain, tenderness, erythema of the overlying mucosa, ulceration, loose teeth, epistaxis, hemorrhage, nasal obstruction, exophthalmos, trismus, and blindness. Hypoesthesia has also been reported in cases where peripheral nerves have become involved.

Imaging Features

Location. The mandible is more commonly affected than the maxilla. Although the lesion can occur in any part of either jaw, the posterior mandibular alveolar process, angle, and ramus are most commonly affected. The molar areas are also more commonly affected in the maxilla, with the most frequent sites being the alveolar ridge, antrum, and palate (Fig. 24.11). In the anterior parts of the jaws, the lesion may cross the midline.

Periphery. Osteosarcoma has a poorly defined border with no cortex.

Internal structure. Osteosarcoma may be entirely radiolucent, mixed radiolucent–radiopaque, or radiopaque, depending on the ability of the malignant cells to produce a mineralized matrix. The internal structure may have the appearance of granular- or sclerotic-appearing bone, cotton, wisps of bone, or honeycombs with adjacent destruction of the normal osseous architecture. Whatever the resultant internal structure, the normal trabecular structure of the jaws is lost.

Effects on adjacent structures. Mandibular lesions may destroy the cortex of the mandibular canal, and the walls of the maxillary sinus or nasal fossa may be lost with maxillary lesions. Alternatively, the canal

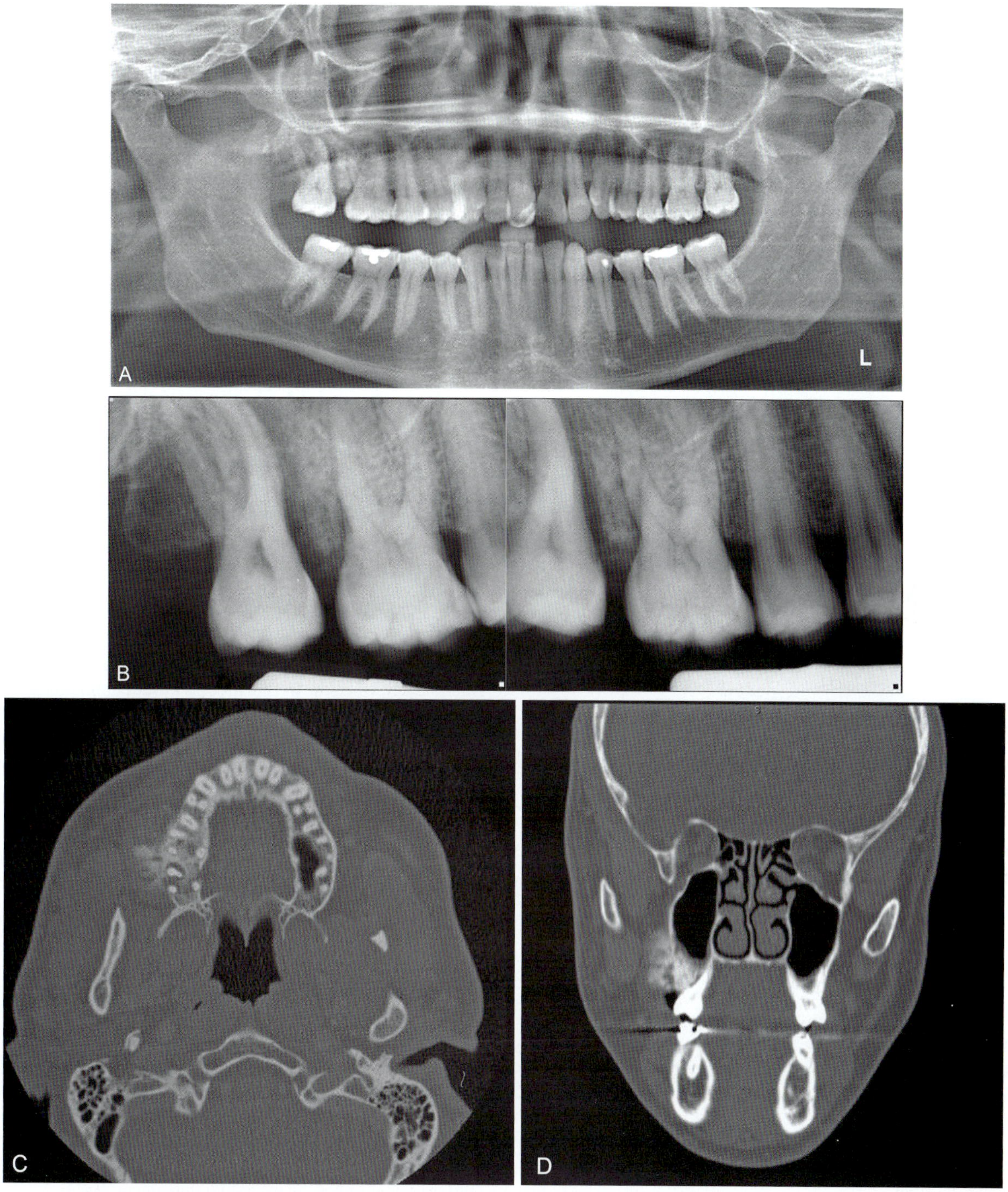

Fig. 24.11 Panoramic (A) and periapical images (B) of an osteosarcoma involving the right posterior maxilla. Note the noncontentric widening of the periodontal ligament space around the maxillary right second molar. Axial (C) and coronal (D) multidetector computed tomographic images demonstrating the spiculated bone response emanating from the buccal surface of the maxilla. (Courtesy Dr. M. Dagenais, Ottawa, ON.)

may be symmetrically widened and enlarged if the malignant cells invade this space. If the lesion extends to the bone surface, a soft tissue mass may be seen emanating from the bone. Should the overlying periosteum be lifted and displaced, a mineralized triangle called a Codman triangle may be seen at the periphery of the elevated periosteum. Also, a sunray or hair-on-end appearance, caused by mineralization of Sharpey fibers and/or small vessels, may also be seen within the adjacent soft tissues (Figs. 24.11 and 24.12).

Effects on adjacent teeth. Nonconcentric widening of the periodontal ligament space is associated with osteosarcoma (Fig. 24.11A and B) but is also seen in other malignancies, including chondrosarcoma. This appearance, sometimes referred to as "Garrington sign," arises when malignant cells invade the periodontal ligament space (Fig. 24.11A and B and 24.12), destroying the adjacent lamina dura and alveolar process and producing external resorption of the tooth root.

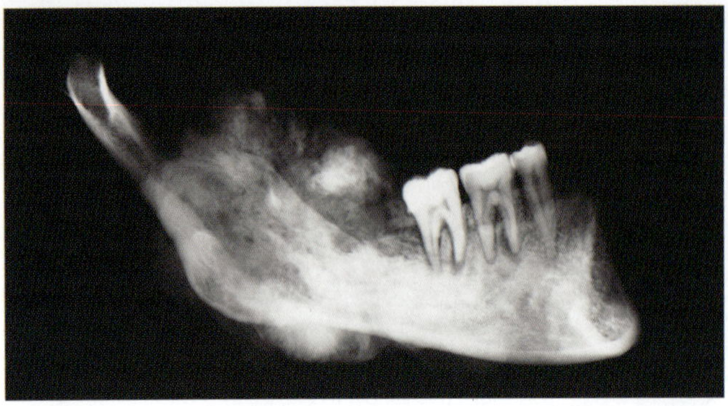

Fig. 24.12 Lateral planar image of an excised specimen of an osteosarcoma of the mandible. Note the mineralization of the mass and the spiculated bone emanating from the inferior border of the lesion. As well, nonconcentric periodontal ligament space widening can be seen around the molar roots closer to the epicenter of the neoplasm. (Courtesy Dr. K.C. Chan, New York, NY.)

Differential Interpretation

It is impossible to differentiate osteosarcoma from chondrosarcoma. If no osseous structure is visible, the practitioner should also consider fibrosarcoma. If the sunray or spiculated bone pattern is seen at the bone surface, prostate and breast metastases should also be considered. A comprehensive examination and laboratory testing may be useful in differentiating a primary bone-forming malignancy from metastatic disease.

Benign neoplasms, such as ossifying fibroma, and fibrous dysplasia, are better demarcated than osteosarcoma. In general, they are more uniform in their internal structure and both lack invasive, destructive characteristics. The histopathology of a biopsy specimen of osteosarcoma may be interpreted as a bone dysplasia, and the correct diagnosis in these cases may rely on the imaging characteristics. Ewing sarcoma, solitary plasmacytoma, and osteomyelitis share some of the radiographic characteristics of osteosarcoma, although osteosarcoma is generally not associated with signs of infection.

Management

The management of osteosarcoma is resection with a large border of adjacent normal bone. Such resection may be possible in orthopedic cases but may be complicated by the myriad of important adjacent anatomic structures in the head and neck. Generally, radiation therapy and chemotherapy are used only for controlling metastatic spread or for palliation.

Chondrosarcoma

Disease Mechanism

Chondrosarcoma is a malignant neoplasm of mesenchymal origin where the malignant cells produce cartilage. These neoplasms may occur centrally within bone, on the bone surface, or, less commonly, in soft tissue. Some form directly from malignant mesenchymal cells and some from preexisting cartilaginous lesions. In the case of the latter, they are termed secondary chondrosarcomas.

Clinical Features

Chondrosarcomas are quite rare in the facial bones, accounting for about 10% of all cases. Generally, these neoplasms occur at any age, although they are more common in adults with a mean age of 47 years. Males and females are affected equally. A patient with chondrosarcoma may have a firm or hard mass of relatively long duration. Enlargement of these lesions may cause pain, headache, and deformity. Less frequent signs and symptoms include hemorrhage from the neoplasm or from the supporting structures around teeth. As with osteosarcoma, there may also be sensory nerve deficits, proptosis, and visual disturbances. The neoplasms invariably are covered with normal overlying skin or mucosa unless secondarily ulcerated. If chondrosarcoma occurs in or near the temporomandibular joint region, trismus or abnormal joint function may result.

Imaging Features

Location. Chondrosarcomas occur in the mandible and maxilla with equal frequency. Maxillary lesions typically occur in the anterior region in areas where cartilage may be present, while mandibular lesions involve the coronoid process, condylar head and neck (Fig. 24.13B and C), and occasionally the symphysis.

Periphery. Chondrosarcomas are slow-growing neoplasms, and their radiologic signs may be misleading and appear benign in nature. The lesions are generally round, ovoid, or lobulated. Their borders are generally well defined and at times corticated. Sometimes, however, the periphery can blend with the adjacent normal bone. Occasionally, a sunray or hair-on-end appearance may be seen. Uncommonly, these lesions have more aggressive appearances, and their peripheries may appear poorly defined and infiltrative with noncorticated borders.

Internal structure. Chondrosarcomas are rarely radiolucent but usually exhibit some form of internal calcification, giving them a mixed radiolucent and radiopaque appearance. The internal pattern may be quite variable. The appearance can take the form of moth-eaten bone alternating with islands of residual bone unaffected by neoplasm. Alternatively, when the malignant cells produce mineralization, the central radiopaque pattern has been described as "flocculent," having the appearance of flakes of snow. This type of diffuse calcification may be superimposed on a background that resembles granular or ground-glass–appearing abnormal bone (see Fig. 24.13A). Careful examination of these areas of flocculence may reveal a central radiolucent nidus, which is probably cartilage surrounded by calcification.

Effects on adjacent structures. Chondrosarcoma, being relatively slow growing, often expands normal cortical boundaries rather than rapidly destroying them. In mandibular cases, the inferior border or alveolar process may be grossly expanded, while still maintaining its cortical covering. Maxillary lesions may displace the walls of the maxillary sinus or nasal fossa and impinge on the infratemporal fossa. Lesions of the mandibular condyle may cause expansion and remodel the adjacent glenoid fossa and articular eminence. If lesions encroach on the articular disk region, a widened joint space may be present with corresponding remodeling of the condylar neck. Erosion of the articular fossa may also occur.

Effects on adjacent teeth. When chondrosarcoma develops near teeth, external root resorption and tooth displacement may occur, as may the widening of the periodontal ligament space.

Differential Interpretation

Chondrosarcoma is indistinguishable from osteosarcoma on diagnostic images. Although the calcifications may be absent from osteosarcoma, the neoplasms share many other radiologic features. Fibrous dysplasia may have a similar internal pattern to chondrosarcoma, although generally, the periphery of fibrous dysplasia is more well defined without signs of bone destruction, and its borders with adjacent teeth differ from chondrosarcoma. For instance, fibrous dysplasia alters the bone pattern up to and including the lamina dura, leaving a normal or thin periodontal ligament space. Because chondrosarcomas may be slow growing and displace teeth and other surrounding structures, these characteristics may be misinterpreted as benign features.

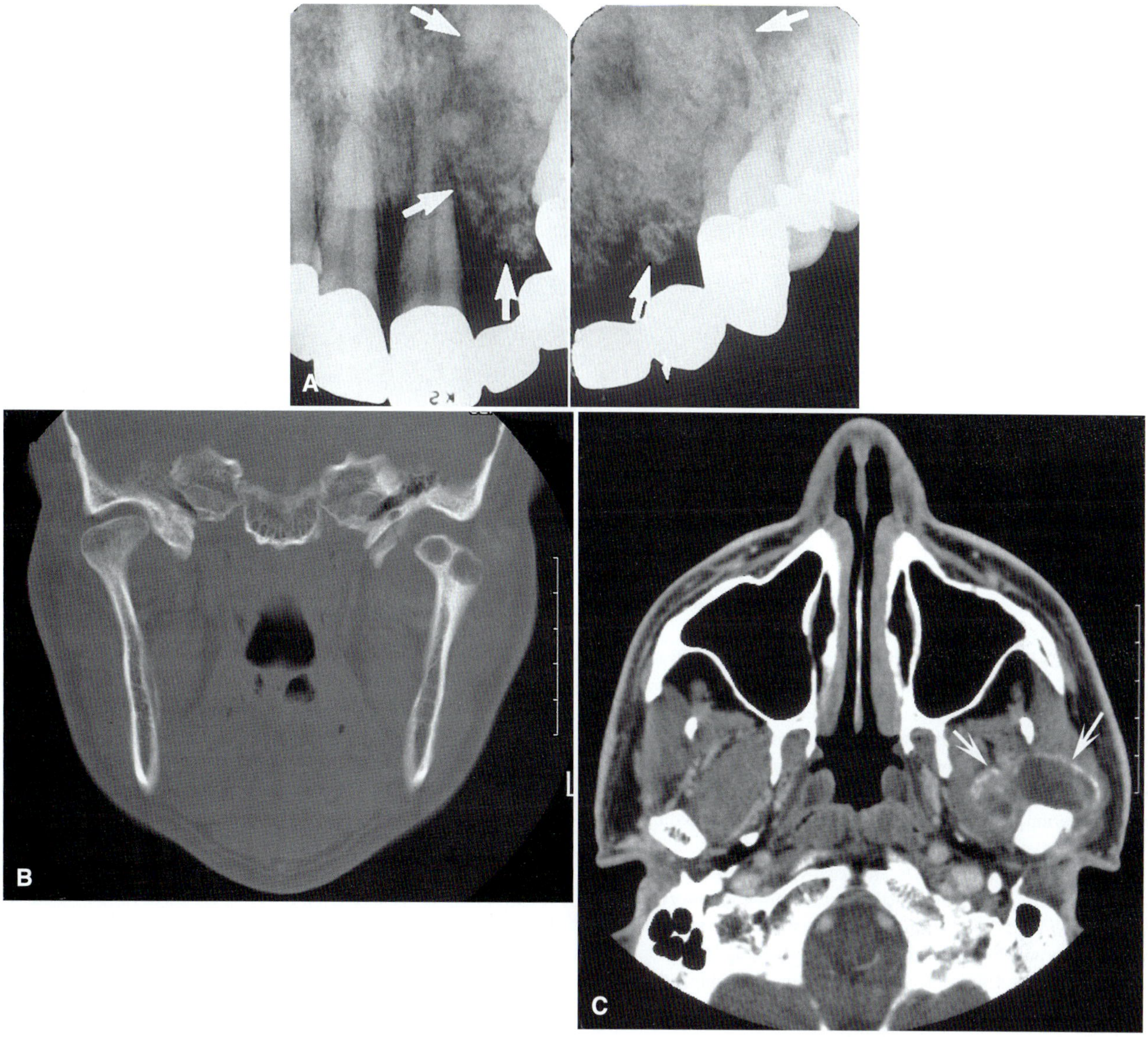

Fig. 24.13 Chondrosarcoma of the anterior maxilla, with sparse, irregular areas of mineralization within the neoplasm *(arrows)* (A). Coronal multidetector computed tomographic image (B) of a chondrosarcoma involving the mandibular condyle (note the two areas of bone destruction). Axial soft tissue window multidetector computed tomographic image demonstrating the soft tissue component *(arrows)* of a chondrosarcoma, which cannot be appreciated on the bone window multidetector computed tomographic image (C). (A, Courtesy Dr. L. Hollender, Seattle, WA.)

Management

The management of chondrosarcoma is surgical. Radiation therapy and chemotherapy generally have no role to play. Patients with chondrosarcomas have a relatively good 5-year survival rate, but 10-year survival is poor.

Ewing Sarcoma

Disease Mechanism

Ewing sarcoma is a small round cell neoplasm that appears to have a common origin with primitive neuroectodermal neoplasms. It is a neoplasm of long bones and very rarely occurs in the jaws. Lesions arise in the medullary portion of the bone and spread to the endosteal, and later periosteal, surfaces.

Clinical Features

Ewing sarcoma is malignancy of the young, with most arising in the second decade of life. Males are twice as likely to develop the disease as females. The patient's signs and symptoms may include, in descending frequency, swelling, pain, loose teeth, paresthesia, exophthalmos, ptosis, epistaxis, ulceration, displaced teeth, trismus, and sinusitis. Multicentric lesions have been reported, as has cervical lymphadenopathy.

Imaging Features

Location. Mandibular cases outnumber maxillary cases by about 2:1, with the highest frequency found in the posterior areas of both jaws. Generally, the lesions develop centrally within the marrow spaces and expand to the adjacent bone cortices.

Periphery. Ewing sarcoma may be round or ovoid in shape with a poorly defined periphery that is never corticated. Its advancing edge destroys bone in an uneven fashion, resulting in a ragged border. The neoplasm can cause jaw fracture with an adjacent radiographically visible soft tissue mass (Fig. 24.14).

Internal structure. Ewing sarcoma is primarily osteolytic, with little internal bone formation. Because the neoplasm grows from within the

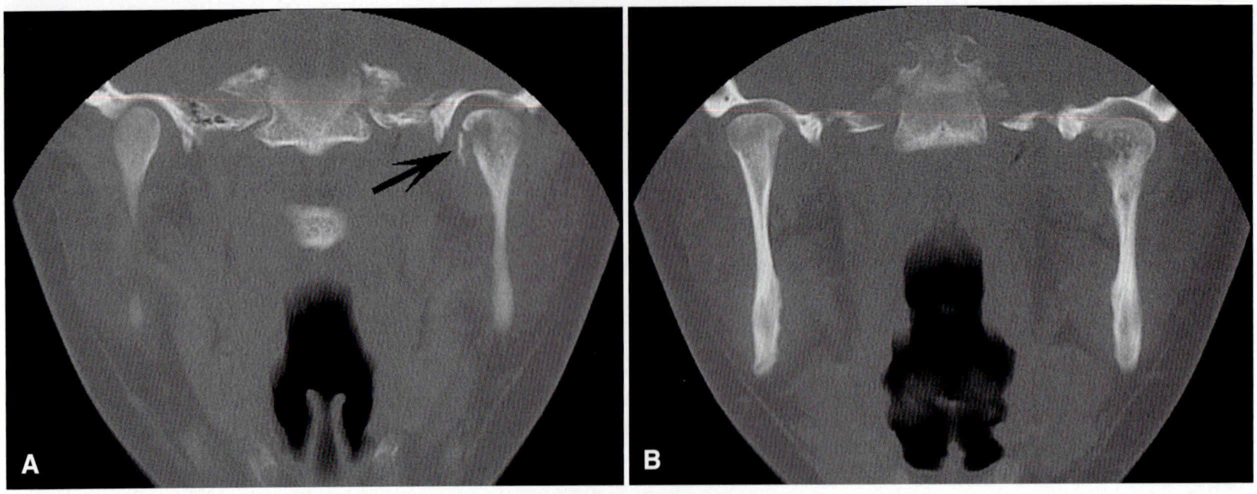

Fig. 24.14 Coronal multidetector computed tomographic images (A and B) demonstrate a Ewing sarcoma involving the left mandibular condyle. Note the irregular borders of the lesion, destruction of the medial cortex of the condyle, and a small fracture fragment *(arrow)*.

bone and only involves the endosteal and periosteal surfaces as it increases in size, it is usually entirely radiolucent.

Effects on adjacent structures. Ewing sarcoma grows rapidly and can engage the bone surface and periosteum quickly. This may produce a sunray or hair-on-end appearance that is similar to osteosarcoma with formation of a Codman triangle. Laminar periosteal new bone formation, similar to that seen in osteomyelitis, has also been reported to occur, but this is more common in the long bones. Adjacent normal structures, including the inferior alveolar canal, inferior border of the mandible, and alveolar cortices, may be lost. If the lesion abuts teeth or tooth follicles, the lamina dura and follicular cortices are destroyed, as is the supporting bone. This neoplasm does not characteristically cause root resorption.

Effects on adjacent teeth. If the lesion abuts teeth or tooth follicles, the lamina dura and follicular cortices are destroyed. This neoplasm does not characteristically cause root resorption, although it does destroy the supporting bone of adjacent teeth.

Differential Interpretation

Osteomyelitis can share some of the radiographic features of Ewing sarcoma. Although both lesions are radiolucent, osteomyelitis will show some evidence of reactive bone formation (sclerosis). As well, osteomyelitis will show demonstrable sequestra within the confines of the lesion, whereas Ewing sarcoma does not.

Chronic localized Langerhans cell histiocytosis of the jaw is also a destructive process. This disease process can be associated with laminar periosteal new bone formation, whereas Ewing sarcoma in the jaws may not. Other central primary malignancies of bone, such as osteosarcoma, chondrosarcoma, and fibrosarcoma, may be difficult to differentiate from Ewing sarcoma.

Management

Too few cases of maxillofacial Ewing sarcoma are available at any single treatment center for any specific treatment policy to have been adopted. Surgery, radiation therapy, and chemotherapy may be used alone or in combination.

Fibrosarcoma

Disease Mechanism

Fibrosarcoma is a neoplasm composed of malignant fibroblasts that produce collagen and elastin. The etiology is unknown, although mutations may develop in cells that have received therapeutic levels of radiation.

Clinical Features

These lesions occur equally in males and females with a mean age in the fourth decade. Fibrosarcoma can develop within the bone or in the adjacent soft tissues. If the fibrosarcoma develops centrally, it is usually accompanied by pain. Peripheral lesions or those lesions that grow out of the bone into the adjacent soft tissues can produce a bulky swelling. If such lesions reach a large size, jaw fracture may occur. If fibrosarcoma involves the course of peripheral nerves, sensorineural abnormalities may arise. Overlying mucosa, although initially normal, may become erythematous or ulcerated. Involvement of the temporomandibular joint or the muscles of mastication is often accompanied by trismus.

Imaging Features

Location. Most cases of fibrosarcoma of the jaws occur in the mandible, with the greatest number of these occurring in the premolar and molar region.

Periphery. Fibrosarcoma has a noncorticated, poorly defined border that is best described as being ragged (Fig. 24.15). Intraosseous neoplasms are generally shaped in a fashion that suggests that they are growing along or through a bone and so they can appear somewhat elongated. The radiographic border may underestimate the extent of the neoplasm because they exhibit a typically infiltrative periphery. If a fibrosarcoma is arising in the soft tissues adjacent to bone, it may cause a saucer-like depression similar to squamous cell carcinoma. Finally, sclerosis may occur in the adjacent normal bone.

Internal structure. A centrally growing fibrosarcoma is radiolucent. If the lesion has been present for some time and is not overly aggressive, either residual jawbone can be seen or reactive bone formation can occur.

Effects on adjacent structures. The most common effect on adjacent structures is destruction. In the mandible, the alveolar process, the inferior border of the jaw, and the cortices of neurovascular canal are lost. In the maxilla, the floor of the maxillary sinus, posterior wall of the maxilla, and floor of the nasal fossa can be destroyed. If the lesion grows aggressively, distending the periosteum, a Codman triangle or sunray or hair-on-end type of spiculation may be evident.

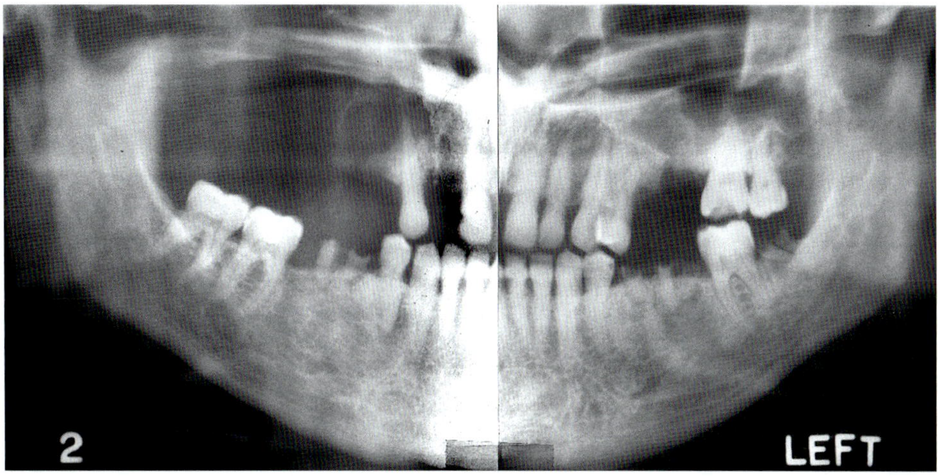

Fig. 24.15 A panoramic image of a fibrosarcoma involving the right maxillary sinus. The lesion has destroyed the floor of the maxillary sinus, the zygomatic process of the maxilla, the hard palate, and the alveolar process.

Effects on adjacent teeth. Widening of the periodontal ligament space occurs should the malignant cells invade the periodontal ligament space of teeth, although root resorption is rare. Lamina dura and follicular cortices are obliterated, and teeth will lose their support and appear to be floating in space with destruction of the supporting bone.

Differential Interpretation

Fibrosarcoma is difficult to differentiate from other central malignancies. If the lesion does not cause enlargement of the jaw, the practitioner must rule out metastatic carcinoma, multiple myeloma, and primary or secondary intraosseous carcinoma. Squamous cell carcinoma and Ewing sarcoma share many imaging characteristics with fibrosarcoma and, therefore, may not be distinguishable. If there is substantial enlargement of the jaw with an associated soft tissue mass, other sarcomas such as chondrosarcoma and osteosarcoma should be considered, although both usually have some internal structure.

Management

The management of fibrosarcoma is primarily surgical. A wide margin of adjacent normal bone is taken if anatomically possible. Radiation therapy and chemotherapy are usually palliative treatments.

MALIGNANCIES OF THE HEMATOPOIETIC SYSTEM

Plasmacytoma and Multiple Myeloma

Disease Mechanism

Plasmacytoma and multiple myeloma are malignant neoplasms of cells derived from plasma cells. A solitary lesion is referred to as a plasmacytoma, while multiple lesions are called multiple myeloma. These neoplasms may arise as a result of the partial deletion of chromosome 13, although chromosomal translocations have also been reported.

Clinical Features

Multiple myeloma, in particular, is the most common malignancy arising in bone. Most patients are male between 35 and 70 years of age, with a mean age of 60 years. The patient may complain of fatigue, weight loss, fever, and bone pain; a typical presenting feature is low back pain. Patients may also complain of tooth pain, swelling, hemorrhage, dysesthesia, or paresthesia. Secondary systemic signs may include anemia, amyloidosis, and hypercalcemia. In half of all patients, the characteristic Bence-Jones protein can be detected in the patient's urine, which causes the urine to foam. When this clonal proliferation of plasma cells occurs, the cells first occupy cancellous bone spaces, and later cortical bone as the population of cells increases. These abnormal cells accumulate in the bone marrow and interfere with normal hematopoiesis.

Imaging Features

Location. Plasmacytoma and multiple myeloma are more frequently seen in the mandible than in the maxilla. In the mandible, lesions are more commonly seen in the posterior body, ramus, and condyle. Maxillary lesions usually appear in more posterior sites.

Periphery. Solitary plasmacytoma has an oval or round shape; however, untreated or aggressive areas of bone destruction may develop confluence, giving the appearance of multilocularity. Although some lesions of plasmacytoma and multiple myeloma may have ragged borders and even appear infiltrative, more commonly, the periphery of the lesions are well defined but noncorticated (Fig. 24.16). The lack of cortication or any response of the adjacent bone to the lesion results in a nonexistent zone of transition between the lesion and the normal adjacent bone. Consequently, these appearances have led to the adaptation of the descriptor "punched out" to describe the lesions (Fig. 24.17). In older patients who may be osteopenic, lesions may be difficult to detect.

Internal structure. Lesions of plasmacytoma and multiple myeloma are radiolucent. Occasionally islands of residual bone, yet unaffected by the neoplasm, may give the appearance of mineralization with the radiolucency.

Effects on adjacent structures. The borders of the mandibular canal may become less clear as it loses its cortical border, in whole or in part. Mandibular lesions can produce a localized "cookie bite" or scallop of the endosteal inner surface of the cortex, and this cortex may be lost if lesions grow larger. Periosteal reaction is uncommon, but if present, it takes the form of a single radiopaque line oriented parallel to the bone surface.

Effects on adjacent teeth. If a good deal of bone is lost, teeth may appear relatively radiopaque and may stand out conspicuously against the osteopenic background of the bone. Lamina dura and the follicles of impacted teeth may lose their corticated peripheries in a manner analogous to that seen in hyperparathyroidism. In rare cases, there may be irregular root resorption.

Differential Interpretation

The most likely differential interpretation is metastasis, particularly when the metastases are osteolytic. Knowledge of a prior malignancy

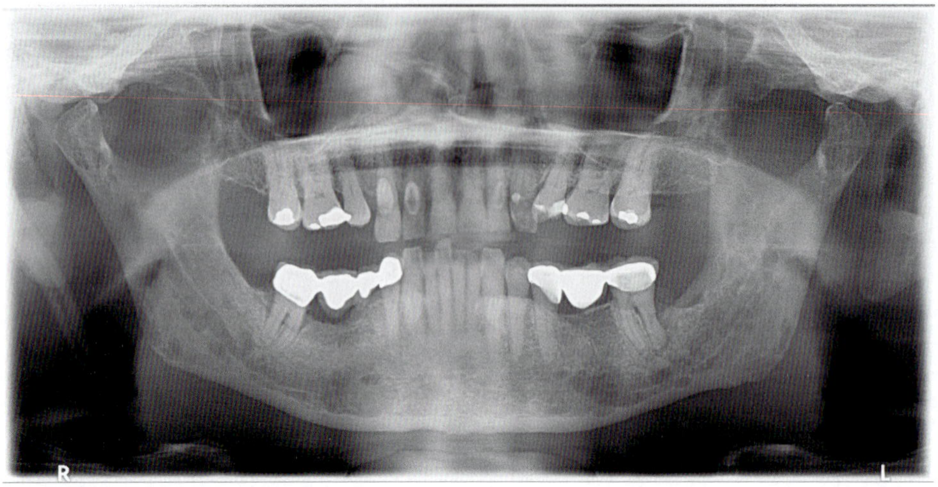

Fig. 24.16 Multiple myeloma lesions in the mandible showing the "punched-out" nature of the lesions. Note the absence of any bone reaction at the peripheries of the lesions. (Courtesy Dr. L. Lee, Toronto, ON.)

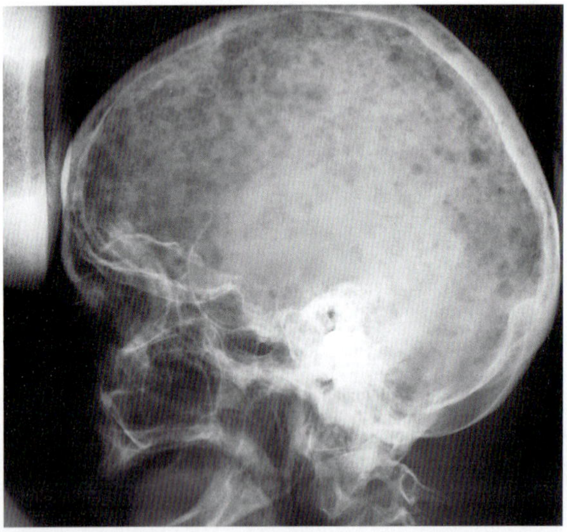

Fig. 24.17 A lateral planar image of the skull shows multiple circular radiolucent lesions of multiple myeloma.

in a patient will help differentiate multiple myeloma from metastatic disease. Osteomyelitis may appear similar to multiple myeloma; however, a visible cause for the inflammatory response usually exists. Furthermore, inflammatory disease is generally accompanied by a wide zone of transition due to sclerosis, which is not the case with multiple myeloma. The simple bone cavity (SBC) may be mistaken for multiple myeloma, although SBCs are usually delicately corticated and characteristically scallop between the roots of the teeth in a much younger population. Also, on periapical images, the periodontal ligament spaces and lamina dura are preserved adjacent to a simple bone cavity.

Generalized osteopenia of the jaws may be caused by hyperparathyroidism, but this can be differentiated on the basis of abnormal blood chemistry. However, brown tumors of hyperparathyroidism, if present with generalized osteopenia and similar symptoms, can readily be confused with multiple myeloma. Metabolic diseases, such as Gaucher disease or oxalosis, may also cause many changes similar to multiple myeloma, but these are rare.

Management

Should a plasmocytoma be diagnosed, additional investigations should be conducted to rule out other similar lesions in the skeleton. Multiple myeloma is treated with chemotherapy, without or with autologous or allogeneic bone marrow transplantation. Radiation therapy may be used for the treatment of symptomatic osseous lesions when palliation is required.

Lymphoma

Disease Mechanism

Lymphomas are malignant neoplasms of lymphocytes at various levels of maturation. In general, lymphomas arise within lymph nodes; however, extranodal sites, such as bone, skin, gastrointestinal mucosa, and Waldeyer ring, can also be involved. The term non-Hodgkin lymphoma describes a family of heterogeneous neoplasms of varying type and severity, while Hodgkin lymphoma is defined by the identification of the Reid-Sternberg cell in histopathology.

Clinical Features

Lesions occurring outside lymph nodes in the head and neck may be present in approximately 20% of cases. Patients may feel unwell, experience night sweats, pruritus, and weight loss. A palpable, nonpainful swelling, lymphadenopathy, and sensorineural deficits may accompany isolated lesions of the jaws. Lesions present for some time may cause pain and ulceration. In the jaws, the maxillary sinus, palate, tonsillar area, and bone may be sites of lymphoma spread. It is not possible to differentiate non-Hodgkin lymphoma from Hodgkin lymphoma radiographically.

Imaging Features

Location. Extranodal lymphoma is more likely to affect the maxilla, including the maxillary sinus. In the mandible, the posterior mandible is more commonly affected with malignant cells entering the bone via the inferior alveolar canal.

Periphery. When bone is involved, non-Hodgkin lymphomas initially take the shape and form of the host bone. If untreated, the lesions may extend to the bone surface causing destruction of the overlying cortex (Fig. 24.18). Lymphoma lesions may appear round or multiloculated and lack a cortex. The borders are poorly defined, with an invasive quality at the periphery. Occasionally, lymphoma may show multifocal areas of bone destruction, which likely appear as finger-like extensions of malignant neoplasm cells in a buccal or lingual direction (Fig. 24.19). When the lesions involve the soft tissues, their borders are smooth.

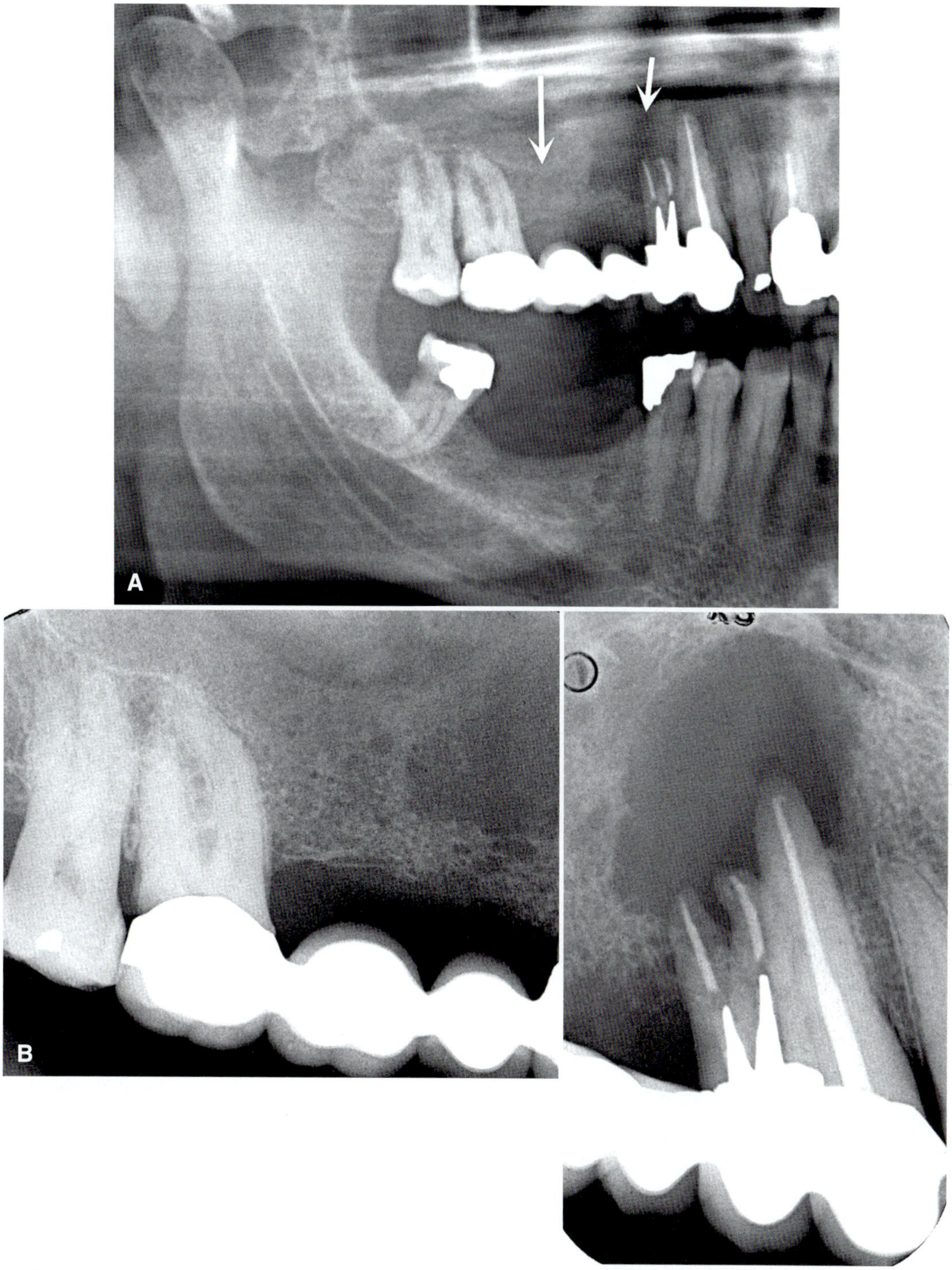

Fig. 24.18 Panoramic image (A) revealing lymphoma invading the right maxilla. Note the bone destruction and the poorly defined periphery of the lesion. Also, there has been destruction of the floor of the maxillary sinus *(arrows)*. Intraoral images also show bone destruction and the lack of any bone reaction surrounding the lesion (B).

Internal structure. The internal structure of lymphoma is almost always entirely radiolucent. It is rare to see internal radiopacities or reactive bone formation at the periphery of lesions.

Effects on adjacent structures. In the maxillary sinus, a soft tissue mass may be visible on imaging, and sinus borders may be lost. Lesions developing within the mandible will destroy the cortices of the inferior alveolar canal and the bone. Bone surface reactions are uncommon, but when seen, there may be a lamellar periosteal reaction or delicate spiculation (Fig. 24.19A and B). With the advent of MRI, it has become apparent that lymphoma has a tendency of growing along fat planes and along the surface of bone.

Effects on adjacent teeth. Lymphoma has a propensity to grow into the periodontal ligament space of erupted teeth producing nonconcentric enlargement of the ligament space (Fig. 24.19A). In developing teeth, the cortex of the crypts may be lost when the malignant cells infiltrate the developing papilla, and the developing

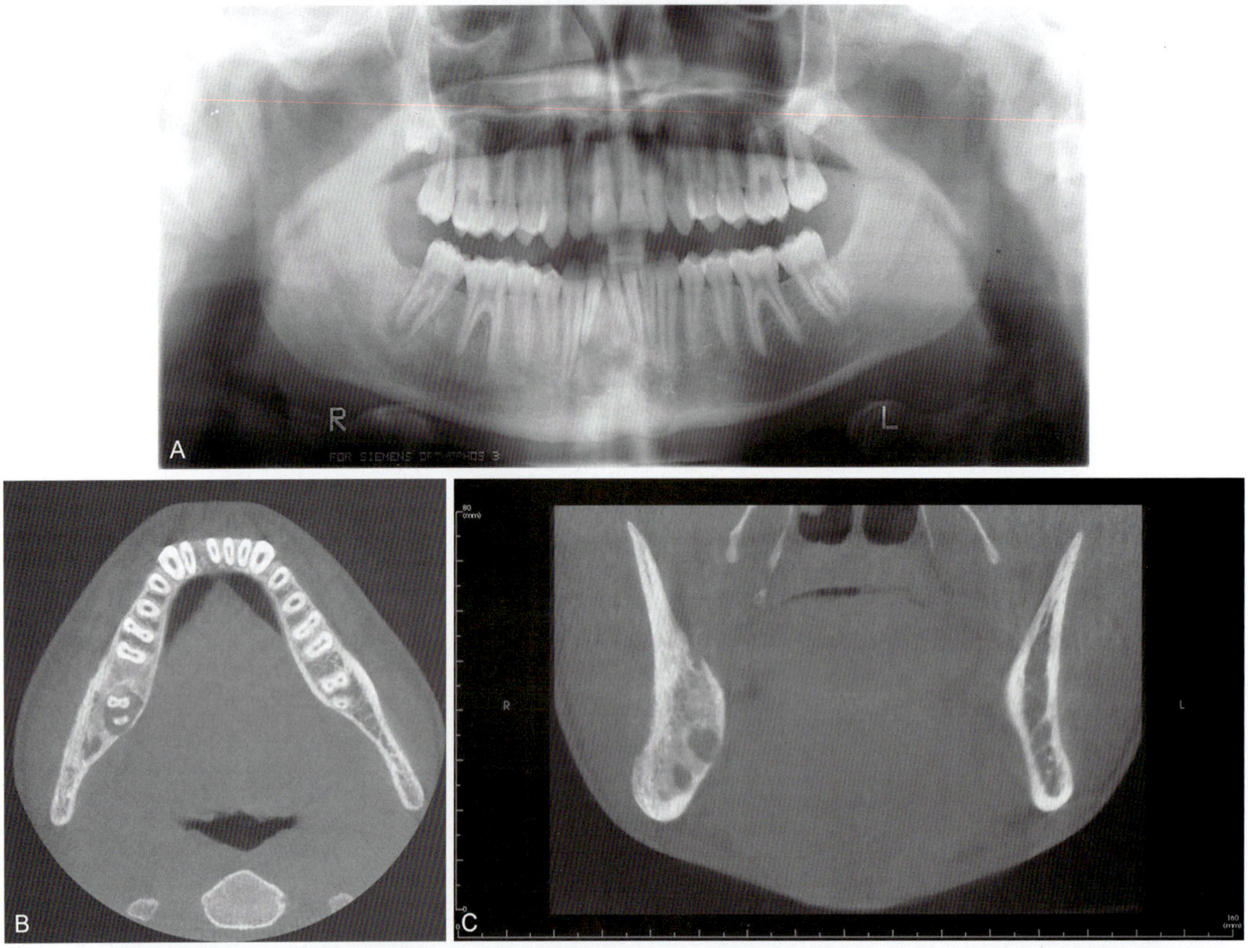

Fig. 24.19 Panoramic image (A) reveals lymphoma invading the right posterior body of the mandible. Note the poorly defined periphery of the lesion as well as the nonconcentric widening of the periodontal ligament space involving the mesial root of the mandibular right first molar. Axial (B) and coronal (C) cone beam computed tomographic images of the same case show the alteration of the bone pattern on the right side compared to the left and the buccal spiculations. (Courtesy Dr. D. Turgeon, Montreal, QC.)

tooth crown may be displaced in an occlusal direction and exfoliated from its follicle.

Differential Interpretation

Lymphoma is indistinguishable from other blood-borne malignancies radiologically. Metastatic disease can be easily confused with lymphoma when it arises in the jawbones. However, Ewing sarcoma and Langerhans cell histiocytosis, although also capable of producing the same effects, occur in a slightly younger age group. Osteosarcoma or chondrosarcoma without an internal pattern and any of the central carcinomas may not be distinguishable from lymphoma on imaging examinations. Squamous cell carcinoma arising in the maxillary sinus may be difficult to differentiate from lymphoma involving the maxillary sinus. Other lesions that can displace developing teeth in an occlusal direction include leukemia and Langerhans cell histiocytosis. Differentiation from rarefying osteitis may be difficult; however, careful inspection of the image may reveal the presence of an infiltrative border with adjacent bone destruction not seen in inflammation.

Management

The management is radiation therapy and/or chemotherapy. Treatment depends on the histopathologic variant and the location and extent of disease.

Burkitt Lymphoma

Disease Mechanism

Burkitt lymphoma is a high-grade B-cell lymphoma that differs from other B-cell lymphomas with respect to its histologic appearance and clinical behavior. First described in East Africa as African jaw lymphoma, two types of the disease have now been described: the endemic African Burkitt lymphoma and the non-African form, although the African form has also been described outside of Africa. The African form is linked to previous infections of malaria parasites and Epstein–Barr virus; however, the role of this virus in the non-African form is uncertain. The infections are believed to facilitate a well-described translocation of chromosome 8 that involves the *Myc* oncogene, which controls cell function and proliferation. The non-African form rarely involves the jaws, but there is involvement of abdominal viscera. African Burkitt lymphoma affects young children, whereas the non-African form affects adolescents and young adults.

Clinical Features

Burkitt lymphoma is a disease of the young. It affects more males than females, and clinically, the hallmark of this disease is rapid growth with a neoplasm doubling time of less than 24 hours. Consequently, facial deformity can develop very early in the disease course and block nasal passages, displace orbital contents, and ulcerate through skin.

The African type can also cause pain and paresthesia, with paresthesia of the inferior alveolar nerve or other sensory facial nerves being more common.

Imaging Features

Location. Extranodal disease is the norm in Burkitt lymphoma. African cases may involve one jaw or both, primarily affecting the posterior parts of the jaws.

Periphery. The lesions may begin as multiple, poorly defined, noncorticated radiolucencies, which later coalesce into larger areas. The lesions may be of no specific shape; however, they can expand bone rapidly, producing a balloon-like growth. This type of expansion can thin and breach bone cortices, growing into the adjacent soft tissues. Lesions that abut the orbital contents or the maxillary sinus may radiologically show a smooth surface soft tissue mass.

Internal structure. Burkitt lymphoma developing in the bone is radiolucent in children; however, in older patients, there may be production of reactive bone.

Effects on adjacent structures. Cortical boundaries, such as the maxillary sinus, nasal floor, orbital walls, and inferior border of the mandible, are thinned and later destroyed. The cortex of the mandibular canal is lost, although the canal cortex may be difficult to evaluate in children. If the lesion extends to the bone surface, sunray spiculations, although rare, can be seen. Cases that impinge on the orbit can displace the orbital contents, and this may be seen both clinically and radiologically.

Effects on adjacent teeth. Erupted teeth adjacent to a Burkitt neoplasm are grossly displaced, as are developing tooth crypts. Neoplastic cells invading the crypts of developing tooth crowns may displace the developing tooth bud to one side of the crypt or superiorly. A neoplasm that is located apical to a developing tooth may cause the tooth to be displaced so it appears to erupt with little if any root formation. After neoplasm involvement of the developing dental structures occurs, root development ceases. Lamina dura of teeth in the area are destroyed.

Differential Interpretation

Burkitt lymphoma is indistinguishable from other blood-borne malignancies radiologically or osteosarcoma and chondrosarcoma in the absence of mineralization. Non-Hodgkin lymphoma must be considered, although it occurs in a much older age group in most cases. Cherubism is bilateral, has more internal structure, does not breach bony borders, and grows much more slowly.

Management

Burkitt lymphoma is treated with chemotherapy.

Leukemia

Disease Mechanism

Leukemia is a malignant neoplasm of hematopoietic stem cells and is associated with a number of nonrandom chromosomal abnormalities. A number of histopathologic subtypes have been defined based on their cell of origin. These malignant cells displace normal bone marrow constituents and spill out into the peripheral blood. Acute leukemias occur with a bimodal age distribution in very young patients and very old patients. Most cases of leukemia are associated with nonrandom chromosomal abnormalities, although the exact etiology is not known.

Clinical Features

Leukemia is broadly classified as being either acute or chronic. Patients with acute leukemia generally feel unwell with weakness and bone pain. They may exhibit pallor, spontaneous hemorrhage, hepatomegaly, splenomegaly, lymphadenopathy, and fever. Oral symptoms are generally absent, but if present, they include loose teeth, petechiae, ulceration, and boggy enlarged gingiva. A patient with chronic leukemia may have no presenting signs or complaints.

Imaging Features

Radiologic signs associated with chronic leukemia are comparatively rare.

Location. Leukemia affects the entire body, as the malignant cells are disseminated throughout the bone marrow via the circulating blood, with jaw involvement seen more often in areas of developing teeth.

Periphery. As leukemia is a systemic malignancy, its radiologic features may be present bilaterally as poorly defined, radiolucent areas. With time and lack of treatment, these smaller, patchy areas of disease may coalesce to form larger areas radiolucent regions within the bone (see Fig. 24.20).

Internal structure. The internal structure of leukemia is radiolucent, and there is generalized radiolucency of the bone as the leukemic cell

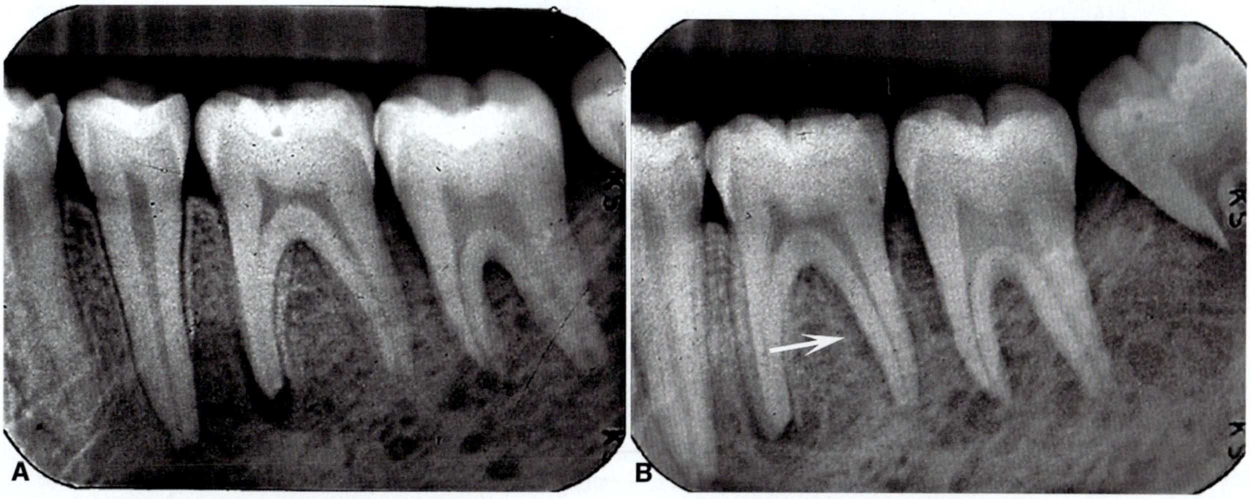

Fig. 24.20 Periapical images (A and B) of the left posterior mandible demonstrate multifocal areas of bone destruction and widening of portions of the periodontal ligament spaces *(arrow)* in leukemia. Note the infiltrative appearance of the bone destruction.

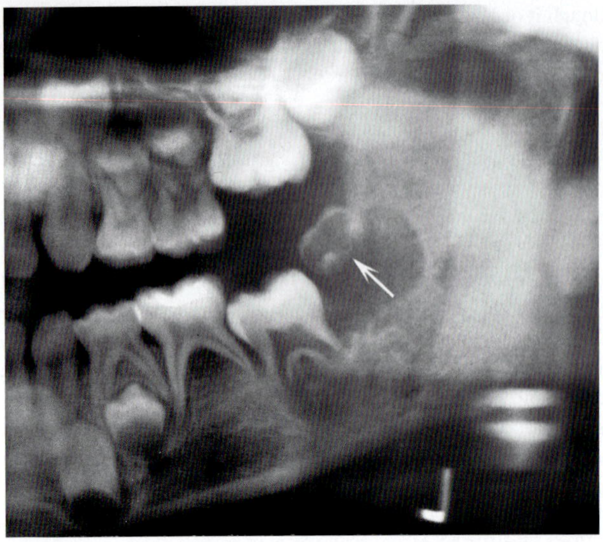

Fig. 24.21 Cropped panoramic image demonstrates unusual occlusal displacement of the developing mandibular second molar from its follicle *(arrow)*.

infiltrate expands within the marrow spaces. Ultimately, this leads to a loss of the trabecular pattern in the bone. Occasionally, foci of leukemic cells may be present outside of the jaws as a mass called a chloroma, which may behave like a solitary, localized, and malignant neoplasm.

Effects on surrounding structures. Leukemia does not cause expansion of bone, although occasionally a single layer of periosteal new bone may be seen in association with this disease; however, this is uncommon in the chronic form. If lesions affect the periodontal structures, the crestal bone may be lost.

Effects on adjacent teeth. The teeth may appear to stand out conspicuously from the surrounding bone as the leukemic infiltrate spreads. Should the lesions involve the periodontal ligament space, there may be nonconcentric widening (Fig. 24.20). Developing teeth in their crypts and teeth undergoing eruption may be displaced in an occlusal direction (Fig. 24.21) or into the oral cavity before root development is completed. Less commonly, developing teeth may be displaced from their normal position. The result of this is premature loss of teeth. The lamina dura and cortical outlines of follicles may also be lost.

Differential Interpretation

Leukemia is indistinguishable from other blood-borne malignancies radiologically. Generally, a medical diagnosis has been reached by the time radiologic signs of leukemia are present in the jaws. However, the development of radiologic changes may be the first indication of the relapse of disease. Metabolic disorders may be considered in cases in which generalized rarefaction of bone is seen; however, these conditions can be excluded on the basis of blood testing. Rarefying osteitis can be excluded following careful clinical and radiologic examination of the involved tooth.

Management

The management of leukemia is primarily through a combination of chemotherapy with or without allogeneic or autologous bone marrow transplantation. Some chronic leukemias are managed with low-dose chemotherapy.

Langerhans Cell Histiocytosis

Disease Mechanism

Langerhans cells are specialized cells of the histiocytic cell line that normally are found in the skin. The disorders results from the abnormal proliferation of Langerhans-like cells or their precursors due to mutations affecting the proto-oncogene *BRAF*^{V600E}. This proto-oncogene encodes a protein, B-Raf, which plays a role in the control of cell proliferation.

The abnormal proliferation of Langerhans cells and eosinophils results in a spectrum of clinical diseases; chronic localized histiocytosis (eosinophilic granuloma), chronic disseminated histiocytosis (Hand-Schüller-Christian disease), and acute disseminated histiocytosis (Letterer-Siwe disease). More recently, a newly proposed classification scheme designates two types: nonmalignant unifocal or multifocal eosinophilic granuloma; and malignant Letterer-Siwe disease and variants of histiocytic lymphoma. Although lesions often have a prominent inflammatory component, more recently, all forms of this malignancy have been shown to be clonal and of a neoplastic nature.

Clinical Features

Langerhans cell histiocytosis usually involves the skeleton (ribs, pelvis, long bones, skull, and jaws) and rarely soft tissue. Approximately 10% of all patients have oral lesions. This condition occurs most commonly in older children and young adults.

The lesions often form quickly and may cause a dull, steady pain. In the jaws, lesions may cause bony swelling, a soft tissue mass, gingivitis, bleeding gingiva, and ulceration. There may have a single focus or may develop into a multifocal, more aggressive disease. The chronic disseminated form (Hand-Schüller-Christian disease) may involve multiple bone lesions, diabetes insipidus, and exophthalmos.

The acute disseminated form (Letterer-Siwe disease) is the most aggressive form and most often occurs in children younger than 3 years of age. Soft tissue granulomatous reactions disseminate throughout the body, and the condition is marked by intermittent fever, hepatosplenomegaly, anemia, lymphadenopathy, hemorrhage, and failure to thrive. Bone lesions are rare. Sadly, patients succumb to the disease within several weeks of onset.

Imaging Features

Location. Langerhans cell histiocytosis developing within the alveolar processes commonly involve multiple sites, whereas intraosseous lesions usually are solitary. The mandible is a more commonly affected site than the maxilla, and the posterior regions are more involved than the anterior regions (Fig. 24.22). The mandibular ramus is a common site of intraosseous lesions. Solitary lesions of the jaws may be accompanied by lesions in other bones.

Periphery. The periphery of the lesions varies from moderately well defined to well defined but without cortication. In some cases, the periphery can appear punched out with a nonexistent zone of transition (Fig. 24.23). The borders may be smooth or irregular. Lesions within the alveolar processes have an epicenter in the middle thirds of the roots, and bone destruction progresses in an oval or round shape until the alveolar process appears scooped out (Figs. 24.24 and 24.25).

Internal structure. The internal structure usually is radiolucent.

Effects on adjacent structures. Langerhans cell histiocytosis destroys bone. These lesions are able to stimulate periosteal new bone formation; this occurs more commonly with the intraosseous type of lesion (Fig. 24.26). The periosteal new bone formation is indistinguishable from the lamellar appearance seen with inflammatory lesions of the jaws. This lesion can destroy the outer cortical plate and in rare cases extends into the surrounding soft tissues in the multidetector CT examination.

Effects on adjacent teeth. With lesions centered in the alveolar processes, the bone around teeth, including the lamina dura, is destroyed, and the teeth appear to be floating in space. The lesion does not displace teeth, although teeth may move because they are bereft of bone support (see Fig. 24.25). Only minor root resorption has been reported.

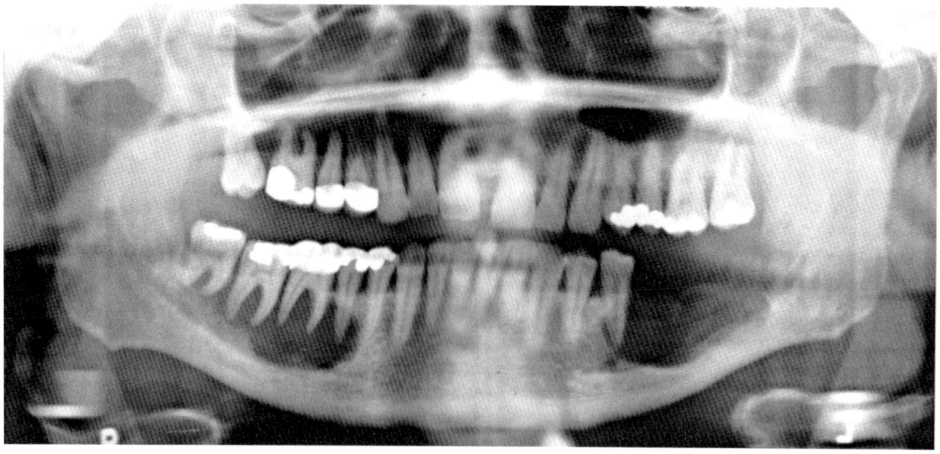

Fig. 24.22 Panoramic image of multiple lesions of Langerhans cell histiocytosis. Note the "scooped-out" shape of the bone destruction, as well as the destruction of the floor of the right maxillary sinus.

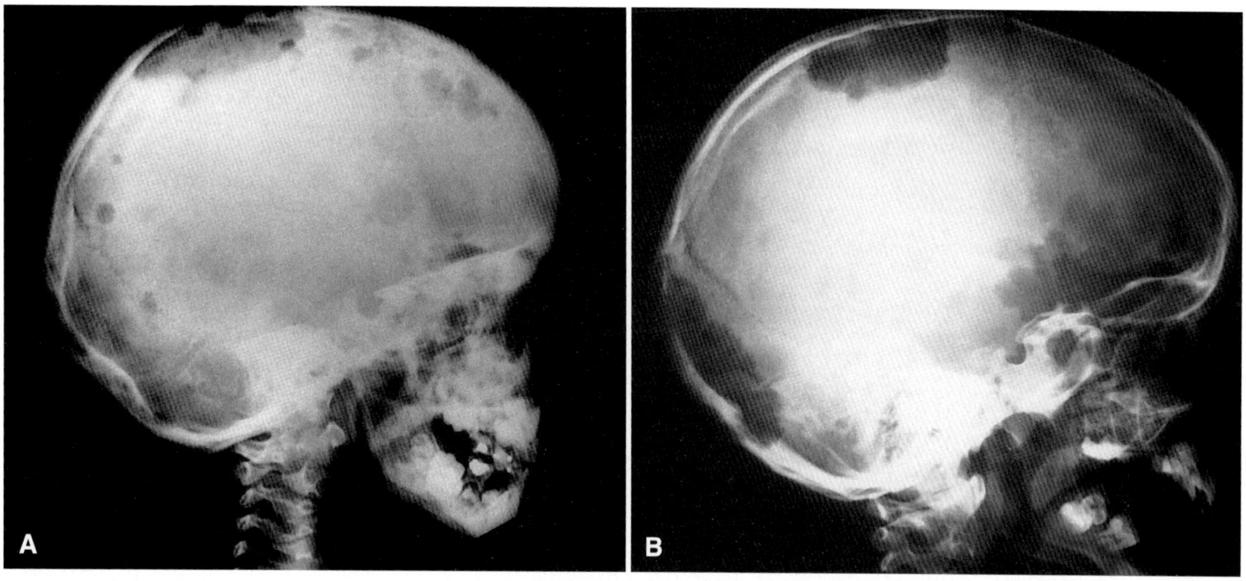

Fig. 24.23 Skull involvement of Langerhans cell histiocytosis showing the variably sized radiolucent lesions (A and B).

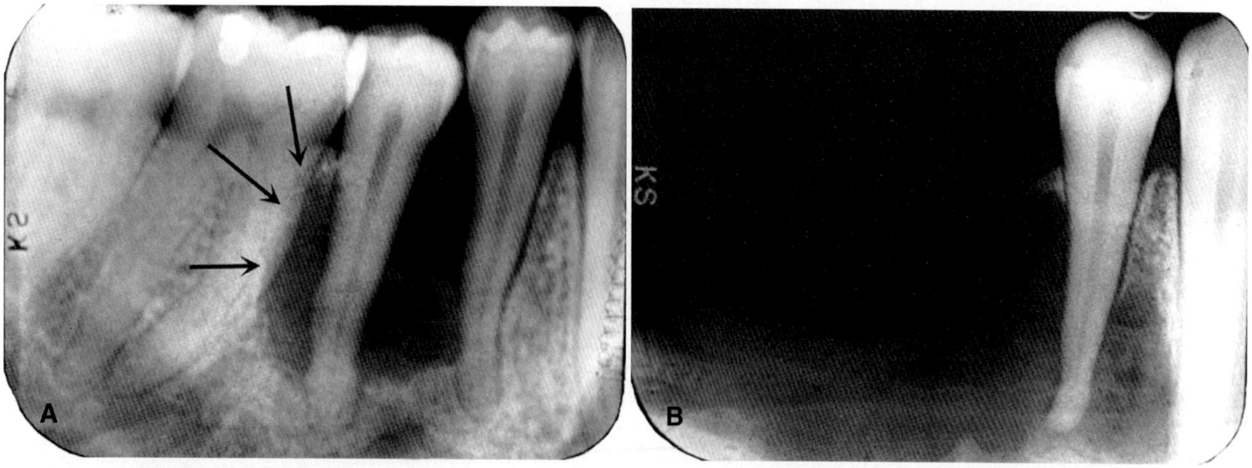

Fig. 24.24 Periapical images of the same region of the mandible approximately 1 year apart. The earlier image (A) shows the scooped-out appearance of the lesion with an epicenter near the mid-root level of the involved teeth (in contrast to periodontal disease). The later image (B) shows much more extensive bone destruction and the loss of teeth. (Courtesy Dr. D. Stoneman, Toronto, ON.)

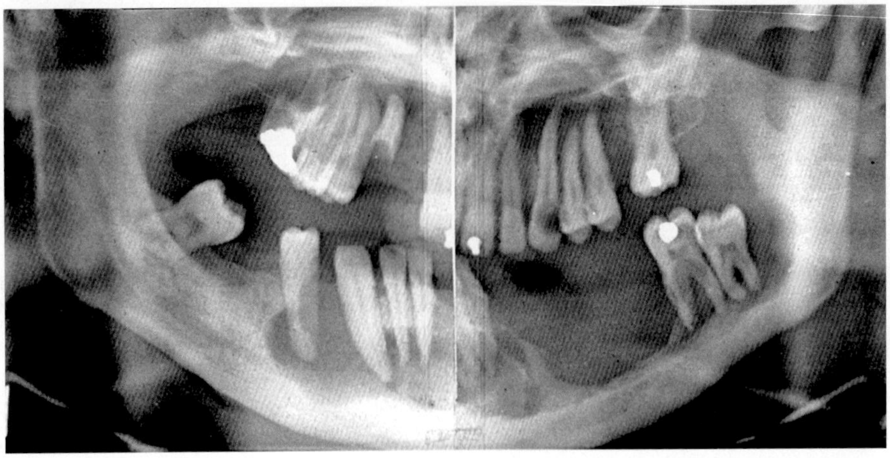

Fig. 24.25 Panoramic image shows the bone extensiveness of the bone destruction that can occur with Langerhans cell histiocytosis and the appearance of the remaining teeth to be floating in space. (Courtesy Dr. D. Stoneman, Toronto, ON.)

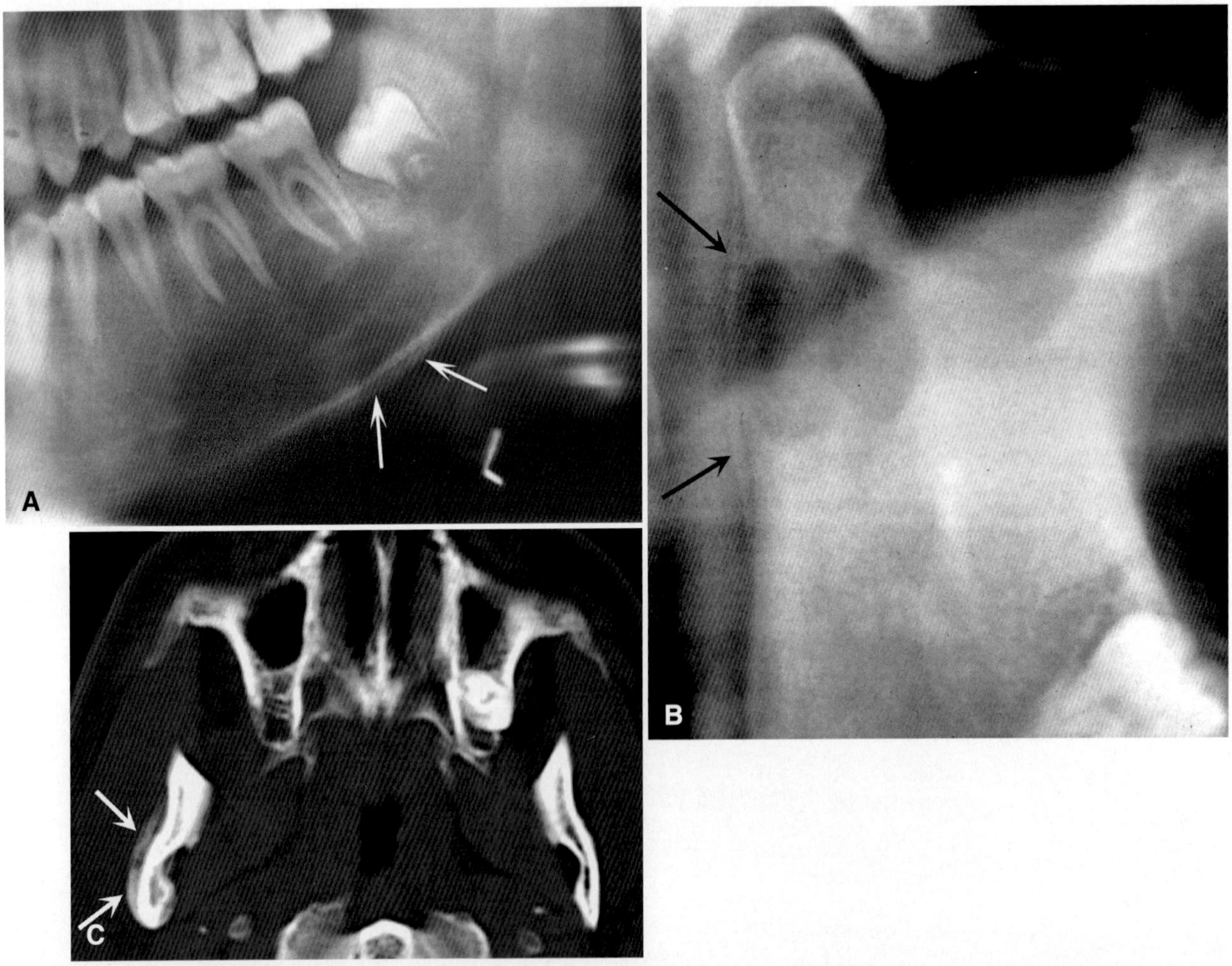

Fig. 24.26 Periosteal new bone formation in Langerhans cell histiocytosis. Note the early destruction of bone around the molar teeth on the cropped panoramic image (A) and the lamellar periosteal new bone formation adjacent to the inferior cortex of the mandible *(arrows)*. A similar appearance can be seen along the posterior border of the right ramus (B). Axial multidetector computed tomographic image (C) shows the lamellar periosteal new bone formation along the lateral surface of the right mandibular ramus.

Differential Interpretation

The most important differential interpretation is advanced stage and grade periodontitis. Important characteristics that can be used to differentiate this disease from periodontitis is that the epicenter of the bone destruction in Langerhans cell histiocytosis is located in the middle third of the tooth roots and the scooped-out appearance. In contrast, the bone destruction in periodontal disease begins at the alveolar crest and extends apically along the root surface. Differentiation of a squamous cell carcinoma may be impossible based on the imaging characteristics alone, although the borders of Langerhans cell histiocytosis are typically better defined. Multiple lesions in a younger age group (usually the first three decades) are more likely to be Langerhans cell histiocytosis than squamous cell carcinoma, which typically appears as a single lesion in middle-aged or elderly patients.

The differential interpretation of solitary intraosseous lesions includes metastatic disease and malignant neoplasms extending into bone from adjacent soft tissues. However, the well-defined borders and the periosteal reaction seen in Langerhans cell histiocytosis help in the differential interpretation.

Management

Patients suspected to have Langerhans cell histiocytosis should be referred to an oral and maxillofacial radiologist for an initial workup and to their physician for nuclear medicine imaging to detect other bone lesions in the skeleton and biopsy. Because the histopathologic appearance of histiocytosis may be hidden by changes caused by secondary infection from the oral cavity in alveolar lesions, it is important to correlate the radiologic and histopathologic findings from the biopsy.

Management of localized lesions usually consists of surgical curettage or limited radiation therapy. Surgical management of jaw lesions usually is preferable because these lesions have a low recurrence rate. The earlier lesions of the mandible are diagnosed and controlled, and fewer teeth are lost to bone destruction. Disseminated disease is treated with chemotherapy.

ORAL AND MAXILLOFACIAL IMAGING FOR CANCER SURVIVORS

Patients who have survived cancer treatment require dental treatment just like any other patient. For a cancer survivor, an oral and maxillofacial radiologic examination may be more important than for a healthy patient to receive a recall examination. Some patients who have received a full course of radiation therapy are concerned about the additional radiation dose from an oral and maxillofacial radiologic examination. Such patients should be reassured that the radiation dose associated with oral and maxillofacial radiologic imaging examinations is relatively minuscule compared to the dose received from radiation therapy.

A patient treated for head and neck malignancy with radiation therapy—even with today's advanced radiotherapeutic methods—is prone to develop postradiation dental caries and radiation-induced bone necrosis. Careful clinical examination and a thorough oral and maxillofacial radiologic examination may be periodically required to ensure that the remaining dentition and periodontium are disease free.

Radiation caries occurs in many patients and appears clinically different from typical dental caries. If untreated, these carious teeth can develop nonvital pulps, and there may be extension of the inflammatory response to the jaw more widely. If such a patient requires tooth extraction, healing can be expected to be slow, and occasionally osteoradionecrosis may result. Also, bisphosphonates and other related therapies are now used extensively with some chemotherapy regimens, as in multiple myeloma. Changes seen with either radiation therapy or medication may mimic odontogenic inflammatory disease and should be differentiated to avoid unnecessary treatment and secondary osteonecrosis (see Chapter 20).

The role of oral and maxillofacial radiology in these patients should not be restricted to examination only of the teeth and supporting structures. Equally important is monitoring of the outcome of treatment and specifically the examination of oral and maxillofacial images for evidence of neoplasm recurrence and the development of metastases and osteonecrosis.

BIBLIOGRAPHY

Central Squamous Cell Carcinoma

de Morais EF, Carlan LM, de Farias Morais HG, et al. Primary intraosseous squamous cell carcinoma involving the jaw bones: a systematic review and update. *Head Neck Pathol.* 2021;15:608-616.

Chondrosarcoma

de Souza LL, Pontes FSC, Fonseca FP, et al. Chondrosarcoma of the jaw bones: a review of 224 cases reported to date and an analysis of prognostic factors. *Int J Oral Maxillofac Surg.* 2019;48:452-460.

Garrington GE, Collett WK. Chondrosarcoma. I. A selected literature review. *J Oral Pathol.* 1988;17:1-11.

Garrington GE, Collett WK. Chondrosarcoma. II. Chondrosarcoma of the jaws: analysis of 37 cases. *J Oral Pathol.* 1988;17:12-20.

Ewing Sarcoma

Becker M, Stefanelli S, Rougemont AL, et al. Non-odontogenic tumors of the facial bones in children and adolescents: role of multiparametric imaging. *Neuroradiology.* 2017;59(4):327-342. doi:10.1007/s00234-017-1798-y.

Guimarães JB, Rigo L, Lewin F, et al. The importance of PET/CT in the evaluation of patients with Ewing neoplasms. *Radiol Bras.* 2015;48:175-180.

Fibrosarcoma

Pereira CM, Jorge J Jr, Di Hipólito O Jr, et al. Primary intraosseous fibrosarcoma of jaw. *Int J Oral Maxillofac Surg.* 2005;34:579-581.

Langerhans Cell Histiocytosis

Dagenais M, Pharoah MJ, Sikorski PA, et al. The radiographic characteristics of histiocytosis X. *Oral Surg Oral Med Oral Pathol Oral Radiol Endod.* 1992;74:230-236.

Faustino ISP, Fernandes PM, Pontes HAR, et al. Langerhans cell histiocytosis in the oral and maxillofacial region: an updated. *J Oral Pathol Med.* 2021;50:565-571.

Leukemia

Curtis AB. Childhood leukemias: initial oral manifestations. *J Am Dent Assoc.* 1971;83:159-164.

Gomes NR, Lima LA, Morais-Perdigão AL, et al. Radiological aspects of lymphomas and leukemias affecting the jaws: a systematic review. *J Oral Pathol Med.* 2023;52:315-323.

Lymphoma

Burkitt DA. Sarcoma involving the jaws in African children. *Br J Surg.* 1958;46:218-223.

Gomes NR, Lima LA, Morais-Perdigão AL, et al. Radiological aspects of lymphomas and leukemias affecting the jaws: a systematic review. *J Oral Pathol Med.* 2023;52:315-323.

MacDonald D, Martin M, Savage K. Maxillofacial lymphomas. *Br J Radiol.* 2021;94:20191041.

Maxymiw WG, Goldstein M, Wood RE. Extranodal non-Hodgkin's lymphoma of the maxillofacial region: analysis of 88 consecutive cases. *SADJ.* 2001;56:524-527.

"Malignant Ameloblastoma" and Ameloblastic Carcinoma

Dissanayake RK, Jayasooriya PR, Siriwardena DJ, et al. Review of metastasizing (malignant) ameloblastoma (METAM): pattern of metastasis and treatment. *Oral Surg Oral Med Oral Pathol Oral Radiol Endod.* 2011;111:734-741.

Yunaev M, Abdul-Razak M, Coleman H, et al. A rare case of ameloblastic carcinoma. *Ear Nose Throat J*. 2014;93:E34-E36.

Metastatic Neoplasms

D'Silva NJ, Summerlin DJ, Cordell KG, et al. Metastatic neoplasms in the jaws: a retrospective study of 114 cases. *J Am Dent Assoc*. 2006;137:1667-1672.

Fidler IJ. The pathogenesis of cancer metastasis: the 'seed and soil' hypothesis revisited. *Nat Rev Cancer*. 2003;3:453-458.

Gupta S, Jawanda MK, Ganganna A. Jaw bone metastasis from lunch cancer as sole primary source: a systematic review. *J Clin Exp Dent*. 2022;14:e573-e593.

Mucoepidermoid Carcinoma

Chan KC, Pharoah M, Lee L, et al. Intraosseous mucoepidermoid carcinoma: a review of diagnostic imaging features of four jaw cases. *Dentomaxillofac Radiol*. 2013;42:20110162.

Inagaki M, Yuasa K, Nakayama E, et al. Mucoepidermoid carcinoma in the mandible. *Oral Surg Oral Med Oral Pathol Oral Radiol Endod*. 1998;85:613-618.

Raut D, Khedkar S. Primary intraosseous mucoepidermoid carcinoma of the maxilla: a case report and review of the literature. *Dentomaxillofac Radiol*. 2009;38:163-168.

Multiple Myeloma

Lombardo EM, Maito FLDM, Heitz C. Solitary plasmacytoma of the jaws: therapeutical considerations and prognosis based on a case reports systematic survey. *Braz J Otorhinolaryngol*. 2018;84:790-798.

Raza S, Leng S, Lentzsch S. The critical role of imaging in the management of multiple myeloma. *Curr Hematol Malig Rep*. 2017;12(3):168-175. doi:10.1007/s11899-017-0379-9.

Osteosarcoma

Gardner DG, Mills DM. The widened periodontal ligament of osteosarcoma of the jaws. *Oral Surg Oral Med Oral Pathol*. 1976;41:652-656.

Ricotta F, Bassi M, Tomasetti N, et al. Osteosarcoma of the jaws: a literature review. *Curr Med Imaging*. 2021;17:225-235.

Squamous Cell Carcinoma

Brown JS, Lowe D, Kalavrezos N, et al. Patterns of invasion and routes of neoplasm entry into the mandible by oral squamous cell carcinoma. *Head Neck*. 2002;24:370-383.

Czerwonka L, Bissada E, Goldstein DP, et al. High-resolution cone-beam computed tomography for assessment of bone invasion in oral cancer: comparison with conventional computed tomography. *Head Neck*. 2017;39:2016-2020.

Rao LP, Das SR, Mathews A, et al. Mandibular invasion in oral squamous cell carcinoma: investigation by clinical examination and orthopantomogram. *Int J Oral Maxillofac Surg*. 2004;33:454-457.

Squamous Cell Carcinoma Originating in a Cyst

Cavalcanti MGP, Veltrini VC, Ruprecht A, et al. Squamous-cell carcinoma arising from an odontogenic cyst—the importance of computed tomography in the diagnosis of malignancy. *Oral Surg Oral Med Oral Pathol Oral Radiol Endod*. 2005;100:365-368.

Kaffe I, Ardekian L, Peled M, et al. Radiological features of primary intraosseous carcinoma of the jaws: analysis of the literature and report of a new case. *Dentomaxillofac Radiol*. 1998;27:209-214.

van der Wal KG, de Visscher JG, Eggink HF. Squamous cell carcinoma arising in a residual cyst. A case report. *Int J Oral Maxillofac Surg*. 1993;23:350-352.

Trauma

Sanjay M. Mallya

Radiologic examination is essential in the evaluation of the patient who has experienced trauma to the teeth and jaws. Imaging provides necessary information about the presence, location, and orientation of fracture planes and fragments; the involvement of adjacent vital anatomic structures; and the presence of foreign objects that may have become embedded within the soft tissues. Posttreatment imaging allows for the monitoring of healing and the detection of long-term changes resulting from the trauma.

APPLIED DIAGNOSTIC IMAGING

The initial assessment of a patient with craniofacial trauma is directed toward developing a prioritized treatment plan based on the presence of any life-threatening injuries and the severity and extent of injuries sustained. The American College of Surgeons Committee on Trauma triage guidelines are used worldwide to recognize and assess the severity and urgency of injury. These guidelines use standard scales such as the Glasgow Coma Scale, Revised Trauma Score, and Injury Severity Score to identify patients that will likely benefit from referral to a level I trauma center for prompt care.

Decisions regarding management of maxillofacial injuries are made once the patient's airway, breathing, and circulation have stabilized, and diagnostic imaging contributes essential information to guide this process. Depending on the extent of the injuries and the clinical context, the imaging examination may encompass the brain, facial bones, dentoalveolar arches, and cervical spine. In acute trauma settings, this is typically accomplished with multidetector computed tomography (MDCT) and may be supplemented with targeted dentoalveolar imaging.

The design of the imaging examination may be limited by the patient's ambulatory status; for example, unconscious patients or nonambulatory patients cannot be imaged in an imaging device that requires the patient to be seated or standing. The availability of imaging equipment at the treatment facility may also limit radiologic evaluation. Finally, treatment priorities developed during the initial systematic assessment will guide the order in which imaging examinations need to be performed for timely interventions.

Radiologic Signs of Fracture

Fractures are often erroneously referred to as "lines," despite their three-dimensional nature. Fractures represent planes of cleavage through a tooth or bone, and these planes can extend deep into the tissues. A fracture may be missed if the plane of the fracture is not aligned with the orientation of the incident x-ray beam on a single planar image.

The following are general radiologic signs that may indicate the presence of a fracture of a tooth or bone:

1. **The presence of one or two usually sharply defined radiolucent lines within the anatomic boundaries of a structure.** Radiolucent lines that extend beyond the boundaries of the bone most likely represent a superimposed structure. If the line extends beyond the boundaries of a tooth root, it may represent a superimposed neurovascular canal.
2. **A change in the normal anatomic outline or shape of the structure.** A change in the contour of an object, the normal, gentle curvature of the occlusal plane, or an asymmetry may indicate the presence and location of a fracture plane.
3. **A loss of continuity of a surface.** This may appear as a gap in the continuity of an otherwise smooth tooth surface or cortical border. Such a gap may also produce a "step-type defect," where the two fragments have become displaced relative to one another.
4. **An increase in the radiopacity of a structure.** When two fragments of tooth or bone overlap, that region may appear "doubly" radiopaque. The region adjacent to this radiopaque zone must be scrutinized for a change to the normal anatomical outline, or a border discontinuity, as described earlier.

DENTOALVEOLAR TRAUMA

Dentoalveolar injuries can affect all age groups and can be caused by falls, sporting and playground activities, fights, and abuse. Injuries may also occur as part of more extensive facial trauma caused by motor vehicle accidents. Trauma to the teeth may be iatrogenic; indeed, dental trauma is a frequent general anesthesia-related claim in litigation. Andreasen's classification system of dentoalveolar injuries is widely used to facilitate communication and treatment planning of injuries to the primary and permanent dentitions. The system categorizes these injuries into three groups: tooth fractures, periodontal tissue injury, and injuries to the supporting bone (Box 25.1).

Imaging of the teeth and supporting alveolar processes is necessary prior to definitive management, especially in pediatric patients where manipulation of a root of a traumatized deciduous tooth could inadvertently damage the underlying permanent tooth bud. Guidelines to manage traumatic dental injuries have been developed by the International Association of Dental Traumatology, American Academy of Pediatric Dentistry, and the American Association of Endodontists.

Clinical indicators of dentoalveolar injury:

- Tooth fracture with or without loss of tooth structure.
- Mobile teeth.
- Empty sockets from avulsed teeth.
- Tooth displacement, including intrusion into socket.
- Altered occlusion or step deformity in occlusal plane.

Imaging objectives:

- Locate and define extent of damage to dental hard tissues and alveolar processes.
- Assess potential pulp involvement.
- Assess periodontal ligament injury.

BOX 25.1 Classification of Dentoalveolar Injuries

Dental Fractures
Crown infraction
Crown fracture, uncomplicated
Crown fracture, complicated
Fracture of enamel, dentin, and cementum, uncomplicated
Fracture of enamel, dentin, and cementum, complicated
Root fracture

Periodontal Tissue Injury
Concussion
Subluxation
Luxation

Injuries to Supporting Bone
Comminution of alveolar bone
Single-wall alveolar fracture
Fracture of the alveolar process
Fracture of the maxilla or mandible

- Assess impact of injury on restorability and retention of the involved teeth.
- Monitor responses to treatment and sequelae to injury.

Imaging approaches:

Patients with isolated dentoalveolar trauma are often first evaluated in a dental clinic. Here, intraoral imaging is the best approach for the initial diagnostic evaluation. To effectively identify tooth fractures, at least three periapical images should be made; one with a standard projection geometry and two images at different horizontal angulations of the x-ray beam, mesial and distal to the standard projection. Furthermore, the examination can include periapical images of teeth in the opposing arch and at multiple angles if fractures of these teeth are also suspected. When mouth opening is limited because of trauma, occlusal images (see Chapter 6) may be used in place of periapical projections. In pediatric patients, an American National Standards Institute size 2 receptor may be used to obtain occlusal images of the anterior maxilla and mandible. Often, information on periapical radiographs is adequate for management.

Panoramic imaging is a convenient approach to examine a broad anatomic region in order to localize dentoalveolar injuries and detect concomitant mandibular fractures. However, image distortion, particularly in the anterior region, limits critical evaluation of the teeth and periodontal ligament spaces. If the x-ray beam is not projected through the fracture plane, root and alveolar process fractures may also be masked.

Limited field of view (FOV) cone-beam computed tomography (CBCT) can be used to create multiplanar images that overcome the limitations of two-dimensional imaging, thereby enhancing the detection of fractures of the teeth and alveolar processes. The American Association of Endodontists and the American Academy of Oral and Maxillofacial Radiology recommend that "limited FOV CBCT should be considered the imaging modality of choice for diagnosis and management of limited dentoalveolar trauma, root fractures, luxation, and/or displacement of teeth and localized alveolar fractures, in the absence of other maxillofacial or soft tissue injury that may require other advanced imaging modalities."

Patients with concomitant midface or mandibular trauma are imaged with MDCT or craniofacial FOV CBCT as these examinations may provide information on the integrity of dentoalveolar structures. However, the resolution of these imaging protocols is often inadequate to detect involvement of the teeth or their supporting structures.

If a tooth or a large fragment of a tooth is missing, a chest or abdominal image can provide information on accidental aspiration or ingestion. If there are lacerations in the lips or cheek, the soft tissues must be evaluated for potential embedded foreign bodies or tooth fragments. This can be accomplished relatively simply by exposing an intraoral receptor placed adjacent to the traumatized soft tissue. If the laceration is in the tongue, an imaging examination can be accomplished with a mandibular occlusal projection image. Alternatively, the tongue can be protruded and then imaged with a receptor placed adjacent to the laceration site.

DENTAL FRACTURES

Dental Crown Fractures

Definition

Fractures of the dental crown account for approximately 25% of traumatic injuries to the permanent teeth and 40% of injuries to the deciduous teeth. The most common event responsible for the fracture of permanent teeth is a fall, followed by accidents involving vehicles (e.g., bicycles, motorcycles, and automobiles) and impacts from foreign objects striking the teeth. Fractures involving only the crown are divided into three categories:

1. **Crown infraction:** Fractures and cracks confined to enamel without the loss of enamel substance (Fig. 25.1A).
2. **Uncomplicated crown fractures:** Fractures confined to enamel or enamel and dentin with no pulp exposure (Fig. 25.1B).
3. **Complicated crown fractures:** Fractures that involve enamel, dentin, and pulp (Fig. 25.1C).

Clinical Features

Fractures of the dental crowns most frequently involve anterior teeth, especially maxillary incisors. Infractions and cracks in the enamel are best detected by indirect light or transillumination. Histopathologic studies have shown that such cracks extend through the enamel but do not involve dentin. Teeth are not sensitive to percussion or palpation and respond positively to pulp vitality testing.

Uncomplicated crown fractures that involve dentin can be recognized by the contrast in color between dentin and the peripheral layer of enamel. The exposed dentin is usually sensitive to chemical, thermal, or mechanical stimulation. In the permanent dentition, uncomplicated crown fractures are more common than complicated ones. In contrast, complicated and uncomplicated fractures occur with nearly equal frequencies in deciduous teeth. When the fracture extends deeper into the tooth, the pink blush of the pulp may be evident through the thin remaining dentin wall. Complicated crown fractures are distinguishable by bleeding from the exposed pulp or by droplets of blood forming from pinpoint exposures. The pulp is visible and may extrude from the open pulp chamber if the fracture is not recent. The exposed pulp is sensitive to most forms of stimulation.

Imaging Features

The objectives of imaging are to identify the location and extent of tooth fracture and its relationship to the pulp chamber, the status of root development, and involvement of the periodontal ligament. Imaging also provides a baseline record for comparison with future images made to monitor the development of the pathologic consequences of dental trauma, such as inflammatory disease, disruption of root development, and root resorption. The initial assessment of tooth trauma is usually made with intraoral imaging (Fig. 25.2). CBCT imaging of complicated and potentially complicated fractures will

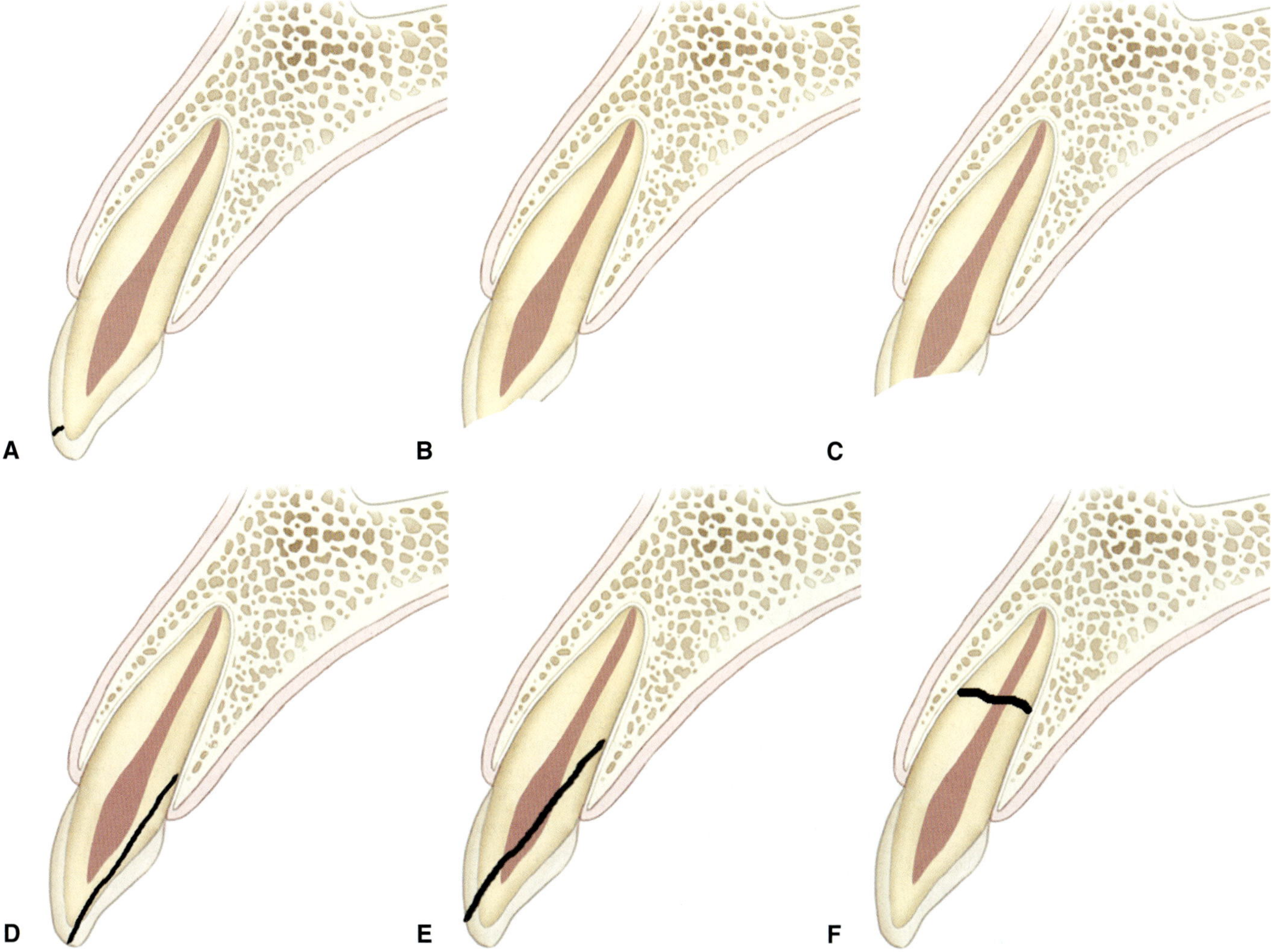

Fig. 25.1 Classification of dental fractures. (A) Crown infraction. (B) Uncomplicated crown fracture. (C) Complicated crown fracture. (D) Uncomplicated crown-root fracture. (E) Complicated crown-root fracture. (F) Horizontal root fracture.

identify the presence of pulp involvement and whether the fracture is more extensive than clinically apparent. Imaging of the adjacent soft tissues may be needed to locate embedded tooth fragments or foreign objects (Fig. 25.3).

Management

Crown infractions typically do not require management beyond smoothing of rough edges or restoration of form and function to the damaged tooth. The vitality of the tooth pulp should be determined at the initial visit and after approximately 6–8 weeks and 1 year following an injury. The prognosis for teeth with fractures limited to the enamel is good, and pulpal necrosis develops in less than 2% of such cases. If a fracture involves both dentin and enamel, the frequency of pulpal necrosis is approximately 3%. Oblique fractures have a worse prognosis than horizontal fractures because potentially a greater amount of dentin is exposed. Concomitant concussion and luxation increase the risk of subsequent pulpal necrosis to 15% and 30%, respectively.

When complicated crown fractures occur in permanent teeth where root formation has yet to be completed, attempts should be made to maintain pulp vitality to support the completion of root formation. If development of the root apex has completed, orthograde endodontic therapy is typically the treatment of choice, although pulp capping and partial pulpectomy (Cvek pulpotomy) may be acceptable depending on the size of the pulp exposure and the amount of elapsed time since the injury. In the primary dentition, complicated crown fractures are managed by pulp capping and pulpectomy in an attempt to retain apical pulp vitality. Depending on the child's maturity and their ability to cooperate during treatment, extraction may, however, be an acceptable option.

Dental Crown and Root Fractures

Definition

Fractures involving both the crown and roots (crown-root fractures) are most often complicated by pulp exposure (Fig. 25.1D and E). The permanent teeth are affected about twice as frequently as deciduous teeth. Most crown and root fractures of the anterior teeth are the result of direct trauma, whereas posterior teeth may be predisposed to fractures because of extensive caries or large restorations.

Clinical Features

The fracture plane of a typical crown-root fracture of an anterior tooth extends obliquely from the labial surface near the gingival third of the

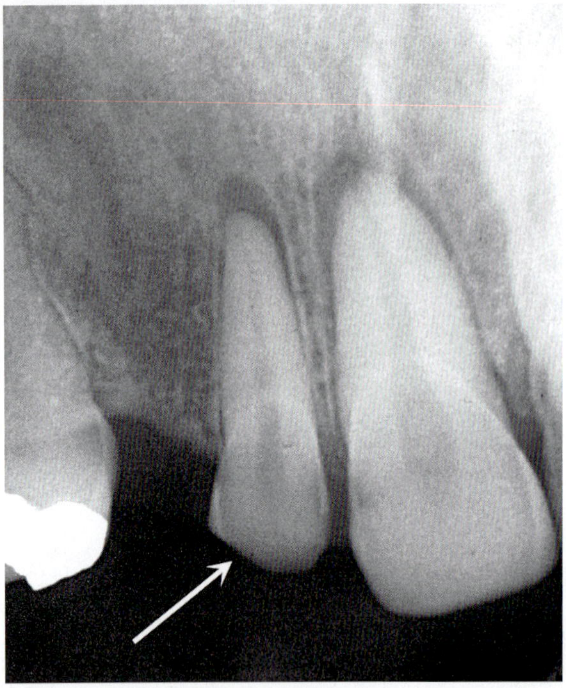

Fig. 25.2 Incisal-edge fracture involving the right maxillary lateral incisor *(arrow)* and subluxation of both the central and the lateral incisors. Note the increases to the widths of the apical periodontal ligament spaces.

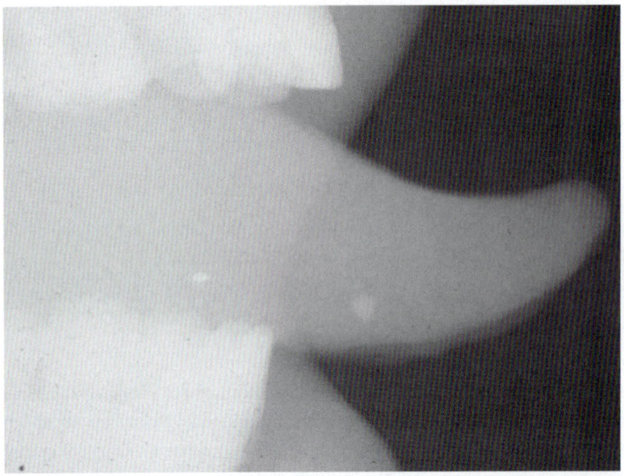

Fig. 25.3 Image of the tongue to locate fractured tooth fragments embedded in the soft tissue. The image is underexposed to highlight contrast between the small radiopaque fragments and the soft tissue of the tongue. (Courtesy Dr. A. Tadinada, Farmington, CT.)

crown to a position apical to the gingival attachment on the palatal or lingual surface. The apical extension of the fracture plane is usually subgingival and, therefore, not visible. The involved tooth is tender to percussion, and the patient may experience pain with separation of the fractured tooth fragments when the tooth is loaded (e.g., during biting or mastication). Displacement of the fragments is usually minimal, and the coronal fragment may be mobile. Crown-root fractures occasionally manifest with bleeding from the pulp.

Imaging Features

Manifestation of a fracture on planar two-dimensional imaging depends on the relative angulation of the incident x-ray beam to the

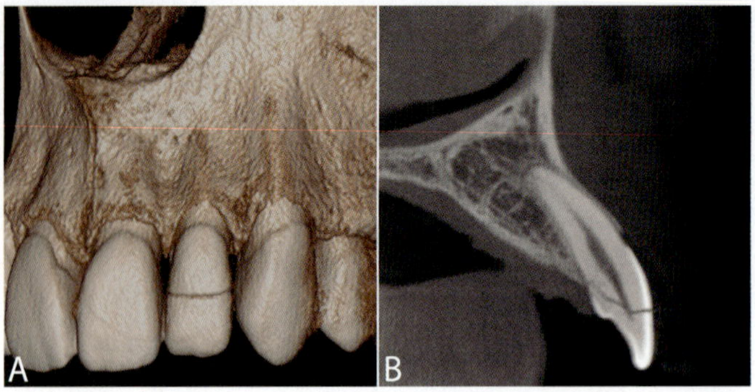

Fig. 25.4 Cone-beam computed tomographic images of a dental crown-root fracture. (A) 3D surface rendered image. A horizontal fracture plane is seen across the crown of the maxillary lateral incisor. (B) Corrected sagittal section through the lateral incisor. The fracture plane traverses to the palatal root surface at the level of the alveolar crest. Note the involvement of pulp and the intact dentoalveolar cortical boundaries.

fracture plane and the degree of separation of the fragments. If the x-ray beam is aligned along the fracture plane, the root fracture is depicted as a single well-defined radiolucent line confined to the anatomic limits of the root. However, if the x-ray beam traverses the fracture plane in a more oblique manner, the root fracture appears as a poorly defined single line or as two discrete lines that converge at the mesial and distal surfaces of the root.

The demarcation of crown-root fractures can be challenging. Although multiple periapical images may be made at different horizontal and vertical angulations to detect these fractures, limited FOV CBCT imaging is now the more preferred modality. CBCT can depict the apical extent of a fracture and the coexistence of periodontal ligament involvement (Fig. 25.4), which is an important consideration in management and prognosis.

Management

Emergency management involves temporary stabilization of the involved teeth. Management options include fragment removal and restoration, often after endodontic therapy. If the tooth pulp is not exposed and the fracture does not extend more than 3–4 mm below the gingival attachment, restorative treatment is likely to be successful. Orthodontic extrusion and crown lengthening may be necessary. In teeth where root development has yet to be completed, apexogenesis can be performed to encourage further root development and apex formation if the tooth pulp is vital. Otherwise, apexification can be performed if the tooth pulp has lost vitality. If only a small amount of root is lost with the coronal fragment but the pulp has been compromised, it is likely that the tooth can be restored after endodontic treatment. Fractures that extend deeper into the root, especially in the vertical direction, have a poor prognosis and are managed by extraction, with subsequent implant-supported or conventional prosthetic rehabilitation.

Dental Root Fractures

Root fractures are categorized as horizontal or vertical, depending on the orientation of the fracture plane, and they all involve the pulp.

Horizontal Root Fractures

Definition

With horizontal fractures, the plane of cleavage is horizontal or oblique through the thickness of the root.

Clinical Features

Horizontal root fractures occur more commonly in maxillary central incisors and are usually the result of a direct application of traumatic force to the face, alveolar processes, or teeth. The coronal root fragmenl may be displaced, but the stable apical fragment retains vitality. The mobility of the tooth relates to the level of the root fracture. When the fracture plane is located toward the apex, the tooth is relatively less mobile. The mobility of a traumatized tooth is tested by placing a finger firmly over the alveolar process; if movement of only the crown is detected, a root fracture is likely. Fractures of the root may occur with fractures of the alveolar process and are often not detected. This situation is most commonly observed in the anterior region of the mandible, where root fractures are infrequent. Although root fracture is usually associated with temporary loss of sensitivity (by all usual criteria), the sensitivity of most teeth returns to normal within about 6 months.

Imaging Features

Without imaging, horizontal root fractures may be undetectable. As described earlier, visualization of a root fracture on planar two-dimensional imaging depends on the relative angulation of the incident x-ray beam to the fracture plane and the degree of separation of the fragments. On periapical images, a root fracture may manifest as a single well-defined radiolucent line, a poorly defined single line, or as two discrete lines that converge at the mesial and distal surfaces of the root. A root fracture that is comminuted (i.e., there is more than one fracture plane generating multiple fragments) may also be less well defined. Horizontal root fractures may occur at any level and involve one (Fig. 25.5) or more roots of a multirooted tooth. Most of the fractures occur in the apical and middle thirds of the root. The fracture plane is often oriented diagonally through the root.

The imaging appearance of nondisplaced root fractures is usually subtle and may necessitate making two to three images at different horizontal x-ray beam angles. These fractures may, however, not be evident on periapical images, particularly immediately following the traumatic episode. Subsequent inflammation of the periodontal ligament at the site of fracture or resorption may increase the visible separation between the fragments and facilitate image detection. In some instances when the fracture plane is not visible, the only evidence of a fracture may be a localized increase in the width of the periodontal ligament spacc adjacent to the fracture site (Fig. 25.6A). With longer-standing fractures, the width of the fracture plane tends to increase with movement of the more coronal fragment or resorption of the fracture surfaces (see Fig. 25.6B). Over time, calcification and obliteration of the pulp chamber and root canal may be seen.

Nondisplaced fractures and fractures oriented in the mesiodistal plane are often undetectable on periapical images and pose a diagnostic challenge. Limited FOV CBCT imaging is recommended to evaluate teeth with suspected root fractures (Fig. 25.7). CBCT shows the angulation of the fracture plane and the extent of dislocation of the more coronal fragment. When the separation is more, the prognosis is poor. Delineation of the fracture relative to the alveolar crest is also important (Fig. 25.7). Prognosis of root fractures that extend to or above the alveolar crest is poor.

Fracture healing must be radiographically monitored. Healing may take the form of calcified material so that with time, the fracture plane may become barely perceptible. More often, healing occurs with connective tissue interspersed between the fractured segments. The fracture fragment margins will appear rounded with resorption and become separated by a zone of new trabecular bone (Fig. 25.8). The development of a radiolucency at the fracture site suggests inflammation, which usually develops secondary to pulp necrosis in the coronal fragment (Fig. 25.8).

Differential Interpretation

On periapical images, superimposition of the image of a fracture involving the alveolar process, small neurovascular canals, or soft tissue structures such as the lip, ala of the nose, or nasolabial fold over the image of a root may mimic a root fracture.

Management

Horizontal root fractures are managed by approximation of the fractured tooth fragments as closely as possible. The fractured tooth is splinted to adjacent teeth for 2–4 weeks. Horizontal fractures at or

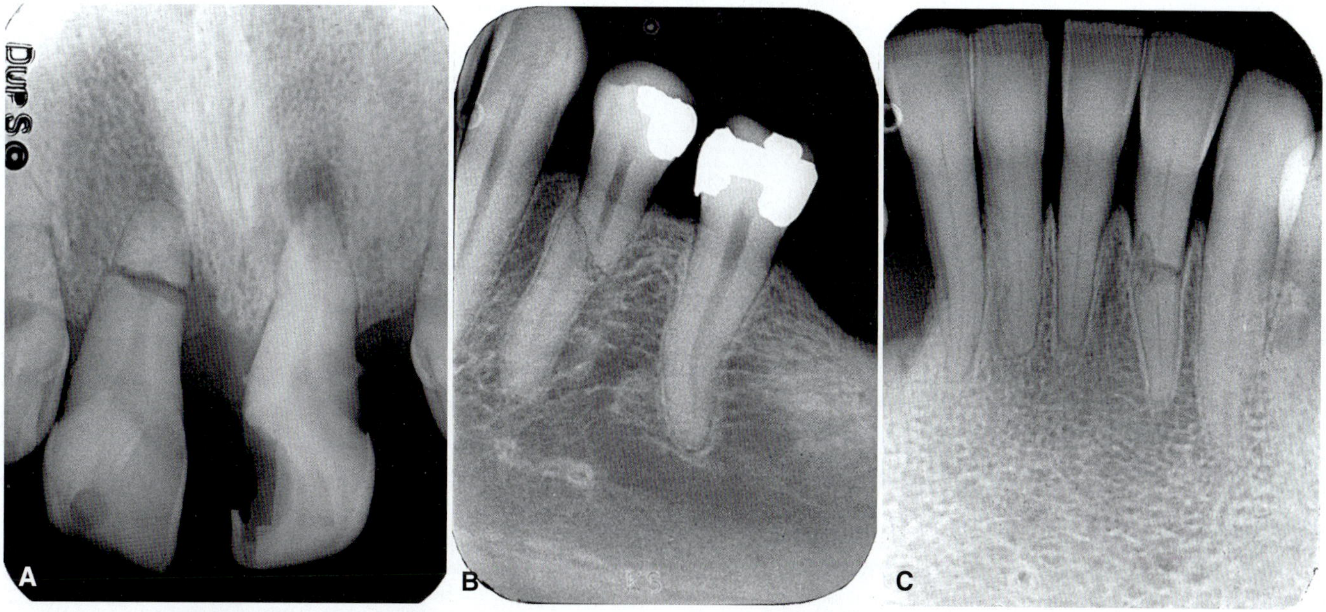

Fig. 25.5 (A) Recent horizontal fracture of the right maxillary central incisor and periapical rarefying osteitis involving the adjacent left central incisor. (B) Healed fracture with slight displacement of the fragments. (C) Healed fracture with root resorption and separation of the fractured segments.

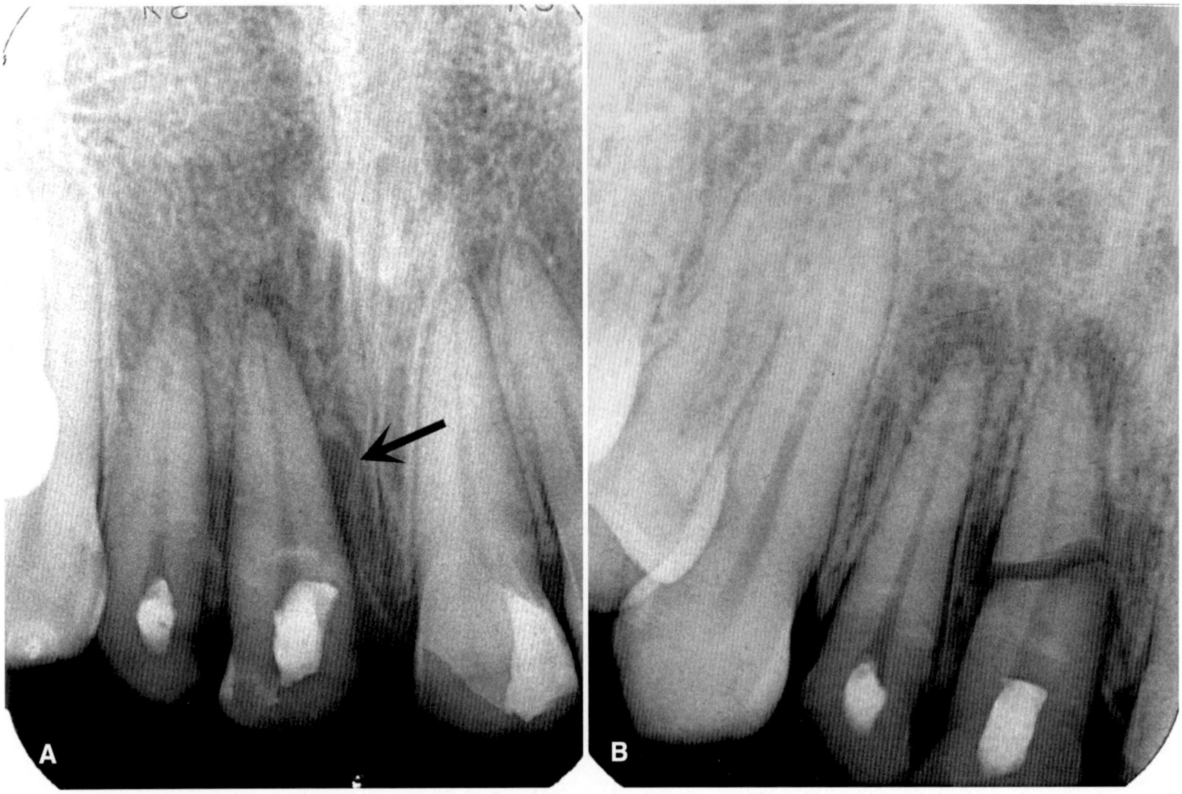

Fig. 25.6 (A) Subtle evidence of a root fracture involving the root of the maxillary right central incisor. Although a fracture plane is not apparent on the mesial aspect of the root because of malalignment of the x-ray beam, there is widening of the periodontal membrane space on the mesial surface *(arrow)* at the site of the fracture. (B) Later dislocation of the root fragments.

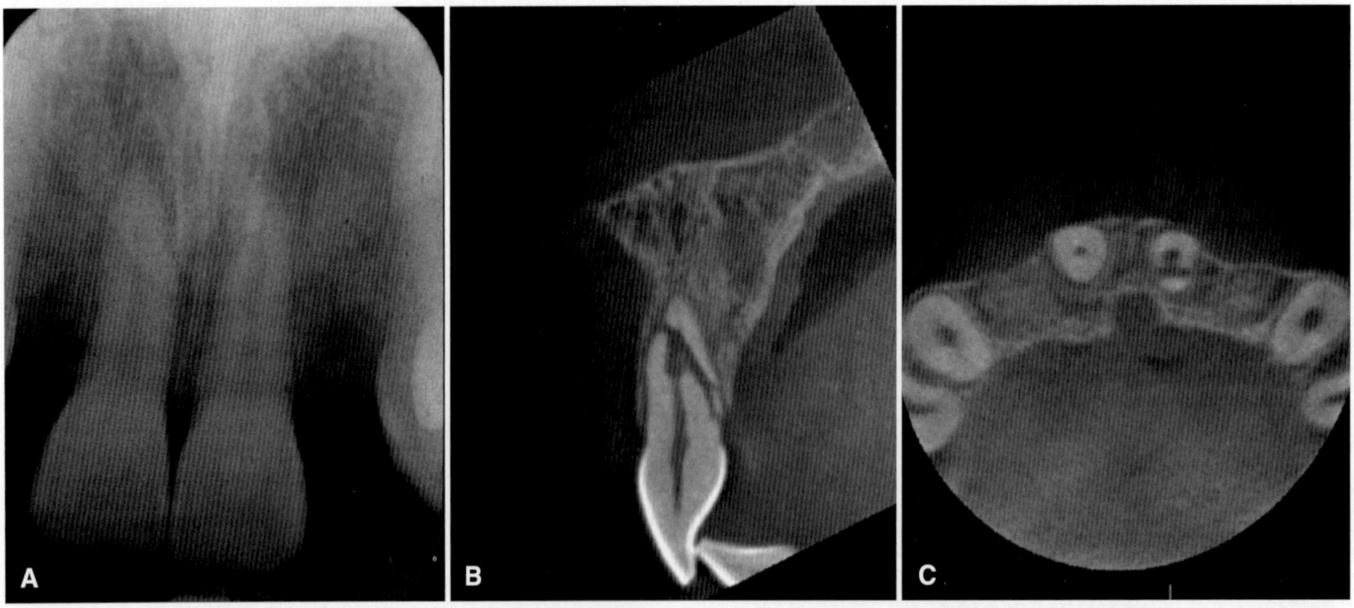

Fig. 25.7 (A) Periapical image of the maxillary central incisors with no evidence of a root fracture. In the same patient, corrected sagittal (B) and axial (C) cone-beam computed tomographic images through the maxillary left central incisor show a transverse fracture through the root, extending to the level of the alveolar crest. Resorption of the fractured edges has caused separation of the fragments. Resorption of the pulp canal in the distal fragment is evident.

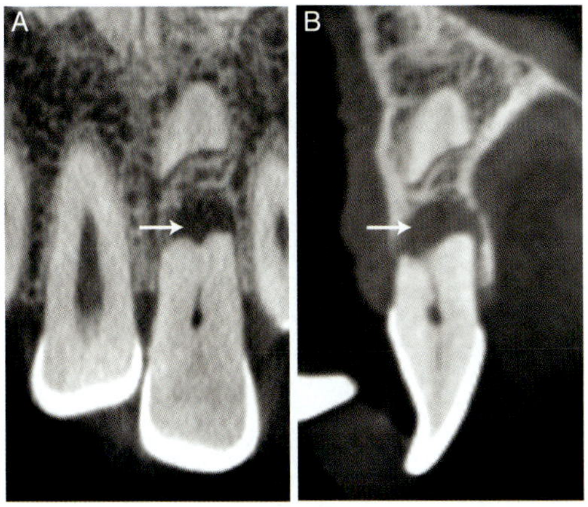

Fig. 25.8 Cone-beam computed tomography employed to monitor root fracture healing. (A) Coronal and (B) sagittal images through the central incisor show the coronal and apical fragments separated by bone. The fragment edges are resorbed and a radiolucency is present at the fracture site associated with the coronal fragment (arrows), a consequence of pulp necrosis in the coronal fragment.

above the alveolar crest have a poor prognosis. Fractured deciduous tooth roots may be retained with the expectation that they will be normally resorbed, as attempts at removal may result in damage to the developing permanent tooth.

It is important to determine pulp vitality on follow-up visits. Notably, false-negative responses may persist for as long as 3 months. Approximately 25% teeth with horizontal root fractures will develop pulp necrosis and require endodontic treatment (Fig. 25.8).

Vertical Root Fractures

Definition

In vertical root fracture, the fracture plane extends longitudinally along the root length. Fractures may be *complete* (extend through the full root diameter) or *incomplete* (extend partially through the root diameter). Vertical root fractures most commonly occur in endodontically treated premolar and molar teeth. They may also be iatrogenic following the insertion of retention screws or pins into teeth, or they may develop as a result of high occlusal forces, particularly in teeth with large restorations. Unlike other traumatic dental injuries, vertical root fractures develop slowly and their consequences manifest in subsequent months to years.

Clinical Features

Approximately 86%–97% of teeth with vertical root fractures are endodontically treated, with fractures typically occurring 2–5 years after endodontic treatment. The fractures do not propagate from coronal cracks but originate de novo within the root. These fractures are more frequent in premolars, mandibular molars, and maxillary molars. Large restorations and posts inserted into root canals increase the risk of a vertical fracture. Roots with two canals connected by an isthmus or with excessive dentin removal during canal preparation are at higher risk to fracture.

Vertical root fractures develop slowly, and most are undetectable in the early stages of their development, so they may not manifest clinically. As the fracture propagates, the separation of tissue becomes a conduit between the periodontal ligament, the root canal, and the oral environment, eventually causing periradicular inflammation at the fracture site. The periodontal inflammation will manifest as tenderness to palpation or percussion of the tooth, and a dull pain may be elicited on biting, which is often the patient's presenting symptom. The breakdown of the periodontal ligament where the fracture plane extends to the root surface may manifest as a deep narrow periodontal pocket. Localized pocket formation with a depth of 5 mm or more is considered pathognomonic of a vertical root fracture and is observed in 60%–67% of teeth with a vertical root fracture. A coronally located sinus tract or fistula, another characteristic feature, is noted in 13%–35% of cases. Despite the presence of these features, the clinical presentation can be nonspecific, posing a diagnostic challenge. The identification of a vertical root fracture is essential to clinical decision making. Although a vertical fracture involving a multirooted tooth may be managed by root amputation of the fracture root, a single-rooted tooth with a vertical root fracture necessitates extraction.

Imaging Features

Most frequently, patients presenting with clinical or radiographic findings suggestive of vertical root fracture are imaged with periapical images. Unlike horizontal root fractures that occur after trauma, vertical root fractures are rarely perceptible on periapical radiographs unless there has been separation of the root fragments (Fig. 25.9). At this point, the clinical consequences are straightforward and do not pose a challenge to management. More commonly, the fracture plane cannot be visualized on imaging; however, in such instances, a vertical root fracture may be inferred from the pattern of periradicular bone loss.

Early in the development of a vertical root fracture, there may be no radiographically evident periradicular bone loss. Even as bone loss become more apparent, early changes can often be misdiagnosed as periodontitis or persistent periapical inflammatory disease, which can lead to inappropriate management. Most vertical root fractures develop along the buccal-lingual plane of the tooth, and any bone loss along these surfaces is often masked by density of the tooth itself. As more bone resorption occurs adjacent to the fracture plane, the change will be seen as a radiolucent halo encircling the affected root (Fig. 25.10). More than 50% of vertical root fractures manifest this appearance. This appearance may, however, also develop from periapical inflammatory disease and periodontitis, and periapical images may be inconclusive. Another pattern of bone loss that is often seen is a "J-shaped" radiolucent pattern that extends from the bone crest along the length of the involved root to a focus of rarefying osteitis at the root apex.

The American Association of Endodontists and the American Academy of Oral and Maxillofacial Radiology have written guidelines that recommend limited FOV CBCT imaging when clinical examination and two-dimensional intraoral images are inconclusive in the detection of a vertical root fracture. The sensitivity and specificity of CBCT for detection of vertical root fractures is higher than that of periapical imaging; however, the detection accuracy is influenced by the width of fragment separation, imaging artifacts from endodontic filling material, metal restorative materials, and the extent of periradicular bone loss. Despite its higher accuracy, CBCT imaging does not significantly increase detection of the fracture plane per se, and the diagnosis of a vertical root fracture may still rely on the pattern of periradicular bone loss. The characteristic appearances of vertical root fractures on CBCT examination are listed below:

A. ***Perceptible fracture plane:*** Longstanding fractures with root resorption and fragment separation along the fracture plane may be evident (Fig. 25.11A). Bone loss, typically with buccal dehiscence, is usually evident.

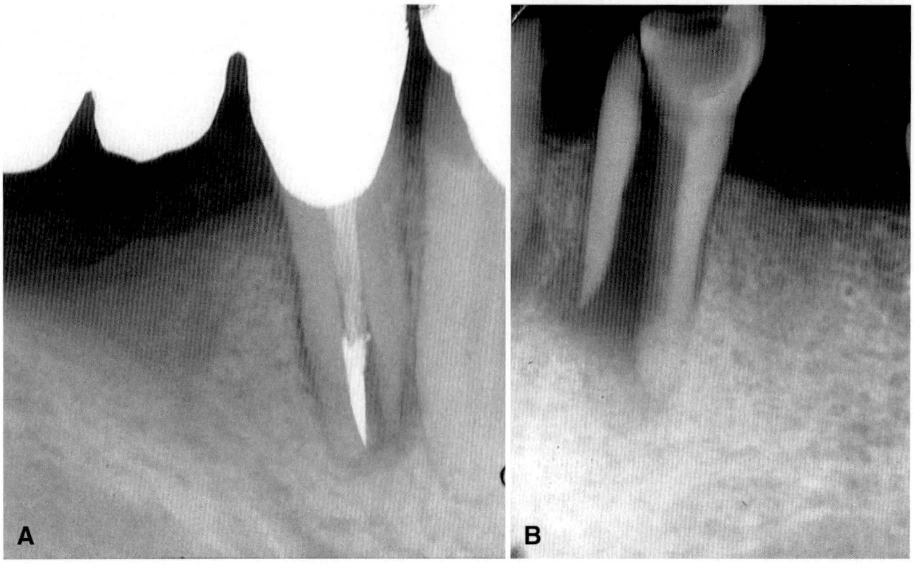

Fig. 25.9 (A) Vertical fracture through the root of a mandibular first premolar that has been endodontically treated. The fracture plane extends through the root canal, and there is more displacement between the root fragments at the apex of the root. (B) Vertical root fracture through the root of a mandibular canine with significant displacement of the fragments.

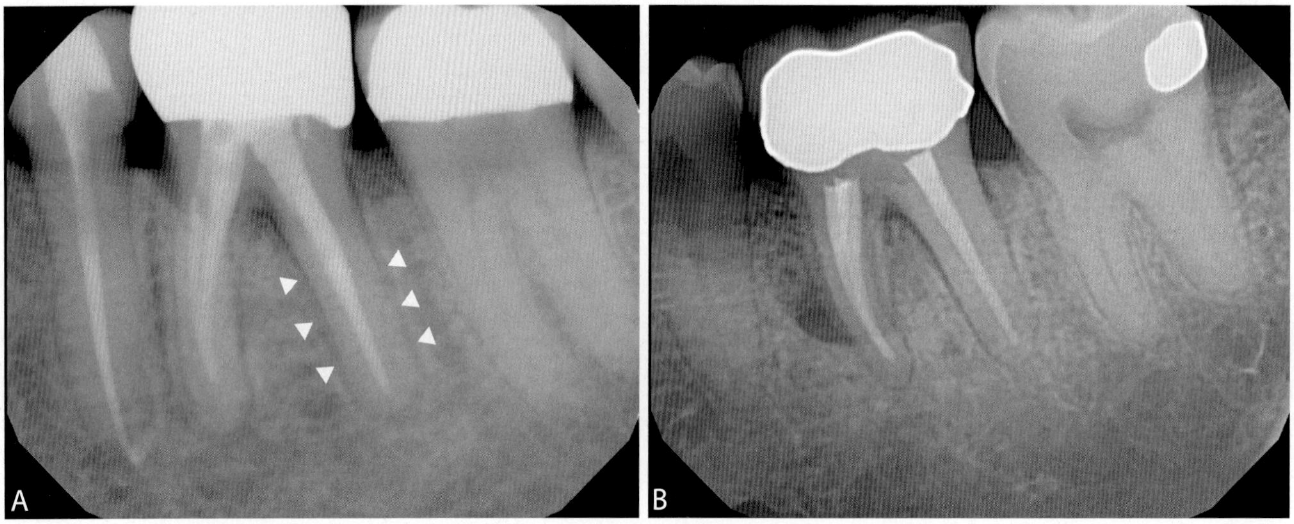

Fig. 25.10 Manifestations of vertical root fracture on periapical radiographs. (A) Radiolucent halo along the length of the distal root of the mandibular first molar. Note the rarefaction in the furcation. (B) Localized mid-root radiolucency that extends into the furcation.

B. ***Asymmetrically wide periodontal ligament:*** Incomplete root fractures that involve only one root surface will result in a localized focus of inflammation. This is best evaluated on axial images rendered perpendicular to the long axis of the root (Fig. 25.11B).

C. ***Diametrically opposite wide periodontal ligament:*** With complete root fractures, more than one root surface is involved and inflammatory changes will manifest on opposite ends of the fracture plane (Fig. 25.11C).

D. ***Mid-root level bone loss:*** Approximately 70% of root fractures involve the middle third of the root. Localized periodontal ligament space widening at the mid-root level is an indication of inflammation at the interface between the fracture plane and the periodontal ligament (Fig. 25.11D).

E. ***Circumferential bone loss along the root length:*** With complete fractures that involve most of the root length, bone loss may encompass the root circumference. In multiroot teeth, the bone loss may extend into the furcation. The presence of this isolated pattern of bone loss in the absence of local periodontal bone loss is key in differentiating this from periodontal disease or persistent periapical inflammatory disease (Fig. 25.11E).

F. ***Trough-like bone loss with or without dehiscence:*** Periradicular bone loss along the root length is often limited by the lingual or buccal cortex, creating a trough-like appearance along the root (Fig. 25.11F, *arrowhead*) Often, this pattern of bone loss can produce a dehiscence of the adjacent cortex (Fig. 25.11F, *arrow*). The isolated presence of this change around a single root can differentiate vertical root fracture from periodontitis.

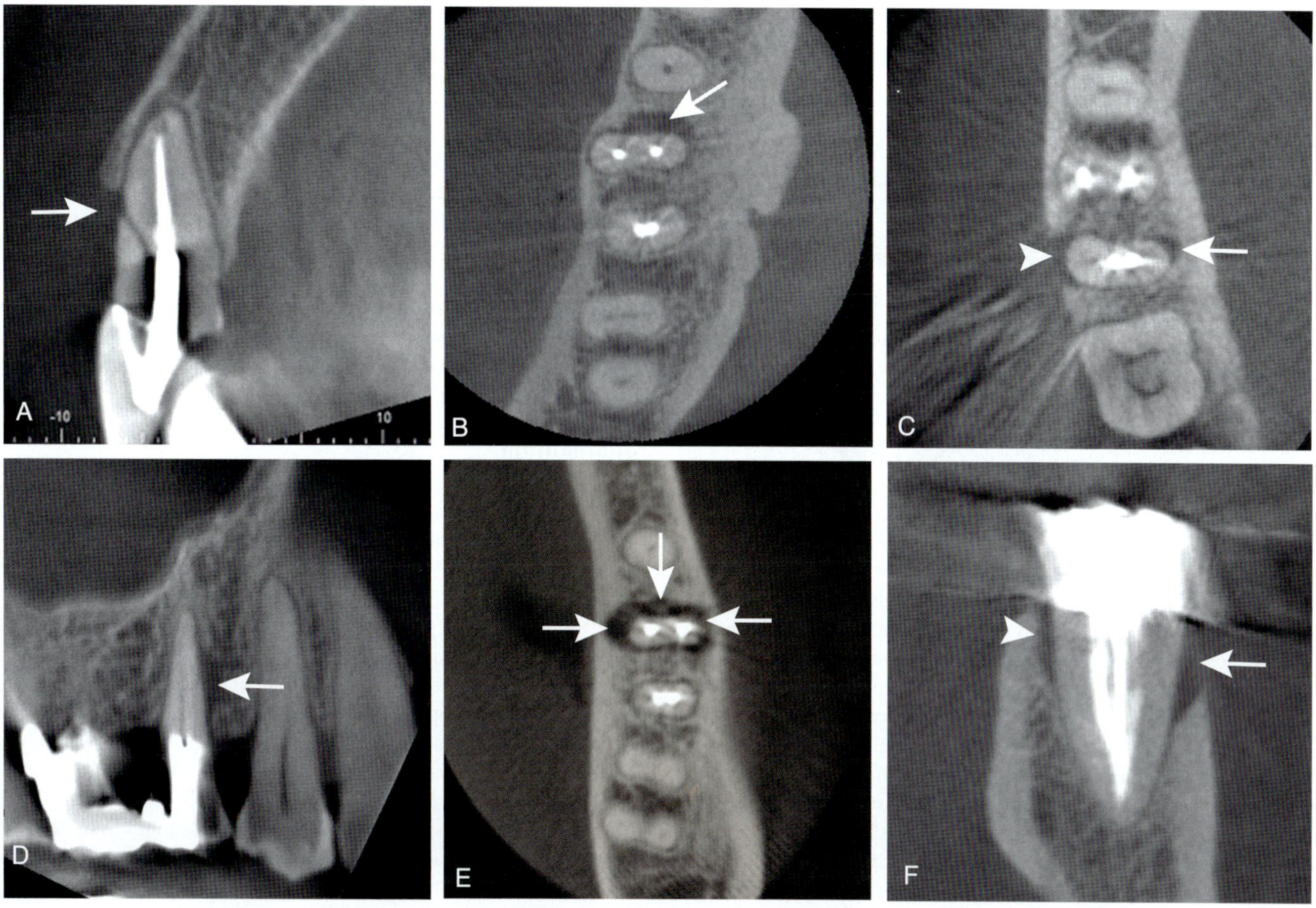

Fig. 25.11 Appearances of vertical root fracture on cone-beam computed tomography imaging. (A) Fractured maxillary central incisor with a visible fracture plane. The fracture plane starts at the base of the restorative post and extends to the buccal surface. Note dehiscence of buccal bone and periapical radiolucency. (B) Asymmetrically wide periodontal ligament around the mesiolingual line angle of the mesial root of the mandibular first molar. Note normal periodontal ligament width and intact lamina dura around the remainder of the root and the adjacent roots. (C) Periodontal ligament is wide on opposing ends of the root diameter indicating a complete fracture of the distal root of the mandibular first molar. Note buccal dehiscence *(arrowhead).* (D) Fractured maxillary second premolar with radiolucency at mid-root level. Note intact alveolar crest on the mesial and distal surfaces of the tooth. (E) Circumferential bone loss around the mesial root of the mandibular first molar. Note periodontal ligament of normal width with intact lamina dura around the remainders of visible roots. (F) Periradicular bone loss with a trough-like pattern between the root and lingual cortex *(arrowhead).* Note dehiscence of buccal cortex adjacent to root surface *(arrow).*

Management

Single-rooted teeth with vertical root fractures cannot be salvaged and must be extracted. For multirooted teeth, the decision to extract only the fractured root while maintaining the nonfractured roots may be considered. Early detection of a vertical root fracture is important to minimize the extent of bone loss, which can compromise future prosthetic restorations, especially implant-supported restorations.

PERIODONTAL TISSUE INJURY

Patients with dentoalveolar trauma must be examined clinically and radiologically to assess involvement of the periodontal tissues.

Concussion

Definition

The term *concussion* refers to a crush injury to the vascular structures at the tooth root apex and the periodontal ligament, resulting in inflammatory edema. The affected tooth is minimally loosened with no displacement. The injury may result in mild extrusion of the tooth from its socket, causing its occlusal surface to make premature contact with an opposing tooth during mandibular closing.

Clinical Features

The patient usually complains that the traumatized tooth is tender to touch, and this can be confirmed by gentle horizontal or vertical percussion of the tooth. The tooth may also be sensitive to biting forces, although patients usually try to modify their occlusion to avoid contacting the traumatized tooth.

Imaging Features

The imaging appearance of a dental concussion may be subtle. No changes may be visible, or there may be localized widening of the apical periodontal ligament space (Fig. 25.12). Changes to the size of the pulp chamber and root canals may develop in the months and years after traumatic

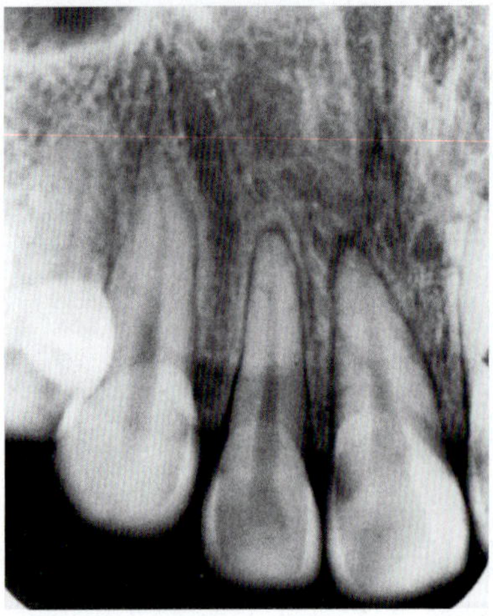

Fig. 25.12 Widening of the periodontal ligament spaces of the incisors after dental concussion.

injury to a tooth, and this may be particularly evident in a tooth that is still developing. Should pulpal necrosis occur after trauma, there may be no further deposition of (secondary) dentin as the odontoblasts, as well as the pulpal and pulpal stem cell populations will have necrosed.

Teeth that have undergone trauma before apical closure may develop a morphologically abnormal apex called an osteodentin cap. As the process of pulpal necrosis begins coronally and progresses apically, vital odontoblasts may remain at the developing root apex and tertiary dentin (osteodentin) may be deposited ahead of the advancing front of pulpal necrosis. This disorganized and irregularly mineralized matrix may resemble bone in structure and morphologically "caps" the end of the root. The osteodentin cap may appear on an image to be continuous with the developing root apex, or it may appear separate from it. In contrast to the pattern of internal resorption, where the root canal is focally widened (Fig. 25.13), the root canal seen in association with a tooth that has developed an osteodentin cap appears uniformly widened from the pulp chamber to the apex (Fig. 25.14). The development of the canal and deposition of dentin can appear "frozen in time" at the developmental stage at which pulpal necrosis occurred. When the image of the cap is covered or "hidden" from view, the apex of the root resembles that of a developing tooth (see Fig. 25.14C).

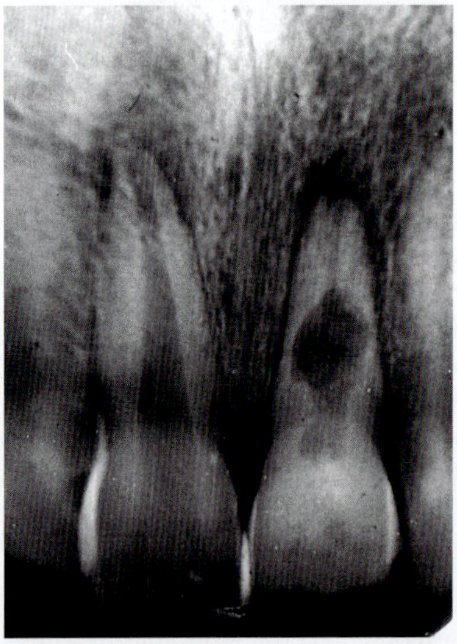

Fig. 25.13 Consequences of dental trauma. An incisal fracture of the maxillary left central incisor is present. Note obliteration of the pulp chamber but not the root canal and internal root resorption. Also note the periapical radiolucency involving the maxillary right central incisor and the widened pulp chamber and canal.

Management

Because significant displacement of the concussed tooth or teeth does not occur, the appropriate treatment is conservative and may include occlusal adjustment of the opposing tooth or teeth (if necessary) or the application of a flexible splint. Notably approximately 4% of teeth with concussion will develop pulp necrosis by 1 year. Monitoring after 4 weeks and 1 year with repeated vitality testing and radiographic images is indicated. Should pulp necrosis develop, endodontic treatment is appropriate. The management of a tooth with an osteodentin cap is orthograde endodontic treatment.

Subluxation

Definition

The term *subluxation* refers to periodontal tissue injury that causes a greater amount of abnormal tooth loosening than concussion but with no displacement.

Clinical Features

The traumatized tooth is tender to horizontal or vertical percussion and is sensitive to biting forces. Bleeding at the gingival crevice is indicative of the damage to the periodontal tissues. There is increased mobility but no displacement of teeth.

Imaging Features

As with dental concussion, the imaging manifestations are subtle, with no visible changes or with localized widening of the apical periodontal ligament space.

Management

Treatment is conservative, with occlusal adjustments of the opposing dentition and a splint as needed. There is periodic monitoring after 2 weeks, 12 weeks, 6 months, and 1 year, with repeated vitality testing and imaging when indicated. Approximately 10% of teeth with subluxation develop pulpal necrosis within 1 year of the trauma.

Luxation

Definition

Luxation is a dislocation of the tooth from its socket after severing of the periodontal attachment. Such teeth are abnormally mobile and displaced.

Depending on their magnitude and direction, traumatic forces can cause intrusive luxation (displacement of a tooth into the alveolar process), extrusive luxation (partial displacement of a tooth out of its socket), or lateral luxation (movement of a tooth in a direction other than intrusive or extrusive displacement). In intrusive and lateral luxation, comminution or crushing of the alveolar process may accompany tooth dislocation.

The movement of the apex and disruption of the circulation to the traumatized tooth that accompanies luxation can produce either temporary or permanent changes to the dental pulp, and these changes may result in pulpal necrosis. If the pulp survives the traumatic incident, the rate of dentin formation may accelerate and continue until it obliterates the pulp chamber and root canal. This process may occur in both permanent and deciduous teeth.

Clinical Features

Clinical history is helpful in identifying luxation. The clinical crowns of intruded teeth may appear reduced in height. Maxillary incisors may be

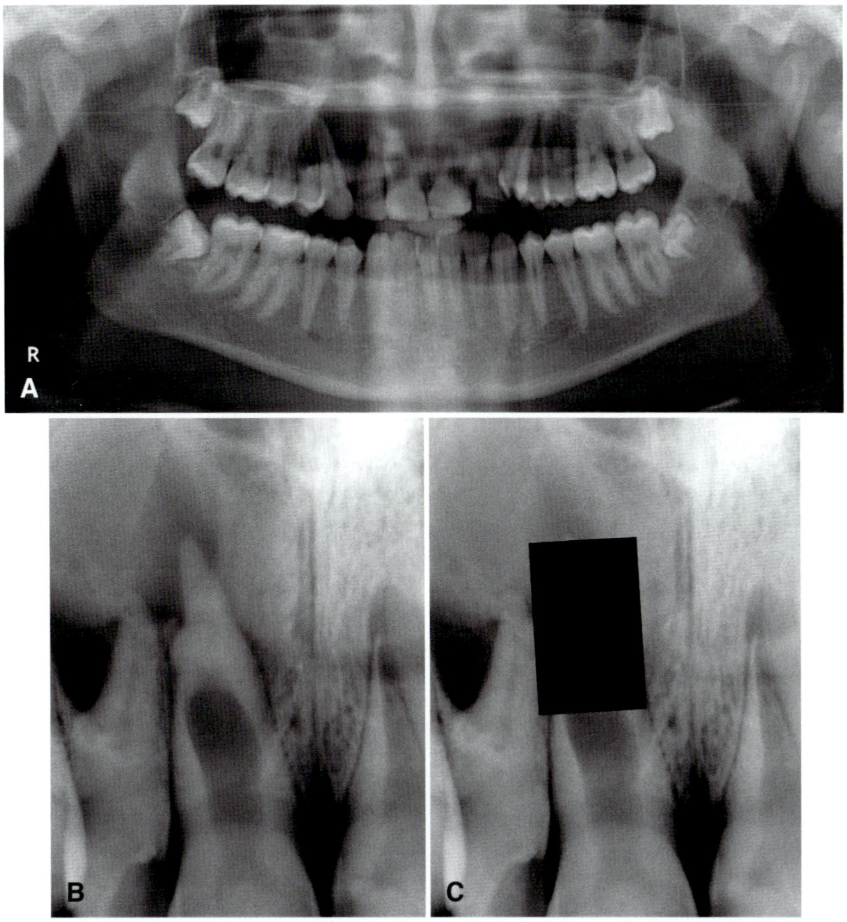

Fig. 25.14 Panoramic (A) and periapical (B) images showing an osteodentin cap associated with the maxillary right central incisor. There is a large area of rarefying osteitis extending from the maxillary midline to the mesial surface of the maxillary right canine. Note the uniformly wide root canal of the incisor. When the osteodentin cap is "obscured," the apex of the root is reminiscent of a developing root apex (C).

intruded so deeply into the alveolar process that they may appear to be avulsed or lost. The displaced tooth may cause some damage to adjacent teeth and particularly to underlying developing permanent teeth.

Depending on the orientation and magnitude of the force and the shape of the root, the tooth may be displaced through the buccal or, less commonly, the lingual cortex of the alveolar process, where it may be seen and palpated. On repeated vitality testing, the sensitivity of a luxated tooth may be temporarily decreased or undetectable, especially shortly after the injury. Vitality may return weeks or several months later.

Usually two or more teeth are involved in luxation injuries, and the teeth most frequently affected are the deciduous and permanent maxillary incisors. The mandibular teeth are seldom affected. The type of luxation appears to vary with age; this may reflect changes to the nature of maturing bone. Both intrusions and extrusions occur in the deciduous dentition. In the permanent dentition, the intrusive type of luxation is less frequent.

Imaging Features

Imaging examinations of luxated teeth demonstrate the extent of injury to the root and alveolar process, as well as the involvement of the periodontal ligament. An image made at the time of injury can serve as a valuable reference point for comparison with subsequent images. Luxation injuries are often accompanied by damage to the bony socket and alveolus.

The depressed position of the crown of an intruded tooth is often apparent on an image (Fig. 25.15), although a minimally intruded tooth may be difficult to demonstrate. Intrusion may result in partial or total obliteration of the apical periodontal ligament space. Multiple radiologic projections, including occlusal views, may be necessary to show the direction of tooth displacement and the relationship of the displaced tooth to adjacent teeth and the outer cortex of bone.

A tooth that has been extruded may demonstrate varying degrees of apical widening of the periodontal ligament space, depending on the magnitude of the extrusive force (Fig. 25.16). A laterally luxated tooth with some degree of extrusion may show a widened periodontal ligament space with greater width on the side of impact.

Management

Management of intrusive luxation is dictated by root development. Teeth with partially developed roots can be repositioned through guided orthodontic extrusion as needed. Teeth with completely developed roots may be repositioned and stabilized. Pulp necrosis is likely, and endodontic treatment is initiated 2 weeks following trauma.

Teeth with extrusive luxation may be gently repositioned and splinted. Pulp necrosis is a common sequela, occurring in approximately 65% of teeth with such injuries. Thus, periodic vitality testing and follow-up imaging are essential and are continued up to 5 years.

Lateral luxation is managed by digital manipulation to reposition the displaced teeth to reestablish occlusion, with splinting as needed.

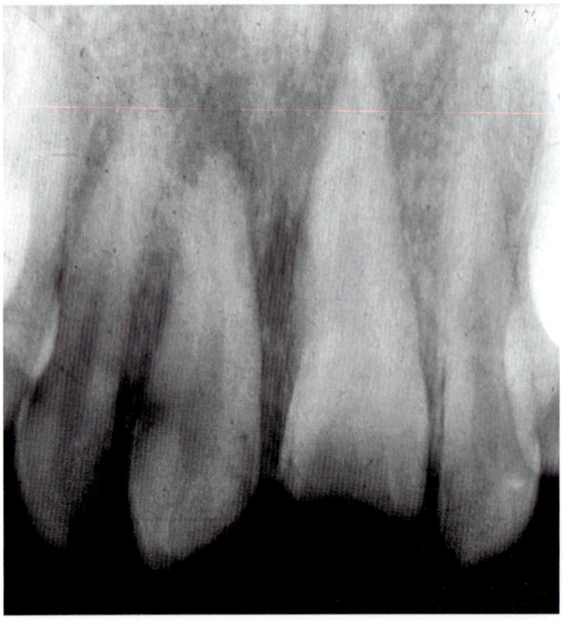

Fig. 25.15 Intruded maxillary central incisor after trauma. Note the fractured incisal edges of both central incisors.

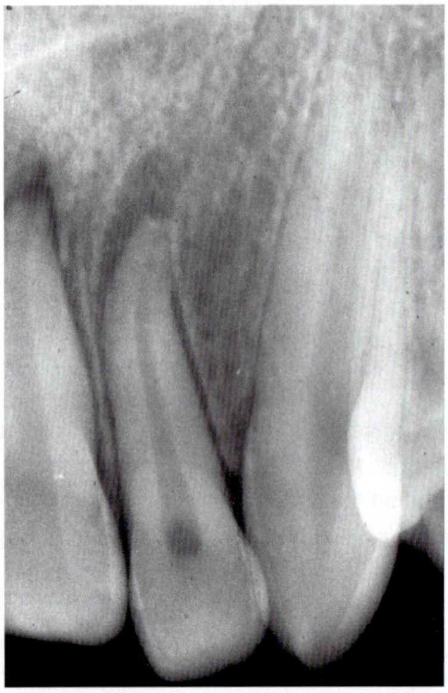

Fig. 25.16 Extruded maxillary lateral incisor after trauma. Note the localized increase to the width of the apical periodontal ligament space.

Approximately 44% teeth with lateral luxation undergo pulp necrosis. Follow-up imaging and vitality testing of the traumatized tooth and adjacent teeth are continued up to 5 years.

Avulsion

Definition

The term *avulsion* refers to complete displacement of a tooth from the alveolar process. Teeth may be avulsed when a force is applied directly to the tooth or by indirect trauma, such as a force applied as a result of sudden jaw closure. Avulsion occurs in approximately 15% of traumatic injuries to the teeth, with fights being responsible for the avulsion of most permanent teeth and accidental falls accounting for the traumatic loss of most deciduous teeth.

Clinical Features

Maxillary central incisors are the most commonly avulsed teeth from both dentitions. Most often only a single tooth is lost. This injury typically occurs in a relatively young age group when the permanent central incisors are just erupting. Fractures of the alveolar process and lip lacerations may also be seen with an avulsed tooth.

Imaging Features

In a recent avulsion, the lamina dura of the empty socket is apparent and usually persists for several months. The missing tooth may be displaced into the adjacent soft tissue and its image may project over the image of the alveolar process on planar imaging, giving the false impression that it lies within the bone. To differentiate between an intruded tooth and an avulsed tooth lying within the adjacent soft tissues, a soft tissue image of the lacerated lip or tongue should be made. In some instances, new bone within the healing socket may be very dense and resemble a retained root tip (Fig. 25.17).

Management

If the avulsed tooth cannot be found by clinical or radiologic examination, a chest or abdominal image may be considered to localize it within the airway or gastrointestinal tract. Although an avulsed teeth can be reimplanted into its dentoalveolar socket, the success of reimplantation is determined by the viability of the periodontal tissues that remain attached to the tooth surface, the condition of the tooth, and the length of time it is out of its socket. Optimally, teeth must be reimplanted within 2 hours of avulsion. Commercially available solutions, such as Hank's balanced salt solution provide a compatible osmolality and pH to store teeth for as long as 96 hours. Pasteurized milk has often been used as a medium to store avulsed teeth but is effective for only approximately 6 hours.

Endodontic treatment may be necessary following reimplantation. In teeth with completed root development, endodontic treatment may be performed ex vivo prior to implantation. Complications following reimplantation include ankylosis and external root resorption. Avulsed deciduous teeth are not reimplanted, as the procedure can damage the underlying developing permanent tooth.

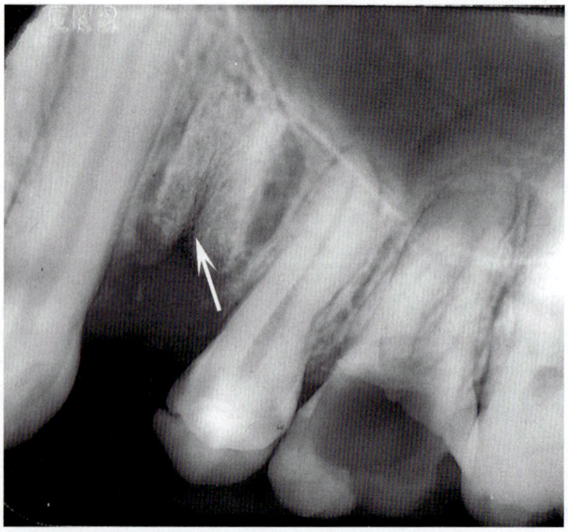

Fig. 25.17 Bone formation during healing of a first premolar tooth socket. Note how the bone is developing from the lateral walls of the socket. The central radiolucent line *(arrow)* may have a similar appearance to that of a root canal, falsely giving the impression of a retained tooth fragment.

ALVEOLAR PROCESS INJURY

Definition

Simple fractures of the alveolar process may involve the buccal or lingual cortical plates of the maxillae or mandible. These fractures are commonly associated with luxation injuries with or without dislocation. Several teeth are usually affected, and the fracture plane is most often horizontal in orientation. The fracture may involve a single cortical plate or extend through the entire alveolar process; the fracture plane may also be located apical to the teeth or involve the tooth socket. Alveolar process injuries are commonly associated with luxation injuries, often with tooth fractures.

Clinical Features

Alveolar fractures are more common in the anterior and premolar regions and are relatively rare in the posterior segments of the arches. The attached gingiva may be lacerated. In the posterior maxilla, fracture of the buccal plate can occur during removal of a maxillary posterior tooth. A characteristic feature of an alveolar process fracture is marked malocclusion with displacement and mobility of the fragment. Any teeth contained within the fragment will have a recognizable dull sound when percussed and move as a block. The detached bone may include the floor of the maxillary sinus, in which case bleeding from the nose on the involved side may occur as well as ecchymosis of the buccal vestibule. Misalignment or displacement of the fractured segments may result in altered occlusion.

Imaging Features

Patients with limited dentoalveolar trauma are often imaged with periapical and occlusal images. These images may show radiolucent fracture planes located at any level between the crest of the alveolar process and the periapical regions of the teeth. Fractures of a single cortical plate are difficult to detect, especially when the fractured segments are nondisplaced. However, a fracture of the anterior labial cortical plate may be apparent on an occlusal image if bone displacement has occurred and the x-ray beam is oriented at nearly right angles to the direction of bone displacement. Fractures of both cortical plates of the alveolar process are usually apparent (Fig. 25.18). When the fracture plane is in contact with the tooth root apices, the risk of root resorption is high.

Small FOV CBCT imaging can more reliably depict the location, extent, and displacement of the fracture plates (Fig. 25.19). Imaging guidelines recommend that in the absence of other maxillofacial or soft tissue injuries that may require other advanced imaging modalities, limited FOV CBCT should be considered the imaging modality of choice for the diagnosis of limited dentoalveolar trauma.

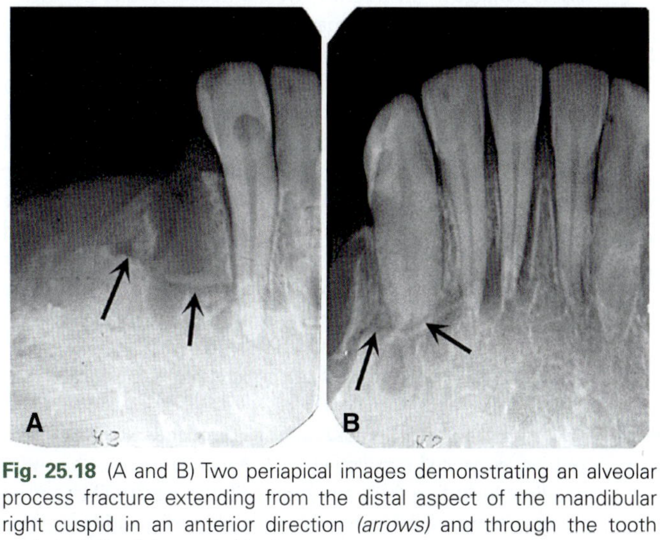

Fig. 25.18 (A and B) Two periapical images demonstrating an alveolar process fracture extending from the distal aspect of the mandibular right cuspid in an anterior direction *(arrows)* and through the tooth socket of the right central incisor.

When the fracture is close to the alveolar crest, the possibility that a root fracture is also present is high. On planar imaging, it may be difficult to differentiate a root fracture from an overlapping fracture plane involving the alveolar process. Multiple images made at different projection angles may help with this differentiation; if the fracture plane is truly associated with the tooth, the radiolucent line should not shift relative to the tooth. Fractures of the posterior alveolar process may involve the floor of the maxillary sinus and result in abnormal thickening of the sinus mucosa or the accumulation of blood and sinus secretions, in which case an air-fluid level may be apparent.

Management

Treatment of limited injury to the alveolar process is directed toward fracture reduction and stabilization. Closed reduction by digital manipulation and rigid splints are often adequate. Fracture segments that are markedly displaced may need open reduction.

TRAUMATIC INJURIES TO THE FACIAL BONES

Facial fractures most frequently affect the mandible and midface and, to a lesser extent, the maxillae. Imaging plays a crucial role in the diagnosis and management of traumatic injuries to these and other facial bones. Superficial signs of injury, such as soft tissue swelling, hemorrhage, or hematoma formation from a laceration or abrasion, may focus the radiologic examination. Imaging evaluation of maxillofacial trauma is conducted primarily using MDCT.

Mandibular Fractures

The mandible is the second most commonly fractured facial bone after the nasal bones. Assaults, motor vehicle accidents, and falls are the most frequent causes of injury. Most mandibular fractures occur in the 18–54 year age group and 80% of mandibular fractures occur in males. Fractures of the symphysis, body, and angle are most frequent, followed by the condyle, condylar neck, and ramus. Fractures of the alveolar and coronoid processes are less frequent. Fractures are more likely to occur on weekend days than on other days of the week. Trauma to the mandible is often associated with other injuries, most commonly concussion (loss of consciousness) and other fractures, usually of the maxillae, zygomatic bones, and cranial vault.

The locations and patterns of the fractures can vary with the mechanism of injury and the direction the force of impact. Depending on its anatomic location, fractures of the mandible are classified as dentoalveolar, symphyseal, parasymphyseal, body, angle, ramal, coronoid, or condylar (Fig. 25.20). A second clinically relevant categorization is based on the pattern of the fracture. *Simple fractures* consist of a single fracture plane that does not communicate with the external environment. In contrast, *compound fractures* communicate with the exterior, either via the periodontal ligament space or through lacerations of the oral mucosa or facial skin. *Comminuted fractures* involve multiple fracture planes creating multiple bone fragments at one fracture site and are often the consequence of a higher-impact force. *Greenstick fractures* are incomplete fractures that involve only one cortical plate leading to a distortion of the bone shape without separation of bone fragments. The term *complex fracture* or *complicated fracture* is used to describe fractures with damage to adjacent major vessels and nerves (e.g., the inferior alveolar neurovascular bundle).

Fractures that arise distant to the site of direct traumatic impact are called *indirect fractures*. Indirect fractures may occur in the mandible because of its unique morphology; the bone is curved and there are

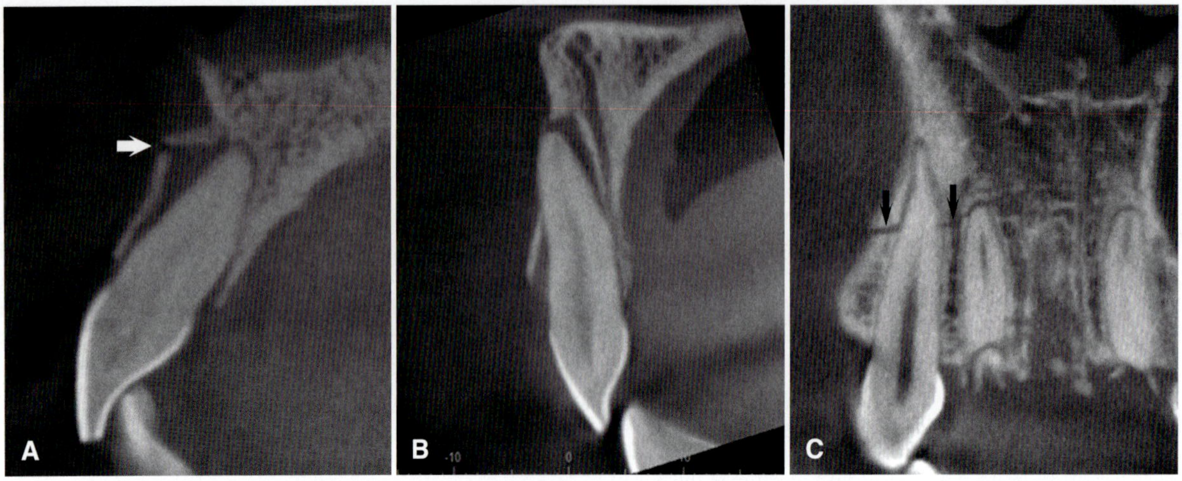

Fig. 25.19 Cone-beam computed tomographic images through the long axes of the maxillary central incisors showing fractures of the buccal cortical plate *(white arrow)* and asymmetric widening of the periodontal ligament spaces, indicating luxation injuries and alveolar fractures. (C) Coronal cone-beam computed tomographic image through the maxillary anterior region shows an alveolar fracture *(black arrows)*.

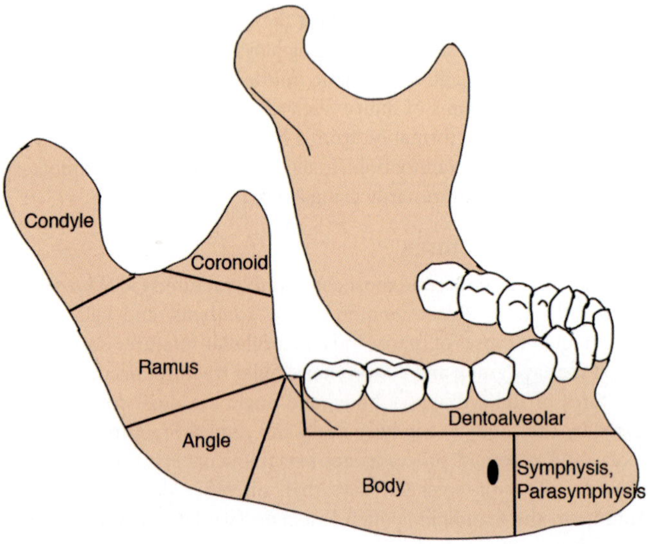

Fig. 25.20 Classification of mandibular fractures based on anatomic location.

regional differences in cortical thickness and buccolingual width. Consequently, tensile forces from an impact can be transmitted through the bone to sites that are distant from the site of primary impact. For example, a fracture of the mandibular body on one side can be accompanied by a fracture of the condylar neck on the opposite side. Likewise, trauma to the anterior mandible can result in unilateral or bilateral fractures of the condylar necks. When a localized heavy force is directed posteriorly to the mandible, there may be fractures of the angle, ramus, or coronoid process. In children, fractures of the mandibular body usually occur in the anterior region. A "pathologic fracture" is one that has developed in a bone that has been compromised by a pathologic process, despite the bone being able to withstand normal functional forces or from minimal traumatic forces. For example, inflammation, cysts, or tumors arising in the mandible can be extensive and compromise the structural integrity of the bone.

Mandibular fractures can also be classified as being either favorable or unfavorable, depending on the orientation of the fracture plane and the displacement of the bone fragments (Fig. 25.21). Unfavorable fractures are those in which the contractile action of the adjacent muscles displaces the fragments away from one another, causing the fracture plane to increase in width. In favorable fractures, the muscle action tends to reduce the fracture, drawing the fragments together. Fractures may be further categorized as being vertically or horizontally favorable or unfavorable. In a vertically favorable fracture, the orientation of the fracture plane resists the medial displacement of the more posterior fragment by the medial pterygoid muscle. In contrast, a horizontally favorable fracture resists displacement of the more posterior fragment by the contractile action of the masseter muscle (see Fig. 25.21).

Clinical indicators of mandible injury:

- Altered occlusion or step deformity in the mandibular occlusal plane.
- Tenderness to palpation.
- Mobility of fractured fragments on bimanual palpation.
- Trismus or deviation of mandible on opening.
- Ecchymosis on the floor of the mouth.

Imaging objectives:

- Locate and define the extent of the fracture(s).
- Detect displacement of the fractured segments.
- Assess damage to the inferior alveolar neurovascular bundle.
- Monitor responses to treatment.

Imaging approaches:

- Panoramic imaging is often the initial examination performed to evaluate suspected or clinically evident mandibular fractures in a conscious patient. Isolated mandible fractures in the ramus and body are mostly detected on panoramic imaging. However, the sensitivity of panoramic imaging in the detection of condylar head and/or neck fractures is lower. Similarly, nondisplaced and minimally displaced symphysis fractures are often masked by superimposition from the cervical spine. The open-mouth Towne view (see Chapter 7) has been used in the past to supplement panoramic imaging to evaluate the mandibular condylar heads and necks, especially in cases of suspected nondisplaced greenstick fractures of the condylar neck.
- The American College of Radiology recommends the use of noncontrast–enhanced maxillofacial CT that encompasses the entire mandible including the temporomandibular joints (TMJs) as an appropriate examination to evaluate suspected mandibular fractures. The sensitivity of CT for detection of mandibular fractures

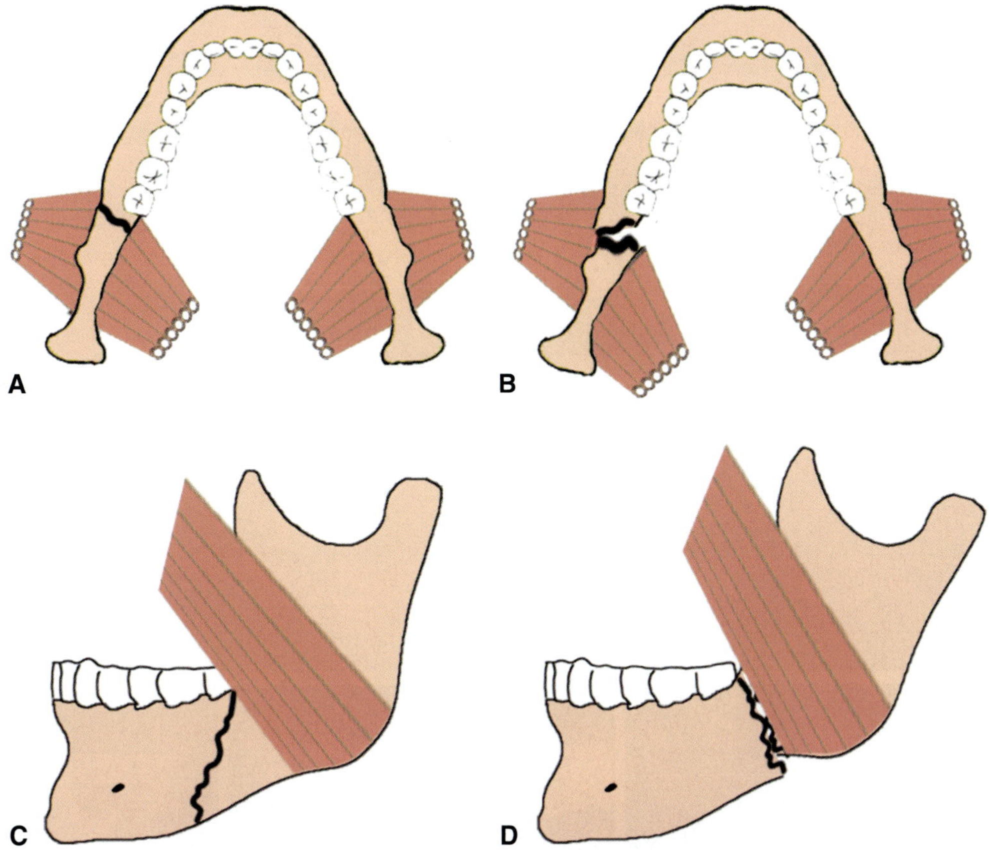

Fig. 25.21 (A) Vertically favorable fracture. (B) Vertically unfavorable fracture, with the medial pterygoid muscle pull causing separation of the fragments. (C) Horizontally favorable fracture of the mandibular body. (D) Horizontally unfavorable fracture, with the masseter muscle pull causing separation of the fragments.

is 100%, whether MDCT or CBCT. In comparison, the sensitivity of panoramic imaging is approximately 86%.

- Magnetic resonance imaging is not required in most cases of mandibular trauma. It may be of value in specific situations to evaluate trauma complications such as TMJ disk displacement or inferior alveolar nerve injury.

Fractures of the Mandibular Symphysis, Body, Angle, and Ramus

Definition. Most mandibular fractures involve the symphysis, body, and ramus. Should these fractures involve teeth (which they often do), they should be considered compound fractures. Most mandibular fractures alter the occlusion, so appropriate correction of the occlusal discrepancy is an important outcome from fracture reduction.

Clinical features. Traumatic injury is typically substantiated by evidence of injury to the overlying skin. The patient frequently has swelling and a deformity that is accentuated when the patient opens their mouth. The patient may report a discrepancy involving their occlusion or a TMJ abnormality such as crepitus or a change in their normal jaw mobility. Intraoral examination may reveal ecchymosis in the floor of the mouth. In the case of bilateral fractures to the mandible, a risk exists that the digastric, mylohyoid, and omohyoid muscles will displace the anterior mandibular fragment posteriorly and inferiorly, causing impingement on the airway.

Imaging features. Suspected mandibular fractures may be evaluated with panoramic or CT imaging. In cooperative and conscious patients with suspected dentoalveolar fractures, intraoral imaging and limited FOV CBCT may be beneficial, given their higher spatial resolution.

The margins of fracture planes usually appear as sharply defined radiolucent planes of separation that are confined to the structure of the mandible (Fig. 25.22). Nondisplaced or minimally displaced fractures may be difficult to detect. Sites of occlusal discrepancy should be closely examined on imaging to aid in fracture detection (Fig. 25.23). Displaced fracture fragments result in a cortical discontinuity or "step-type" defect or an irregularity in the normal curvature of the occlusal plane. Should the x-ray beam not be directed through the fracture plane, the radiolucent lines in the buccal and lingual plates will not superimpose over one another, and two lines may appear that converge at the periphery (Fig. 25.23). Occasionally, the margins of the adjacent fracture fragments may overlap, resulting in an area of increased radiopacity at the fracture site on panoramic images (Fig. 25.22A). Fractures with this appearance may be missed on panoramic imaging but are clearly seen on CT imaging (Fig. 25.22B–D). Displacement of fractured segments in the symphysis may be difficult to detect on panoramic imaging (Figs. 25.23A and 25.24A). CT imaging may demonstrate the displacement of fractions from muscle traction (Fig. 25.24B–D), which may contribute to management decisions (i.e., closed vs. open reduction of the fractures).

Differential interpretation. The superimposition of images of soft tissue on a panoramic image of the mandible may simulate a fracture. A narrow airspace between the dorsal surface of the tongue and the soft palate superimposed across the angle of the mandible on a panoramic image may simulate a fracture. The airspace between the dorsal surface of the tongue and the posterior pharyngeal wall can mimic a fracture on lateral views of the mandible. Similar appearances can occur in the region of the soft palate where it is superimposed on the ramus.

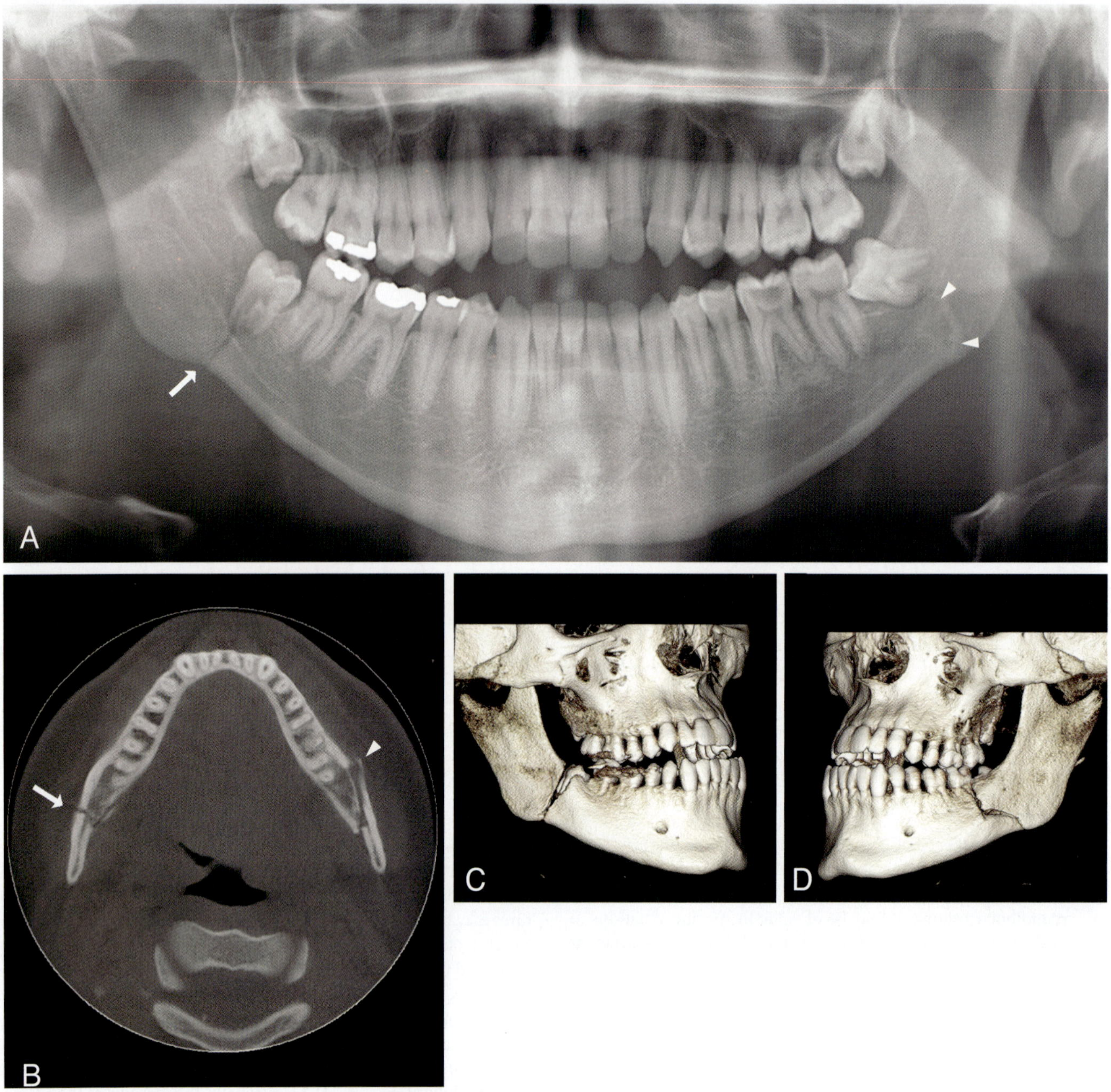

Fig. 25.22 Bilateral fractures of the mandibular angles. (A) Panoramic image shows a radiolucent fracture plane *(arrow)* at the right mandibular angle, extending to involve the periodontal ligament space of the mandibular third molar. A second fracture is present at the left mandibular angle and appears radiopaque due to fragment superimposition *(arrowheads)*. Note open bite. (B) Axial cone-beam computed tomographic image shows a fracture involving the right mandibular angle with minimal displacement of the fractured segments. Displacement of the ramus *(arrowhead)* is evident at the left angle of the mandible. (C) Surface rendered image shows fracture at the right angle of the mandible. (D) Surface rendered image shows fracture at the left angle of the mandible.

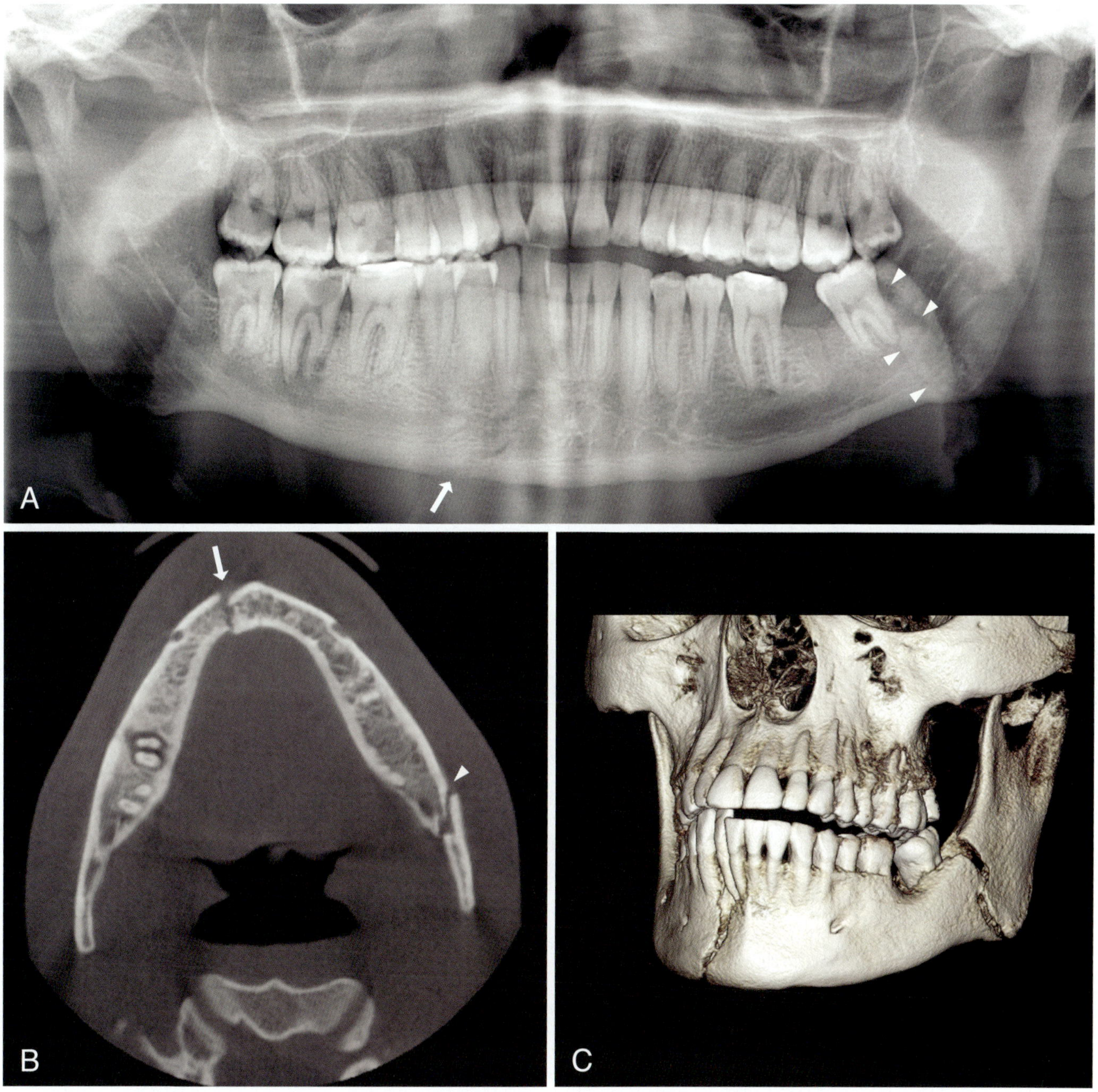

Fig. 25.23 Fracture of the mandibular symphysis and angle. (A) Panoramic image shows a fracture of the left mandibular angle *(arrowheads)* with involvement of the left mandibular third molar. Note the two radiolucent lines converging toward the inferior border; an appearance caused when the x-ray beam is oblique to the fracture plane. A second fracture is present at the right mandibular symphysis *(arrow)* and appears as a faint radiolucent line that extends from the inferior border to the alveolar crest. There is minimal deformity perceptible at the inferior border. Note sharp "step-deformity" in mandibular occlusal plane with an open bite from the right mandibular central incisor to the left mandibular third molar. (B) Axial CT section showing fractures with displacement in the right symphysis and left mandibular angle. (C) Surface rendered image shows fractures at the right symphysis and left angle of the mandible.

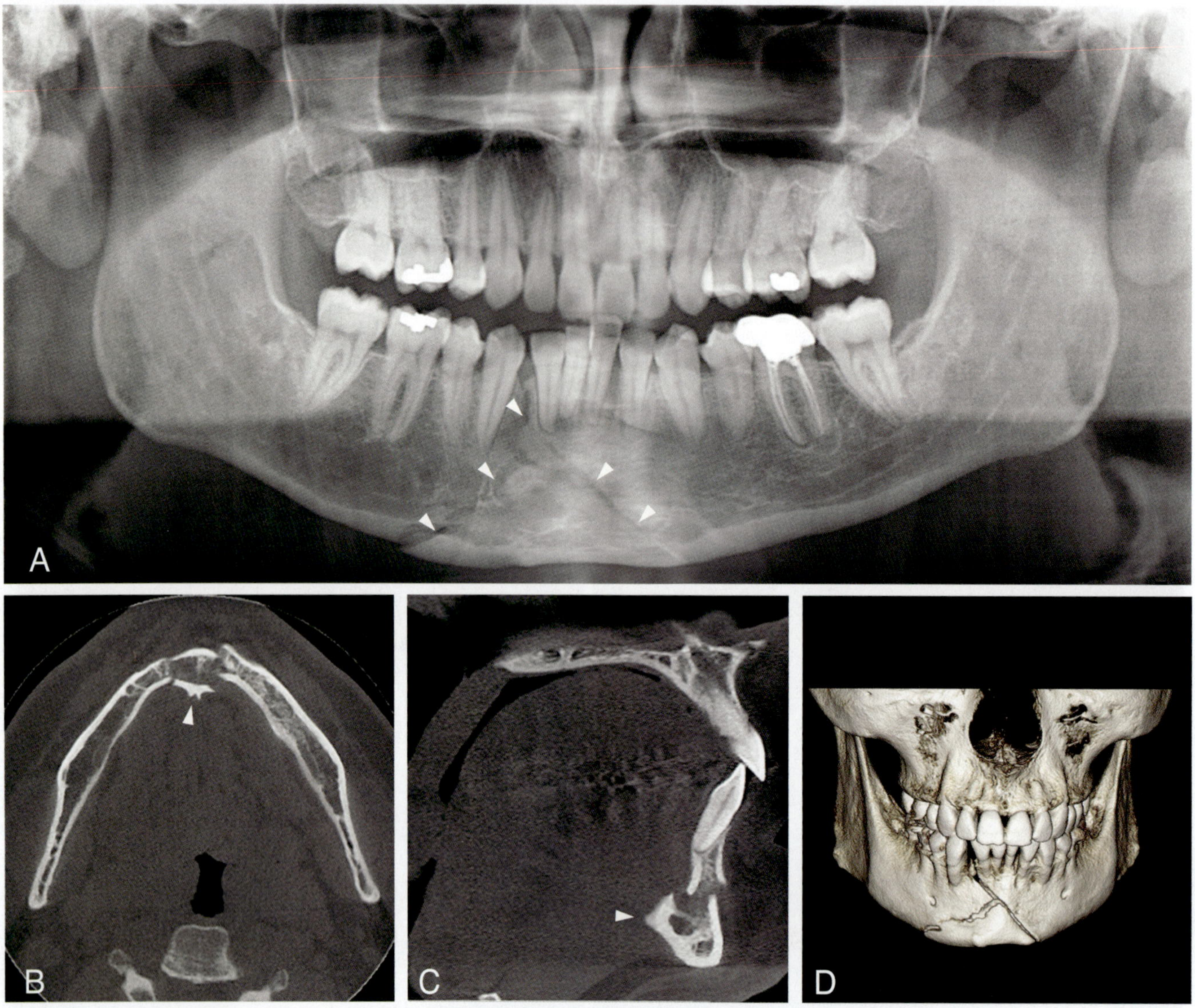

Fig. 25.24 Comminuted fracture of the mandibular symphysis. (A) Panoramic image shows discrete fracture lines in the mandibular symphysis *(arrowheads)* extending from the alveolar crest to the inferior border of the mandible. Axial (B) and sagittal (C) cone-beam computed tomographic images depicting fractures of the symphysis. The genial tubercles *(arrowhead)* are shown on the central fragment which is displaced by muscles attached to the genial tubercle. The fractured symphysis is displaced in a lingual direction. (D) 3D surface rendered image shows a comminuted fracture of the mandibular symphysis. The fracture plane extends into the interdental space between the right mandibular lateral incisor and canine.

Management. The management goals of a mandibular symphysis or body fracture are to restore a stable occlusion and the range of mandibular opening and excursive movements. Most mandibular fractures can be managed by closed reduction and intermaxillary fixation. Fractures with more severely displaced fragments may require open reduction. When the fracture plane involves one or more severely mobile teeth, or if there is significant root exposure within the fracture plane, the involved teeth are often extracted to reduce the risk of infection and problems with fixation. Should management include retaining these teeth, antibiotic therapy is often included.

Mandibular Condyle Fractures

Definition. Fractures of the mandibular condylar process may involve the condylar neck or the condylar head. Condylar neck fractures are more common and typically result in displacement of the condylar head in a medial, inferior, and anterior direction as a result of the contractile action of the lateral pterygoid muscle (Fig. 25.25). Condylar head fractures may include a single vertically oriented plane or cleft separating the condylar head into two fragments, or multiple fragments may be generated in a compression-like injury (Fig. 25.26). Almost half of patients with condylar fractures also have fractures in the mandibular body.

Clinical features. The clinical symptoms of a fractured mandibular condylar head are not always apparent, so the preauricular area must be carefully examined and palpated. The patient may have pain on opening or closing the mouth or trismus from local swelling. An anterior open bite may be present with only distal molar contacts, and there may be deviation of the mandible on opening. A significant feature may be the patient's inability to protrude the mandible because the lateral pterygoid muscle is attached to the condyle.

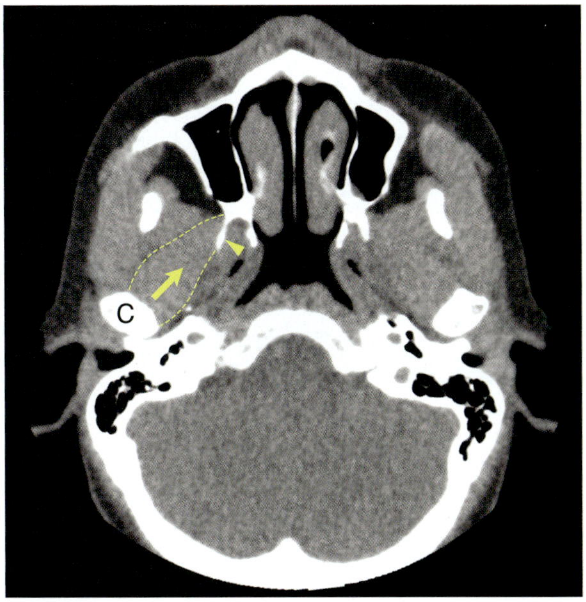

Fig. 25.25 Axial multidetector computed tomographic image shows the lateral pterygoid muscle *(yellow dashed lines)* extending from the lateral pterygoid plate *(arrowhead)* to the condyle, *C*. The *yellow arrow* denotes the anterior and medial direction of the muscle traction.

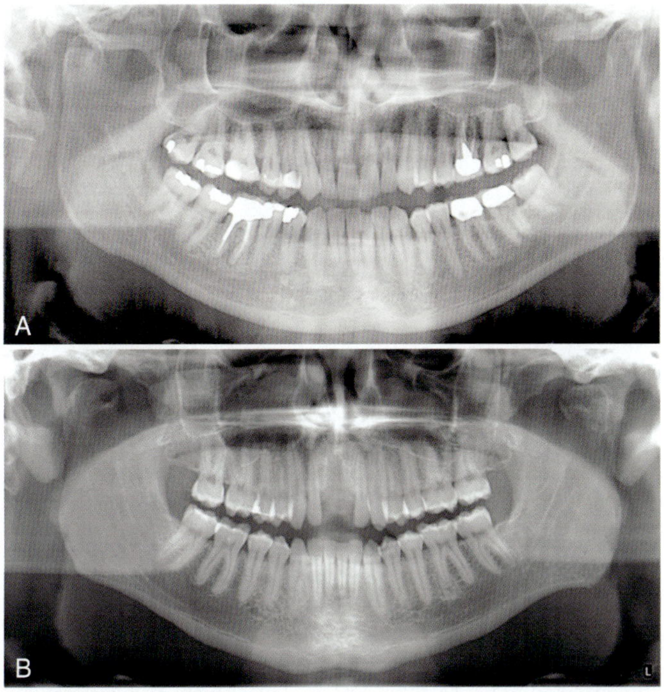

Fig. 25.26 (A) Panoramic image showing right condyle fracture with anterior displacement of the fractured condylar fragment. (B) Panoramic image showing bilateral condylar fractures with anterior and inferior displacement of the fractured condylar fragments.

Imaging features. Nondisplaced or minimally displaced fractures of the mandibular condylar head may be difficult or often impossible to detect on a panoramic image (Fig. 25.26). CT imaging is the modality of choice because it depicts the three-dimensional spatial relationship of the displaced condylar head to the glenoid fossa and to the adjacent anatomic structures in the skull base and infratemporal fossa (Figs. 25.27, 25.28, and 25.29).

Children and adolescents have much greater bone remodeling potential than adults. In children younger than 12 years, most fractured condyles regain normal morphology after healing, whereas the remodeling is less complete in teenagers. In adults, only minor remodeling is observed. The extent of remodeling is also greater with fractures of the condylar head than with condylar neck fractures with condylar head displacement. The most common deformities are medial inclination of the condyle, abnormal shape of the condyle, shortening of the neck, erosion, and flattening. Early condylar fractures commonly result in hypoplasia of the ipsilateral mandible.

Management. Condylar fractures can be successfully managed by closed reduction in both adults and children. This is accomplished with a period of intermaxillary fixation to reestablish the occlusion. Factors that dictate treatment decisions include whether one or both condyles are involved, the extent of displacement, and the occurrence and severity of other associated fractures. The treatment is directed to relieve acute symptoms, restore proper anatomic relationships, and prevent bony ankylosis. If a malocclusion develops, intermaxillary fixation may be provided to restore proper occlusion. Open reduction of condylar neck fractures is limited by the risk of procedure-related morbidity and the size and position of the fracture fragments.

Midfacial Fractures Including Maxillary Fractures

Midface fractures are caused by falls, motor vehicle accidents, and assaults, and they can involve one or multiple bones in the midface skeleton. The midface comprises the nasal, lacrimal, ethmoid, sphenoid, maxillary, zygomatic, and palatine bones. Fractures involving the frontal bone and midface are often complex, involve multiple bones, and have potentially serious complications from intracranial involvement.

Clinical indicators of midface injury:

- Periorbital ecchymosis.
- Infraorbital nerve paresthesia.
- Facial swelling.
- Visible or palpable nasal deformity.
- Epistaxis with or without evidence of cerebrospinal fluid leakage.
- Zygomatic deformity or facial elongation.
- Vestibular and palatal ecchymosis.
- Malocclusion or step deformity of the maxillary occlusal plane.

Imaging objectives:

- Locate and define fracture patterns.
- Assess intracranial involvement.
- Assess involvement of orbits, paranasal sinuses, and dentition.
- Monitor responses to treatment.

Imaging approaches:

- CT is the method of choice for imaging fractures of the maxillofacial skeleton, particularly when they involve multiple bones. The American College of Radiology recommends maxillofacial CT without contrast as an appropriate examination to evaluate suspected fractures of the frontal bone and midface. Because of its superior soft tissue contrast, MDCT is preferred to CBCT. The examination must encompass the region from the frontal bone to past the maxillary occlusal plane. Axial and coronal plane images provide optimal views of the anatomy.

Orbital Fractures

Definition. Orbital fractures are present in 10%–30% patients with facial fractures. Eighty percent of orbital fractures are blowout fractures caused by direct trauma to the orbit by an object that is too large to enter the orbital cavity, such as a fist or a baseball. The force of the impact travels through the orbital cavity or bone, and this is transferred to one or more of the very thin walls of the orbit. By definition,

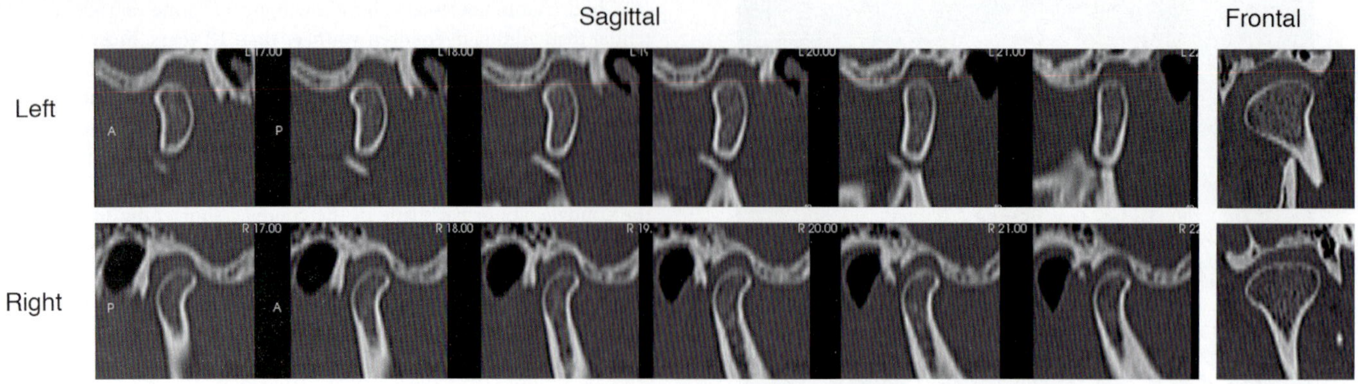

Fig. 25.27 Corrected sagittal and coronal cone-beam computed tomographic images through the right and left temporomandibular joints show a condylar neck fracture. The corrected sagittal images of the left temporomandibular joint *(top panel)* show anterior and slight inferior displacement of the condylar head. The coronal images show medial rotation of the condylar head. Sections through the contralateral side *(bottom panel)* show normal condylar morphology.

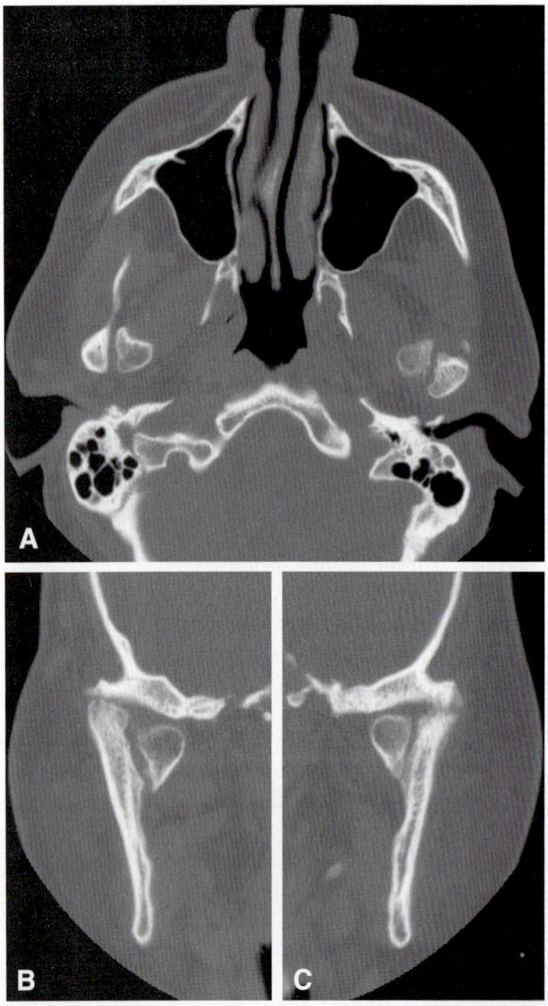

Fig. 25.28 Multidetector computed tomographic images of bilateral condylar neck fractures showing medial displacement of the condylar heads in line with the lateral pterygoid muscles in the axial image (A) and medial displacement in the coronal images (B and C); also, in (C), there is osseous ankylosis between the residual condylar neck and the temporal bone.

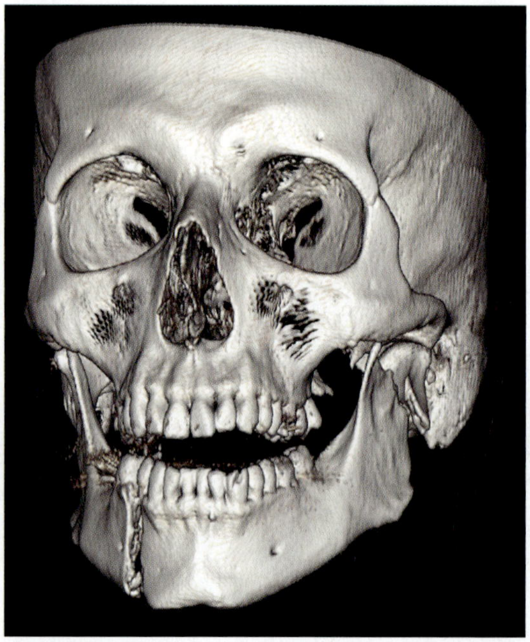

Fig. 25.29 Surface rendered image shows fractures of the left condylar neck and the right mandibular body.

the orbital rim remains intact in a blowout fracture. The most common fractures involve the medial wall, which is formed by the lamina papyracea of the ethmoid bone and the floor of the orbit which separates this space from the maxillary antrum. Involvement of the lateral wall of the orbit may suggest a zygomatic complex fracture. When the orbital roof is involved, the orbital rim is almost always displaced requiring surgical repositioning.

Clinical features. Periorbital edema is a common feature of the orbital blowout fracture, as is enophthalmos. Eye movements may be restricted if one or more of the periorbital muscles become entrapped in the bony defect created by the fracture. If the ethmoid air cells are involved, there may be epistaxis.

Imaging features. The imaging modality of choice to evaluate orbital blowout fractures is thin-section MDCT with multiplanar coronal and sagittal reconstructed images in bone and soft tissue kernels. Coronal reconstructions best demonstrate discontinuities of the lamina papyracea in a medial wall or the orbital floor. In orbital floor blowout fractures, herniation of the orbital cavity soft tissues can be seen through the roof of the maxillary sinus. Coronal CT imaging may show the classic "trapdoor" appearance of the displaced orbital floor (Fig. 25.30A). MDCT imaging may also show soft tissue densities and air-fluid levels in the adjacent ethmoid air cells or maxillary sinus (see Fig. 25.30B) or herniation of periorbital fat through the bony defect in the orbital floor (see Fig. 25.30C).

Management. Surgical repair may be attempted for patients who have severely affected eye movements because of muscle entrapment or unacceptable enophthalmos.

Zygomatic Fractures

Definition. Fractures involving the zygomatic bone may include tripod and zygomatic arch fractures and Le Fort type II and III fractures. Tripod fractures may also involve adjacent areas of the maxillary, frontal, sphenoid, and temporal bones, while zygomatic arch fractures can involve the zygomatic process of the temporal bone. Injuries to the zygomatic bone or arch usually result from a forceful blow to the cheek or side of the face. Although a zygomatic bone fracture may rotate or displace the fragments medially, support by the adjacent temporalis and masseter muscles may limit displacement.

Clinical features. Flattening of the upper cheek with tenderness and dimpling of the skin over the side of the face may occur, although

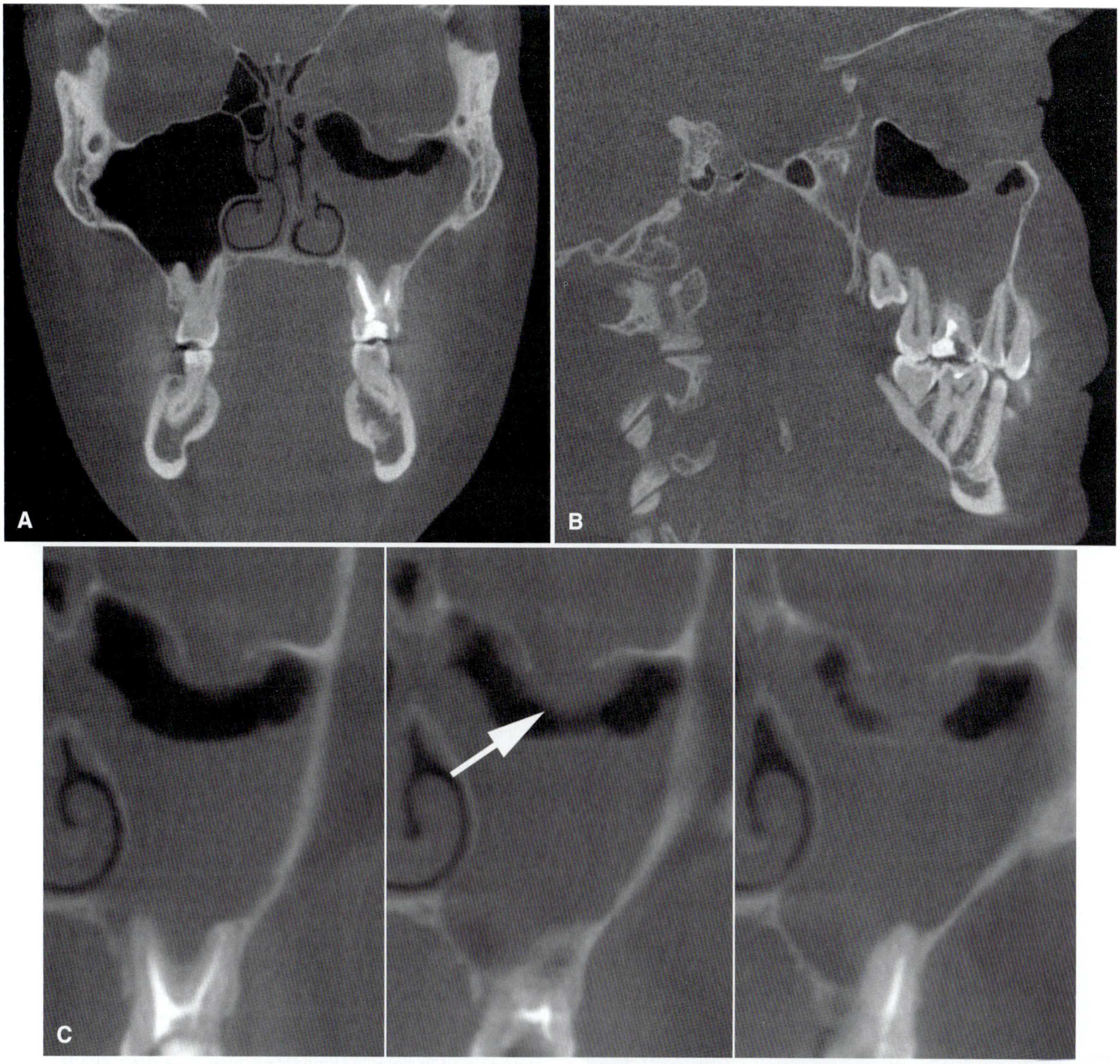

Fig. 25.30 Cone-beam computed tomographic images show an orbital blowout fracture involving the lamina papyracea of the left ethmoid bone and the orbital floor in the coronal (A) and sagittal (B) planes. Note the fluid/soft tissue densities in the adjacent ethmoid air cells and the air-fluid level in the left maxillary sinus. (C) Coronal cone-beam computed tomographic images show the "trapdoor" appearance of the orbital floor blowout fracture with herniation of soft tissue into the maxillary sinus *(arrow)*.

some of the clinical characteristics of zygomatic fractures may not be apparent much longer than an hour after trauma because they may be masked by edema. In most cases, periorbital ecchymosis and hemorrhage into the sclera (near the outer canthus of the eye) occur. Additional symptoms may include unilateral epistaxis for a short time after the injury, anesthesia or paresthesia of the cheek, and compromised eye movements. The presence of diplopia suggests a significant injury to the floor of the orbit. Mandibular movement may be limited if the displaced zygomatic bone impinges on the coronoid process.

Imaging features. Because of edema obscuring the clinical features, the imaging examination may provide the only means of determining the presence and extent of the injury. MDCT is the modality of choice for imaging these fractures (Fig. 25.31).

The zygomatic arch may fracture at its weakest point, about 1 cm posterior to the zygomaticotemporal suture (Fig. 25.32). Separation or fracture through the frontozygomatic suture may also occur. Fractures do not usually occur through the zygomaticomaxillary suture; however, in some cases, a fracture plane may extend obliquely, involving the inferior rim of the orbit and the lateral wall of the maxilla. If the fracture plane involves the maxillary sinus, the sinus may exhibit increased radiopacity subsequent to accumulation of blood and mucous secretions or an air-fluid level.

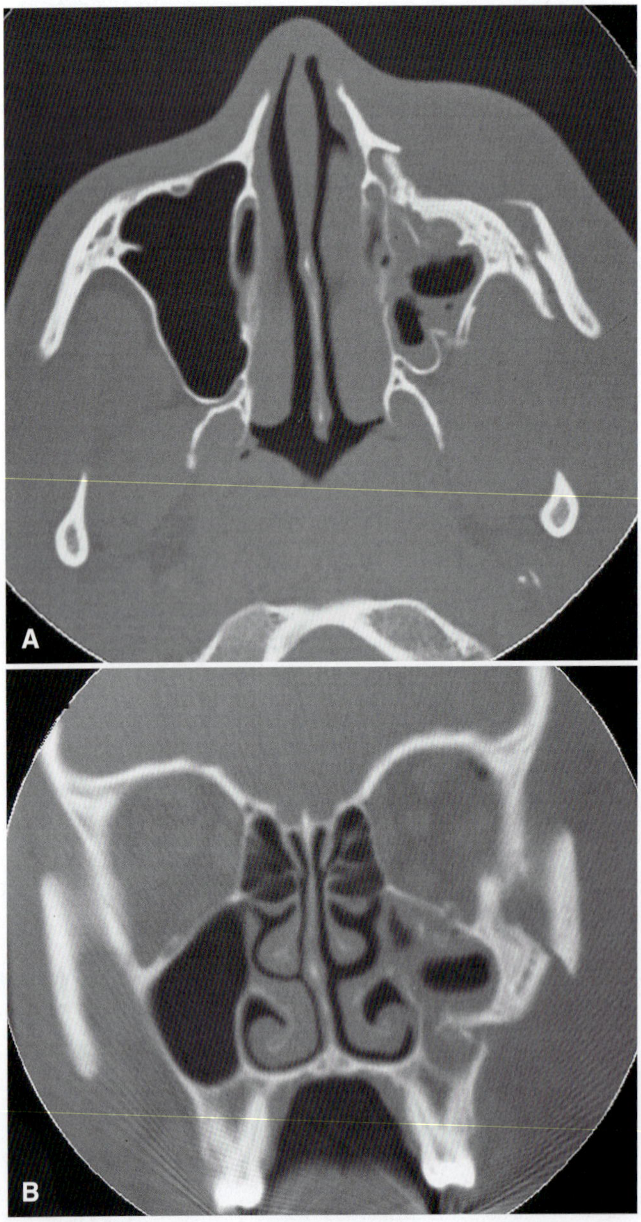

Fig. 25.31 Axial (A) and coronal (B) multidetector computed tomographic images show depression and rotation of a left tripod fracture. An air-fluid level is also visible in the left maxillary sinus.

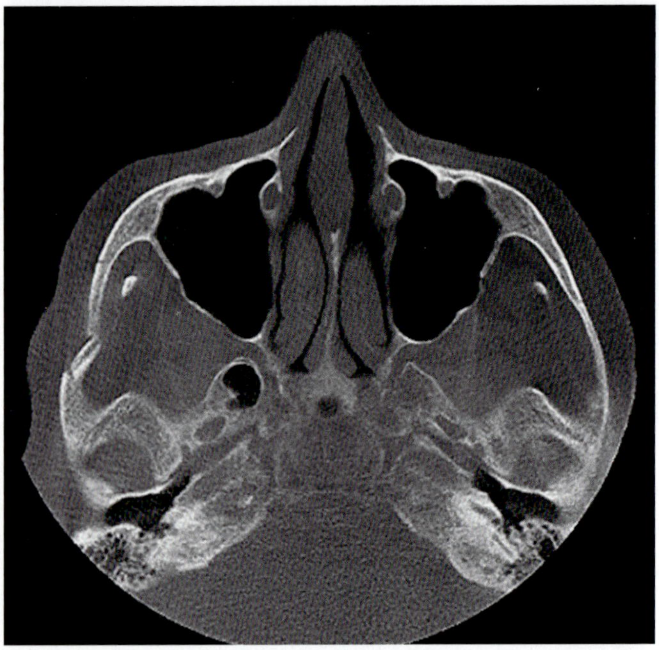

Fig. 25.32 Axial multidetector computed tomographic image shows fracture of the right zygomatic arch with depression of the fractured fragment.

It is important to consider that on panoramic images, the zygomaticotemporal suture appears as a radiolucent line that may have the appearance of a discontinuity in the inferior border. This is a variation of normal anatomy and should not be misinterpreted as a fracture.

Management. When there has been minimal displacement of the zygomatic arch without cosmetic deformities or impairment of eye movement, no treatment may be required. Otherwise reduction is usually indicated. Fractures of the zygomatic bone and arch may be reduced through an intraoral or extraoral approach.

Le Fort Fractures

Complex fractures involving multiple facial bones may be quite variable but often follow general patterns described by the French surgeon René Le Fort. By definition, all Le Fort fractures include fractures of one or more of the pterygoid plates of the sphenoid bone. Although Le Fort fractures may be bilateral, they are most often unilateral.

The detection of fractures of the midface in images is difficult because of the complex anatomy and the multiple superimpositions of structures. MDCT is the diagnostic imaging modality of choice for complex facial fractures because it generates multiple image slices in orthogonal planes through the face, displaying osseous structures without the complication of overlapping anatomy, which is problematic with planar imaging. MDCT also provides suitable soft tissue image detail to detect secondary changes associated with trauma, including herniation of orbital fat and extraocular muscle, soft tissue swelling or emphysema, and blood or fluid accumulation. As an aid in determining the spatial orientation of fractures or bone fragments, MDCT image data can be used to produce three-dimensional surface renderings.

Le Fort I (Horizontal Fracture)

Definition. The Le Fort I fracture plane extends through the maxillary body in a relatively horizontal orientation that results in detachment of the alveolar process and adjacent bone of the maxilla from the midface. This fracture is the result of a horizontally directed traumatic force directed posteriorly at the base of the nose. The fracture plane passes superior to the roots of the teeth and nasal floor and posteriorly through the base of the maxillary sinus and the tuberosity to the pterygoid processes (Fig. 25.33). In the unilateral fracture, there is an auxiliary fracture in the midline of the palate. The unilateral fracture must be distinguished from a fracture within the alveolar process (discussed previously) that does not extend to the midline or involve the pterygoid plates posteriorly. Concomitant fractures of the mandible (54%) and zygomatic bone (23%) are frequent in these patients.

Clinical features. If the fragment is not distally impacted, it can be manipulated by holding on to the teeth. If the fracture plane is at a high level, the fragment may include the pterygoid muscle attachments, which will pull the fragment posteriorly and inferiorly. As a result, the posterior maxillary teeth will contact the mandibular teeth first, resulting in an anterior open bite, a retruded chin, and an elongated face. If the fracture is at a low level, no displacement will occur. Other symptoms may include associated swelling and bruising around the eyes, pain over the nose and face, deformity of the nose, and flattening of the middle of the face. Epistaxis is inevitable, and occasionally, double vision and varying degrees of paresthesia over the distribution of the infraorbital nerve may occur. Manipulation may reveal a mobile maxilla and crepitation.

Imaging features. MDCT imaging reveals an air-fluid level or radiopacification in the maxillary sinus (Fig. 25.34A). Coronal images may reveal the plane of the fracture extending posteriorly through the maxilla, whereas coronal or axial images together may reveal involvement of the pterygoid plates posteriorly. Three-dimensional reconstructions of the MDCT dataset may show the plane of the fracture to the greatest advantage (see Fig. 25.34B).

Management. If the fracture is not displaced and is at a relatively low level in the maxilla, it can be treated by intermaxillary fixation. Fractures that are high, with the fragment displaced posteriorly or with pronounced separation, require craniomaxillary fixation in addition to intermaxillary fixation.

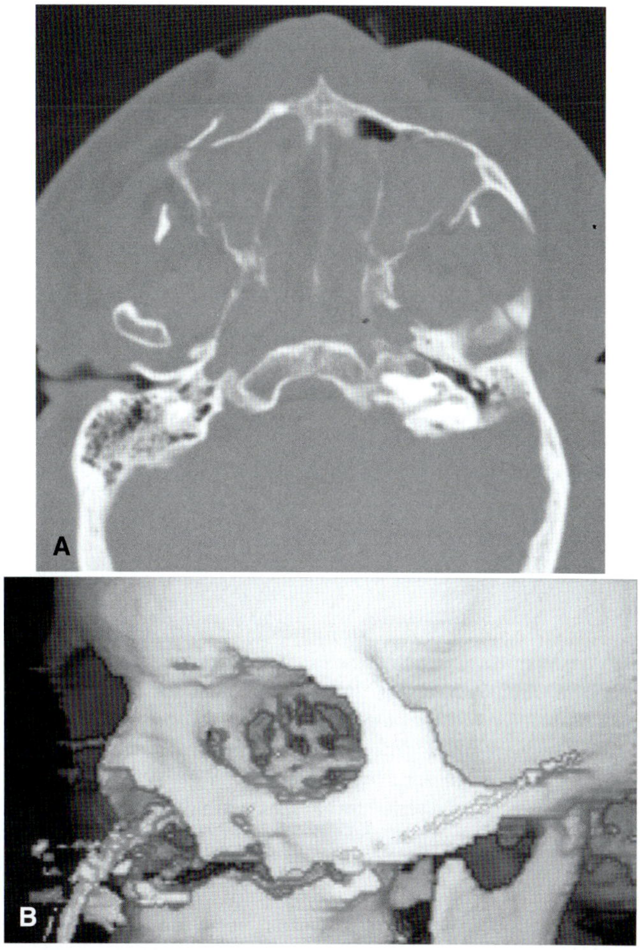

Fig. 25.34 (A) Axial multidetector computed tomographic image of a Le Fort I fracture involving the anterior and posterolateral walls of the right and left maxilla and the pterygoid plates. Opacification of the maxillary sinuses is also seen, with a small retained collection of air in the left maxillary sinus. (B) Three-dimensional surface reconstruction of the image data shows extension of the fracture plane from above the base of the nose posteriorly through the maxillary tuberosity.

Le Fort II (Pyramidal Fracture)

Definition. A Le Fort II fracture has a pyramidal shape on planar posteroanterior skull images and hence the name. This fracture pattern results from a violent force applied posteriorly and superiorly through the base of the nose, separating the maxilla from the base of the skull. The fracture plane extends from the bridge of the nose inferiorly, laterally, and posteriorly through the nasal and lacrimal bones, the orbital floor and inferior rim obliquely, inferiorly across the maxilla, and posteriorly to the pterygoid processes (Figs. 25.35 and 25.36). The frontal and ethmoid sinuses are involved in about 10% of cases, especially in severe comminuted fractures.

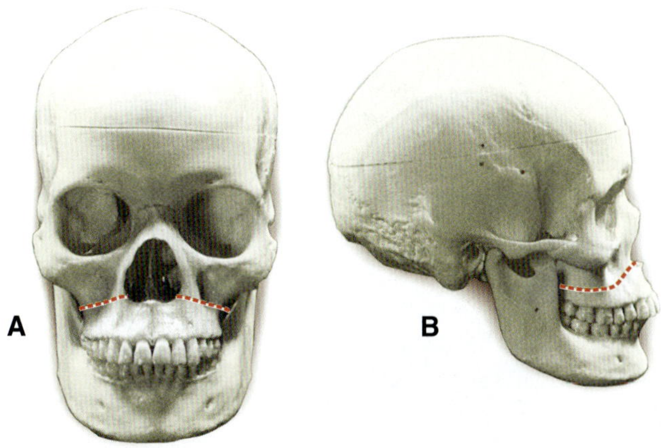

Fig. 25.33 Usual position of a Le Fort I fracture on frontal (A) and lateral (B) views.

Clinical features. In contrast to the Le Fort I fracture, which may be characterized by only slight swelling about the upper lips, a Le Fort II fracture results in massive edema and marked swelling of the middle third of the face. Typically ecchymosis develops around the eyes within minutes of the injury. The edema is likely to be so severe that it is impossible to see the globes. The conjunctivae over the inner quadrants of the eyes are bloodshot; if the zygomatic bones are involved, this ecchymosis will extend to the outer quadrant.

The broken nose is displaced because the face has fallen, and the nose and face are elongated. An anterior open bite occurs. Epistaxis is inevitable, and cerebrospinal fluid rhinorrhea may occur. Palpation reveals the discontinuity of the lower borders of the orbits. By applying pressure between the bridge of the nose and the palate, the "pyramid"

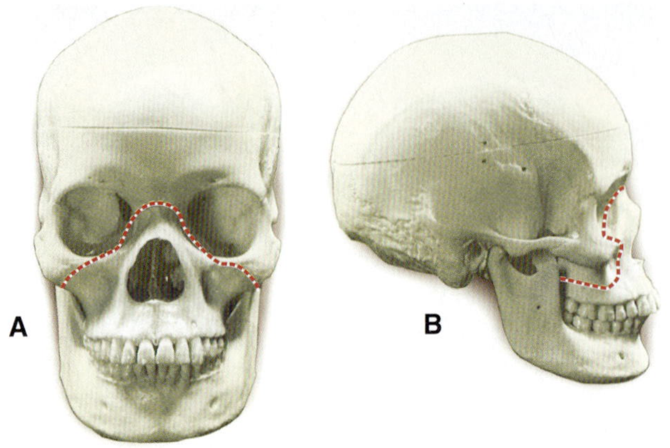

Fig. 25.35 Usual position of the Le Fort II fracture on frontal (A) and lateral (B) views.

of bone can be moved. Other common symptoms include double vision and variable degrees of paresthesia over the distribution of the infraorbital nerve.

Imaging features. MDCT is the modality of choice for imaging such complex fractures. The radiologic examination reveals fractures of the nasal bone, frontal process of the maxilla, infraorbital rim, and orbital floor. More inferiorly and posteriorly, there is involvement of the zygomatic bone or zygomatic process of the maxilla, separation of the zygomaticomaxillary suture, and fracture of the lateral wall of the maxillary sinus and the pterygoid plates. Involvement of the ethmoid air cells and frontal and maxillary sinuses would result in thickening of the sinus mucosa or the accumulation of blood-fluid levels in the airspaces.

Management. Le Fort II fractures are managed by reduction of the displaced maxilla via intermaxillary fixation, open reduction, and interosseous wiring of the infraorbital rims as well as plating of the accompanying fractures of the nose, nasal septum, and orbital floor. Repair of the detached medial canthal ligaments may also be required. Leakage of cerebrospinal fluid requires neurosurgical intervention if the posterior or superior walls of the frontal sinuses are involved.

Le Fort III (Craniofacial Disjunction)

Definition. A Le Fort III midface fracture results when the traumatic force is of sufficient magnitude to separate the middle third of the facial skeleton completely from the cranium. The fracture plane usually extends from the nasal bone and frontal process of the maxilla or nasofrontal and maxillofrontal sutures across the orbital floor, through the ethmoid air cells and sphenoid sinus, to the zygomaticofrontal sutures (Fig. 25.37). More posteriorly and inferiorly, the fracture plane passes across the pterygomaxillary fissure and separates the bases of the pterygoid plates from the sphenoid bone. If the maxilla is displaced and freely movable, a fracture must also have occurred at the zygomaticotemporal suture. Because the zygomatic bone or zygomatic arch is involved, these injuries are associated with multiple other maxillary fractures. Mandibular fractures are also observed in half the cases.

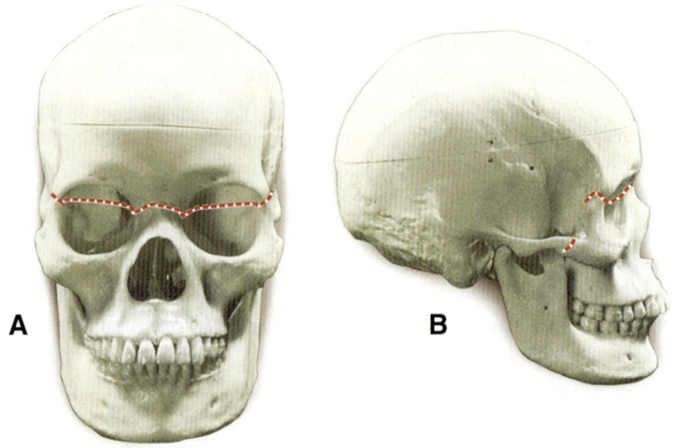

Fig. 25.37 Usual position of a Le Fort III fracture on frontal (A) and lateral (B) views.

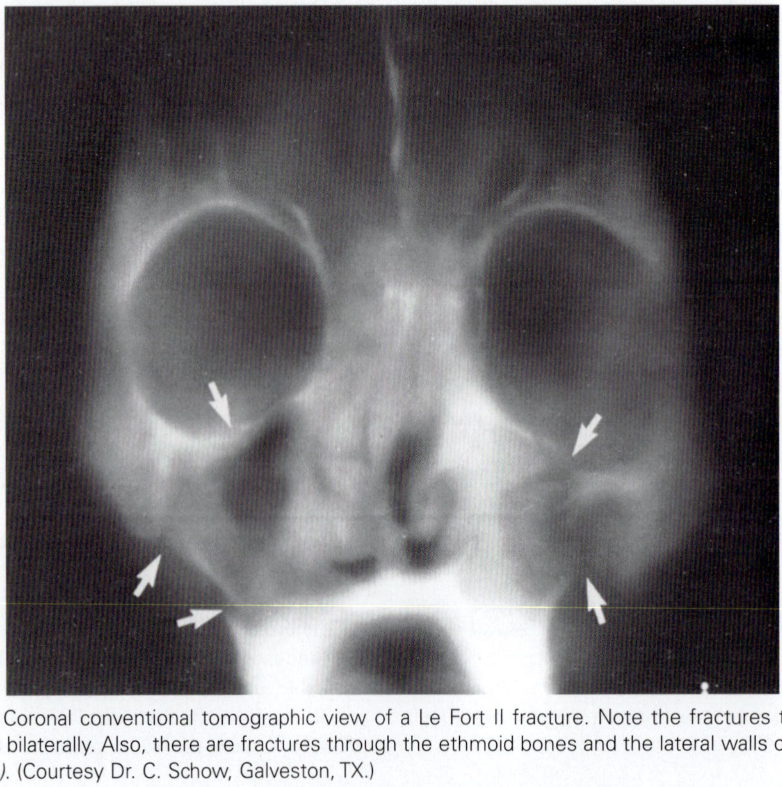

Fig. 25.36 Coronal conventional tomographic view of a Le Fort II fracture. Note the fractures through the orbital rims bilaterally. Also, there are fractures through the ethmoid bones and the lateral walls of the maxillae *(arrows)*. (Courtesy Dr. C. Schow, Galveston, TX.)

Clinical features. Craniofacial disjunction produces a clinical appearance similar to that of a pyramidal fracture; however, this injury is considerably more extensive. The soft tissue injuries are severe, with massive edema. The nasal cavity may be obstructed by blood or blood clot, or cerebrospinal fluid rhinorrhea may be present. Bleeding may occur into the periorbital tissues and the conjunctiva, and numerous eye signs of neurologic importance are likely to be present. A "dished-in" or concave deformity of the face is characteristic of this fracture pattern, as is an anterior open bite because of the retroclined positions of the maxillary incisors with only the posterior teeth in occlusion. Even on mandibular opening, the patient is unable to separate the molars. Intraoral and extraoral palpation reveals irregular contours and step deformities, and crepitation is apparent when the fragments are moved.

Imaging features. It is virtually impossible to document these multiple fractures with planar imaging, and MDCT imaging in concert with the clinical information is required. The main radiologic findings are distractions of the frontonasal, frontomaxillary, zygomaticofrontal, and zygomaticotemporal sutures and fractures through the nasal bone, frontal process of the maxilla, orbital floor, and pterygoid plates (Fig. 25.38). Associated fractures involving the walls of all the paranasal sinuses result in radiopaque air-fluid levels with mucosal thickening. Three-dimensional reconstructions of MDCT data show the fracture planes and large bone fragments (see Fig. 25.38D and E).

Management. The associated severe soft tissue injury necessitates airway management, initial hemorrhage control, and repair of lacerations. Surgery may be delayed until the edema has sufficiently resolved. Fixation of the loose middle third of the facial skeleton is difficult due to concurrent fractures of the zygomatic arch. The only possibilities are external immobilization or immobilization within the tissues. In the former, the loose maxilla is suspended by wires through the cheeks from a metal head frame (halo) or fixed by external pins anchored in bone. The other possibility is immobilization within the tissues by using internal wiring to the closest solid bone superior to the fracture. Many complications may develop during or after this treatment.

MONITORING THE HEALING OF FRACTURES

The goals of imaging following management of facial trauma are to confirm the adequate reduction of fracture planes and to monitor the continued immobilization of the fracture site during healing. Typically, monitoring of this type is accomplished by the use of planar imaging and is directed to the evaluation of the alignment of the cortical plates of the involved bone(s) and remodeling and remineralization of the fracture site. During normal healing, the fracture plane increases in width about 2 weeks after reduction of the fracture. This change develops as a result of resorption of the fractured ends and small sequestered fragments of bone. Early evidence of remineralization usually occurs 5–6 weeks after treatment. In contrast to the long bones of the skeleton, callus formation during healing of jaw fractures is rare. The complete remodeling of the fracture site with obliteration of the fracture plane may take several months. Rarely, fracture planes may persist for years, even after the patient has made a complete clinical recovery. Possible complications of healing can include malalignment of fracture segments, inflammatory lesions related to teeth that have developed

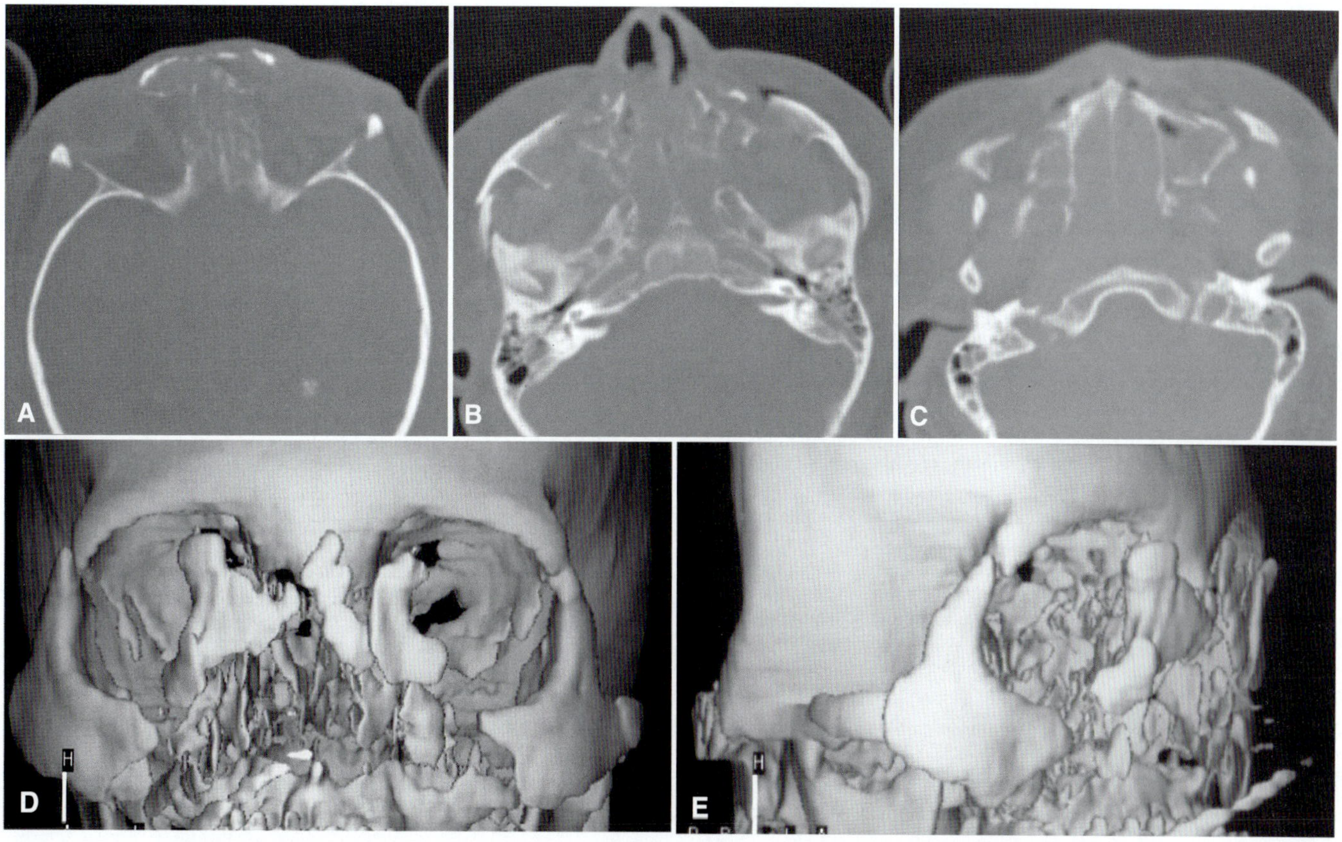

Fig. 25.38 Axial multidetector computed tomographic images show a bilateral Le Fort III fracture with distractions of the frontonasal (A), frontomaxillary, zygomaticofrontal, and zygomaticotemporal sutures (B) and fractures of the nasal bone, frontal process of the maxilla, orbital floor, and pterygoid plates (C). Note the near-total radiopacification of the maxillary sinuses. Frontal (D) and lateral (E) views of the three-dimensional surface reconstructions revealing substantial fragmentation of the periorbital bones, zygomatic bone, and arch posteriorly.

nonvital pulps near or in the plane of the fracture, nonunion of fracture fragments, and secondary infection of the fracture. Nonunion may be seen as an increase in the width of the radiolucent fracture plane, cortication of the fractured surfaces, and rounding of the sharp edges of the fragment edges. The development of osteomyelitis at the fracture site appears as an increase in sclerosis of the adjacent bone, inflammatory periosteal new bone formation, and the development of sequestra.

BIBLIOGRAPHY

Guidelines and General Assessment

American Association of Endodontists. The Treatment of Traumatic Dental Injuries. https://www.aae.org/specialty/wp-content/uploads/sites/2/2019/02/19_TraumaGuidelines.pdf. Accessed September 6, 2023.

American College of Surgeons Trauma Quality Improvement Program. Best Practices Guidelines in Imaging. https://www.facs.org/media/oxdjw5zj/imaging_guidelines.pdf. Accessed September 7, 2023.

Bourguignon C, Cohenca N, Lauridsen E, et al. International Association of Dental Traumatology guidelines for the management of traumatic dental injuries: 1. Fractures and luxations. *Dent Traumatol.* 2020;36:314-330.

Day PF, Flores MT, O'Connell AC, et al. International Association of Dental Traumatology guidelines for the management of traumatic dental injuries: 3. Injuries in the primary dentition. *Dent Traumatol.* 2020;36:343-359.

Expert Panel on Neurological I, Parsons MS, Policeni B, et al. ACR Appropriateness Criteria® Imaging of Facial Trauma Following Primary Survey. *J Am Coll Radiol.* 2022;19:S67-S86.

Fouad AF, Abbott PV, Tsilingaridis G, et al. International Association of Dental Traumatology guidelines for the management of traumatic dental injuries: 2. Avulsion of permanent teeth. *Dent Traumatol.* 2020;36:331-342.

Krishnan DG. Systematic assessment of the patient with facial trauma. *Oral and Maxillofac Surg Clin North Am.* 2013;25(4):537-544. https://doi.org/10.1016/j.coms.2013.07.009

Levin L, Day PF, Hicks L, et al. International Association of Dental Traumatology guidelines for the management of traumatic dental injuries: general introduction. *Dent Traumatol.* 2020;36:309-313.

Boffano P, Kommers SC, Karagozoglu KH, et al. Aetiology of maxillofacial fractures: a review of published studies during the last 30 years. *Br J Oral Maxillofac Surg.* 2014;52:901-906.

Brook IW, Wood N. Aetiology and incidence of facial fractures in adults. *Int J Oral Surg.* 1983;12:293-298.

Dental Fractures

Andreasen JO, Bakland L, Flores M, et al. *Traumatic Dental Injuries: A Manual, 3rd Edition.* Wiley-Blackwell (STMS); 2011.

Bissinger R, Muller DD, Reymus M, et al. Treatment outcomes after uncomplicated and complicated crown fractures in permanent teeth. *Clin Oral Investig.* 2021;25:133-143.

Ravn JJ. Follow-up study of permanent incisors with enamel fractures as a result of acute trauma. *Scand J Dent Res.* 1981;89:213-217.

Ravn JJ. Follow-up study of permanent incisors with enamel-dentin fracture after acute trauma. *Scand J Dent Res.* 1981;89:355-365.

Ravn JJ. Follow-up study of permanent incisors with complicated crown fractures after acute trauma. *Scand J Dent Res.* 1982;90:363-372.

Tooth Root Fracture

Abbott PV. Diagnosis and management of transverse root fractures. *J Endod.* 2019;45:S13-S27.

Cvek M, Mejare I, Andreason JO. Healing and prognosis of teeth with intra-alveolar fractures involving the cervical part of the root. *Dent Traumatol.* 2002;18:57-65.

Edlund M, Nair MK, Nair UP. Detection of vertical root fractures by using cone-beam computed tomography: a clinical study. *J Endod.* 2011;37:768-772.

Majorana A, Pasini S, Bardellini E, et al. Clinical and epidemiological study of traumatic root fractures. *Dent Traumatol.* 2002;18:77-80.

Patel S, Bhuva B, Bose R. Present status and future directions: vertical root fractures in root filled teeth. *Int Endod J.* 2022;55(suppl 3):804-826.

Sim IG, Lim TS, Krishnaswamy G, et al. Decision Making for Retention of Endodontically Treated Posterior Cracked Teeth: a 5-year Follow-up Study. *J Endod.* 2016;42:225-229.

Walton RE, Michelich RJ, Smith GN. The histopathogenesis of vertical root fractures. *J Endodont.* 1984;10:48-56.

Fractures of the Alveolar Process

Andreasen JO. Fractures of the alveolar process of the jaw: a clinical and radiographic follow-up study. *Scand J Dent Res.* 1970;78:263-272.

Susarla HK, Sheller B. Dental and Dentoalveolar Injuries in the Pediatric Patient. *Oral Maxillofac Surg Clin North Am.* 2023;35(4):543-554.

Luxation

Andreasen JO. Luxation of permanent teeth due to trauma: a clinical and radiographic follow-up study of 189 injured teeth. *Scand J Dent Res.* 1970;78:273-286.

Avulsion

Donaldson M, Kinirons MJ. Factors affecting the time of onset of resorption in avulsed and replanted incisor teeth in children. *Dent Traumatol.* 2001;17:205-209.

Trauma to the Mandible

Afrooz PN, Bykowski MR, James IB, et al. The epidemiology of mandibular fractures in the United States, part 1: a review of 13,142 cases from the US National Trauma Data Bank. *J Oral Maxillofac Surg.* 2015;73:2361-2366.

Braasch DC, Abubaker AO. Management of mandibular angle fracture. *Oral Maxillofac Surg Clin North Am.* 2013;25:591-600.

Escott EJ, Branstetter BF. Incidence and characterization of unifocal mandible fractures on CT. *AJNR Am J Neuroradiol.* 2008;29:890-894.

Dreizin D, Nam AJ, Tirada N, et al. Multidetector CT of mandibular fractures, reductions, and complications: a Clinically Relevant Primer for the Radiologist. *Radiographics.* 2016;36(5):1539-1564.

Goodday RHB. Management of fractures of the mandibular body and symphysis. *Oral Maxillofac Surg Clin North Am.* 2013;25:601-616.

Kaeppler G, Cornelius CP, Ehrenfeld M, et al. Diagnostic efficacy of cone-beam computed tomography for mandibular fractures. *Oral Surg Oral Med Oral Pathol Oral Radiol.* 2013;116:98-104.

Condylar Fractures

Consensus Conference on Open or Closed Management of Condylar Fractures, 12th ICOMS, Budapest, 1995. *Int J Oral Maxillofac Surg.* 1998;27:243-267.

Dahlström L, Kahnberg KE, Lindahl L. 15 years follow-up on condylar fractures. *Int J Oral Maxillofac Surg.* 1989;18:18-23.

Davis B. Late reconstruction of condylar neck and head fractures. *Oral Maxillofac Surg Clin North Am.* 2013;25:661-681.

Dimitroulis G. Condylar injuries in growing patients. *Aust Dent J.* 1997;42:367-371.

Kisnisci R. Management of fractures of the condyle, condylar neck, and coronoid process. *Oral Maxillofac Surg Clin North Am.* 2013;25:573-590.

Trauma to the Maxilla

Ceallaigh PO, Ekanaykaee K, Beirne CJ, et al. Diagnosis and management of common maxillofacial injuries in the emergency department. Part 4: orbital floor and midface fractures. *Emerg Med J.* 2007;24:292-293.

Dreizin D, Nam AJ, Diaconu SC, et al. Multidetector CT of midfacial fractures: classification systems, principles of reduction, and common complications. *Radiographics.* 2018;38:248-274.

Hopper RA, Salemy S, Sze RW. Diagnosis of midface fractures with CT: what the surgeon needs to know. *Radiographics.* 2006;26:783-793.

Winegar BA, Murillo H, Tantiwongkosi B. Spectrum of critical imaging findings in complex facial skeletal trauma. *Radiographics.* 2013;33:3-19.

Zygomatic Complex Fractures

Kochhar A, Byrne PJ. Surgical management of complex midfacial fractures. *Otolaryngol Clin North Am.* 2013;46:759-778.

Moreira Marinho RO, Freire-Maia B. Management of Fractures of the Zygomaticomaxillary Complex. *Oral Maxillofac Surg Clin North Am.* 2013;25:617-636.

Paranasal Sinus Abnormalities

Mohammed A. Husain, Sotirios Tetradis

The paranasal sinuses are the four paired sets of air-filled cavities of the maxillofacial complex, and they consist of the maxillary, frontal and sphenoid sinuses, and the ethmoid air cells. The maxillary sinuses are of particular importance to the dentist because of their proximity to the teeth and their associated structures. Abnormalities arising from within the maxillary sinuses can cause symptoms that may mimic diseases of odontogenic origin, and conversely, abnormalities that arise in and around the teeth may affect the sinuses or mimic the symptoms of sinus disease. Because the paranasal sinuses may appear on many diagnostic images used in the practice of dentistry, the dentist should be familiar with variations in the normal appearance of the sinuses and the more common diseases that may affect them.

NORMAL DEVELOPMENT AND VARIATIONS

The paranasal sinuses develop as invaginations from the nasal fossae into their respective bones (maxillary, frontal, sphenoid, and ethmoid), and they continue to enlarge until skeletal maturity. Like the nasal cavities, the paranasal sinuses are lined with respiratory mucosa composed of pseudostratified ciliated columnar epithelium. The cilia move sinus secretions through the ostia (narrow openings of the sinuses) into the nasal fossae. The maxillary sinuses or antra are the first to develop in the second month of intrauterine life. An invagination develops in the lateral wall of the nasal fossa in the middle meatus, and the sinus cavity enlarges laterally into the body of the maxilla. At birth, each sinus is a thin, small slit, no more than 8 mm in length in its anteroposterior dimension. With time, the maxilla becomes progressively more pneumatized as the air cavity expands further into the bone both laterally under the orbits toward the zygomatic process and inferiorly into the alveolar process. Pneumatization into the alveolar process drapes the maxillary sinus floor over the roots of the premolar or molar teeth to varying degrees. The imaging appearance of the floor of the maxillary sinus is a thin, well-defined corticated line. If the alveolar process of the maxilla is not well pneumatized, the floor of the sinus may not be visible on periapical images (Fig. 26.1A), or it may be seen superior to the roots of the maxillary premolar or molar teeth (see Fig. 26.1B). With greater pneumatization, the floor of the sinus may appear to undulate around or drape over the roots of the teeth or be superimposed over the tooth roots, giving the false impression that the roots have penetrated the sinus floor (see Fig. 26.1C and D). Closer examination of the periapical areas reveals intact laminae dura and periodontal ligament spaces.

In patients with considerable pneumatization of the alveolar process of the maxilla, the lamina dura of a premolar or molar tooth may be continuous with the sinus floor, forming a portion of it. Maxillary pneumatization may also extend into the palatal, zygomatic, and frontal processes of the maxilla; this can be appreciated on planar images as well as cone beam computed tomography (CBCT), multidetector computed tomography (MDCT) (Fig. 26.2A), and magnetic resonance imaging (MRI). In some instances, the appearance of the normally pneumatized maxilla may be mistakenly confused with a benign space-occupying lesion, particularly on planar images (Fig. 26.3).

Hypoplasia of the maxillary sinuses occurs unilaterally in approximately 1.7% of patients (see Fig. 26.4A) and bilaterally in 7.2%. In planar imaging, the involved sinus may appear more radiopaque than normal because of the relatively large amount of surrounding maxillary bone. The configuration of the maxillary sinus walls frequently helps to distinguish between a hypoplastic sinus and a sinus that is pathologically radiopaque. Asymmetry in the size of the right and left maxillary sinuses is seen not only in the presence of a unilateral hypoplastic sinus but can also appear in silent sinus syndrome (SSS) (see Fig. 26.2B).

SSS is a rare pathologic entity believed to be caused by sinus hypoventilation due to obstruction of the ostium of the involved maxillary sinus, eventually leading to a decrease in sinus volume. SSS is associated with clinical symptoms such as enophthalmos and hypoglobus. Radiographically, SSS is characterized by reduced sinus size with bowing of the sinus walls and an inferiorly displaced orbital floor with increased orbital content.

The frontal sinus is the last of the paranasal sinuses to develop, with development initiated usually around the fifth or sixth year of postpartum life. This sinus develops either directly by extension from the nasal fossae or from the anterior ethmoid air cells (Fig. 26.5B). In approximately 4% of the population, the frontal sinuses fail to develop. As with the other paranasal sinuses, the right and left frontal sinus cavities develop independently; however, as they expand, they approach each other in the midline. In such instances, a thin bony septum may partially or completely separate the two asymmetric cavities. In adults, frontal sinus pneumatization may also extend posteriorly into the orbital roofs.

The sphenoid sinus develops during the fourth fetal month from invaginations of the spheno-ethmoidal recesses of the nasal fossae. Located in the body of the sphenoid bone, there is usually a partial or complete bony septum separating the left airspace from the right, and these are often asymmetric in size and shape. As with the other sinuses, the sphenoid sinuses may hyperpneumatize, extending beyond the sphenoid body into the dorsum sella, the clinoid processes, the greater or lesser wings, and the pterygoid processes. The ostium of the sphenoid sinus is a relatively large-diameter opening; this may explain why blockages of the sphenoid sinus ostium are uncommon (see the section on mucoceles later in this chapter).

The ethmoid air cells extend into the developing ethmoid bones during the fifth fetal month. They consist of multiple separate or interconnected air-filled chambers that usually border the medial aspect of the orbital cavities (see Fig. 26.5A and B). At times, ethmoid air cells develop inferior to the orbit, in which case they may be referred to as

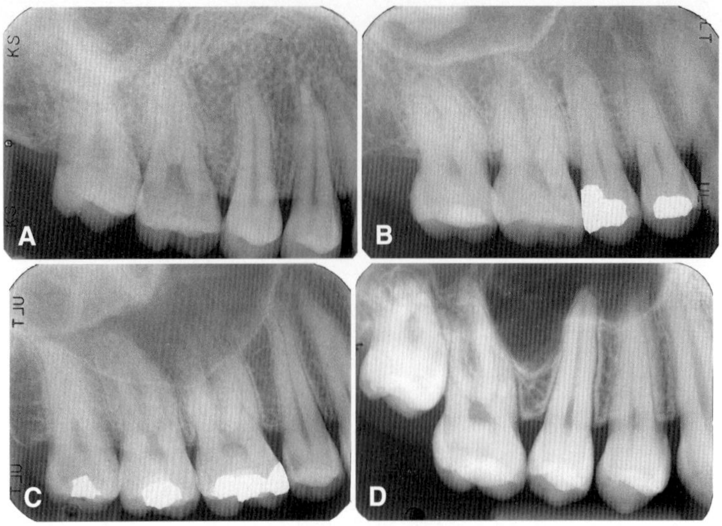

Fig. 26.1 (A–D) The range of the normal positions of the maxillary sinus floor relative to the premolar and molar teeth is shown in periapical images. There is no visible floor in (A), with progressively more pneumatization of the alveolar process in (B) and (C); draping of the maxillary sinus border over the apices of the teeth is particularly evident in (D).

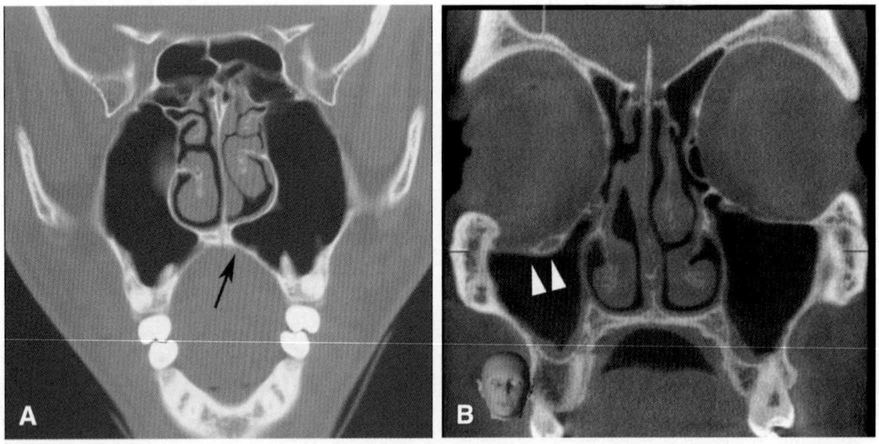

Fig. 26.2 (A) Pneumatization of the palatal process of the maxilla *(arrow)* by the maxillary sinus in a coronal multidetector computed tomographic image. (B) Coronal cone beam computed tomographic image of a patient with silent sinus syndrome. Note the inferiorly positioned floor of the right orbit *(arrowheads)* and the enlarged size of the orbit.

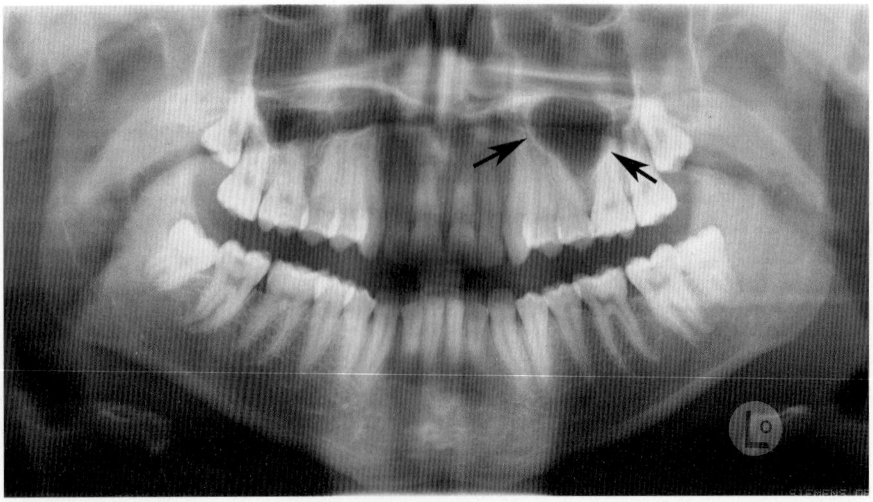

Fig. 26.3 Panoramic image of a locule *(arrows)* of the left maxillary sinus draping over the tooth roots, mimicking a benign space-occupying lesion.

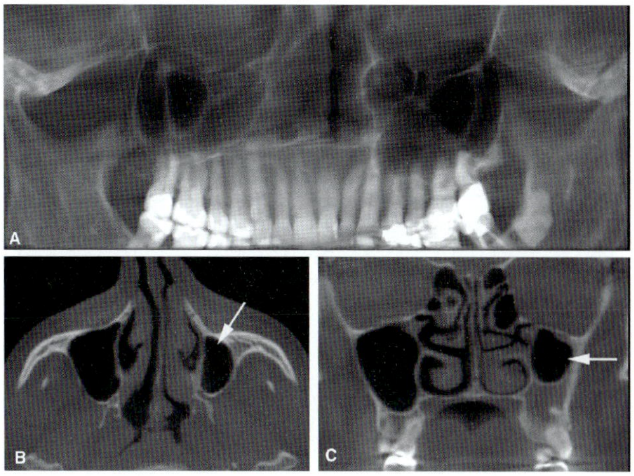

Fig. 26.4 (A) Panoramic reconstruction showing right-sided maxillary sinus hypoplasia. (B) Axial and (C) coronal cone beam computed tomographic images demonstrating a hypoplastic left maxillary sinus *(arrows)*.

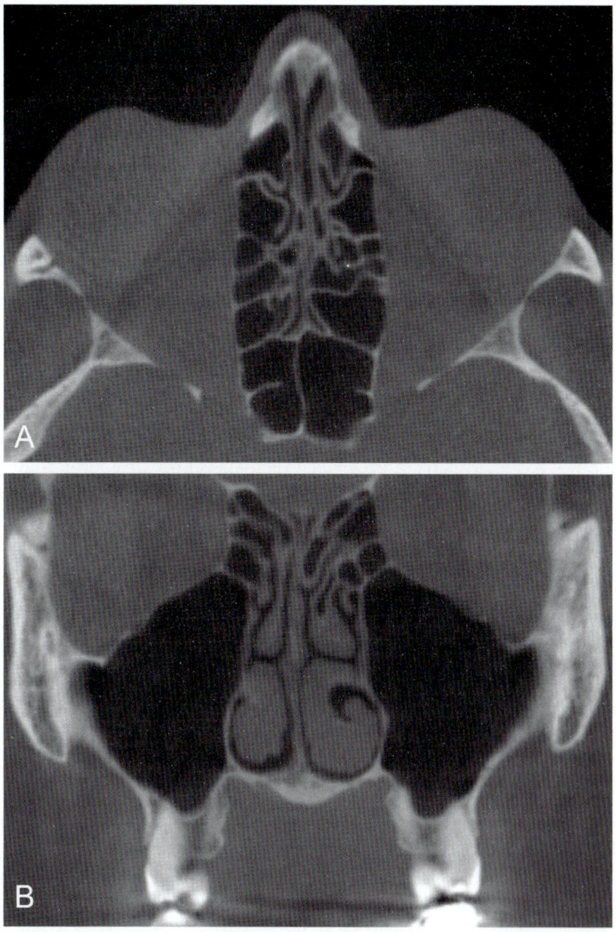

Fig. 26.5 (A) Axial cone beam computed tomographic image of normal ethmoid and sphenoid sinuses. (B) Coronal cone beam computed tomographic image of normal maxillary and ethmoid sinuses.

Haller cells or infraorbital ethmoid air cells. The total number of air cells varies considerably, with each ethmoid bone containing 8–15 cells. In some cases, the ethmoid air cells may encroach into the neighboring maxillary, lacrimal, frontal, sphenoid, and palatine bones.

The function of the paranasal sinuses has been controversial. Some authorities believe the role of the paranasal sinuses is to insulate and protect deeper vital structures from external trauma. Others have cited a possible role of the sinuses in the humidification and warming of inspired air or in the overall lightening of the weight of the skull bones. More recently, the epithelium of the paranasal sinuses has been shown to play an important role in upper airway nitric oxide (•NO) production, which may have both a local antimicrobial effect and a downstream role of pulmonary vasodilation and improved blood oxygen exchange.

DISEASES OF THE PARANASAL SINUSES

The maxillary sinuses are of greatest concern to the dentist because of their proximity to the teeth and supporting structures. Therefore, the emphasis in this chapter is on diseases related to the maxillary sinus.

Definition

Diseases associated with the maxillary sinuses include those originating primarily from tissues within the sinus (intrinsic diseases) and those originating outside the sinus (commonly of odontogenic origin) that either impinge on or infiltrate the sinus (extrinsic diseases).

Clinical Features

The clinical signs and symptoms of maxillary sinus disease include pain and a sensation of pressure, altered voice characteristics, pain with head movement, percussion sensitivity of the teeth, regional dysesthesia, paresthesia or anesthesia, and swelling and tenderness of the facial structures adjacent to the maxilla.

Applied Diagnostic Imaging

When maxillary sinus disease is suspected, it may be reasonable for the dentist to proceed with an initial radiologic investigation. A periapical image provides a detailed view of the periapical structures of the teeth and their relationships to the alveolar recess and floor of the maxillary antrum. If an abnormality is suspected, a panoramic radiograph image depicts a greater region of the sinus as well as parts of the inferior, posterior, and anteromedial walls. In some cases, it may be difficult to compare the floors of the right and left sinuses on a panoramic image because of the superimposition of adjacent anatomic structures or ghost images. If there are positive findings, consultation with an oral and maxillofacial radiologist should be considered to determine the need for additional imaging and for appropriate interpretation of the radiologic finding.

Advanced imaging has become increasingly important in the evaluation and management of complicated sinus disease such as in cases of chronic or recurrent sinusitis, odontogenic diseases encroaching on the sinus, or when cysts or neoplasms are suspected to be present. In such cases, CBCT and MDCT depict sinus anatomy, delineate the extent and character of the disease process, and establish or eliminate a possible odontogenic etiology.

Coronal CBCT and MDCT images, in particular, provide superior visualization of the ostiomeatal complex (the region of the ostia of the maxillary sinus and ethmoid air cells) and nasal cavities and demonstrate any reaction in the adjacent bone to sinus disease. MRI provides superior visualization of the soft tissues, especially the extension of neoplasms developing within or infiltrating into the sinuses or surrounding soft tissues or the differentiation of retained fluid secretions from soft tissue masses in the sinuses.

INTRINSIC DISEASES OF THE PARANASAL SINUSES

This section describes abnormalities that originate from tissues within the sinuses.

Inflammatory Disease

Inflammation may result from various causes, such as infection, chemical irritation, allergy, introduction of a foreign body, or facial trauma. These conditions can produce thickening of the sinus mucosa, which can be captured on imaging. Viral infections may, however, not produce any imaging change to a sinus.

Mucositis

Disease mechanism. The mucosal lining of the paranasal sinuses is normally less than 1 mm thick and cannot be visualized on imaging. However, when the mucosa becomes thickened due to inflammation, it may increase in thickness 10–15 times, and this may be seen with imaging. Localized inflammatory change is referred to as mucositis.

Clinical features. Many patients may be unaware of a change to their sinus mucosa, and these changes are often discovered as incidental findings on images made for other purposes. Consequently, the discovery of thickened mucosa in an individual who is otherwise asymptomatic does not imply that further investigations are warranted or that treatment is required.

Imaging features. Thickened mucosa is readily detectable on imaging as a well-defined, noncorticated radiopaque band of soft tissue density that conforms to the contour of the bony wall of the sinus (Fig. 26.6).

Rhinosinusitis

Disease mechanism. Rhinosinusitis is a generalized inflammatory condition of the mucosa of the sinuses and nasal cavity caused by an allergen, bacterium, or virus. Inflammatory changes may lead to ciliary dysfunction and the retention of sinus secretions, as well as, on occasion, blockage of the ostiomeatal complex (Fig. 26.7B). The term *pansinusitis* refers to rhinosinusitis with involvement of all the paranasal sinuses. In children with pansinusitis, the possibility of cystic fibrosis should be considered. Rhinosinusitis is often categorized as acute or chronic based on the length of time the disease has been present. If the disease has been present for 4 weeks or less, it is termed *acute rhinosinusitis.* If sinus disease has been present for more than 12 consecutive weeks, it is considered *chronic.* For rhinosinusitis lasting from more than 4 weeks up to 12 weeks, the term *subacute* may be used.

Clinical features. Acute rhinosinusitis is the most common of the sinus conditions that can cause pain and is often a complication of the common cold. After a few days, nasal congestion accompanied by a clear discharge can increase, and the patient may complain of pain and tenderness to pressure or swelling over the involved sinus. Pain may also be referred to the premolar and molar teeth on the affected side, and these teeth may develop sensitivity to percussion. In the case of a bacterial rhinosinusitis, a green or greenish-yellow discharge may accompany the other aforementioned signs and symptoms. In such circumstances, it is important that the dentition be ruled out as a possible source of the pain or infection.

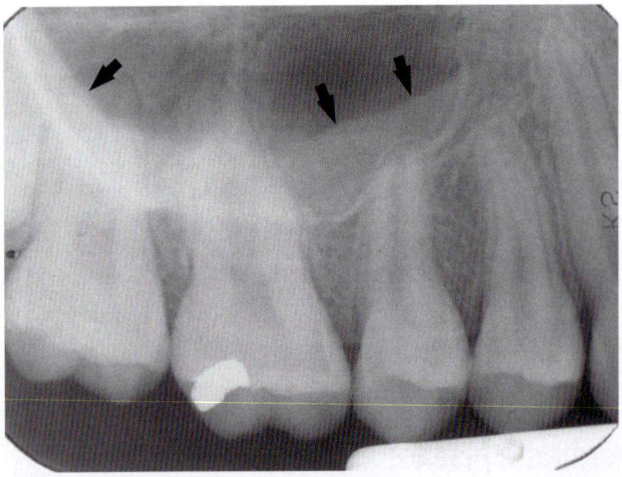

Fig. 26.6 Thickened sinus mucosa *(arrows)* is portrayed as a radiopaque ribbon of soft tissue that parallels the contour of the maxillary sinus floor.

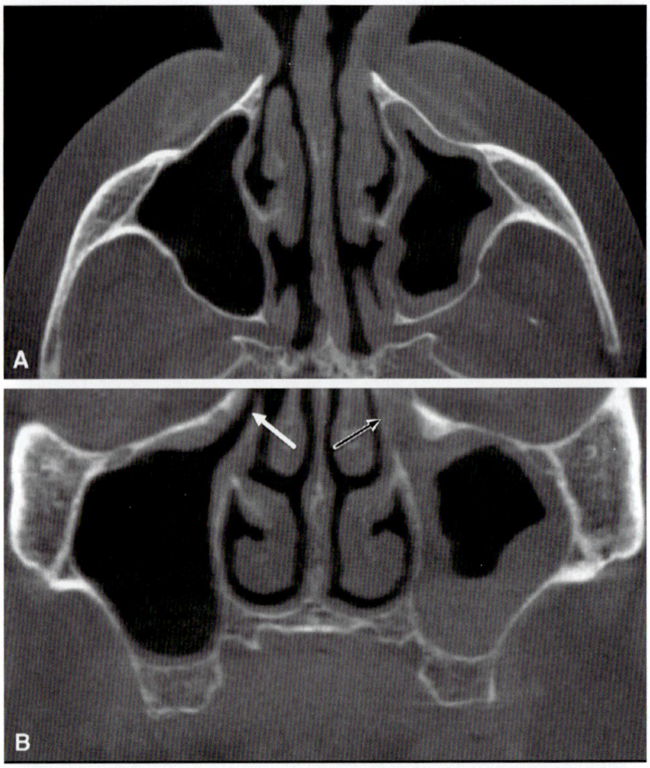

Fig. 26.7 (A) Axial cone beam computed tomographic image showing a circumferential pattern of mucosal thickening in the left maxillary sinus. (B) Coronal cone beam computed tomographic image of an obstructed ostiomeatal complex on the left side *(black and white arrow).* On the right side, the ostiomeatal complex is patent *(white arrow).*

Chronic maxillary rhinosinusitis is a sequela of an acute infection that fails to resolve by 12 weeks. Generally, no external signs occur except during periods of acute exacerbation, when increased pain and discomfort become apparent. Chronic rhinosinusitis may develop in association with anatomic derangements, including deviation of the nasal septum and the presence of concha bullosa (pneumatization of the middle concha), which inhibit the outflow of mucus. It may also occur secondary to allergic rhinitis, asthma, cystic fibrosis, and odontogenic infections.

Imaging features. Thickening of the sinus mucosa and the accumulation of secretions, both of which accompany rhinosinusitis, reduce the sinus airspace, and cause the sinus cavity to become increasingly radiopaque. The most common patterns are generalized thickening of the mucosal lining around the sinus cavity wall (Fig. 26.7) to nearly complete or complete radiopacification of the sinus (Fig. 26.8). Mucosal thickening, when present, may cause blockage of the sinus ostium (Fig. 26.7B). Mucosal thickening limited to the base of the sinus may not represent rhinosinusitis, particularly in asymptomatic patients. Rather, it may represent the more localized thickening or mucositis that is commonly found incidentally or can sometimes occur in association with rarefying osteitis from a maxillary posterior tooth. In the latter scenario, if the tooth is left untreated, the condition may progress to involve the entire sinus.

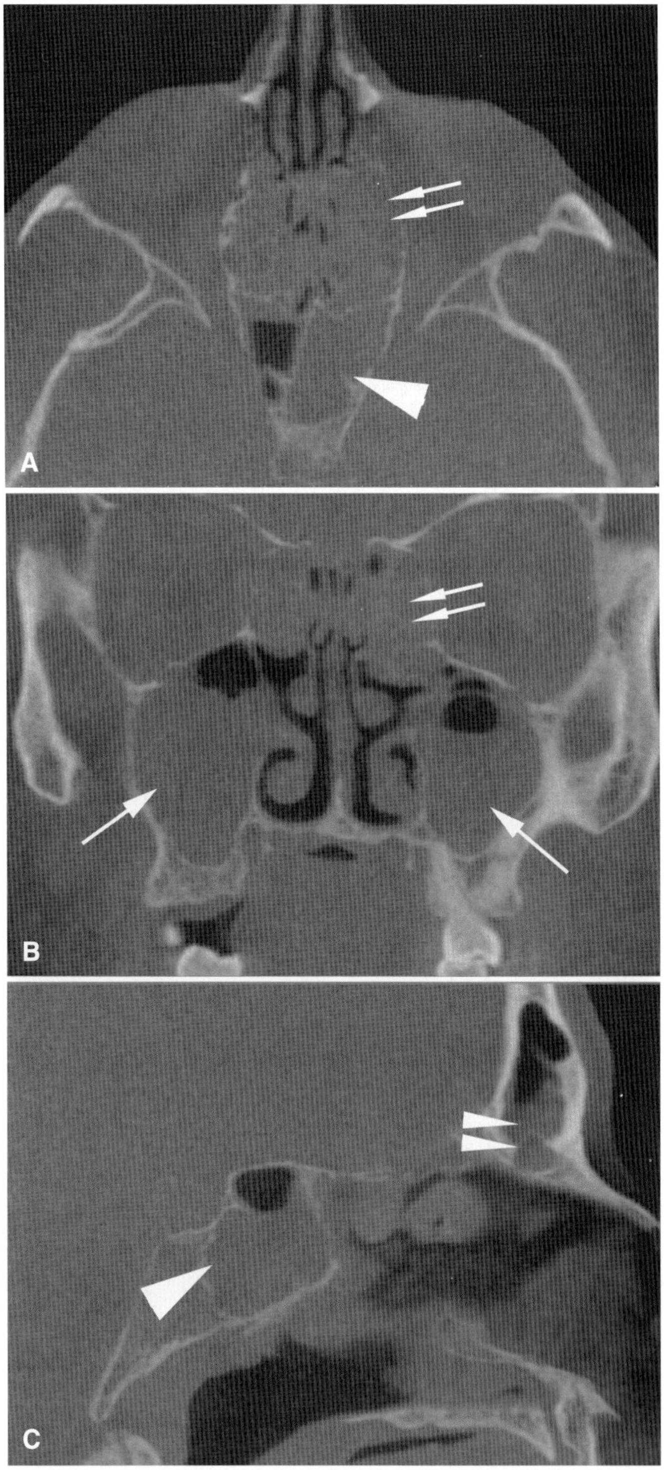

Fig. 26.8 (A) Axial, (B) coronal, and (C) sagittal cone beam computed tomographic images showing opacification of the maxillary *(arrows)*, ethmoid *(double arrows)*, sphenoid *(arrowheads)*, and frontal *(double arrowheads)* paranasal sinuses.

The image of thickened sinus mucosa may be uniform or polypoid. In the case of an allergic reaction, the mucosa tends to be more lobulated. In contrast, in cases of infection, the thickened mucosal outline tends to be smoother, with its contour following that of the sinus wall. The inability to perceive the delicate walls of the ethmoid air cells is a particularly sensitive sign of ethmoid sinusitis.

An air-fluid level resulting from the accumulation of secretions may also be present (Fig. 26.9). Because the radiopacities of transudates, exudates, blood, and pathologically altered mucosa are similar, differentiation among them relies on their shape and distribution. When present, fluid appears radiopaque and occupies the inferior or so-called dependent region of the sinus. The border between the radiopaque fluid and the relatively radiolucent air in the antrum is horizontal and straight, and a meniscus may be seen at the periphery where the fluid meets the sinus wall (see Fig. 26.9). Chronic rhinosinusitis may result in persistent opacification of the sinus with sclerosis and thickening of the bony walls as osteoblasts in the periosteum respond to inflammatory mediators and lay down new bone (Fig. 26.10).

Resolution of acute rhinosinusitis becomes apparent on the image as a gradual increase in the airspace within the sinus. This can first be recognized when a small clear area appears within the sinus; the thickened mucosa gradually thins until it begins to mirror the outline of the bony wall. In time, the image of the mucosa becomes invisible and the

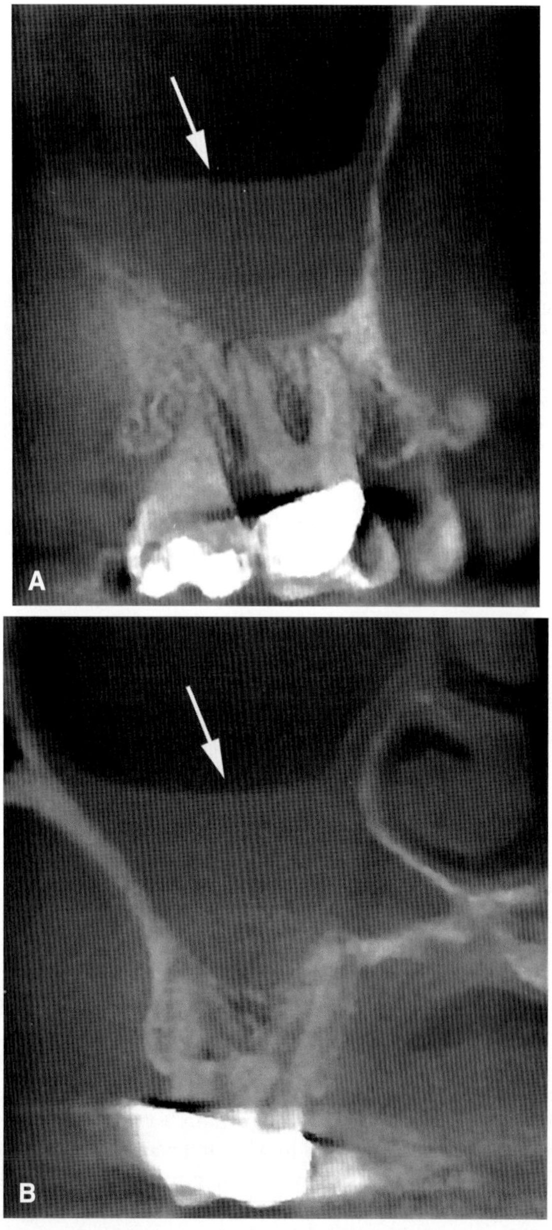

Fig 26.9 (A) Sagittal and (B) coronal cone beam computed tomographic images demonstrating an air-fluid level in the right maxillary sinus *(arrows)*.

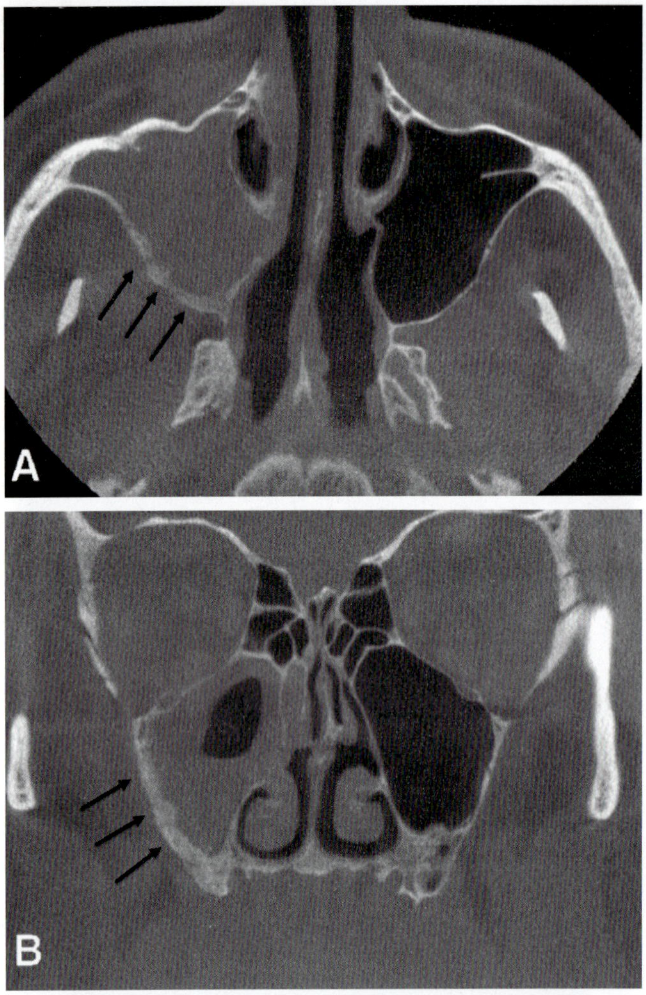

Fig. 26.10 Axial (A) and coronal (B) cone beam computed tomographic images show opacification of the lumen of the right maxillary sinus and bony thickening of the sinus walls *(arrows)* secondary to chronic rhinosinusitis.

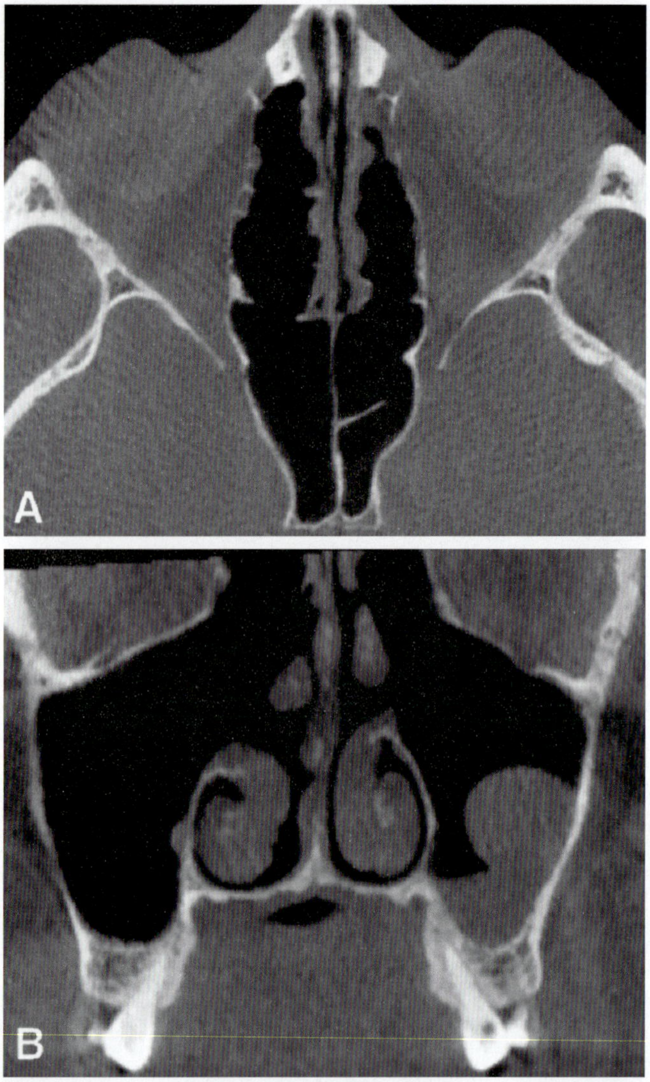

Fig. 26.11 (A) Axial cone beam computed tomographic image showing surgical changes from prior endoscopic sinus surgery, including bilateral ethmoidectomy (removal of the partitions between the ethmoid air cells to facilitate sinus drainage). (B) Coronal cone beam computed tomographic image on the same patient showing further changes of endoscopic sinus surgery, specifically bilateral maxillary antrostomy (enlargement of the maxillary ostium) and middle turbinectomy (reduction or removal of the turbinate).

sinus returns to a normal appearance. In chronic rhinosinusitis, the changes to the sinus wall may persist (Fig. 26.10).

Management. The treatment goals of rhinosinusitis are to control the infection, promote drainage, and relieve pain. Acute rhinosinusitis is usually treated pharmacologically with decongestants to reduce mucosal swelling and with antibiotics in the case of bacterial rhinosinusitis. Chronic rhinosinusitis is primarily a disease of obstruction of the ostia; therefore, the goal is ventilation and drainage. Endoscopic sinus surgery (ESS) is often performed to enlarge obstructed ostia or to establish an alternative path of drainage (Fig. 26.11).

Retention Pseudocyst

Disease mechanism. The term *retention pseudocyst* is used to describe several related conditions that result in the development of cyst-like lesions that lack an epithelial lining. The pathogenesis of these lesions is controversial, but because their clinical and imaging features are similar, no attempt is made to distinguish between them. As such, many synonyms have been used for this entity: antral pseudocyst, benign mucous cyst, mucous retention cyst, mucous retention pseudocyst, mesothelial cyst, pseudocyst, interstitial cyst, lymphangiectatic cyst, false cyst, retention cyst of the maxillary sinus, benign cyst of the antrum, benign mucosal cyst of the sinus, serous nonsecretory retention pseudocyst, and mucosal antral cyst.

One etiology suggests that blockage of the secretory ducts of seromucous glands in the sinus mucosa may result in a pathologic submucosal accumulation of secretions, resulting in swelling of the tissue. A second theory suggests that the serous nonsecretory retention pseudocyst arises as a result of cystic degeneration within an inflamed, thickened sinus lining.

Clinical features. Retention pseudocysts can be found in any of the sinuses at any time of the year, although they may occur more often in the early spring or fall. This occurrence suggests that the development of retention pseudocysts may be related to changes in seasonal allergies, colds, humidity, or temperature. Most studies have found that retention pseudocysts are more common in males.

A retention pseudocyst rarely causes any signs or symptoms, and the patient is usually unaware of the entity. It is often noticed as an incidental finding on images obtained for other purposes. Retention pseudocysts may range widely in size—from very small to a size large enough to fill the sinus cavity completely, making it appear radiopaque.

However, when a pseudocyst completely fills the maxillary sinus cavity, it may prolapse (extrude) through the ostium and cause nasal obstruction. The retention pseudocyst may also rupture as a result of abrupt pressure changes caused by sneezing or blowing of the nose, producing postnasal discharge. These symptoms may be the only clinical evidence of the presence of the retention pseudocyst. The retention pseudocyst may be present on an imaging examination of the maxillary sinus and be absent only a few days later, only to reappear on subsequent examinations.

The maxillary sinus is the most common site of retention pseudocysts, although these are found occasionally in the sphenoid sinus and less often in the frontal sinus and ethmoid air cells. Antral retention pseudocysts are not related to dental extractions or associated with periapical inflammatory disease.

Imaging features.

Location. Partial images of retention pseudocysts of the maxillary antrum may appear on maxillary posterior periapical images (Fig. 26.12A), but they are best demonstrated on views acquired extraorally (see Fig. 26.12B). One or more pseudocysts may occur within the same or different sinus cavities. Retention pseudocysts usually develop on the floor of the sinus (see Fig. 26.12A and B), although they may form on any wall or the roof, or they may fill most of the sinus cavity (see Fig. 26.12C–E).

Periphery. Retention pseudocysts usually appear as well-defined mostly sessile radiopaque masses that are noncorticated, smooth, and dome shaped. Because the lesion originates from within the sinus, it lacks a radiopaque corticated border.

Internal structure. The internal structure is homogeneous and more radiopaque than the surrounding air of the sinus cavity (see Fig. 26.12). The radiopacity of the lesion is caused by the accumulation of fluid in the soft tissue lining of the sinus together with the thickened mucosa, both of which are relatively more radiopaque than air.

Effects on adjacent structures. There are no effects on the surrounding structures. The adjacent sinus floor is always intact.

Effects on adjacent teeth. When a retention pseudocyst occurs adjacent to the root of a tooth, the lamina dura surrounding the root is intact and the width of the periodontal ligament space is unaffected.

Differential interpretation. It is important to distinguish retention pseudocysts from antral polyps or odontogenic cysts or neoplasms arising in the maxilla adjacent to the sinus. In contrast, the floor of the maxillary sinus may be displaced by a developing odontogenic cyst or neoplasm as the border of the lesion becomes coincident with the bony sinus floor. In some instances, periodic fenestrations can be seen through the bony sinus floor, depending on the growth rate or aggressiveness of the cyst or neoplasm. The retention pseudocyst is dome shaped but lacks the thin marginal radiopaque line representing the corticated border characteristic of an odontogenic cyst or neoplasm.

Antral polyps of infectious or allergic origin may be difficult to distinguish from retention pseudocysts, but when there is concurrent mucositis and multiple soft tissue masses, the possibility of polyps should be considered. Retention pseudocysts most often are not associated with thickened mucosal lining of the remaining sinus. Benign neoplasms may also mimic retention pseudocysts though are more

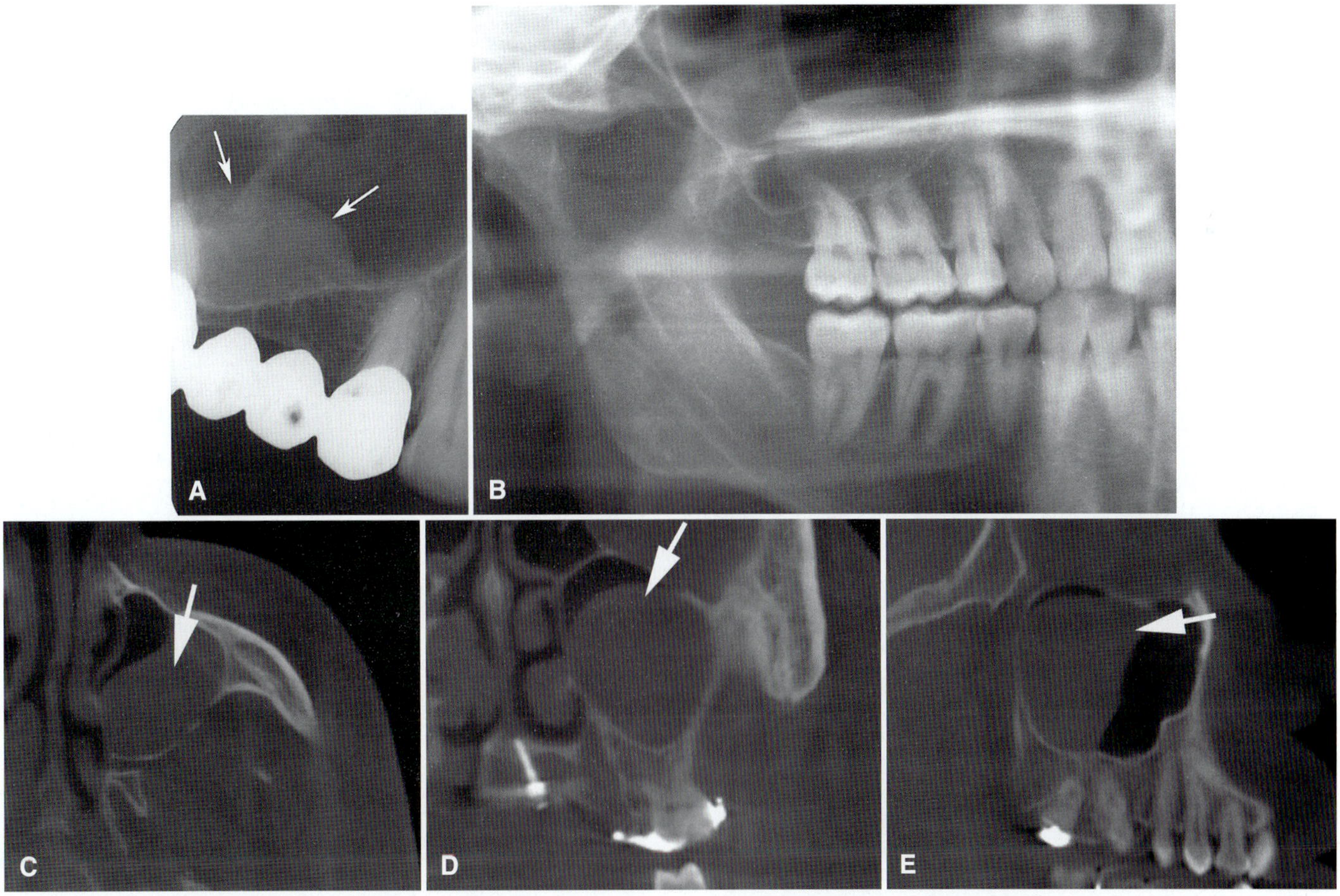

Fig. 26.12 Noncorticated dome-shaped retention pseudocysts *(arrows)* seen in periapical (A) and panoramic (B) images and axial (C), coronal (D), and sagittal (E) cone beam computed tomographic images. Retention pseudocysts have noncorticated borders, indicating that they arise from within the sinus. They can reach various sizes and can occupy most of the sinus cavity.

likely to demonstrate mass effect. If benign neoplasms originate from outside the sinus, they are separated from the cavity of the sinus by a radiopaque border, similar to odontogenic cysts. Malignant neoplasms may destroy the osseous border of the sinus, whether they arise from within the sinus or from the alveolar process. However, a malignant neoplasm is less likely to appear as dome shaped as a retention pseudocyst.

Management. Retention pseudocysts in the maxillary sinus require no treatment because they customarily resolve spontaneously without any residual effect on the antral mucosa.

Polyps

Disease mechanism. The chronically inflamed sinonasal mucosa frequently forms into irregular folds called *polyps*. Polyposis of the mucosa (Fig. 26.13) may develop in an isolated area or in many areas throughout the sinus and nasal cavity.

Clinical features. Polyps may cause displacement or destruction of bone. In the ethmoid air cells, polyps may cause destruction of the medial wall of the orbit (lamina papyracea of the ethmoid bone) and produce ipsilateral proptosis (protrusion of the globe of the eye).

Imaging features. A polyp may be differentiated from a retention pseudocyst on an image by noting that a polyp occurs with a thickened mucosal lining because the polypoid mass is no more than an accentuation of mucosal thickening. In the case of a retention pseudocyst, the adjacent mucosa is usually not apparent. If multiple retention pseudocysts are seen within a sinus, the possibility of sinus polyposis should be considered.

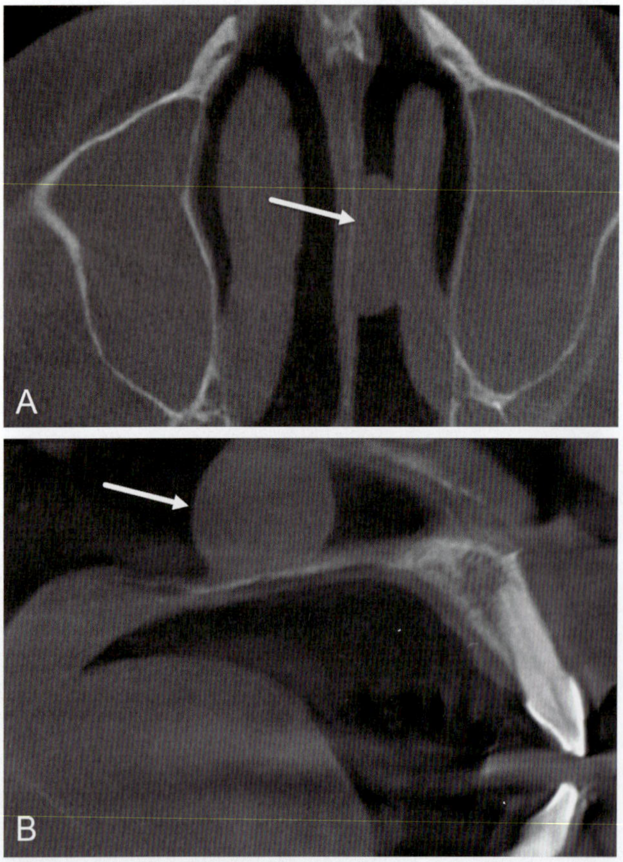

Fig. 26.13 Axial (A) and sagittal (B) cone beam computed tomographic images showing a nasal polyp medial to the inferior turbinate within the left nasal cavity *(arrows)*. Note the maxillary sinus opacification consistent with rhinosinusitis.

The image of the bone displacement or destruction associated with polyps may mimic a benign or malignant neoplasm. Because many sinus neoplasms are asymptomatic, examination of a paranasal sinus that reveals bone destruction associated with a soft tissue mass is an indication for additional imaging and biopsy; management should not be delayed by initial conservative treatment.

Antrolith

Disease mechanism. Antroliths occur within the maxillary sinuses and are the result of the deposition of mineral salts—such as calcium phosphate, calcium carbonate, and magnesium—around a nidus. An antrolith may be intrinsic when masses of stagnant or inspissated mucus or cellular debris collect at sites of previous inflammation. Alternatively, an antrolith may be extrinsic when extrinsic material is introduced into the sinus.

Clinical features. Small antroliths are usually asymptomatic and discovered incidentally on an imaging examination done for another purpose. If they continue to enlarge, the patient may have associated rhinosinusitis, a blood-stained nasal discharge, nasal obstruction, or facial pain.

Imaging features.

Location. Antroliths occur within the maxillary sinus above the floor of the maxillary antrum in either periapical, panoramic, or CBCT images that include the maxillary sinuses (Fig. 26.14).

Periphery. Antroliths have a well-defined periphery and may have a smooth or irregular shape.

Internal structure. The internal pattern may vary from a barely perceptible radiopacity to an extremely radiopaque structure. The internal radiopacity may be homogeneous or heterogeneous. In some

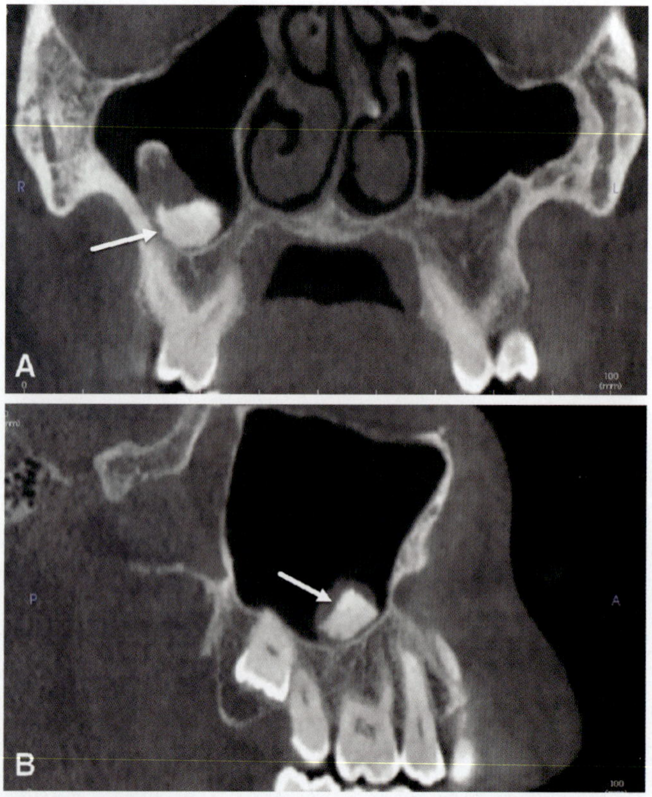

Fig. 26.14 (A) Coronal, and (B) sagittal cone beam computed tomographic images showing an amorphous radiopacity of homogenous attenuation near the floor of the right maxillary sinus embedded in an area of localized mucositis *(arrows)*.

instances, alternating layers of concentric radiolucency and radiopacity in the form of laminations may be seen.

Differential interpretation. Antroliths may be distinguished from root fragments in the sinus by inspection of the mass for the usual root anatomy, such as the presence of a root canal. Unless it is lodged between the bone and the sinus lining, a displaced root fragment in the sinus may move when imaging is performed with the head in different positions. Rhinoliths are similar calcifications found within the nasal fossae.

Management. An otolaryngologist may have to remove symptomatic antroliths.

Mucocele

Disease mechanism. A mucocele is an expanding, destructive lesion that results from a blocked sinus ostium. The blockage may result from intraantral or intranasal inflammation, polyp, odontogenic cyst, or neoplasm, and the entire sinus becomes the pathologic cavity. As the air cavity accumulates mucous secretions and fills, the increase in pressure within the cavity results in thinning and displacement of the sinus walls and, in some cases, sinus wall destruction. When the cavity is filled with pus, it is termed an empyema, pyocele, or mucopyocele.

Clinical features. A mucocele in the maxillary sinus may exert pressure on the superior alveolar nerves and cause radiating pain. The patient may first complain of a sensation of fullness in the cheek, and the area may swell. This swelling may first become apparent over the anteroinferior aspect of the antrum—the area where the wall is thin or destroyed. If the lesion expands inferiorly, it may cause loosening of the adjacent posterior teeth. If the medial wall of the sinus is expanded, the lateral wall of the nasal cavity deforms and the nasal airway may become obstructed. If the lesion expands into the orbit, it may cause diplopia (double vision) or proptosis.

Imaging features.

Location. About 90% of mucoceles occur in the ethmoid air cells and frontal sinuses; they are rarely found in the maxillary and sphenoid sinuses.

Periphery. The normal shape of the sinus is changed into a more circular, "hydraulic" shape as the mucocele enlarges.

Internal structure. Internally, the air cavity is uniformly radiopaque (Fig. 26.15).

Effects on adjacent structures. The shape of the sinus changes as its borders are displaced outward and the bone expands. Septa and the bony walls may be severely thinned. When the mucocele is associated with the maxillary antrum, teeth may be displaced or roots resorbed. In the frontal sinus, border scalloping is lost due to the expanding mucocele, and any septa may be displaced. The superomedial border of the orbit may be displaced or destroyed. In the ethmoid air cells, displacement of the lamina papyracea may occur, displacing the contents of the orbit. In the sphenoid sinus, the sinus border may expand in a superior direction.

Differential interpretation. Although it may be impossible to distinguish between a mucocele in the maxillary antrum and a cyst or neoplasm, any suggestion that the lesion is associated with an occluded ostium should strengthen the likelihood of a mucocele. Blockage of the ostium is usually the result of a previous surgical procedure, although a deviated nasal septum or polyps may be a factor. A large odontogenic cyst displacing the maxillary sinus floor may mimic a mucocele. One should look for any remnants of an airspace between the wall of the cyst and the walls of the antrum. CBCT or MDCT is the imaging method of choice for making these distinctions.

Management. Treatment of the mucocele is usually surgical through a transnasal endoscopic or a Caldwell-Luc approach to allow excision of the lesion. The prognosis is excellent.

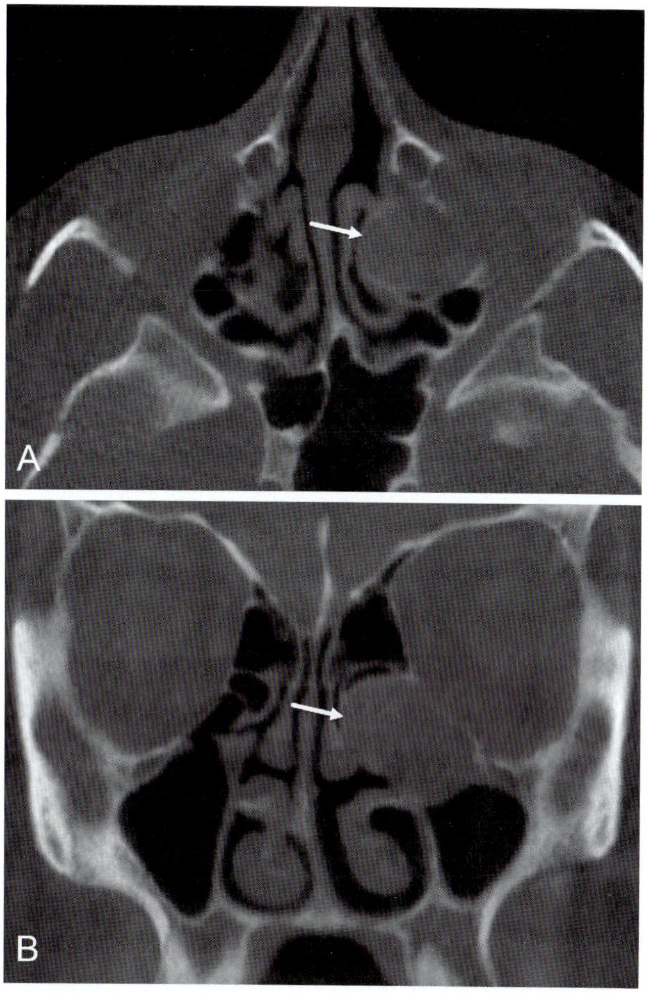

Fig. 26.15 (A) Axial and (B) coronal cone beam computed tomographic images demonstrating a mucocele within a left anterior ethmoid air cell *(arrows)*. Note the opacification and expansion of the air cell and its encroachment upon the superior aspect of the left maxillary sinus lumen.

Fungus Balls

Disease mechanism. Fungus balls are considered a noninvasive form of mycosis and are commonly referred to as fungal rhinosinusitis, aspergillosis, or mycetoma. They develop from the entrapment and growth of fungal hyphae and spores within the sinus and are associated with abnormal function of mucosal cilia. *Aspergillus fumigatus, Aspergillus flavus, Alternaria* spp., and *Pseudallescheria boydii* are the most common associated fungi. Interestingly, the presence of fungus balls in the maxillary sinus has been associated with endodontic treatment of maxillary teeth and the use of zinc containing endodontic sealers.

Clinical features. Usually, fungus balls are seen in older individuals (60–70 years of age), although the age range is wide (28–86 years). They usually affect only one sinus and are more commonly found in the maxillary and less frequently in the sphenoid sinuses. The symptoms are similar to those of chronic rhinosinusitis and include nasal discharge, pain, and nasal obstruction. Sometimes, the patient may be asymptomatic and the diagnosis may be an incidental finding.

Imaging features.

Location. Fungus balls usually affect the maxillary sinuses and, less commonly, the sphenoid sinus. The ethmoid air cells may be affected by extension of the maxillary sinus disease.

Periphery. Fungus balls may cause partial or complete opacification of the maxillary sinus (Fig. 26.16). Thickening of the anterior, lateral, and posterior walls of the affected sinus is commonly seen.

Internal structure. Most of the sinus demonstrates a uniform opacification with soft tissue density. Central, focal areas of increased attenuation may be visible within the fungus ball, representing calcified fungal debris, hyphae, or heavy metal metabolites (Fig. 26.16).

Effects on adjacent structures. Erosion of the medial wall of the maxillary sinus with extension of the mass into the nasal cavity may occur. Thickening of the other involved sinus walls is often present.

Differential interpretation. The differential interpretation of fungus balls includes other forms of rhinosinusitis or a mucocele. The presence of central, internal calcifications, and/or hyperintense areas on imaging aids in the diagnosis. The presence of fungi is confirmed by biopsy.

Management. Treatment usually involves the surgical removal of the fungus ball via ESS and includes reestablishment of sinus drainage by middle meatus antrostomy.

Neoplasms

Benign neoplasms of the paranasal sinuses are rare. The imaging features of such benign neoplasms are nonspecific. The involved portion of the sinus cavity appears radiopaque because of the presence of a mass, and there may be displacement of adjacent sinus borders.

The most common malignant neoplasms of the paranasal sinuses are squamous cell carcinoma and, to a lesser extent, malignant salivary gland neoplasms. Of all carcinomas that originate in the paranasal sinuses, 74% arise in the maxillary sinus. Although sinus opacification is a feature of both inflammatory conditions and neoplasms, bone destruction is more common with malignant neoplasms.

Benign Neoplasms of the Paranasal Sinuses

Inverted Papilloma

Disease mechanism. Inverted papilloma is a rare neoplasm of respiratory epithelium that originates in the nasal cavity and often extends into the adjacent paranasal sinuses. It occurs predominantly in men.

Clinical features. Unilateral nasal obstruction, nasal discharge, pain, and epistaxis may occur. The patient may have complained of recurring rhinosinusitis for years, and subsequent nasal obstruction on the same side as the rhinosinusitis may develop. The inverted papilloma, although benign, has a 10% incidence of malignant transformation.

Imaging features. Imaging features are nonspecific; the diagnosis can be made only by histopathologic examination of the tissue.

Location. The inverted papilloma may appear as an isolated polyp in the nose. However, it commonly extends to and involves the maxillary sinus or ethmoid air cells.

Internal structure. This neoplasm appears as a homogeneous radiopaque mass of soft tissue density.

Effects on adjacent structures. If bone destruction is apparent, it is the result of pressure erosion.

Osteoma

Disease mechanism. The osteoma is the most common mesenchymal neoplasm in the paranasal sinuses. For a detailed description, see Chapter 22.

Clinical features. Osteomas are almost twice as common in males than females and typically arise in the second, third, and fourth decades. Most are slow growing, self limiting, and asymptomatic and are usually detected incidentally in an examination performed for another purpose. However, some lesions may demonstrate greater growth potential and cause obstruction of the ostiomeatal complex, bone erosion

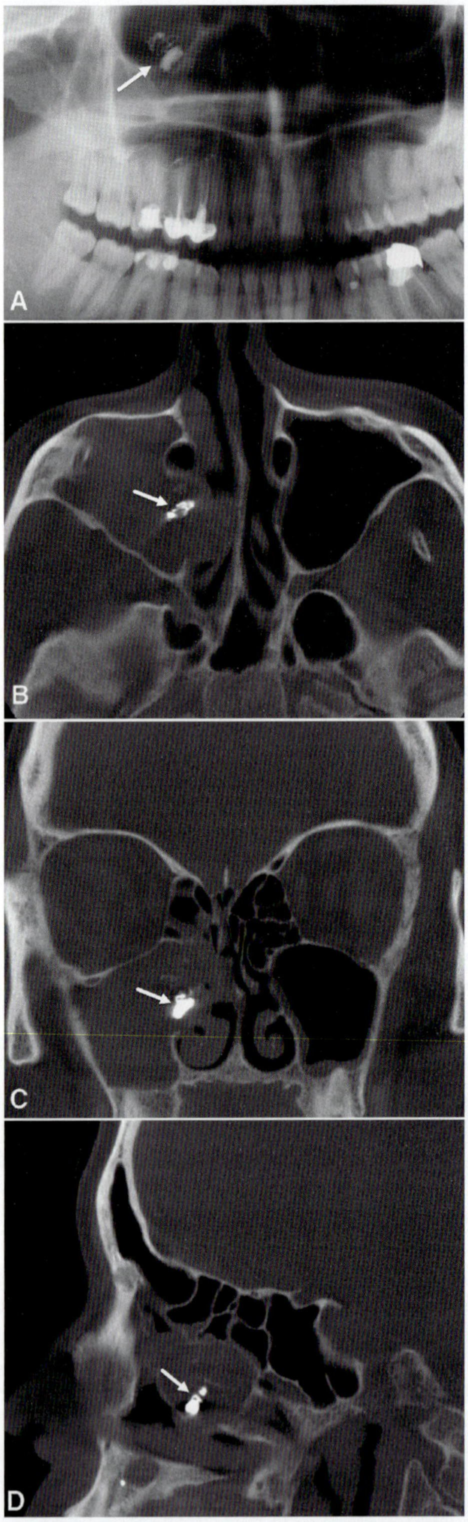

Fig. 26.16 (A) Panoramic image showing generalized opacification of the right maxillary sinus relative to the left side. Additionally, discrete radiopacities, suggestive of calcified material, are noted in the superior aspect of the sinus lumen *(arrow)*. Axial (B), coronal (C), and sagittal (D) cone beam computed tomographic images of the same patient demonstrating complete radiopacification of the right maxillary sinus, erosion of the medial wall of the maxillary sinus, and extension of the lesion into the nasal cavity. Furthermore, the discrete radiopacities previously seen on the panoramic radiograph now appear to have a metal-like attenuation, consistent with calcified fungal debris and heavy metal metabolites in a patient with a fungus ball.

and deformity, orbital involvement or intracranial extension. Osteomas growing in the maxillary sinus may extend into the nose and cause nasal obstruction or swelling of the side of the nose. They may also expand the sinus and produce swelling of the cheek or hard palate. In cases extending to the orbit, the patient may have proptosis.

Imaging features.

Location. Osteomas more often occur in the frontal sinus and ethmoid air cells and are less frequent in the maxillary sinus. The incidence in the maxillary antrum ranges from 3.9% to 28.5% of the incidence in all paranasal sinuses.

Periphery. An osteoma is usually round or lobulated and has a well-defined border (Fig. 26.17).

Internal structure. The internal pattern is homogeneous and extremely radiopaque.

Differential interpretation. The differential interpretation includes an antrolith, mycolith, tooth, odontome, or odontogenic neoplasm, although these entities are usually not as homogeneous in appearance as an osteoma.

Malignant Neoplasms of the Paranasal Sinuses

Malignant neoplasms of the paranasal sinuses are exceptionally rare, accounting for less than 1% of all malignancies in the body. Squamous cell carcinoma accounts for 80%–90% of the cancers in this site and is the most common primary malignant neoplasm of the paranasal sinuses. Other primary neoplasms include adenocarcinoma, carcinomas of salivary gland origin, soft and hard tissue sarcomas, melanoma, and lymphoma. Factors that contribute to a poor prognosis for cancers of the paranasal sinuses include the advanced stage of the disease when it is finally diagnosed and the close proximity to vital anatomic structures.

The clinical signs and symptoms of a sinus malignancy may masquerade as inflammatory rhinosinusitis. An early primary lesion may appear only as a soft tissue mass in the sinus before it causes bone destruction. The lesion may become extensive, involving the entire sinus, with evidence of bone destruction before symptoms become apparent. Therefore, any suggestion of bone erosion or destruction involving the paranasal sinuses should be investigated thoroughly.

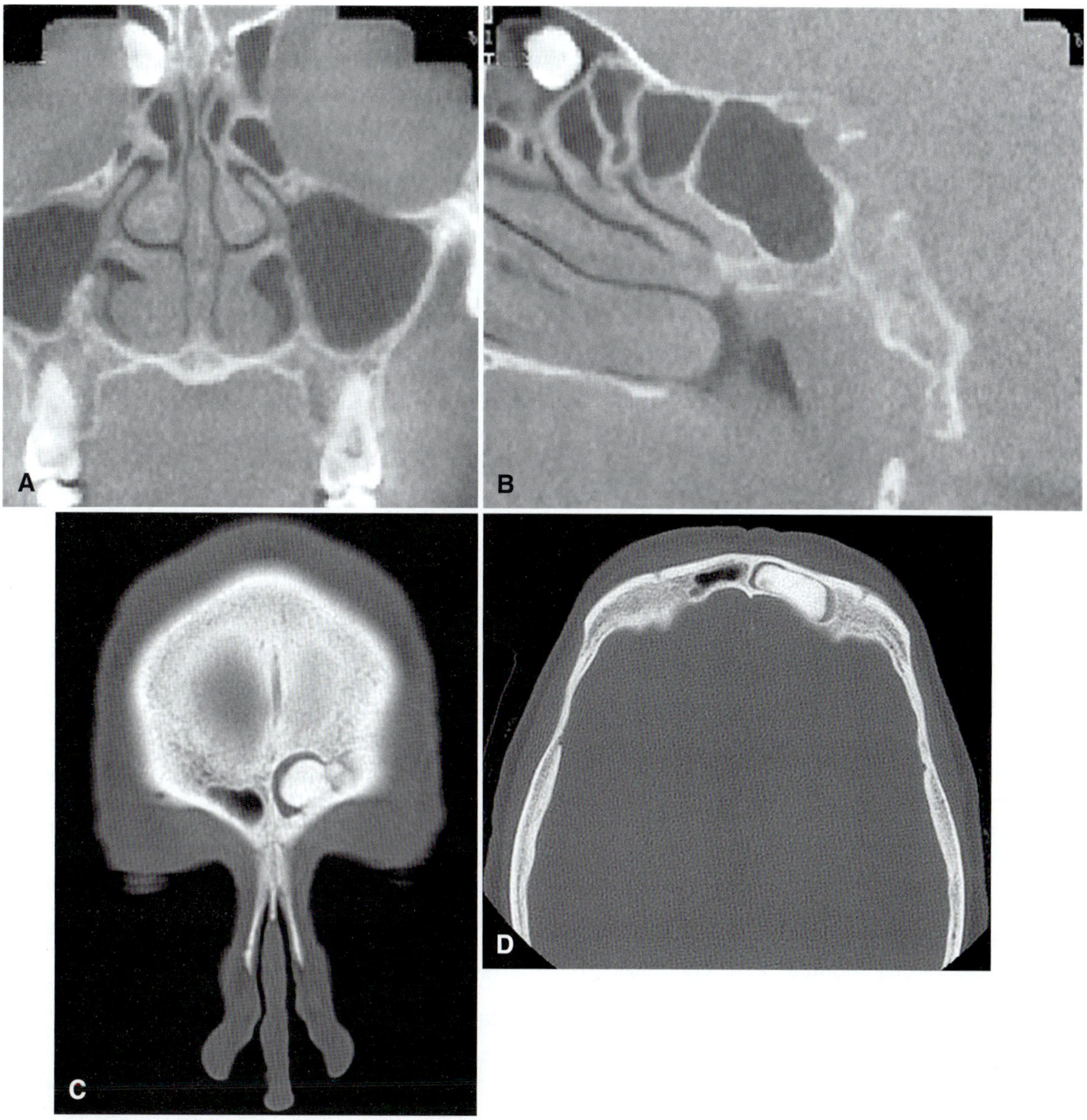

Fig. 26.17 Coronal (A) and sagittal (B) cone beam computed tomographic images show an osteoma attached to the lateral wall of an anterior ethmoid air cell. Coronal (C) and axial (D) computed tomography images of an osteoma in the frontal sinus. (Courtesy Dr. E. Yu, Toronto, ON.)

Squamous Cell Carcinoma

Disease mechanism. Squamous cell carcinoma originates from cells in the epithelium of the sinus mucosa.

Clinical features. The most common symptoms of cancer in the maxillary sinus are facial swelling, epistaxis, dysesthesia, paresthesia, nasal obstruction, and the presence of a lesion in the oral cavity. The mean patient age is 60 years (range, 25–89 years). Twice as many men are affected than women. Lymph nodes are involved in about 10% of cases, and symptoms are present for approximately 5 months before diagnosis.

The symptoms produced by malignant neoplasms in the maxillary sinus depend on which wall of the sinus is involved. The medial wall is usually the first to become eroded, leading to nasal signs and symptoms such as obstruction, discharge, bleeding, and pain. These symptoms may appear trivial and their significance may be unappreciated. Lesions that arise on the floor of the sinus may first produce dental signs and symptoms, including unexplained pain or altered sensation of the teeth, loose teeth, expansion or swelling of the palate or alveolar process, and ill-fitting dentures. The neoplasm may erode the sinus floor and penetrate the oral cavity. Such oral manifestations appear in 25%–35% of patients with malignancies developing in the maxillary sinus. When the lesion penetrates the lateral wall, facial and vestibular swelling becomes apparent, and the patient may complain of pain and hyperesthesia of the maxillary teeth. Involvement of the sinus roof and the floor of the orbit causes signs and symptoms related to the eye. These may include diplopia, proptosis, hyperesthesia or anesthesia, and pain over the cheek and maxillary teeth. Invasion through the posterior wall of the antrum can lead to the involvement of the muscles of mastication, causing painful trismus and obstruction of the eustachian tube, resulting in a "stuffy ear." It may also cause referred pain and hyperesthesia over the distribution of the second and third divisions of the fifth cranial nerve.

Imaging features. Sometimes the imaging findings, especially in the early stages of malignant disease of the paranasal sinuses, are nonspecific. It may be impossible to differentiate the early manifestations in images of the maxillary sinus from the radiopacity of the sinus that develops in rhinosinusitis and polyp formation. Evidence relies on changes seen in the surrounding bone, the sinus walls, and the alveolar process.

Location. Most carcinomas occur in the maxillary sinuses, but involvement of the frontal and sphenoid sinuses is also comparatively common.

Internal structure. The internal structure of the maxillary sinus has a soft tissue radiopaque appearance.

Effects on adjacent structures. As the lesion enlarges, it may destroy sinus walls and, in general, cause irregular radiolucent areas in the surrounding bone. A detailed examination of the adjacent alveolar process may reveal bone destruction around the teeth. Frequently the medial wall of the maxillary sinus is thinned or destroyed, although there may also be destruction of the floor or other walls of the sinus. Destruction of the borders of the nasal cavity may also be present. These findings may be detected on panoramic images or periapical images, which encompass the maxillary sinus floor.

Effects on adjacent teeth. A detailed examination of the adjacent alveolar process may reveal irregular widening of the periodontal ligament space and loss of lamina dura.

Additional imaging. If planar imaging of any radiopacified sinus reveals the slightest suggestion of bone destruction, advanced imaging such as CBCT, MDCT, or MRI is imperative (Fig. 26.18). CBCT imaging can confirm the presence and extent of bony destruction and the overall suspicion of malignancy. MDCT and MRI, both offer soft tissue information and are excellent modalities to detect potential invasion of adjacent soft tissue spaces; a hallmark sign of malignancy. Of all imaging modalities, MRI offers the greatest soft tissue detail and is the ideal modality to define the soft tissue extent of paranasal sinus neoplasms, including any involvement of the orbit, infratemporal fossa, or cranial cavity. This information is often critical for the appropriate staging, prognosis, and treatment planning of a malignant neoplasm.

Differential interpretation. The differential interpretation includes all the conditions that may cause radiopacity of the antrum, such as rhinosinusitis, a large retention pseudocyst, and odontogenic cysts or tumors. Bone destruction may also occur in infectious conditions and some benign conditions. A neoplasm should be suspected in any older patient in whom chronic rhinosinusitis develops for the first time without an obvious cause.

Management. Treatment of squamous cell carcinoma in the paranasal sinuses may include radiation therapy, surgery, or a combination of these. Malignant neoplasms in the paranasal sinuses usually have a poor prognosis because they tend to be well advanced by the time of diagnosis. Other factors contributing to the poor prognosis include frequently inaccurate preoperative staging and the complex anatomy of the region.

Pseudotumor

Disease mechanism. *Pseudotumor* is a generic term applied to any nonspecific, chronic inflammatory expansile lesion, which clinically and radiographically simulates a neoplasm. Alternatively, this has been referred to as an inflammatory pseudotumor, plasmocytic cell granuloma, fibroinflammatory pseudotumor, inflammatory myofibroblastic tumor, fibroblastoma, xanthogranuloma, and plasma cell granuloma. These are generally composed of a large number of plasma cells, lymphocytes, fibroblasts, histiocytes, and eosinophils. Although the exact etiopathogenesis is unknown, and as reflected in the multitude of synonyms, the lesion is considered an exaggerated inflammatory reaction.

Clinical features. Pseudotumor often occurs after a series of recurrent infections. The symptoms may not be very specific. There may be recurring pain and a mass simulating a neoplasm. The latter may cause erosion of the walls of the involved sinus and proptosis if the orbit is involved. Altered nerve function resulting from involvement of a nerve or occlusion of blood vessels by the mass has also been reported. Although cases have been documented in otherwise healthy individuals, in many instances, patients may be immunocompromised or have systemic diseases, such as diabetes mellitus, von Willebrand disease, or myelodysplasia.

Imaging features. The imaging findings in pseudotumor include masses simulating malignant neoplasms that cause erosion of bony walls of the involved sinuses.

Differential interpretation. The differential interpretation includes benign and malignant neoplasms.

Management. The treatment of pseudotumor, which can include debridement of the sinuses by a Caldwell-Luc surgical approach or pharmacologic management (e.g., corticosteroid), reflects differences in etiopathogenesis of the specific lesions included under the term *pseudotumor of the sinuses*, the exact location of the disease, the organism involved, and the medical status of the patient.

EXTRINSIC DISEASES INVOLVING THE PARANASAL SINUSES

Inflammatory Diseases

Perhaps 10% of inflammatory episodes of the maxillary sinuses develop as a result of dental infections, often referred to as odontogenic sinusitis. Inflammatory lesions such as periodontal disease or periapical inflammatory disease may cause a localized mucositis in the adjacent floor of the maxillary antrum. This mucositis that develops is a result of the inflammatory mediators diffusing beyond the floor of the antrum,

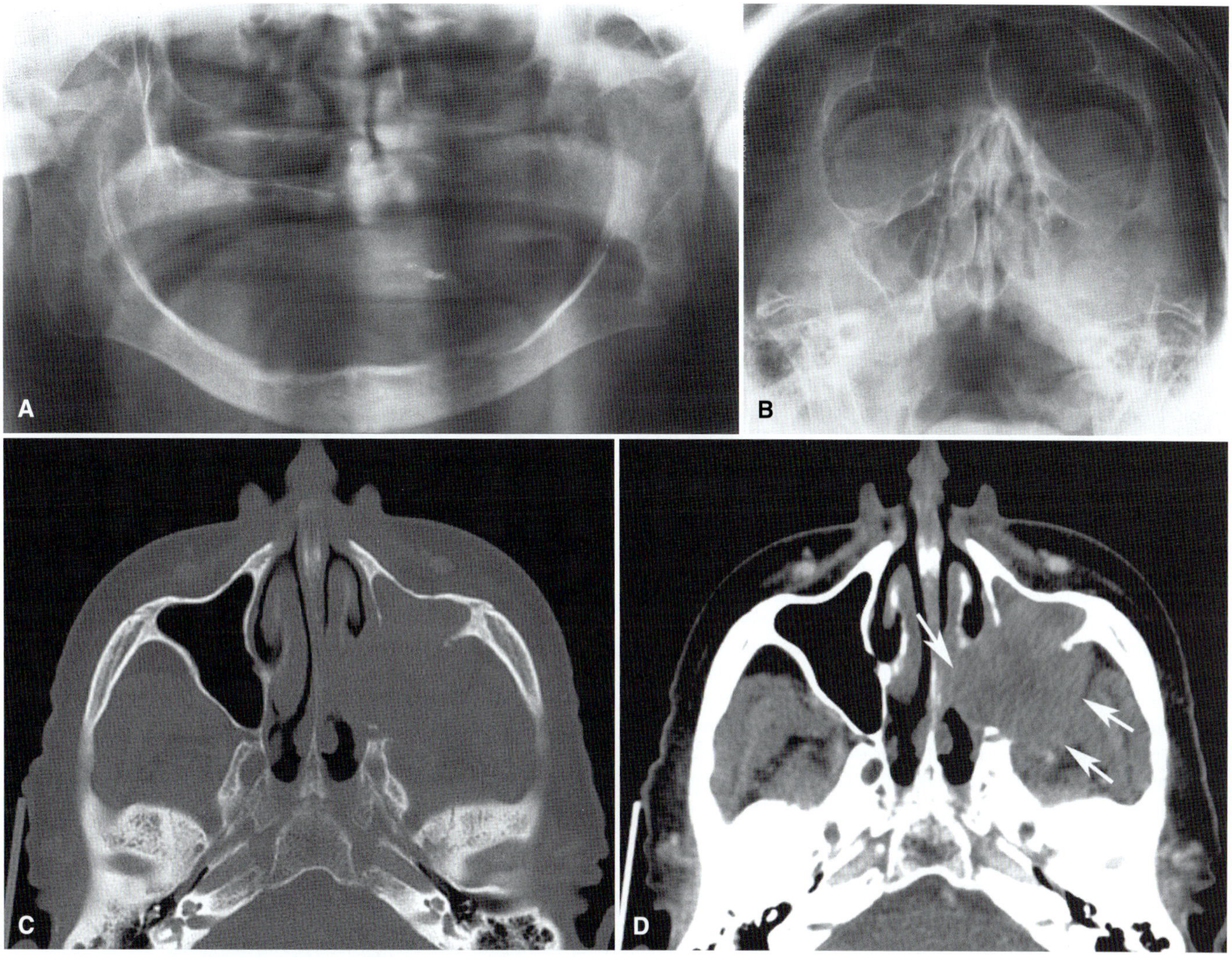

Fig. 26.18 (A) Panoramic image of a squamous cell carcinoma shows loss of definition of the cortex of the left maxillary sinus, nasal floor, and alveolar crest. (B) Water view of the same patient shows a similar loss of cortical integrity to the lateral wall of the left maxilla and opacification of the left maxillary sinus. (C) Axial bone algorithm multidetector computed tomographic image of a squamous cell carcinoma of the left maxillary sinus shows destruction of the posterolateral and medial walls of the sinus. (D) Same axial image slice with soft tissue algorithm demonstrates extension of the malignant neoplasm into the surrounding soft tissues *(arrows)*. (B, Courtesy Dr. K. Dolan, Iowa City, IA.)

into the periosteum and the mucosal lining of the sinus. This latter change can manifest as a homogeneous radiopaque, ribbon-like thickening of the soft tissue that follows the contour of the maxillary sinus (Fig. 26.6), and usually resolves in days or weeks after successful treatment of the underlying cause. The thickened mucosa is usually centered immediately superior to the inflammatory lesion.

Periosteal New Bone Formation

Disease mechanism. As previously described, the exudate from an inflammatory lesion can diffuse through the cortical boundary of the antral floor. These products can strip and elevate the periosteal lining of the cortical bone of the floor of the maxillary antrum, stimulating the differentiation of pluripotential stem cells found within the osteoprogenitor layer of the periosteum, producing one or more elevated, thin layers of new bone adjacent to the root apex of the involved tooth (Fig. 26.19). The presence of one or more halo-like layers of new bone is a characteristic feature of periosteal new bone formation due to inflammation.

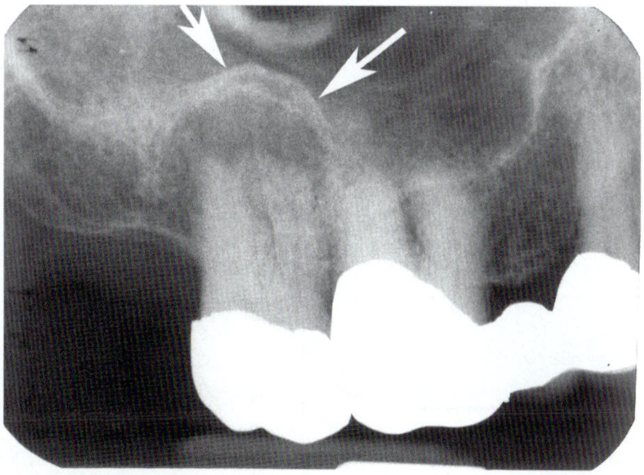

Fig. 26.19 The halo-like appearance of bone surrounding the roots of a maxillary second molar is the result of periosteal new bone formation and displacement of the adjacent maxillary sinus floor *(arrows)*.

Imaging features. Although the periosteum is not visible on the image *per se,* this process is referred to as periosteal new bone formation. Such new bone may take the form of one or more thin radiopaque lines, or the line may be thick. The new bone should be centered just superior to the inflammatory lesion.

Benign Odontogenic Cysts and Neoplasms

The effects of odontogenic cysts and benign neoplasms on the maxillary sinuses may be similar. Periapical inflammatory disease and odontogenic cysts, such as dentigerous cysts, are the most common extrinsic lesions that encroach on the maxillary sinuses. For detailed descriptions of specific odontogenic cysts and benign neoplasms, see Chapters 21 and 22, respectively. With continued growth, these lesions can encroach on the space of the sinus, displacing its borders and reducing the volume of the air-filled space. Should the lesion grow large enough, the lesion's border can become indistinguishable from the sinus border, and only a thin radiopaque line may divide the contents of the lesion from the sinus cavity (Fig. 26.20). This appearance is in contrast to intrinsic sinus lesions which do not show a cortex around their periphery.

Imaging Features

Periphery. The enlarging cyst or benign neoplasm can have a round or oval shape with a curved or "hydraulic" contour. Both groups of lesions may have well-defined thin cortical borders, although more aggressively growing lesions may lack areas of cortication.

Internal structure. The internal structure of the cyst is homogeneous and radiopaque relative to the air-filled sinus cavity. Some neoplasms may also develop fine or coarse internal septation and appear multilocular or have regions of dystrophic calcification, depending on the histopathologic nature of the neoplasm. CBCT or MDCT may be particularly useful in such situations to differentiate the area of increased radiopacity from bone.

Effects on adjacent structures. Both odontogenic cysts and neoplasms may displace the floor of the maxillary sinus and cause thinning of the peripheral cortex. These lesions may enlarge to the point where they almost completely encroach on the sinus airspace. This residual airspace may appear as a thin crescent or saddle over the cyst or neoplasm (see Fig. 26.20).

Effects on adjacent teeth. A cyst or benign neoplasm can cause displacement of adjacent teeth as well as external resorption of roots, often producing a sharp, curved edge that mirrors the growth front of the cyst or neoplasm. Also, the lamina dura and periodontal ligament space may be lost.

Differential interpretation. An antral loculation may occasionally have a round shape and sometimes appear to have a cortex. However, because it contains air, the loculation appears as radiolucent as the surrounding sinus or more so.

Odontogenic cysts, in particular, must be differentiated from the common retention pseudocyst. Although odontogenic cysts may have a shape that is similar to that of a retention pseudocyst, only odontogenic cysts should demonstrate a peripheral cortex (Fig. 26.21). If the

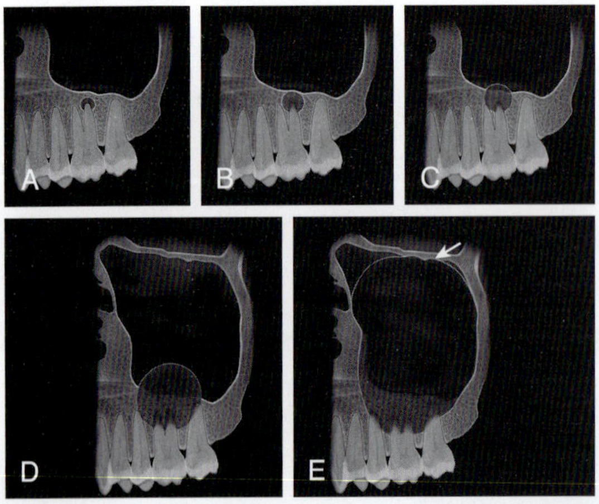

Fig. 26.20 An odontogenic cyst or neoplasm develops adjacent to the floor of a sinus. (A). As the lesion enlarges (B), it abuts the maxillary sinus floor. As it continues to enlarge (C and D), it displaces the maxillary sinus floor further superiorly, ultimately encroaching on almost all the space of the sinus (E), leaving a small crescent-shaped or salle-like remnant *(arrow).* The appearance may mimic rhinosinusitis.

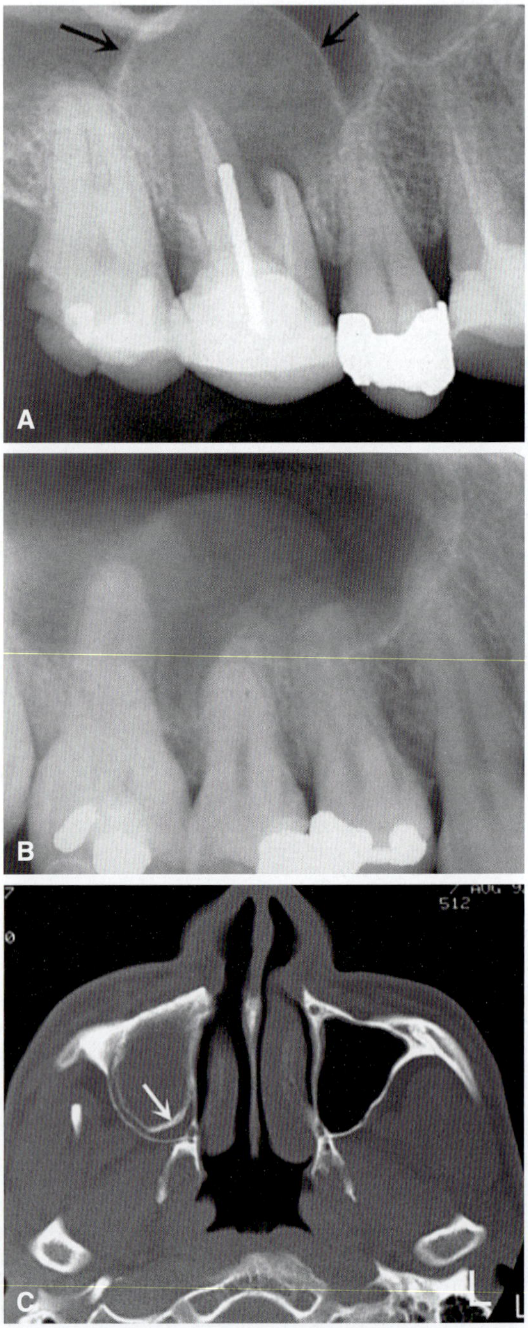

Fig. 26.21 (A) Periapical image of rarefying osteitis associated with a maxillary molar tooth. Note the peripheral cortex *(arrows).* (B) Periapical image of a pseudocyst; note the lack of a peripheral cortex. (C) Axial multidetector computed tomographic image showing the "double cortex" sign. Note the lesion cortex *(arrow)* within the cortex of the sinus border.

odontogenic cysts were to become infected, the cortex may become thickened, developing a sclerotic periphery, or it may be lost. Should the cortex become lost, it may be difficult to determine whether the lesion has arisen from outside or from within the sinus. However, in most cases, careful scrutiny of the lesion periphery can reveal some remaining cyst cortex, and the relationship to neighboring teeth may help to make this decision (Fig. 26.22). It may be difficult to differentiate a dentigerous cyst from an odontogenic keratocyst if the latter develops in a pericoronal relationship to a tooth. The differentiation may be aided by visualizing the association of the lesion with a tooth's cementoenamel junction on CBCT or MDCT.

Large cysts or neoplasms can completely efface the sinus cavity. When this occurs, little or no imaging evidence of residual airspace may exist, and it may appear as if the cyst had developed within the sinus. In this case, because of the radiopacity of the cyst, the appearance may resemble rhinosinusitis with opacification of the sinus. Evaluation of such a situation is aided by locating a region where both the displaced sinus floor and the unaffected sinus wall are in close proximity to one another; this is known as the "double cortex" sign (see Fig. 26.21C). Additionally, the wall of the cyst often has a more "hydraulic" contour than the wall of the sinus. A cyst that has effaced the entire sinus cavity usually causes expansion of the medial wall in the area of the middle meatus. As well, the normal sigmoid contour of the posterolateral wall of the sinus may be altered, as viewed in axial CBCT or MDCT images.

With or sometimes without treatment, an odontogenic cyst abutting the sinus may "collapse" and heal. The end result is the appearance of an irregularly shaped bone formation with a lower attenuation center projecting superiorly from the floor of the sinus (Fig. 26.23). This bone formation should be differentiated from a bone-forming neoplasm, such as an osteoma or ossifying fibroma.

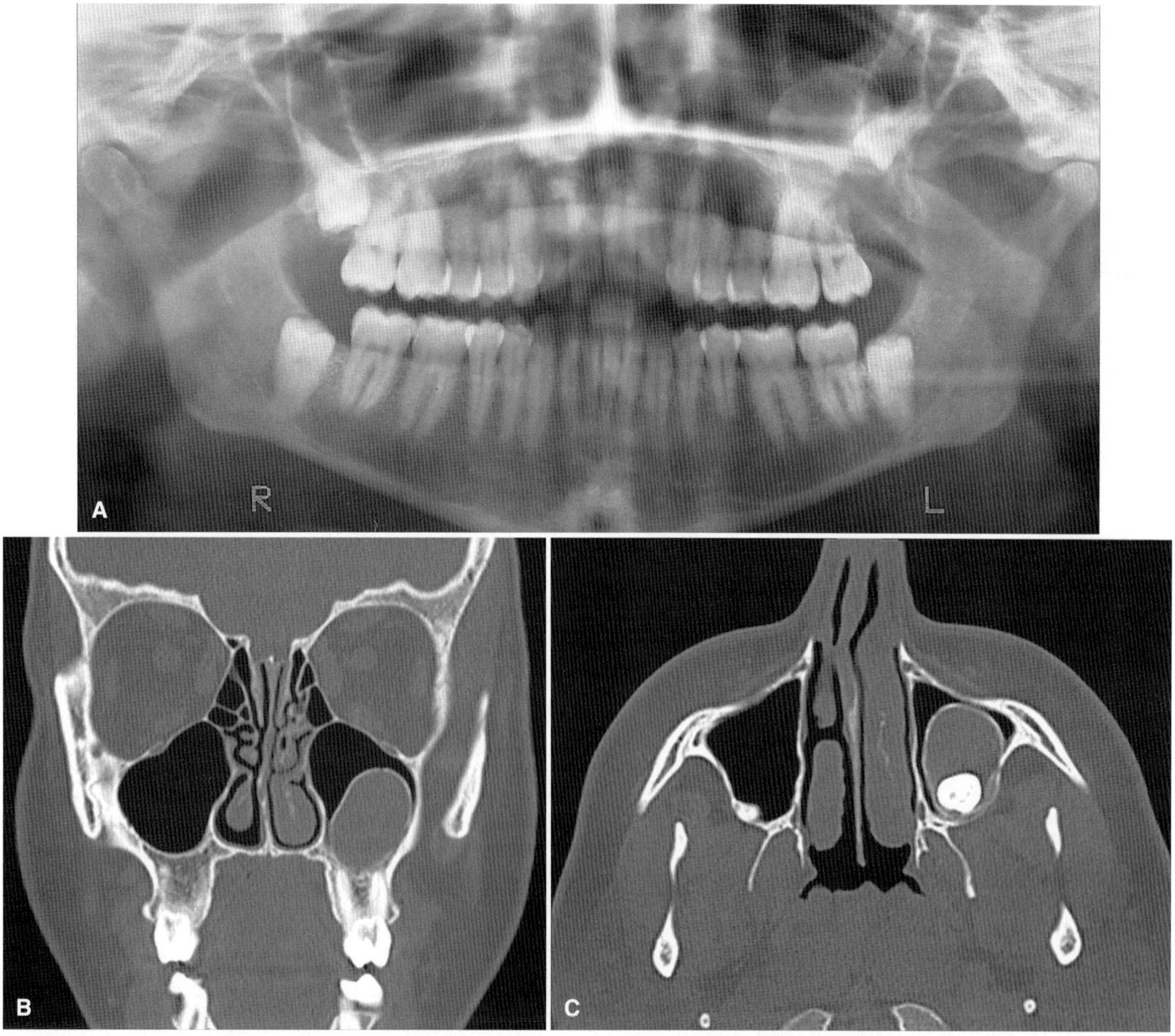

Fig. 26.22 Series of images showing displacement of the left maxillary sinus floor as a result of a developing dentigerous cyst associated with the maxillary left third molar. (A–C) The corticated periphery of the cyst is well seen in the panoramic image (A). (B) Coronal multidetector computed tomographic image shows the displaced floor of the left maxillary sinus. (C) Axial multidetector computed tomographic image shows the bowing of the posterior sinus wall and the adjacent impacted tooth.

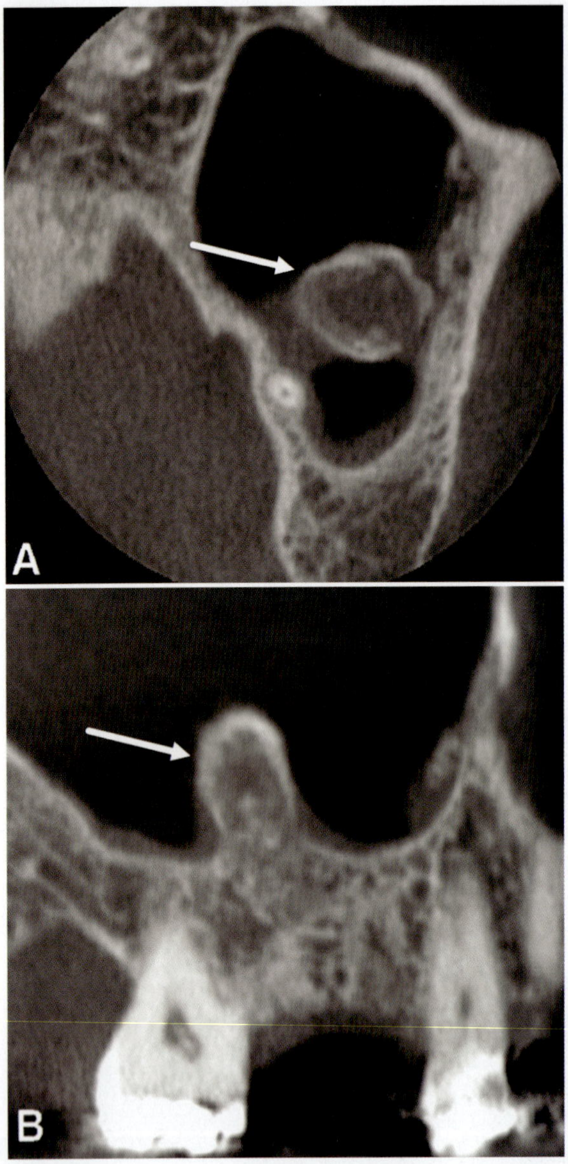

Fig. 26.23 (A) Axial and (B) sagittal cone beam computed tomographic images showing bone formation within a "collapsed" cyst that had invaginated into the maxillary sinus lumen *(arrows)*.

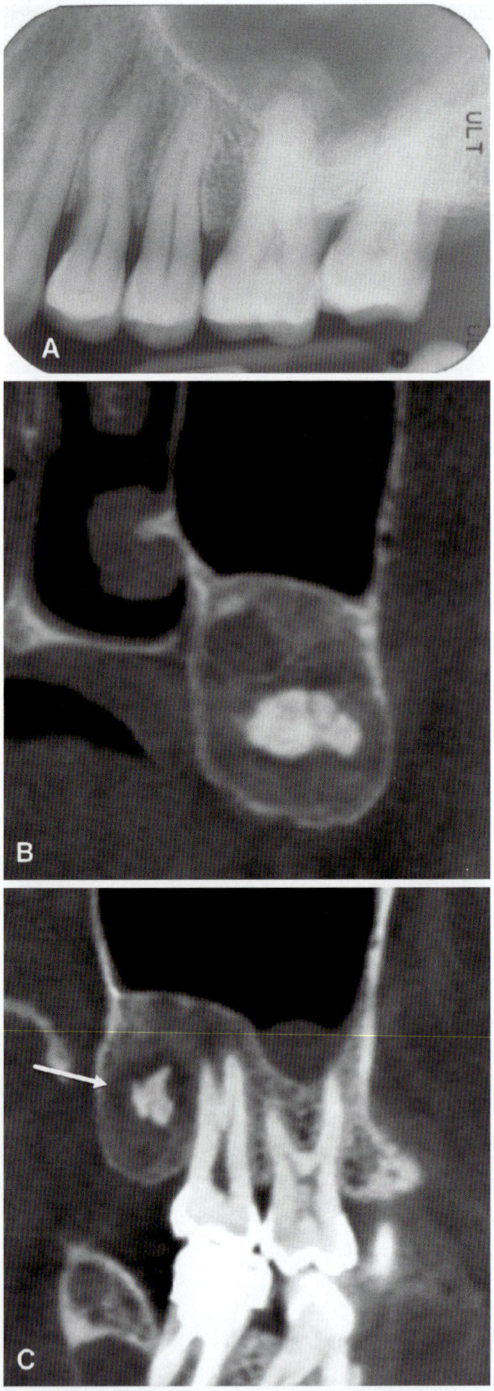

Fig. 26.24 (A) Periapical image demonstrates elevation of the maxillary sinus floor by a focus of periapical cemento-osseous dysplasia located at the apices of the maxillary left first molar. (B) Coronal and (C) sagittal cone beam computed tomographic images showing a focal area of cemento-osseous dysplasia at the no. 16 edentulous site. Note the displacement of the sinus floor and the overall anatomic expansion of the alveolar process.

Bone Dysplasias

Periapical and florid cemento-osseous dysplasias, when they develop near the root apices of the maxillary premolar and molar teeth, may displace the floor of the maxillary antrum in a similar way as cysts or benign neoplasms (Fig. 26.24). Fibrous dysplasia, when arising adjacent to any of the paranasal sinuses, may have greater mass effect, causing enlargement of the bone and more notable displacement of sinus borders, resulting in a substantially smaller sinus on the affected side (Fig. 26.25). For a detailed description of bone dysplasias, see Chapter 23.

Clinical Features

Involvement of the facial skeleton with fibrous dysplasia can result in facial asymmetry, nasal obstruction, proptosis, pituitary gland compression, impingement on cranial nerves, or sinus obliteration. Obliteration of the airspace results when the expanding dysplastic bone encroaches on it. The lesion may displace the roots of teeth and cause teeth to separate or migrate, but it usually does not cause root resorption. Fibrous dysplasia is more common in children and young adults, and growth of the dysplastic bone usually ceases at the age of skeletal maturity.

Imaging Features

Location. In the maxilla, the posterior maxilla is the most common location for fibrous dysplasia.

Periphery. The periphery is usually poorly defined, and the dysplastic bone pattern tends to blend into the normal surrounding bone. The external cortex of the bone and the sinus border are intact but displaced.

Internal structure. The normal radiolucent maxillary sinus may be partially or totally replaced by the increased radiopacity of this lesion. The degree of radiopacity depends on its stage of development and the relative amounts of bone and connective tissue present. Often, fibrous dysplasia presents with a homogenous, fine, granular appearance, characteristically described as resembling ground glass or the texture of an orange peel (Fig. 26.25). However, more coarse heterogeneous mixed attenuation presentations of this lesion do occur.

Effects on adjacent structures. Fibrous dysplasia may cause enlargement of the alveolar process, with superior displacement of the sinus floor. The dysplastic bone may encroach on the dimensions of the air cavity, causing it to appear smaller in size while maintaining a relatively normal shape.

Effects on adjacent teeth. There may be little to no effect on the dentition. Mild splaying of the roots of the involved teeth is common. In some cases, when the radiopacity of the dysplastic bone increases, definition of the lamina dura may be lost as it assumes the pattern of the dysplastic bone. Narrowing of the PDL space is also commonly encountered.

Differential Interpretation

The diagnosis of fibrous dysplasia in a relatively young person is usually not difficult. In some cases, however, differentiating cemento-ossifying fibroma involving the antrum from fibrous dysplasia can be difficult, so attention to periphery as well as the pattern of lesional expansion is helpful. The border of fibrous dysplasia is more poorly defined, blending into the normal adjacent bone, whereas cemento-ossifying fibroma displays a well-defined corticated border with an internal radiolucent periphery. Cemento-ossifying fibroma, being a benign neoplasm, more frequently displays a concentric or more spherical growth pattern, while fibrous dysplasia usually causes more uniform anatomic enlargement of the bone. When both lesions involve the maxillary alveolar process, both may encroach on the sinus resulting in a smaller airspace. However, in instances of fibrous dysplasia, the relatively normal shape of the airspace is typically maintained. In contrast, Paget's disease of bone occurs in an older age group and does not usually obliterate the sinus.

Iatrogenic Effects of Dental Procedures on the Maxillary Sinus

Mechanism

Dental procedures involving the posterior maxilla may have adverse effects on the appearance and function of the maxillary sinuses (Fig. 26.26).

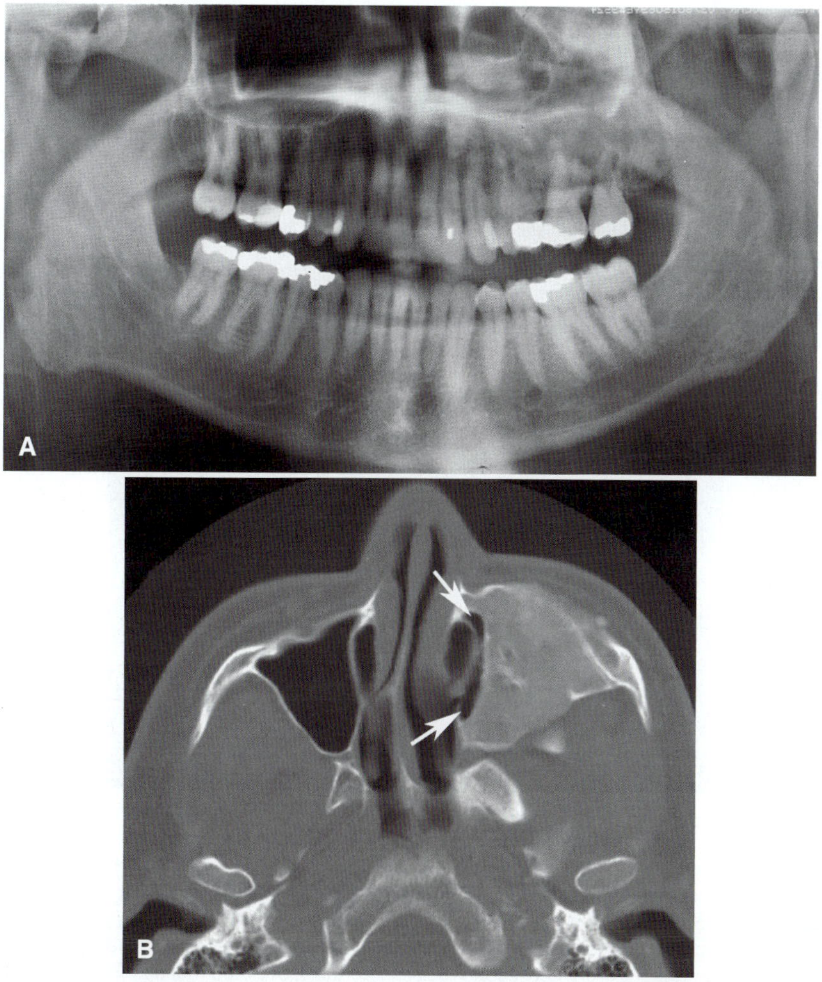

Fig. 26.25 (A) Panoramic image of involvement of the left maxillary sinus with fibrous dysplasia. Note the opacification of the left maxillary sinus compared to the right sinus. (B) Axial multidetector computed tomographic image of the same case reveals almost complete encroachment on the sinus; a small portion of the medial airspace remains *(arrows)*. Note the very fine homogeneous bone pattern of fibrous dysplasia.

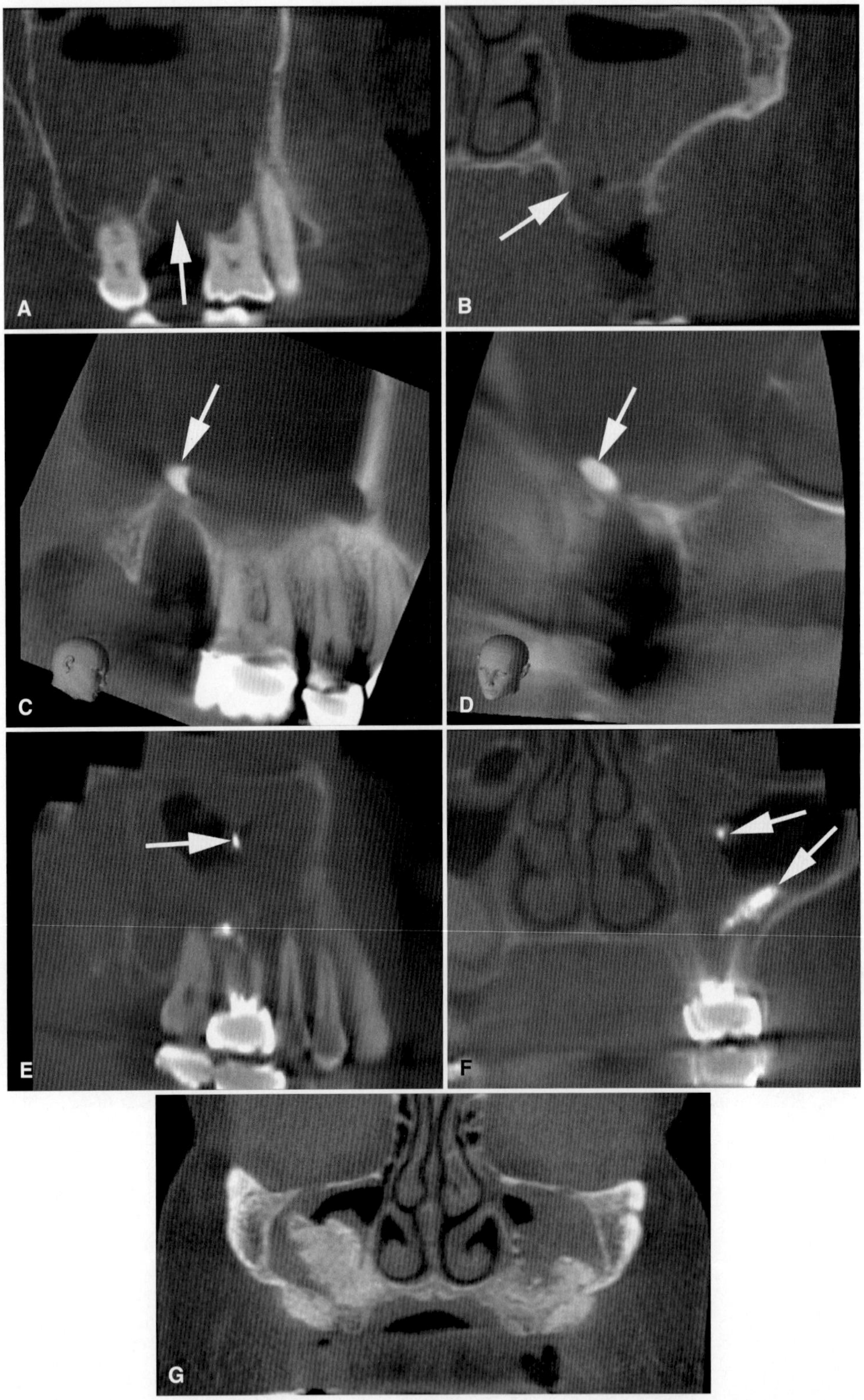

Fig. 26.26 Sagittal (A) and coronal (B) cone beam computed tomographic images demonstrating loss of the continuity of the sinus floor *(arrow)* after extraction of the maxillary left second molar. Note the presence of air collections and the air-fluid level. Sagittal (C) and coronal (D) cone beam computed tomographic images showing a root fragment *(arrows)* intruding through the base of the extraction socket of the maxillary right second molar and displacement through the floor of the maxillary sinus. Sagittal (E) and coronal (F) cone beam computed tomographic images of endodontic material *(arrows)* displaced into the maxillary sinus after endodontic treatment of the maxillary left second molar. Note the associated mucosal thickening. Coronal (G) cone beam computed tomographic image of bone graft material within the right and left maxillary sinuses after an alveolar ridge augmentation procedure. Note the nearly complete radiopacification of both sinuses and the punctate spicules of the graft in the left sinus.

The continuity of the maxillary sinus floor may be lost during tooth extraction, resulting in an oroantral communication. Tooth roots may be fractured as a result of various forms of trauma, including tooth extraction, and may be displaced into the airspace of the sinus. Exuberant extrusion of restorative material during endodontic treatment of posterior maxillary teeth may lead to the deposition of these materials in the maxillary sinus. Finally, ridge augmentation procedures during implant placement may disrupt the integrity of the sinus mucosal lining and result in the intrusion of bone graft material into the sinus cavity.

Clinical Features

No specific clinical features may be present if the integrity of the sinus wall has been acutely violated. However, in cases of tooth extraction, the dentist may note the absence of the root fragment on examining the extracted tooth and may be unable to locate it anywhere else. Sometimes asking the patient to hold his or her nose while attempting to breathe out, similar to a Valsalva maneuver, causes bubbles to appear within the blood contained within the fresh extraction socket. If the insult has occurred in the more distant past, the presenting symptom may be that of rhinosinusitis (see the previous discussion of rhinosinusitis).

Imaging Features

Location. Teeth, root fragments (Fig. 26.27A), endodontic filling material, dental implants (Fig. 26.28), or osseous grafts may be

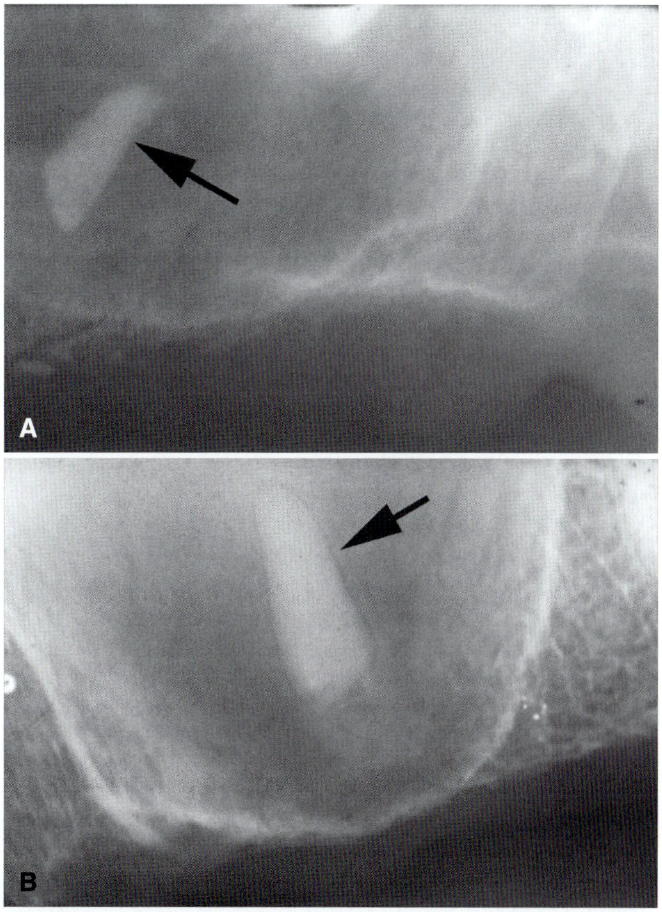

Fig. 26.27 (A) Periapical image revealing a portion of tooth root *(arrow)* within the maxillary sinus. (B) Another periapical image of a retained root tip outside the sinus, but its image is superimposed over the sinus *(arrow)*. The presence of a periodontal ligament space indicates that it is in the alveolar process and not in the sinus.

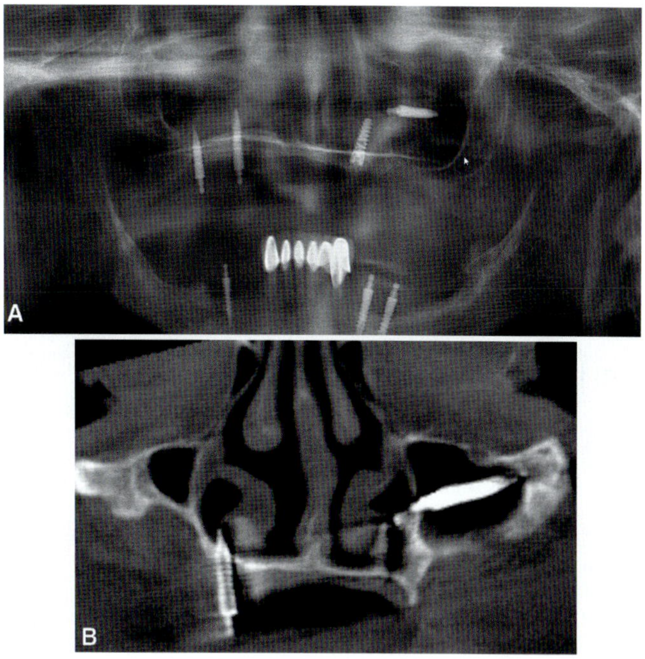

Fig. 26.28 (A) Panoramic radiograph of a partially edentulous patient showing displacement of an implant fixture into the left maxillary sinus. (B) Coronal cone beam computed tomographic image on the same patient showing the implant fixture in a horizontal orientation within the left maxillary sinus lumen.

displaced into the sinus. These may be found anywhere within the sinus but are more often located near the floor of the sinus because of gravity. Sometimes they may be located submucosally, between the osseous wall of the sinus and the mucoperiosteum.

Periphery. Disruption of the sinus wall may be difficult to see on planar images. CBCT avoids superimposition of anatomic structures and is ideal for assessment of the integrity of the sinus walls.

Internal structure. Most displaced objects are radiopaque and, if large enough, can be seen on an imaging examination. However, owing to the limitations of two-dimensional images, their exact location can be difficult to identify.

Effects on adjacent structures. Usually, no effect on surrounding structures is noted other than the altered anatomy caused by the dental procedure or the violation of the sinus floor's integrity from the intrusion of a tooth fragment. At later stages and if rhinosinusitis ensues, partial or complete opacification of the involved sinus might be present.

Differential Interpretation

In most cases, the history of a surgical procedure and the relevant clinical symptoms and signs lead to the correct diagnosis. However, the diagnostic challenge focuses on identifying the exact location of the displaced objects, their relation to anatomic landmarks such as the sinus ostium, and the possible concomitant sinus inflammation.

Bony masses that represent hyperostosis of the sinus wall or floor or septa within the sinus may mimic tooth root fragments or even whole teeth. Antroliths may also have a similar appearance. The shape of the radiopacity, the presence of a pulp chamber or root canal, a layer of enamel, or the dense radiopacity of endodontic materials may help in the differential interpretation. If the root tip remains in its socket, it may be superimposed over the maxillary sinus, but the presence of a lamina dura and periodontal ligament space indicates a position within the alveolar process (see Fig. 26.22B).

Management

Management ranges from follow up with the patient to see whether the object will be removed from the sinus through the ostium by ciliary action to entering the sinus surgically by a Caldwell-Luc procedure. Rhinosinusitis may develop and should be managed with the appropriate treatment. Defects in the sinus floor from oral-antral communication may heal with soft tissue and not osseous closure. In these cases, the cortication of the sinus floor will remain disrupted even after resolution of sinus inflammation.

For other trauma involving the paranasal sinuses, see Chapter 25.

BIBLIOGRAPHY

Normal Development and Variations

Bazak R, Elwany S, Mina A, Donia M. Nitric oxide unravels the enigmatic function of the paranasal sinuses: a review of literature. *Egypt J Otolaryngol.* 2020;36:1-5.

Cobb AR, Murthy R, Cousin GC, et al. Silent sinus syndrome. *Br J Oral Maxillofac Surg.* 2012;50:e81-e85.

DuBrul EL. *Sicher's Oral Anatomy.* 7th ed. Mosby; 1980.

Grant JCB. *A Method of Anatomy.* Williams & Wilkins; 1958.

Guillen DE, Pinargote PM, Guarderas JC. The silent sinus syndrome: protean manifestations of a rare upper respiratory disorder revisited. *Clin Mol Allergy.* 2013;11:5.

Hengerer AS. Embryonic development of the sinuses. *Ear Nose Throat J.* 1984;63:134-136.

Karmody CS, Carter B, Vincent ME. Developmental anomalies of the maxillary sinus. *Trans Sect Otolaryngol Am Acad Ophthalmol Otolaryngol.* 1977;84:723-728.

Keir J. Why do we have paranasal sinuses? *J Laryngol Otol.* 2009;123:4-8.

Lusted LB, Keats TE. *Atlas of Roentgenographic Measurement.* 3rd ed. Year Book Medical Publishers; 1972.

Moore K, Ross A. Frontal sinus development and juvenile age estimation. *Anat Rec (Hoboken).* 2017;300:1609-1617.

Pula JH, Mehta M. Silent sinus syndrome. *Curr Opin Ophthalmol.* 2014;25:480-484.

Ritter FN. *The Paranasal Sinuses: Anatomy and Surgical Technique.* Mosby; 1973.

Scuderi AJ, Harnsberger HR, Boyer RS. Pneumatization of the paranasal sinuses: normal features of importance to the accurate interpretation of CT scans and MR images. *AJR Am J Roentgenol.* 1993;160:1101-1104.

Shapiro R. *Radiology of the Normal Skull.* Year Book Medical Publishers; 1981.

Som PM. The paranasal sinuses. In: Bergeron RT, Osborn AG, Som PM, eds. *Head and Neck Imaging: Excluding the Brain.* Mosby; 1984.

Stryjewska-Makuch G, Goroszkiewicz K, Szymocha J, et al. Etiology, early diagnosis and proper treatment of silent sinus syndrome based on review of the literature and own experience. *J Oral Maxillofac Surg.* 2022;80:113.e1-113.e8.

Takahashi R. The formation of the human paranasal sinuses. *Acta Otolaryngol Suppl.* 1984;408:1-28.

Zinreich SJ. Imaging of chronic sinusitis in adults: X-ray, computed tomography, and magnetic resonance imaging. *J Allergy Clin Immunol.* 1992;90:445-451.

Inflammatory Changes

Nurbakhsh B, Friedman S, Kulkarni GV, et al. Resolution of maxillary sinus mucositis after endodontic treatment of maxillary teeth with apical periodontitis: a cone beam computerized tomography pilot study. *J Endod.* 2011;37:1504-1511.

Robinson K. Roentgenographic manifestations of benign paranasal disease. *Ear Nose Throat J.* 1984;63:144.

Yeung AW, Hung KF, Li DT, Leung YY. The use of CBCT in evaluating the health and pathology of the maxillary sinus. *Diagnostics.* 2022;12:2819.

Thickened Mucous Membrane—Mucositis

Chen HH, Yi CA, Chen YC, Huang HH. Anatomical characteristics of maxillary sinus antroliths and their influence on sinus membrane thickness: a retrospective cone beam computed tomography analysis. *Int J Oral Maxillofac Surg.* 2021;50:1107-1112.

Dolan K, Smoker W. Paranasal sinus radiology. Part 4A: maxillary sinuses. *Head Neck Surg.* 1983;5:345-362.

Killey HC, Kay LA. *The Maxillary Sinus and Its Dental Implications.* John Wright; 1975.

Rhinosinusitis

Druce HM. Diagnosis and medical management of recurrent and chronic sinusitis in adults. In: Gershwin ME, Incaudo GA, eds. *Diseases of the Sinuses.* Humana Press; 1996.

Fireman P. Diagnosis of sinusitis in children: emphasis on the history and physical examination. *J Allergy Clin Immunol.* 1992;90:433-436.

Frerichs N, Brateanu A. Rhinosinusitis and the role of imaging. *Cleve Clin J Med.* 2020;87(8):485-492.

Incaudo G, Gershwin ME, Nagy SM. The pathophysiology and treatment of sinusitis. *Allergol Immunopathol (Madr).* 1986;14:423-434.

Killey HC, Kay LA. *The Maxillary Sinus and Its Dental Implications.* John Wright; 1975.

Palacios E, Valvassori G. Computed axial tomography in otorhinolaryngology. *Adv Otorhinolaryngol.* 1978;24:1-8.

Paparella MM. Mucosal cyst of the maxillary sinus. *Arch Otolaryngol.* 1963;77:650-670.

Psillas G, Papaioannou D, Petsali S, Dimas GG, Constantinidis J. Odontogenic maxillary sinusitis: a comprehensive review. *J Dent Sci.* 2021;16(1):474-481.

Reilly JS. The sinusitis cycle. *Otolaryngol Head Neck Surg.* 1990;103:856-861.

Zinreich SJ. Imaging of chronic sinusitis in adults: X-ray, computed tomography, and magnetic resonance imaging. *J Allergy Clin Immunol.* 1992;90:445-451.

Zhu J, Lin W, Yuan W, Chen L. New insight on pathophysiology, diagnosis, and treatment of odontogenic maxillary sinusitis. *J Nanomater.* 2021;2021:1-6.

Empyema

Ash JE, Raum M. *An Atlas of Otolaryngic Pathology.* American Registry of Pathology; 1956.

Groves J, Gray RF. *A Synopsis of Otolaryngology.* John Wright; 1985.

Polyps

Hopkins C. Chronic rhinosinusitis with nasal polyps. *N Engl J Med.* 2019;381:55-63.

Potter GD. Inflammatory disease of the paranasal sinuses. In: Valvassori GE, Potter GD, Hanefee WN, eds. *Radiology of the Ear, Nose and Throat.* Saunders; 1982.

Retention Pseudocysts

Allard RH, van der Kwast WA, van der Waal JI. Mucosal antral cysts: review of the literature and report of a radiographic survey. *Oral Surg Oral Med Oral Pathol.* 1981;51:2-9.

Anitua E, Alkhraisat MH, Torre A, Eguia A. Are mucous retention cysts and pseudocysts in the maxillary sinus a risk factor for dental implants? A systematic review. *Med Oral Patol Oral Cir Bucal.* 2021;26:e276.

Dolan K, Smoker W. Paranasal sinus radiology. Part 4A: maxillary sinuses. *Head Neck Surg.* 1983;5:345-362.

Kaffe I, Littner MM, Moskona D. Mucosal-antral cysts: radiographic appearance and differential diagnosis. *Clin Prev Dent.* 1988;10:3-6.

Kim SB, Yun PY, Kim YK. Clinical evaluation of sinus bone graft in patients with mucous retention cyst. *Maxillofac Plast Reconstr Surg.* 2016;38:35.

Ruprecht A, Batniji S, el-Neweihi E. Mucous retention cyst of the maxillary sinus. *Oral Surg Oral Med Oral Pathol.* 1986;62:728-731.

Mucocele—Fungus Balls

Abdel-Aziz M, El-Hoshy H, Azooz K, et al. Maxillary sinus mucocele: predisposing factors, clinical presentations, and treatment. *Oral Maxillofac Surg.* 2017;21:55-58.

Atherino C, Atherino T. Maxillary sinus mucopyoceles. *Arch Otolaryngol.* 1984;110:200.

Hathiram BT, Khattar VS. Fungus balls of the paranasal sinuses. *Otolaryngol Clin North Am.* 2009;1:33-35.

Jones JL, Kaufman PW. Mucopyocele of the maxillary sinus. *J Oral Surg.* 1981;39:948.

Nicolai P, Mensi M, Marsili F, et al. Maxillary fungus ball: zinc-oxide endodontic materials as a risk factor. *ACTA Otorhinolaryngol Ital*. 2015;35:93-96.

Tomazic PV, Dostal E, Magyar M, et al. Potential correlations of dentogenic factors to the development of clinically verified fungus balls: a retrospective computed tomography–based analysis. *Laryngoscope*. 2016;126:39-43.

Odontogenic Cysts

Killey HC, Kay LA. *The Maxillary Sinus and Its Dental Implications*. John Wright; 1975.

Xu GZ, Jiang Q, Yang C, Yu CQ, Zhang ZY. Clinicopathologic features of dentigerous cysts in the maxillary sinus. *J Craniofac Surg*. 2012;23:e226-e231.

Odontogenic Keratocysts

MacDonald-Jankowski DS. The involvement of the maxillary antrum by odontogenic keratocysts. *Clin Radiol*. 1992;45:31-33.

Walsh M, Hussein MA, Carter M, Abdulrahman S. Maxillary odontogenic keratocyst. *J Surg Case Rep*. 2022;2022:rjac078.

Neoplasms

Goepfert H, Luna MA, Lindberg RD, et al. Malignant salivary gland tumors of the paranasal sinuses and nasal cavity. *Arch Otolaryngol*. 1983;109:662-668.

Loevner LA, Sonners AI. Imaging of neoplasms of the paranasal sinuses. *Neuroimaging Clin N Am*. 2004;14:625-646.

St-Pierre S, Baker SR. Squamous cell carcinoma of the maxillary sinus: analysis of 66 cases. *Head Neck Surg*. 1983;5:508-513.

Inverted Papilloma

Lisan Q, Laccourreye O, Bonfils P. Sinonasal inverted papilloma: From diagnosis to treatment. *Eur Ann Otorhinolaryngol Head Neck Dis*. 2016;133:337-341.

Miyazaki T, Haku Y, Yoshizawa A, et al. Clinical features of nasal and sinonasal inverted papilloma associated with malignancy. *Auris Nasus Larynx*. 2018;45:1014-1019.

Rogers JH, Fredrickson JM, Noyek AM. Management of cysts, benign tumors, and bony dysplasia of the maxillary sinus. *Otolaryngol Clin North Am*. 1976;9:233-247.

Wang MJ, Noel JE. Etiology of sinonasal inverted papilloma: a narrative review. *World J Otorhinolaryngol Head Neck Surg*. 2017;3:54-58.

Wood JW, Casiano RR. Inverted papillomas and benign nonneoplastic lesions of the nasal cavity. *Am J Rhinol Allergy*. 2012;26:157-163.

Osteoma

Arslan HH, Tasli H, Cebeci S, Gerek M. The management of the paranasal sinus osteomas. *J Craniofac Surg*. 2017;28:741-745.

Dolan K, Smoker W. Paranasal sinus radiology. Part 4B: maxillary sinuses. *Head Neck Surg*. 1983;5:428-446.

Goodnight J, Dulguerov P, Abemayor E. Calcified mucor fungus ball of the maxillary sinus. *Am J Otolaryngol*. 1993;14:209-210.

Lee DH, Jung SH, Yoon TM, et al. Characteristics of paranasal sinus osteoma and treatment outcomes. *Acta Otolaryngol*. 2015;135:602-607.

Reuben BM. Odontoma of the maxillary sinus: a case report. *Quintessence Int Dent Dig*. 1983;14:287-290.

Samy LL, Mostofa H. Osteoma of the nose and paranasal sinuses with a report of twenty-one cases. *J Laryngol Otol*. 1971;85:449-469.

Ameloblastoma

Hames RS, Rakoff SJ. Diseases of the maxillary sinus. *J Oral Med*. 1972;27:90-95.

Reaume C, Wesley RK, Jung B, et al. Ameloblastoma of the maxillary sinus. *J Oral Surg*. 1980;38:520-521.

Sehdev MK, Huvos AG, Strong EW, Gerold FP, Willis GW. Ameloblastoma of maxilla and mandible. *Cancer*. 1974;33:324-333.

Malignant Neoplasms of the Paranasal Sinuses

Kilic S, Shukla PA, Marchiano EJ, et al. Malignant primary neoplasms of the nasal cavity and paranasal sinus. *Curr Otorhinolaryngol Rep*. 2016;4:249-258.

Taylor MA, Saba NF. Cancer of the paranasal sinuses. *Hematol Oncol Clin*. 2021;35:949-962.

Squamous Cell Carcinoma

Bridger M, Beale F, Bryce D. Carcinoma of the paranasal sinuses: a review of 158 cases. *J Otolaryngol*. 1978;7:379-388.

Eddleston B, Johnson R. A comparison of conventional radiographic imaging and computed tomography in malignant disease of the paranasal sinuses and the post-nasal space. *Clin Radiol*. 1983;34:161-172.

Hasso AN. CT of tumors and tumor-like conditions of the paranasal sinuses. *Radiol Clin North Am*. 1984;22:119-130.

Larheim TA, Kolbenstvedt A, Lien H. Carcinoma of maxillary sinus, palate and maxillary gingiva, occurrence of jaw destruction. *Scand J Dent Res*. 1984;92:235-240.

Pałasz P, Adamski Ł, Górska-Chrząstek M, et al. Contemporary diagnostic imaging of oral squamous cell carcinoma–a review of literature. *Pol J Radiol*. 2017;82:193-202.

St-Pierre S, Baker SR. Squamous cell carcinoma of the maxillary sinus: analysis of 66 cases. *Head Neck Surg*. 1983;5:508-513.

Tiwari R, Hardillo JA, Mehta D, et al. Squamous cell carcinoma of maxillary sinus. *Head Neck*. 2000;22:164-169.

Tsaknis PJ, Nelson JF. The maxillary ameloblastoma: an analysis of 24 cases. *J Oral Surg*. 1980;38:336-342.

Weber A, Tadmore R, Davis R, et al. Malignant tumors of the sinuses: radiologic evaluation, including CT scanning, with clinical and pathologic correlation. *Neuroradiology*. 1978;16:443-448.

Pseudotumor

Huang WH, Dai YC. Inflammatory pseudotumor of the nasal cavity. *Am J Otolaryngol*. 2006;27:275-277.

Muzaffar M, Hussain SI, Chughtai A. Plasma cell granuloma: maxillary sinuses. *J Laryngol Otol*. 1994;108:357-358.

Naveen J, Sonalika W, Prabhu S, et al. Inflammatory pseudotumor of maxillary sinus: Mimicking as an aggressive malignancy. *J Oral Maxillofac Pathol*. 2011;15:344-345.

Newlin HE, Werning JW, Mendenhall WM. Plasma cell granuloma of the maxillary sinus: a case report and literature review. *Head Neck*. 2005;27:722-728.

Ozhan S, Araç M, Isik S, et al. Pseudotumor of the maxillary sinus in a patient with von Willebrand's disease. *AJR Am J Roentgenol*. 1996;166:950-951.

Som PM, Brandwein MS, Maldjian C, et al. Inflammatory pseudotumor of the maxillary sinus: CT and MR findings in six cases. *AJR Am J Roentgenol*. 1994;163:689-692.

Fibrous Dysplasia

MacDonald-Jankowski D. Fibrous dysplasia: a systematic review. *Dentomaxillofac Radiol*. 2009;38:196-215.

Sontakke SA, Karjodkar FR, Umarji HR. Computed tomographic features of fibrous dysplasia of maxillofacial region. *Imag Sci Dent*. 2011;41:23-28.

Cemento-ossifying Fibroma

Malcolmson KG. Ossifying fibroma of the sphenoid. *J Laryngol Otol*. 1967;81:87-92.

Thomas GK, Kasper KA. Ossifying fibroma of the frontal bone. *Arch Otolaryngol*. 1966;83:43-46.

27

Craniofacial Anomalies

Carol Anne Murdoch-Kinch

Developmental disturbances can affect the normal differentiation and growth of craniofacial structures, and these can result in observable craniofacial anomalies. Developmental craniofacial anomalies are usually first discovered in infancy or childhood. Some are caused by known genetic mutations, others result from environmental factors that may affect the epigenome, and a third group are multifactorial. These conditions are manifested by a variety of abnormalities of the face and jaws, including abnormalities of structure, shape, organization, and function of the hard and soft tissues. A multitude of conditions affect the morphogenesis of the face and jaws, many of which are rare syndromes. This chapter briefly reviews more common or significant craniofacial developmental anomalies that may be encountered in dental practice.

CLEFT LIP AND PALATE

Disease Mechanism

Facial clefts of various types are caused by a failure of fusion of the developmental processes of the face during fetal development. Cleft lip and cleft palate (CL/P), cleft lip (CL), and cleft palate (CP) together are the most common developmental craniofacial anomalies worldwide. Their incidence varies with geographic location, race, and socioeconomic status. Worldwide, the average birth prevalence of all orofacial clefts is 0.45 per 1000 live births. In White populations, the incidence of CL is 1:800 to 1:1000 live births, and the incidence of CP is approximately 1:1000. CL with or without CL/P and CP are two different conditions with different embryonic origins.

CL/P results from a failure of fusion of the medial nasal process with the maxillary process in the developing embryo, and can range in severity from a unilateral CL to bilateral complete clefting through the lip, maxillary alveolar processes, and hard and soft palate in the most severe cases. CP develops from a failure of fusion of the lateral palatal shelves. The minimal manifestation of CP is a submucous cleft in which the palate appears to be intact except for notching of the uvula (bifid uvula) or notching in the posterior border of the hard palate, detectable by palpation. The most severe presentation of CP is complete clefting of the hard and soft palate. The precise etiology of orofacial clefting is not yet completely understood. However, most cases of nonsyndromic CL/P and CP are considered to follow a multifactorial threshold model, with environmental risk factors and a strong genetic component.

Several genes are associated with orofacial clefting. CL/P and CP each can be associated with other abnormalities as part of a genetic malformation syndrome. Deletion of genetic material at position 11 on the long arm of chromosome 22 can result in CP with facial and cardiac abnormalities. This is referred to as 22q.11 deletion syndrome or velocardiofacial syndrome. CL or CP, or both, and lip pits can develop in van der Woude syndrome, which is caused by a mutation of the interferon regulatory factor 6 *(IRF6)* gene. This gene has a role in the development of the head and face. Other factors that have been implicated in the development of orofacial clefts include nutritional disturbances (prenatal folate deficiency), environmental teratogenic agents (maternal smoking, in utero exposure to anticonvulsants), stress (which results in increased secretion of hydrocortisone), defects of vascular supply to the involved region, and mechanical interference with the fusion of the embryonic processes (CP in Pierre Robin sequence). Clefts involving the lower lip and mandible are extremely rare.

Clinical Features

The frequency of CL/P and CP vary with sex and race, but in general CL/P is more common in males, whereas CP is more common in females. Both conditions are much more common in east Asian and Indigenous American populations than those with European, south Asian, and African ancestry, which have lower birth prevalence rates. The severity of CL/P can vary from a notch in the upper lip, to a cleft involving only the lip, to an extension of the soft tissue cleft into the nostril resulting in deformity of the ala of the nose. As CL/P increases in severity, the cleft can include the alveolar process and palate. Bilateral CL is more frequently associated with CP.

CP can also vary in severity, ranging from involvement of only the uvula or soft palate to complete extension through the palate to include the alveolar process in the region of the lateral incisor on one or both sides. With involvement of the alveolar process, there is an increase in frequency of dental anomalies in the region of the cleft, including missing, hypoplastic, and supernumerary teeth and enamel hypoplasia. Dental anomalies are also more prevalent in the mandible in these patients. In both CL/P and CP, the palatal defects interfere with speech and swallowing. Affected individuals with palatal clefts are also at increased risk for recurrent middle ear infections because of the abnormal anatomy and function of the eustachian tube. A recent systematic review and meta-analysis has also confirmed that children with orofacial clefts have higher caries experience and risk than children without.

Imaging Features

The typical imaging appearance is a well-defined vertical radiolucent defect in the alveolar process and numerous associated dental anomalies (Fig. 27.1). These anomalies may include the absence of the maxillary lateral incisor, and the presence of supernumerary teeth in this region. Teeth adjacent to the cleft often are malformed and poorly positioned. In patients with CL/P, there may also be a mild delay in the development of maxillary and mandibular teeth, and an increased incidence of hypodontia in both arches. The osseous defect may extend to include the floor of the nasal cavity (Fig. 27.2). In patients with a repaired cleft, instead of a well-defined osseous defect, a vertically short alveolar process may be apparent at the cleft site.

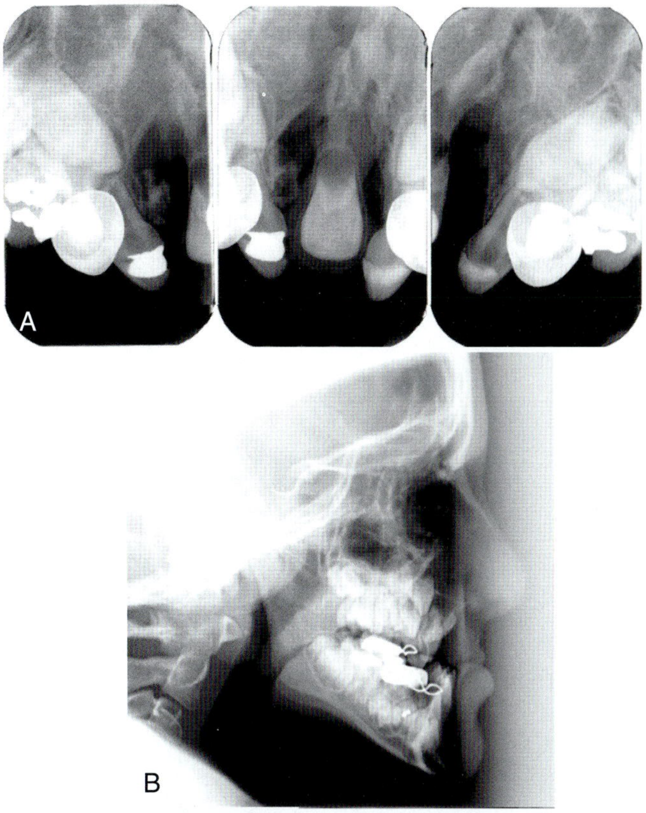

Fig. 27.1 Cleft lip/palate results in defects in the alveolar ridge and abnormalities of the dentition. (A) Bilateral clefts of the maxilla in the lateral incisor regions and defects of the dentition. (B) Lateral cephalometric skull image shows underdevelopment of the maxilla.

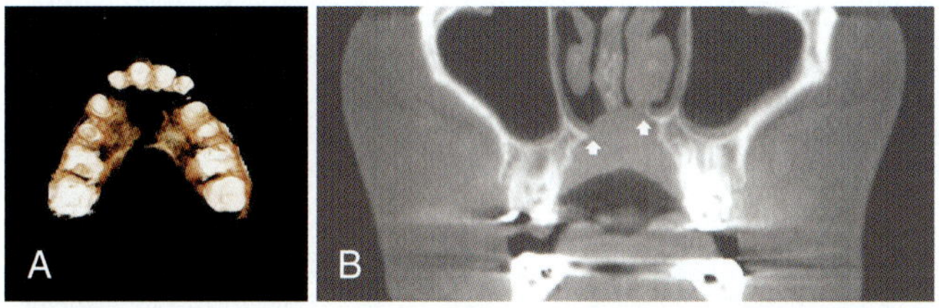

Fig. 27.2 (A) Three-dimensional reconstruction from a cone beam computed tomography study shows bilateral clefts of the maxillary alveolar processes. (B) Coronal image shows discontinuities of the nasal floors *(arrows)*.

Management

Management of CL/P and CP is complex, requiring the coordinated efforts of a multidisciplinary team known as a CP/craniofacial anomalies team. This team usually includes a plastic and reconstructive surgeon, an oral and maxillofacial surgeon, an otolaryngologic surgeon, an orthodontist, a dentist, a speech therapist, an audiologist, psychologist/behaviorist, a nutritionist, and a social worker. Clefts of the palate are usually surgically repaired within the first year of life, whereas clefts of the lip are usually repaired within the first 3 months to aid in feeding and maternal–infant bonding. The bone in the cleft site is often augmented with bone graft material before replacement of missing teeth with either fixed or removable partial denture prostheses, or dental implants. Orthodontic treatment, without or with orthognathic surgery, is usually necessary to recreate a normal arch form and functional occlusion. The increased caries risk associated with orofacial clefts necessitates regular dental care aimed at preventing and treating caries.

CRANIOFACIAL DYSOSTOSIS (CROUZON SYNDROME)

Disease Mechanism

Craniofacial dysostosis (syndromic craniostenosis, premature craniostenosis) or Crouzon syndrome is an autosomal-dominant skeletal dysplasia characterized by variable expressivity and almost complete penetrance. It is one of many diseases characterized by premature closure of cranial sutures (craniosynostosis), and has an incidence estimated at 1:25,000 births. Of these cases, 33%–56% may arise as a consequence of spontaneous mutations, with the remaining being familial.

Craniofacial dysostosis is caused by a mutation of the fibroblast growth factor receptor 2 *(FGFR2)* gene on chromosome 10. Mutations at this site are also responsible for other craniosynostosis syndromes with similar facial features but clinically visible limb abnormalities. In patients with this syndrome, the coronal suture usually closes first, and eventually all cranial sutures close early. There is also premature fusion of the synchondroses of the cranial base. The subsequent lack of bone growth perpendicular to the synchondroses and cranial coronal sutures produces the characteristic cranial shape and facial features.

Clinical Features

Patients characteristically have a shorter than normal anterior to posterior skull dimension (brachycephaly), increased distance between the eyes (hypertelorism), and protruding eyes (orbital proptosis) (Fig. 27.3A and B). In familial cases, the minimal criteria for diagnosis are hypertelorism and orbital proptosis. Patients may become blind because of early suture closure and increased intracranial pressure. The nose often appears prominent and pointed because the maxilla is narrow and short in its vertical and anteroposterior dimensions. The anterior nasal spine is hypoplastic and retruded, failing to provide adequate support to the soft tissue of the nose. The palatal vault is high, and the maxillary arch is narrow and retruded, resulting in crowding of the dentition.

Imaging Features

The earliest radiologic features of craniosynostosis involve the cranial sutures. Sutures that should normally appear radiolucent on a planar skull image are not detectable, or show sclerotic changes. Rarely, the facial features may manifest before evidence of sutural synostosis. Premature fusion of the cranial base leads to diminished downward and forward facial growth. In some cases, prominent cranial markings are noted, which can also be seen in normal growing patients, but are more prominent because of an increase in intracranial pressure from the growing brain. These markings are seen as multiple radiolucencies appearing as depressions (so-called digital impressions) of the inner surface of the cranial vault, which results in a "beaten metal" or "beaten copper" appearance (Fig. 27.3C–E).

In the jaws, the lack of growth of the cranial base in the anteroposterior direction results in maxillary hypoplasia, creating an Angle Class III malocclusion in some patients. The maxillary hypoplasia contributes to the characteristic orbital proptosis because the maxilla forms the inferior orbital rim and, if severely hypoplastic, fails to support the orbital contents adequately. The mandible is typically smaller than normal but appears prognathic in relation to the severely hypoplastic maxilla.

Differential Diagnosis

Premature craniosynostosis, either isolated or as part of a genetic syndrome, is a common disorder. The incidence of craniofacial dysostosis is reported to range from 1:2100 to 1:2500 births. Other causes of craniosynostosis must be differentiated from craniofacial dysostosis,

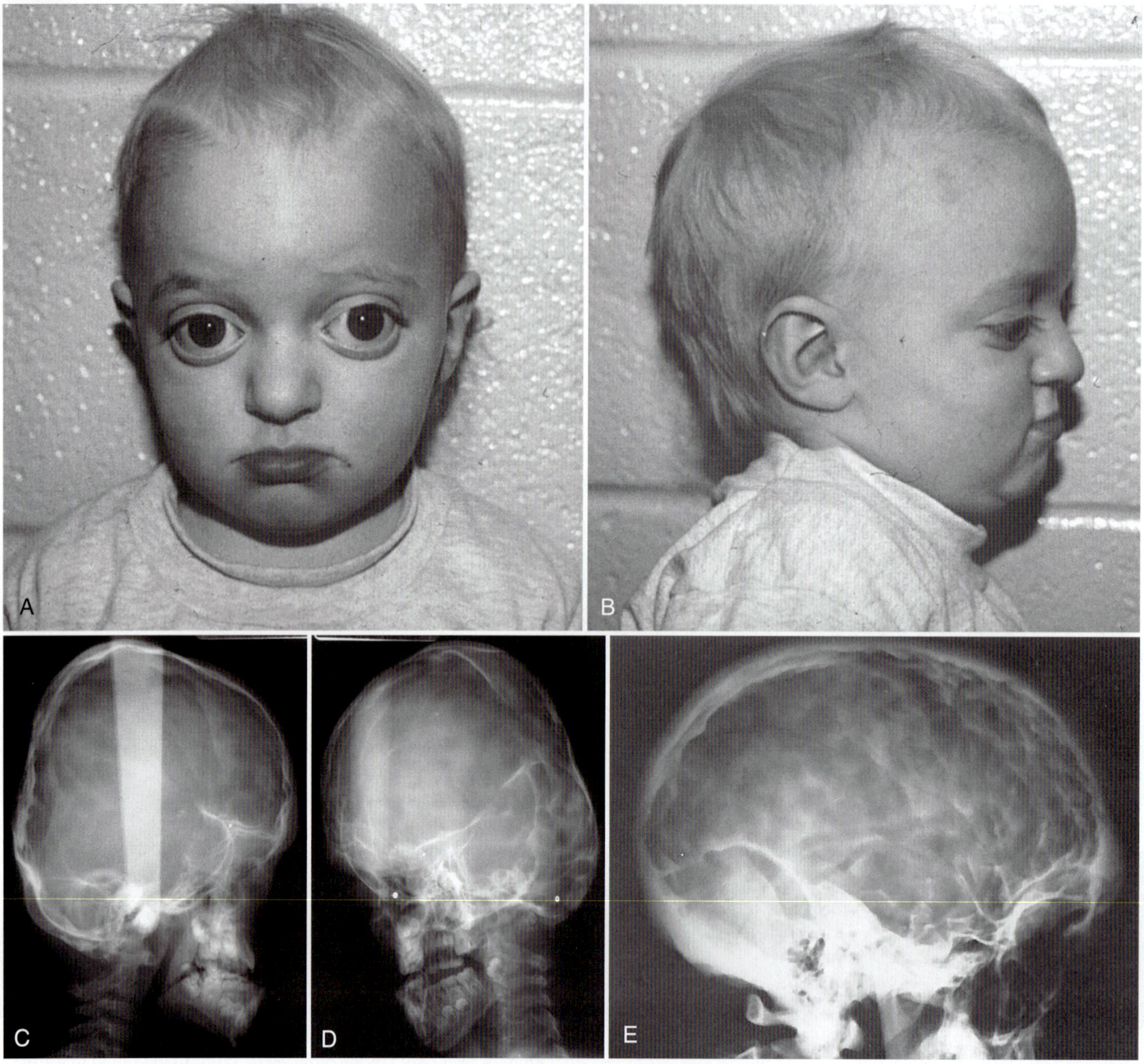

Fig. 27.3 (A and B) Characteristic facial features of craniofacial dysostosis (Crouzon syndrome) in this 2-year-old patient include orbital proptosis, hypertelorism, and midfacial hypoplasia. Rarely do these facial features precede the radiographic signs of sutural synostosis. (C) Mandibulofacial dysostosis results in early closure of the cranial sutures and depressions (digital impressions) on the inner surface of the calvarium from growth of the brain. (D and E) Closure of the cranial sutures in another patient. Note also the prominent digital markings. (D and E, Courtesy Department of Radiology, Baylor University Hospital, Dallas, TX.)

including other syndromic forms of craniosynostosis and nonsyndromic coronal craniosynostosis. The characteristic facial features must be present to suggest Crouzon syndrome.

Management

The craniofacial features of craniofacial dysostosis worsen over time because of the abnormal craniofacial growth. Early diagnosis permits surgical and orthodontic treatment from infancy through adolescence, coordinated by a multidisciplinary craniofacial anomalies team. The objectives of these treatments are to allow normal brain growth and development by preventing increased intracranial pressure, protect the eyes by providing adequate bony support, and improve facial esthetics and occlusal function. Because of early diagnosis and improvements in medical and dental care, most patients have good functional outcomes, normal intelligence, and they can expect a normal lifespan.

HEMIFACIAL MICROSOMIA

Hemifacial microsomia is known by several different terms, including hemifacial hypoplasia, craniofacial microsomia, lateral facial dysplasia, Goldenhar syndrome, and oculoauriculovertebral (OAV) dysplasia spectrum.

Disease Mechanism

Hemifacial microsomia is a common birth defect involving the first and second branchial arches. It is the second most common developmental craniofacial anomaly after CL/P and affects approximately 1:5600 live births. Hemifacial microsomia is a feature of Goldenhar syndrome. This syndrome can also include a broader array of anomalies within the OAV dysplasia complex. Patients with hemifacial microsomia typically display reduced growth and development of half of the face owing to abnormal development of the branchial arches. Although this malformation sequence is usually unilateral, it may occasionally be bilateral (craniofacial microsomia). When the whole side of the face is involved, the mandible, maxilla, zygomatic bone, external and middle ear, hyoid bone, parotid gland, vertebrae, fifth and seventh cranial nerves, musculature, and other soft tissues are reduced in size, and sometimes fail to develop. Delayed eruption of teeth and hypodontia on the affected side also have been reported. Most cases occur spontaneously, but familial cases demonstrating autosomal-dominant inheritance, and occasionally, autosomal recessive inheritance have also been reported. There is a male predominance of 3:2 and a right-side predominance of 3:2. Cases have been reported with epibulbar dermoids, preauricular skin appendages, preauricular fistulas, additional vertebral anomalies, as well as cardiac, cerebral, and renal malformations (Goldenhar syndrome and OAV complex).

Genetic mutations involving the long arm of chromosome 14 at region 32 (14q32) and microdeletions at 22q11 subregion 2 (22q11.2) have been associated with some cases of Goldenhar syndrome. In most cases, however, a clear genetic cause cannot be found. The pathogenesis is not known; however, hemifacial microsomia is thought to be caused by a disruption of vascular supply during embryonic development. There is some limited evidence that assisted reproductive technologies are associated with an increased risk of OAV dysplasias, including patients with hemifacial macrosomia. A recent large study demonstrated that systemic malformations including vertebral, genitourinary, cardiovascular, and cerebral anomalies were common, and seen in a total of 73/86 patients in one institution; therefore, multidisciplinary team-based care is essential.

Clinical Features

Hemifacial microsomia is usually apparent at birth. Patients with this condition have facial asymmetry and ear malformations. Aplasia or hypoplasia of the external ear (microtia) is common, and the ear canal is often missing. In some patients, the skull is diminished in size. In about 90% of cases, there is malocclusion on the affected side. The midsagittal plane of the patient's face is curved toward the affected side. The occlusal plane often is canted cranially (i.e., superiorly) to the affected side.

Imaging Features

The primary radiologic finding is a reduction in the sizes of the bones on the affected side. This change is clearest in the mandible, which may show a reduction in the size or, in severe cases, lack of any development of the condyle, coronoid process, or ramus. The mandibular body is also reduced in size, and a portion of the bone may be missing (Fig. 27.4). The dentition on the affected side may show a reduction in the number or size of the teeth. Multidetector computed tomography (MDCT) shows a reduction in the sizes of the muscles of mastication and muscles of facial expression, and hypoplasia or atresia of the auditory canal and ossicles of the middle ear. The course of the facial nerve is often shown to be abnormal on an MDCT examination of the temporal bone. Magnetic resonance imaging (MRI) can also be useful in demonstrating the extent of inner ear abnormalities, and involvement of the facial nerve and other soft tissues of the mouth and eyes. Thin-section MDCT imaging of the temporal bone is often performed to assess the degree of stenosis of the external auditory meatus, as well as middle and inner ear malformations to plan treatment; these may include cochlear implants, bone-anchored hearing aids, or implant-retained ear prostheses. This type of imaging is particularly important for patients with Goldenhar syndrome and the broader OAV complex. A multimodality approach to imaging is optimal, and these may include panoramic images to investigate dental development, planar skull cephalometric images and cone beam computed tomography (CBCT) to assess the facial asymmetry and to plan orthognathic and orthodontic treatment, MDCT imaging of the temporal bones to assess the external and internal ear anatomy, and 3D volumetric reconstructions of MDCT images for surgical treatment planning.

Differential Interpretation

The features of hemifacial microsomia are characteristic. Condylar hypoplasia, especially caused by a fracture at birth or progressive condylar resorption may be similar, but it does not produce the ear changes. Exposure of the face of a child to radiation therapy during growth also may result in underdevelopment of the irradiated tissues. In progressive hemifacial atrophy (Parry–Romberg syndrome), the changes become more severe over time but are generally not present at birth, and the ears are normal.

Management

The mandibular abnormalities may be corrected by conventional orthognathic surgery or distraction osteogenesis to lengthen the ramus on the affected side. Orthodontic intervention may correct or prevent malocclusion. The external ear abnormalities may be repaired by plastic surgery or corrected with prosthetic ears, and the hearing loss may be partly corrected by bone-anchored hearing aids. In bilateral cases (Goldenhar syndrome and OAV complex), cochlear implants may be used to correct profound hearing loss. Because of the range of craniofacial anomalies as well as systemic anomalies associated with this condition, management by a multidisciplinary team is recommended.

MANDIBULOFACIAL DYSOSTOSIS (TREACHER COLLINS SYNDROME)

Disease Mechanism

Mandibulofacial dysostosis or Treacher Collins syndrome is an autosomal-dominant disorder of craniofacial development. It is the most common type of mandibulofacial dysostosis, with an incidence of 1:50,000. Mandibulofacial dysostosis is caused by a mutation of the treacle ribosome biogenesis factor 1 gene *(TCOF1)*, which encodes a protein that is important in the development of facial structures, including the bones. Mandibulofacial dysostosis has variable expressivity and complete penetrance. Approximately half of cases arise as the result of sporadic mutation, and the rest are familial.

Clinical Features

Individuals with mandibulofacial dysostosis have a wide range of anomalies depending on the severity of the condition. The most common clinical findings are relative underdevelopment or absence of the zygomatic bones resulting in a small, narrow face, a downward inclination of the palpebral fissures, underdevelopment of the mandible resulting in a downturned, wide mouth, malformation of the external ears, absence of the external auditory canal, and occasional facial clefts (Fig. 27.5A and B). The palate develops with a high arch or cleft in 30% of cases. Hypoplasia of the mandible and a steep mandibular angle results in an Angle Class II malocclusion with anterior open bite. Hypoplasia or atresia of the external ear, auditory canal, and ossicles of the middle ear may result in partial or complete deafness.

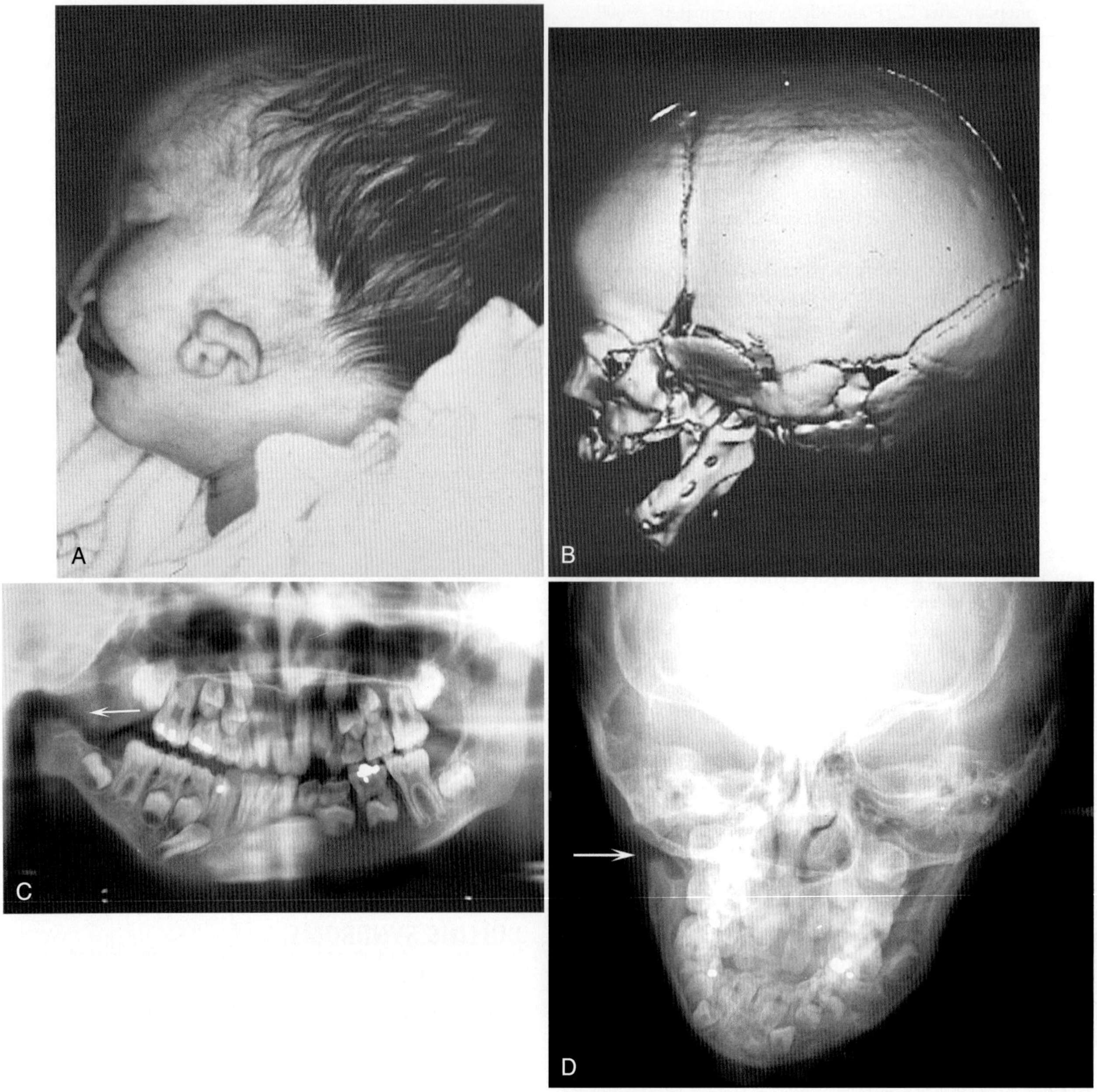

Fig. 27.4 (A and B) Hemifacial microsomia showing reduced size and malformation of the left ear and left side of the mandible. (A) Clinical photograph of an infant with hemifacial microsomia. (B) Three-dimensional multidetector computed tomographic reconstruction of the affected side shows the extent of the bony malformation. Note the complete absence of the temporomandibular joint and coronoid process as well as auditory canal atresia. Panoramic image (C) and posteroanterior skull image (D) of other cases show lack of development of the ramus, coronoid process, and condyle *(arrows)*. (A and B, Courtesy Dr. A. Rozzelle, Detroit, MI.)

Imaging Features

A striking finding is the hypoplastic or absent zygomatic bones, and hypoplasia of the lateral aspects of the orbits. The auditory canal, mastoid air cells, and articular eminence often are smaller than normal or absent. The maxilla and especially the mandible are hypoplastic, showing accentuation of the antegonial notch and a steep mandibular angle, which gives the impression that the body of the mandible is bending in an inferior and posterior direction (Fig. 27.5C–F). The ramus is especially short. The condyles are positioned posteriorly and inferiorly. The maxillary sinuses may be underdeveloped or absent.

Cervical spine anomalies have also been reported in 18% of patients with mandibulofacial dysostosis, including spina bifida occulta, dysmorphic C1, and reduced C2–C3 space. In one case series, five of seven patients with cervical spine anomalies also had CP. This finding suggests that patients with mandibulofacial dysostosis and CP may be at higher risk for cervical spine anomalies and should be targeted for assessment. A more recent study has also reported dysplasia or aplasia of major salivary glands, as detected by ultrasound imaging, in half of patients with mandibulofacial dysostosis followed at a major craniofacial anomalies center. This finding is important because these salivary gland anomalies could significantly increase risk for dental caries in patients with this syndrome.

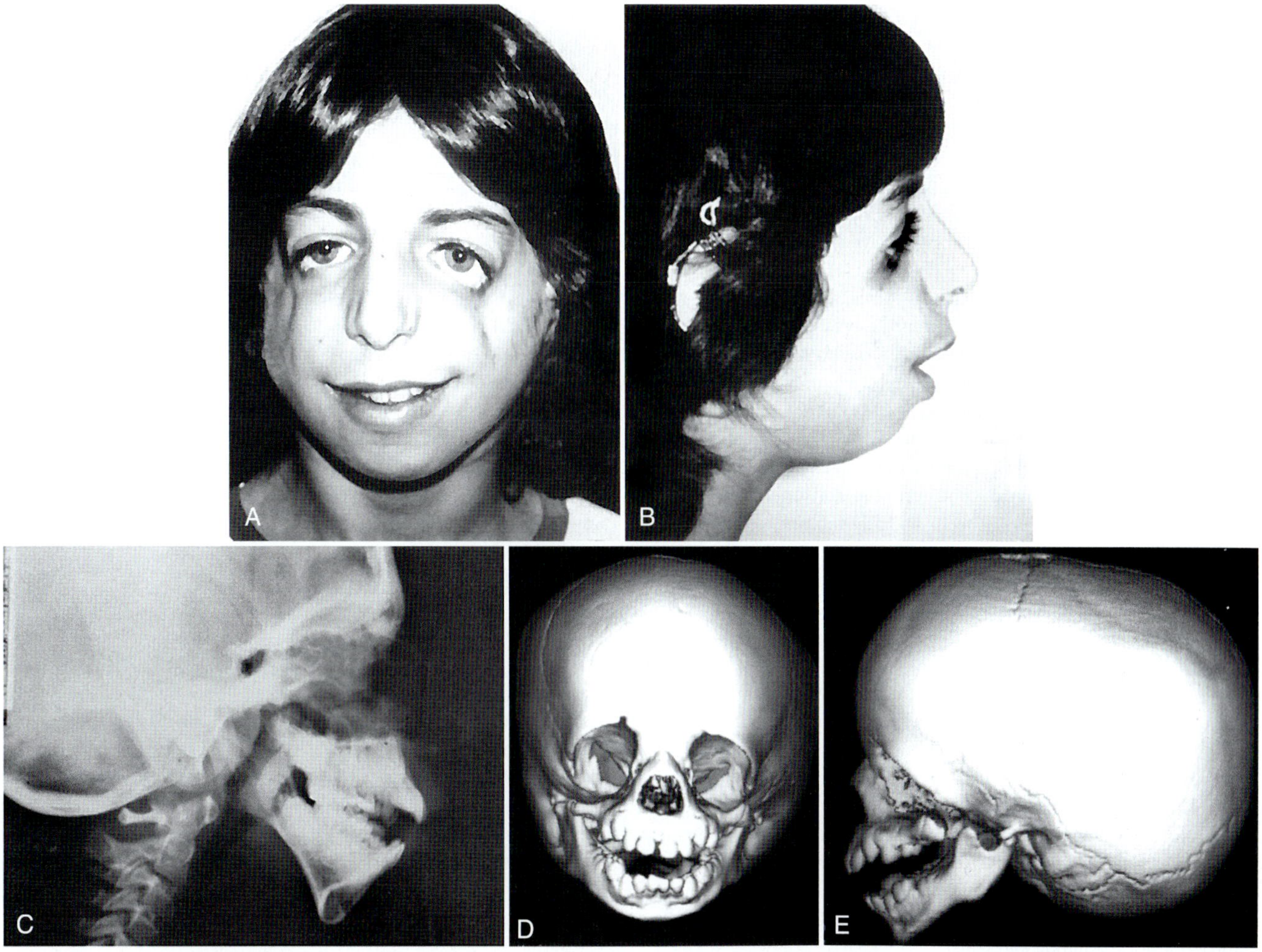

Fig. 27.5 Mandibulofacial dysostosis (Treacher Collins syndrome). (A and B) Note the characteristic facies: downward-sloping palpebral fissures, colobomas of the outer third of the lower lids, depressed cheekbones, receding chin, little if any nasofrontal angle, and a nose that appears relatively large. (C) Correlation of radiographic features with clinical features: short mandibular rami, steep mandibular angle, and anterior open bite. The zygomatic bones are poorly formed. (D and E) Three-dimensional multidetector computed tomographic reconstruction of a young patient with mandibulofacial dysostosis shows the extent of the bony abnormalities, including bilateral auditory canal atresia, aplasia of the zygomatic arch, and hypoplasia of the mandibular ramus with characteristic "curved" shape of the mandibular body and pronounced antegonial notching.

Differential Interpretation

Other disorders that may result in severe hypoplasia of the entire mandible include condylar agenesis, Hallermann–Streiff syndrome, Nager syndrome, and Pierre Robin sequence, which can be a part of several other genetic syndromes or an isolated anomaly.

Management

Comprehensive treatment of patients with mandibulofacial dysostosis is optimally provided by a multidisciplinary craniofacial anomalies team. Growth of the facial bones during adolescence may result in some cosmetic improvement. Surgical intervention, including bilateral distraction osteogenesis of the mandible, may improve the osseous defects. Treatment of the external ear defects may involve plastic and reconstructive surgery, prostheses, or both. Hearing aids or cochlear implants may be used to treat the hearing loss, depending on the severity. Coordinated orthodontics and orthognathic surgery are often used to treat malocclusion and improve function and esthetics.

CLEIDOCRANIAL DYSPLASIA

Disease Mechanism

Cleidocranial dysplasia is an autosomal-dominant malformation syndrome affecting bones and teeth. The prevalence is estimated at 1:1 million, and it affects both sexes equally. Cleidocranial dysplasia is caused by a mutation in the *RUNX2* gene that encodes a protein which is responsible for the development of the hard tissues. The mutation has variable expressivity and almost complete penetrance, and can be inherited or arise because of sporadic mutation.

Clinical Features

Although the disease affects the entire skeleton, cleidocranial dysplasia primarily affects the dentition, skull, and clavicles. Affected individuals have been shown to be of shorter stature than unaffected relatives but not short enough for this to be considered a form of dwarfism. The face appears small in contrast to the cranium because of hypoplasia of the maxilla, and the skull demonstrates a reduced anteroposterior dimension (brachycephaly). As well, the presence of frontal, and in particular, parietal bossing can increase skull width. The paranasal sinuses may be underdeveloped and there is an increased risk of sinusitis. Hearing loss and recurrent otitis media have also been reported. There is delayed closure of the cranial sutures, and the fontanels may remain patent years beyond the normal time of closure. The bridge of the nose may be broad and depressed, with excessive distance between the eyes (hypertelorism). The complete absence (aplasia) or reduced size (hypoplasia) of the clavicles allows excessive mobility of the shoulder girdle (Fig. 27.6A and B).

The dental abnormalities produce most of the morbidity associated with cleidocranial dysplasia, and are often the reason for diagnosis in mildly affected individuals. Characteristically, patients show prolonged retention of the primary dentition and delayed eruption of the permanent dentition. Extraction of primary teeth does not adequately stimulate eruption of underlying permanent teeth. A study of teeth from patients with cleidocranial dysplasia revealed a paucity or complete absence of cellular cementum on both erupted and unerupted teeth. Often unerupted supernumerary teeth are present, and considerable crowding and disorganization of the developing permanent dentition may occur. The number of supernumerary teeth has been correlated with a reduction in skeletal height in these patients.

Imaging Features

The characteristic skull findings are brachycephaly, delayed or failed closure of the fontanels, open skull sutures including a persistent open metopic suture, and multiple wormian bones (small, irregular bones in the sutures of the skull that are formed by secondary centers of ossification in the suture lines) (Figs. 27.6C–G and 27.7). In the most severe cases, very little formation of the parietal and frontal bones may occur. Typically, the clavicles are underdeveloped to varying degrees, and they are completely absent in approximately 10% of cases. Other bones also may be affected, including the long bones, vertebral column, pelvis, and bones of the hands and feet.

In the jaws, the maxilla and paranasal sinuses are characteristically hypoplastic and the mandible is usually normal in size giving the appearance of relative mandibular prognathism. A persistent (i.e., open) mandibular symphyseal suture has also been reported in 3% of adults and 64% of children. Several investigators have described the alveolar processes overlying unerupted teeth as being denser than usual with a coarse trabecular pattern in the mandible. This finding correlates to the histologic findings of decreased resorption and multiple reversal lines, which may account for the delayed eruption of teeth not mechanically obstructed by supernumerary and other unerupted teeth.

Characteristically, there is prolonged retention of the primary dentition and multiple unerupted permanent and supernumerary teeth (Fig. 27.8A and B). The number of supernumerary teeth can vary, with as many as 63 having been reported in one individual with the disorder. The unerupted teeth develop most commonly in the anterior maxilla and premolar regions of the jaws. Many resemble premolars, and these unerupted teeth may develop dentigerous cysts. The supernumerary teeth develop, on average, 4 years later than the corresponding normal teeth. Because of this delayed development, it has been proposed that the supernumerary teeth represent a third dentition.

Differential Interpretation

Cleidocranial dysplasia may be identified by the family history, medical genetics, excessive mobility of the shoulders, clinical and radiographic morphometric examination of the skull, and the pathognomonic findings of prolonged retention of the primary teeth with multiple unerupted supernumerary teeth on imaging. Other conditions associated with multiple unerupted and supernumerary teeth, such as pyknodyostosis and familial adenomatous polyposis (Gardner syndrome) must be considered in the differential interpretation.

Management

Patients should be identified early (before age 5 years) to take advantage of combined orthodontic and surgical treatment, as well as address other problems including hearing loss. Dental care should include the removal of primary and supernumerary teeth and guided eruption of the permanent teeth. Autotransplantation of teeth has been shown to be a successful strategy to treat older patients. Prosthodontic rehabilitation with dental implants has been used in some cases. Patients should be monitored for development of distal molars and cysts until late adolescence. Surgical treatment of the bony defects of the skull is often performed to address esthetic concerns. In those cases, CT imaging is used to visualize the size and thickness of such defects and plan for harvesting of bone graft material from other parts of the skull (Fig. 27.7A–C). As with other complex craniofacial anomalies, management is best provided by an experienced multidisciplinary craniofacial anomalies team.

HEMIFACIAL HYPERPLASIA

Disease Mechanism

Hemifacial hyperplasia (hemifacial hypertrophy, hemihyperplasia) is a condition in which there is unilateral enlargement of the region of the face, extending from the frontal bone to the inferior border of the mandible, and from the midline to the pinna of the ear. There is enlargement of teeth, bone, and soft tissues within the affected region. This condition can be associated with enlargement of other parts of the body as well. The cause of this condition is unknown. Some cases are associated with genetic diseases such as Beckwith–Wiedemann syndrome.

Clinical Features

Hemifacial hyperplasia begins at birth and usually continues throughout the growing years, although in some cases, it may not be recognized until it becomes more apparent with growth. The condition often occurs with other abnormalities, including mental deficiency, skin abnormalities, compensatory scoliosis, genitourinary tract anomalies, and various neoplasms, including Wilms tumor of the kidney, adrenocortical tumor, and hepatoblastoma (Beckwith–Wiedemann syndrome). Females and males are affected with approximately equal frequency. The dentition of affected individuals may show unilateral enlargement, accelerated development, and premature loss of primary teeth. The tongue and alveolar bone enlarge on the involved side.

Imaging Features

Radiologic examination of the skull reveals enlargement of the bones on the affected side, including the mandible (Fig. 27.8), maxilla, zygomatic, frontal, and temporal bones. A few cases have been reported involving only one side of the maxilla or one side of the mandible.

Differential Diagnosis

The differential diagnosis should consider hemifacial hypoplasia of the opposite side, arteriovenous malformation, hemangioma, and congenital lymphedema. Also, severe condylar hyperplasia that may involve half of the mandible should be considered. The presence of enlarged teeth together with rapid eruption of the dentition suggests hemifacial hyperplasia. Cases limited to one side of the maxilla must be differentiated from monostotic fibrous dysplasia and segmental odontomaxillary dysplasia, both of which have characteristic changes

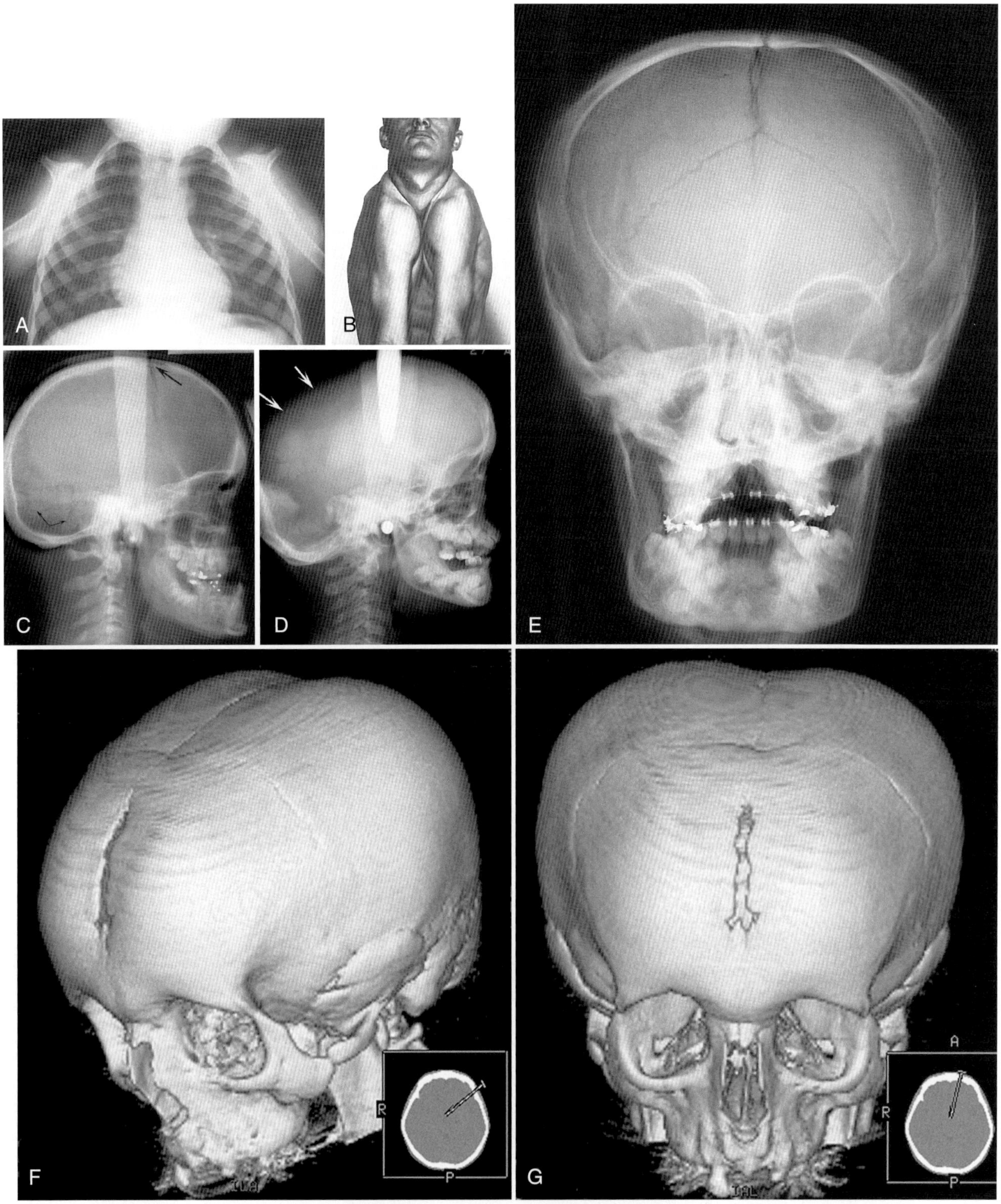

Fig. 27.6 Cleidocranial dysplasia. (A) Note the absence of clavicles on the chest image. (B) The result is excessive mobility of the shoulders. Note also the frontal bossing and hypoplastic maxilla. (C) Lateral cephalometric skull image shows wormian (sutural) bones in the occipital region *(small arrows)* and the open fontanel *(large arrow)*. (D) Lateral cephalometric skull image shows a lack of development of the parietal bones *(arrows)*. (E) Posteroanterior cephalometric skull image showing a brachycephalic skull and the "light bulb" shape to the images of the skull and mandible. (F) Oblique orientation of a three-dimensional reconstruction from a multidetector computed tomographic study shows the typical skull shape seen in this condition. Note the parietal and frontal bossing, and the open metopic suture in this patient. (G) Direct frontal view of the same 3D reconstruction showing the "light bulb" shape of the skull and the open metopic suture. (A, Courtesy Department of Radiology, Baylor University Hospital, Dallas, TX.)

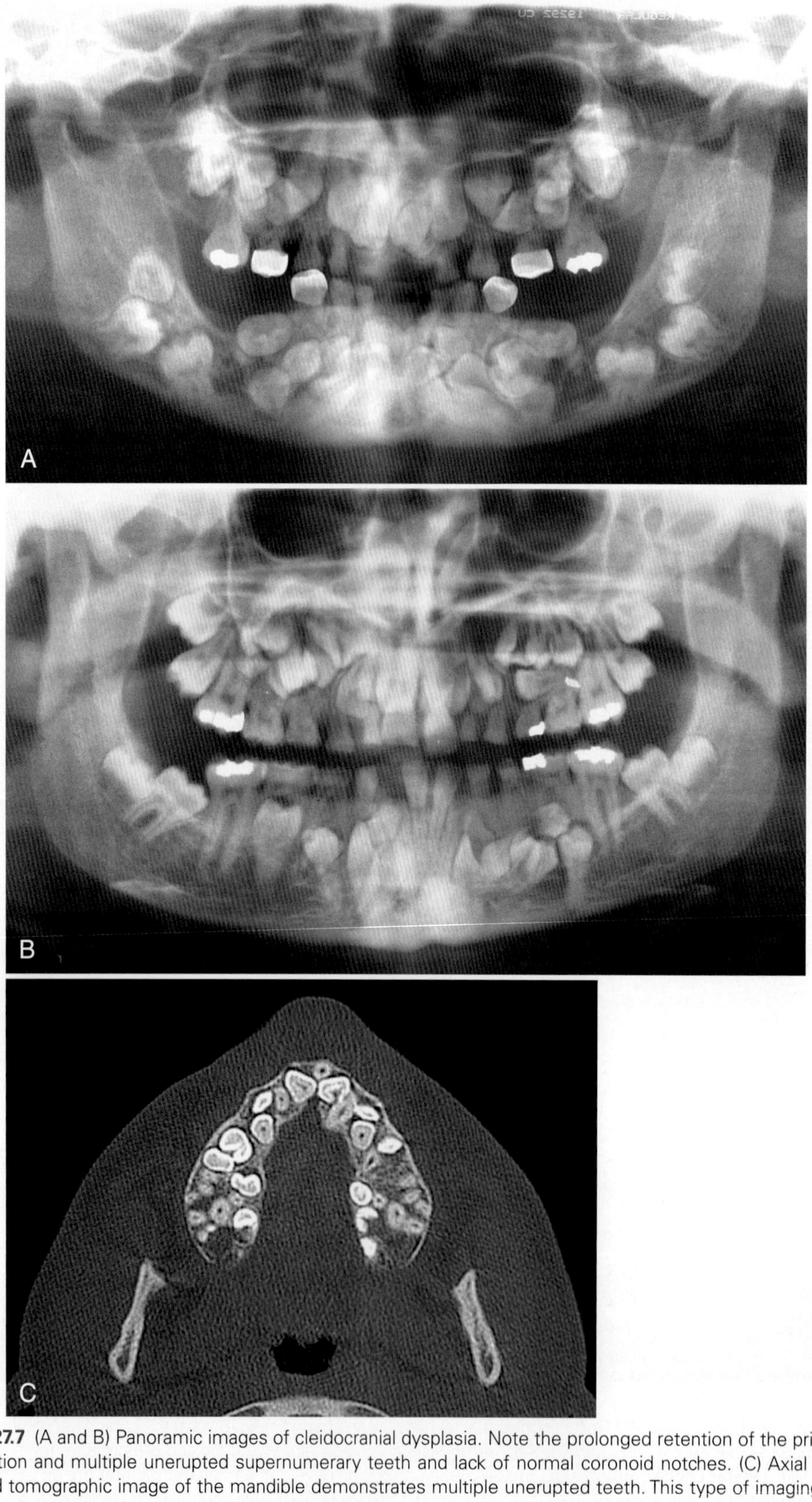

Fig. 27.7 (A and B) Panoramic images of cleidocranial dysplasia. Note the prolonged retention of the primary dentition and multiple unerupted supernumerary teeth and lack of normal coronoid notches. (C) Axial computed tomographic image of the mandible demonstrates multiple unerupted teeth. This type of imaging can be used to localize the unerupted teeth to assist in treatment planning of extractions and orthodontic tooth movement. (Courtesy Dr. S. Edwards, Ann Arbor, MI.)

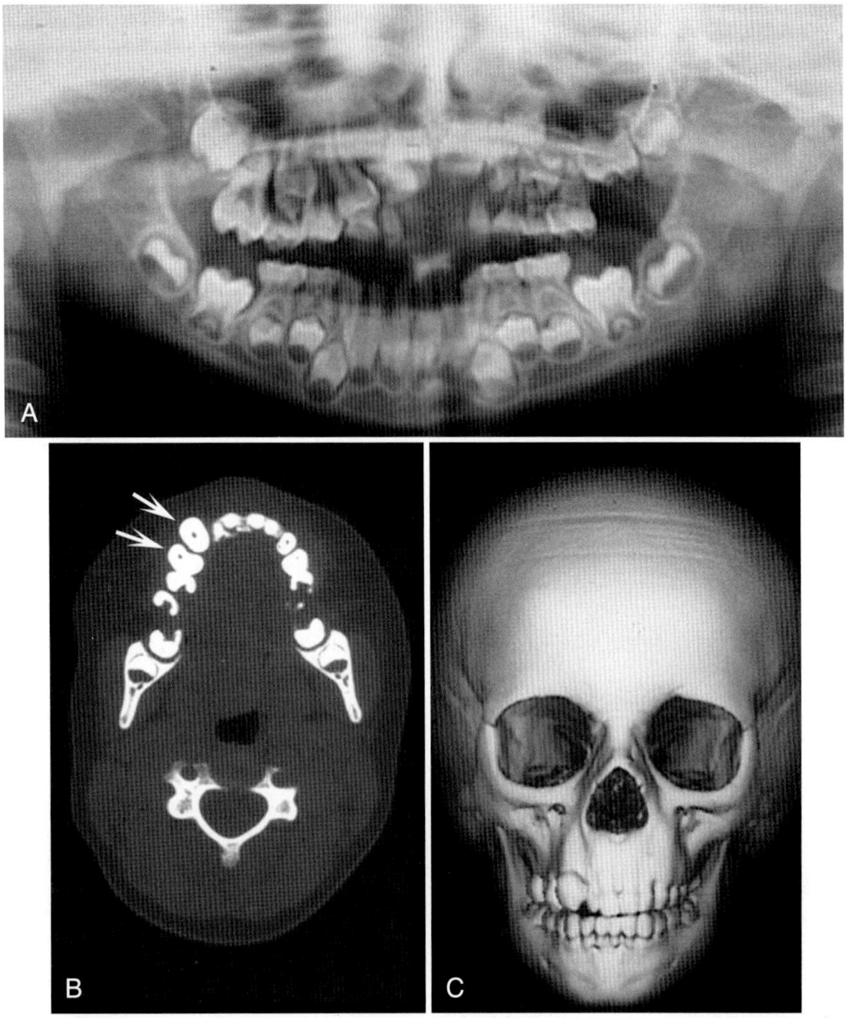

Fig. 27.8 Hemifacial hyperplasia revealing enlargement of the right maxilla only. (A) Panoramic image shows accelerated dental development limited to the right maxilla in a 5-year-old patient. (B) Bone algorithm axial multidetector computed tomographic image of the same patient demonstrates enlargement of the maxillary canine and first premolar *(arrows)* compared with the contralateral side. (C) Three-dimensional multidetector computed tomographic reconstruction shows subtle bony enlargement of the right maxilla and the right canine.

in the radiographic appearance of the alveolar bone, not present in hemifacial hyperplasia.

Management

An insufficient number of cases of hemifacial hyperplasia with long-term follow up have been reported to make definitive recommendations for treatment. Although most cases are isolated, a child with suspected hemifacial hyperplasia should be referred to a medical geneticist for diagnosis and early detection of one of several genetic syndromes that can be associated with this condition.

SEGMENTAL ODONTOMAXILLARY DYSPLASIA

Disease Mechanism

Segmental odontomaxillary dysplasia or hemimaxillofacial dysplasia is a developmental abnormality of unknown etiology that affects the posterior alveolar process of one side of the maxilla, including the teeth and attached gingiva. It has recently been included as a "fibro-osseous lesion" in the fifth edition of the World Health Organization Classification of Head and Neck Tumors (2022).

Clinical Features

The abnormality is always unilateral and results in enlargement of the alveolar process, without or with enlargement of the gingiva, and dental anomalies. Teeth are frequently missing (most commonly the premolars) or hypoplastic, and some of the teeth that remain are unerupted. Ipsilateral hypertrichosis and other skin anomalies, including closely packed sebaceous glands in the upper lip, hypo- or hyperpigmentation, and Becker nevus have also been found. Mild facial enlargement has been found in a few cases, and clefting has been reported in 23% of cases. Most cases are detected in childhood because a parent notices the lack of tooth eruption or mild facial asymmetry, or the dentist notices missing premolars on diagnostic images.

Imaging Features

The density of the maxillary alveolar process is increased, with a greater number of thick trabeculae that appear to be aligned in a vertical orientation (Fig. 27.9). There have been some reports of missing buccal cortical plate, but this is not a consistent feature. The roots of the deciduous teeth are larger than on the unaffected side and usually are splayed in shape. The crowns of the deciduous teeth and sometimes

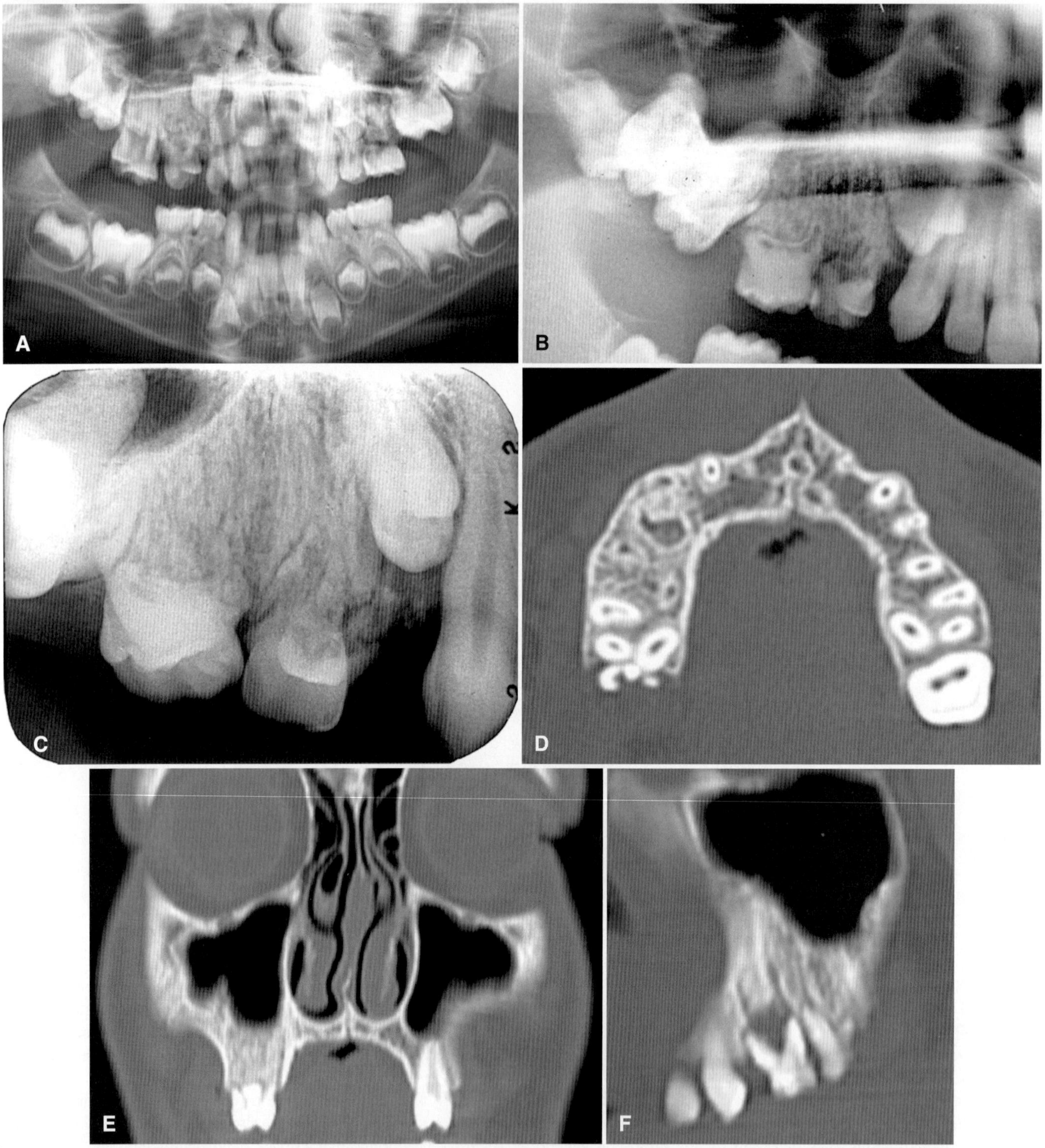

Fig. 27.9 (A) Panoramic image of segmental odontomaxillary dysplasia. Note the large left maxillary deciduous molars compared with the right side and the lack of formation of the premolars, delayed eruption of the first molar, and the dense bone pattern of the left maxillary alveolar process. (B and C) A second case demonstrating the coarse trabecular pattern of the right maxillary alveolar process and delayed eruption of the maxillary right first premolar and molars. Cone beam computed tomographic images of another case involving the right maxilla. (D) Axial image shows an increase in internal bone density within the right maxilla. (E) Coronal image shows an increase in the width of the alveolar process. (F) Sagittal image shows multiple vertical, radiolucent linear structures, which likely represent nutrient canals.

the permanent teeth are enlarged. Enlargement of pulp chambers and irregular resorption of the roots of deciduous teeth also may be seen. The alveolar process is not pneumatized by the maxillary sinus and appears smaller than on the contralateral side. There is often delayed eruption of the first and second permanent molars.

Differential Interpretation

Other conditions that must be differentiated from segmental odontomaxillary dysplasia include segmental hemifacial hyperplasia, monostotic fibrous dysplasia, and regional odontodysplasia. Hemifacial hyperplasia is not associated with coarse vertically oriented trabeculae in the bone. Monostotic fibrous dysplasia is not typically associated with missing teeth and, in contrast to segmental odontomaxillary dysplasia, will continue to show disproportionate growth of the affected side. Regional odontodysplasia is typically associated with "ghost teeth," and is not associated with expansion and alteration in trabecular pattern in the alveolar bone.

BIBLIOGRAPHY

Cohen MM Jr, McLean RE. *Craniosynostosis: Diagnosis, Evaluation, and Management.* 2nd ed. Oxford University Press; 2000.

Gorlin RJ, Cohen MM Jr, Hennekam RCM. *Syndromes of the Head and Neck.* 4th ed. Oxford University Press; 2001.

Neville BW, Damm DD, Allen CM, et al. *Oral and Maxillofacial Pathology.* 5th ed. Saunders; 2023.

Cleft Lip and Cleft Palate

Babai A, Irving M. Orofacial clefts: genetics of cleft lip and palate. *Genes (Basel).* 2023;14(8):1603. doi:10.3390/genes14081603.

Beaty TH, Marazita ML, Leslie EJ. Genetic factors influencing risk to orofacial clefts: today's challenges and tomorrow's opportunities. F1000Res. 2016;5:2800. doi:10.12688/f1000research.9503.1.g.

Grewcock RE, Innes NPT, Mossey PA, et al. Caries in children with and without orofacial clefting: a systematic review and meta-analysis. *Oral Dis.* 2022;28(5):1400-1411. doi:10.1111/odi.14183.

Habel A, Sell D, Mars M, et al. Management of cleft lip and palate. *Arch Dis Child.* 1996;74:360.

Harris EF, Hullings JG. Delayed dental development in children with isolated cleft lip and palate. *Arch Oral Biol.* 1990;35:469.

Honein MA, Rasmussen SA, Reefhuis J, et al. Maternal and environmental tobacco smoke exposure and the risk of orofacial clefts. *Epidemiology.* 2007;18:226-233.

Craniofacial Dysostosis (Crouzon Syndrome)

Murdoch-Kinch CA, Bixler D, Ward RE. Cephalometric analysis of families with dominantly inherited Crouzon syndrome: an aid to diagnosis in family studies. *Am J Med Genet.* 1998;77:405-411.

Tuite GF, Evanson J, Chong WK, et al. The beaten copper cranium: a correlation between intracranial pressure, cranial radiographs, and computed tomographic scans in children with craniosynostosis. *Neurosurgery.* 1996;39:691-699.

Hemifacial Microsomia

AlHadidi A, Cevidanes LHS, Mol A, et al. Comparison of two methods for quantitative assessment of mandibular asymmetry using cone beam computed tomography image volumes. *Dentomaxillofac Radiol.* 2011;40:351-357.

Cohen N, Cohen E, Gaiero A, et al. Maxillofacial features and systemic malformations in expanded spectrum hemifacial microsomia. *Am J Med Genet.* 2017;173:1208-1218.

Johnson JM, Moonis G, Green GE, et al. Syndromes of the first and second branchial arches, part 2: syndromes. *AJNR Am J Neuroradiol.* 2011;32: 230-237.

Maruko E, Hayes C, Evans CA, et al. Hypodontia in hemifacial microsomia. *Cleft Palate Craniofac J.* 2001;38:15-19.

Monahan R, Seder K, Patel P, et al. Hemifacial microsomia: etiology, diagnosis and treatment. *J Am Dent Assoc.* 2001;132:1402-1408.

Senggen E, Laswed T, Meuwly J-Y, et al. First and second branchial arch syndromes: multimodality approach. *Pediatr Radiol.* 2011;41:549-561.

Mandibulofacial Dysostosis (Treacher Collins Syndrome)

Osterhus IN, Skogedal N, Akre H, et al. Salivary gland pathology as a new finding in Treacher Collins syndrome. *Am J Med Genet A.* 2012;158A:1320-1325.

Posnick JC. Treacher Collins syndrome: perspectives in evaluation and treatment. *J Oral Maxillofac Surg.* 1997;55:1120.

Pun AHY, Clark BE, David DJ, et al. Cervical spine in Treacher Collins syndrome. *J Craniofac Surg.* 2012;23:218-220.

Cleidocranial Dysplasia

Dalessandri D, Laffranchi L, Tonni I, et al. Advantages of cone beam computed tomography (CBCT) in the orthodontic treatment planning of cleidocranial dysplasia patients: a case report. *Head Face Med.* 2011;7:6.

Golan I, Baumert U, Hrala BP, et al. Dentomaxillofacial variability of cleidocranial dysplasia: clinicoradiological presentation and systematic review. *Dentomaxillofac Radiol.* 2003;32:347-354.

Kreiborg S, and Jensen BL. Tooth formation and eruption-lessons learnt from cleidocranial dysplasia. *Eur J Oral Sci.* 2018;126(suppl 1):72-80. doi:10.1111/eos.12418.

Seow WK, Hertzberg J. Dental development and molar root length in children with cleidocranial dysplasia. *Pediatr Dent.* 1995;17:101-105.

Yoshida T, Kanegane H, Osata M, et al. Functional analysis of RUNX2 mutations in Japanese patients with cleidocranial dysplasia demonstrates novel genotype-phenotype correlations. *Am J Hum Genet.* 2002;71:724-738.

Shi Y, Ye Z, Liu Y et al. Detection and diagnosis of cleidocranial dysplasia by panoramic radiography: a retrospective review. *BMC Oral Health.* 2022;22:558. doi:10.1186/s12903-022-02610-7.

Hemifacial Hyperplasia

Fraumeni JF, Geiser CF, Manning MD, et al. Wilms' tumor and congenital hemihypertrophy: report of five new cases and review of the literature. *Pediatrics.* 1967;40:886.

Hoyme HE, Seaver LH, Procopio F, et al. Isolated hemihyperplasia (hemihypertrophy): report of a prospective multicenter study of the incidence of neoplasia and review. *Am J Med Genet.* 1998;79:274-278.

Kogon SL, Jarvis AM, Daley TD, et al. Hemifacial hypertrophy affecting the maxillary dentition: report of a case. *Oral Surg Oral Med Oral Pathol.* 1984;58:549-553.

Segmental Odontomaxillary Dysplasia

Danforth RA, Melrose RJ, Abrams AM, et al. Segmental odontomaxillary dysplasia: report of eight cases and comparison with hemimaxillofacial dysplasia. *Oral Surg Oral Med Oral Pathol.* 1990;70:81.

Miles DA, Lovas JL, Clhen MM, et al. Hemimaxillofacial dysplasia: a newly recognized disorder of facial asymmetry, hypertrichosis of the facial skin, unilateral enlargement of the maxilla, and hypoplastic teeth in two patients. *Oral Surg Oral Med Oral Pathol.* 1987;64:445.

Minett CP, Daley TD. Hemimaxillofacial dysplasia (segmental odontomaxillary dysplasia): case study with 11 years of follow-up from primary to adult dentition. *J Oral Maxillofac Surg.* 2012;70:1183-1191.

Packota GV, Pharoah MJ, Petrikowski CG, et al. Radiographic features of segmental odontomaxillary dysplasia: a study of 12 cases. *Oral Surg Oral Med Oral Pathol Oral Radiol Endod.* 1996;82:577.

Vered M, Wright JM. Update from the 5th edition of the World Health Organization classification of head and neck tumors: odontogenic and maxillofacial bone tumors. *Head and Neck Pathology.* 2022;16:63-75.

Whitt JC, Rokos JW, Dunlap CL, et al. Segmental odontomaxillary dysplasia: report of a series of 5 cases with long-term follow-up. *Oral Surg Oral Med Oral Pathol Oral Radiol Endod.* 2011;112:e29-e47.

28

Temporomandibular Joint Abnormalities

Susanne E. Perschbacher

DISEASE MECHANISM

Disorders of the temporomandibular joint (TMJ) include all abnormalities that interfere with the normal form or function of the TMJ. These disorders include developmental abnormalities that can result in an abnormal form of the osseous or soft tissue structures of the joint, as well as acquired ones, such as dysfunction of the articular disk and associated ligaments, the muscles of mastication, joint arthritides, inflammatory lesions, trauma, and neoplasia.

CLINICAL FEATURES

A wide range of conditions can elicit disorders of the TMJ, and these may manifest with an extensive assortment of clinical features. Dysfunction of the joint is the most common disorder, and is most likely to manifest with pain in the TMJ or ear, or both; headache; muscle tenderness; joint stiffness; clicking or other joint noises; reduced range of motion; and locking and subluxation. Careful clinical examination can help identify which structures are likely contributing to the joint dysfunction. For example, pain to palpation of the muscles of mastication and headache suggest a myofascial pain disorder, while clicking or popping sounds in the joint, locking, or reduced range of motion are often associated with disk abnormalities. Crepitus and pain over the joint itself can commonly indicate arthritic involvement.

A higher incidence of TMJ dysfunction has been reported in females, particularly during childbearing and peri-menopause years, and this is believed to be due to changes in estrogen signaling. In most cases, the clinical signs and symptoms are transient, and often treatment is not indicated beyond patient reassurance and education. However, a small percentage (5%) of patients have severe dysfunction (e.g., severe pain, marked functional impairment, or both), which requires a thorough diagnostic workup, including diagnostic imaging, before treatment.

Other disorders of the TMJs are less common. A neoplasm may manifest with swelling of the area surrounding the joint, whereas redness and heat over the joint may indicate an inflammatory condition. Developmental abnormalities are most likely to be unilateral and manifest with facial asymmetry. Changes in occlusion also may be a sign of an abnormality in one or both of the TMJs.

IMAGING ANATOMY OF THE TEMPOROMANDIBULAR JOINT

A thorough understanding of the anatomy and morphology of the TMJ is essential so that disruptions in anatomy can be identified as potential disease, and a normal variant is not mistaken for an abnormality. Each joint is formed by the articulating components of the mandible and the temporal bone. The mandible is unique because the two TMJs must function together in a coordinated fashion as part of a single unit in order to facilitate mandibular movements. An articular disk composed of fibrocartilage is interposed between the articulating surfaces of the mandibular condylar head and the glenoid fossa of the temporal bone of each joint, and retrodiscal tissues and ligamentous attachments help maintain the normal position of the disk. A fibrous joint capsule lined with a synovial membrane surrounds and encloses the joint. Synovial tissue is present on non-load–bearing surfaces which secretes synovial fluid that lubricates the joint. The muscles of mastication allow movement of the condyle, but the ligaments limit the extent of this movement.

Mandibular Component

The mandibular condyle is the mandibular component of the TMJ. The condyle is a bony ellipsoid process of the mandible that extends superiorly from the mandibular ramus by way of a narrow neck (Fig. 28.1). The condyle is approximately 20 mm in width mediolaterally and 8–10 mm in dimension, anteroposteriorly. The shape of the condyle varies considerably; the superior surface may be flat, round, or markedly convex, whereas the mediolateral contour is usually only mildly convex. These variations in shape may cause difficulty with radiographic interpretation, and it is this that underlines the importance of understanding the range of normal appearances (Fig. 28.2).

The extreme medial and lateral surfaces of the condyle are called the medial and lateral poles. The long axis of the condyle is formed by an imaginary line connecting these poles, and is slightly rotated on the condylar neck so that the medial pole is angled posteriorly, forming an angle of between 15 and 33 degrees with respect to the midsagittal plane. The two condylar axes typically intersect near the anterior border of the foramen magnum in the axial or horizontal plane of the skull.

Most condyles have a pronounced ridge oriented mediolaterally on the anterior surface, marking the anteroinferior limit of the articulating area. This ridge is the upper limit of the pterygoid fovea, a small depression on the anterior surface at the junction of the condyle and condylar neck, which is the insertion site of the lateral pterygoid muscle. The ridge should not be mistaken for an osteophyte (spur), which is a sign of degenerative joint disease (DJD).

Although the mandibular and temporal components of the TMJ are calcified by 6 months of age, complete calcification of the cortical borders may not be completed until age 20. As a result, images of the mandibular condyles in children may show little or no evidence of a cortical border. In the absence of disease, the cortical borders in adults are visible in the diagnostic image. The layer of fibrocartilage overlying the condyle is not visible in planar imaging or computed tomography (CT). In magnetic resonance imaging (MRI), the cortical border and fibrocartilage are both imaged as a single low-signal (i.e., dark) structure.

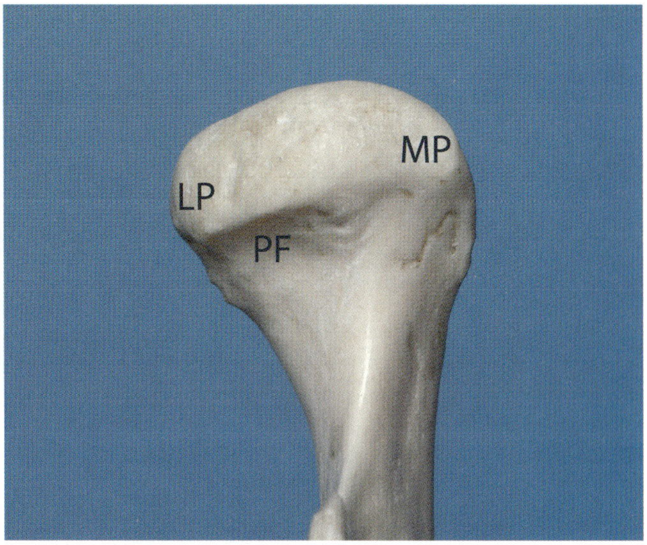

Fig. 28.1 Anterior view of the mandibular condyle. *LP,* Lateral pole; *MP,* medial pole; *PF,* pterygoid fovea.

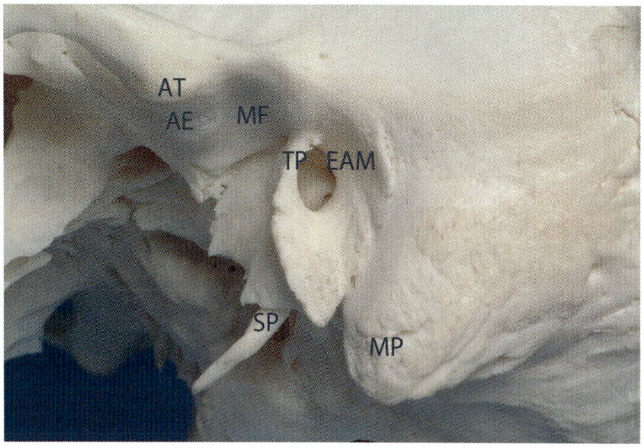

Fig. 28.3 Lateral and inferior view of the skull showing the temporal component of the temporomandibular joint. *AE,* Articular eminence; *AT,* articular tubercle; *EAM,* external auditory meatus; *MF,* mandibular fossa; *MP,* mastoid process; *SP,* styloid process; *TP,* tympanic plate.

Temporal Component

The articular component of the temporal bone is formed by the inferior surface of the squamous process, and is composed of the glenoid or mandibular fossa posteriorly and the articular eminence and tubercle anteriorly (Fig. 28.3). As with the condyle, the mandibular fossa is covered with a thin layer of fibrocartilage. The posterior surface of the articular eminence is convex in shape, and its most inferior point is called the summit, apex, or crest. In the normal TMJ, the roof of the glenoid fossa, the posterior slope of the articular eminence and the summit form a gentle "S-shape" curve when viewed in the sagittal plane (Fig. 28.4A). The squamotympanic fissure and its medial extension, the petrotympanic fissure, form the posterior border of the glenoid fossa. The roof of the glenoid fossa forms a small portion of the floor of the middle cranial fossa, and here, only a thin layer of cortical bone separates the joint cavity from the intracranial space. The spine of the sphenoid forms the medial limit of the fossa. Glenoid fossa depths vary, and the development of the articular eminence relies on a functional stimulus from the condyle. For example, the mandibular fossa is very shallow and underdeveloped in patients with micrognathia or condylar

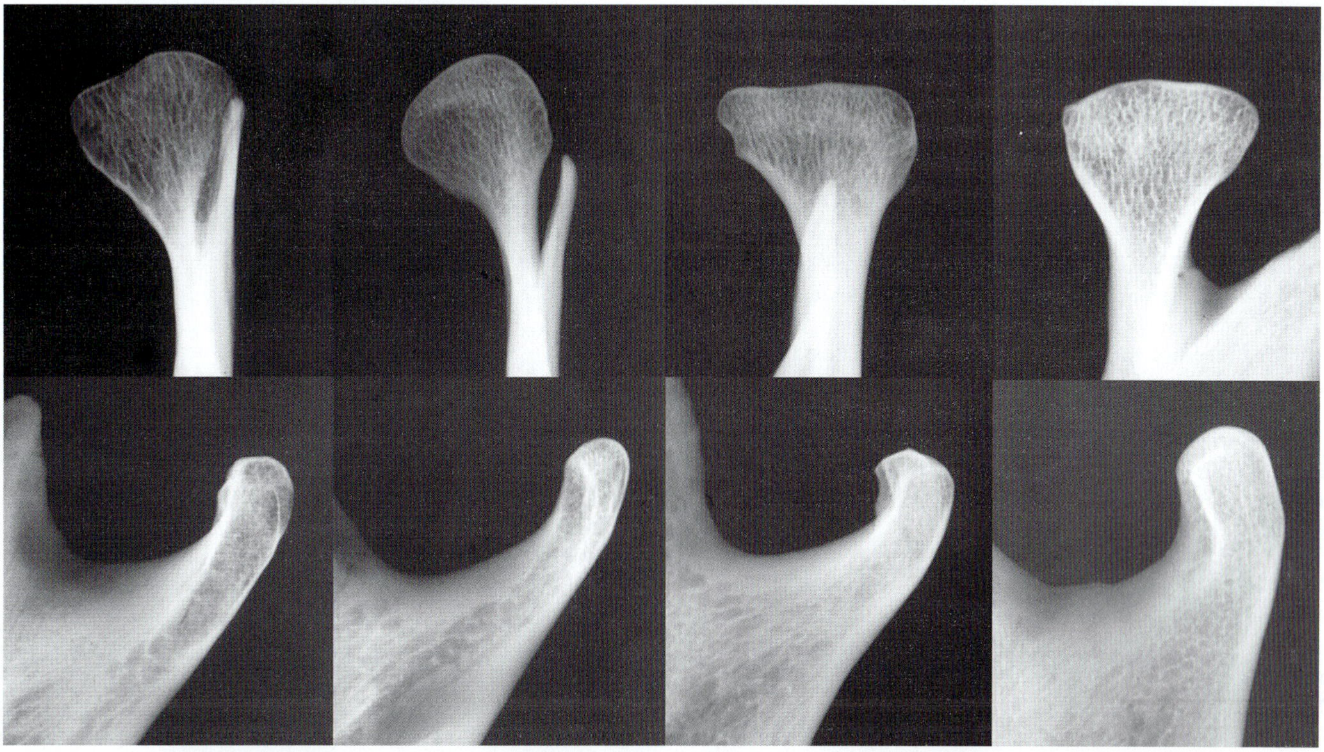

Fig. 28.2 Composite of images of normal mandibular condyles demonstrates the extensive variability in condylar shape: heart shaped, round, flat, and with large medial and lateral poles. The upper row are coronal views with the corresponding lateral views immediately below.

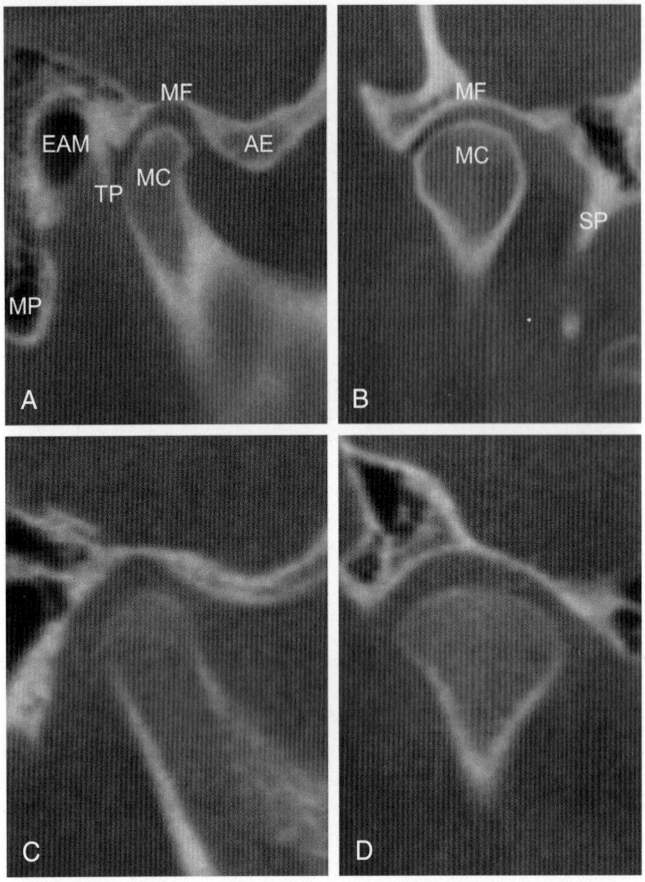

Fig. 28.4 Corrected sagittal (A) and coronal (B) reconstructed cone beam computed tomographic images of a normal temporomandibular joint (TMJ) in an adult. Note the thick regular cortication of all articulating surfaces and development of the glenoid fossa and articular eminence. *AE,* Articular eminence; *EAM,* external auditory meatus; *MC,* mandibular condyle; *MF,* mandibular fossa; *MP,* mastoid process; *SP,* styloid process; *TP,* tympanic plate. Corrected sagittal (C) and coronal (D) reconstructed cone beam computed tomographic images of a normal TMJ in a 7-year-old child. Note the thin cortication of the articulating surfaces, shallow glenoid fossa, and short articular eminence.

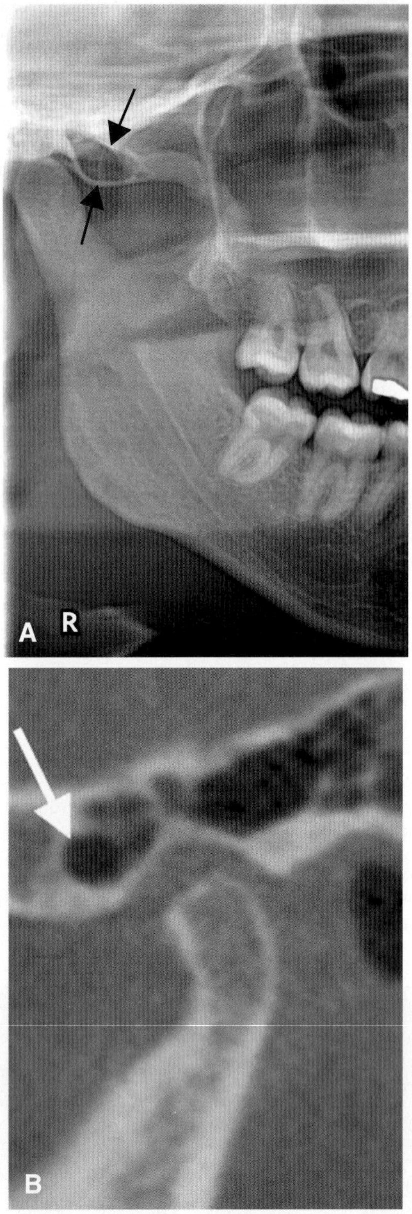

Fig. 28.5 (A) Cropped panoramic shows a large mastoid air cell within the articular eminence *(arrows).* This is a variation of normal. (B) Note the pneumatization of the articular eminence by mastoid air cells on this reconstructed corrected sagittal cone beam computed tomographic image *(arrow).*

agenesis. Young infants also lack a definitive fossa and articular eminence. In this age group, the fossa and articular eminence develop during the first 3 years of life and reach a mature shape by age 4 years, although the cortices may remain indistinct until adulthood (Fig. 28.4C and D, compared to A and B).

All aspects of the temporal bone, including the temporal component of the TMJ, may be pneumatized by small air cells derived from the mastoid air cell complex (Fig. 28.5A and B). Pneumatization of the articular eminence is seen radiographically in approximately 2% of patients.

Interarticular Disk

The interarticular disk (sometimes referred to as a meniscus) is composed of avascular fibrocartilage, and is positioned between the condylar and temporal components of the joint. The disk divides the joint cavity into two compartments; the inferior (lower) and superior (upper) joint spaces, which are located below and above the disk, respectively (Fig. 28.6). The normal disk has a biconcave shape with a thick anterior band, a thicker posterior band, and a thin middle or intermediate zone. The disk is also thicker medially than laterally. In the normal joint, the thin central portion serves as the articulating portion of the disk, acting as a cushion between the convex articulating surfaces of the condyle and articular eminence. In the closed mouth position, the posterior band is located adjacent to the superior surface of the condyle, or slightly anterior to it, in the 11 o'clock position. The periphery of the disk blends with fibers of the inner surface of the joint capsule. Medial and lateral collateral ligaments also anchor the disk under the medial and lateral poles of the condyle. The anterior band attaches to some fibers of the superior head of the lateral pterygoid muscle, while the posterior band attaches to the retrodiscal tissues.

During mandibular opening, as the condyle rotates and translates anteriorly and inferiorly, the disk is also carried forward under load from the adjacent bones so that its thin biconcave intermediate zone remains interposed between the articulating convexities of the condylar

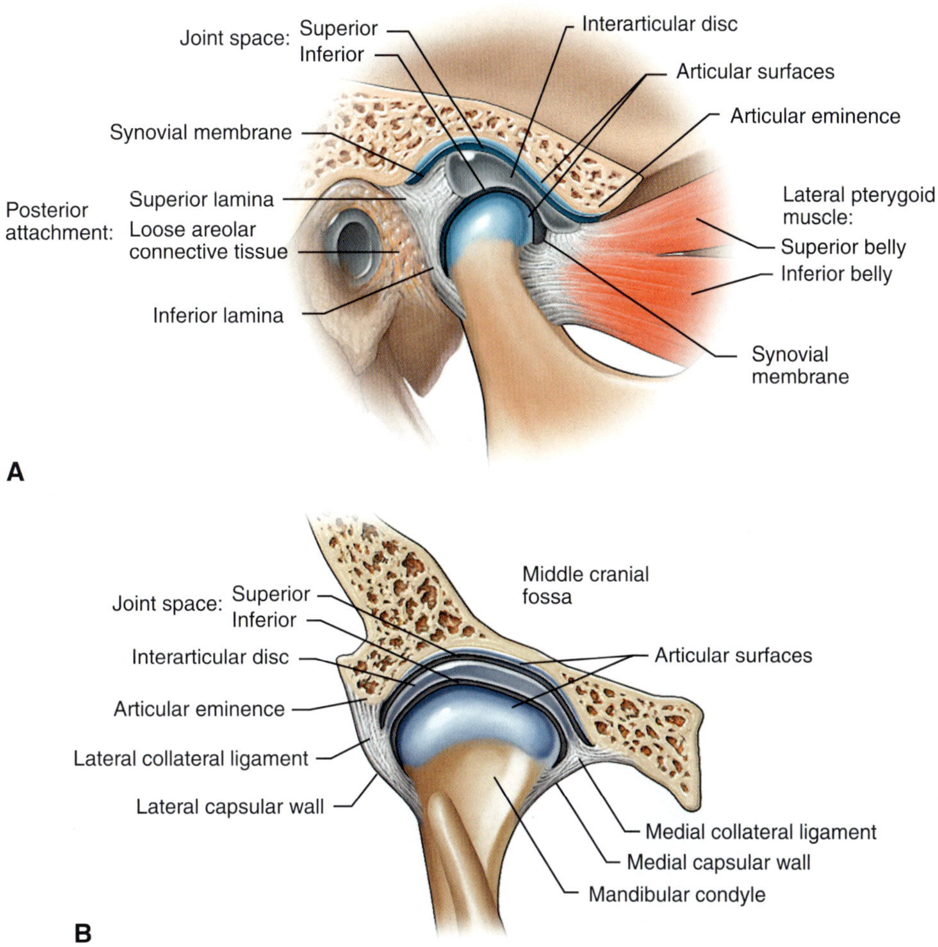

Fig. 28.6 Lateral (A) and coronal (B) views of normal temporomandibular joint anatomy.

head and articular eminence. The disk attachments to the condylar neck laterally and medially by the collateral ligaments help to ensure positional stability of the disk during jaw movements. On mandibular closing, this process reverses, with the disk moving posteriorly and superiorly with the condyle into the mandibular fossa.

Retrodiscal Tissues (Posterior Disk Attachment)

The retrodiscal tissues consist of superior and inferior lamellae enclosing a region of loose vascular tissue, often referred to as the bilaminar zone. The superior lamina, which is rich in elastin, inserts into the tympanic plate at the posterior wall of the mandibular fossa. During opening movements of the jaw, the superior lamina distends, and allows the disk to move anteriorly with condylar translation. On closing, the superior lamina allows for the smooth recoil of the disk posteriorly. The inferior lamina attaches more tightly to the posterior surface of the condyle. As the condyle moves anteriorly and inferiorly, the retrodiscal tissues expand in volume, primarily as a result of venous distention, to fill the void created by the translated condyle. The retrodiscal tissues are well innervated and may be the source of pain when the posterior attachment becomes trapped between the condyle and articular eminence in cases of anterior disk displacement.

Temporomandibular Joint Bony Relationships

Joint space is a general term used to describe the radiolucent or low-attenuation space located between the condyle and temporal component of the joint seen in planar diagnostic images and CT. The radiographic joint space contains the articular disk and its attachments. This term should not be confused with the terms *superior joint space* and *inferior joint space* described earlier, which refer to soft tissue spaces located superior and inferior to the disk. The anteroposterior position of the condyle within the glenoid fossa can be determined by examining the dimensions of the radiographic joint space viewed on lateral imaging projections of the joint that have been corrected for the angulation of the condylar head. Under normal conditions, the condyle is positioned centrally when the anterior and posterior spaces are uniform in width. The condyle is considered to be retruded when the anterior joint space width is greater than the posterior, and it is considered to be protruded when the anterior joint space is narrower than the posterior. However, because the surface contours of the glenoid fossa and the condyle do not necessarily mirror one another as a perfect "ball and socket," the dimensions of the joint spaces often vary from the medial to the lateral aspects of the normal joint (Fig. 28.7).

The diagnostic significance of mild or moderate condylar eccentricity is unclear. Condylar eccentricity is seen in one-third to one-half of asymptomatic individuals, and is not a reliable indicator of the soft tissue status of the joint, particularly because the shape of the condylar head does not always mirror the concavity of the fossa. Markedly eccentric condylar positioning usually represents an abnormality. For example, inferior positioning of the condyle where the joint space is widened superoinferiorly may be seen in cases involving fluid or blood

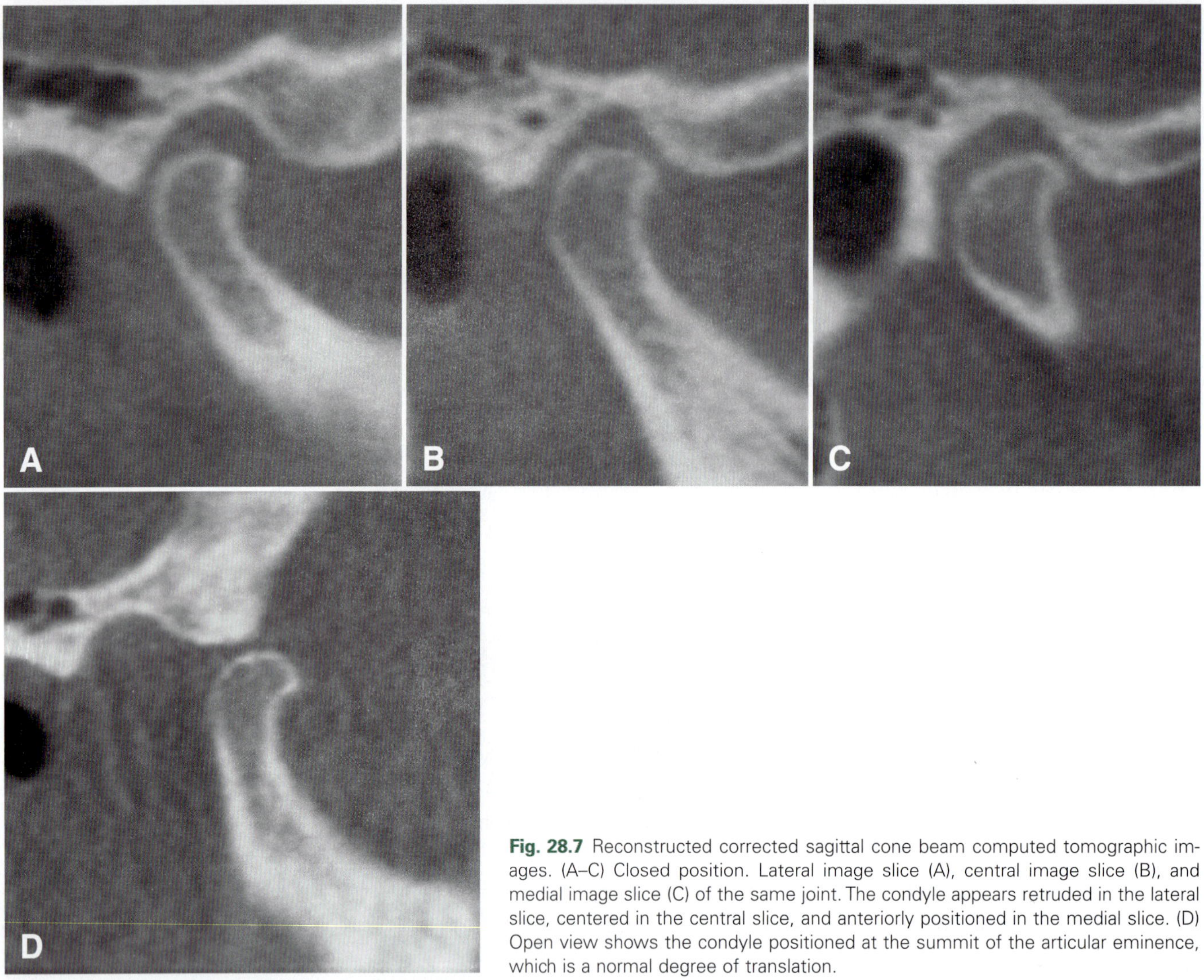

Fig. 28.7 Reconstructed corrected sagittal cone beam computed tomographic images. (A–C) Closed position. Lateral image slice (A), central image slice (B), and medial image slice (C) of the same joint. The condyle appears retruded in the lateral slice, centered in the central slice, and anteriorly positioned in the medial slice. (D) Open view shows the condyle positioned at the summit of the articular eminence, which is a normal degree of translation.

accumulation within the joint. In contrast, superior positioning of the condyle where this space is narrowed or not visible, with apparent contact of the osseous components, may indicate loss, displacement, or perforation of the disk or its attachments. Marked posterior condylar positioning is seen in some cases of anterior disk displacement, and pronounced anterior condylar positioning may be seen when there has been destruction of the articular eminence, such as in juvenile idiopathic arthritis (JIA).

Condylar Movement

The condyle undergoes complex rotational and translational movements during mandibular opening. A hinge-like, rotational movement of the condylar head occurs between the superior surface of the condyle and the inferior surface of the disk (in the inferior joint space), and this is followed by inferior and anterior translation (sliding) of the condyle, which occurs between the superior surface of the disk and the articular eminence (in the superior joint space). The extent of normal condylar translation varies considerably. In most individuals, at maximal opening, the condyle translates to the summit of the articular eminence or slightly anterior to it (see Fig. 28.7D). The condyle typically is found within a range of 2–5 mm posterior and 5–8 mm anterior to the crest of the eminence. Reduced condylar translation, in which the condyle has little or no downward and forward movement and does not leave the mandibular fossa, is seen in patients who clinically have a reduced degree of mouth opening. Hypermobility of the joint may be suspected if the condyle translates more than 5 mm anterior to the eminence. If a superior movement also occurs anterior to the articular eminence, anterior locking or dislocation of the condyle may occur.

APPLICATION OF DIAGNOSTIC IMAGING

Imaging of the TMJ may be necessary to supplement information obtained from the clinical examination. Diagnostic imaging should be considered when an osseous abnormality or infection is suspected, in patients with a history of trauma, significant dysfunction, alteration in range of motion, sensory or motor abnormalities, or significant changes in occlusion. TMJ imaging is not indicated for joint sounds if other signs or symptoms are absent, or for asymptomatic patients, particularly children and adolescents, before orthodontic treatment. The purpose of TMJ imaging is to evaluate the integrity and relationships of the hard and soft tissues, confirm the extent or stage of progression of disease, and evaluate the effects of treatment. There is often poor correlation between the severity of findings on TMJ imaging and the severity of the patient's clinical signs and symptoms. For example, severe degenerative changes may be noted on an imaging examination, but the patient has only mild discomfort, or vice versa. The clinician must correlate the imaging information with the patient's history and clinical findings to arrive at a final diagnosis and to plan the management of the underlying disease process.

TEMPOROMANDIBULAR JOINT IMAGING MODALITIES

Several variables must be considered when selecting the type of imaging to order, including the specific clinical problem to be addressed; whether the imaging of hard or soft tissues is desired; the benefits and limitations of the modalities being considered; the cost of the examination; and the radiation dose. Both joints should be imaged during the examination for comparison. Images of the osseous structures of the joints may be obtained using panoramic imaging, cone beam computed tomography (CBCT) or multidetector computed tomography (MDCT). The soft tissues of the joints are best imaged with MRI. The application of these techniques to the diagnosis of TMJ dysfunction is discussed further in the following sections.

Osseous Structures

Panoramic Imaging

The panoramic image is a useful tool for broadly examining the anatomic structures of, and around, the TMJs. This form of imaging allows the clinician to rule out gross disease, and for some patients, it is the only imaging required before conservative therapy is initiated. Gross osseous changes involving the condyles may be identified, such as asymmetries, extensive erosions, large osteophytes, neoplasms, or fractures; however, panoramic imaging is less reliable for more subtle changes (Fig. 28.8). The panoramic image also provides a means of comparing left and right sides of the mandible, and can reveal odontogenic diseases and other disorders that may be the source of TMJ symptoms. However, no reliable information about condylar position or function is provided because the mandible is partially opened and protruded when this image is made. Also, mild osseous changes may be obscured, and only marked changes in articular eminence morphology can be seen as a result of superimposition by the skull base and zygomatic processes of the temporal bones. Some panoramic imaging devices offer TMJ algorithms; however, these do not provide the views required because of thick image layers and oblique, distorted views. For these reasons, when a detailed assessment of the joint structures is desired, the panoramic image should be supplemented.

Cone Beam Computed Tomography

CBCT creates image volumes that allow the user to reconstruct thin section views of anatomy in multiple, customizable planes. Thin sections allow the structures of the joints to be assessed without superimposition of surrounding anatomy. Classically, the joints are viewed in coronal and sagittal planes, corrected along the long axes of the condylar heads (Fig. 28.9). These "corrected" views provide the least distorted representations of the condylar and temporal components of the joint, and their relationship to one other. Other renderings of the jaws also can be created from a CBCT volume, and these may be useful for assessing skeletal asymmetries or other osseous deformities.

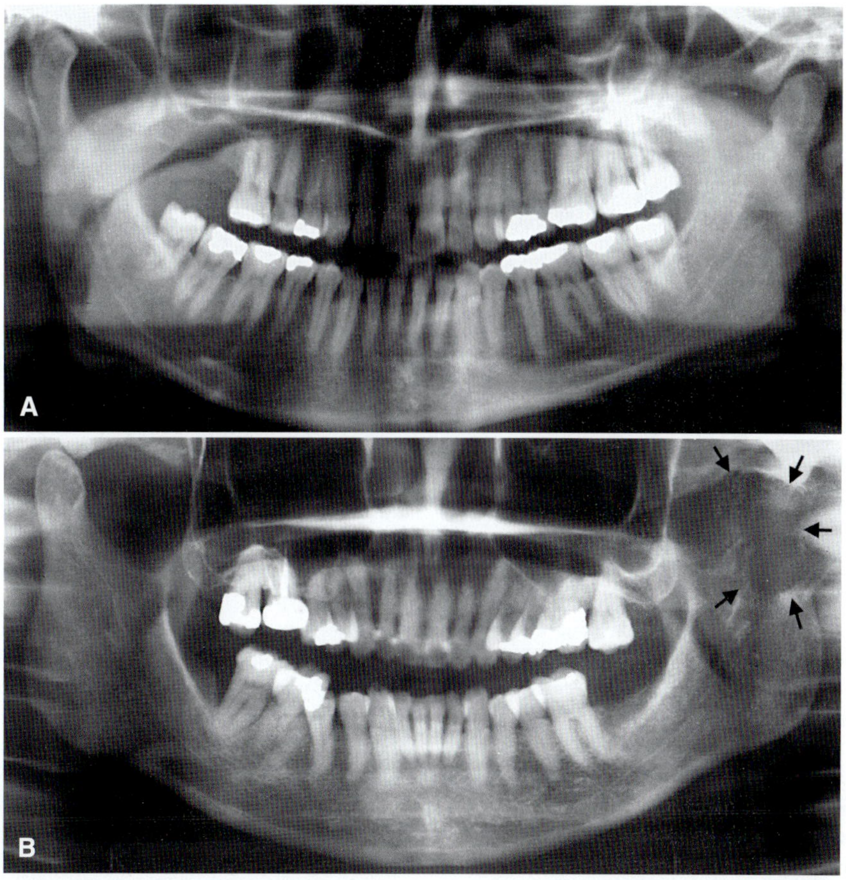

Fig. 28.8 Panoramic images reveal right condylar hyperplasia (A) and destruction of the condyle by a malignant tumor (B) *(arrows)*.

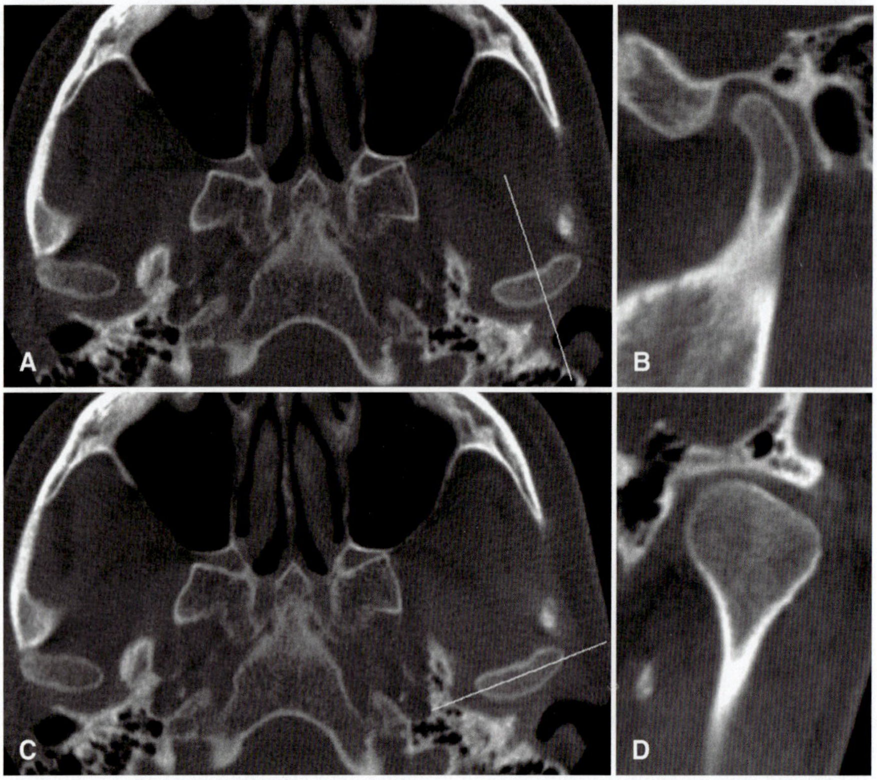

Fig. 28.9 Cone beam computed tomographic images show reconstruction planes for evaluating the temporomandibular joints. (A) Axial image with line indicating the corrected sagittal plane. (B) Resulting corrected sagittal image. (C) Axial image with a line indicating the corrected coronal plane. (D) Resulting corrected coronal image.

A CBCT examination is usually acquired with the patient in the closed mouth position with the teeth in maximal intercuspation. Some CBCT systems allow low-resolution image acquisitions to be done in the open mouth or other positions (see Chapter 9) to evaluate range of motion. CBCT has the advantage of reduced radiation dose to the patient compared with MDCT. This reduced dose makes CBCT imaging ideal for imaging of osseous changes associated with DJD. CBCT imaging is also useful for determining the presence and extent of ankylosis and neoplasms, characterizing fractures, evaluating complications from the use of polytetrafluoroethylene or silicon sheet implants, and identifying heterotopic bone growth. Soft tissue structures including the disks cannot be visualized with CBCT imaging. Metallic implants in or around the joints may create significant image artifacts, which can obscure the joint structures.

Multidetector Computed Tomography

MDCT (see Chapter 9) is capable of providing the same information as CBCT imaging, but additionally, it allows some—albeit limited—visualization of the soft tissues. This additional visualization is required only in a few situations, such as when a neoplasm arising within the bone is suspected to extend beyond the bone borders. The articular disk cannot be visualized with this modality, and patients are exposed to higher radiation doses than CBCT imaging.

Soft Tissue Structures

The most common indication for soft tissue imaging is when clinical findings suggest disk displacement with symptoms such as TMJ pain and dysfunction, and when symptoms do not respond to conservative therapy. Soft tissue imaging also may be required to supplement osseous imaging in rare cases where infection or a neoplasm is suspected. As with any other modality, imaging should be prescribed only when the anticipated results are expected to influence patient management. MRI is the modality of choice for visualizing the disk and other soft tissues of the TMJ.

Magnetic Resonance Imaging

MRI uses static and gradient magnetic fields, and nonionizing electromagnetic radiation in the form of radiofrequency pulses to produce multiplanar images (see Chapter 10). Specialized surface coils placed on the skin surface over the patient's TMJs improve image signal to noise, and therefore image quality. Depending on the radiofrequency pulse sequence selected, MRI creates contrast between different soft tissues, and this feature can be used to differentiate the articular disk from the other soft tissue components of the joint. Joint effusions can also be detected with MRI. MRI imaging displays the osseous structures of the TMJ but not with the detail comparable to CBCT or MDCT. TMJ MRI examinations may be performed with the use of T_1-weighted, proton density or T_2-weighted pulse sequences, depending on the type of information required. T_1-weighted or proton density sequences are shown to best demonstrate the discal and osseous tissues in cases of joint dysfunction, while T_2-weighted images can demonstrate inflammation and joint effusion. MRI allows the acquisition of images in the corrected sagittal and coronal planes without repositioning the patient (Fig. 28.10). These images usually are acquired in closed and opened mouth positions, with the aid of a bite block. Cinematic or cine MRI studies during opening and closing can be obtained by having the patient open the jaw incrementally, and using rapid image acquisition ("fast scan") techniques.

MRI is contraindicated in patients who have pacemakers or other devices such as intracranial vascular clips or metal particulate matter

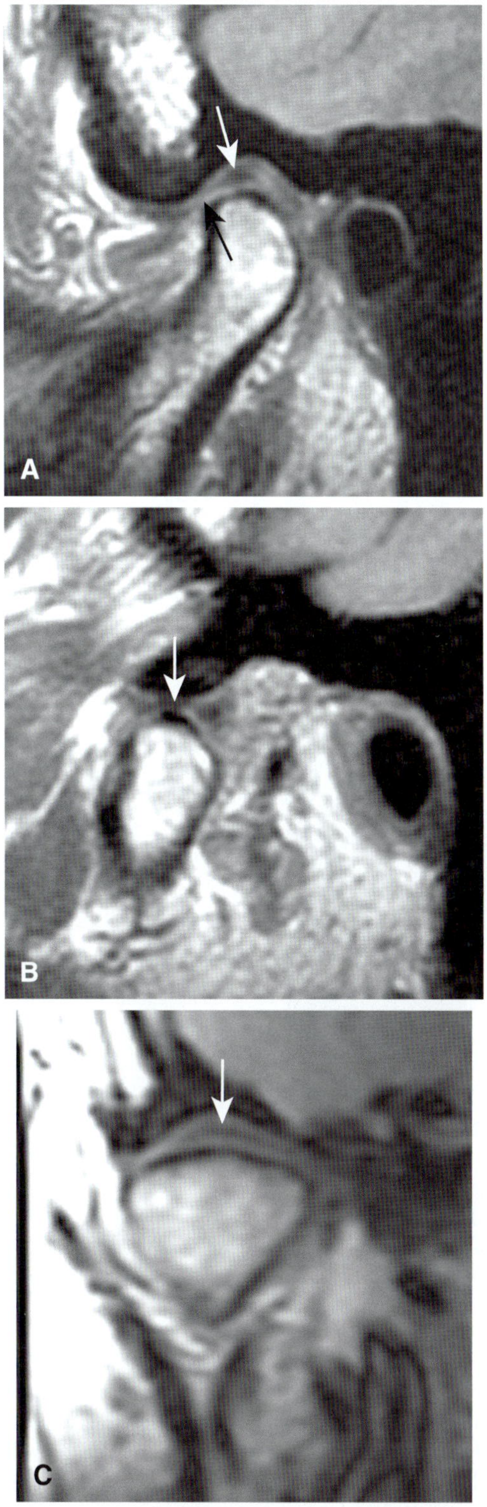

Fig. 28.10 Magnetic resonance imaging of a normal temporomandibular joint. (A) Corrected sagittal image in the closed mouth position shows the condyle and temporal component. The biconcave disk is located with its posterior band *(white arrow)* directly superior to the condyle and the thin intermediate part interposed between the articulating surfaces *(black arrow)*. (B) Corrected sagittal image in the open mouth position shows the condyle positioned at the summit of the articular eminence with the articular disk normally positioned between the osseous components *(white arrow)*. (C) Corrected coronal image in the closed mouth position shows the osseous components and disc *(white arrow)* superior to the condyle.

implanted in vital structures. Dental materials that contain ferromagnetic materials, including stainless steel or its component metals such as orthodontic hardware, may create image artifacts over the jaws, and in some cases, may obscure the joints. Some patients may be unable to tolerate the procedure because of claustrophobia or an inability to remain motionless.

ABNORMALITIES OF THE TEMPOROMANDIBULAR JOINT

Developmental Abnormalities

Disease Mechanism

Developmental abnormalities are the result of disturbances in the normal growth and development of the TMJ. These abnormalities may affect the form or size of the joint components, most commonly the mandibular condyle. Because the condylar articular cartilage is considered a growth center for the mandible, disturbances involving this cartilage can result in altered growth of the mandibular condyle, ramus, body, and alveolar process on the affected side.

Condylar Hyperplasia

Disease mechanism. Condylar hyperplasia is a developmental abnormality that results in enlargement and occasionally deformity of the condylar head; this may have a secondary effect on the mandibular fossa as it remodels to accommodate the abnormal condyle. Proposed etiologic factors include hormonal influences, trauma, infection, heredity, intrauterine factors, and hypervascularity. The mechanism may involve overactive cartilage or persistent cartilaginous rests; islands of active cartilage have been identified in specimens of hyperplastic condyles. This condition usually is unilateral and may be accompanied by varying degrees of hyperplasia of the ipsilateral mandible.

Clinical features. Condylar hyperplasia is more common in females and is most frequently discovered before 20 years of age. The condition is self-limiting and tends to arrest with the termination of skeletal growth; however, a few cases continue to grow, and adult onset has been reported. The condition may progress slowly or rapidly. Patients have mandibular asymmetry that varies in severity, depending on the degree of condylar enlargement. The chin may be deviated to the unaffected side, or it may remain unchanged but with an increase in the vertical dimension of the ramus, mandibular body, or alveolar process of the affected side. As a result of this growth pattern, patients may develop a posterior open bite on the affected side or a crossbite on the contralateral side with resultant problems with mastication or speech. Patients may also have symptoms related to TMJ dysfunction and may complain of a limited or deviated mandibular opening caused by restricted mobility of the enlarged condyle.

Imaging features. The hyperplastic condyle may have a relatively normal shape but be enlarged, or its form could be altered (e.g., conical, spherical, elongated, lobulated) or irregular. It may appear to be more radiopaque on planar images because of the additional bone volume present. However, the cortical thickness and trabecular pattern of the enlarged condyle are usually normal, which helps to distinguish hyperplasia from a neoplasm. The glenoid fossa may be enlarged to accommodate the larger condylar head, usually as a result of remodeling of the posterior slope of the articular eminence. Secondary degenerative changes may be present because of the altered forces on the joint. The condylar neck also may be longer and thickened. Forward bending of the elongated condylar head and neck, to compensate for the increased bone volume, may result in an inverted "L-shape" to these structures. Lateral bowing of the condylar neck and canting of the occlusal plane may be seen in anteroposterior views (Fig. 28.11).

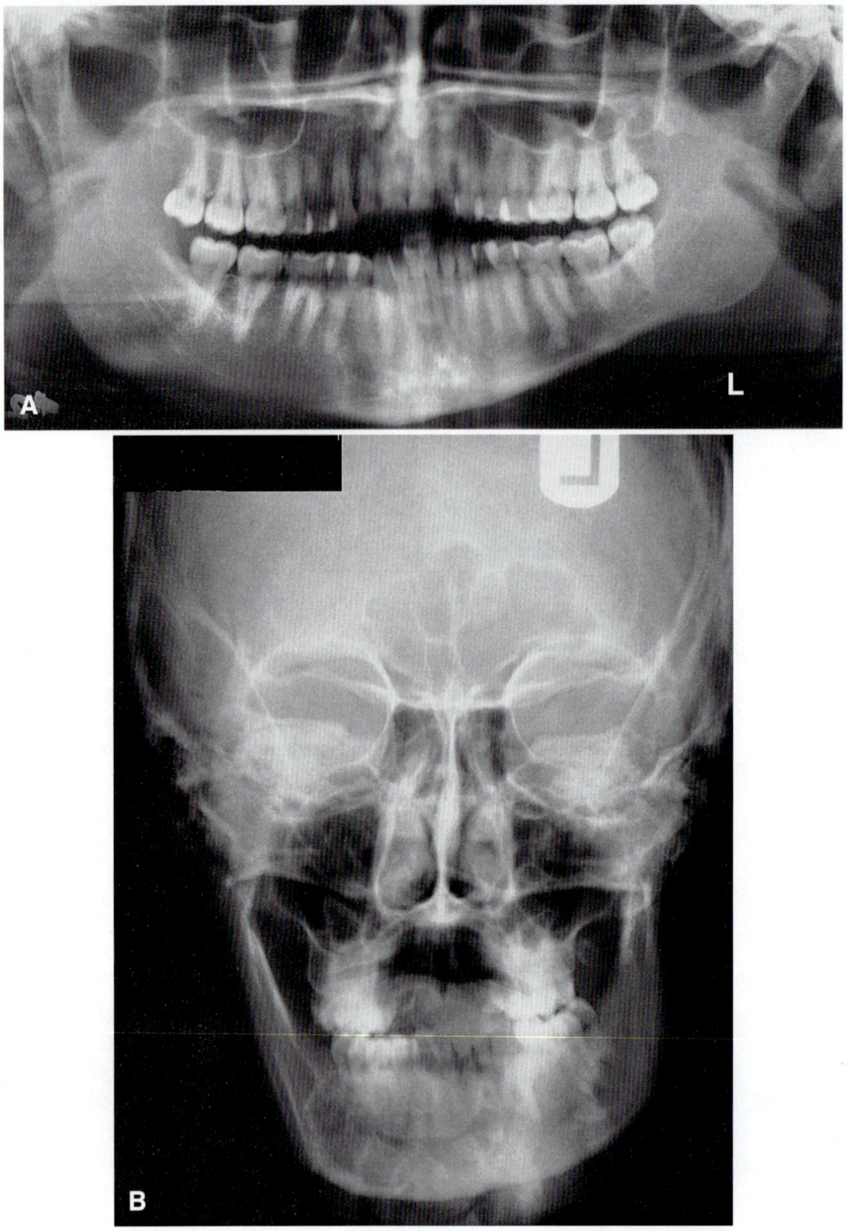

Fig. 28.11 (A) Panoramic image of condylar hyperplasia causing enlargement of the right condyle, ramus, and body of the mandible. (B) The resulting asymmetry of the mandible and associated occlusal plane cant is apparent in the posteroanterior skull view.

Secondary enlargement of the ramus and mandibular body also may result in a characteristic downward bowing of the inferior mandibular border on the affected side. The ramus may have increased vertical and anteroposterior dimensions.

Differential interpretation. A condylar neoplasm, most notably an osteochondroma, is included in the differential interpretation. An osteochondroma usually results in a condyle with a more lobular and irregular shape compared with a hyperplastic condyle because this neoplasm creates a more localized, protruding growth. However, coexistent mandibular hyperplasia may be seen with osteochondroma. Surface irregularities and continued growth after cessation of skeletal growth should increase suspicion of neoplasia. Occasionally, a condylar osteoma or a large osteophyte occurring in chronic DJD may simulate condylar hyperplasia. Associated ipsilateral hyperplasia of the mandible would not be seen in these other conditions.

Management. The management of condylar hyperplasia consists of a combination of condylectomy, orthognathic surgery, and orthodontics. Condylectomy removes the source of abnormal growth, whereas orthognathic surgery and orthodontics aim to correct any resultant functional and esthetic deficits. The initiation of treatment before condylar growth is complete helps limit the severity of mandibular deformation and compensatory changes in the maxilla and dentoalveolar structures. Management also may be delayed until growth is completed to avoid relapse and the need for additional interventions. A nuclear medicine examination (single-photon emission computed tomography or SPECT) with the radionuclide technetium (^{99m}Tc) may be helpful in determining if condylar growth is still active or if it has ceased. However, nuclear medicine may be misleading because of its poor specificity, and particularly if there is increased activity secondary to concurrent remodeling or degenerative changes.

Condylar Hypoplasia

Disease mechanism. Condylar hypoplasia is an undersized mandibular condyle, which may be the result of congenital, developmental, or acquired diseases that affect condylar growth. Severe congenital malformations may result in complete lack of formation of the condyle (aplasia). Rare congenital conditions causing hypoplasia of the condyle often also present with abnormalities of other structures of the face, such as the ear, eye, and zygomatic arch (see Chapter 27). Trauma, infection, and therapeutic radiation exposure to the condyle during growth are potential acquired causes of hypoplasia.

Clinical features. Condylar hypoplasia is more commonly unilateral, unless it is a feature of a syndrome (e.g., mandibulofacial dysostosis or Treacher Collins syndrome, Pierre Robin sequence). The condyle is a mandibular growth center; therefore, condylar hypoplasia is usually associated with some degree of unilateral mandibular hypoplasia and facial asymmetry. Deviation of the mandibular midline to the affected side and accentuation of this deviation on mandibular opening and malocclusion may develop. The amount of growth disturbance of the mandible is related to how early the onset of the disturbance to condylar growth occurs; earlier onset results in more severe underdevelopment of the ramus and mandibular body. Patients with condylar hypoplasia may develop symptoms of TMJ dysfunction.

Imaging features. The condyle may be normal in shape and structure but is diminished in size, and the mandibular fossa is proportionally small. The condylar neck is thinner and may appear short or elongated. The coronoid process is usually slender. The posterior border of the ramus and condylar neck may have a posterior (dorsal) inclination, creating a concavity in the outline of the posterior surface of the mandibular ramus in the panoramic image. If there is an associated mandibular hypoplasia, it manifests with a deepened antegonial notch and decreased vertical height of the mandibular body (Fig. 28.12). Occasional dental crowding may also result. Degenerative changes in the affected joint may be detected (Fig. 28.13).

Differential interpretation. JIA may cause damage to the condyle, resulting in hypoplasia. However, other signs of joint destruction would also be seen. An examination of other joints or testing for rheumatoid factor may be helpful if there is uncertainty. Changes in condylar morphology in severe DJD or other arthritic conditions also may mimic a hypoplastic condyle, but other signs of arthritis are usually visible in the affected joint. Additionally, arthritis does not cause mandibular hypoplasia of the affected side unless it occurs during growth. Occasionally, it is difficult to determine if there is condylar hypoplasia or if the contralateral side is enlarged. Careful examination of the inferior border for a pronounced antegonial notch (hypoplasia) versus downward bowing (hyperplasia) is helpful.

Treatment. Orthognathic surgery, bone grafts, and orthodontic therapy may be considered.

Coronoid Hyperplasia

Disease mechanism. Coronoid hyperplasia results from an elongation of the coronoid process of the mandible. The etiology may be acquired or developmental. Conditions that cause an increased activity of the temporalis muscle and tendon, which attach at the coronoid process, are associated with coronoid hyperplasia. Acquired coronoid hyperplasia usually develops secondary to restricted movement of the condyle, such as in ankylosis. The coronoid process may impinge on the posterior surface of the maxilla or zygomatic bone during opening, restricting condylar translation. Sometimes a pseudojoint develops between the hyperplastic coronoid and the posterior surface of the zygomatic bone, a condition called Jacob disease.

Clinical features. The developmental variant of coronoid hyperplasia is more commonly bilateral. This form is most often diagnosed in young men who have a long history of progressive limitation of mouth opening. The resulting restricted opening may simulate the features of an apparent closed lock owing to disk displacement. The condition is generally painless.

Imaging features. Coronoid hyperplasia is best seen in panoramic images and CT examinations. The coronoid processes are elongated, and the tips extend at least 1 cm above the inferior rim of the zygomatic arch (Fig. 28.14). The coronoid processes may have a large but normal shape, or may curve anteriorly and appear very radiopaque. Impingement of the coronoid against the zygomatic bone can be confirmed by performing CT imaging with the patient's mouth opened maximally. Remodeling of the posterior surface of the zygomatic process of the maxilla, to accommodate the enlarged coronoid process during function, also may be seen. Because this condition is often bilateral, both sides should be examined for abnormality. The radiographic appearances of the TMJs are usually normal.

Differential interpretation. Unilateral elongation of the coronoid process should be differentiated from a neoplasm such as an osteochondroma or osteoma. In contrast to coronoid hyperplasia, neoplasms usually have an irregular shape. Clinical presentation of limited opening most often prompts examination of the TMJs for abnormalities that may restrict joint movement, such as internal derangement, neoplasm, or ankylosis. However, inclusion of the coronoid processes during TMJ imaging helps ensure that coronoid hyperplasia is not overlooked.

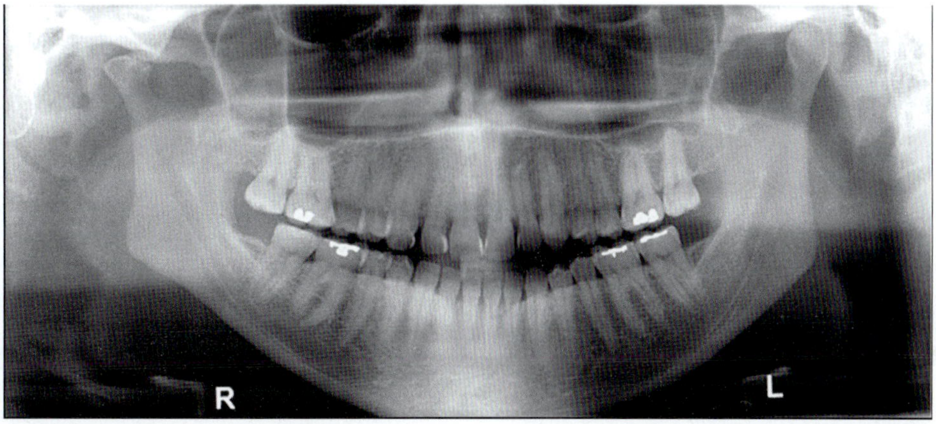

Fig. 28.12 Panoramic image of hypoplasia of the right condyle with the associated short vertical height of the right mandibular ramus and body.

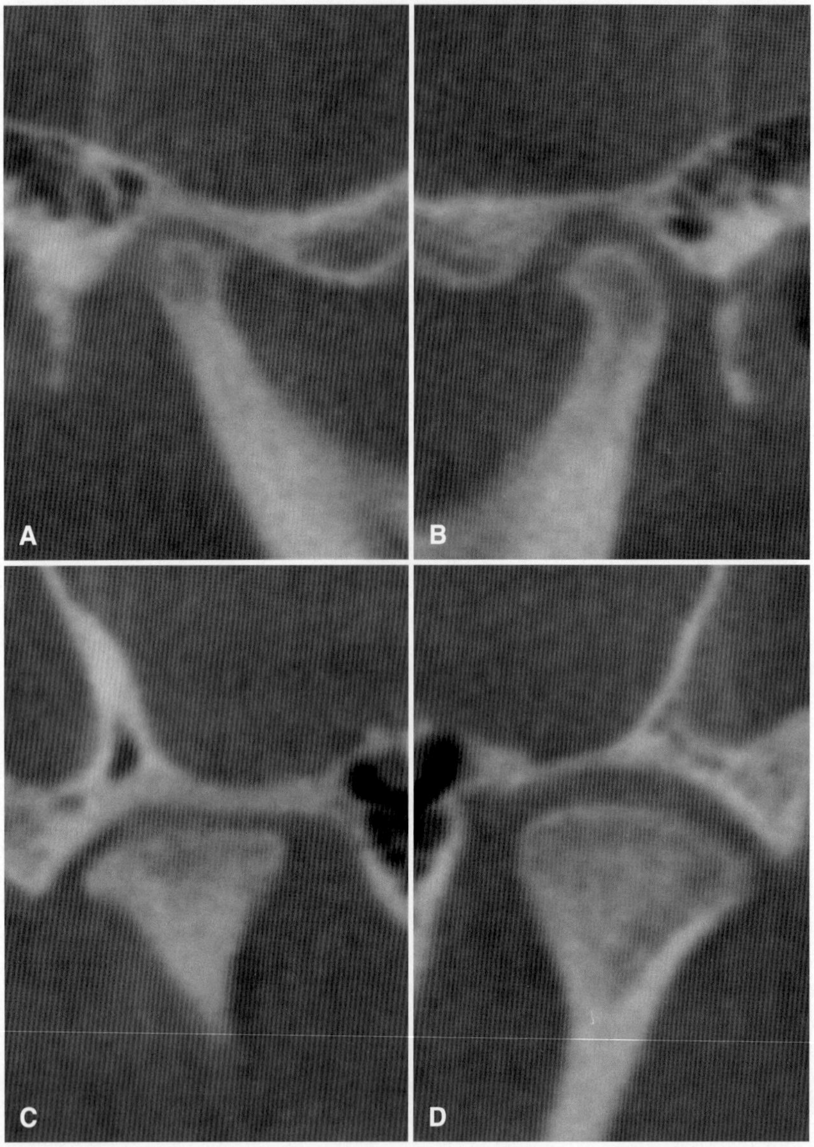

Fig. 28.13 Cone beam computed tomographic images of unilateral condylar hypoplasia. Corrected sagittal (A and B) and coronal (C and D) images. (A and C) The right condyle is hypoplastic, and there is secondary remodeling. The articular surfaces of the condyle and anterior aspect of the glenoid fossa are flattened, and the superior joint space is thinner compared with the left. (B and D) Left side of the same patient showing a normal condyle.

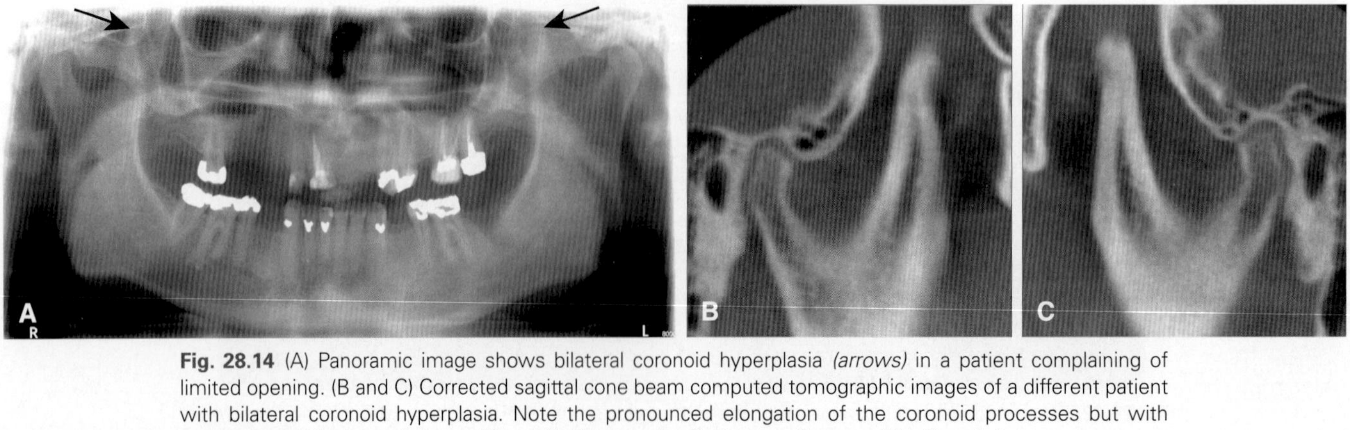

Fig. 28.14 (A) Panoramic image shows bilateral coronoid hyperplasia *(arrows)* in a patient complaining of limited opening. (B and C) Corrected sagittal cone beam computed tomographic images of a different patient with bilateral coronoid hyperplasia. Note the pronounced elongation of the coronoid processes but with maintenance of a normal shape. (B and C, Courtesy Dr. S. Fireman, Toronto, ON, Canada.)

Management. Treatment consists of surgical removal of the coronoid process and postoperative physiotherapy. Regrowth of the coronoid process after surgery has been reported.

Bifid Condyle

Disease mechanism. A condyle that is bifid has a vertical depression, notch, or cleft in the surface of the condylar head. This feature is best seen in the corrected sagittal or coronal plane, and results in the appearance of a "double-headed" condyle. There may be actual duplication of the condyle. Trauma may give rise to a duplicated condyle either by longitudinal fracture or by complete displacement of the original condyle after fracture with remodeling of a second new functional condyle. A retained embryonic fibrous band creating a condylar groove has also been postulated as a developmental etiology.

Clinical features. Bifid condyle is usually an incidental finding in panoramic images or anteroposterior planar imaging. This condition is rare and is more often unilateral, although it may be bilateral. Some patients have signs and symptoms of TMJ dysfunction, including joint noises and pain.

Imaging features. The orientation of the bifid condyle may be anteroposterior or mediolateral; most commonly, a depression or notch is present on the superior condylar surface, giving a heart-shaped outline when viewed in the corrected coronal plane (Fig. 28.15). The depth of the depression is variable. A more remarkable presentation is complete duplication of the condylar head in the sagittal plane. The mandibular fossa may remodel to accommodate the altered condylar morphology.

Differential interpretation. A slight medial depression on the superior condylar surface may be considered a normal variation; the point at which the depth of the depression signifies a bifid condyle is unclear. The differential interpretation also includes a vertical fracture through the condylar head.

Management. Treatment is not indicated unless pain or functional impairment is present.

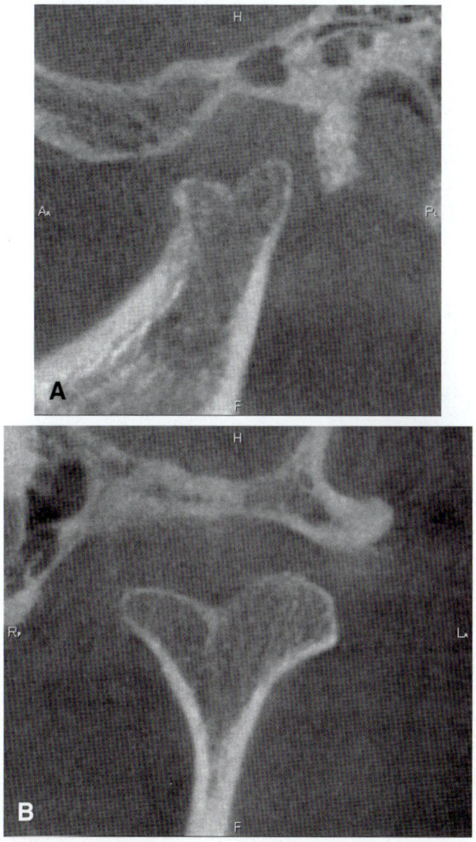

Fig. 28.15 Bifid condyle. Corrected sagittal (A) and coronal (B) cone beam computed tomographic images show a central depression in the superior surface of the mandibular condyle creating a bilobed or heart-shaped outline. The osseous structures in this joint are otherwise normal.

Soft Tissue Abnormalities

Disk Displacement

Disease mechanism. The articular disk may become abnormally positioned or displaced relative to the condylar and temporal components of the TMJ. The disk most often is displaced in an anterior direction, but it may be displaced anteromedially, medially, or anterolaterally. Lateral and posterior displacements are extremely rare. A displaced disk may interfere with normal function of the joint or cause pain, although it can also be a common finding in asymptomatic patients, leading to the hypothesis that disk displacements may represent a normal variation of anatomy. A disk that is displaced in the closed position may resume a normal relationship with the condyle when the mouth is open, or it may remain displaced; the terms *reducing* and *nonreducing* are used to describe these situations, respectively (Fig. 28.16). A displaced disk may become deformed or be associated with other signs of TMJ dysfunction, including DJD, adhesion, effusion, and perforation. The cause of disk displacement is unknown, although parafunction, jaw injuries (e.g., direct trauma), whiplash injury, and forced opening

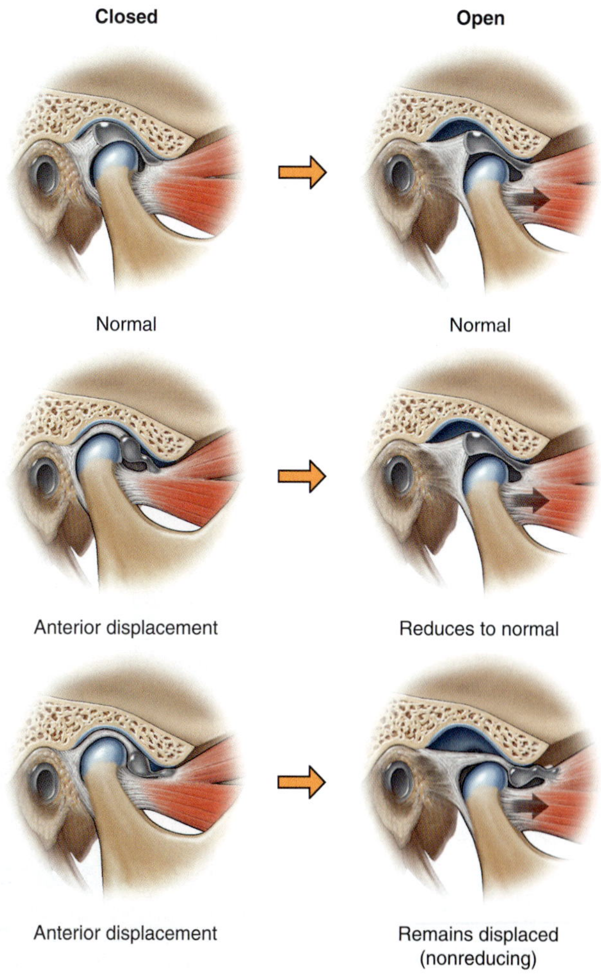

Fig. 28.16 Position and movement of the articular disk during jaw opening. *Top,* Normal position. *Middle,* Partially displaced anteriorly (with reduction). *Bottom,* Severely displaced anteriorly (without reduction).

beyond the normal range have been implicated. The term *internal derangement* is a nonspecific designation for an abnormality in the soft tissue components of the joint resulting in altered function, which may include disk displacement.

Clinical features. Disk displacement has been found both in symptomatic and asymptomatic patients, and it is not known why some individuals progress to more severe dysfunction and others do not. Joint noises, such as popping or clicking, are a common sign of disk displacement but are not usually painful. Crepitus, a crunching or grinding sound, is suggestive of osseous degeneration associated with a long-term, nonreducing disk. Symptoms associated with a displaced disk include pain in the preauricular region, headaches, and closed or open locking of the joint. A decreased range of motion may be present, and when the displacement is unilateral, this may manifest as deviation of the mandible to the affected side on opening.

Imaging features.

Normal disk position. The articular disk cannot be visualized with planar imaging, CBCT, or MDCT; MRI is the technique of choice. On MRI, the normal disk has a low signal intensity relative to the signal from the joint space immediately surrounding it. In other words, the disk signal is lower (i.e., darker). In contrast, the signal intensity of the posterior attachment is usually higher (i.e., brighter).

In a corrected sagittal image, the normal biconcave disk has a "bow tie" shape. In the closed mouth position, the normal disk is positioned with the thick posterior band located either directly superior to or slightly anterior to the condylar head (around the 11 o'clock position). The thin intermediate zone of the disk is located between the anterosuperior surface of the condyle and the posterior surface of the articular eminence (see Fig. 28.10). In all positions of mouth opening, the thin intermediate zone should remain between the condyle and the articular eminence in this location.

Disk displacement. MRI is required for identification of a displaced disk. Although a retruded condylar position, seen in CBCT or MDCT, has been associated with an anteriorly displaced disk, condylar position in maximal intercuspation is an unreliable indicator of disk displacement. Anterior displacement is the most common disk displacement. A disk is considered anteriorly displaced when its posterior band is located anterior to the normal position and the thin intermediate zone is no longer positioned between the condyle and articular eminence (Fig. 28.17A). This displacement may range from partial to

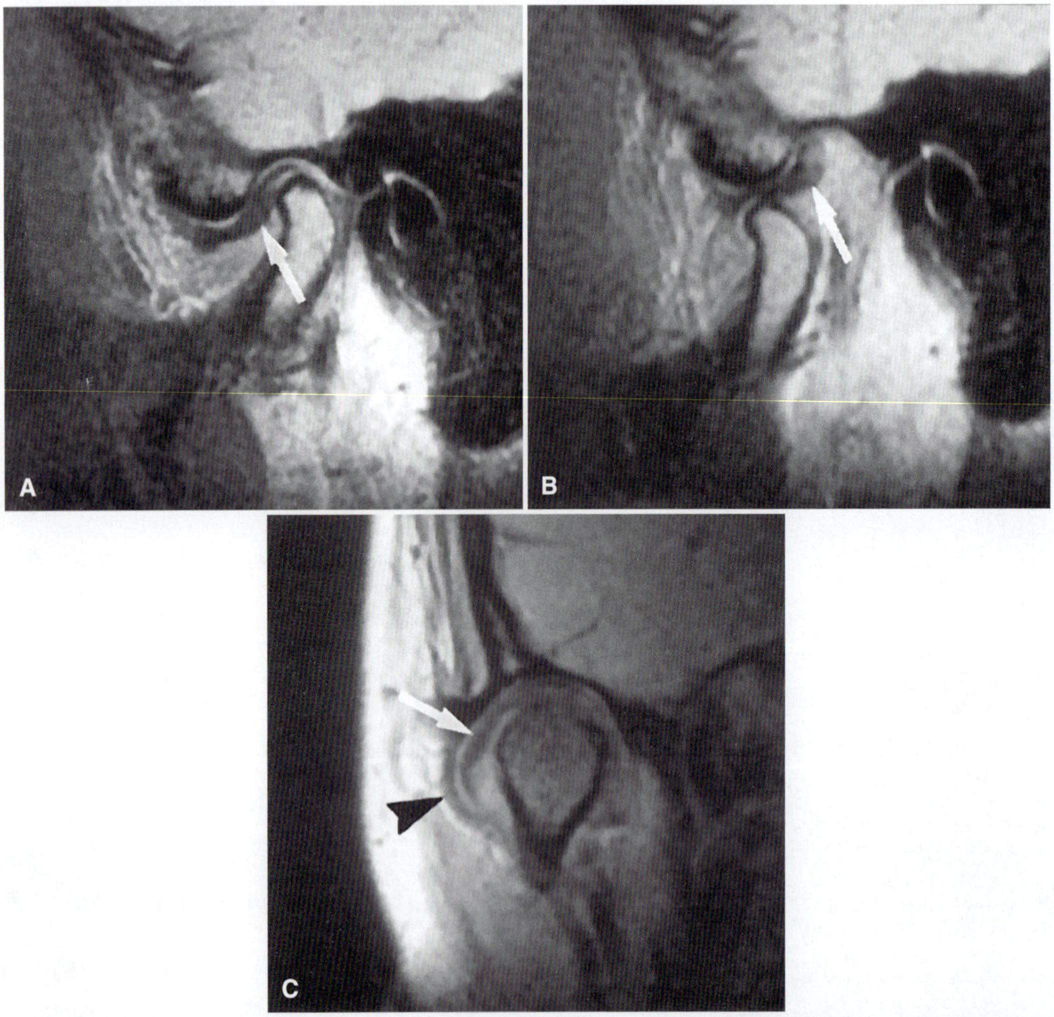

Fig. 28.17 Magnetic resonance imaging of anterior disk displacement with reduction. (A) Corrected sagittal image in the closed mouth position shows the disk with its posterior band *(arrow)* anterior to the condyle. Note the anterior position of the thin intermediate section of the disk. (B) Corrected sagittal image in the open mouth position shows the normal relationship of the disk and condyle and the posterior band of the disk *(arrow)*. (C) Corrected coronal image shows the disk *(arrow)* laterally displaced. The joint capsule *(arrowhead)* bulges laterally. (B, Courtesy Dr. P.-L. Westesson, Rochester, NY.)

full displacement with the posterior band located between the condyle and articular eminence in a mild partial displacement to being located well anterior to the condylar head in a severe, full dislocation. When the disk is severely anteriorly displaced, partial folding of the disk within the anterior joint space may be seen. Sometimes identification of the posterior band is difficult because of deformation of this portion of the disk.

When the disk is chronically anteriorly positioned, the posterior attachment is stretched between the articulating surfaces of the condyle and temporal bone, and owing to resulting fibrosis its MRI signal may become lower and approximate that of the posterior band. It is helpful to identify the position of the thin intermediate part of the disk to determine if it is anteriorly displaced from its normal position between the articulating surfaces of the condyle and articular eminence.

Medial and lateral sideways displacement, and anteromedial and anterolateral rotational displacements also can be identified on MRI (see Fig. 28.17C). Medial or lateral displacement is identified on corrected coronal MRI when the body of the disk is positioned at the medial or lateral aspect of the condyle, respectively. Rotational displacements present with the disk seen in a normal position in corrected sagittal sections through one side of the joint, and anteriorly displaced in the lateral side (in anteromedial rotation) or medial side (in anterolateral rotation). Posterior disk displacement is rare.

Disk reduction and nonreduction. During mouth opening, an anteriorly displaced disk may return to a normal relationship with the condylar head during any part of the opening movement. In motion studies, this is usually seen as a rapid posterior movement of the disk, and it is often accompanied by an audible click as the condylar head contacts the intermediate zone of the disk. This condition is referred to as disk reduction and can be diagnosed on MRI if the disk is anteriorly displaced in corrected sagittal closed mouth views but is in a normal position in open mouth images (see Fig. 28.17). If the disk remains anteriorly displaced on opening, it is interpreted as being nonreducing. A nonreducing disk may appear bent or deformed as the condyle pushes forward against it (Fig. 28.18). Fibrotic changes of the posterior attachment of a displaced disk may alter its tissue signal to approximate the signal of the disk. In such cases, the disk may be erroneously interpreted as occupying a normal position at maximal opening. Identification of excessive tissue with low signal intensity anterior to the condylar head, representing the true disk tissue, should help confirm the nonreducing state of the disk.

Deformities and perforation. If the disk remains chronically displaced, it can undergo permanent deformation, losing its biconcave shape. MRI can demonstrate this change, which may vary from enlargement of the posterior band to a bilinear or biconvex disk outline. In cases of gross deformation or atrophy, visualization of the disk may be difficult or impossible. Disk deformities may be accompanied by changes in its signal intensity, including an increase in signal. Changes to the condyle and temporal component of the joint consistent with DJD often accompany cases with long-standing displaced disks (Fig. 28.19). Perforations between the superior and inferior joint spaces most commonly occur in the retrodiscal tissue, just behind the posterior band of the disk (Fig. 28.20D). Although the loss of the joint space, resulting in bone-to-bone contact between the osseous components, is suggestive of perforation of the disk or its attachment, arthrographic investigations provide more reliable evidence for this.

Fibrous adhesions and effusion. Fibrous adhesions are masses of fibrous tissue or scar tissue that form in the joint space, particularly after TMJ surgery. Adhesions may restrict normal movement of the disk during mandibular opening, resulting in a "stuck disk" and possible closed lock. Adhesions are best identified with arthrography by resistance to injection of contrast agent, or they may be detected on MRI studies as tissue with low signal intensity. Adhesions in the superior joint space also may be suspected when there is no movement of the disk relative to the articular eminence in mandibular open position in MRI. Joint effusion (fluid in the joint) is considered to be an early change that may precede DJD. MRI can detect joint effusion, which appears as an area of high signal intensity in the joint spaces on T_2-weighted images (see Fig. 28.18B and C).

Management. Management of an asymptomatic displaced disk is not indicated. In symptomatic patients, conservative, noninvasive therapy should be initiated first. Most patients' symptoms resolve with time. Arthroscopy or arthrocentesis may be helpful in releasing adhesions and improving joint mobility. Open joint surgery is reserved for refractory cases.

Remodeling and Arthritic Conditions

Remodeling

Disease mechanism. Remodeling is an adaptive response of cartilage and bone to increased or altered loading forces applied to the joint. This adaptive response results in alterations of the shape of the condyle and articular eminence, and may result in the flattening of the normally

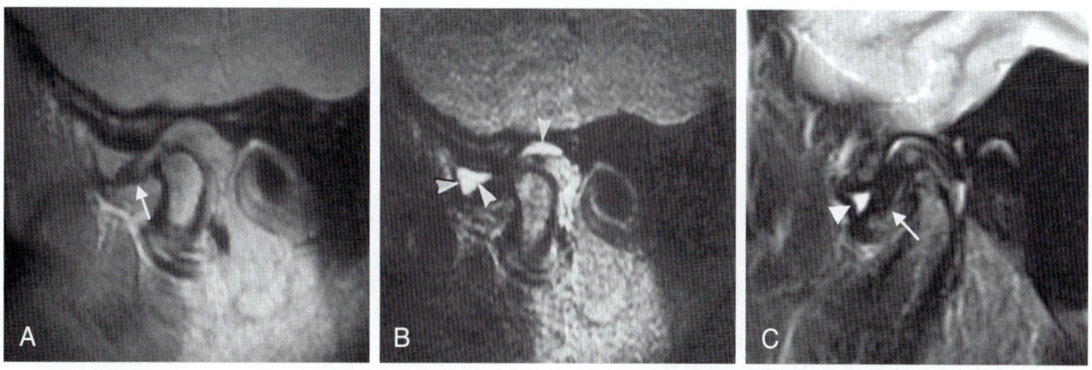

Fig. 28.18 Magnetic resonance imaging of disk displacement without reduction in the presence of joint effusion. (A) T_1-weighted image in the open mouth position shows the disc displaced anterior to the condyle. The posterior band of the disk is indicated with an *arrow*. (B) T_2-weighted image in the open mouth position at the same level as image in (A). Note the joint effusion *(arrowheads)* in the anterior and posterior recesses of the upper joint space. (C) T_2-weighted image of a different joint with anterior disk displacement and effusion in the superior joint space *(arrowhead)* seen as a high-signal collection. The posterior band of the disk is indicated with an *arrow*. (A and B, Courtesy Dr. P.-L. Westesson, Rochester, NY. C, Courtesy Dr. L. Alshafai, Toronto, ON.).

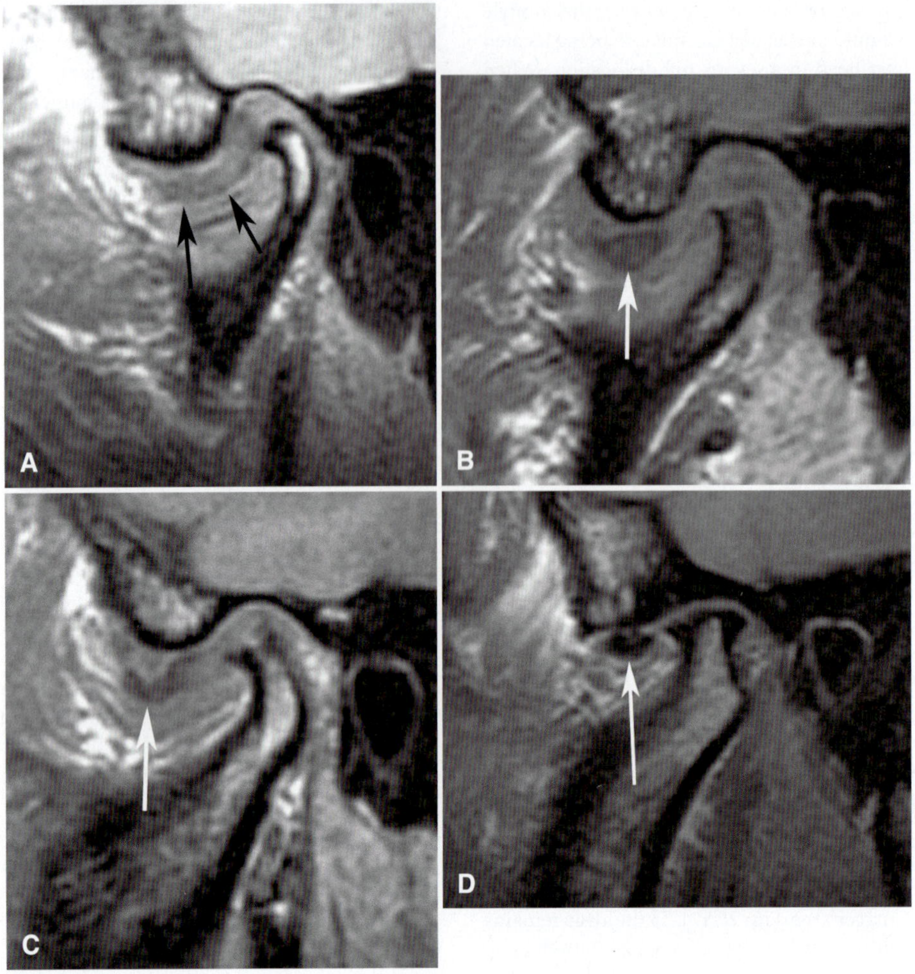

Fig. 28.19 Corrected sagittal magnetic resonance imaging of several cases of anteriorly displaced disks *(arrows)* with various stages of degenerative joint disease. (A) Example of severe deformation of the disk and an increase in the tissue signal. (B) Severe erosions of the superior aspect of the condyle. (C) Erosions involving the condyle and a small osteophyte on the anterior aspect. (D) Example of osteophytes forming on both the anterior and the posterior surfaces of the condyle.

gently curved joint surfaces. Such changes effectively redistribute the loading forces over a greater surface area. The number of trabeculae also increase, thereby increasing the density of subchondral cancellous bone (subchondral sclerosis) to better resist loading forces. No destruction or degeneration of the fibrocartilage articular tissue covering the bony components occurs. TMJ remodeling occurs throughout adult life and is considered abnormal only if it is accompanied by clinical signs and symptoms of pain or dysfunction, or if the degree of remodeling seen on imaging is judged to be severe. Remodeling may be unilateral and does not invariably serve as a precursor to DJD.

Clinical features. Remodeling may be asymptomatic, or patients may have signs and symptoms of TMJ dysfunction that may be related to the soft tissue components, associated muscles, or ligaments. Accompanying disk displacement may be a factor.

Imaging features. Changes noted in the diagnostic images may affect the condyle, temporal bone, or both. Such changes first occur on the anterosuperior surface of the condyle and the posterior slope of the articular eminence. The lateral aspect of the joint also may be affected in the early stages, and the central and medial aspects become involved as the remodeling progresses. These changes may include one or a combination of the following: flattening, thickening of the cortex of the articulating surfaces, and subchondral sclerosis (see Fig. 28.20).

Differential interpretation. It may be difficult to differentiate remodeling changes from early DJD as the microscopic changes associated with bone degeneration occur before the macroscopic changes can be visualized on imaging. The appearance of bone erosions, osteophytes, and loss of joint space in the diagnostic image are the more definitive signs of DJD, however, these may not be present early on. Joints affected by degenerative changes may also remodel to have flattened surfaces during nondestructive phases; significant loss of bone volume of the condyle or eminence suggests previous erosion as opposed to adaptive remodeling.

Management. When no clinical signs or symptoms are present, management is not indicated. Otherwise, management directed to reduce joint loading, such as splint therapy, may be considered. However, this should be preceded by an attempt to discover the cause of the joint overloading, such as parafunctional habits.

Degenerative Joint Disease

Disease mechanism. DJD or osteoarthritis is the breakdown of the fibrocartilaginous covering over the articulating surfaces of the joint that lead to the eventual deterioration of the osseous structures. DJD is thought to occur when the ability of the joint to adapt to excessive loading forces through remodeling is exceeded. Numerous etiologic

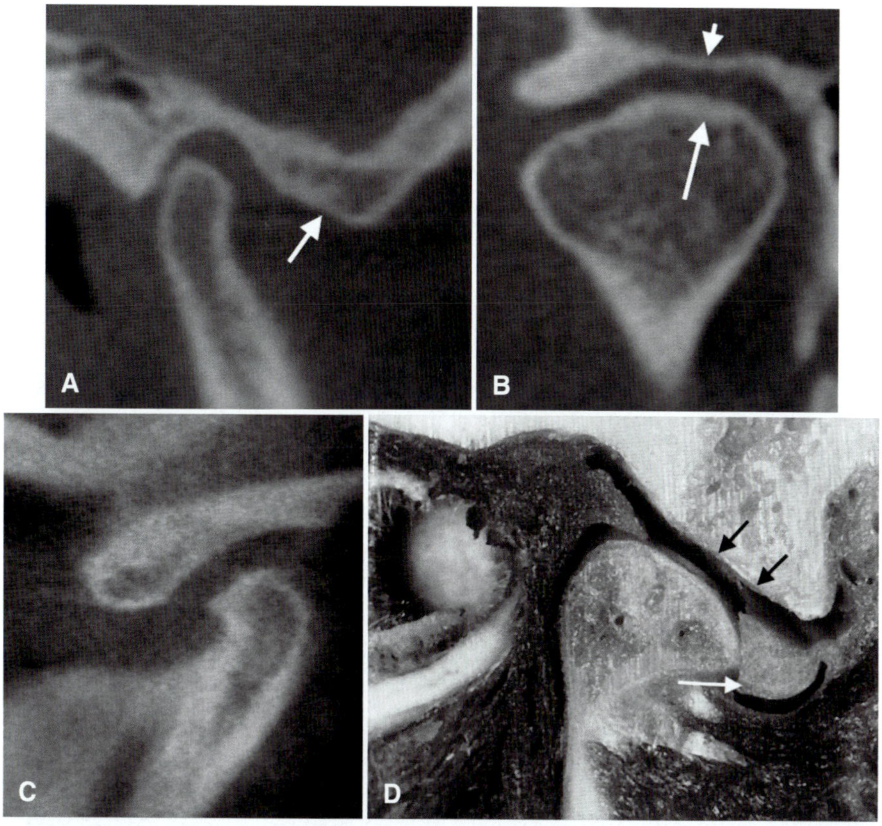

Fig. 28.20 Corrected sagittal (A) and coronal (B) cone beam computed tomographic images of the right temporomandibular joint show remodeling. (A) The right temporal component shows subchondral sclerosis and flattening of the articular eminence *(arrow)*. (B) The right condyle shows mild flattening of the lateral aspect and subchondral sclerosis of the medial aspect *(arrow)*. The right temporal component is also flattened *(arrowhead)*. (C) Reconstructed corrected sagittal CBCT image shows significant flattening of the condylar head. (D) Cadaver specimen. Note the flattening of the temporal component *(black arrows)* and large perforation posterior to a residual deformed disk *(white arrow)*.

factors may be important, including acute trauma, hypermobility, and abnormal loading of the joint that may occur in parafunction. Disk displacement also may be a contributing element, and loss of normal lubrication within the joint has been suggested to play a part at the molecular level. It has been reported that joints with long-term nonreducing disk displacement have a higher incidence of progressive radiographic changes of DJD than joints with no disk displacement or reducing disks.

It should be noted that DJD is a noninflammatory condition characterized by joint deterioration and bony proliferation. Joint deterioration is characterized by bone erosion, whereas new bone formation at the periphery of articular surfaces (osteophyte) and in the subchondral region (sclerosis) represents the proliferative components. Usually a combination of both deterioration and proliferation can occur, but occasionally one response predominates. Generally, deterioration is more common in acute disease, and proliferation predominates in chronic disease.

Clinical features. DJD can occur at any age, although the incidence increases with age. DJD has a female preponderance. The disease may be asymptomatic, or patients may complain of signs and symptoms of TMJ dysfunction, including pain on palpation and movement, joint noises (crepitus), limited range of motion, and muscle spasm or hyperactivity, and pain. The onset of symptoms may be sudden or gradual, and symptoms may disappear spontaneously, only to return in recurring cycles. Some studies report that the disease eventually "burns out," and symptoms disappear or decrease markedly in severity in long-standing cases.

Imaging features. Osseous changes in DJD are more accurately depicted on CT images, although osseous changes also may be seen on MRI; particularly T_1-weighted or proton density images. Erosions of the bone are a sign of the deteriorating component of DJD. These manifest as small to large "bites" or "scoops" within the articulating surfaces of the joint, resulting in loss of the continuity of the cortices and eventual loss of bone volume (Fig. 28.21). In severe DJD, the glenoid fossa may appear grossly enlarged because of erosion of the posterior slope of the articular eminence. If significant enough, these erosions may allow the condylar head to move forward and superiorly into an abnormal anterior position that may result in an anterior open bite. The condyle may also be markedly diminished in size and altered in shape because of severe erosions. In some cases, small, round, radiolucent areas with irregular margins surrounded by a varying area of sclerosis are visible, deep to the articulating surfaces. These lesions, referred to as subchondral or Ely cysts, are not true cysts but rather are areas of degeneration that contain fibrous connective tissue, granulation tissue, and osteoid (see Fig. 28.21A and B). As the bone overlying a subchondral cyst is lost or collapses, it may appear to migrate to the bone surface, and in this situation, the subchondral cyst may be difficult to differentiate from a surface erosion.

In the proliferative phase of the disease, bone formation occurs at the periphery of the articulating surfaces. These projections of new

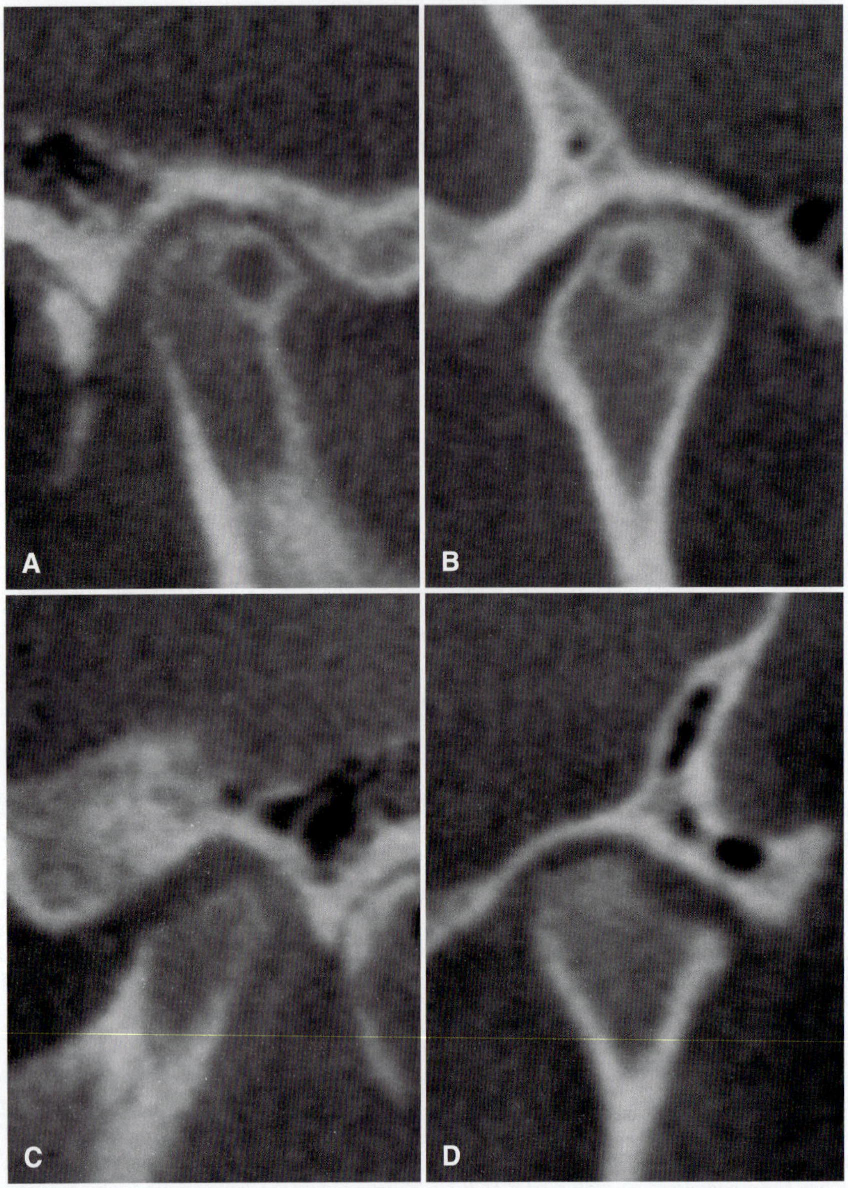

Fig. 28.21 Cone beam computed tomographic image, closed position, depicting various erosions in degenerative joint disease. (A and B) Same patient, right side. Large subchondral cyst-like erosion (Ely cyst) of the condyle surrounded by a broad zone of sclerosis. Note also the thin joint space. (C and D) Same patient, left side. Broad erosion of the anterolateral condylar surface. Note also the lack of cortication of the remaining condylar surface and flattening of the temporal component.

bone are called osteophytes, and although they may form on any part of the joint, they usually emanate from the anterosuperior surface of the condyle, the lateral aspect of the temporal bone, or both (Fig. 28.22). Osteophytes create broader, flatter bony articulating surfaces, and serve to better distribute the biomechanical load on the joint over a greater area. In severe cases, osteophyte formation may extend from the articular eminence almost to encase the condylar head. Osteophytes may also break off and lie free within the joint space. These fragments are known as "joint mice," and they must be differentiated from other conditions that cause joint space radiopacities (Fig. 28.23). Variable degrees of sclerosis of the subchondral bone may accompany any of the changes described.

DJD can also be associated with a narrowing or total absence of the joint space in maximum intercuspation. This finding often correlates with a displaced disk and frequently with a perforation of the disk or posterior attachment, resulting in bone-to-bone contact of the joint components.

Differential interpretation. DJD can have a spectrum of appearances ranging from extensive erosions (degenerative component) to substantial subchondral sclerosis and osteophyte formation (proliferative component). A more erosive appearance may simulate inflammatory arthritides, such as rheumatoid arthritis (RA), whereas a more proliferative appearance with extensive osteophyte formation may simulate a benign neoplasm, such as an osteoma or osteochondroma.

Management. The changes to the joint produced by DJD cannot be reversed by any known treatment. Treatment is directed toward unloading the forces on the abnormally loaded joint, relieving secondary inflammation with antiinflammatory drugs, and increasing joint mobility and function (e.g., physiotherapy). Occlusal splint therapy, intra-articular injections and, in severe refractory cases, joint replacement surgery are all possible treatments.

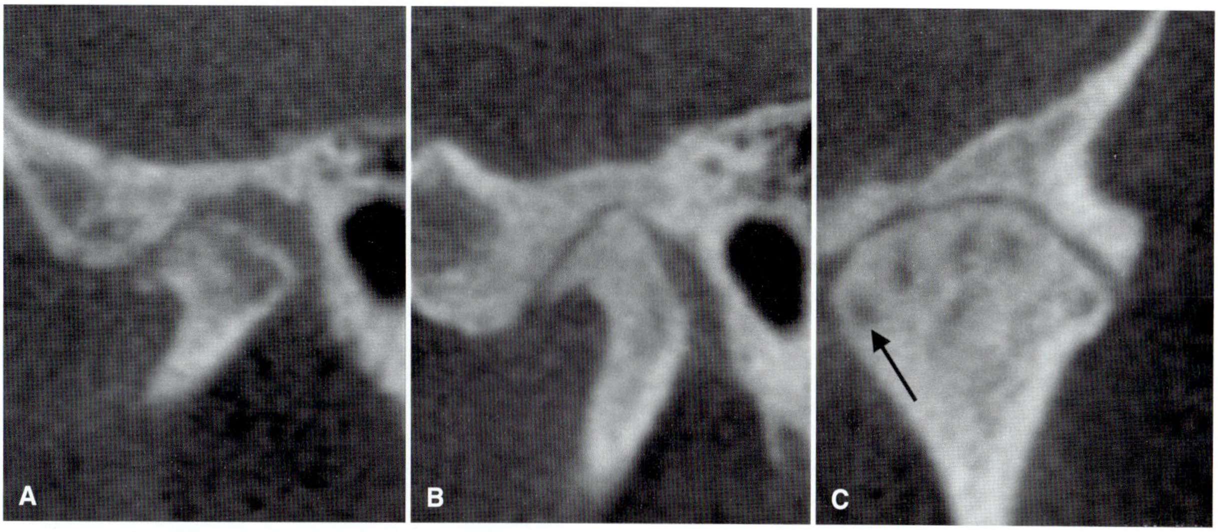

Fig. 28.22 Cone beam computed tomographic image, closed position displaying two cases of degenerative joint disease (different patients). (A) Corrected sagittal reconstruction. Surface erosions and subchondral sclerosis of the condyle and articular eminence. There is also osteophyte formation at the anterior aspect of the condyle. The condyle is anteriorly positioned in the glenoid fossa. (B) Corrected sagittal reconstruction. Prominent osteophyte formation at the anterior aspect of the condyle, flattening, and subchondral sclerosis of all joint components, with decreased width of the joint space. (C) Corrected coronal reconstruction, same patient as (B). Multiple subchondral erosions are seen, which are not visible in the sagittal reformat (one example indicated by *arrow*).

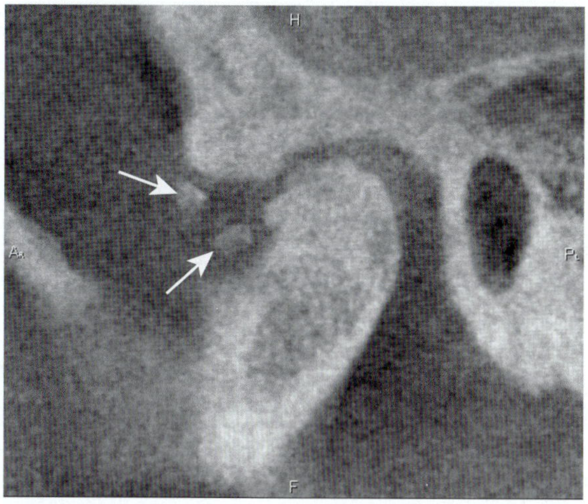

Fig. 28.23 Corrected sagittal reconstructed cone beam computed tomographic image shows detached osteophytes (joint mice) located anterior to the condyle *(arrows)*. Erosions, profound subchondral sclerosis, and osteophyte formation affecting the articulating surfaces are also noted, consistent with degenerative joint disease.

Rheumatoid Arthritis

Disease mechanism. RA is a heterogeneous group of autoimmune systemic disorders that manifests mainly as synovial membrane inflammation and proliferation in several joints. The TMJ becomes involved in approximately half of affected patients. The characteristic imaging findings are a result of inflammation and hypertrophy of the synovium, which becomes a destructive mass (pannus) that grows into the fibrocartilage and subchondral bone of the joint, causing erosion of the articular surfaces and underlying osseous structure.

Clinical features. RA is more common in females and can occur at any age but increases in incidence with age. A juvenile variant is discussed separately. Usually the small joints of the hands, wrists, knees, and feet are affected in a bilateral, symmetric fashion. TMJ involvement is variable, but when affected, involvement is often bilateral and occurs later than in other joints. Patients with TMJ involvement complain of swelling, pain, tenderness, stiffness on opening, limited range of motion, and crepitus. The chin appears receded, and an anterior open bite is a common finding because the condyles settle in an anterosuperior position as the articulating surfaces of the bone are progressively destroyed.

Imaging features. MRI may demonstrate the pannus, joint effusions, marrow edema, and disk abnormalities. These signs may precede changes to the bone. The use of gadolinium as an MRI contrast agent improves detection of a pannus which creates high signal due to hypervascularity of the inflamed tissue. Marrow edema is seen as increased signal in the cancellous bone on T_2-weighted images and may be an early sign of future bone destruction. The pannus may destroy the disk resulting in diminished width of the joint space.

CT imaging allows a more detailed assessment of the osseous changes, including periarticular osteopenia, and bone erosions that most often involve the articular eminence and the anterior aspect of the condylar head due to pannus formation. Erosion of the anterior and posterior condylar surfaces where the synovial lining comes into contact with the bone may result in a "sharpened pencil" appearance of the condyle. Erosive changes may be so severe that the entire condylar head is destroyed, with only the neck remaining as the articulating surface. Similarly, the articular eminence may be destroyed to the extent that a concavity replaces the normally convex eminence. These patterns of erosions may alter the anterosuperior position of the condyle when the teeth are in maximal intercuspation, resulting in an anterior open bite (Fig. 28.24). Joint destruction eventually leads to secondary DJD, and subchondral sclerosis and flattening of articulating surfaces as well as subchondral cyst and osteophyte formation may occur. Fibrous ankylosis or, in rare cases, osseous ankylosis may occur (Fig. 28.25) with reduced mobility related to the duration and severity of the disease.

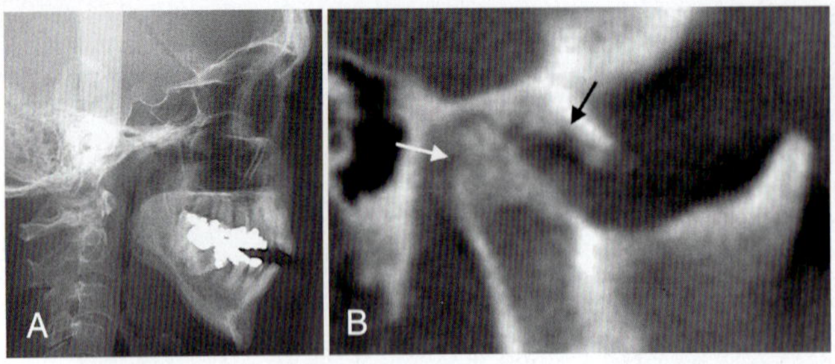

Fig. 28.24 Rheumatoid arthritis. (A) Lateral cephalometric skull image illustrates a steep mandibular plane and anterior open bite due to bone loss in the temporomandibular joints. (B) Corrected sagittal cone beam computed tomographic image showing severe erosions affecting the articular eminence *(black arrow)* and condyle, including the posterior surface *(white arrow)*.

Differential interpretation. The differential interpretation includes severe DJD and psoriatic arthritis. Periarticular osteopenia and severe erosions, particularly of the articular eminence, are more characteristic of RA. Involvement of other joints is also suggestive, and as such, referral to the patient's physician is required when RA is suspected. Psoriatic arthritis may be considered when the patient has a history of skin lesions.

Management. Treatment is directed toward pain relief (analgesics), reduction or suppression of inflammation (e.g., nonsteroidal antiinflammatory drugs [NSAIDs], antirheumatic drugs, corticosteroids), and preservation of muscle and joint function (physiotherapy). Joint replacement surgery may be necessary in patients with severe joint destruction.

Juvenile Idiopathic Arthritis

Disease mechanism. JIA, formerly known as juvenile RA, juvenile chronic arthritis, and Still disease, is a chronic rheumatologic inflammatory disease that manifests before age 16 years with a mean age of 5 years. JIA is characterized by chronic, intermittent synovial inflammation that results in synovial hypertrophy, joint effusion, and swollen, painful joints. As the disease progresses, cartilage and bone are destroyed. The rheumatoid factor may be absent; hence the preferred terminology of JIA rather than juvenile RA. JIA differs from adult RA in that it has an earlier age of onset, and systemic involvement is usually more severe. TMJ involvement occurs in approximately 40% of patients, and may be unilateral or bilateral.

Clinical features. JIA more commonly affects females. Children with JIA may have systemic symptoms, including lethargy and pain. The TMJs in these patients are often asymptomatic, even when active disease affects the joints. When symptoms are present, they include pain in the muscles of mastication, pain and swelling over the joints, and limitations in mandibular movement. Unilateral onset is common, but contralateral involvement may also occur as the disease progresses. Severe TMJ involvement results in the inhibition of mandibular growth. Loss of bone structure in the joints combined with growth inhibition may result in micrognathia and posteroinferior chin rotation, leading to the development of an anterior open bite. The degree of micrognathia is proportional to the severity of joint involvement and is worse with earlier onset of the disease. Additionally, when only one TMJ is involved, or if one side is more severely affected, the patient may have a mandibular asymmetry with the chin deviated to the affected side.

Imaging features. MRI with gadolinium contrast agent is the modality of choice for assessing patients with JIA because it can demonstrate early synovial inflammation, even in asymptomatic patients, before bone destruction occurs. CT imaging can be performed for a more detailed assessment of the osseous changes, whereas panoramic and cephalometric skull images are useful for evaluation of growth disturbances. Osteopenia (decreased density) of the affected TMJ components may be the only initial radiographic finding. Erosion of the articular eminence may result in the appearance of a large glenoid fossa. The condyle may be pointed (pencil shaped) or concave, or completely destroyed. As a result of bone destruction, the condylar head typically is positioned anterosuperiorly in the mandibular fossa (Fig. 28.26).

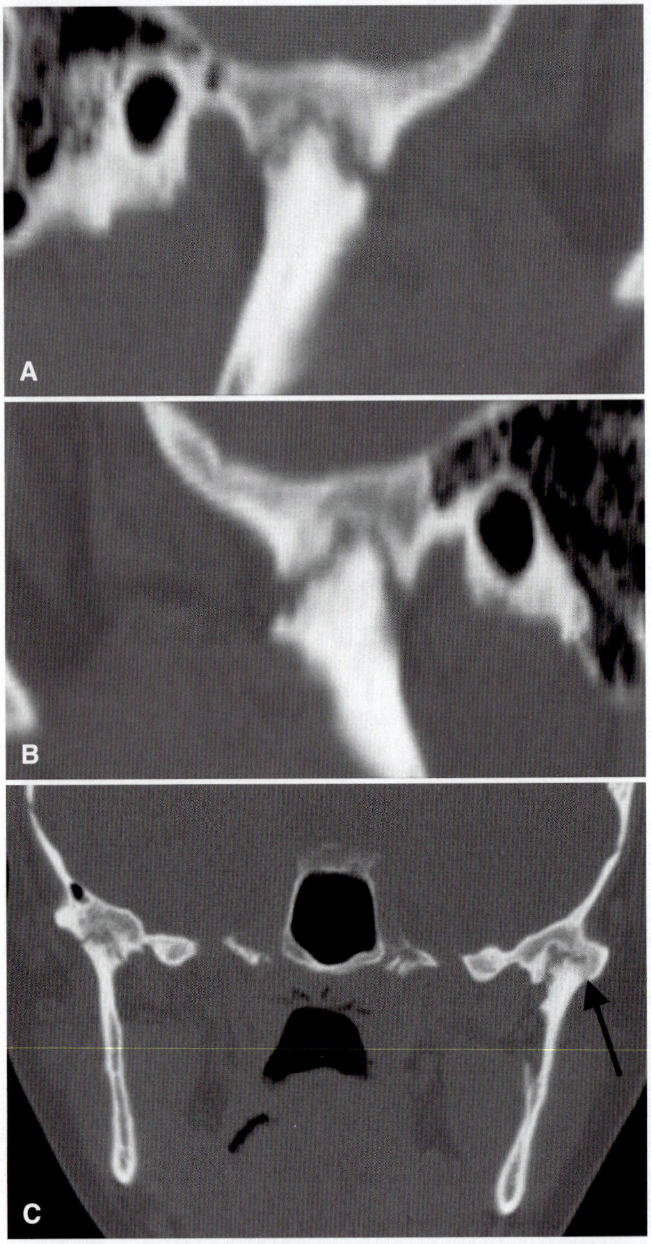

Fig. 28.25 (A and B) Corrected sagittal reconstructed multidetector computed tomographic images with bone algorithm of the right and left joints affected by rheumatoid arthritis. Note the irregular surfaces of the condyle and articular eminence which interdigitate, similar to opposing pieces of a puzzle, suggesting the possibility of fibrous ankylosis. Because of erosion of the articular eminence, the condyles have an abnormal anterior position near the residual articular eminence. (C) Coronal MDCT image of the same patient. Note osseous ankylosis on the lateral aspect of the left joint *(arrow)*.

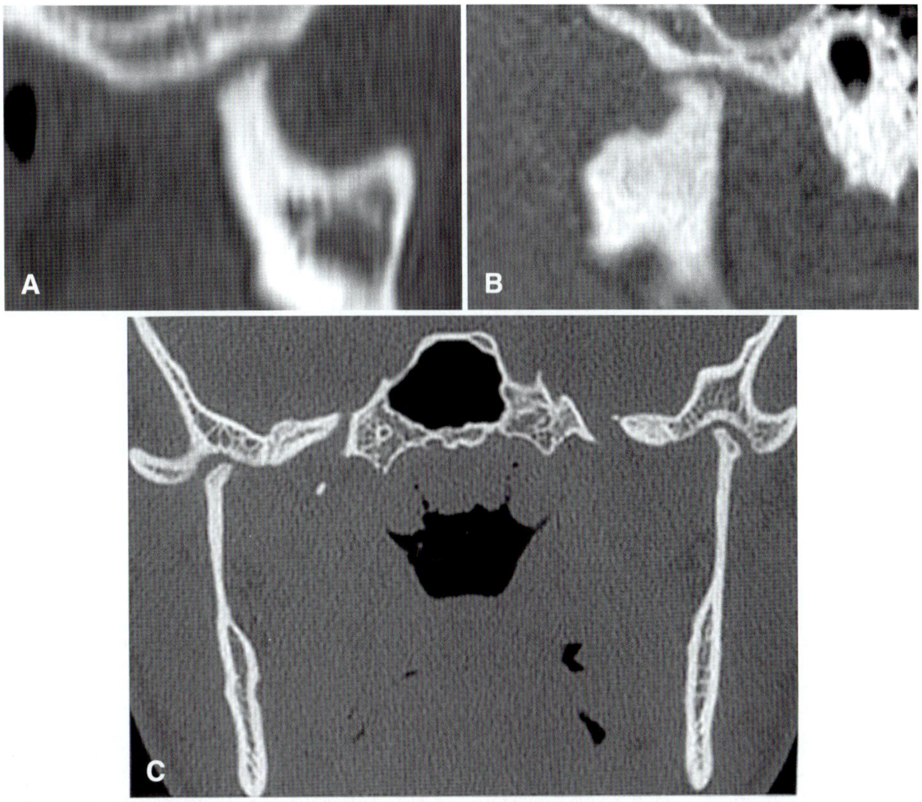

Fig. 28.26 (A and B) Corrected sagittal reconstructed multidetector computed tomographic images of juvenile idiopathic arthritis. Note the severe erosion of the articular eminences and the condyles, and the abnormal anterior positioning of both condyles. (C) Coronal computed tomography image of the same patient shows small remnants of the condylar heads after severe erosion.

Because the inflammatory response is intermittent, the cortex of the joint surfaces may reappear during quiescent periods, and the surfaces appear flattened. Secondary degenerative changes manifesting as sclerosis and osteophyte formation may be superimposed on the rheumatoid changes. Hypomobility at maximal opening is common, and fibrous ankylosis may occur in some cases. An abnormal disk shape is often observed in patients with long-term TMJ involvement. Manifestations of inhibited mandibular growth, such as deepening of the antegonial notch, diminished height of the ramus, and dorsal bending of the ramus and condylar neck, also may occur unilaterally or bilaterally, resulting in an obtuse angle between the mandibular body and the ascending ramus.

Management. Early, aggressive management of JIA has resulted in improved outcomes. Medical treatments include NSAIDs, methotrexate, and biologic agents. Orthodontics and orthognathic surgery are often required to improve dentofacial form and function.

Psoriatic Arthritis and Ankylosing Spondylitis

Psoriatic arthritis and ankylosing spondylitis are seronegative, systemic arthritides that may affect the TMJs. Psoriatic arthritis occurs in patients with psoriasis of the skin, with inflammatory joint disease occurring in 7% of patients. Ankylosing spondylitis occurs predominantly in males and progresses to spinal fusion. TMJ imaging changes seen in these disorders may be indistinguishable from changes caused by RA, although occasionally a profound sclerotic change is seen in psoriatic arthritis.

Idiopathic Condylar Resorption

Disease mechanism. Idiopathic condylar resorption (ICR), otherwise known as progressive condylar resorption or condylosis, is a condition leading to loss of bone mass of the mandibular condyle, not attributable to other destructive conditions (i.e., DJD, RA, or septic arthritis). ICR also may be related to the condition first described in the 1960s by Boering as "Boering's arthrosis."

During the first decade of growth, the mandibular condyle appears normal, but there is significant resorption of the condylar head, typically during adolescence. The etiology of ICR is unknown, although it is theorized to be the result of decreased biologic adaptation to increased mechanical loading in a susceptible population of young females. A hormonal influence has also been postulated, but the role of estrogen has not been established. An association with specific skeletal relationships, namely steep mandibular plane angle and class II jaw relationship, has been noted. Displacement of the articular disk away from its normal position also may be a risk factor. Many cases have been reported to occur after orthognathic surgery.

Clinical features. ICR affects mainly females during the second decade of life. It is usually an incidental finding on a panoramic image, or the patient may develop a mandibular asymmetry, signs and symptoms of TMJ dysfunction, or both. ICR may be unilateral or bilateral. As the condylar changes progress, the patient often develops an anterior open bite.

Imaging features. On a panoramic image, the mandibular condyle often demonstrates flattening and apparent elongation of the

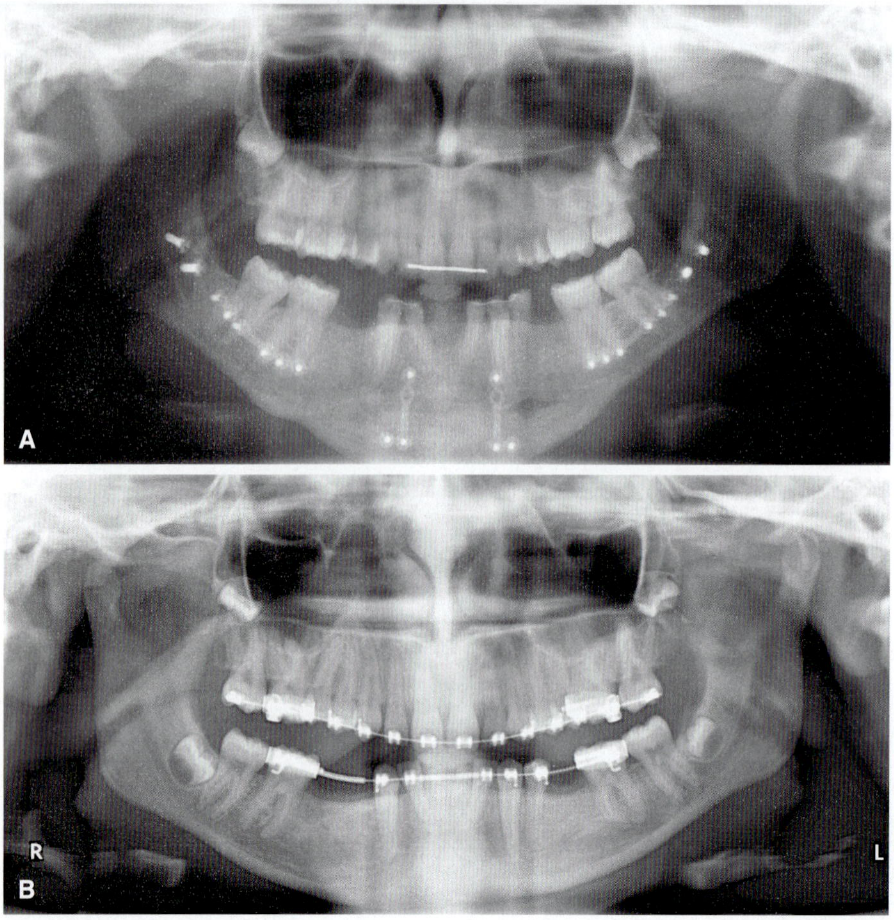

Fig. 28.27 (A) Panoramic image of idiopathic condylar resorption in a young female patient. There is loss of bone structure of the mandibular condyles due to severe resorption. The anterior surfaces of the condyles appear flattened and elongated. (B) Prior panoramic image of the same patient before orthognathic surgery shows normal condylar morphology.

anterior surface with a posterior deflection of the condylar head and neck (Fig. 28.27). In addition, there also may be bowing of the posterior surface of the ramus. Together these features have been described as a "toadstool" appearance. Secondary hypoplasia of the ipsilateral mandible is seen due to loss of the normal growth center within the affected condyle. This is evident by shortening of the ramus and deepening of the antegonial notch. More detailed imaging with CBCT or MDCT may demonstrate erosion of the articulating surface of the condyle. Progressive erosion of bone mass leads to loss of the vertical height of the condyle, and eventual complete resorption of the condyle can occur in some cases. Involvement of the temporal component also may be seen. An anterior open bite can develop as condylar height is lost and the mandible rotates to a retruded chin position.

Differential interpretation. None of the radiologic features of ICR is unique to this condition; rather, they overlap with other arthritic conditions affecting the TMJs. Diagnosis requires consideration of the clinical presentation with the imaging features, and elimination of other possible diagnoses, including resorption secondary to JIA and severe DJD.

Management. The management of ICR is difficult because orthognathic surgery and orthodontic therapy done to correct occlusal discrepancies or asymmetry may exacerbate the condition. Relapse after orthognathic surgery is common. Disk repositioning, costochondral grafts, and alloplastic TMJ replacement also have been advocated.

Septic Arthritis

Disease mechanism. Septic or infectious arthritis is an inflammatory condition involving the TMJ that can result in joint destruction. Compared with the incidence of DJD and RA in the TMJ, septic arthritis is rare. Septic arthritis of the TMJ may be caused by direct spread of bacterial microorganisms from an adjacent cellulitis, or from parotid, otic, or mastoid infections. It also may occur by direct extension of osteomyelitis involving the mandibular body and ramus. Hematogenous spread from a distant, often occult, nidus also has been reported. Trauma and immunosuppression are also potential etiologic factors.

Clinical features. Individuals can be affected at any age but there is a predilection for young males. It usually occurs unilaterally. The patient may have redness and swelling over the joint, trismus, severe pain on opening, inability to occlude the teeth, large, tender cervical lymph nodes, and fever and malaise. The mandible may be deviated to the unaffected side as a result of joint effusion.

Imaging features. CBCT, MDCT, and MRI are most useful for examining cases of suspected septic arthritis. No imaging signs may be present in the acute stages of the disease, although the space between the condyle and the roof of the mandibular fossa may be widened because of inflammatory exudate in the joint spaces. Osteopenic (radiolucent) changes involving the osseous components of the joint as well as the mandibular ramus may be evident. More obvious bony changes

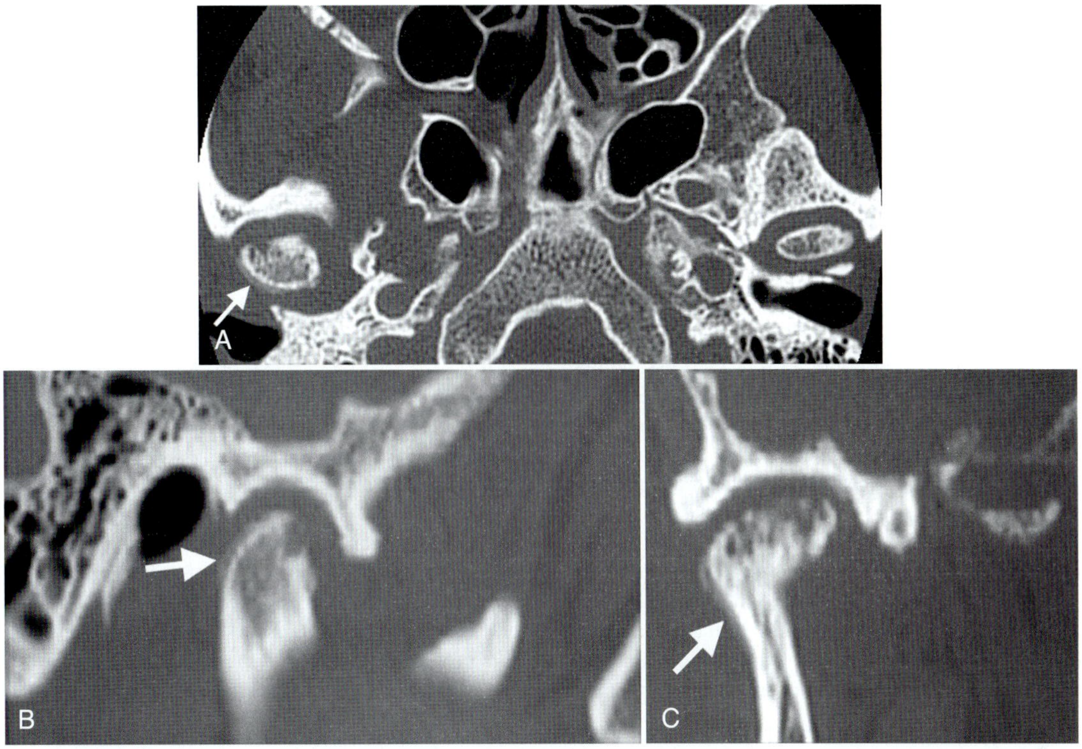

Fig. 28.28 Axial (A), corrected sagittal (B), and coronal (C) multidetector computed tomographic images of septic arthritis involving the right TMJ. Note the erosions, sclerosis, and periosteal reaction that extends along the back of the condyle and lateral condylar neck *(arrows)*.

may be seen approximately 7–10 days after the onset of clinical symptoms. Some of these changes mimic DJD including loss of definition of the articular cortex and erosions of the articulating surfaces of the condyle and articular eminence. Other signs, including sequestra and periosteal new bone formation, are more indicative of the infectious etiology (Fig. 28.28).

Inflammatory changes that may accompany septic arthritis can be seen in CT images, such as opacification of mastoid air cells, osteomyelitis of the mandible, and cellulitis of the surrounding soft tissue. MRI, with T_2-weighted images, may show muscle enlargement and edema, joint effusion, or abscess. Nuclear medicine may have a role in the diagnosis because ^{99m}Tc bone imaging shows increased bone metabolism within the involved osseous components, especially the condyle. Furthermore, a positive nuclear medicine examination with gallium (^{67}Ga) can confirm the presence of infection. As the disease progresses, the condyle and articular eminence, including the disk, may be destroyed. DJD is a common long-term sequela, and fibrous or osseous ankylosis may occur after the infection subsides. If the disease occurs during the period of mandibular growth, manifestations of inhibited mandibular growth may be evident in the diagnostic images.

Differential interpretation. The diagnosis of septic arthritis is ideally made by identification of organisms in joint aspirate, although cultures occasionally remain negative. The imaging changes caused by septic arthritis may mimic the changes of severe DJD or RA, although septic arthritis usually occurs unilaterally. Also, the patient often has an acute onset and clinical signs and symptoms of infection.

Management. Management can include antimicrobial therapy, drainage of effusion, arthrocentesis, and joint rest. Physiotherapy to reestablish joint mobility is initiated after the acute phase of infection has passed.

Articular Loose Bodies

Disease Mechanism

Articular loose bodies are calcifications of varying origin that may be located in the synovium, inside the capsule in the joint spaces, or outside the capsule in soft tissue. They appear on images as radiopaque entities seen around or superimposed over the condylar head. The loose bodies may represent bone that has separated from joint components in DJD (joint mice), hyaline cartilage metaplasia with ossification that occurs in synovial chondromatosis, crystals deposited in the joint space in crystal-associated arthropathy (chondrocalcinosis), or tumoral calcinosis associated with renal disease. In rare cases, chondrosarcoma also may mimic the appearance of articular loose bodies.

Synovial Chondromatosis

Disease mechanism. Synovial chondromatosis, also known as osteochondromatosis or chondrometaplasia, is an uncommon benign disorder characterized by metaplastic formation of multiple cartilaginous and osteocartilaginous nodules within the synovial membrane. Some of these nodules may detach from the synovial tissues and form loose bodies in the joint space where they persist and increase in size, nourished by synovial fluid. This condition is more common in the axial skeleton than in the TMJ. When the cartilaginous nodules ossify, the term *synovial osteochondromatosis* is appropriate. Primary and secondary forms exist. Primary synovial chondromatosis arises in otherwise healthy joints and has an unknown etiology. The secondary form develops in a joint with existing degenerative changes or a history of trauma, as a result of mechanical alterations.

Clinical features. Females are more commonly affected in the TMJ than males. Primary synovial chondromatosis affects younger individuals than the secondary form. Patients may be asymptomatic or may complain of preauricular swelling, pain, a change in occlusion, and a decreased range of motion. Some patients have crepitus or other joint noises. The condition usually occurs unilaterally.

Imaging features. The osseous components may appear normal or may exhibit osseous changes similar to changes in DJD. The joint space may be widened, and if ossification of the cartilaginous nodules has occurred, one or multiple radiopaque loose bodies may be seen surrounding the condylar head (Fig. 28.29). There is considerable variation in the size of these ossified loose bodies. Rounded shapes with smooth borders are highly suggestive of the condition. CT imaging improves localization of the loose bodies, and can demonstrate an internal pattern with osseous architecture. Osseous changes that are reminiscent of DJD may also be seen, which may potentially be due to changes in joint loading caused by the presence of the loose bodies. Occasionally, erosion through the glenoid fossa roof into the middle cranial fossa may occur, which is best detected with CT imaging. MRI can detect joint space effusion and enlargement, and may be useful in defining the tissue planes between the synovial chondromatosis mass and the surrounding soft tissues.

Differential interpretation. The appearance of synovial chondromatosis cannot always be differentiated from chondrocalcinosis; however, the ossified bodies in synovial chondromatosis are often larger and may have a peripheral cortex that identifies their bony nature. Conditions that appear similar include DJD with joint mice (detached osteophytes), or chondrosarcoma or osteosarcoma. Sarcomas may be accompanied by severe bone destruction, which would help in differentiating these tumors from synovial chondromatosis.

Treatment. Treatment consists of removal of the loose bodies and resection of the abnormal synovial tissue in the joint by arthroscopic or open joint surgery.

Chondrocalcinosis

Disease mechanism. Chondrocalcinosis or pseudogout is a condition that is characterized by acute or chronic synovitis and precipitation of calcium pyrophosphate dihydrate crystals in the joint space. It differs from classical gout, in which monosodium urate monohydrate crystals are precipitated; hence the term "pseudogout."

Clinical features. The more commonly affected joints are the knee, wrist, hip, shoulder, and elbow; TMJ involvement is uncommon and the condition occurs unilaterally. Patients most often complain of pain and swelling over the joint; however, some patients are asymptomatic.

Imaging features. The appearance of chondrocalcinosis may simulate synovial chondromatosis, however, the radiopaque loose bodies in chondrocalcinosis are often finer and more evenly distributed than those seen in synovial chondromatosis (Fig. 28.30). Crystal deposition may also extend to tissues surrounding the joint. Bone erosions and profound sclerosis of the osseous components have been described. Erosions of the glenoid fossa may be present, which require

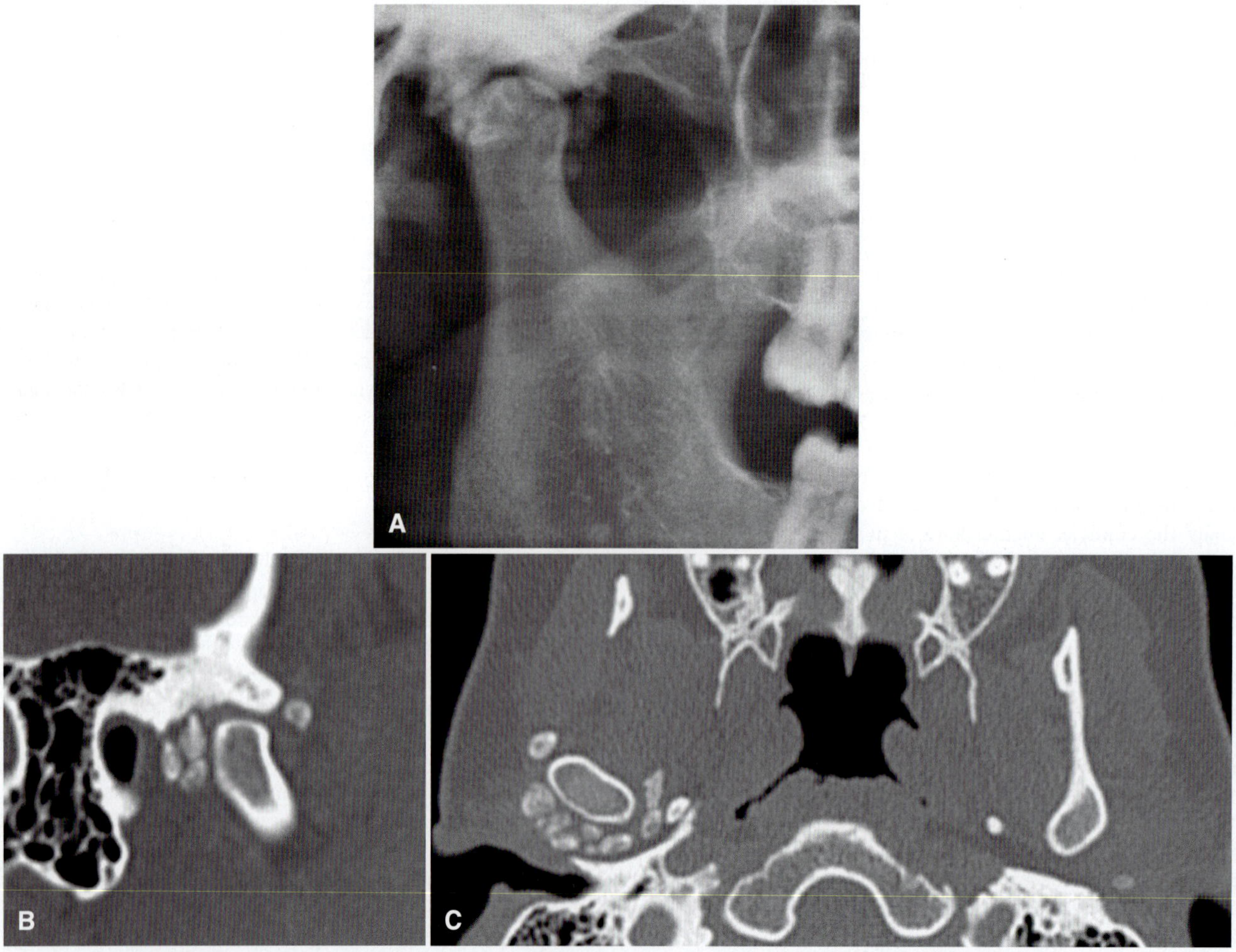

Fig. 28.29 (A) Cropped panoramic image of synovial chondromatosis involving a right TMJ. Sagittal (B) and axial (C) multidetector computed tomographic images revealing multiple loose bodies surrounding the condyle and within the joint capsule.

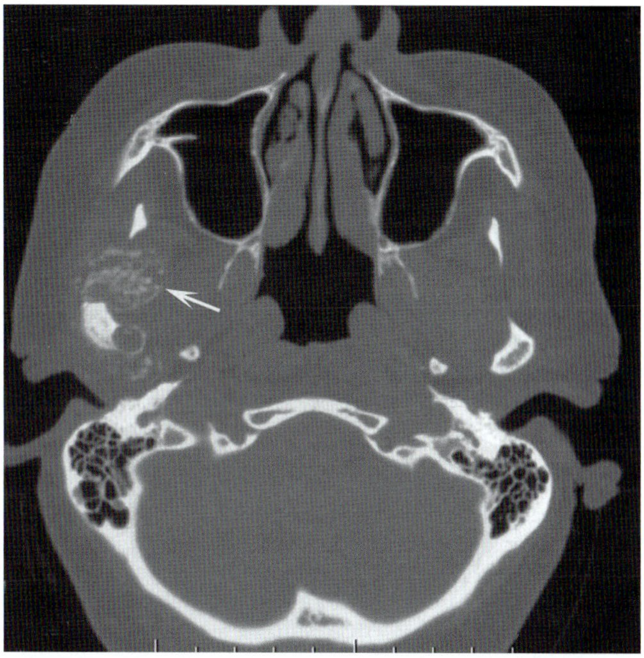

Fig. 28.30 Axial bone algorithm multidetector computed tomographic image of chondrocalcinosis. Note the calcifications anterior to the right condyle *(arrow)* and the large erosion involving the medial pole of the condyle. There is also profound sclerosis of the lateral pole.

CT imaging for detection. Soft tissue swelling and edema of the surrounding muscles may be seen with MRI.

Differential interpretation. The differential interpretation is the same as for synovial chondromatosis.

Management. Management consists of surgical removal of the large crystalline masses. Steroids, aspirin, and NSAIDs may provide relief. Colchicine may be used to alleviate acute symptoms and for prophylaxis.

Trauma

Effusion

Disease mechanism. Effusion is an influx of fluid into the joint and may be associated with trauma, soft tissue abnormalities, such as disk displacement, or arthritic conditions. Effusions within the joint after trauma most often represent hemorrhage into the joint spaces (hemarthrosis).

Clinical features. The patient may have swelling over the affected joint, pain in the TMJ preauricular region or ear, and limited range of motion. Patients may also complain of the sensation of fluid in the ear, tinnitus, hearing difficulties, and difficulty occluding the posterior teeth.

Imaging features. Joint effusions are best seen on T_2-weighted MRI as high signal (bright) areas around the condyle. The involved joint spaces are also increased in width (see Fig. 28.18).

Differential interpretation. Effusion secondary to trauma must be differentiated from other conditions manifesting with effusion, including disk displacement and arthritis. Evidence of condylar fracture may be detected in cases of trauma. Patient history and clinical examination should be helpful.

Management. Treatment may include anti-inflammatory drugs, although surgical drainage of the effusion occasionally is necessary.

Condylar Dislocation

Disease mechanism. Condylar dislocation is abnormal positioning of the mandibular condyle out of the mandibular fossa but within the joint capsule. It usually occurs bilaterally and most commonly, the dislocation is in an anterior direction. Dislocation may be caused by trauma and is often associated with a condylar fracture. Forced mouth opening, such as during an intubation procedure, also may lead to dislocation. Loose ligaments and joint capsule may predispose to chronic TMJ dislocation. Dislocation also may rarely occur superiorly through the roof of the glenoid fossa into the middle cranial fossa as a result of trauma.

Clinical features. In anterior dislocation, patients are unable to close the mandible to maximal intercuspation. Some patients cannot reduce the dislocation, whereas others may be able to reduce the mandible by manipulation. Associated pain and muscle spasm often are present.

Imaging features. CBCT and MDCT are most useful for evaluating the relationships of the osseous structures. Imaging shows the condyle positioned outside the glenoid fossa, most commonly anterior and superior to the summit of the articular eminence. Signs of an associated condylar fracture also may be present.

Differential interpretation. In patients with mandibular hypermobility, the condyles may translate anterior and superior to the articular eminence on opening. Clinical correlation to confirm that the patient cannot close the jaw normally is important to make the diagnosis of dislocation.

Management. Treatment consists of manual manipulation of the mandible to reduce the dislocation. Surgery occasionally is necessary to achieve reduction, especially in protracted cases.

Fracture

Disease mechanism. Fractures of the TMJ may involve the condylar head (intracapsular) or the condylar neck (extracapsular). Condylar neck fractures are most common and are often accompanied by dislocation of the condylar head. Condylar head fractures may be horizontal or vertical, or they may be compression fractures. Rarely does the fracture involve the temporal component. Unilateral fractures, which are more common than bilateral fractures, may be accompanied by a parasymphyseal or mandibular body fracture on the contralateral side.

Clinical features. The patient may have swelling over the TMJ, pain, limited range of motion, deviation to the affected side, and malocclusion or an anterior open bite. Some TMJ fractures may be asymptomatic and may not be discovered at the time of trauma. Instead, such traumatic injuries may come to light as incidental findings at a later time when images are obtained for other purposes. Condylar fractures should be ruled out if the patient has a history of an impact to the mandible, especially to the mental region.

If a condylar fracture occurs during the period of mandibular growth, growth may be disrupted because of damage to the condylar growth center. The degree of subsequent hypoplasia is related to the severity of the injury and the stage of mandibular development at the time of injury (younger patients have more profound hypoplasia). Patients younger than 10 years old have a higher remodeling potential and may have less deformity compared with older patients, although injuries in patients younger than 3 years old tend to produce severe asymmetries. Injury to the joint may result in hemorrhage or effusion into the joint spaces that may eventually form bone during the healing process, and this may result in ankylosis and limited joint function.

Imaging features. In a relatively recent condylar neck fracture, a radiolucent fracture plane limited to the confines of the neck may be visible. This plane may vary in width, depending on the amount of distraction between the fragments. When the bone fragments are well aligned, the width of the plane is narrow. However, when there is greater displacement between the fragments, the plane may appear wider. If the bone fragments overlap, an area of apparent increased radiopacity may be seen (the "overlapping fragment sign") instead of the radiolucent plane (Fig. 28.31). Careful examination of the cortical outline of the condyle and neck may reveal an irregularity to the

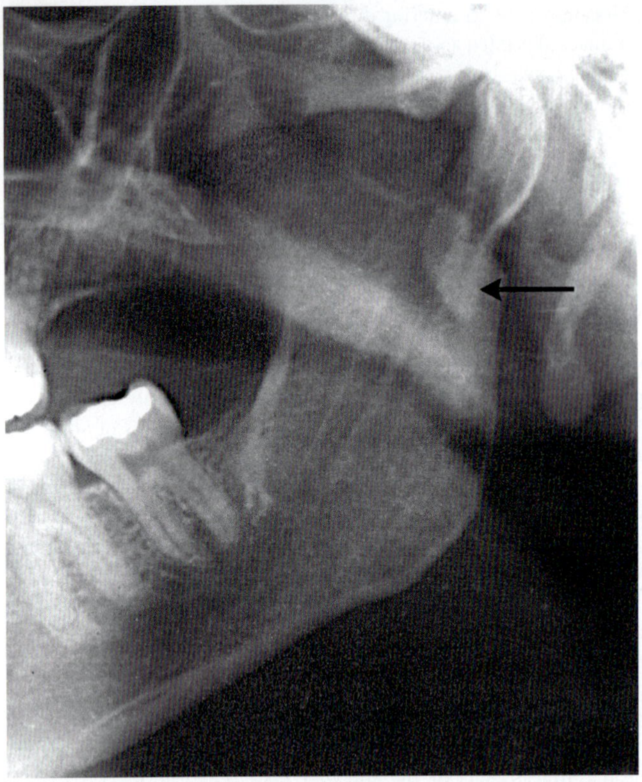

Fig. 28.31 Cropped panoramic image of condylar neck fracture. The *arrow* points to overlapped fragments, as evidenced by the increased radiopacity. There is also a step defect evident along the posterior border of the ramus.

normally smooth outline of the bone surface (i.e., a "step defect"). Approximately 60% of condylar fractures show evidence of fragment angulation and a variable degree of displacement of the fracture fragments. Displacement of the condylar head most commonly occurs in an anteromedial direction due to the action of the lateral pterygoid muscle, which attaches to the pterygoid fovea of the condyle. Fractures of the condylar head are less common and may be horizontal, vertical (responsible for the traumatic type of bifid condyle), or compressive (Fig. 28.32). CBCT is the preferred imaging modality to evaluate condylar fractures because there is no superimposition of adjacent structures, and multiplanar reformatted images can better demonstrate disruption of anatomic boundaries and localize fractured fragment.

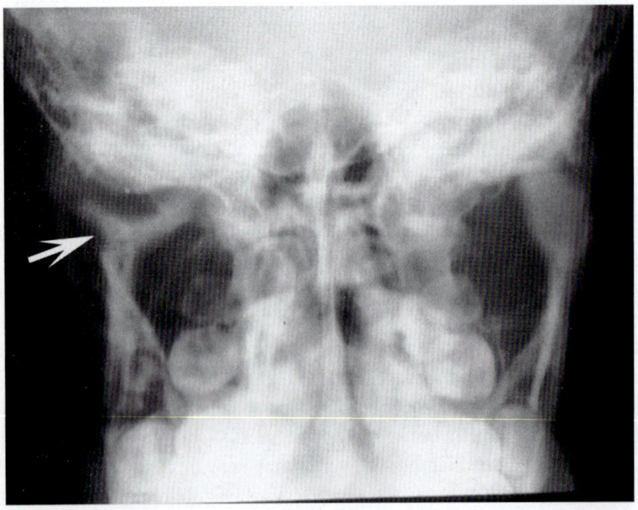

Fig. 28.32 Open mouth Towne image demonstrates a flattened appearance of the right mandibular condyle due to a compression fracture *(arrow)*.

The amount of remodeling seen in the TMJ after a condylar fracture with medial displacement varies considerably. In some cases, the bony fragments may remodel to a form that is essentially normal. Alternatively, the mandibular fossa may remodel, becoming more shallow, to compensate for the new condylar position. The condylar fragment may fuse to the condylar neck or ramus in a new, abnormal position. The condyle eventually may show degenerative changes, including flattening, erosion, osteophyte formation, and ankylosis. These changes are more severe if the condyle is displaced. Condylar fractures also can be associated with damage of the intracapsular soft tissues including the disk, the joint capsule, and the retrodiscal tissues, and with hemarthrosis and joint effusion.

Differential interpretation. The most common difficulty is determining whether a fracture is present or not. Panoramic images made as an initial examination may not disclose a fracture, especially greenstick fractures of the condylar neck, because changes in the coronal plane of the bone cannot be appreciated. Supplementation of the panoramic image with a planar image at right angles such as an open-mouth Towne view or CBCT is often necessary to visualize displacements. Occasionally, prior fractures that have remodeled may be difficult to differentiate from developmental abnormalities of the condyle.

Management. Management may not be indicated if mandibular function is adequate; otherwise, the fracture is reduced surgically. Physiotherapy may be important to maintain mobility and prevent the development of ankylosis.

Neonatal Fractures

Disease mechanism. The use of forceps during delivery of neonates may result in fracture and displacement of the rudimentary condyle, which later manifests as severe mandibular hypoplasia and lack of development of the glenoid fossa and articular eminence. Such cases have a characteristic radiographic appearance in the panoramic image, having the appearance of a partly opened pair of scissors in place of a normal condyle (Fig. 28.33). This presentation results from the overlapping images of the medially displaced carrot-shaped rudimentary condyle and remnants of the condylar neck.

Differential interpretation. This condition often is not diagnosed until later in life, at which time a diagnosis of fracture may be made without a history that the fracture occurred at the time of birth. The condition must be differentiated from developmental hypoplasia of the mandible, which is unrelated to birth injury.

Management. The fracture usually is not treated, but the mandibular asymmetry may be corrected with a combination of orthodontics and orthognathic surgery.

Ankylosis

Disease Mechanism

Ankylosis is a condition in which condylar movement is restricted because of fusion of the intraarticular joint components ("true ankylosis") or a physical impediment caused by structures outside the joint. Intraarticular ankylosis may be bony or fibrous. In bony ankylosis, the condyle or ramus is attached to the temporal or zygomatic bone by an osseous bridge. In fibrous ankylosis, a soft tissue (fibrous) union of joint components occurs. Most unilateral cases are caused by mandibular trauma or infection. Severe arthritis, particularly related to rheumatic conditions, and therapeutic radiation exposure to the joint (for cancer treatment) also may give rise to ankylosis. Extraarticular ankylosis may result from conditions that inhibit condylar movement, such as muscle spasm or fibrosis, myositis ossificans, or coronoid process hyperplasia.

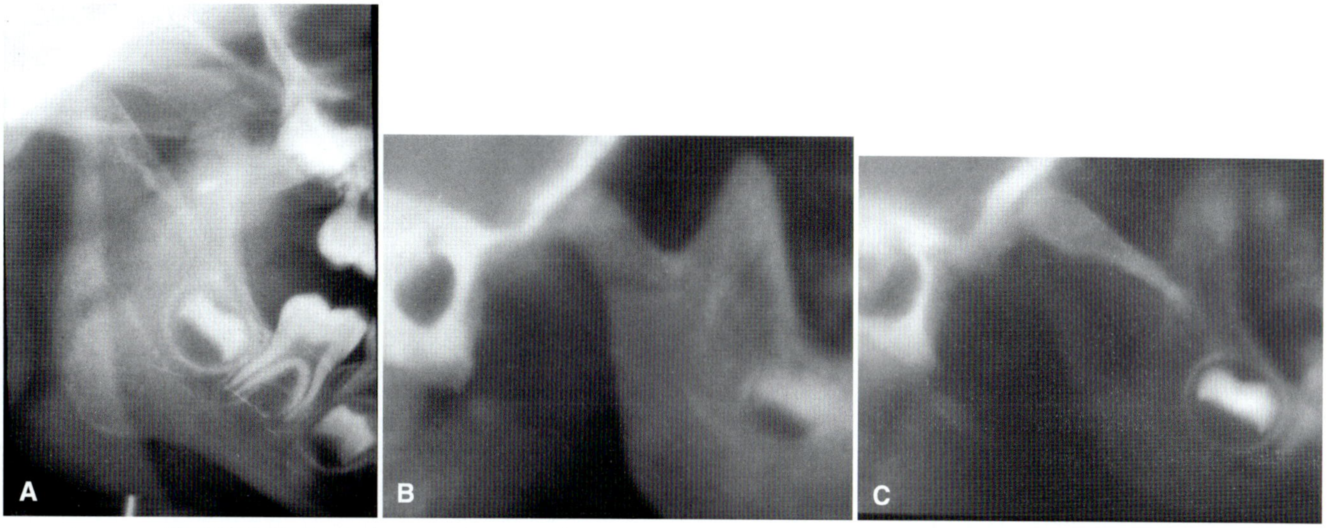

Fig. 28.33 (A) Cropped panoramic image of a neonatal fracture of the right condyle. Note the unusual shape of the coronoid notch, similar to a partially opened pair of scissors. (B) Sagittal conventional tomographic image of the lateral aspect of the same joint. Note the normal-appearing coronoid notch but the lack of formation of the glenoid fossa and eminence, and the abnormal anterior position of the condyle. (C) A more medial sagittal tomographic image of the same case disclosing the fractured segment.

Clinical Features

Patients have a history of progressively restricted jaw opening, or they may have a long-standing history of limited opening. Some degree of mandibular opening usually is possible through flexing of the mandible, although opening may be restricted to only a few millimeters, particularly in the case of bony ankylosis. Patients who develop ankylosis in childhood may have an associated facial asymmetry because of altered growth of the mandible. Pain is not commonly associated with ankylosis.

Imaging Features

In fibrous ankylosis, the articulating surfaces are usually irregular because of erosions. The joint space is very narrow, and although the bones are not fused, the two irregular surfaces may appear to fit one another like two pieces of a jigsaw puzzle (see Fig. 28.25). Little or no condylar movement is seen.

Radiographic signs of remodeling occasionally are visible as the joint components adapt to repeated attempts at mandibular opening. In bony ankylosis, the joint space may be partly or completely obliterated by the osseous bridge, which can vary from a slender segment of bone to a large bony mass (Fig. 28.34). Degenerative changes of the joint components are common. Morphologic changes often occur, such as compensatory progressive elongation of the coronoid processes and deepening of the antegonial notch in the mandibular ramus on the affected side, as a result of muscle function during attempted mandibular opening. Corrected coronal CT images are the best diagnostic imaging method to evaluate ankylosis.

Differential Interpretation

Ankylosis is a sequela to other conditions affecting the joint, and the primary cause must be determined. A history of trauma, infection, arthritis, or previous surgery may help elucidate the etiology and rule out neoplastic disease. Differentiation of fibrous ankylosis from other causes of limited condylar movement is difficult because fibrous tissue is not visible in the diagnostic image.

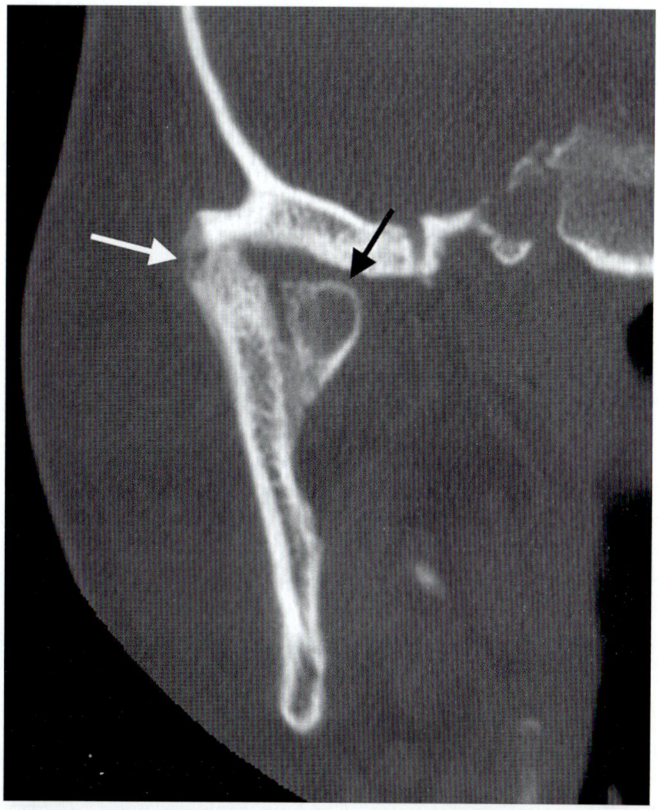

Fig. 28.34 Coronal bone algorithm multidetector computed tomographic image of bony ankylosis. Previous trauma has resulted in fracture and medial displacement of the condyle, which is re-fused to the medial surface of the ramus *(black arrow)*. There is bony ankylosis between the articular eminence and condylar neck in the lateral part of the joint *(white arrow)*.

Management

TMJ ankylosis requires surgical intervention. Gap arthroplasty involves removal of the osseous bridge or creation of a pseudarthrosis below the original joint space. An interpositional arthroplasty involves grafting soft tissue (skin, muscle, fat) between the bony components and is associated with better outcomes. Costochondral grafts and alloplastic joint replacements are also used. Recurrence of ankylosis after surgery may develop.

Neoplasia

Disease Mechanism

Benign and malignant neoplasms originating in or involving the TMJ are rare. Neoplasms affecting the TMJ may be intrinsic to the joint, developing in the condyle, temporal bone or soft tissues of the joint, or they may be extrinsic, developing in the adjacent structures, such as the coronoid process or adjacent soft tissues.

Benign Neoplasia

The most common benign intrinsic tumor involving the TMJ is an osteochondroma. Other rare nonodontogenic entities may also develop in the TMJ, including osteomas, osteoblastomas, chondroblastomas, fibromyxomas, central giant cell lesions, simple bone cavities, aneurysmal bone cysts, and Langerhans cell histiocytosis. Benign neoplasms and cysts of the mandible (e.g., ameloblastomas, odontogenic keratocysts, simple bone cavities) may involve the entire ramus, and in rare cases, may extend into the condyle. In cases of extraarticular ankylosis, in which mandibular movement is restricted but the TMJs appear normal, hyperplasia or a tumor of the coronoid process must be ruled out.

Clinical features. Benign condylar neoplasms grow slowly, and may attain considerable size before becoming clinically noticeable. Patients may complain of TMJ swelling, and this may be accompanied by pain and decreased range of motion. Indeed, the symptoms often mimic TMJ dysfunction. The clinical examination may reveal facial asymmetry, malocclusion, and deviation of the mandible to the unaffected side. Tumors of the coronoid process typically are painless, but patients may complain of progressive limitation of mandibular motion.

Imaging features. A benign neoplasm involving the mandibular condyle usually manifests as an irregularly shaped enlargement of the condylar head. There may be decreased trabecular bone density owing to bony destruction or increased density owing to new, abnormal bone formed by the neoplasm. An osteoma or osteochondroma will have the appearance of being attached to, or growing from, the condyle.

Osteochondromas are benign neoplasms that most often extend from the anterior surface of the condyle near the insertion of the lateral pterygoid muscle. They may have a triangular or lobulated shape and a smooth periphery. To differentiate these from osteomas, it is important to note that the internal cancellous bone of the condyle is continuous with the internal structure of the osteochondroma (Fig. 28.35), while an osteoma arises from the periosteal surface and therefore does not show trabecular continuity. Because benign neoplasms may interfere with normal joint function, secondary bone remodeling or degenerative changes may be seen in the affected joint. Neoplasms involving the coronoid process may also affect TMJ function, which emphasizes the need to image and evaluate the coronoid process when evaluating joint abnormalities.

Differential interpretation. Condylar neoplasms may simulate unilateral condylar hyperplasia because of condylar enlargement. Osteomas and osteochondromas generally create a more irregular appearance, with a bulbous or pedunculated growth pattern, whereas the characteristic condylar shape and proportions are better preserved in condylar hyperplasia. Similarly, hyperplasia of the coronoid process will maintain the regular shape, whereas a neoplasm involving the coronoid would alter the morphology.

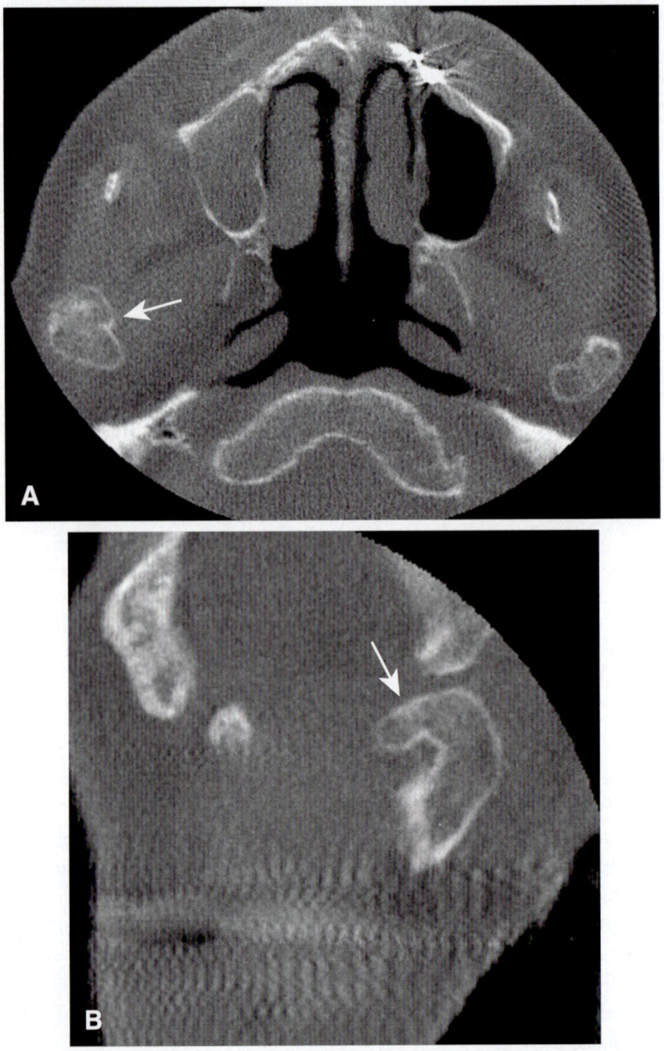

Fig. 28.35 Axial (A) and corrected sagittal (B) cone beam computed tomographic images of an osteochondroma discovered incidentally. Lobulated outgrowth from anterior surface of condyle shows continuity of the cancellous and cortical bone between the normal condyle and the lesion *(arrows)*.

Management. Treatment consists of surgical excision of the neoplasm, and occasionally excision of the condylar head or coronoid process.

Malignant Neoplasia

Disease mechanism. Malignant neoplasms involving the TMJs may be primary or, more commonly, metastatic. Primary intrinsic malignant neoplasms of the condyle are extremely rare and include chondrosarcoma, osteosarcoma, synovial sarcoma, and fibrosarcoma of the joint capsule. Extrinsic malignant neoplasms may represent direct extension of adjacent parotid salivary gland malignancies, rhabdomyosarcoma (particularly in children), or other regional carcinomas from the skin, ear, and nasopharynx. Lesions of Langerhans cell histiocytosis and multiple myeloma may also involve the condyle, as well as metastatic lesions originating in the breast, kidney, lung, colon, prostate, and thyroid gland.

Clinical features. Malignant neoplasms, whether primary or metastatic, may be asymptomatic, or patients may have symptoms of TMJ dysfunction, such as pain, limited mandibular opening, mandibular deviation, and swelling. A patient occasionally is treated for TMJ dysfunction without recognition that the underlying condition is a malignancy.

Imaging features. Malignant primary and metastatic neoplasms involving the TMJ manifest with a variable degree of bone destruction with ill-defined, noncorticated, and irregular borders. Most lack the ability to stimulate new bone formation, with the exception of osteosarcoma and chondrosarcoma, which may demonstrate a radiopaque component. Chondrosarcoma also may appear as an indistinct, essentially radiolucent destructive lesion of the condyle, depending on the ability of the malignant cells to produce a mineralized matrix. In some cases, the pattern of mineralization in chondrosarcoma may simulate the appearances of the articular loose bodies seen in synovial chondromatosis or chondrocalcinosis (Fig. 28.36).

In the case of metastatic neoplasms, the radiographic appearance is usually nonspecific condylar destruction. Rarely, when a metastatic malignancy has the ability to stimulate bone cells locally, an osteoblastic reaction may be seen (Fig. 28.37). Fracture of the condyle may be seen as a sequela of destruction of the bony structure of the joint (Fig. 28.38). CT imaging is the imaging modality of choice to view bone involvement. Malignancies are more likely to involve soft tissues beyond the joint which are best visualized with MRI.

Differential interpretation. Joint destruction caused by a malignant neoplasm must be differentiated from the osseous destruction seen in severe DJD. Malignant neoplasm causes profound central bone destruction, whereas the bone resorption seen in DJD is more peripheral, originating at the articulating surfaces. Also, no soft tissue mass is seen in association with DJD but would be expected when a malignant neoplasm is present. Malignancies capable of stimulating local bone

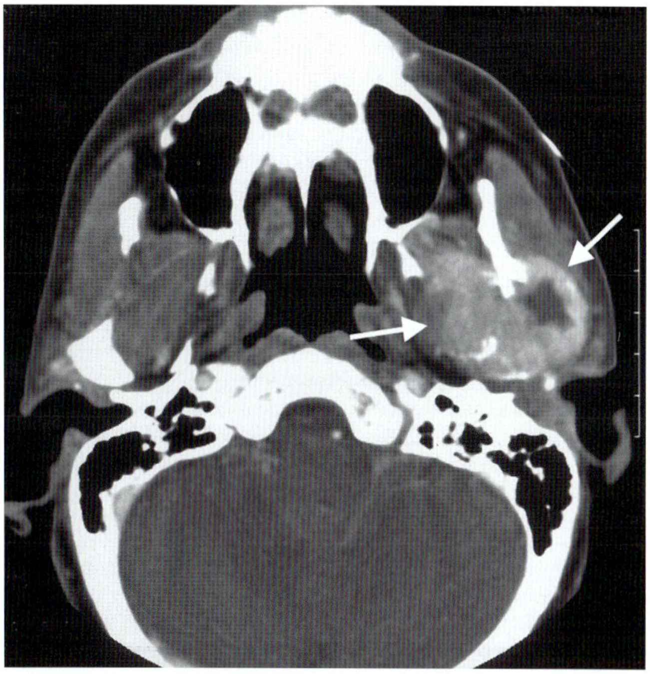

Fig. 28.37 Axial soft tissue algorithm multidetector computed tomographic image of a metastatic lesion from a thyroid gland carcinoma that has destroyed all of the left mandibular condyle. A large soft tissue mass is also seen *(arrows)*.

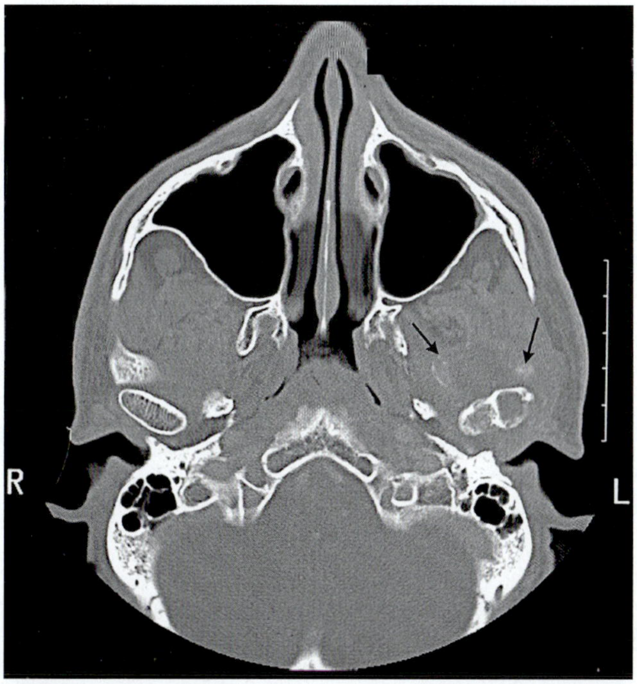

Fig. 28.36 Axial bone algorithm multidetector computed tomographic image of a chondrosarcoma. A radiolucent destructive lesion is present in the left condylar head, and faint radiopacities (soft tissue calcifications) are visible anterior to the condylar head *(arrows)*.

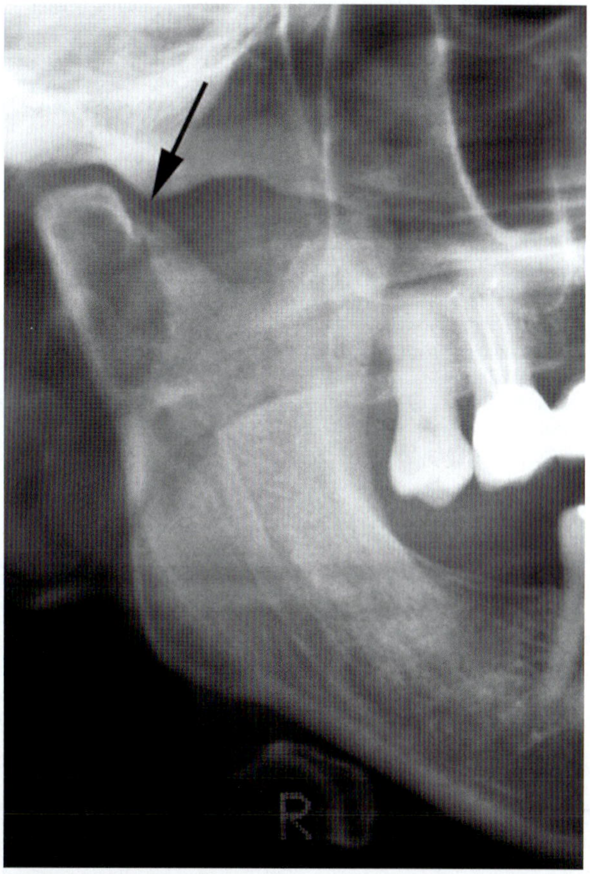

Fig. 28.38 Cropped panoramic image shows destruction of the right condyle from a metastatic lung carcinoma with a secondary fracture *(arrow)*.

cells to deposit a mineralized matrix may simulate joint space calcifications, but they are also associated with severe bone destruction, in contrast to other conditions forming loose joint bodies.

Management. In the case of primary malignant neoplasms, management consists of wide surgical removal of the tumor. Tumor extension to vital anatomic structures may compromise survival. Metastatic lesions involving the TMJ rarely are treated surgically; treatment may include radiotherapy and chemotherapy.

BIBLIOGRAPHY

Disorders of the Temporomandibular Joint

Mallya SM, Ahmad M, Cohen JR, et al. Recommendations for imaging of the temporomandibular joint. Position statement from the American Academy of Oral and Maxillofacial Radiology and the American Academy of Orofacial Pain. *Oral Surg Oral Med Oral Pathol Oral Radiol.* 2022;134:639-648.

Li DTS, Leung YY. Temporomandibular disorders: current concepts and controversies in diagnosis and management. *Diagnostics (Basel).* 2021;11:459. doi:10.3390/diagnostics11030459.

Petrikowski CG, Grace MG. Temporomandibular joint radiographic findings in adolescents. *Cranio.* 1996;14:30-36.

Robinson JL, Johnson PM, Kister K, et al. Estrogen signaling impacts temporomandibular joint and periodontal disease pathology. *Odontology.* 2020;108(2):153-165.

Whyte A, Boeddinghaus R, Bartley A, et al. Imaging of the temporomandibular joint. *Clin Radiol.* 2021;76:76.e21-76.e35.

Anatomy of the Temporomandibular Joint

Drace JE, Enzmann DR. Defining the normal temporomandibular joint: closed, partially open, and open mouth MR imaging of asymptomatic subjects. *Radiology.* 1990;177:67-76.

Hansson LG, Hansson T, Petersson A. A comparison between clinical and radiologic findings in 259 temporomandibular joint patients. *J Prosthet Dent.* 1983;50:89-94.

Ingervall B, Carlsson GE, Thilander B. Postnatal development of the human temporomandibular joint. II. A microradiographic study. *Acta Odont Scand.* 1976;34:133-139.

Larheim TA. Radiographic appearance of the normal temporomandibular joint in newborns and small children. *Acta Radiol Diagn (Stockh).* 1981;22:593-599.

Ten Cate AR. Gross and micro anatomy. In: Zarb GA, Carlsson BJ, Mohl ND, eds. *Temporomandibular Joint and Masticatory Muscle Disorders.* 2nd ed. Munksgaard; 1994.

Westesson PL, Kurita K, Eriksson L, et al. Cryosectional observations of functional anatomy of the temporomandibular joint. *Oral Surg Oral Med Oral Pathol.* 1989;68:247-251.

Yale SH, Allison BD, Hauptfuehrer JD. An epidemiological assessment of mandibular condyle morphology. *Oral Surg.* 1966;21:169-177.

Imanimoghaddam M, Madani AS, Mahdavi P, et al. Evaluation of condylar positions in patients with temporomandibular disorders: a cone-beam computed tomographic study. *Imaging Sci Dent.* 2016;46:127-131.

Diagnostic Imaging of the Temporomandibular Joint

Bag AK, Gaddikeri S, Singhal A, et al. Imaging of the temporomandibular joint: an update. *World J Radiol.* 2014;28:567-582.

Katzberg RW. Temporomandibular joint imaging. *Radiology.* 1989;170:297-307.

Diagnostic Imaging of the Temporomandibular Joint—*Hard Tissue Imaging*

Christiansen EL, Chan TT, Thompson JR, et al. Computed tomography of the normal temporomandibular joint. *Scand J Dent Res.* 1987;95:499-509.

Tsiklakis K, Syriopoulos K, Stamatakis HC. Radiographic examination of the temporomandibular joint using cone beam computed tomography. *Dentomaxillofac Radiol.* 2004;33:196-201.

Diagnostic Imaging of the Temporomandibular Joint—*Soft Tissue Imaging*

Hansson LG, Westesson PL, Eriksson L. Comparison of tomography and midfield magnetic resonance imaging for osseous changes of the temporomandibular joint. *Oral Surg Oral Med Oral Pathol Oral Radiol Endod.* 1996;82:698-703.

Moses JJ, Salinas E, Goergen T, et al. Magnetic resonance imaging or arthrographic diagnosis of internal derangement of the temporomandibular joint. *Oral Surg Oral Med Oral Pathol.* 1993;75:268-272.

Tomas X, Pomes J, Berenquer J, et al. MR imaging of temporomandibular joint dysfunction: a pictorial review. *Radiographics.* 2006;26:765-781.

Radiographic Abnormalities of the Temporomandibular Joint—*Condylar Hyperplasia*

Gray RJM, Sloan P, Quayle AA, et al. Histopathological and scintigraphic features of condylar hyperplasia. *Int J Oral Maxillofac Surg.* 1990;19:65-71.

Kün-Darbois JD, Bertin H, Mouallem G, et al. Bone characteristics in condylar hyperplasia of the temporomandibular joint: a microcomputed tomography, histology, and raman microspectrometry study. *Int J Oral Maxillofac Surg.* 2023;52:543-552.

Radiographic Abnormalities of the Temporomandibular Joint—*Condylar Hypoplasia*

Jerell RG, Fuselier B, Mahan P. Acquired condylar hypoplasia: report of a case. *ASDC J Dent Child.* 1991;58:147-153.

Worth HM. Radiology of the temporomandibular joint. In: Zarb GA, Carlsson BJ, Mohl ND, eds. *Temporomandibular Joint Function and Dysfunction.* Munksgaard; 1979.

Radiographic Abnormalities of the Temporomandibular Joint—*Coronoid Hyperplasia*

McLoughlin PM, Hopper C, Bowley NB. Hyperplasia of the mandibular coronoid process: an analysis of 31 cases and a review of the literature. *J Oral Maxillofac Surg.* 1995;53:250-255.

Mulder CH, Kalaykova SI, Gortzak RA. Coronoid process hyperplasia: a systematic review of the literature from 1995. *Int J Oral Maxillofac Surg.* 2012;4:1483-1489.

Radiographic Abnormalities of the Temporomandibular Joint—*Bifid Condyle*

Daniels JSM, Ali I. Post-traumatic bifid condyle associated with temporomandibular joint ankylosis: report of a case and review of the literature. *Oral Surg Oral Med Oral Pathol Oral Radiol Endod.* 2005;99:682-688.

Loh FC, Yeo JF. Bifid mandibular condyle. *Oral Surg Oral Med Oral Pathol.* 1990;69:24-27.

Soft Tissue Abnormalities

Helms CA, Kaban LB, McNeill C, et al. Temporomandibular joint: morphology and signal intensity characteristics of the disc at MR imaging. *Radiology.* 1989;172:817-820.

Katzberg RW, Tallents RH, Hayakawa K, et al. Internal derangements of the temporomandibular joint: findings in the pediatric age group. *Radiology.* 1985;154:125-127.

Larheim TA. Role of magnetic resonance imaging in the clinical diagnosis of the temporomandibular joint. *Cells Tissues Organs.* 2005;180:6-21.

Rammelsberg P, Pospiech PR, Jäger L, et al. Variability of disc position in asymptomatic volunteers and patients with internal derangements of the TMJ. *Oral Surg Oral Med Oral Pathol Oral Radiol Endod.* 1997;83:393-399.

Sano T, Westesson PL. Magnetic resonance imaging of the temporomandibular joint: increased T2 signal in the retro-discal tissue of painful joints. *Oral Surg Oral Med Oral Pathol Oral Radiol Endod.* 1995;79:511-516.

Wilkes CH. Internal derangements of the temporomandibular joint: pathological variations. *Arch Otolaryngol Head Neck Surg.* 1989;115:469-477.

Remodeling and Arthritic Conditions—*Remodeling*

Brooks SL, Westesson PL, Eriksson L, et al. Prevalence of osseous changes in the temporomandibular joint of asymptomatic persons without internal derangement. *Oral Surg Oral Med Oral Pathol.* 1992;73:118-122.

Moffett BC, Johnson LC, McCabe JB, et al. Articular remodeling in the adult human temporomandibular joint. *Am J Anat.* 1964;115:119-141.

Remodeling and Arthritic Conditions—*Degenerative Joint Disease*

Palconet G, Ludlow JB, Tyndall DA, et al. Correlating cone beam CT results with temporomandibular joint pain of osteoarthritic origin. *Dentomaxillofac Radiol.* 2012;41:126-130.

Helenius LMJ, Tervahartiala P, Helenius I, et al. Clinical, radiographic and MRI findings of the temporomandibular joint in patients with different rheumatic diseases. *Int J Oral Maxillofac Surg.* 2006;35:983-989.

Mélou C, Pellen-Mussi P, Jeanne S, et al. Osteoarthritis of the temporomandibular joint: a narrative overview. *Medicina (Kaunas).* 2022;59:8. doi:10.3390/medicina59010008.

Remodeling and Arthritic Conditions—Rheumatoid Arthritis

Gynther GW, Tronje G, Holmlund AB. Radiographic changes in the temporomandibular joint in patients with generalized osteoarthritis and rheumatoid arthritis. *Oral Surg Oral Med Oral Pathol Oral Radiol Endod.* 1996;81:613-618.

Larheim TA, Smith HJ, Aspestrand F. Rheumatic disease of the temporomandibular joint: MR imaging and tomographic manifestations. *Radiology.* 1990;175:527-531.

Remodeling and Arthritic Conditions—*Juvenile Idiopathic Arthritis*

Hu YS, Schneiderman ED. The temporomandibular joint in juvenile rheumatoid arthritis. I: computed tomographic findings. *Pediatr Dent.* 1995;17:46-53.

Hu YS, Schneiderman ED, Harper RP. The temporomandibular joint in juvenile rheumatoid arthritis. II: relationship between computed tomographic and clinical findings. *Pediatr Dent.* 1996;18:312-319.

Karhulahti T, Ylijoki H, Rönning O. Mandibular condyle lesions related to age at onset and subtypes of juvenile rheumatoid arthritis in 15-year-old children. *Scand J Dent Res.* 1993;101:332-338.

Stoll ML, Sharpe T, Beukelman T, et al. Risk factors for temporomandibular joint arthritis in children with juvenile idiopathic arthritis. *J Rheumatol.* 2012;39:1880-1887.

Remodeling and Arthritic Conditions—*Psoriatic Arthritis*

Koorbusch GF, Zeitler DL, Fotos PG, et al. Psoriatic arthritis of the temporomandibular joints with ankylosis. *Oral Surg Oral Med Oral Pathol.* 1991;71:267-274.

Wilson AW, Brown JS, Ord RA. Psoriatic arthropathy of the temporomandibular joint. *Oral Surg Oral Med Oral Pathol.* 1990;70:555-558.

Remodeling and Arthritic Conditions—*Ankylosing Spondylitis*

Locher MC, Felder M, Sailer HF. Involvement of the temporomandibular joints in ankylosing spondylitis (Bechterew's disease). *J Craniomaxillofac Surg.* 1996;24:205-213.

Ramos-Remus C, Major P, Gomez-Vargas A, et al. Temporomandibular joint osseous morphology in a consecutive sample of ankylosing spondylitis patients. *Ann Rheum Dis.* 1997;56:103-107.

Remodeling and Arthritic Conditions—*Septic Arthritis*

Leighty SM, Spach DH, Myall RW, et al. Septic arthritis of the temporomandibular joint: review of the literature and report of two cases in children. *Int J Oral Maxillofac Surg.* 1993;22:292-297.

Sembronio S, Albiero AM, Robiony M, et al. Septic arthritis of the temporomandibular joint successfully treated with arthroscopic lysis and lavage: case report and review of the literature. *Oral Surg Oral Med Oral Pathol Oral Radiol Endod.* 2007;103:e1-e6.

Idiopathic Condylar Resorption

Kobayashi T, Izumi N, Kojima T, et al. Progressive condylar resorption after mandibular advancement. *Br J Oral Maxillofac Surg.* 2012;50:176-180.

Nicolielo LFP, Jacobs R, Ali Albdour E, et al. Is oestrogen associated with mandibular condylar resorption? A systematic review. *Int J Oral Maxillofac Surg.* 2017;46:1394-1402.

Sansare K, Raghav M, Mallya SM, et al. Management-related outcomes and radiographic findings of idiopathic condylar resorption: a systematic review. *Int J Oral Maxillofac Surg.* 2015;44:209-216.

Wolford LM, Gonçalves JR. Condylar resorption of the temporomandibular joint: how do we treat it? *Oral Maxillofac Surg Clin North Am.* 2015;27:47-67.

Articular Loose Bodies

Ardekian L, Faquin W, Troulis MJ, et al. Synovial chondromatosis of the temporomandibular joint: report and analysis of eleven cases. *J Oral Maxillofac Surg.* 2005;63:941-947.

Dijkgraaf LC, Liem RS, de Bont LG, et al. Calcium pyrophosphate dihydrate crystal deposition disease: a review of the literature and a light and electron microscopic study of a case of the temporomandibular joint with numerous intracellular crystals in the chondrocytes. *Osteoarthr Cartil.* 1995;3:35-45.

Pynn BR, Weinberg S, Irish J. Calcium pyrophosphate dihydrate deposition disease of the temporomandibular joint: a case report and review of the literature. *Oral Surg Oral Med Oral Pathol Oral Radiol Endod.* 1995;79:278-284.

Yu Q, Yang J, Wang P, et al. CT features of synovial chondromatosis in the temporomandibular joint. *Oral Surg Oral Med Oral Pathol Oral Radiol Endod.* 2007;97:524-528.

Trauma—*Effusion*

Emshoff R, Brandimaier I, Bertram S, et al. Magnetic resonance imaging findings of osteoarthrosis and effusion in patients with unilateral temporomandibular joint pain. *Int J Oral Maxillofac Surg.* 2002;31:598-602.

Westesson PL, Brooks SL. Temporomandibular joint: relationship between MR evidence of effusion and the presence of pain and disc displacement. *AJR Am J Roentgenol.* 1992;159:559-563.

Trauma—*Dislocation*

Kai S, Kai H, Nakayama E, et al. Clinical symptoms of open lock position of the condyle: relation to anterior dislocation of the temporomandibular joint. *Oral Surg Oral Med Oral Pathol Oral Radiol.* 1992;74:143-148.

Wijmenga JP, Boering G, Blankestijn J. Protracted dislocation of the temporomandibular joint. *Int J Oral Maxillofac Surg.* 1986;15:380-388.

Trauma—*Fracture*

Choi J, Oh IK. A follow-up study of condyle fracture in children. *Int J Oral Maxillofac Surg.* 2005;34:851-858.

Dahlström L, Kahnberg KE, Lindahl L. Fifteen years follow-up on condylar fractures. *Int J Oral Maxillofac Surg.* 1989;18:18-23.

Gerhard S, Ennemoser T, Rudisch A, et al. Condylar injury: magnetic resonance imaging findings of the temporomandibular joint soft tissue changes. *Int J Oral Maxillofac Surg.* 2007;36:214-218.

Zachariades N, Mezitis M, Mourouzis C, et al. Fractures of the mandibular condyle: a review of 466 cases. Literature review, reflections on treatment and proposals. *J Craniomaxillofac Surg.* 2006;34:421-432.

Trauma—*Neonatal Fractures*

Pharoah MJ. Radiology of the temporomandibular joint. In: Zarb GA, Carlsson BJ, Mohl ND, eds. *Temporomandibular Joint and Masticatory Muscle Disorders.* 2nd ed. Munksgaard; 1994.

Worth HM. Radiology of the temporomandibular joint. In: Zarb GA, Carlsson GE, eds. *Temporomandibular Joint Function and Dysfunction.* Munksgaard; 1979.

Ankylosis

Ferretti C, Bryant R, Becker P, et al. Temporomandibular joint morphology following post-traumatic ankylosis in 26 patients. *Int J Oral Maxillofac Surg.* 2005;34:376-381.

Rowe NL. Ankylosis of the temporomandibular joint. *J R Coll Surg Edinb.* 1982;27:67-79.

Upadya VH, Bhat HK, Rao BHS, Reddy SG. Classification and surgical management of temporomandibular joint ankylosis: a review. *J Korean Assoc Oral Maxillofac Surg.* 2021;47:239-248.

Wood RE, Harris AM, Nortje CJ, et al. The radiologic features of true ankylosis of the temporomandibular joint: an analysis of 25 cases. *Dentomaxillofac Radiol.* 1988;17:121-127.

Tumors—*Benign Tumors*

Chen MJ, Yang C, Qiu YT, Zhou Q, Huang D, Shi HM. Osteochondroma of the mandibular condyle: a classification system based on computed tomographic appearances. *J Craniofac Surg.* 2014;25:1703-1706.

Pharoah MJ. Radiology of the temporomandibular joint. In: Zarb GA, Carlsson BJ, Mohl ND, eds. *Temporomandibular Joint and Masticatory Muscle Disorders.* 2nd ed. Munksgaard; 1994.

Svensson B, Isacsson G. Benign osteoblastoma associated with an aneurysmal bone cyst of the mandibular ramus and condyle. *Oral Surg Oral Med Oral Pathol.* 1993;76:433-436.

Worth HM. Radiology of the temporomandibular joint. In: Zarb GA, Carlsson GE, eds. *Temporomandibular Joint Function and Dysfunction.* Munksgaard; 1979.

Tumors—*Malignant Tumors*

Jang BG, Huh KH, Kang JH, et al. Imaging features of chondrosarcoma of the temporomandibular joint: report of nine cases and literature review. *Clin Radiol.* 2020;75:878.e1-878.e12.

Oliver C, Mouallem G, Dutot-Philipeau N, et al. A case report of condyle metastasis and a review of the literature. *J Stomatol Oral Maxillofac Surg.* 2022;123(3):360-363. doi:10.1016/j.jormas.2021.04.013.

Rubin MM, Jui V, Cozzi GM. Metastatic carcinoma of the mandibular condyle presenting as temporomandibular joint syndrome. *J Oral Maxillofac Surg.* 1989;47:507-510.

Takehana dos Santos D, Cavalcanti MGP. Osteosarcoma of the temporomandibular joint: report of 2 cases. *Oral Surg Oral Med Oral Pathol Oral Radiol Endod.* 2002;94:641-647.

29

Soft Tissue Calcifications and Ossifications

Laurie C. Carter

DISEASE MECHANISMS

The deposition of calcium salts in an unorganized fashion in soft tissue is referred to as heterotopic calcification. These can develop in a variety of unrelated disorders and degenerative processes and may be divided into dystrophic calcification, dystrophic mineralization, and metastatic calcification.

Clinical Features

Heterotopic calcification and ossification may be asymptomatic and are most often detected as incidental findings during imaging studies made for other purposes.

Imaging Features

The goal of imaging is to correctly identify the mineralization and to determine whether further investigation, and possibly intervention, is required. Therefore, meticulous assessment of the entirety of all images obtained is paramount. Some soft tissue mineralizations do not require long-term surveillance or treatment, while others may be life threatening and require intervention. Important criteria to consider in arriving at the correct interpretation are the anatomic location, number, distribution, and shapes of the mineralizations. Determination of the location requires knowledge of the soft tissue anatomy such as the locations of lymph nodes, ligaments, blood vessels, cartilage, and the major salivary glands and their ducts.

Radiopaque entities occurring in the soft tissues are common and can be found in about 4% of panoramic images (Fig. 29.1). Cone beam computed tomography (CBCT) and multidetector computed tomography (MDCT) offer 3D visualization with no magnification, distortion, or overlap, which helps reveal the precise locations of the mineralizations, facilitating diagnosis, albeit at potentially higher radiation doses and financial costs. As some soft tissue mineralizations are lightly mineralized, it is critical that clinicians minimize peripheral lighting, employ magnification, and adjust filters and contrast settings when reviewing imaging studies.

HETEROTOPIC CALCIFICATIONS

Dystrophic Calcification

Disease Mechanism

In dystrophic calcification, calcium salts are precipitated at sites of chronic inflammation or into damaged tissue despite normal serum calcium and phosphate levels. This is associated with high local phosphatase activity, an increase in local pH, and anoxic conditions within the dead or dying tissue.

Clinical Features

Common soft tissue locations include the lymph nodes, tonsils, muscles, neck, cheeks, and tongue. Dystrophic calcifications may be asymptomatic, although the precipitated calcium salts may be palpated as a solid mass, and occasionally, there may be enlargement and ulceration of overlying soft tissues.

Imaging Features

The radiographic appearance of dystrophic calcifications varies from being barely perceptible, punctate radiopaque grains to larger, irregular, radiopaque structures. One or more of these radiopaque entities may be seen, and the calcifications may be homogeneous or heterogeneous internally. Common sites are long-standing, chronically inflamed cysts (Fig. 29.2) and soft tissues (Fig. 29.3).

Calcified Lymph Nodes

Disease mechanism. Dystrophic calcification occurs in chronically inflamed lymph nodes where the lymphoid tissue is replaced by hydroxyapatite-like calcium salts, effacing nodal architecture. The presence of calcifications in lymph nodes implies either active disease or disease that has since resolved. The etiology of nodal calcification includes granulomatous diseases such as tuberculosis (scrofula or tuberculous cervical lymphadenitis), sarcoidosis, cat scratch disease, bacille Calmette-Guérin vaccination, as well as rheumatoid arthritis and systemic sclerosis, lymphoma previously treated with radiation therapy, fungal infections, and malignancy, including metastases from distant calcifying neoplasms (most notably metastatic papillary thyroid carcinoma).

Clinical features. Calcified lymph nodes are generally asymptomatic and discovered as incidental findings on extraoral planar images. When these nodes can be palpated, they are hard, lumpy, and round to oblong masses.

Imaging features.

Location. The most commonly involved nodes are located within the submandibular and superficial and deep cervical node chains. Less commonly, the preauricular and submental nodes are involved. In the submandibular region, the nodes may be located either at or inferior to the inferior border of the mandible near the angle where the image of the calcified node is sometimes superimposed over the inferior portion of the ramus. Lymph node calcifications may affect a single node or a linear series of nodes in a phenomenon known as lymph node "chaining," typically seen in scrofula (Fig. 29.4).

Periphery. The periphery is well defined and usually irregular. Occasionally, the calcified node may have a cauliflower-like, lobulated appearance. This irregularity of shape is of great significance in distinguishing node calcifications from other potential soft tissue calcifications in the area.

Internal structure. The internal structure may vary in the degree of radiopacity, giving the impression of a collection of smaller, spherical, or irregular masses. Occasionally, the calcified node may have a lamellar appearance, or the radiopacity may appear only on the surface of the node. This latter appearance has been called an eggshell calcification.

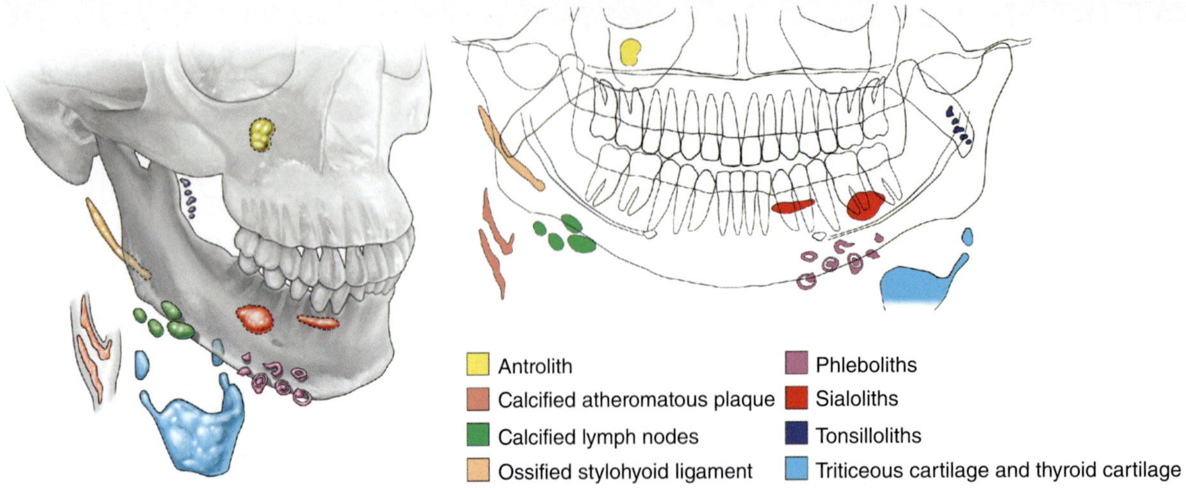

Fig. 29.1 Schematic of the head and neck and panoramic rendering demonstrating the typical geometry and locations of selected soft tissue calcifications and ossifications.

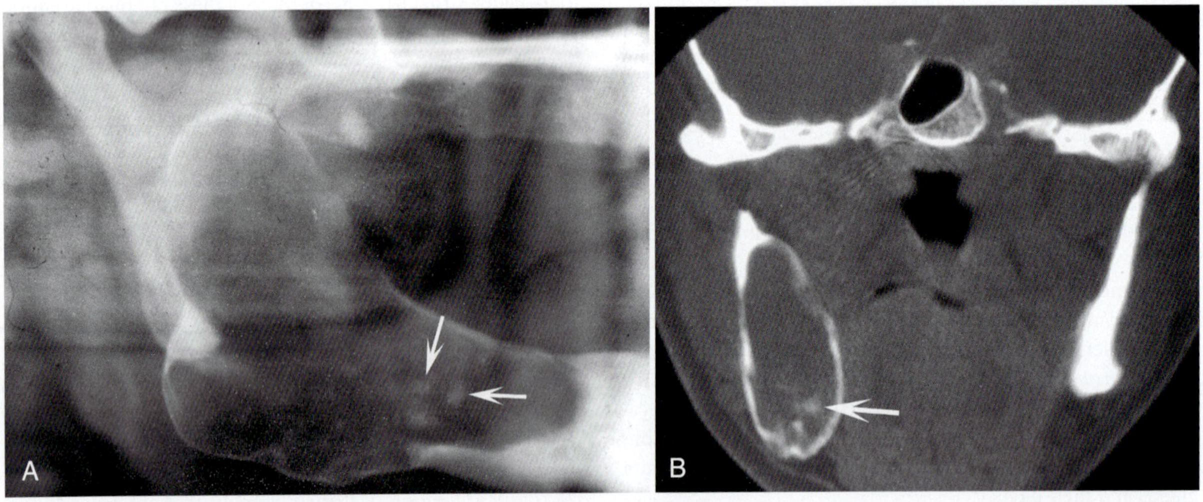

Fig. 29.2 (A) Large residual cyst with poorly defined calcifications seen in a panoramic image *(arrows)*. (B) Coronal multidetector computed tomography image with bone algorithm of the same case, which demonstrates the dystrophic calcification within the cyst *(arrow)*.

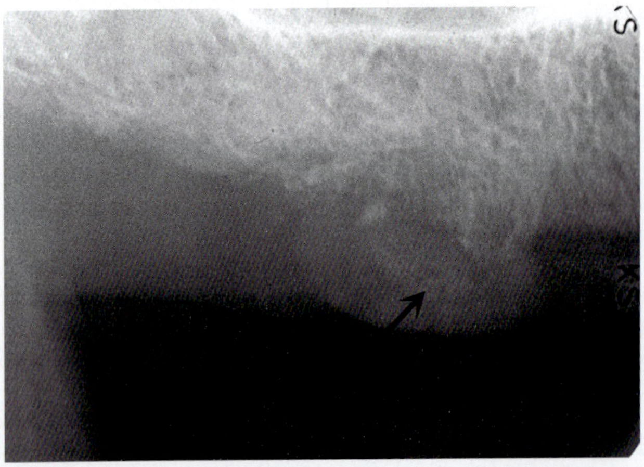

Fig. 29.3 Periapical image shows the soft tissue mass, inflammatory fibrous hyperplasia, emanating from the edentulous ridge. This soft tissue mass contains a dystrophic calcification *(arrow)*.

The pattern of nodal calcification does not reliably distinguish between benign and malignant disease.

Differential interpretation. Differentiation between a single calcified lymph node and a sialolith in the hilar region of the submandibular gland may be difficult because both may appear near or adjacent to the inferior cortex of the mandible just anterior to the angle. Usually a sialolith has a smooth outline, whereas a calcified lymph node is usually irregular and sometimes lobulated. The differentiation can be made if the patient has symptoms related to the submandibular salivary gland (see Chapter 30). Occasionally, sialography may be necessary to facilitate the differentiation. Fine-needle aspiration cytology is a simple, cost effective, sensitive, and specific tool for diagnosis of scrofula. Another calcification that may have a similar appearance in this region is a phlebolith. However, phleboliths are usually smaller and multiple, with concentric radiopaque and radiolucent rings, and their shape may mimic the cross section of a blood vessel.

Management. Calcified lymph nodes usually do not require treatment; however, should the cause be related to an underlying disease process, that disease should be diagnosed and managed.

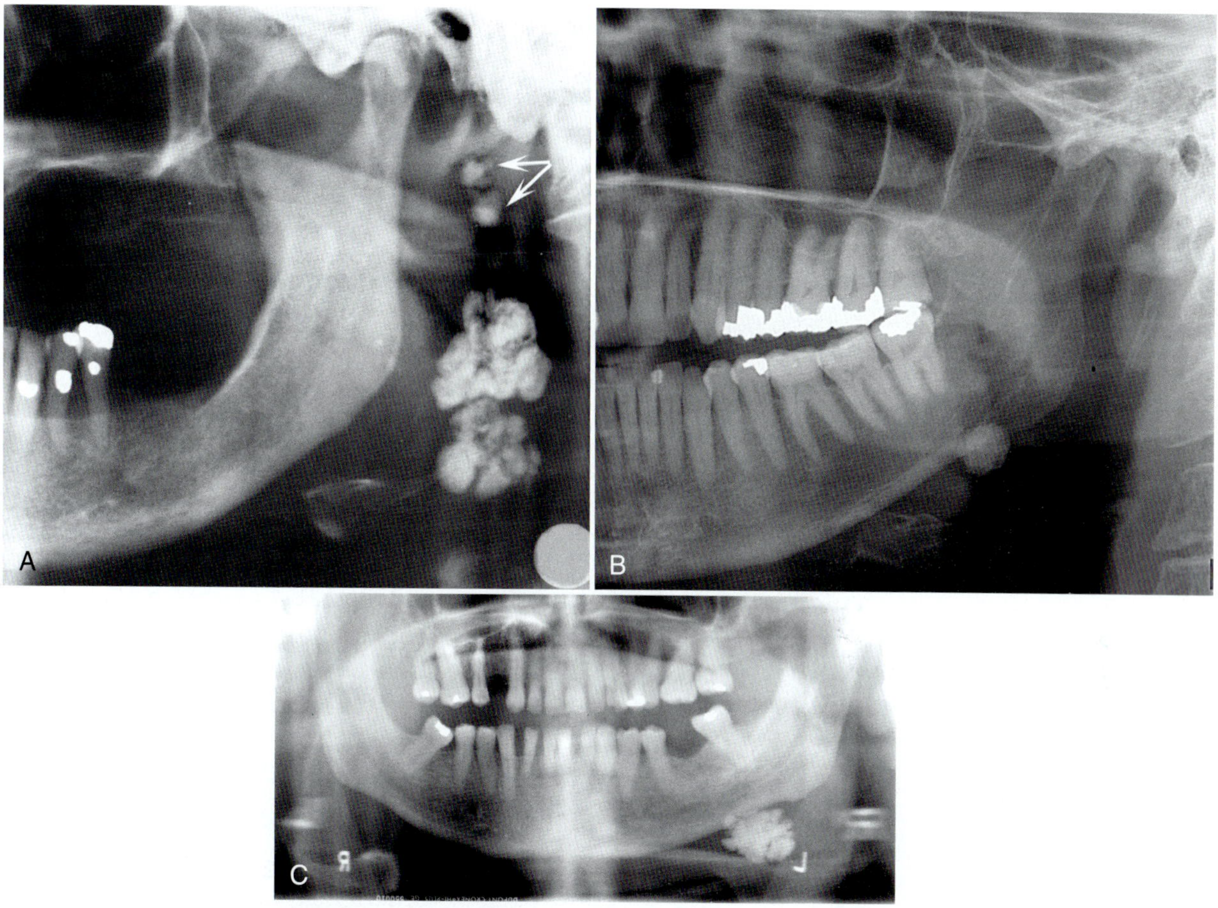

Fig. 29.4 Examples of dystrophic calcification in the lymph nodes. (A) Two large examples positioned behind the ramus with a cauliflower-like shape and two smaller examples in a more superior position *(arrows)*. (B) Submandibular lymph node superimposed on antegonial notch. (C) Larger example.

Dystrophic Calcification in the Tonsils

Disease mechanism. Tonsilloliths or tonsillar calculi are formed when repeated episodes of inflammation enlarge the tonsillar crypts. Incomplete resolution of organic debris (e.g., bacterial biofilms and pus, epithelial cells and food) can serve as the nidus for dystrophic calcification.

Clinical features. Tonsilloliths usually manifest as hard, round, white or yellow objects projecting from the tonsillar crypts, usually of the palatine tonsil. Small calcifications usually produce no clinical signs or symptoms. However, sore throat, dysphagia, otalgia, halitosis, and social embarrassment due to the production of volatile sulfur compounds or a foreign body sensation on swallowing have been reported with larger calcifications. Giant tonsilloliths distending lymphoid tissue, resulting in ulceration and extrusion, are much less common. Tonsilloliths may occur at any age, although they are more commonly found in older age groups.

Imaging features.

Location. On a panoramic image, tonsilloliths appear as single or multiple radiopaque entities that are superimposed over the mid portion of the mandibular ramus, the dorsal surface of the tongue, and the oropharyngeal airspaces. Tonsilloliths may also frequently appear immediately inferior to the mandibular canal on a panoramic image (Fig. 29.5). On axial CBCT or MDCT images, tonsilloliths appear in the soft tissues medial to the mandibular ramus and adjacent to the lateral wall of the oropharyngeal airspace.

Periphery. The most common appearance of tonsilloliths is a cluster of multiple small, ill-defined radiopaque entities of varying sizes. Rarely, these calcifications may attain a large size.

Internal structure. Tonsilloliths appear somewhat more radiopaque than cancellous bone and are approximately the same density as cortical bone.

Differential interpretation. The differential interpretation is a radiopaque entity located within the mandibular ramus, such as a dense bone island. When in doubt, a posteroanterior skull or mandible image, or an open-mouth reverse Towne image, may show that the calcification lies adjacent to the medial surface of the ramus. Rarely, CBCT or MDCT is necessary to precisely localize the entity for diagnosis.

Management. No management is usually required for most tonsillar calcifications. In symptomatic patients, tonsilloliths may be expressed manually, possibly with the patient under sedation to suppress the gag reflex. Large calcifications with associated symptoms require tonsillectomy. Treatment of asymptomatic tonsilloliths may be considered in elderly patients with mechanical deglutition disorders and immunocompromised patients because of the risk for aspiration pneumonia.

Cysticercosis

Disease mechanism. Cysticercosis is acquired through a fecal-oral route, either by eating fecally contaminated vegetables or consuming infected pork. When humans unknowingly ingest eggs or gravid proglottids from the parasite *Taenia solium* (the pork tapeworm), the

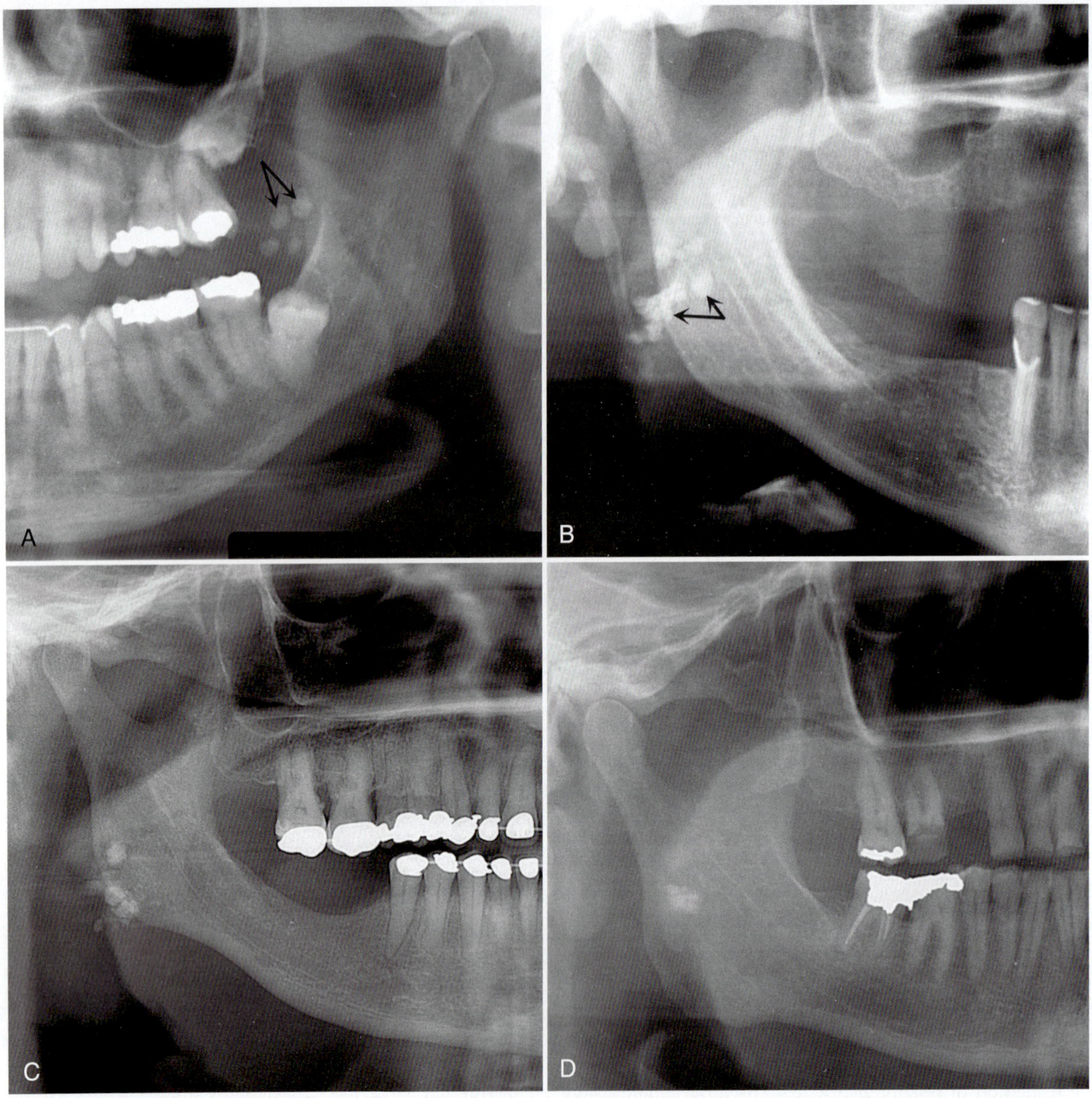

Fig. 29.5 Dystrophic calcification of the tonsils. (A and B) These two examples show positions anterior to the ramus (A) and overlapping the posterior aspect of the ramus (B; *arrows*). Note the calcified stylohyoid ligament. (C and D) Clusters of tonsilloliths superimposed on mandibular ramus.

covering of the eggs is digested in the stomach, and the larval form *(Cysticercus cellulosae)* of the parasite is hatched. The larvae penetrate the mucosa, enter the blood vessels and lymphatics, and are distributed as cysticerci in tissues throughout the body, notably in the brain, muscle, skin, liver, lungs, subcutaneous tissues, and heart. They may also be found in oral and perioral tissues, especially the muscles of mastication. Although the glycoprotein-rich cyst wall is greater than 100 μm thick, it rarely elicits any host response when intact. However, in tissues other than the intestinal mucosa, the larvae eventually die years after infection and are treated as foreign bodies, eliciting a strong inflammatory reaction causing granuloma formation, scarring, and calcification. There is currently an increased incidence of cysticercosis in the southwestern and urban northeastern United States, and the problem is endemic in developing countries in Central and South America, Asia, and Africa.

Clinical features. Cysticercosis is a potentially fatal parasitic disease and an important cause of morbidity globally. Mild cases are asymptomatic. The intensity of the signs and symptoms depends on the number of invasive tapeworm larvae (oncospheres) present, their location, and the immune response mounted by the host on the parasites. More severe cases have symptoms that range from gastrointestinal upset with severe nausea and vomiting. Invasion of the brain may result in seizures, headache, visual disturbances, acute obstructive hydrocephalus, irritability, loss of consciousness, and death. Examination of the oral mucosa may disclose palpable, well circumscribed, soft, fluctuant swellings, which may resemble a mucocele or benign mesenchymal neoplasm.

Imaging features. While alive, the larvae are not visible radiographically. Death of the parasites and development of calcifications in subcutaneous and muscular sites occurs years after the initial infection.

Ultrasound and MRI are gold standard imaging modalities for confirming clinical suspicion of live larvae, with findings reinforced by fine needle aspiration cytology.

Location. The oral locations of calcified cysticerci include the muscles of mastication and facial expression, the suprahyoid muscles, and the postcervical musculature as well as the oral mucosa.

Periphery and shape. Multiple well-defined elliptical entities that resemble grains of rice are seen.

Internal structure. The internal structure is homogeneous and radiopaque.

Differential interpretation. Cysticercus may appear similar to a sialolith. However, the small size of the calcified nodules of cysticerci and their widespread dissemination, particularly in brain and muscles, are highly suggestive of the diagnosis.

Management. Basic sanitation and proper preparation of pork are needed to eliminate this source of infection. Surgical excision of solitary maxillofacial parasitic cysts is recommended. The symptoms that accompany the initial infestation are best treated by a physician using anthelmintic drugs. Adjunctive corticosteroids help stem the inflammatory reaction, and anticonvulsants may prevent epileptic seizures. After the larvae have settled and calcified in the oral tissues, they are harmless. However, it is important to carry out a detailed investigation in each patient to rule out the presence of the parasite in other locations and to perform serologic testing on close contacts to identify a possible source of infection.

Arterial Calcifications

Two distinct patterns of arterial calcification can be identified in imaging examinations and histopathologically: medial calcific sclerosis and calcified atherosclerotic plaque.

Medial Calcific Sclerosis

Disease mechanism. Medial calcific sclerosis or Mönckeberg medial calcinosis (arteriosclerosis) is an age-related degenerative process. The hallmark of this condition is the fragmentation, degeneration, and eventual loss of elastic fibers in the tunica media of medium and small muscular arteries, followed by dystrophic deposition of calcium in the form of crystalline hydroxyapatite. Patients with encephalotrigeminal angiomatosis (Sturge-Weber syndrome) also develop intracranial arterial calcifications.

Clinical features. Mönckeberg medial calcinosis is an occult finding in middle aged and elderly adults. The vascular calcifications are an independent marker of cardiovascular risk and often serve as a harbinger of diseases like diabetes mellitus and hyperparathyroidism. Most patients are asymptomatic initially, although increased blood pressure and reduced arterial compliance may incite peripheral arterial occlusive disease leading to vascular insufficiency, below the knee amputation, or sudden cardiac death.

Imaging features

Location. In the head and neck, medial calcinosis most frequently involves the facial artery but may affect the maxillary and infraorbital arteries as well.

Periphery. The calcific deposits in the artery wall outline the image of the artery. A lateral projection of the artery may show a pair of thin, parallel running, radiopaque lines (Fig. 29.6). The course of these lines may be straight, described as a "pipe stem" or "tram-track," which is pathognomonic for medial calcinosis. In cross section, the calcified artery has a well defined, circular, or ring-like pattern.

Internal structure. There is no internal structure because the diffuse, finely divided calcium deposits occur solely in the medial wall of the vessel.

Differential interpretation. The radiographic appearance of medial calcific sclerosis is so distinctive as to be pathognomonic of the condition.

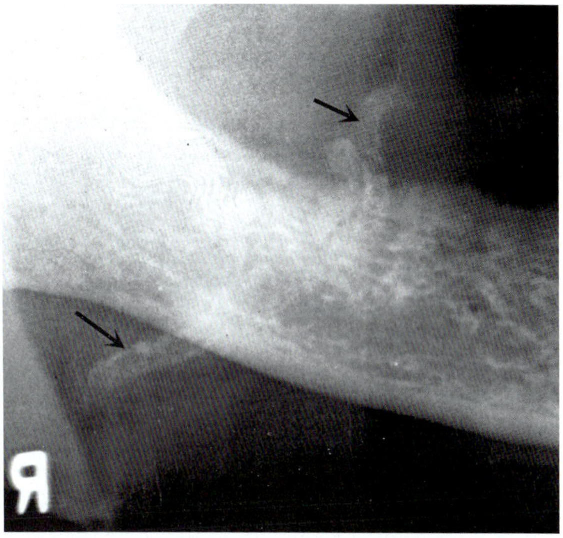

Fig. 29.6 Cropped panoramic image shows calcification of a blood vessel, probably the facial vein *(arrows).*

Clinically, hyperparathyroidism may be considered because medial calcific sclerosis frequently develops as a metastatic calcification in patients with this condition.

Management. Dentists should be vigilant for radiographic features of medial calcinosis, especially in their older population. Immediate referral to a physician is indicated for comprehensive evaluation to identify the etiology and institute risk reduction strategies to mitigate effects of comorbidities and improve patient outcomes.

Calcified Atherosclerotic Plaque

Disease mechanism. Stenotic atheromatous plaque in the extracranial carotid vasculature is the major contributing source of cerebrovascular embolic and occlusive disease. Dystrophic calcification can develop in the evolution of plaque within the intimal layer of the involved vessel.

Imaging findings.

Location. Atherosclerosis develops as a result of increased endothelial damage from shear forces at the arterial bifurcation of the vessel. When calcification has occurred, these may be visible in panoramic images in the soft tissues of the neck, either superior or inferior to the greater cornu of the hyoid bone (where the common carotid artery bifurcates into the external and internal carotid arteries) and adjacent to the third and fourth cervical vertebrae or the intervertebral space between them (Fig. 29.7).

Periphery. These soft tissue calcifications are usually multiple, irregular in shape, and well defined from the surrounding soft tissues, and they have a vertical linear distribution.

Internal structure. The internal structure is heterogeneously radiopaque with radiolucent voids.

Differential interpretation. Calcified triticeous cartilage and the superior cornu of the thyroid cartilage may be mistaken for an atheromatous plaque, although the uniform size, shape, and location of the calcified laryngeal cartilage skeleton identify these as normal anatomy.

Management. Patients with calcified carotid atheromas are at a heightened risk for a cerebrovascular incident. Referral to a physician for Doppler ultrasonography is indicated to assess risk, as the increased risk can be significant.

Calcified plaques on panoramic images of elderly males are associated with elevated neutrophil count. Heightened numbers of neutrophils and the cytokines they elaborate are critical for the initiation and propagation of the low-grade inflammatory process underlying

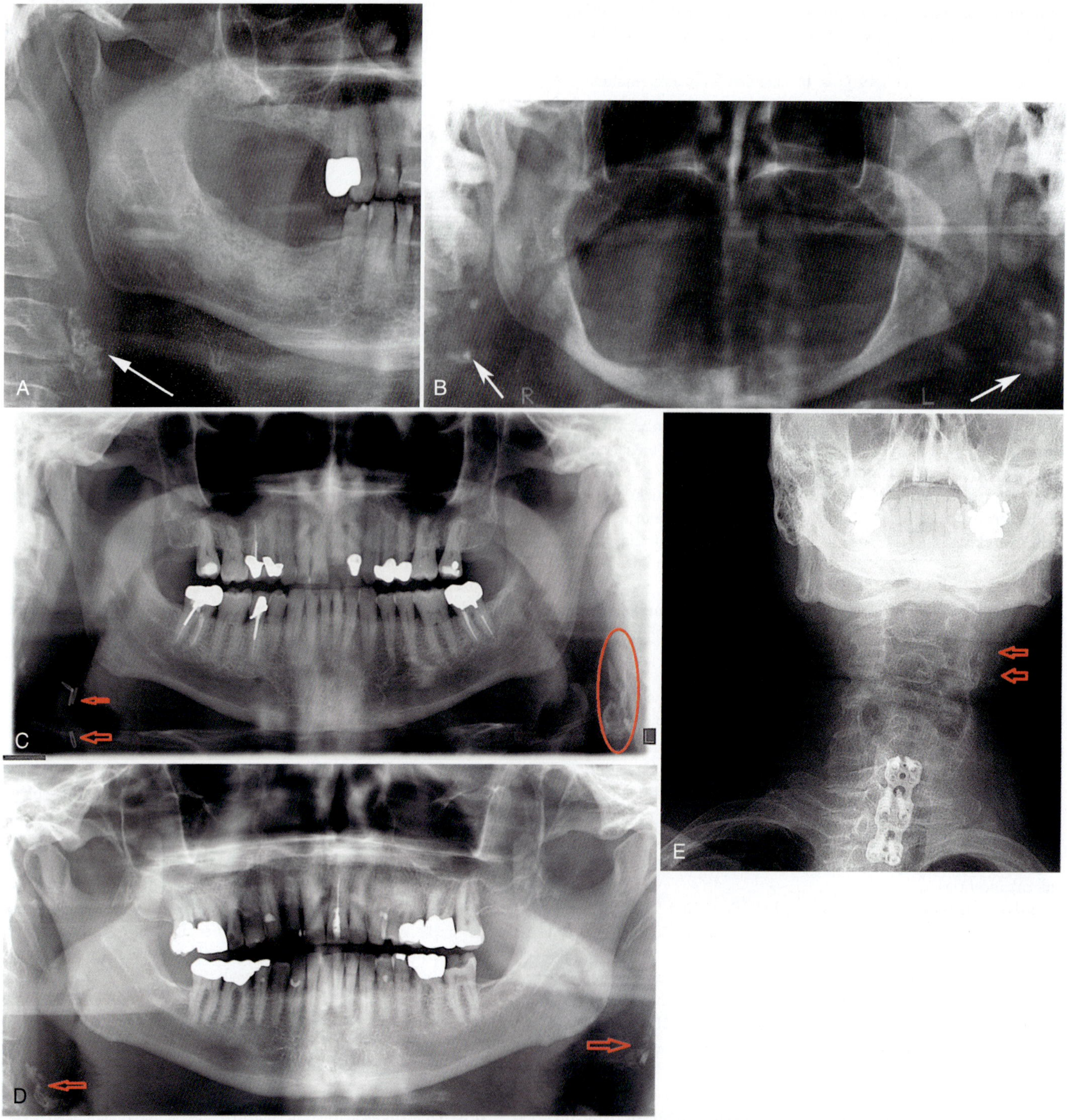

Fig. 29.7 (A) Cropped panoramic image shows calcifications related to the carotid artery. (B) Panoramic image with bilateral examples of calcifications associated with the carotid arteries *(arrows)*. (C) Calcified atheromatous plaque in the left extracranial carotid vasculature at the level of the bulb *(oval)*. Vascular staples in the right side of the neck from prior carotid endarterectomy *(arrows)*. (D) Bilateral calcified carotid atheromata *(arrows)* in a 63-year-old male with type 2 diabetes mellitus. (E) Anteroposterior cervical spine projection in the same case shown in B, displaying calcification in vascular tree *(arrows)*. The patient had fusion of the cervical vertebrae.

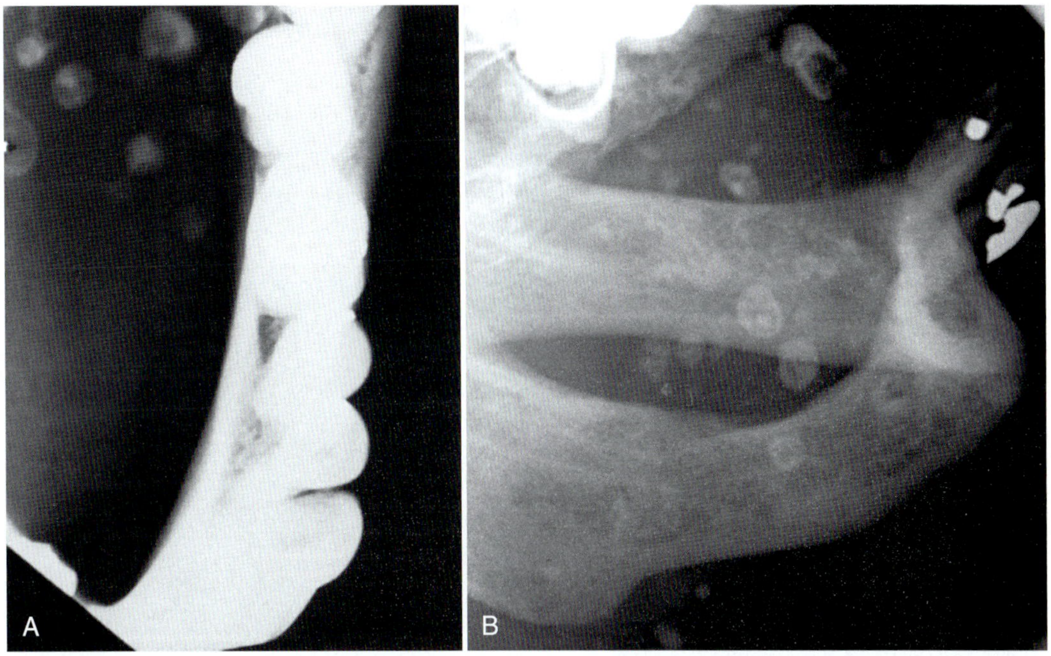

Fig. 29.8 (A and B) Phleboliths are soft tissue dystrophic calcifications found in veins. They are usually associated with hemangiomas.

atherogenesis in the coronary and carotid vasculature and serve as a strong predictor of future adverse events. As such, medical consultation is recommended prior to invasive dental procedures.

Idiopathic Calcification

Idiopathic calcification (or calcinosis) results from deposition of calcium in normal tissue despite normal serum calcium and phosphate levels. They are fairly common in the head and neck.

Sialolith

Sialoliths are calcifications found within the salivary glands, and they will be discussed in Chapter 30.

Phleboliths

Disease mechanism. Phleboliths are calcified thrombi, which develop from blood stagnation in veins, venulae, or the sinusoidal vessels of hemangiomas (especially the cavernous type). Mineralization of thrombi begins in the core of the thrombus and consists of crystals of calcium carbonate-fluorohydroxyapatite.

Clinical features. Phleboliths are pathognomonic for hemangioma or vascular malformation in the maxillofacial region. In an adult, phleboliths may be the sole residua of a childhood hemangioma that has long since regressed. The involved soft tissue may be swollen, throbbing, or discolored by the presence of veins. Hemangiomas often fluctuate in size, associated with changes in body position or during a Valsalva maneuver. Applying pressure to the involved tissue should cause a blanching or change in color if the lesion is vascular in nature. Auscultation may reveal a bruit in cases of cavernous hemangioma but not in the capillary type.

Imaging features

Location. Phleboliths are found in hemangiomas and vascular malformations (see Chapter 22).

Periphery. In cross section, the shape of a phlebolith is round or oval, and they typically measure up to 6 mm in diameter with a smooth periphery. If the involved blood vessel is viewed from the side, the phlebolith may resemble a straight or slightly curved sausage.

Internal structure. The internal structure has a mixed radiolucent and radiopaque appearance and is characterized by concentric laminations, giving phleboliths a bull's eye or target-like appearance. Radiolucent flow voids may be seen, which may represent the remaining patent portions of the vessel (Fig. 29.8).

Differential interpretation. A phlebolith may have a shape similar to that of a sialolith. However, submandibular sialoliths usually occur as single entities. If more than one sialolith is present, they are usually oriented in a single line. In contrast, phleboliths are usually multiple and have a more random, clustered distribution. The importance of correctly identifying phleboliths lies in the identification of a hemangioma or vascular malformation. This is critical if surgical procedures are contemplated.

Laryngeal Cartilage Calcifications

Disease mechanism. The epiglottis and vocal processes of the arytenoid cartilages are fibroelastic cartilages, whereas all the remaining laryngeal cartilages are made of hyaline cartilage. Endochondral calcification and ossification of hyaline laryngeal cartilages may begin at the age of skeletal maturity and progress thereafter as a physiologic process.

Clinical features. Calcified laryngeal cartilages are incidental findings on extraoral planar images, and the calcified triticeous and thyroid cartilages are the laryngeal cartilages that are most frequently seen.

Imaging features.

Location. The small, paired triticeous cartilages are found within the lateral thyrohyoid ligaments. The cartilages can be seen on lateral skull or panoramic images within the soft tissues of the pharynx, inferior to the greater cornu of the hyoid bone, and adjacent to the superior border of the fourth cervical vertebra (C4). The superior cornu of the calcified thyroid cartilage appears medial to C4 and is superimposed on the prevertebral soft tissue (Fig. 29.9).

Periphery. The word *triticeous* means "grain of wheat," and the cartilage measures approximately 7–9 mm in length and 2–4 mm in width. The periphery of the calcified triticeous cartilage is well defined and smooth, and the geometry is exceedingly regular. Usually only the

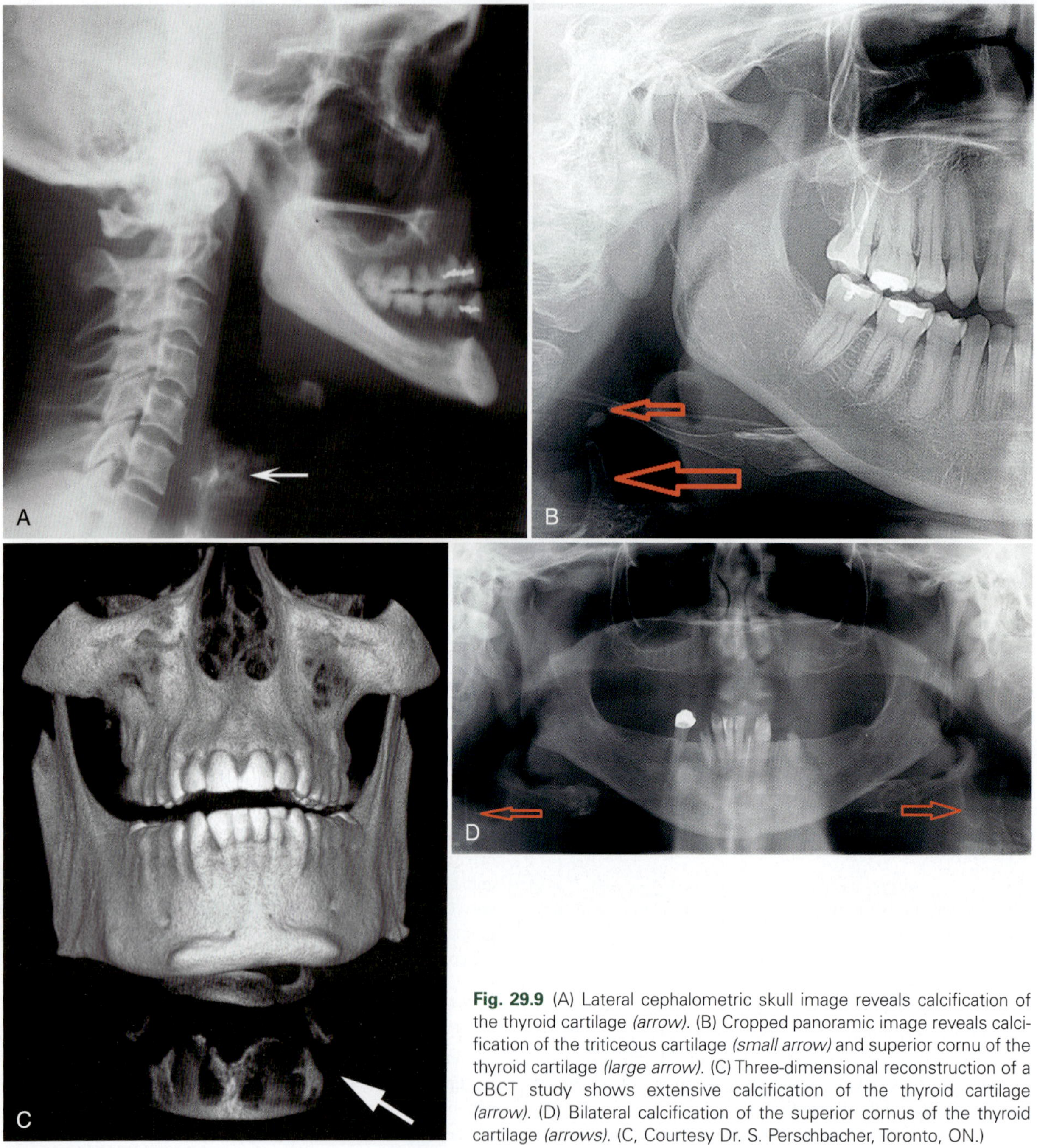

Fig. 29.9 (A) Lateral cephalometric skull image reveals calcification of the thyroid cartilage *(arrow)*. (B) Cropped panoramic image reveals calcification of the triticeous cartilage *(small arrow)* and superior cornu of the thyroid cartilage *(large arrow)*. (C) Three-dimensional reconstruction of a CBCT study shows extensive calcification of the thyroid cartilage *(arrow)*. (D) Bilateral calcification of the superior cornus of the thyroid cartilage *(arrows)*. (C, Courtesy Dr. S. Perschbacher, Toronto, ON.)

top 2–3 mm of a calcified thyroid cartilage is visible at the lower edge of a panoramic image. Depending on the amount of calcification of the surface, a continuous cortex may or may not be visible.

Internal structure. Calcified triticeous cartilages are generally homogeneously radiopaque, but occasionally, a peripheral cortex can be identified.

Differential interpretation. Calcified triticeous cartilage may be confused with calcified atheromatous plaque in the carotid bifurcation. The solitary nature of the cartilage and its extremely uniform size and shape should allow the dentist to differentiate between the two.

Management. No management is needed for the calcified laryngeal cartilages, but careful attention to the differences in morphology and location enables the clinician to distinguish between calcified triticeous cartilage and calcified carotid atheromas.

Rhinoliths and Antroliths

Disease mechanism. Calcareous concretions that occur in the nasal fossa (rhinoliths) or the maxillary sinus (antroliths) arise from the slow accretion of nasal, lacrimal, and inflammatory mineral salts such as calcium phosphate, calcium carbonate, and magnesium around a nidus. Rarely, concretions form in the frontal sinus or ethmoid air cells.

In the case of a rhinolith, the nidus is usually a forgotten exogenous foreign body (e.g., coins, beads, seeds, plastic), especially in pediatric patients. Drug smugglers who carry contraband packets in the nose sometimes forget to remove one, and a rhinolith develops around it over time. The route of entry of the foreign body is usually anterior, but some may enter the choana posteriorly during sneezing, coughing, or emesis.

The nidus for an antrolith is usually endogenous (e.g., root tip, bone fragment, blood clot, inspissated mucus, ectopic tooth), especially in adults. Dystrophic calcification may also occur within chronically inflamed maxillary sinus mucosa in long-standing sinusitis. These may appear as usually small scattered and faint calcifications in the thickened mucosal lining. Occasionally, a noninvasive aspergillosis mycetoma may develop in the antrum, especially in patients with chronic sinus disease. This mycetoma may manifest as a muddy, necrotic fungus ball, or calcareous deposits that may transform it into a hard mycolith.

Clinical features. Rhinoliths take approximately 15 years to form and may initially be asymptomatic. As the expanding mass begins to impinge on the mucosa, there may be pain, congestion, and ulceration. The patient may experience facial pain, nasal obstruction, septal erosion, fetid unilateral purulent or blood-stained rhinorrhea, sinusitis, headache, epistaxis, anosmia, fetor, and fever.

Imaging features.

Location. Rhinoliths develop in the nose in the inferior meatus where the passage is narrowest (Fig. 29.10A). In contrast, antroliths develop in the antrum, in the molar region adjacent to the sinus floor (Fig. 29.10C).

Periphery. These stones have various shapes and sizes, depending on the nature of the nidus, but all have well-defined peripheries.

Internal structure. Rhinoliths and antroliths may manifest as mixed radiolucent and radiopaque entities, depending on the nature of the nidus, and sometimes may have laminations. Occasionally, these rhinoliths and antroliths may be homogeneously radiopaque, sometimes exceeding the density of the surrounding bone.

Differential interpretation. Diagnosis is usually made radiographically or through clinical visualization via nasal endoscopy. The differential interpretation includes osteoma, calcified polyp, odontoma, and surgical ciliated cyst.

Management. Patients should be referred to an otorhinolaryngologist for endonasal or sinus endoscopic surgical removal of the calcification. In some cases, lithotripsy has been used to debulk large rhinoliths.

Metastatic Calcification

Metastatic calcification of the soft tissues in the oral region is caused by conditions that produce elevated serum calcium and phosphate levels, such as hyperparathyroidism (see Chapter 23) or hypercalcemia of malignancy. In addition, metastatic calcification can arise from high

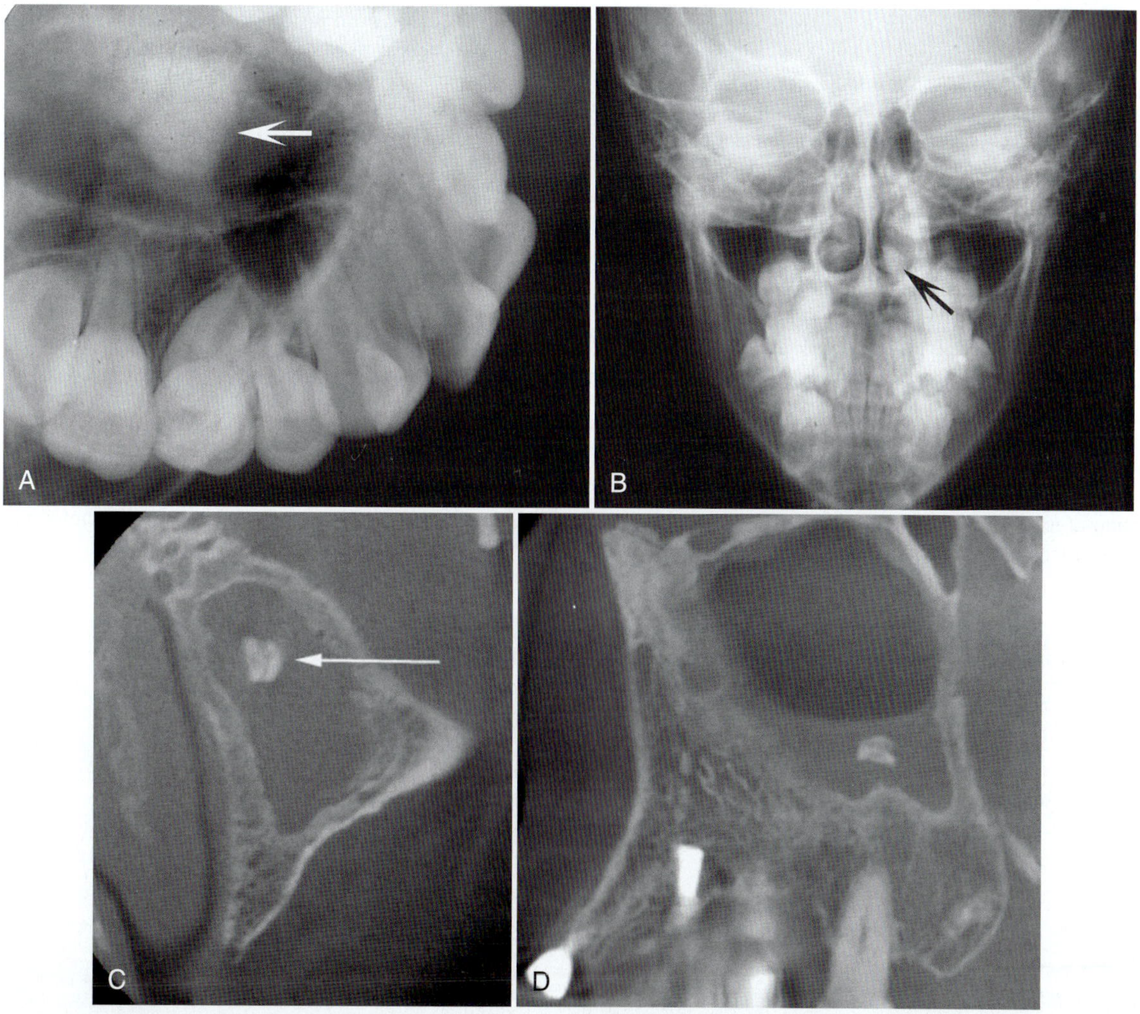

Fig. 29.10 (A) Lateral occlusal film shows a rhinolith *(arrow)* positioned above the floor of the nose. (B) Posteroanterior skull image of the same case shown in A demonstrates that the rhinolith is positioned within the nasal fossa *(arrow)*. (C) Axial cone beam computed tomography (CBCT) image reveals the presence of an antrolith *(arrow)*. (D) Coronal CBCT of the same case shown in C demonstrates the antrolith above the floor of the maxillary sinus.

serum phosphate concentrations that may be seen in chronic renal failure. Metastatic calcifications usually occur bilaterally and symmetrically, and they are extremely rare.

HETEROTOPIC OSSIFICATIONS

Ossification of the Stylohyoid Ligament

Disease Mechanism

Embryologically, the styloid process arises from the second branchial arch (Reichert cartilage), which consists of four sections that give rise to the styloid process and ossified ligament (the stylohyoid complex). Ossification of the stylohyoid ligament usually extends downward from the base of the skull and commonly occurs bilaterally. However, in rare cases, the ossification begins at the lesser horn of the hyoid bone, and in fewer cases still, in a central area of the ligament.

Clinical Features

The elongated styloid process may be detected by palpation over the tonsil as a hard, pointed structure. Symptoms occur in approximately 4% of patients with an elongated styloid process or ossified ligament, and there is little correlation between the extent of ossification and the intensity of the accompanying symptoms. Symptoms related to the elongated styloid process, which includes the ossified ligament, are termed Eagle syndrome, and they can be related to cranial nerve impingement (classic Eagle syndrome) or impingement of the carotid sinus complex (carotid artery syndrome). Affected individuals are usually older than 40 years.

When the symptoms are related to a recent history of neck trauma (typically tonsillectomy), the condition is classic Eagle syndrome. The ossified stylohyoid complex and local scar tissue are thought to cause symptoms by impinging on cranial nerves V, VII, IX, X, XI, or XII, all of which pass in close proximity to the styloid process. Symptoms may include vague, nagging to intense pain in the pharynx on speaking, chewing, swallowing (eliciting a foreign body sensation in the throat), turning the head, or opening the mouth widely, especially on singing or yawning, tinnitus or otalgia.

Clinical findings without a history of neck trauma constitute carotid artery syndrome, and the patient may describe referred pain along the distribution of the internal or external carotid artery. The pain is the result of mechanical impingement of the involved artery and stimulation of its sympathetic nerve plexus. Symptoms when the internal carotid artery is affected may include eye pain, temporal or parietal headache, migraines, aphasia, visual symptoms, weakness, and transient hemispheric ischemia with vertigo or syncope, notably on turning the head to the ipsilateral side. When the external carotid artery is impinged and stimulated, the patient may feel suborbital facial pain. Pain arises by mechanical irritation of the periarterial sympathetic nerve plexus overlying the artery, which produces regional carotidynia; this may occur even in the absence of ossification of the stylohyoid complex. Only deviation of the styloid process, usually medially, is required for the tip of the process to impinge an artery. Carotid artery syndrome is more prevalent than classic Eagle syndrome.

Imaging Features

Ossification of the stylohyoid ligament is detected commonly as an incidental feature on panoramic images. CT is the gold standard for radiographic detection and evaluation of the proximity of an elongated styloid process or ossified ligament to critical neuronal and vascular structures.

Location. On a panoramic image, the linear ossification extends forward from the region of the mastoid process and crosses the posteroinferior aspect of the ramus toward the hyoid bone. The hyoid bone is positioned roughly parallel to, or superimposed over, the posterior aspect of the inferior cortex of the mandible.

Shape. The styloid process appears as a long, tapering, thin, radiopaque process that is thicker at its base and projects downward and forward to an almost needle-like point (see Fig. 29.11). It normally ranges from about 0.5 to 2.5 cm in length. The ossified ligament has roughly a straight outline, but in some cases, some surface irregularity may be seen. The farther the radiopaque ossified ligament extends toward the hyoid bone, the more likely it will be interrupted by radiolucent, joint-like junctions (pseudoarticulations) (Fig. 29.12).

Internal structure. Small ossifications of the stylohyoid ligament appear homogeneously radiopaque. As the ossification increases in length and girth, the outer cortex of this bone becomes evident as a radiopaque band at the periphery.

Differential Interpretation

When the symptoms accompanying stylohyoid complex ossification do occur, there is distinctive evidence of ligament ossification in the diagnostic images. There is little chance that the complaint will be confused with another entity.

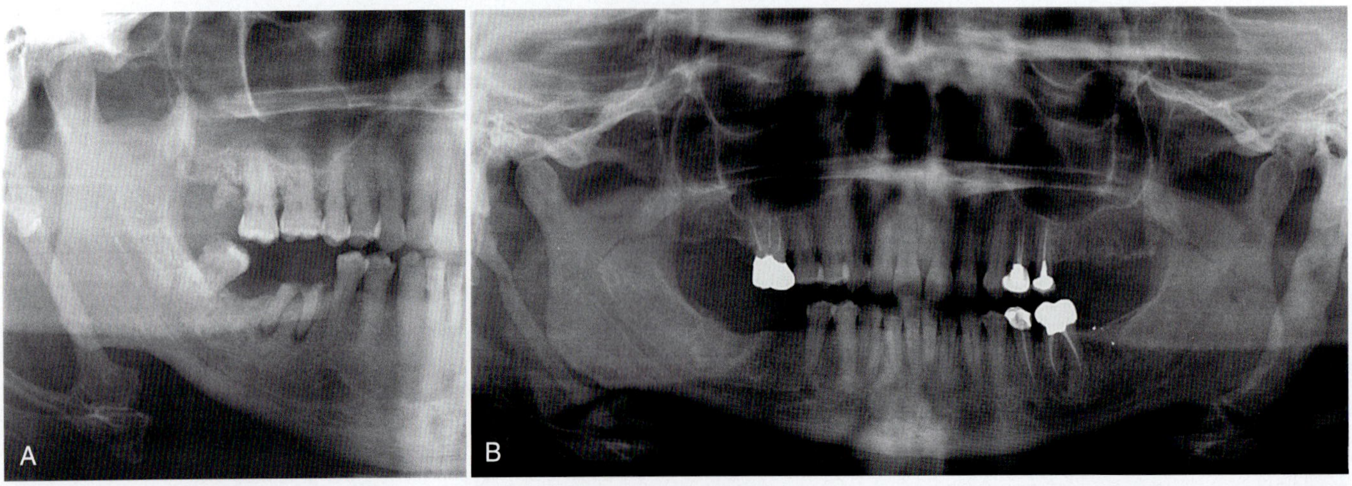

Fig. 29.11 (A and B) Examples of prominent ossification of the stylohyoid ligament. These individuals did not have any symptoms.

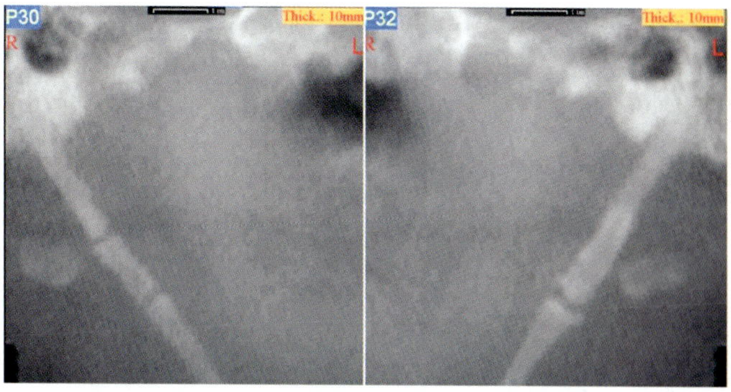

Fig. 29.12 Oblique sagittal cone beam computed tomographic images of a patient with bilateral ossified stylohyoid ligaments. Note the pseudojoint formation between the ossification centers.

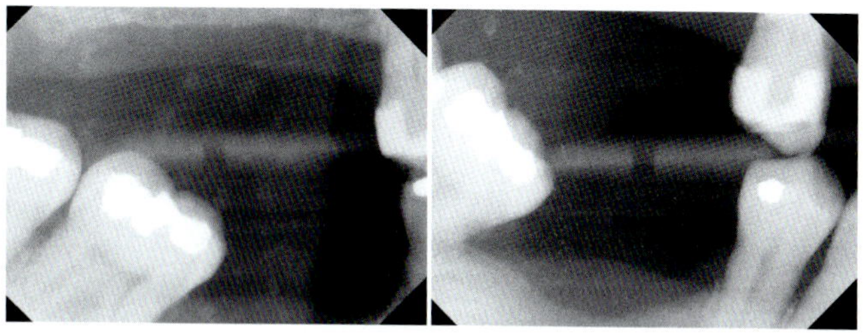

Fig. 29.13 Osteoma cutis is seen as a cluster of donut-like radiopaque calcifications in the soft tissues of the right cheek. (Courtesy Dr. O. Yeung, Chicago, IL.)

Management

Most patients with ossification of the stylohyoid ligament are asymptomatic, and no management is required. With topical anesthesia to suppress the gag reflex, palpation of the tonsillar fossa to reproduce the symptoms and detect the hard submucosal mass may serve as diagnostic confirmation. For mildly symptomatic patients, steroid injection under ultrasound guidance may be recommended initially. For patients with severe or persistent symptoms, transcranial styloidectomy or transoral robotic surgery are recommended. 3D printed models can provide perioperative assistance in determining the extent and direction of the surgical site to permit removal of the offending structure without damaging surrounding anatomical structures.

Osteoma Cutis

Disease Mechanism

Osteoma cutis is a rare soft tissue ossification in the skin or subcutaneous tissues that manifests as focal development of bone within the dermis physically removed from any original osseous tissue. Osteoma cutis may be primary, occurring in normal tissue without any preexisting condition; or secondary, developing in damaged or disrupted skin. Approximately 85% of cases are secondary and occur in long-standing, scarred acne, triggering osteoblastic metaplasia. Alternatively, the lesions can arise within chronic inflammatory, traumatic, or neoplastic dermatosis. They occasionally are found in diffuse scleroderma, replacing the altered collagen in the dermis and subcutaneous septa.

Clinical Features

Osteoma cutis can occur anywhere, but the face is the most common site. The tongue is the most common intraoral site (osteoma mucosae or osseous choristoma). Osteoma cutis does not cause any visible change in the overlying skin other than an occasional color change, which may appear yellowish white. If the lesion is large, the individual osteoma may be palpated. A needle inserted into one of the papules is met with stone-like resistance. Some patients have numerous (dozens to hundreds) lesions, usually on the face in female patients and on the scalp or chest in male patients. This form is known as multiple miliary osteoma cutis.

Imaging Features

Location. Radiographically, osteoma cutis most commonly appears in the cheek and lip regions (Fig. 29.13). In this location, the ossified area can be superimposed over a tooth root or alveolar process, giving the appearance of an area of dense bone. Accurate localization can be achieved by placing an intraoral receptor between the cheek and alveolar process to image the cheek alone. Alternatively, a soft tissue, low (60) kilovoltage (kVp) posteroanterior skull image with the cheek blown outward can localize these entities in the skin.

Periphery. Osteoma cutis are radiopaque, washer-shaped entities with smooth peripheries. These single or multiple radiopaque masses are usually very small, although the size can range from 0.1 to 5 cm.

Internal structure. The internal structure may be homogeneously radiopaque, but usually, a radiolucent center representing normal fatty marrow may be visualized, giving the lesion a donut-like appearance radiographically. Trabeculae occasionally develop in the marrow cavity of larger osteomas. Individual lesions of calcified cystic acne resemble a snowflake-like radiopacity, which corresponds to the clinical location of the scar.

Differential interpretation. The differential interpretation should include myositis ossificans, calcinosis cutis, and osteoma mucosae. Dermal fillers and subcutaneous volume enhancers may have the same radiographic manifestations. If the blown-out cheek technique is used, the lesions of osteoma cutis appear much more superficial than mucosal lesions. Myositis ossificans is of greater proportions, in some cases causing noticeable deformity of the facial contour.

Management. No management is required, but primary osteoma cutis is occasionally removed for cosmetic reasons. Laser resurfacing of the skin with a retinoic acid cream or curettage have been successful in treating osteoma cutis. More recently, good cosmetic results have been reported with a needle microincision-extirpation technique in patients with multiple miliary osteoma cutis.

Myositis Ossificans

In myositis ossificans, fibrous tissue and heterotopic bone form within the interstitial tissue of muscle and associated tendons and ligaments. Secondary destruction and atrophy of the muscle occur as this fibrous tissue and bone interdigitate and separate the muscle fibers. Two principal forms have been described: localized and progressive.

Localized (Traumatic) Myositis Ossificans

Disease mechanism. Localized myositis ossificans develops from trauma or heavy muscle strain caused by certain occupations and sports. Skeletal muscle has limited regenerative capacity after significant physical trauma, and muscle contusion leads to considerable hemorrhage into the muscle or associated tendons and fascia. The fibrous tissue and bone form within the interstitial tissue of the muscle; no actual ossification of the muscle fibers occurs. It has been proposed that exuberant proliferation of vascular granulation tissue subsequently undergoes metaplasia to cartilage and bone during the healing process. Muscle injury from multiple injections (occasionally from the delivery of dental anesthesia) may also be a cause.

Clinical features. Localized myositis ossificans can develop at any age in either sex but occurs most often in young men who engage in vigorous activity. The site of the precipitating trauma remains swollen, tender, and painful for a period of time much longer than expected.

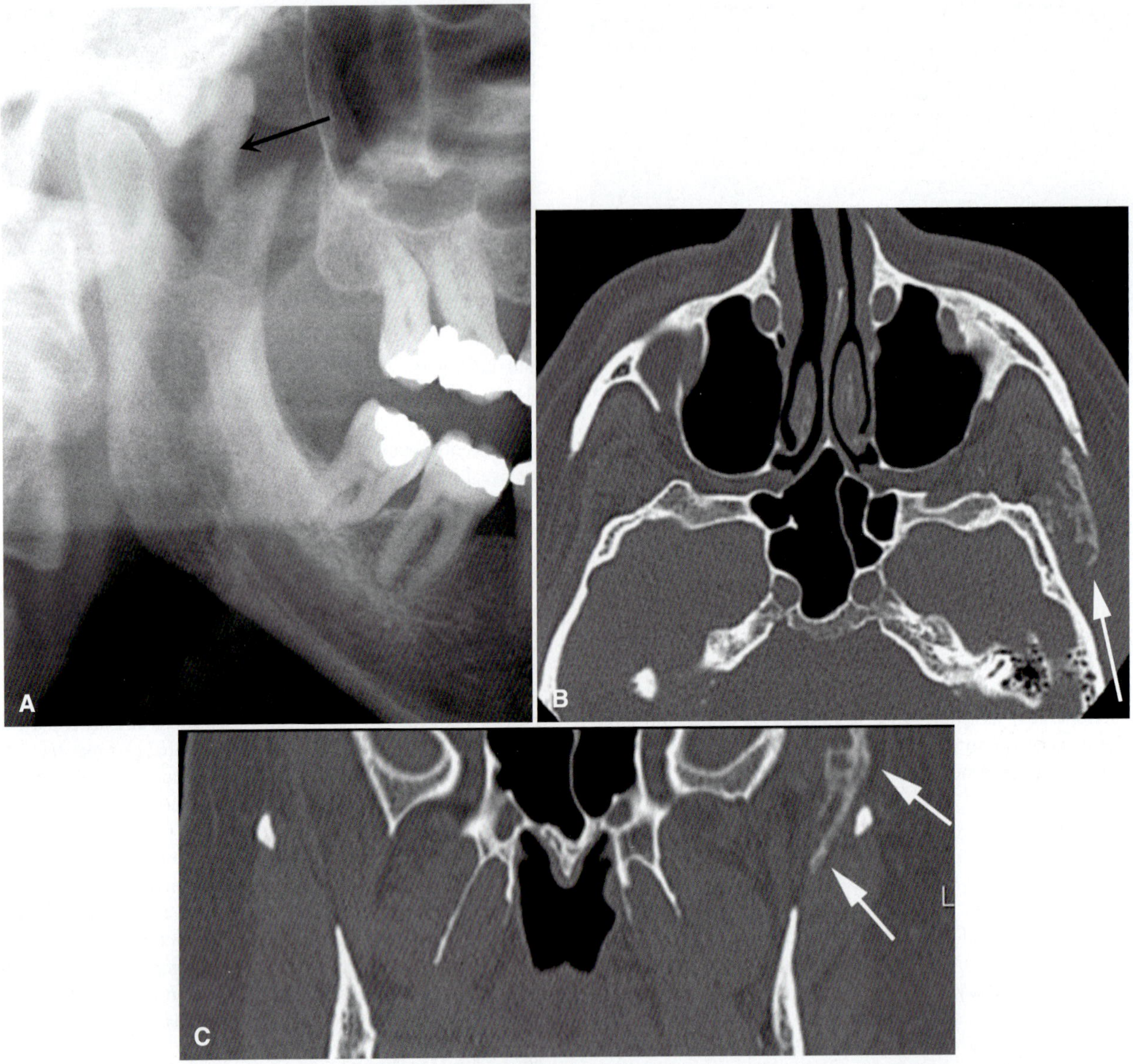

Fig. 29.14 (A) Soft tissue ossification extending from the coronoid process in a superior direction following the anatomy of the temporalis muscle *(arrow)*. This condition arose after several attempts were made to provide a submandibular nerve block, leaving the patient unable to open the mandible. (B) Axial multidetector computed tomography (MDCT) image of ossification along the temporalis muscle *(arrow)* after a surgical procedure. (C) Coronal MDCT image of the same case shown in B reveals the calcifications *(arrows)*.

The overlying skin may be red and inflamed, and when ossification involves a muscle of mastication, opening the jaws may be difficult. After about 2 or 3 weeks, the area of ossification becomes apparent in the tissues, and a firm intramuscular mass can be palpated. The localized lesion may enlarge slowly, but eventually it stops growing. The entity may appear fixed, or it may be freely movable on palpation.

Imaging features.

Location. While this condition most commonly affects the extremities, the most commonly involved muscles of the head and neck are the masseter and sternocleidomastoid. However, the other muscles of mastication may also be involved. The anterior attachments of the temporalis and the medial pterygoid muscles are at risk of injury during the administration of mandibular block anesthesia. The ossified masses generally measure less than 6 cm in greatest dimension.

Periphery. The periphery commonly is more radiopaque than the internal structure. There is a variation in shape from irregular oval to linear streaks (pseudotrabeculae) running in the same direction as the normal muscle fibers. A radiolucent band can usually be seen between the area of ossification and adjacent bone, and heterotopic bone may lie along the long axis of the muscle (Fig. 29.14). These pseudotrabeculae are characteristic, if not pathognomonic of myositis ossificans.

Internal structure. The internal structure varies with time. By 3–4 weeks after injury, the radiographic appearance is faint and homogeneously radiopaque. This radiopacity organizes further, and by 2 months, a delicate lacy or feathery radiopaque internal pattern develops. These changes indicate the formation of bone; however, this bone does not have a normal-appearing trabecular pattern. Gradually, the image of this entity becomes more dense, more homogeneous, and better defined, maturing fully in about 5–6 months. Some lesions may progress more slowly and do not reach maturation until 12 months. After this period, the lesion may shrink.

Differential interpretation. The differential interpretation of localized myositis ossificans includes ossification of the stylohyoid ligament and other soft tissue calcifications. However, the form and location of myositis ossificans are often enough to make a diagnosis. Other lesions to consider are bone-forming tumors. Although tumors, such as osteosarcoma, can form a linear bone pattern (see Chapter 24), the tumor is contiguous with the bone, and signs of bone destruction often are present.

Management. Microinjury and subsequent muscle necrosis attract macrophages, which elaborate the osteogenic growth factors. One strategy during the evolution of the lesion is bone morphogenic protein type I receptor inhibition to reduce the heterotopic ossification. Rest and limitation of use are recommended to diminish the extent of the calcific deposit. For lesions that cause a functional restriction or neurologic impairment, surgical excision of the entire calcified mass with intensive physiotherapy to minimize postsurgical scarring is the recommended treatment. Complete maturation of myositis ossificans occurs between 6 and 12 months. Incomplete excision or excision at an immature stage can result in recurrence.

Progressive Myositis Ossificans

Disease mechanism. Progressive myositis ossificans or *fibrodysplasia ossificans progressiva* is a rare genetic anomaly with an autosomal dominant transmission pattern. Less commonly, it arises as a result of spontaneous mutation. The cause is a gain-of-function mutation in the bone morphogenic protein activin A receptor type 1/activin-like kinase 2. It is more common in males and causes symptoms from early infancy. Progressive formation of heterotopic endochondral bone occurs within the interstitial tissue of muscles, tendons, ligaments, and fascia and the involved muscles atrophy.

Clinical features. Patients display a congenital big toe deformity (hallux valgus). In most cases, catastrophically disabling heterotopic ossification starts in the muscles of the neck and upper back and moves to the extremities. The disease commences with an inflamed soft tissue swelling. The acute symptoms subside, and a firm mass remains in the tissues. This condition may affect tendons, ligaments, striated muscles, the heart, and diaphragm. Ossification spreads extensively, affecting almost all of the large muscles of the body. Trismus, stiffness, and limitation of motion of the neck, chest, back, and extremities (especially the shoulders) gradually increase. Functional deficits are progressive and handicapping. Advanced stages of the disease result in the "petrified man" condition with immobility through a progressive metamorphosis of skeletal muscle into a second skeleton of heterotopic bone. Most patients die during the third or fourth decade, usually due to respiratory embarrassment or infection.

Imaging features. The radiographic appearance of progressive myositis ossificans is similar to that of the localized form. The heterotopic bone more commonly is oriented along the long axis of the involved muscle (Fig. 29.15). Osseous malformation of the regions of muscle attachment, such as the mandibular condyles, also may be seen.

Differential interpretation. In the initial stages of the disease, distinguishing between progressive myositis ossificans and rheumatoid arthritis may be difficult. However, the presence of specific anomalies suggests the diagnosis. In the case of calcinosis, the deposits of amorphous calcium salts frequently resorb, but in progressive myositis ossificans, the bone never disappears.

Management. No effective treatment exists for progressive myositis ossificans. Atraumatic, noninvasive dental procedures are indicated, with avoidance of nerve block anesthesia, instead employing subcutaneous local infiltration anesthesia. Interference with respiration or respiratory infection occurs in the later stages of the disease, so supportive therapy may be required. Currently, drug development is aimed at the activin A receptor mutation, which is a highly conserved target.

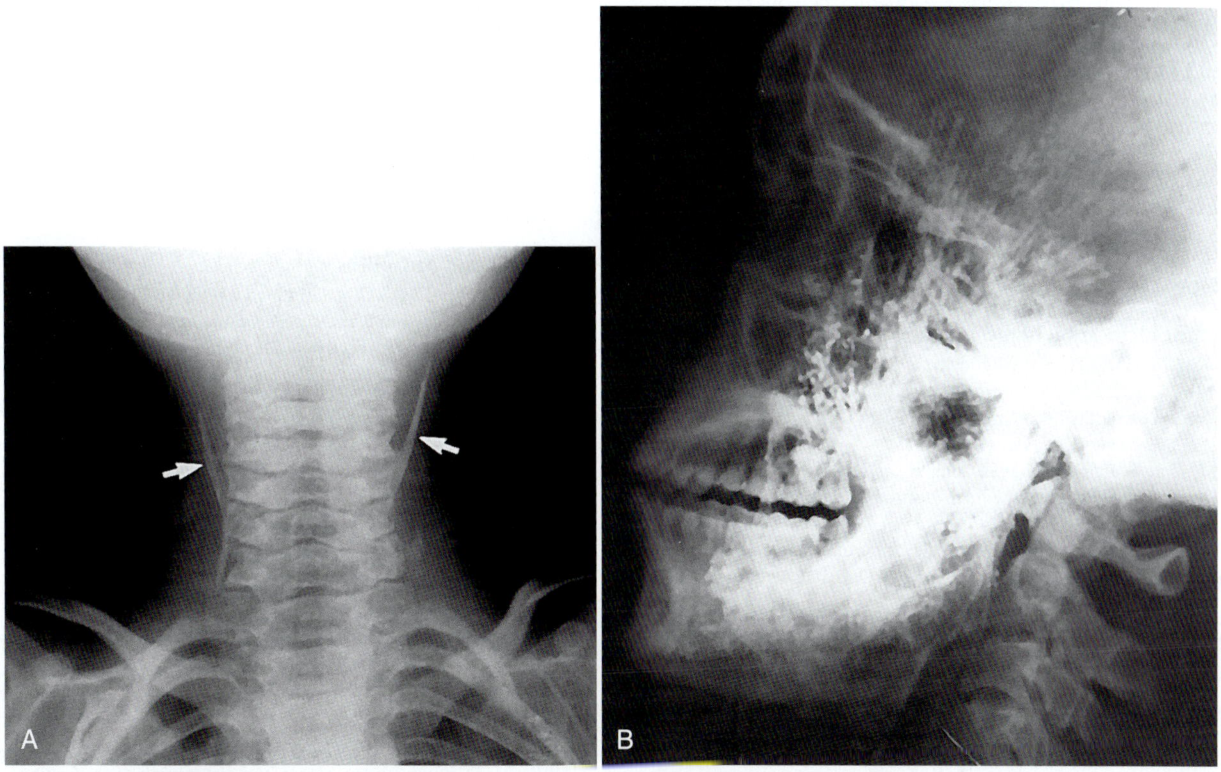

Fig. 29.15 (A) Myositis ossificans, seen as bilateral linear calcifications *(arrows)* of the sternohyoid muscle. (B) Extensive ossification of the masseter and temporalis muscles.

Continued

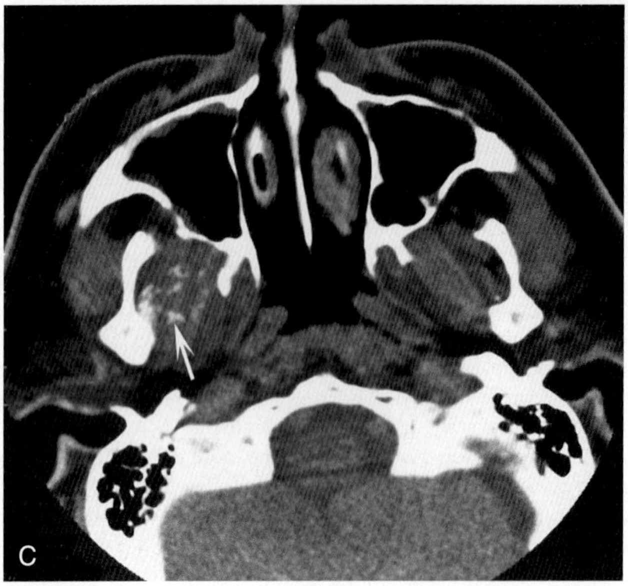

Fig. 29.15, cont'd (C) Axial computed tomography scan with soft tissue algorithm demonstrates calcifications in the lateral pterygoid muscle *(arrow)*. (A, Courtesy Dr. H. Worth, Vancouver, BC.)

BIBLIOGRAPHY

Maia P, Tomaz A, Maia E, et al. Prevalence of soft tissue calcifications in panoramic radiographs of the maxillofacial region of older adults. *Gerodontology*. 2022;39:266-272.

Togan B, Gander Y, Lanzer M, et al. Incidence and frequency of nondental incidental findings on cone-beam computed tomography. *J Craniomaxillofac Surg*. 2016;44:1373-1380.

Yilmaz Z, Tekin A. Relationship between the prevalence of soft tissue radiopacities on panoramic radiographs and medical conditions. *Minerva Stomatol*. 2020;69:235-244.

Calcified Lymph Nodes

Cruz A, Hernandez J. Tuberculosis cervical denitis. *Pediatr Infect Dis J*. 2016;35:1154-1156.

Michaelides SA, Bablekos GD, Michallidis AR, et al. Left lateral cervical mass with draining sinuses. *Case Rep Med*. 2019;2019:7838596. htpps://doi.org/10.1155/2019/7838596.

Rammeh S, Romdhane E, Toumi A, et al. Efficacy of fine-needle aspiration cytology in the diagnosis of tuberculous cervical lymphadenitis. *Acta Cytol*. 2018;62:99-103.

Dystrophic Calcification in the Tonsils

Kim MJ, Kim JE, Huh KH, et al. Multidetector computed tomography imaging characteristics of asymptomatic palatine tonsilloliths: a retrospective study on 3886 examinations *Oral Surg Oral Med Oral Pathol Oral Radiol*. 2018;125:693-698.

Ozdede M, Akay G, Karadag O, et al. Comparison of panoramic radiography and cone-beam computed tomography for the detection of tonnsilloliths. *Med Princ Pract*. 2020;29:279-284.

Patel S, Daher G, Engle L, et al. Adult tonsillectomy: an evaluation of indications and complications. *Am J Otolaryngol*. 2022;43:103403 https://doi.org/10.1016/j.amjoto.2022.103403.

Cysticercosis

Bansal N, Mohanty S, Kadanthode M, et al. Review of cysticercosis of maxillofacial region and report of two cases. *J Stomatol Oral Maxillofac Surg*. 2022;123:e760-e769.

Gupta S, Gupta S, Sharma R, et al. Imaging findings of orofacial cysticercosis: report of 5 cases with review of literature. *Oral Radiol*. 2024;40(1):81-91. doi:10.1007/s11282-022-00651-w.

Manikandan G, James V, Chandrasekaran C, et al. An atypical case of cutaneous cysticercosis in the buccal mucosa. *J Oral Maxillofac Pathol*. 2020;24:591.

Calcified Blood Vessel

Berrgian K, Rao S, Francis J, et al. Monckeberg arteriosclerosis of the facial vasculature presentation on CBCT: a case report. *Compend Contin Educ Dent*. 2021;42:242-246.

Brooks J, Shin K, Price J. Occult Monckeberg medial calcinosis of the facial and infraorbital arteries in an elderly edentulous patient. *Spec Care Dentist*. 2022;42:642-645.

Chang TI, Wu X, Boström KI, et al. Panoramic imaged carotid atheromas are associated with increased neutrophil count: both validated, independent predictors of near-term myocardial infarction. *Dentomaxillofac Radiol*. 2021;50:20210045 https://doi.org/10.1259/dmfr.20210045.

Mupparapu M, Nath S. Calcified carotid artery atheroma and stroke risk assessment. Use of Doppler ultrasonography as a secondary marker: a meta-analysis. *Quintessence Int*. 2021;52:348-359.

Rhinoliths and Antroliths

Chen HH, Yi CA, Chen YC, et al. Influence of maxillary antroliths on the clinical outcome of implants placed simultaneously with osteotome sinus floor elevation: a retrospective radiographic study. *Clin Implant Dent Relat Res*. 2021;23:833-841.

Yildiz E, Kuzu S, Ulu S, et al. Rhinoliths: analysis of 24 interesting forgotten foreign body cases. *Ear Nose Throat J*. 2021;100:570-573.

Phleboliths

Park J, Kim CH, Moon C. Intramuscular hemangioma in buccal cheek: a case report. *J Korean Assoc Oral Maxillofac Surg*. 2017;43:262-266.

Nagaraja A, Kumar N, Kumar B, et al. A solitary phlebolith in the buccal mucosa: report of a rare entity and clinicopathologic correlation. *J Contemp Dent Pract*. 2016;17:706-710.

Uzun C, Celenk P, van der Stelt P. Venous malformation with multiple phleboliths: a case report. *Quintessence Int*. 2017;48:51-56.

Calcified Laryngeal Cartilages

Alqahtani E, Marrero D, Champion W, et al. Triticeous cartilage CT imaging characteristics, prevalence, extent, and distribution of ossification. *Otolaryngol Head Neck Surg*. 2016;154:131-137.

de-Azevedo-Vas S, Machado I, Pereira T, et al. More frequent detection of calcified carotid atherosclerotic plaques and mineralized laryngeal cartilages on digital than on film-based panoramic radiographs. *Imaging Sci Dent.* 2019;49:65-70.

Emre E, Akkoc RF, Ogeturk M. Prevalence and distribution of triticeal cartilage. *Folio Morphol (Warsz).* 2022;81:150-156.

Ossified Stylohyoid Ligament

Cartwright J, Moreno F. Presentation of Eagle syndrome following radiation therapy to carcinoma of the larynx. *Clin Case Rep.* 2022;10:e05325.

Czako L, Simko K, Thurzo A, et al. The syndrome of elongated styloid process, the Eagle's syndrome – from anatomical, evolutionary and embryological backgrounds to 3D printing and personalized surgery planning. report of five cases. *Medicina.* 2020;56:458 https://doi.org/10.3390/medicina 56090458

Lee Y, Chung J. Eagle syndrome after a fracture of complete ossified stylohyoid ligament from indirect trauma treated using local steroid injection. A case report. *Medicine.* 2020;99:e20818.

Osteoma Cutis

Alhazmi D, Badr F, Jadu F, et al. Osteoma cutis of the face inn CBCT images. *Case Rep Dent.* 2017;2017:8468965. https://doi.org/10.1155/8468965.

Safi Y, Valizadeh S, Vasegh Z, et al. Prevalence of osteoma cutis in the maxillofacial region and classification of its radiographic pattern in cone beam CT. *Dermatol Online J.* 2016;22:13030/qt1x769989.

Myositis Ossificans

Jo GD, Kang JH, Kim JE, et al. Head and neck manifestations of fibrodysplasia ossificans progressive: clinical and imaging findings in 2 cases. *Imaging Sci Dent.* 2023;53:257-264 https://doi.org/10.5624/isd.20230069.

Karimi A, Tavakoli I, Jalilimanesh K, et al. Myositis ossificans traumatica: an unusual cause of mandibular hypomobility. *J Craniofac Surg.* 2021;32: e539-e541.

Sharifi R, Hakim L, Mehraban S, et al. Non-traumatic myositis ossificans of the right masseter muscle: a case report and review of the literature. *Clin Case Rep.* 2021;9:e04608.

30

Salivary Gland Diseases

Fatima M. Jadu

Salivary glands and their secretions play a significant role in preserving the overall health of oral structures. Accordingly, conditions that affect the salivary glands and their function also directly affect the teeth and mucosa. These conditions often drive patients to seek care from their dentists. Therefore, it is of paramount importance that dentists understand the pathophysiology of the salivary glands and be aware of the various diagnostic and management methods in order to provide optimal care for their patients.

DISEASE MECHANISM

The salivary glands are the exocrine glands that produce and secrete saliva. There are three pairs of major salivary glands located outside the oral cavity, and numerous minor salivary glands can be found within the mouth, scattered throughout the oral submucosa (Fig. 30.1). Both the major and minor salivary glands can be affected by a variety of inflammatory and noninflammatory conditions and space-occupying masses. Imaging plays a major role in the diagnosis, management, and follow-up of these conditions.

CLINICAL SIGNS AND SYMPTOMS

The clinical signs and symptoms of salivary gland diseases depend on the disease process and the gland affected, although swelling and pain are the two most common symptoms. Xerostomia, or the subjective feeling of dry mouth, is another symptom that is often associated with diseases of the salivary glands, and patients may complain of a burning sensation or soreness of the mouth, as well as altered taste or difficulty swallowing. Signs of xerostomia can include an erythematous fissured tongue, cervical caries, and recurrent *Candida albicans* infections. The objective decrease in the quantity of saliva or hyposalivation can be confirmed through specific tests.

DIAGNOSTIC IMAGING

Imaging is often used to diagnose and to plan management and follow-up of patients with salivary gland disorders. It can provide crucial information regarding the nature of the disease affecting the salivary glands, the extent and severity of glandular involvement, and effects on the surrounding structures. Many imaging modalities have been used to image the salivary glands including planar imaging, high-resolution ultrasonography (HRUS), multidetector computed tomography (MDCT), magnetic resonance imaging (MRI), nuclear medicine, sialography, and, most recently, sialendoscopy.

Planar Imaging

Planar images, whether intraoral or extraoral, are helpful in identifying calcified sialoliths. Panoramic images may be used to demonstrate parotid and submandibular sialoliths; however, cross-sectional mandibular occlusal images are often more effective in the identification and localization of submandibular duct sialoliths (Fig. 30.2). On panoramic images, parotid sialoliths can appear superimposed over the mandibular rami superior to the occlusal plane, whereas submandibular sialoliths, particularly those located within the gland parenchyma, appear superior to the hyoid bone near the antegonial notch of the mandible (Fig. 30.3). Planar images should be considered first when

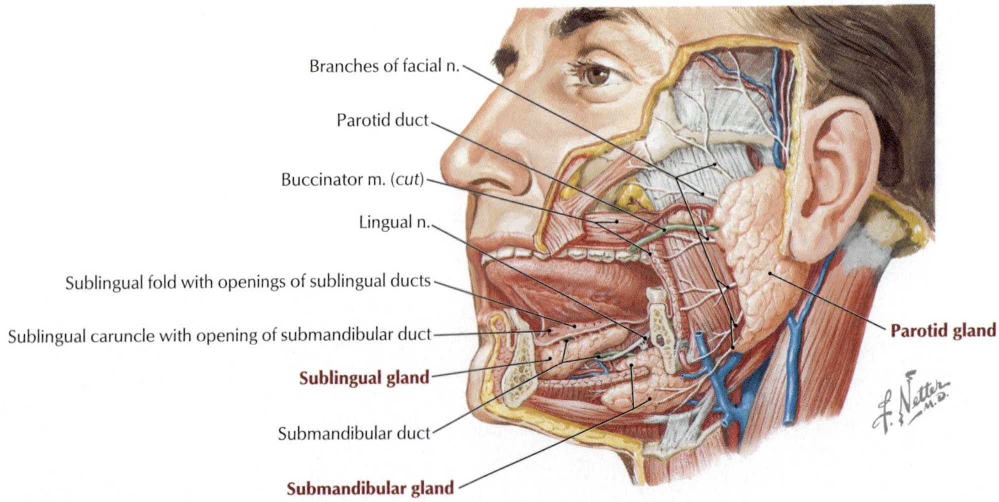

Fig. 30.1 The sizes and locations of the major salivary glands relative to the oral cavity. (Courtesy Netter Images.)

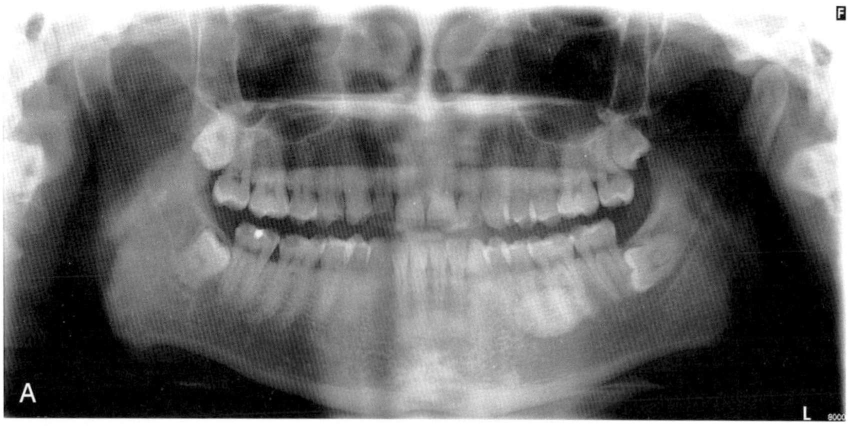

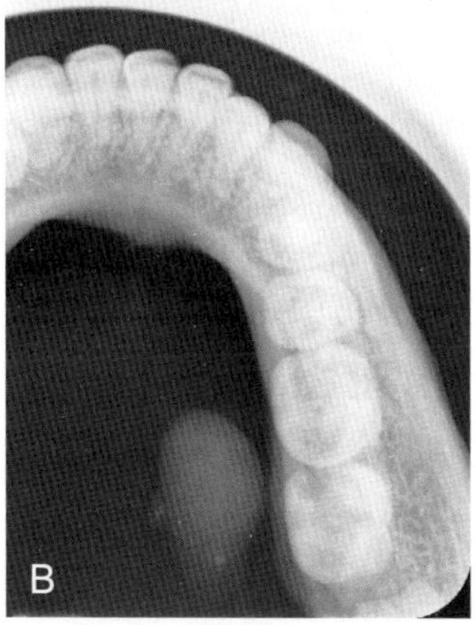

Fig. 30.2 (A) Panoramic and (B) cross-sectional occlusal images demonstrating an oval-shaped radiopaque sialolith in a submandibular salivary gland duct.

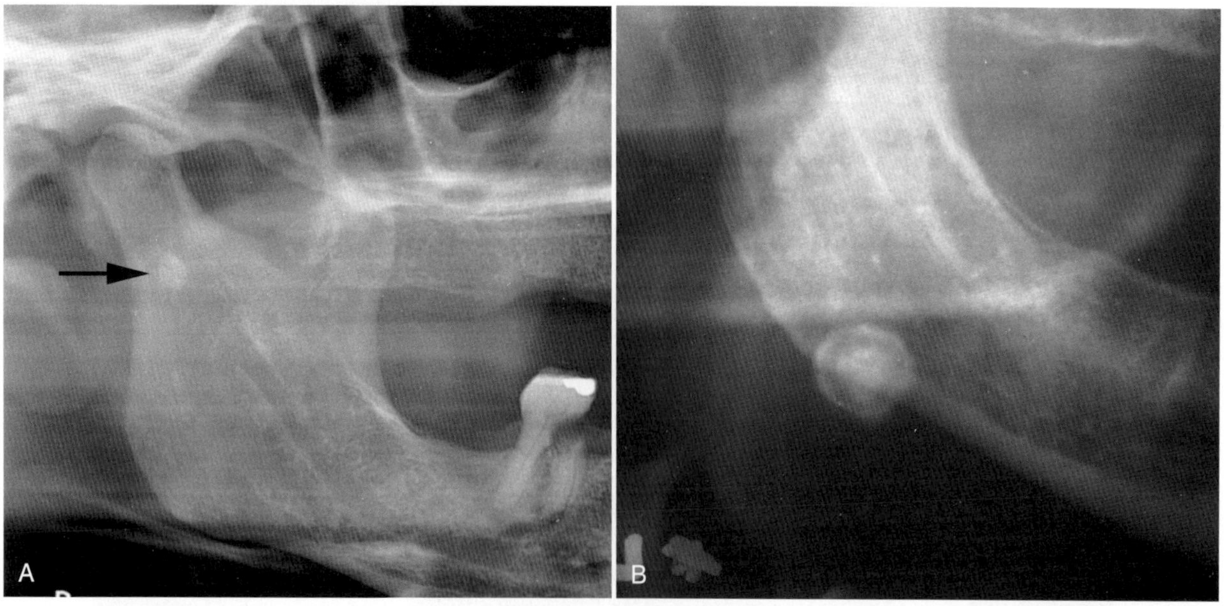

Fig. 30.3 Cropped panoramic images of (A) a parotid sialolith superimposed over condylar neck *(arrow)* superior to the plane of occlusion and (B) a submandibular sialolith near the antegonial notch of the mandible. Note the concentric lamellar pattern charachteristic of sialoliths.

the patient presents with the signs and symptoms of salivary gland obstruction, which can include swelling and pain just prior to or during mealtime. Some of the advantages of planar imaging is that it is readily available, inexpensive, and subjects the patient to a relatively low dose of radiation. In addition, planar images allow the dentist to assess the osseous structures adjacent to the salivary glands. Planar images do, however, fail to identify noncalcified sialoliths, which are estimated to account for approximately 40% of all parotid sialoliths and 20% of all submandibular sialoliths.

High-Resolution Ultrasonography

This technique may be useful in the initial assessment of the major salivary glands, especially when the suspected abnormality is located superficially. High-resolution ultrasonography (HRUS) may be helpful

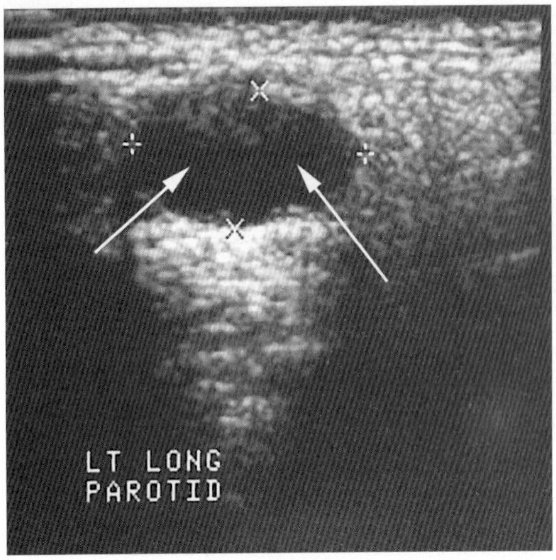

Fig. 30.4 High-resolution ultrasonography image of the parotid gland demonstrating a hypoechoic (echo-free) mass with well-defined margins, which is typical of a cystic mass *(arrows)*. (Courtesy Department of Radiology, Baylor University Medical Center, Dallas, TX.)

in differentiating cysts from neoplasms, and those that are benign from those that may be malignant (Fig. 30.4). Moreover, HRUS may also be used to guide biopsy and inform subsequent imaging choices. HRUS has become useful in identifying salivary gland changes associated with Sjögren syndrome, but it lacks the ability to detect sialoliths. Although a major advantage of HRUS is its relative safety because it does not use ionizing radiation, a major disadvantage lies in its inability to detect deep salivary gland lesions.

Multidetector Computed Tomography

MDCT with its ability to display both hard- and soft-tissue anatomy is useful in evaluating the salivary glands as well as the structures surrounding them (Fig. 30.5). This is especially true when the images are acquired after intravenous administration of a contrast agent that renders glandular tissues hyperdense relative to the surrounding fat and muscle.

MDCT is used in cases when inflammation of the salivary glands is suspected because it demonstrates characteristic features such as peripheral enhancement, thickening of the subcutaneous tissue, and lymph node involvement. Sialoliths can be depicted on MDCT images but only if they are relatively large and significantly calcified. Smaller, less-calcified sialoliths and changes to salivary gland ductal morphology are not well depicted given the resolution constraints of MDCT. MDCT imaging is excellent for detecting cysts and neoplasms but may not be reliable at distinguishing benign from malignant tumors.

Magnetic Resonance Imaging

Although indications for MRI occasionally overlap with those of MDCT, MRI is the imaging method of choice for assessment of space-occupying lesions (cyst and neoplasms) involving the salivary glands because of its superior soft-tissue contrast resolution (Fig. 30.6). Fat suppression sequences in MRI are often used to improve lesion contrast and demarcation with adjacent glandular tissue. In addition, the use of intravenous gadolinium as a contrast agent makes MRI the imaging modality of choice for evaluation of intracranial and perineural spread of salivary gland disease. Detection of sialoliths, particularly when calcified, is problematic in MRI because these calcified entities create low signal areas or signal voids. Other disadvantages of MRI include long acquisition times, relatively poor spatial resolution, cost, and accessibility.

Nuclear Medicine

Nuclear medicine examinations are functional examinations that takes advantage of the selective uptake of specific radiopharmaceuticals such as technetium 99m (^{99m}Tc)-pertechnetate (TPT) by the salivary glands when injected intravenously. The injection is followed by administration of a sialagogue to evaluate the secretory capacity of the salivary glands. Pathosis is determined on the basis of variations in the rate of TPT uptake or clearance. For example, Warthin tumor distinctively demonstrates reduced TPT clearance (Fig. 30.7).

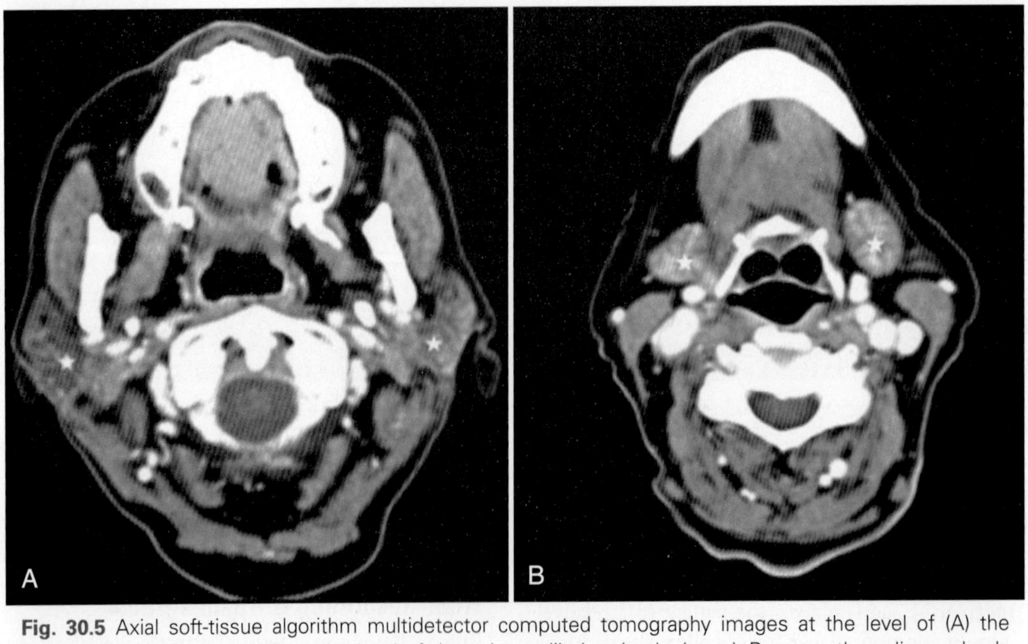

Fig. 30.5 Axial soft-tissue algorithm multidetector computed tomography images at the level of (A) the parotid glands *(stars)* and (B) at the level of the submandibular glands *(stars)*. Because the salivary glands have more fatty stroma than muscles, they appear less dense than adjacent muscles. (Courtesy Dr. K. Khashoggi, Jeddah, KSA.)

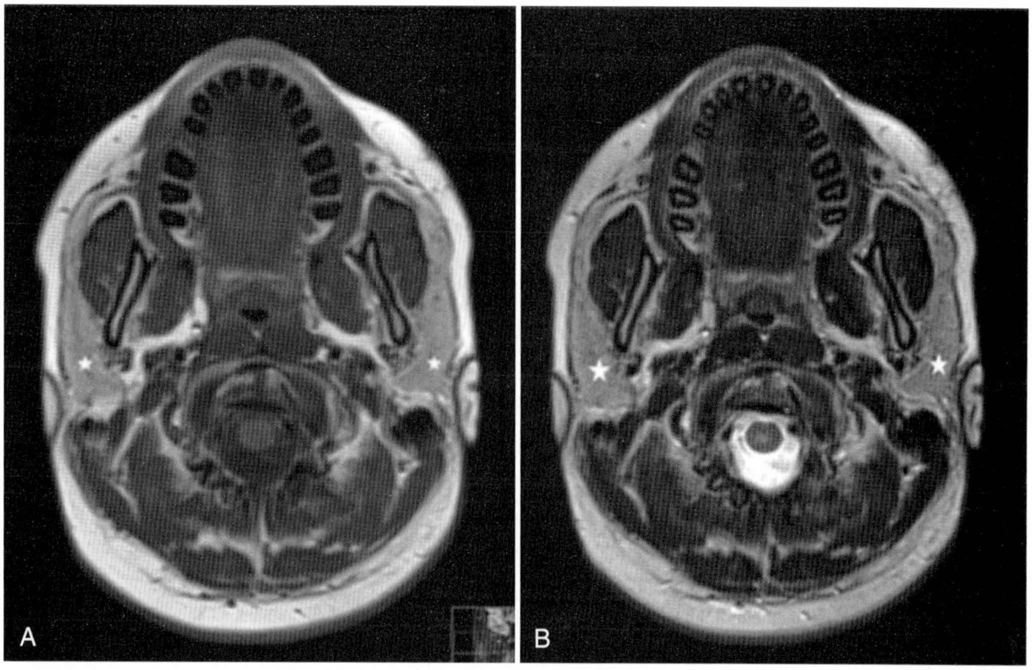

Fig. 30.6 Magnetic resonance imaging of normal parotid glands. (A) T_1-weighted image and (B) T_2-weighted image displaying the hyperintense signal of the parotid glands *(stars)* relative to the adjacent muscle. (Courtesy Dr. K. Khashoggi, Jeddah, KSA.)

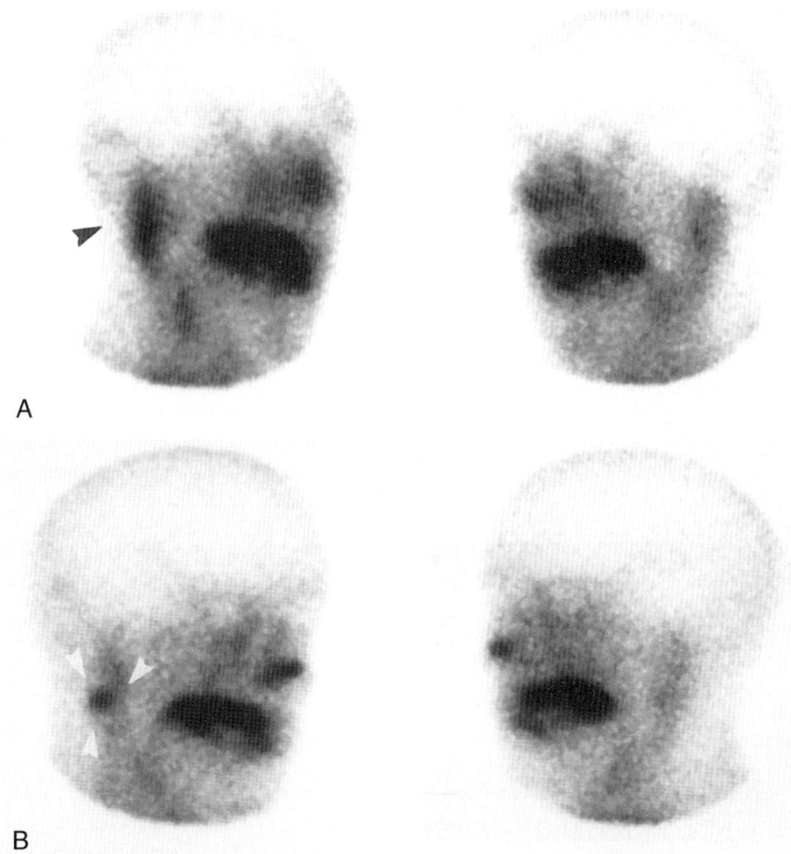

Fig. 30.7 Nuclear medicine technetium 99m (^{99m}Tc) pertechnetate (TPT) images of the salivary glands (right and left anterior oblique views) (A) demonstrate increased uptake in the right parotid gland *(black arrowhead).* (B) Nuclear medicine images obtained after administration of a sialagogue (lemon juice) demonstrate retention of TPT in the right parotid gland *(white arrowheads).* This is a typical presentation of a Warthin tumor.

Nuclear medicine is a highly sensitive technique that allows examination of all the major salivary glands at once; however, it lacks diagnostic specificity and poor image resolution makes assessment of the delicate gland morphology difficult.

Sialography

First performed in 1902, sialography is an imaging technique exclusively used for the major salivary glands. The technique involves infusion of the gland ductal system with an iodinated contrast agent and then imaging the gland with planar imaging, fluoroscopy, MDCT, or cone beam computed tomography (CBCT). The coupling of sialography with CBCT has resulted in three-dimensional images with submillimeter resolution and multiplanar capabilities that have revolutionized the visualization of the parotid and submandibular glands (Fig. 30.8). MRI may also be combined with sialography, but in these cases, the patients' own saliva is used as a contrast agent and the imaging is done using heavily weighted T_2 protocols.

Sialography is the only imaging technique that can assess the morphology of the glands as well as their function. The rate of clearance of the contrast agent from the gland at the conclusion of the procedure, especially when prolonged, is used as an indirect indicator of reduced secretory function. The primary indication for sialography is chronic inflammatory conditions, especially when obstruction is suspected. There are, however, two contraindications for sialography. The first of these is acute infection arising from the dispersal of the infection into otherwise unaffected regions within the gland as the contrast agent is introduced. This may also cause additional patient discomfort. The second contraindication is an immediately anticipated thyroid function test because the iodine in the contrast agent may concentrate in the thyroid gland and interfere with the results of the test.

Sialendoscopy

This examination involves direct visualization of the major salivary gland duct (Fig. 30.9), and since its first use in the 1990s, this technique has transformed the diagnosis and management of obstructive conditions of the glands. This minimally invasive technique introduces an endoscope into the orifice of a major salivary gland duct that can also be equipped with sialolith retrieval and stricture dilation tools. The technique has enabled management of these common conditions with reported success rates greater than 95%. Acute inflammation is the only known contraindication for this technique.

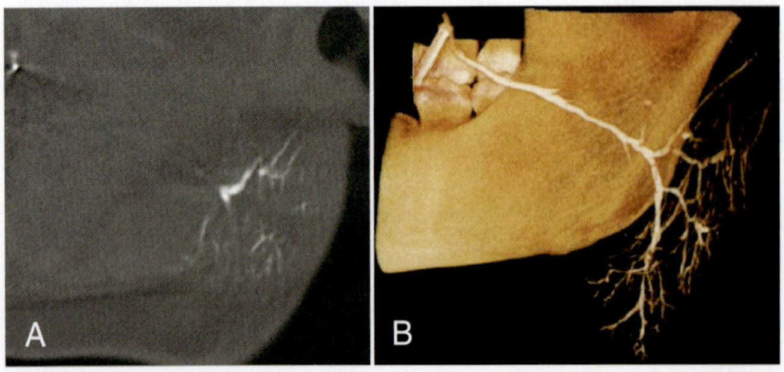

Fig. 30.8 Normal parotid gland sialography coupled with cone beam computed tomography. (A) Corrected sagittal image of a left parotid gland illustrating the branching pattern of the ductal structures. (B) Three-dimensional rendering of the ductal system of the gland showing the delicate branching pattern of the ducts.

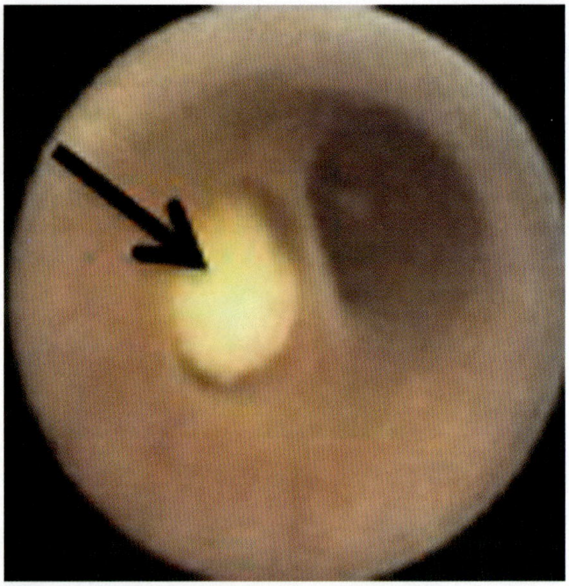

Fig. 30.9 Sialendoscopy allows direct visualization of the parotid and submandibular gland ducts. This particular image demonstrates a sialolith *(arrow)* in one of the branching ducts. (Courtesy Dr. F. Marchal, Geneva, Switzerland.)

CONDITIONS AFFECTING THE SALIVARY GLANDS

Inflammatory Conditions

Inflammation is by far the most common disorder to affect the salivary glands in both adults and children, although the cause of the inflammation differs between these two populations of patients. In adults, the inflammatory condition most often arises due to local obstruction, whereas in children, it is often due to a viral infection. In general, inflammatory conditions of the salivary glands are either acute or chronic. Causes of acute inflammation are typically bacterial or viral infections, whereas chronic inflammation can be caused by chronic local obstruction, autoimmune disorders, and systemic diseases.

Acute Bacterial Infections

Disease mechanism. Inflammation of the parenchymal portion of the salivary gland is termed sialadenitis, whereas inflammation of the ductal structures is termed sialodochitis or ductal sialadenitis.

Inflammation that results from an acute bacterial infection commonly results from reduced salivary secretion and subsequent retrograde infection of the glands by oral bacterial microorganisms (in particular, *Staphylococcus aureus, Streptococcus viridans,* and *Streptococcus pneumoniae*). Reduced salivary flow may be more common in the elderly, patients in postoperative care, and patients who may be dehydrated, diabetic, bulimic, or use medications such as diuretics and antidepressants.

Clinical features. The parotid glands are most commonly affected because the Stensen duct orifice is larger than that of other salivary gland orifices, making it more permissible to retrograde infection. In addition, parotid secretions are not as rich as other salivary gland secretions with respect to antibacterial substances such as immunoglobulin A. Unilateral involvement is more common than bilateral involvement, and the usual presenting sign is that of a tender swelling of both the infected gland and its draining lymph nodes. A purulent discharge may also be noted at the orifice of the gland duct.

Imaging features. Contrast-enhanced MDCT is the imaging of choice when acute inflammation of the major salivary glands is

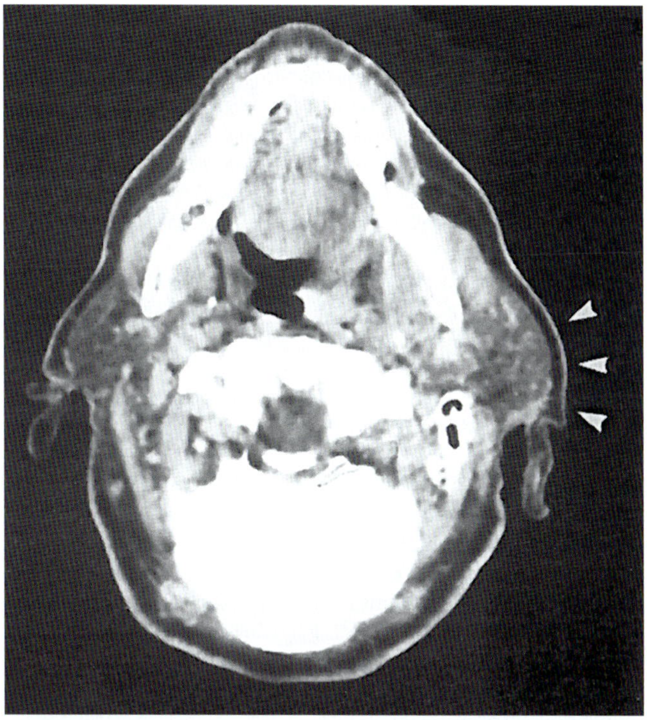

Fig. 30.10 Contrast-enhanced multidetector computed tomographic image depicting enhancement of the left parotid gland *(arrows)*, which is larger than the right, with no suggestion of abscess formation. This appearance is consistent with acute sialadenitis. (Courtesy Department of Radiology, Baylor University Medical Center, Dallas, TX.)

suspected. This type of imaging demonstrates the pathognomonic features of the condition, such as enlargement and enhancement of the affected gland, streaking of the adjacent fat tissue, and thickening of the subcutaneous tissues (Fig. 30.10). Involved lymph nodes may appear enlarged with a higher attenuation than normal. These imaging features are a reflection of the increased vascularity and exudate associated with the inflammatory process. If present, abscesses appear as well-defined areas of low attenuation with peripheral enhancement. MRI is the next imaging modality of choice for acute inflammation because it is unparalleled in its ability to differentiate edema from inflammatory infiltrate. Inflamed glands are usually enlarged and demonstrate a lower signal on T_1-weighted images and a higher signal on T_2-weighted images compared to the surrounding muscle.

Ultrasonography may also be helpful in distinguishing between diffuse inflammation and suppuration. HRUS may also demonstrate abscess cavities if present in the superficial lobes of the major salivary glands. Both sialography and scintigraphy are contraindicated in cases of acute inflammation because they may exacerbate the patient's pain and increase the risk of introducing the infective bacterial organism further into the involved gland.

Management. Treatment of bacterial sialadenitis is typically an appropriate antibiotic regimen. This should be combined with conservative measures such as good oral hygiene and increased fluid intake. Care must be taken not to delay treatment or treat inadequately because this may result in intraglandular abscess formation and the subsequent need for more aggressive treatment and surgical intervention.

Acute Viral Infections

Disease mechanism. A number of viruses may infect the salivary glands, including Epstein–Barr virus, cytomegalovirus, coxsackievirus, parainfluenza viruses, and herpes virus, but the mumps virus is by far the most common. Mumps is an illness that usually affects children between the ages of 5 and 9 years and is caused by a paramyxovirus infection. Epidemics of this infection became known by the term "epidemic parotitis" and were common before the advent of the measles, mumps, and rubella vaccine. Infected individuals usually go through an incubation period that ranges between 2 and 4 weeks and are considered contagious from 1 day before appearance of the clinical symptoms until approximately 14 days after resolution of the symptoms.

Clinical features. Approximately 70% of mumps cases are symptomatic and are preceded by a prodromal period of malaise, myalgia, anorexia, and low-grade fever. This is then followed by enlargement of the parotid glands primarily and intense pain, especially during chewing. The enlargement starts unilaterally but soon after can involve the contralateral side. Approximately 25% of cases demonstrate unilateral involvement, and 25% of cases develop complications such as epididymo-orchitis, meningoencephalitis, pancreatitis, thyroiditis, oophoritis, mastitis, and unilateral hearing loss.

Imaging features. Imaging findings are nonspecific, and the diagnosis is usually made on the basis of the clinical findings and the presence of serum antibodies to the mumps virus in the blood. MDCT images of the infected salivary glands demonstrate enlargement of the glands and with a slightly higher attenuation than normal. The enlarged glands also appear to have a slightly higher T_2-weighted MRI signal than normal.

Management. Treatment of mumps is palliative in nature and involves the administration of analgesics and antipyretics with bed rest. However, the best therapy is prevention, and vaccination is strongly recommended.

Chronic Inflammation

Disease mechanism. As with acute inflammation, *sialadenitis* and *sialodochitis* are used in a similar manner in chronic inflammation. Two thirds of all cases of chronic inflammation in the salivary glands are caused by chronic obstruction of the gland. The causes of obstruction may be further subdivided into primary and secondary causes. The primary causes include salivary stones (sialoliths), ductal narrowing (strictures), and mucous plugs, whereas secondary causes include trauma to the ductal structures or space-occupying lesions impinging on the ductal structures.

Sialoliths are not only the most common cause of chronic inflammation, but they are also the most common condition to affect the salivary glands in adults. Although the development of sialoliths is not well understood, sialoliths may begin as a nidus of inorganic calcium and phosphorus crystals, organic material, or necrotic cell material upon which organic and inorganic substances from the saliva are deposited. Strictures are the second most common cause of chronic inflammation, and although their etiology is still unknown, ductal narrowing is thought to be the result of fibrosis that occurs secondary to sialoliths, recurrent infections, or minor trauma.

Clinical features. It is estimated that approximately 1% of the population have sialoliths, but the peak incidence occurs between the fourth and sixth decades of life. Approximately 83% of sialoliths form in the ducts of the submandibular glands because of their tortuous upward pathway that ends in a relatively narrow orifice. This, in addition to the viscous nature of submandibular saliva, its high pH, and its high mineral content, is believed to contribute to the higher incidence of sialoliths in the submandibular gland ducts.

Obstruction generally results in the accumulation of the saliva produced by the affected gland, proximal to (i.e., closest to the gland parenchyma) the obstruction site, leading to dilatation of that segment of the salivary duct. This dilatation reaches a maximum size during mealtimes when large amounts of saliva are rapidly produced and excreted. Shortly after the meal, the saliva slowly finds its way around the point of obstruction and into the oral cavity. It is thought that this repeated process of saliva obstruction and buildup results in permanent dilatation of the salivary ducts (sialectasia). Stagnation of saliva in these distended portions of ducts may predispose the gland to repeated retrograde entry of oral bacterial microorganisms. Therefore, patients with chronic obstruction usually present with a history of unilateral intermittent tender swelling in the area of the affected salivary gland, especially during mealtimes.

Imaging features. Planar images such as panoramic images are used to identify sialoliths, which appear as well defined, mixed radiolucent and radiopaque, or completely radiopaque entities in the vicinity of the involved salivary gland. Unfortunately, up to 40% of sialoliths may not be calcified enough to be visible on planar images.

Sialography is the imaging modality of choice for chronic inflammation because of its ability to depict sialoliths (even small noncalcified ones), strictures, and subtle changes in the delicate ductal structures of glands. The injection of contrast agent into the ductal system is meant to replicate the patient's symptoms; however, the procedure must be performed during a quiescent period of inflammation so as not to exacerbate the patient's symptoms. One of the typical appearances of chronic inflammation is the "sausage-like" appearance of the salivary gland duct that represents alternating regions of stricture (i.e., obstruction) and sialectasia (Fig. 30.11). Another typical appearance is of globular collections of contrast that represent abscess formation (Fig. 30.12). These differ from the globular collections of contrast encountered in autoimmune sialadenitis by being variable in size and nonuniform in distribution throughout the gland parenchyma. MDCT and MRI may also be used in cases of chronic inflammation, but their sensitivity for detecting small sialoliths and strictures is inferior to sialography. Sialendoscopy is quickly becoming the preferred imaging method for obstructive conditions of the salivary glands because of the added advantage it offers in terms of managing these conditions.

Management. Management of chronic inflammation depends on the type of obstruction causing it, its location, and its effect on the surrounding salivary gland structures. In general, patients are instructed to remain hydrated and to stimulate salivary production and secretion to encourage spontaneous discharge. If conservative methods fail, more invasive methods are used, such as endoscopic basket retrieval of sialoliths and balloon ductoplasty. The last resort is complete surgical removal of the affected salivary gland.

Noninflammatory and Inflammatory-Like Conditions

Three particular conditions (sialadenosis, autoimmune sialadenitis, postirradiation sialadenitis) are of interest because they often present with signs and symptoms that are similar to obstructive conditions of the salivary glands and thus must be differentiated from them.

Sialadenosis

Disease mechanism. Sialadenosis or sialosis is a nonneoplastic, noninflammatory enlargement of the salivary gland, primarily the parotid glands. Causes of this condition include a variety of endocrine disorders such as diabetes mellitus, alcohol use disorder, and certain medications such as nonsteroidal antiinflammatory drugs. The enlargement itself is due to hypertrophy of the salivary acini.

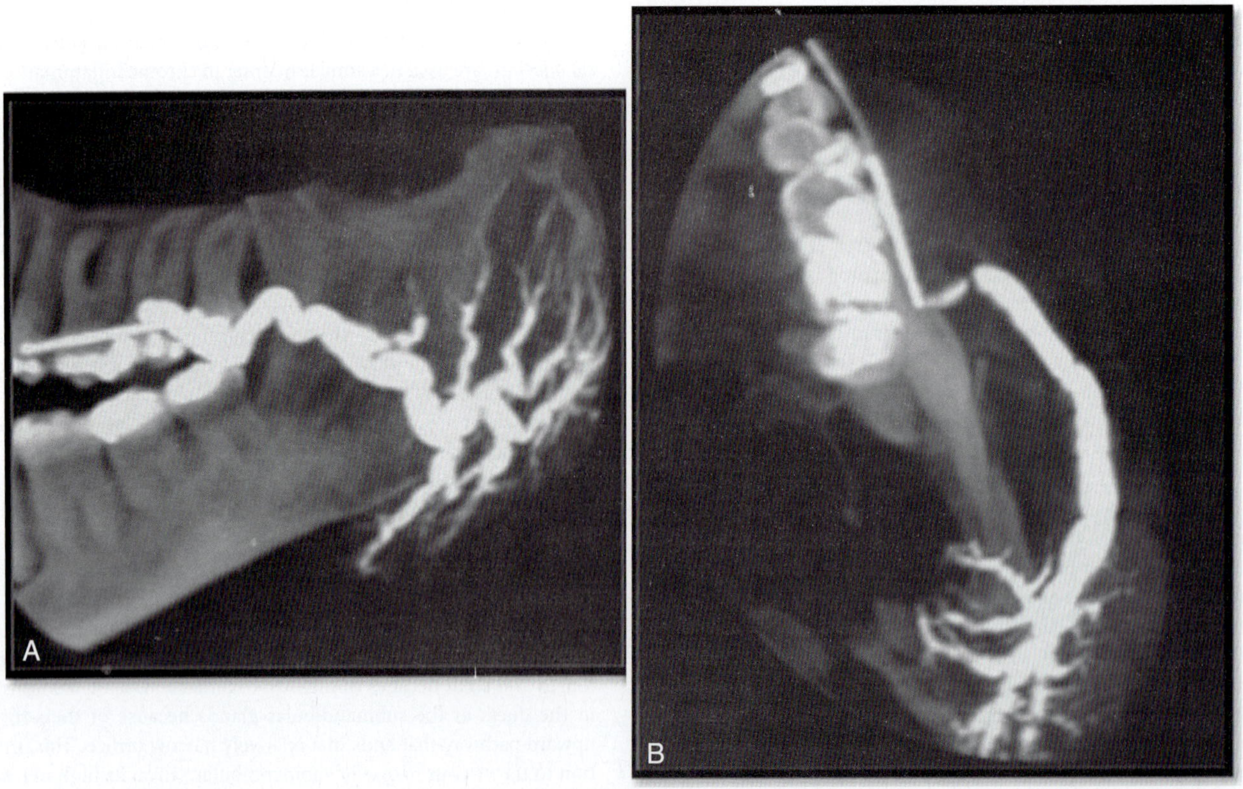

Fig. 30.11 Sialography of the left parotid gland imaged with cone beam computed tomography. Three dimensional reconstructions viewed from the lateral (A) and inferior (B) perspectives of the dilated ducts. A filling defect in the proximal portion of the Stensen duct (B) suggests a minimally calcified sialolith. Intermittent strictures and dilatation of the main and secondary ducts are typical of sialodochitis.

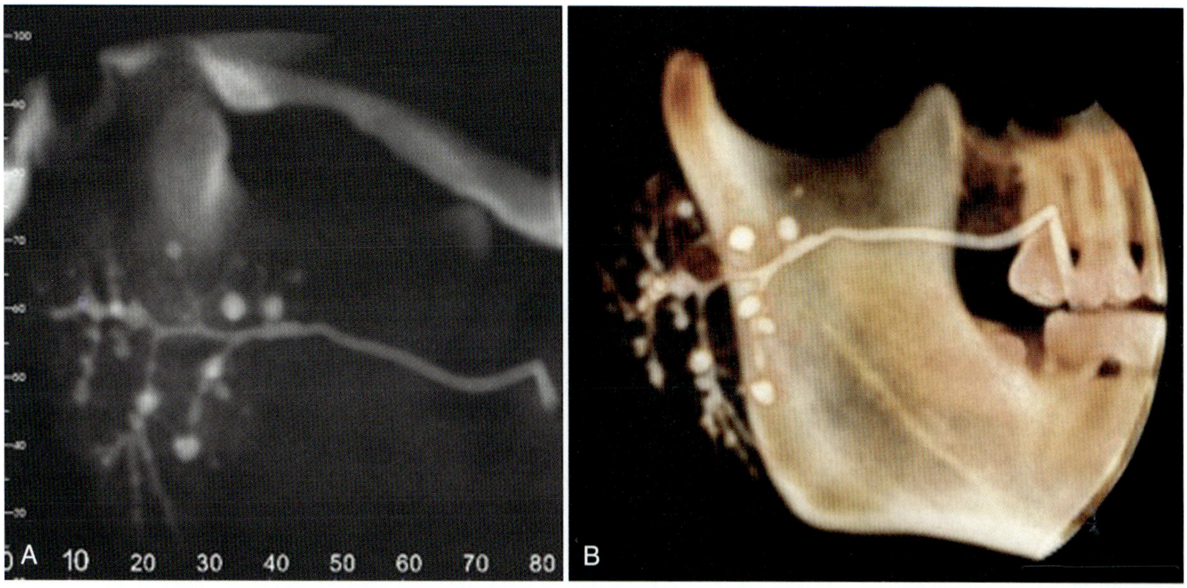

Fig. 30.12 Cone beam computed tomography sialography of the right parotid gland. (A) Sagittal and (B) three-dimensional reconstructed images showing several variably sized globular collections of contrast material. These represent abscesses in a case of chronic sialadenitis.

Clinical features. Because this condition is systemic in nature, bilateral involvement of the salivary glands is common. The enlargement is usually chronic or recurring and is largely painless. Patients with this condition often complain of xerostomia.

Imaging features. MDCT and MRI can demonstrate the nonspecific enlargement of the affected salivary glands and the fibrous or fatty changes in the salivary glands that may occur during different stages of the disease. Sialography can depict more specific findings such as splaying or displacement of otherwise normal caliber ducts (Fig. 30.13). This appearance is due to the ductal structures being pushed by the hypertrophied parenchyma.

Management. The management of sialadenosis relies on the identification and management of the primary cause of the condition. Local measures that can be taken include increased fluid intake, massage, and the use of sialagogues.

Autoimmune Sialadenitis

Disease mechanism. Sjögren syndrome, otherwise known as sicca syndrome or autoimmune sialosis, is an autoimmune disease of the exocrine glands that primarily affects the salivary and lacrimal glands resulting in a significant reduction in their secretions. The term "sicca" references dry eyes and mouth. The syndrome is characterized by a periductal lymphocytic infiltrate that destroys the acini of exocrine glands. The lymphocytic infiltrate may also produce a solid mass within the gland parenchyma, usually the parotid, known as a benign lymphoepithelial lesion (BLEL).

Clinical features. Sjögren syndrome is the second most common autoimmune condition after rheumatoid arthritis. Approximately 90% of cases are diagnosed in females between the fourth and sixth decades of life. There are two forms of the syndrome, a primary form that involves only the salivary and lacrimal glands (also known as sicca syndrome) and a secondary form that is associated with other connective tissue autoimmune conditions such as rheumatoid arthritis or systemic lupus erythematosus. The involved salivary glands are usually enlarged, but the patient's usual complaint is related to xerostomia. Patients with Sjögren syndrome are at a greater risk of developing mucosa-associated lymphoid tissue (MALT) lymphoma, a subtype of non-Hodgkin lymphoma.

Imaging features. Sialography, in the early stages of the disease, demonstrates a normal ductal system and numerous punctate (<1 mm in diameter) collections of contrast material distributed evenly throughout the gland (Fig. 30.14). These early changes are not evident on MDCT or MRI. As the disease progresses, the ducts become narrow and the collections of contrast material become larger (1–2 mm in diameter) and more globular. This appearance is pathognomonic and is termed "pruning of the tree" or "leafless fruit-laden tree" (Fig. 30.15). Typically, these collections of contrast material remain after administration of a sialagogue, which is an indication that the material is pooled extraductally. MDCT imaging in the later stages of the disease demonstrates enlarged and dense glands. On MRI, well-defined globular areas with low T_1 signal intensity and high T_2 signal intensity are seen throughout the gland.

Management. The management of autoimmune disorders of the salivary glands is directed toward relief of the patient's symptoms. Salivary stimulants, increased fluid intake, and artificial saliva and tears are some of the measures used to control the symptoms.

Postirradiation Sialadenitis

Disease mechanism. This condition is seen following both external beam radiation therapy of the head and neck and following intravenous delivery of radioactive iodine-131 (^{131}I) for the management of specific thyroid conditions. Following both types of treatment, an intense inflammatory reaction arises in the salivary glands, and parenchymal cell death and ductal fibrosis lead to impingement and obstruction of the ductal structures.

Clinical features. The typical presentation is tender bilateral swelling of the parotid glands because of the large numbers of serous-producing cells, the most radiosensitive secretory cell within the salivary glands. This is usually accompanied by progressive xerostomia and, ultimately, atrophy and fibrosis of the gland.

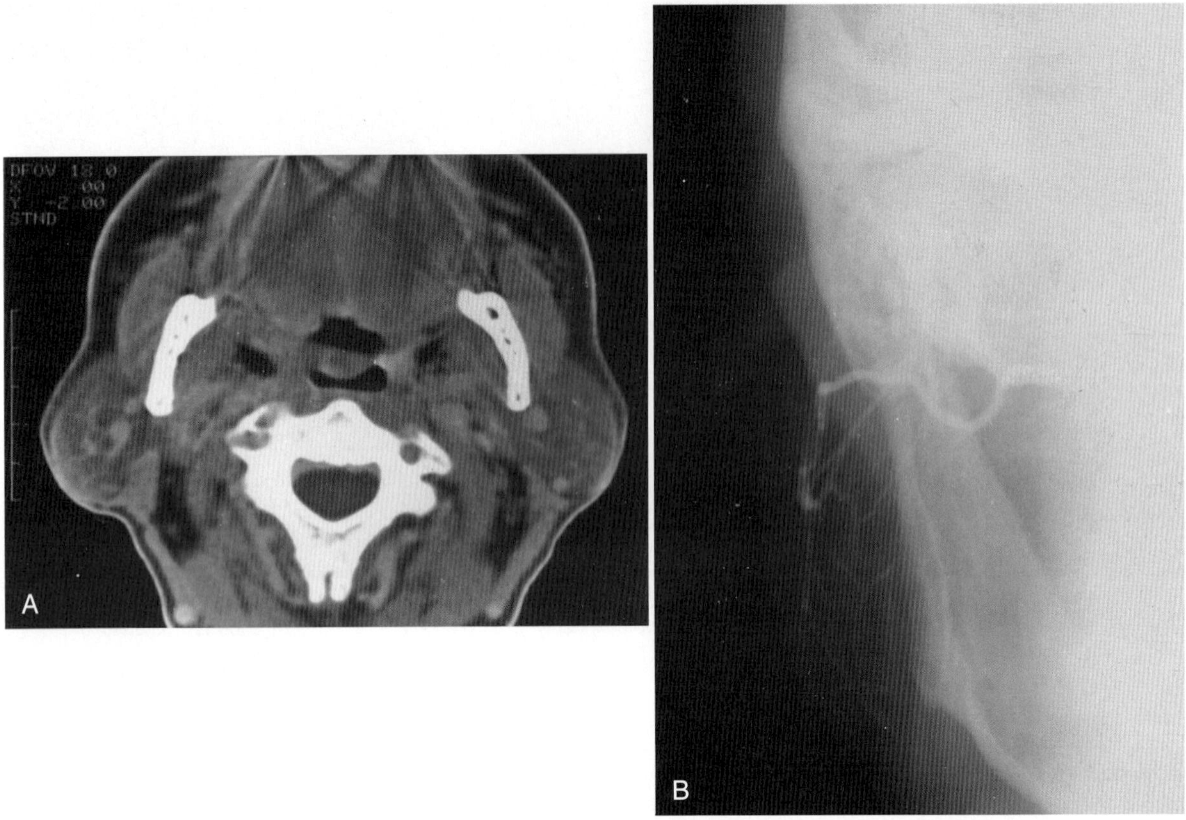

Fig. 30.13 Sialadenosis. (A) Multidetector computed tomographic image demonstrating bilateral enlargement of the parotid glands. The attenuation of the parotid glands appears normal. (B) Anteroposterior skull image of a sialogram of the right parotid gland in the same patient. The size and shape of the ducts appear normal, but they have been splayed and displaced laterally, a finding that is consistent with sialadenosis.

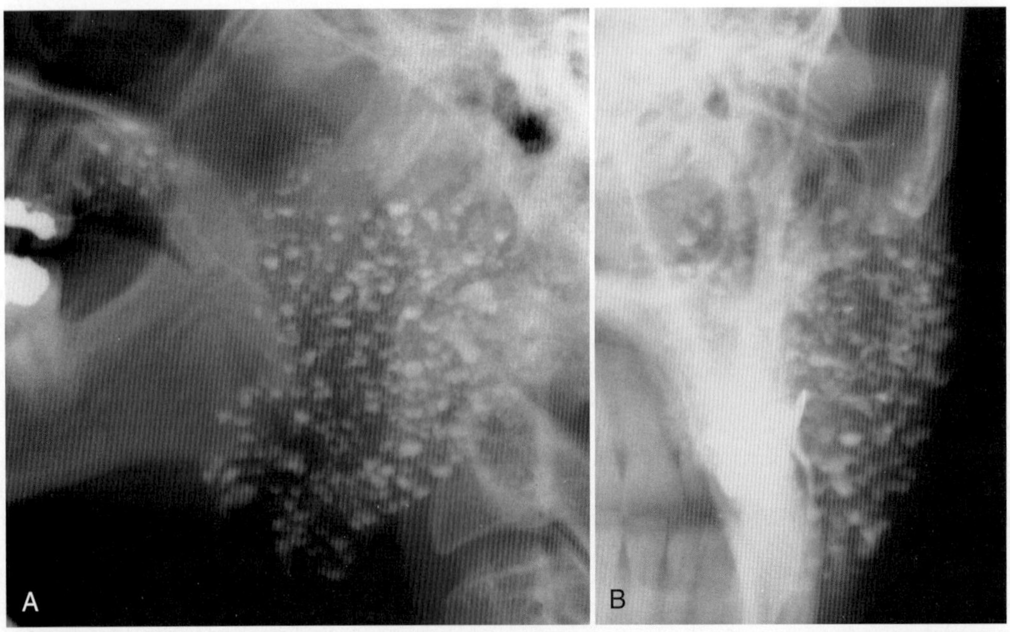

Fig. 30.14 Autoimmune sialadenitis. (A) Lateral skull image and (B) anteroposterior skull image of a left parotid gland sialogram revealing numerous punctate collections of contrast material distributed throughout the gland parenchyma including the accessory lobe, superimposed over the maxillary tuberosity. This appearance is consistent with the early stages of autoimmune sialadenitis.

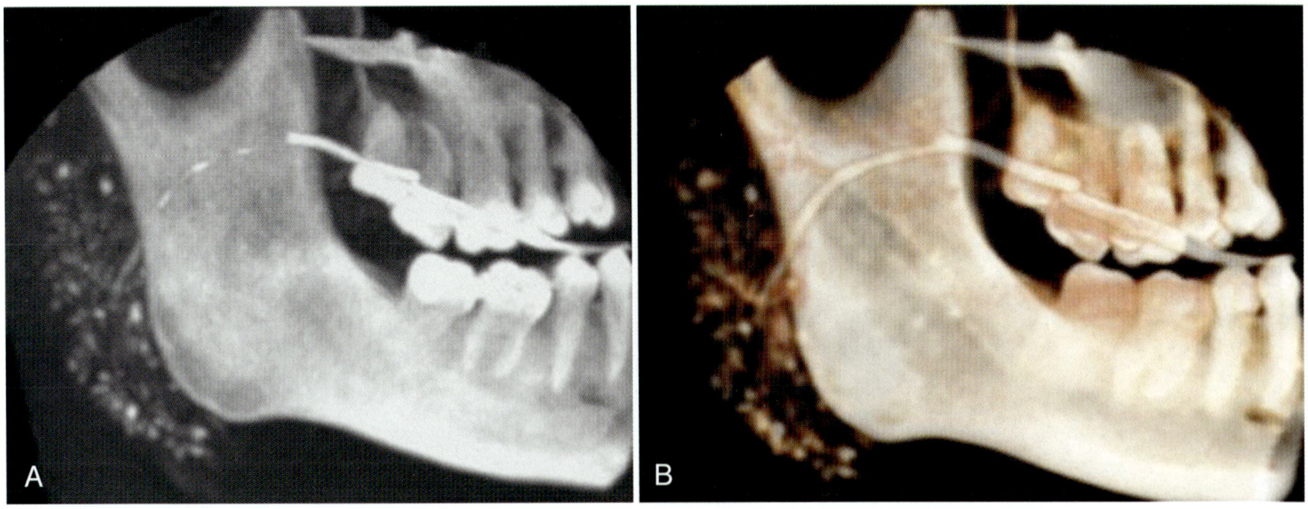

Fig. 30.15 Cone beam computed tomography sialography of the right parotid gland. (A) Sagittal image and (B) three-dimensional reconstruction of the same gland illustrating the typical appearance of autoimmune sialadenitis with multiple equally sized globular collections scattered homogenously throughout the parenchyma of the gland.

Imaging features. The MDCT and MRI findings depend on the stage of the disease at the time of imaging, and these are likely to exhibit varying degrees of gland fibrosis. Early sialogram studies demonstrate flow voids in the parenchyma where atrophy of the acini has started to occur. Sialographic studies in late stages of the disease may not even be possible due to complete obstruction of the ducts due to fibrosis (Fig. 30.16). Nuclear medicine examinations in the early stages reveal normal uptake but delayed excretion of TPT.

Management. The best management for this condition is prevention. In cases of external beam radiation therapy, measures should be taken to shield gland tissue from the tumoricidal dose. These protected areas of the glands may later undergo hypertrophy and compensate for the decrease in salivary flow from the irradiated areas. Unfortunately, shielding is not possible with ^{131}I treatment, but local measures (increased fluid intake, saliva substitutes) are helpful at relieving patients' symptoms.

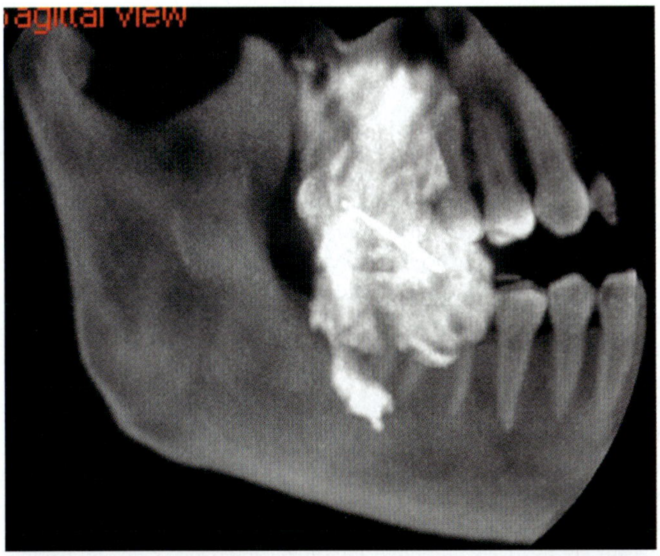

Fig. 30.16 Three-dimensional reconstruction of a right parotid gland sialogram using cone beam computed tomography. The contrast material is seen infusing only the accessory lobe of the parotid but not the ducts or the acini of the superficial and deep lobes of the gland. These findings are consistent with fibrosis because this patient had a history of radioactive iodine therapy. Note the increased size of the accessory lobe due to hypertrophy to compensate for the lack of salivary secretions.

Space-Occupying Conditions

Cystic Lesions

Disease mechanism. Cysts of the salivary glands are rare (<5% of all salivary gland masses). They may be congenital (branchial, lymphoepithelial, dermoid) or acquired (sialocysts and acquired immunodeficiency syndrome [AIDS]-related parotid cysts [ARPCs]).

Sialocysts are true cysts that form in the salivary ducts when obstruction results in dilatation due to retention of saliva within the duct. These are also known as retention cysts, mucous retention cysts, ductal cysts, and salivary ductal cysts. In contrast, a sialocele or mucocoele is a pseudocyst that forms as a result of injury to a salivary duct with extravasation of saliva into the adjacent connective tissue. The terminology of these two conditions (sialocyst and sialocele) is often used interchangeably (and incorrectly) in the literature, but their differing pathophysiologies are well understood and documented. Finally, the term *ranula* is reserved for cysts of the sublingual glands regardless of whether the cyst is a true cyst (usually located in the oral cavity) or a pseudocyst (plunging inferiorly, beyond the mylohyoid muscle).

ARPCs are an important entity for dentists because they may be the first manifestation of an HIV infection. Their pathophysiology is still controversial, but their incidence has decreased with highly active antiretroviral therapy (HAART).

Clinical features. Congenital cysts are usually identified later in life, despite being present at birth. Most cysts are unilateral except for ARPCs, which are bilateral in distribution. Similarly, most cysts affect the parotid salivary glands except for sialoceles, which are more common in minor salivary glands.

Imaging features. Cysts may be indirectly visualized on sialography by an arching displacement of the salivary ducts around the cyst, producing an appearance termed "ball-in-hand." Cystic lesions typically appear as well circumscribed, low attenuation, nonenhancing areas on contrast enhanced MDCT images, whereas by MRI, they appear as

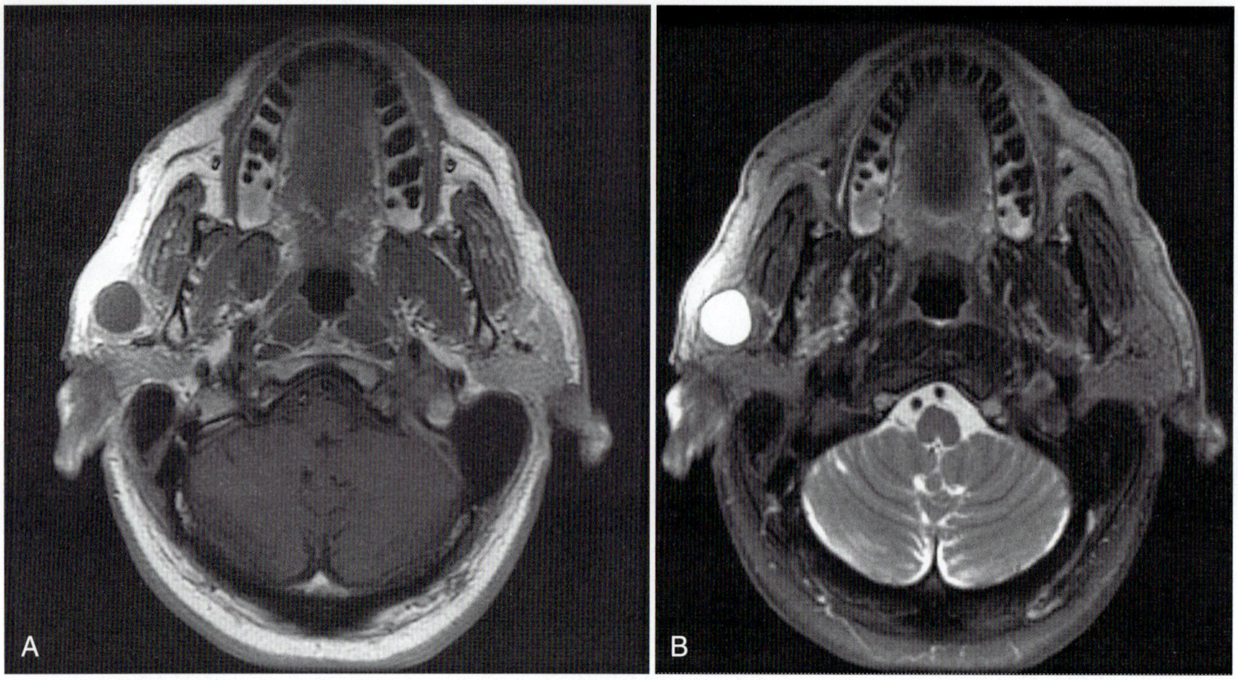

Fig. 30.17 Magnetic resonance imaging reveals a lymphoepithelial cyst involving the right parotid gland. (A) Axial T_1-weighted image depicting a well-defined lesion involving the right parotid gland with an internal signal isointense to muscle. (B) Matching T_2-weighted image depicting the lesion with a high signal intensity because of its fluid content.

well circumscribed, high-signal areas on T2-weighted images, which do not enhance after contrast administration (Fig. 30.17).

Management. Management of cysts of the salivary glands is typically surgical removal of the cyst or the entirety of the involved salivary gland.

Benign Neoplasms

Disease mechanism. Salivary gland neoplasms are uncommon, accounting for less than 3% of all head and neck neoplasms. Approximately 80% of these arise in the parotid gland, 5% arise in the submandibular gland, 1% arise in the sublingual gland, and 10%–15% arise in the minor salivary glands. The likelihood of neoplasms of the salivary glands being benign varies directly with the size of the gland. Therefore, most neoplasms of the salivary glands are benign or low-grade malignancies.

Pleomorphic adenoma is by far the most common neoplasm of the salivary glands, accounting for 75% of all salivary gland neoplasms. It is a benign neoplasm of the salivary ductal epithelium with both epithelial and mesenchymal components and hence is also referred to as a benign mixed tumor. The second most common benign neoplasm is Warthin tumor, more accurately known as papillary cystadenoma lymphomatosum. In children, the most common neoplasm of the salivary glands is hemangioma.

Clinical features. Benign neoplasms typically present as unilateral, slow growing, relatively painless masses. Warthin tumor uniquely affects the salivary glands bilaterally.

Imaging features. MRI is the preferred imaging modality for salivary gland neoplasms because of its superior soft-tissue contrast. MDCT is a reasonable imaging alternative, especially with contrast administration. Benign neoplasms generally appear to have well-defined margins and variable internal signal or attenuation, depending on the predominant tissue of the neoplasm (Fig. 30.18). Intravenous contrast administration causes enhancement of the neoplasm because the vascularity of the neoplasm is greater than that of the adjacent salivary gland tissue. Like cysts, sialography indirectly suggests a space-occupying mass with the ball-in-hand appearance (Fig. 30.19).

Management. The management of benign neoplasms of the major salivary glands is surgical. Benign neoplasms of the parotid gland are usually excised with the intention of preserving the gland to avoid facial nerve deficits. The submandibular and sublingual glands are invariably totally excised with the benign neoplasm.

Malignant Neoplasms

Disease mechanism. Approximately 20% of neoplasms in the parotid glands are malignant compared to 50%–60% of submandibular neoplasms, 90% of sublingual neoplasms, and 60%–75% of minor salivary gland neoplasms. The most common malignant neoplasm of the salivary glands is mucoepidermoid carcinoma, followed by adenoid cystic carcinoma. Mucoepidermoid carcinoma is composed of a variable admixture of mucous and epidermoid cells arising from the ductal epithelium of the salivary glands. Adenoid cystic carcinoma is composed of myoepithelial and ductal cells and has a great propensity to extend along nerves.

Clinical features. The aggressiveness of malignant neoplasms varies with their histopathologic grade. The low-grade variety presents clinically as a slowly growing, painless movable mass. These low-grade malignancies rarely metastasize and have good prognosis, with a 5-year survival rate greater than 95%. In contrast, high-grade neoplasms are relatively immobile and often cause facial pain and paralysis. They also spread locally via nerves, metastasize via blood and lymph, and have high recurrence rates and poor prognosis with a 5-year survival rate of approximately 25%.

Imaging features. The imaging presentation of malignant neoplasms is variable and is related to the grade, aggressiveness, location, and type of neoplasm. In many cases, the low-grade variety has a sialography,

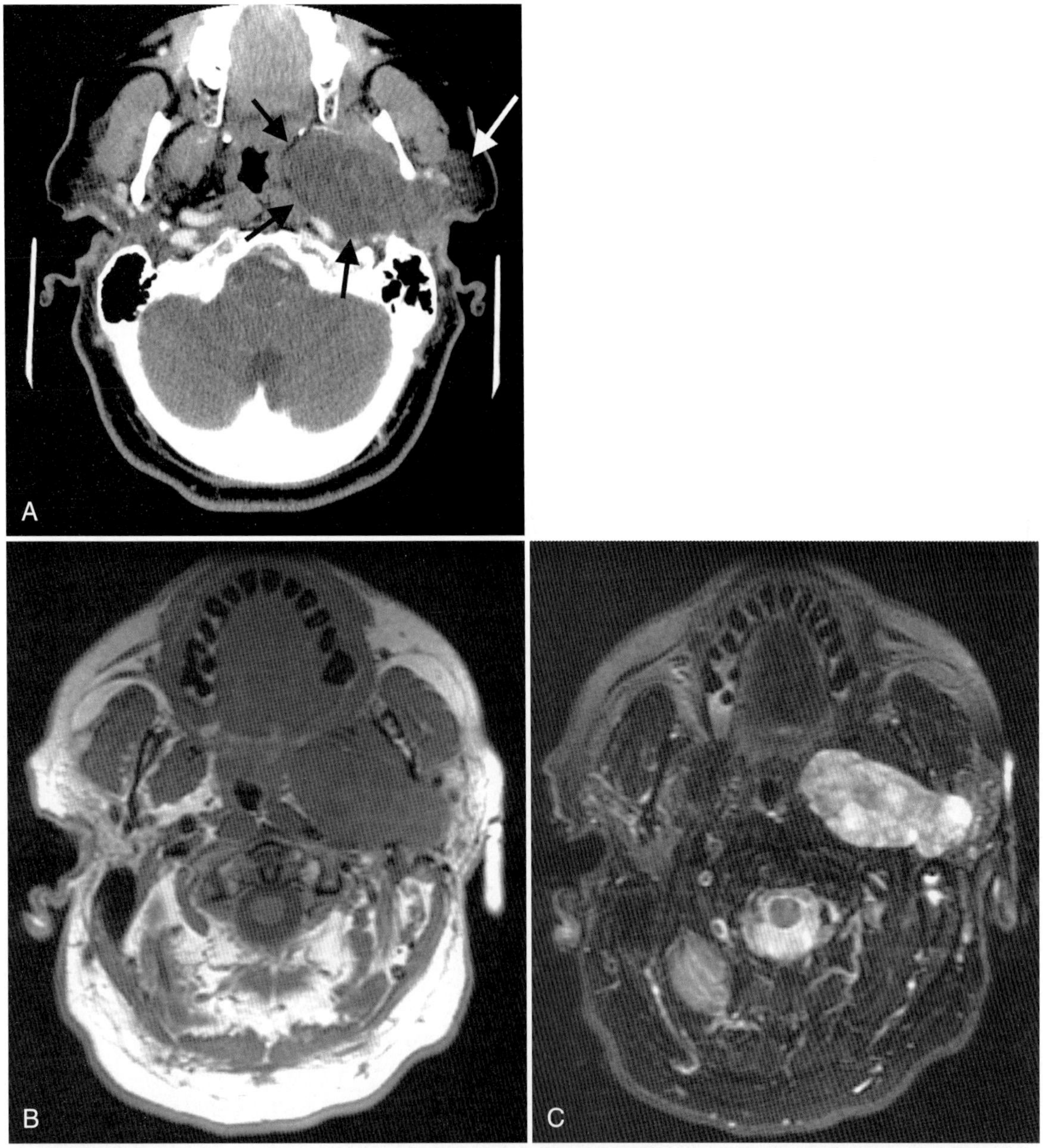

Fig. 30.18 Multidetector computed tomography (MDCT) and magnetic resonance imaging (MRI) of a pleomorphic adenoma in the left parotid gland. (A) Axial soft-tissue algorithm MDCT image. Note the well-defined periphery *(black arrows)* and the internal density that is less than surrounding muscles. The remaining parotid gland *(white arrow)* is displaced laterally. (B) T1-weighted MRI. The tissue signal of the neoplasm is isointense with muscle. (C) T2-weighted MRI. The tissue signal of the neoplasm is heterogenous but generally hyperintense to muscle.

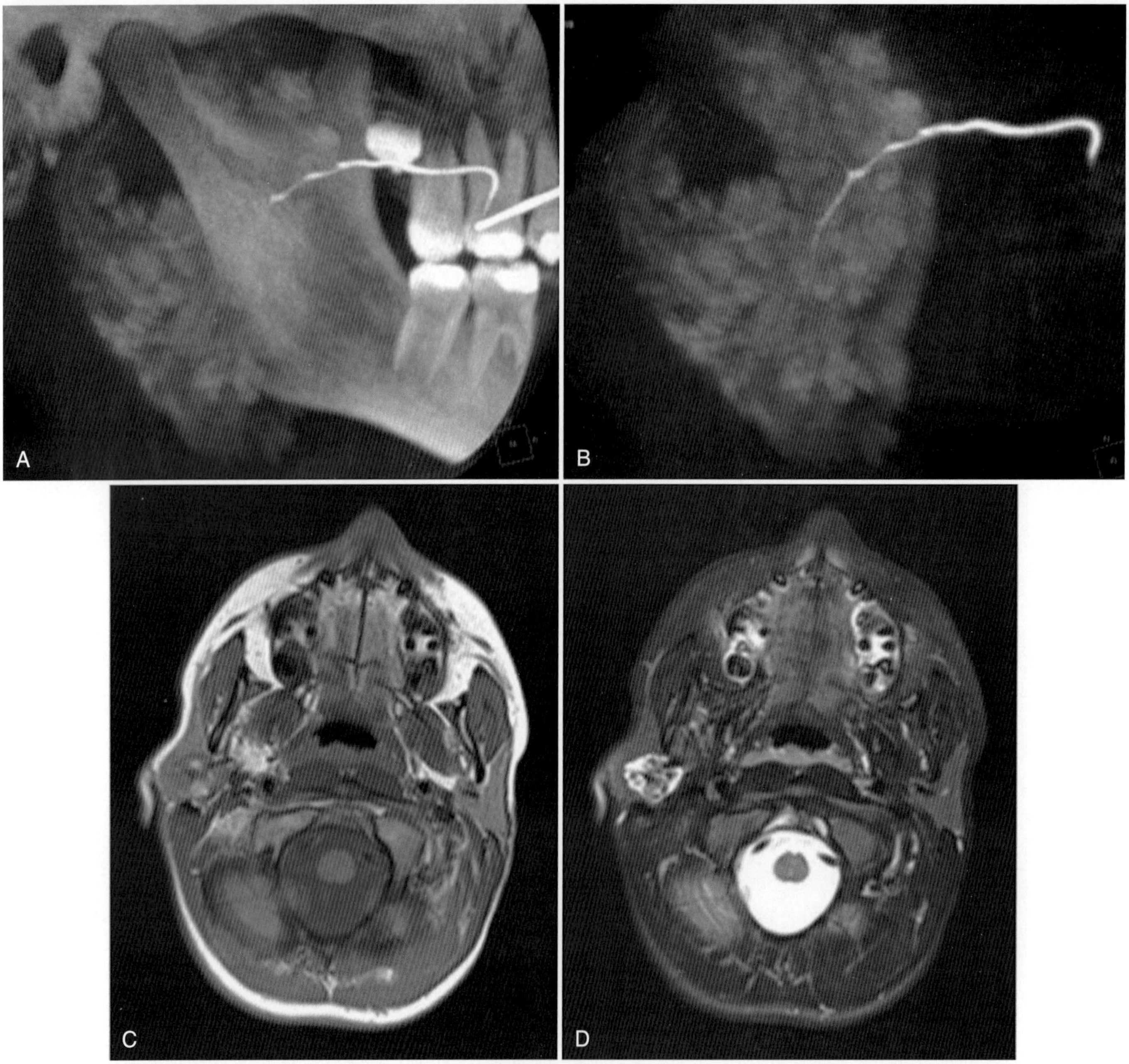

Fig. 30.19 Filling void in these three-dimensional reconstructions from a cone beam computed tomography sialogram of the right parotid gland in a 16-year-old patient with (A) and without (B) the adjacent osseous structures. (C and D) Matched T_1-weighted and T_2-weighted magnetic resonance imaging of the same gland, respectively, demonstrating a vascular neoplasm with flow voids consistent with a hemangioma.

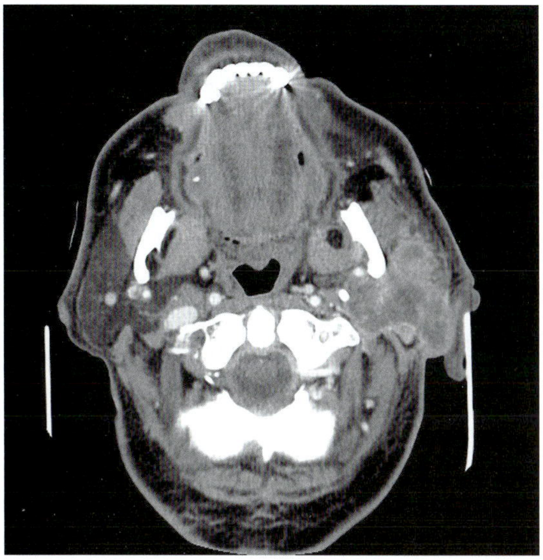

Fig. 30.20 Axial soft-tissue algorithm multidetector computed tomographic image reveals an adenocarcinoma of the left parotid gland. Almost all of the gland has been replaced by this ill-defined neoplasm that has some peripheral enhancement and areas of low density internally, likely representing necrotic regions.

MDCT, MRI, and HRUS presentation that is similar to benign salivary neoplasms. However, features such as ill-defined margins and invasion and destruction of adjacent structures, when seen, are considered to be typical indicators of a high-grade malignancy (Fig. 30.20).

Management. Management of malignant neoplasms of the major salivary glands is typically surgical, often requiring complete excision of the involved gland and a radical neck dissection. Combinations of surgery, therapeutic radiation, and chemotherapy may also be used.

BIBLIOGRAPHY

Douglas DJ, Perschbacher SE, Moayedi M, et al. Optimizing effective dose and image quality in cone beam CT sialography. *Oral Surg Oral Med Oral Pathol Oral Radiol.* 2023;135:686-697.

Drage NA, Brown JE, Escudier MP, et al. Interventional radiology in the removal of salivary calculi. *Radiology.* 2000;214(1):139-142.

Drage NA, Brown JE, Escudier MP, et al. Balloon dilatation of salivary duct strictures: report on 36 treated glands. *Cardiovasc Intervent Radiol.* 2002;25(5):356-359.

El-Khateeb SM, Abou-Khalaf AE, Farid MM, et al. A prospective study of three diagnostic sonographic methods in differentiation between benign and malignant salivary gland tumours. *Dentomaxillofac Radiol.* 2011;40(8): 476-485.

Friedman E, Cai Y, Chen B. Imaging of major salivary gland lesions and disease. *Oral Maxillofac Surg Clin North Am.* 2023;35:435-449.

Jadu FM, Lam EWN. The mystery of meal time swellings revealed. *Oral Health.* 2014;104(2):33-35.

Jadu FM, Jan AM. A meta-analysis of the efficacy and safety of managing parotid and submandibular sialoliths using sialendoscopy assisted surgery. *Saudi Med J.* 2014;35(10):1188-1194.

MacDonald A, Burrell S. Infrequently performed studies in nuclear medicine: part 2. *J Nucl Med Technol.* 2009;37(1):1-13.

Munhoz L, Ramos EADA, Im DC, et al. Application of diffusion-weighted magnetic resonance imaging in the diagnosis of salivary gland diseases: a systemic review. *Oral Surg Oral Med Oral Pathol Oral Radiol.* 2019; 128:280-310.

Nahlieli O, Nazarian Y. Sialadenitis following radioiodine therapy—a new diagnostic and treatment modality. *Oral Dis.* 2006;12(5):476-479.

Ngu RK, Brown JE, Whaites EJ, et al. Salivary duct strictures: nature and incidence in benign salivary obstruction. *Dentomaxillofac Radiol.* 2007;36(2): 63-67.

Turner MD. Sialoendoscopy and salivary gland sparing surgery. *Oral Maxillofac Surg Clin North Am.* 2009;21(3):323-329.

Wang KY, Wintermark M, Penta M. Imaging characteristics of Sjögren's syndrome. *Clin Imaging.* 2022;92:7-18.

Xu MJ, Chang JL. Practical salivary ultrasound imaging tips and pearls. *Otolaryngol Clin North Am.* 2021;54:471-487.

31 Dental Implants

Edwin Chang

Two significant advancements have revolutionized the modern practice of dentistry: the advent and progressive refinement of dental implant-supported protheses and the widespread application of three-dimensional computed tomography (CT) imaging. Oral and maxillofacial radiology plays an increasingly crucial role in the successful planning, placement, and long-term follow-up of dental implants. This chapter provides an overview of imaging techniques used in modern dental implantology and the contribution of radiologic imaging in the preoperative, intraoperative, and postoperative phases of treatment.

IMAGING TECHNIQUES

As with all diagnostic imaging examinations, the radiographic prescription must be guided by a thorough clinical examination and the proposed imaging study must maximize diagnostic benefit while minimizing radiation risk and cost. To aid in this decision-making process, clinicians must be familiar with the indications, advantages, and limitations of imaging techniques used in oral implantology (Table 31.1 and Box 31.1).

Intraoral Radiography

Intraoral radiography is often the first-line imaging modality in the dental setting. This includes periapical, bite-wing, and occlusal images. Periapical imaging is the most commonly used examination in all phases of dental implant evaluation (Fig. 31.1). For preoperative assessment, intraoral radiography provides an evaluation of osseous healing at the edentulous site. It identifies the presence of retained roots, residual periapical pathoses, and variants such as osteosclerosis, all of which complicate implant placement. Periapical radiographs allow adequate assessment of the status of the adjacent teeth and provide approximate mesiodistal and vertical distances to the adjacent anatomic boundaries and vital structures. As they are two-dimensional projection radiographs, periapical images do not provide information on the buccolingual dimension. In the past, occlusal radiographs were used to provide a basic assessment of the buccolingual contour of the mandible. However, the base of the mandibular body usually exhibits a wider buccolingual dimension than the alveolar process, resulting in overestimation of buccolingual bone width (Fig. 31.2). Anatomic limitations make occlusal radiographs ineffective in assessing edentulous sites in the maxilla. The increasing accessibility of three-dimensional CT has progressively reduced the contribution of occlusal images for such purposes.

The major advantages of intraoral radiography are its relatively low cost and near-negligible radiation risk; widespread availability in dental offices; excellent spatial resolution; and, in the case of solid-state–based digital systems, the possibility of instantaneous image generation. However, intraoral imaging is limited by its relatively narrow anatomic coverage and the inability to provide accurate three-dimensional analyses. Superimposition of contiguous structures makes it impractical to analyze the thickness of the buccal and lingual cortical plates and may obscure accurate visualization of crucial anatomic structures such as the inferior alveolar canal. Moreover, periapical imaging is subject to geometric distortion and magnification arising from elongation or foreshortening (see Chapters 5 and 6), which limits its use for linear measurements—a crucial objective of preoperative imaging for implant planning. Overall, intraoral radiography remains a valuable tool in the initial assessment of a single edentulous space or short edentulous span and should be considered as the first-line imaging modality in both intra- and postoperative phases of implant treatment.

Panoramic Imaging

Panoramic imaging is the second most commonly employed dental imaging technique because of its wide anatomic coverage, ease of acquisition, and relatively low cost. It provides a gross overview of the osseous structures of the maxillae and mandible, including the floors of the maxillary sinuses and the inferior alveolar canals—important structural considerations in posterior implant placement (Fig. 31.3). However, major limitations of panoramic imaging are image distortion and superimposition of ghost images. The degree of distortion is unpredictable—it depends on patient positioning and approximation of the patient's jaws within the standardized curvature of the focal trough. Structures located buccal to this predefined focal trough are distorted and appear narrow in the horizontal dimension, whereas structures located lingual to the focal trough will appear horizontally magnified. This nonuniform distortion precludes accurate mesiodistal measurements of the edentulous ridge and cannot be reliably corrected with software. Moreover, a vertical magnification of approximately 15%–30% is present, and the slight negative vertical angulation of the x-ray beam projects images of lingually positioned structures more superiorly on the image. However, much like intraoral imaging, the lack of three-dimensional capabilities precludes accurate assessment of the buccolingual dimension of available bone. Moreover, the resolution of panoramic images is lower than that of intraoral radiographs. Nevertheless, panoramic imaging is of value for the initial examination of a

TABLE 31.1 Commonly Used Imaging Techniques for Implant Placement

Imaging Technique	Advantages	Disadvantages	Recommendation
Periapical imaging	• Readily available • High resolution • Minimal distortion • Lowest financial cost and radiation exposure	• Restricted anatomic coverage • Cannot assess buccolingual dimension • Subject to elongation and foreshortening • Anatomic superimposition • Difficult to reproduce projection geometry • May be limited by patient compliance and anatomy	• Initial assessment of single edentulous space or short edentulous span • Intraoperative imaging during implant placement • Initial postoperative radiograph and recall imaging
Panoramic imaging	• Readily available • Broad anatomic coverage • Low financial cost and radiation exposure	• Image distortion • Anatomic superimposition and ghost images • Lower resolution • Cannot assess buccolingual dimension • Technique sensitive	• Initial examination of multiple edentulous spaces • Radiographic follow-up of multiple implants
CBCT imaging	• Variable field of view: from single edentulous site to full jaws (manufacturer dependent) • 3D tomographic imaging: no superimposition • Dimensionally accurate • Increasingly accessible • Simulate implant surgery with specialized software	• Moderate financial cost and radiation exposure • Susceptible to beam hardening artifacts • Technique sensitive (especially to patient motion) • Special training for interpretation • Not calibrated for bone density measurements (HU) • Poor soft tissue contrast	• Following initial examination, CBCT is recommended for thorough radiologic assessment • Recommended before and after bone augmentation • Postoperatively, recommended for symptomatic implants (implant mobility, altered sensation, displaced implant) • Not appropriate for asymptomatic recall imaging

3D, Three-dimensional; *CBCT,* cone beam computed tomography; *HU,* Hounsfield units.

BOX 31.1 American Academy of Oral and Maxillofacial Radiology Recommendations for Imaging the Dental Implant Patient

Recommendation 1. Panoramic radiography should be used as the imaging modality of choice in the initial evaluation of the dental implant patient.

Recommendation 2. Use intraoral periapical radiography to supplement the preliminary information from panoramic radiography.

Recommendation 3. Do not use cross-sectional imaging, including cone beam computed tomography (CBCT), as an initial diagnostic imaging examination.

Recommendation 4. The radiographic examination of any potential implant site should include cross-sectional imaging orthogonal to the site of interest.

Recommendation 5. CBCT should be considered as the imaging modality of choice for preoperative cross-sectional imaging of potential implant sites.

Recommendation 6. CBCT should be considered when clinical conditions indicate a need for augmentation procedures or site development before placement of dental implants: (1) sinus augmentation, (2) block or particulate bone grafting, (3) ramus or symphysis grafting, (4) assessment of impacted teeth in the field of interest, and (5) evaluation of prior traumatic injury.

Recommendation 7. CBCT imaging should be considered if bone reconstruction and augmentation procedures (e.g., ridge preservation or bone grafting) have been performed to treat bone volume deficiencies before implant placement.

Recommendation 8. In the absence of clinical signs or symptoms, use intraoral periapical radiography for the postoperative assessment of implants. Panoramic radiographs may be indicated for cases requiring more extensive implant therapy.

Recommendation 9. Use cross-sectional imaging (particularly CBCT) immediately postoperatively only if the patient presents with implant mobility or altered sensation, especially if the fixture is in the posterior mandible.

Recommendation 10. Do not use CBCT imaging for periodic review of clinically asymptomatic implants.

Recommendation 11. Cross-sectional imaging, optimally CBCT, should be considered if implant retrieval is anticipated.

From Tyndall DA, Price JB, Tetradis S, et al. Position statement of the American Academy of Oral and Maxillofacial Radiology on selection criteria for the use of radiology in dental implantology with emphasis on cone beam computed tomography. *Oral Surg Oral Med Oral Pathol Oral Radiol.* 2012;113:817-826.

dental implant patient, particularly when multiple implant sites are considered at once, or when intraoral images cannot be made due to difficult patient anatomy or poor patient cooperation. Guidelines from the American Academy of Oral and Maxillofacial Radiology recommend panoramic and intraoral radiography for the initial assessment of the dental implant placement.

Computed Tomography (Multidetector Computed Tomography and Cone Beam Computed Tomography)

CT is an imaging technique that generates three-dimensional cross-sectional views from multiple projections taken at several different angles around the patient. Currently, multidetector CT (MDCT) systems are used worldwide in hospitals and medical imaging centers. MDCT images are acquired with the patient supine on a table that advances through a rotating gantry (see Chapter 9). Although MDCT is used to evaluate several maxillofacial conditions, its higher cost, larger radiation dose, and limited accessibility to dentists have restricted its widespread adoption for the purposes of dental implant planning.

In the last two decades, cone beam CT (CBCT) has evolved to provide high-resolution three-dimensional information; it is now applied to several maxillofacial diagnostic objectives (see Chapter 9). CBCT

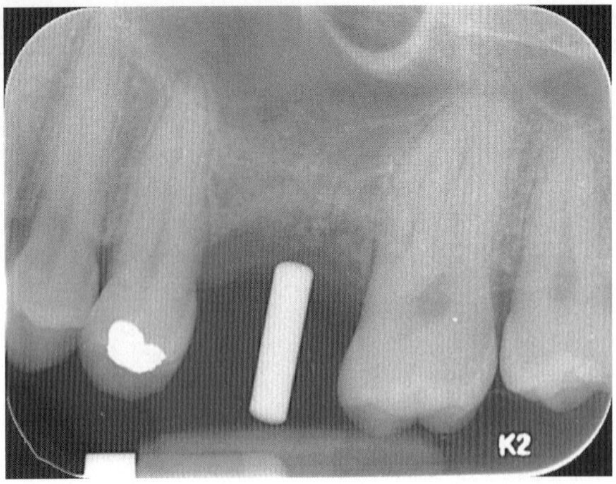

Fig. 31.1 Periapical image of a potential implant site in the posterior left maxilla. An imaging guide containing a cylindrical radiopaque marker has been inserted intraorally to depict the desired angle of implant placement.

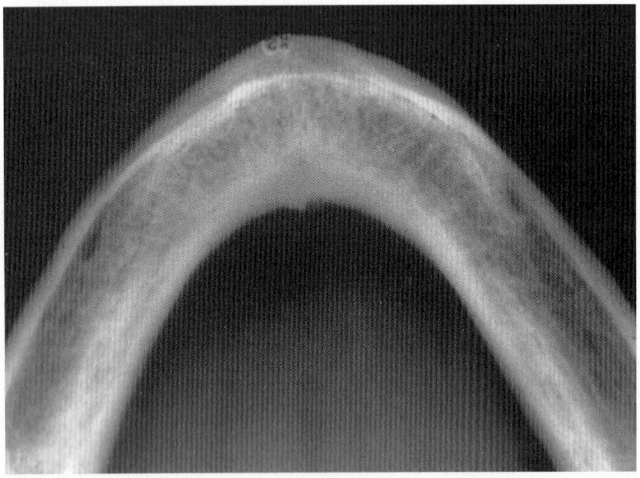

Fig. 31.2 Cross-sectional occlusal radiograph of the edentulous mandible. Note that only the widest buccolingual contours of the mandible are visualized; these are usually located inferior to the desired implant site. This could result in an overestimation of the amount of buccolingual bone available.

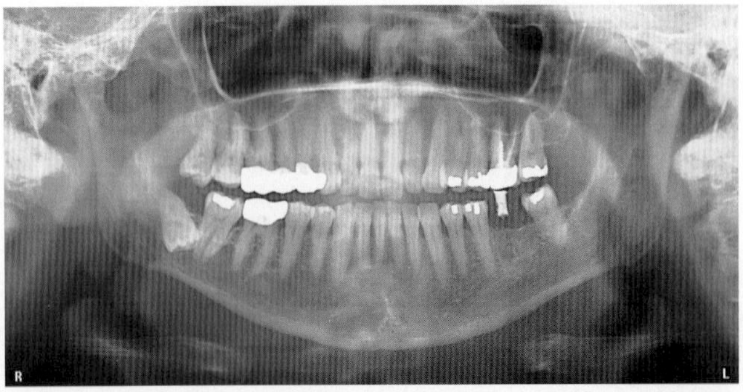

Fig. 31.3 Panoramic radiograph, acquired with an imaging guide, depicting the desired axis of a potential left mandibular first molar implant. Note incidental finding of a full bony impacted mandibular right third molar. The maxillary right third molar is erupted beyond the maxillary occlusal plane.

units acquire images with the patient in a supine, sitting, or standing position, depending on the manufacturer and model of the unit. CBCT imaging offers the advantage of a higher spatial resolution and much lower radiation dose relative to maxillofacial MDCT imaging (see Chapters 3 and 9).

Following a comprehensive patient history, clinical assessment, and initial radiographic examination with periapical and/or panoramic images, CBCT is the imaging modality of choice for the presurgical assessment of an implant site. CBCT allows for accurate, three-dimensional analyses of the quantity of available bone, the thickness of the contiguous cortical plates, the quality and architecture of the trabecular bone, and the proximity to adjacent anatomic structures and boundaries. CBCT is also the modality of choice for preoperative evaluation of the maxillary sinuses prior to sinus floor elevation, the assessment of both donor and recipient sites for autogenous bone grafting procedures, and to evaluate the outcome of these procedures. CBCT datasets are also used to design and fabricate surgical guides using computer-aided design and computer-aided manufacturing (CAD/CAM) technology.

As with all ionizing radiation–based imaging modalities, the use of CBCT should follow responsible and judicious image acquisition protocols. The anatomic field of view should be limited to the region of interest. Depending on the objectives of imaging, the field may be extended beyond the edentulous sites to encompass relevant adjacent anatomy, such as the maxillary sinus ostia prior to sinus lifting, the external oblique ridges for bone harvesting, or the opposing dental crowns for prosthetic planning and surgical guide fabrication. To produce a diagnostically acceptable study using the least amount of ionizing radiation, the exposure parameters should be tailored to the patient's age, size, and anatomy, and efforts should be made during image acquisition to minimize motion. Importantly, given the complexity of three-dimensional imaging volumes and the inclusion of structures beyond the dentoalveolar region, advanced training is necessary to interpret CBCT studies competently.

Image Reconstruction Techniques

Following acquisition of a CBCT volume, the imaged volume must be reconstructed in specific planes to extract the necessary information for implant planning. Owing to the curvature of the dental arch, the orthogonal anatomic planes (axial, coronal, and sagittal) are not optimal for assessing the mesiodistal and buccolingual dimensions of available bone. Therefore curved planar reformatting is applied. This is achieved through first selecting a reference axial slice of the maxillary or mandibular arch, at the midroot level of its teeth. Dedicated software tools are used to define the curve of the dental arch, tailored to the patient's anatomy (Fig. 31.4A), and subsequently to generate a series of cross-sectional images oriented perpendicular to this patient's arch in predefined, equally spaced intervals (typically 1–2 mm). Software tools are used to make measurements of the vertical height and buccolingual width of the edentulous site (see Fig. 31.4B). Pseudopanoramic reconstructions can also be made parallel to this customized arch, and reconstructed at various thicknesses; thinner slices allow localized anatomic visualization that is free of superimposition, whereas a thicker slice will more closely resemble a panoramic radiograph (see Fig. 31.4C). Last, three-dimensional surface and volumetric renderings of the edentulous jaw can be generated to aid in visualizing the overall shape and contour of the edentulous jaw (see Fig. 31.4D). Images of CBCT reconstructions can be delivered in digital format and can be printed life size (i.e., 1:1) on high-quality photographic paper. Some CBCT manufacturers may provide an image processing option that generates a digital imaging and communication in medicine (DICOM) dataset with metal artifact reduction algorithms applied. It should be cautioned that such algorithms may alter the diagnostic information inherent to the original CBCT study, and, if used, they should always be reviewed in conjunction with the native, noncorrected reconstruction to reduce the risk of misinterpretation related to the altered appearance of the algorithmic correction (see Fig. 31.4E).

Other Techniques

Other radiographic imaging techniques that have been used for implant planning include the lateral oblique, lateral cephalometric, and conventional tomographic images. These techniques have been largely replaced by CBCT imaging in contemporary practice for implant treatment planning. Although magnetic resonance imaging (MRI) produces cross-sectional images of the jaws without ionizing radiation, its depiction of the hard tissue structures is inadequate for implant planning.

PREOPERATIVE ASSESSMENT AND TREATMENT PLANNING

Several functional, esthetic, and surgical considerations contribute to successful implant placement. Prior to the widespread availability of CBCT imaging, implant placement was predominantly a surgically driven approach, with the amount of available bone largely dictating the final implant position. However, with the increased accessibility and affordability of three-dimensional imaging, current trends have shifted toward a prosthetically driven approach. CBCT data can be virtually coupled with digital impression models, allowing for greater communication between the surgeon and restorative dentist. The ideal position of the putative implant is first identified based on the functional and esthetic needs of the patient as well as the state of the remaining dentition. This information is then translated into the digital environment and, through specialized software, the implant surgery can be simulated using virtual implant libraries. Based on the amount of available bone and the shape of the residual bony ridge, the need for additional bone grafting and alveoloplasty procedures can be identified and the treatment options provided. This increased transparency and communication between the implant team and the patient allows for a more predictable outcome and keeps expectations earnest through informed decision making.

Radiologic Assessment of Bone Quantity

The principal advantage of CBCT imaging is its ability to accurately assess the quantity of available bone in all three dimensions. It is generally accepted that, ideally, the implant should be placed at least 1.5 mm from the adjacent teeth, 3 mm from an adjacent implant, and 2 mm from vital anatomic structures, such as the inferior alveolar canal. The usual anatomic boundaries are discussed further on for both the maxillae and mandible.

In the anterior maxilla, the absolute vertical limitation is the floor of the nasal fossa. However, the vertical dimension of available bone is often limited by residual ridge atrophy, which can lead to the development of a prominent buccal concavity. CBCT guides the decision for additional buccal bone grafting or restorative compromises for a shorter, more proclined implant (Fig. 31.5). In the maxillary central incisor region, proximity to the nasopalatine canal must be assessed. It is important to recognize that there are large morphologic differences in the dimensions and configuration of the nasopalatine canal; even within the same patient, the diameter of the canal can vary widely across its length (Fig. 31.6). CBCT accurately depicts the canal's topography; it is particularly valuable when there are potential space limitations, as in the case of a mesially positioned lateral incisor.

In the posterior maxilla, the floor of the maxillary sinus is the usual vertical boundary to implant placement. The pneumatization of the alveolar process is a normal physiologic process that is often accelerated by tooth loss. Although the floor of the maxillary sinus can be readily identified in two-dimensional images, the pattern of pneumatization may be variable in the transverse dimension, and the exact position of the sinus floor can be fully appreciated only with three-dimensional

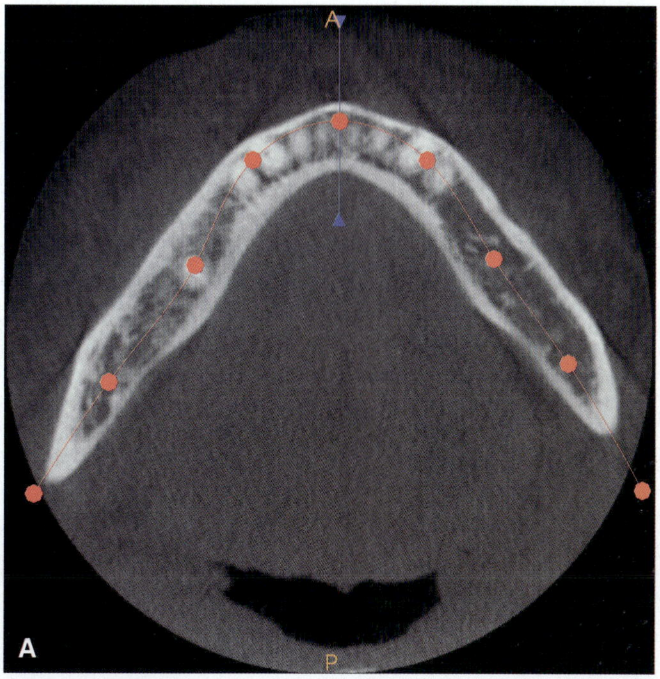

Fig. 31.4 (A) Axial reference cone beam computed tomography image. The curvature of the mandibular arch is approximated through a series of connecting *dots*.

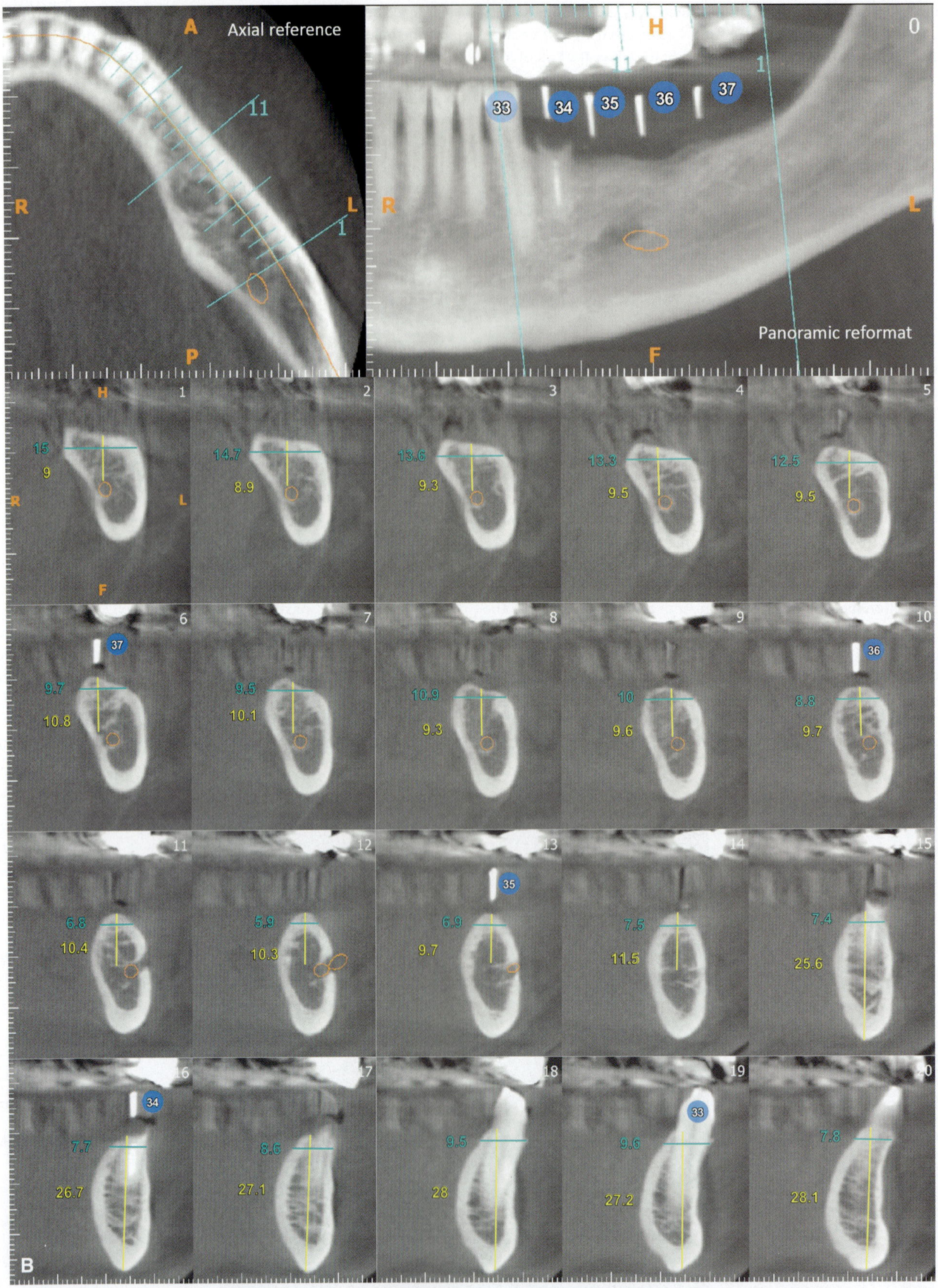

Fig. 31.4, cont'd (B) Sequential cross sections made perpendicular to the curvature of the mandible at 2-mm intervals. The edentulous sites are labeled (in FDI World Dental Federation notation). Vertical and buccolingual measurements are in accordance with the imaging guide. The course of the mandibular canal is outlined in *orange*.

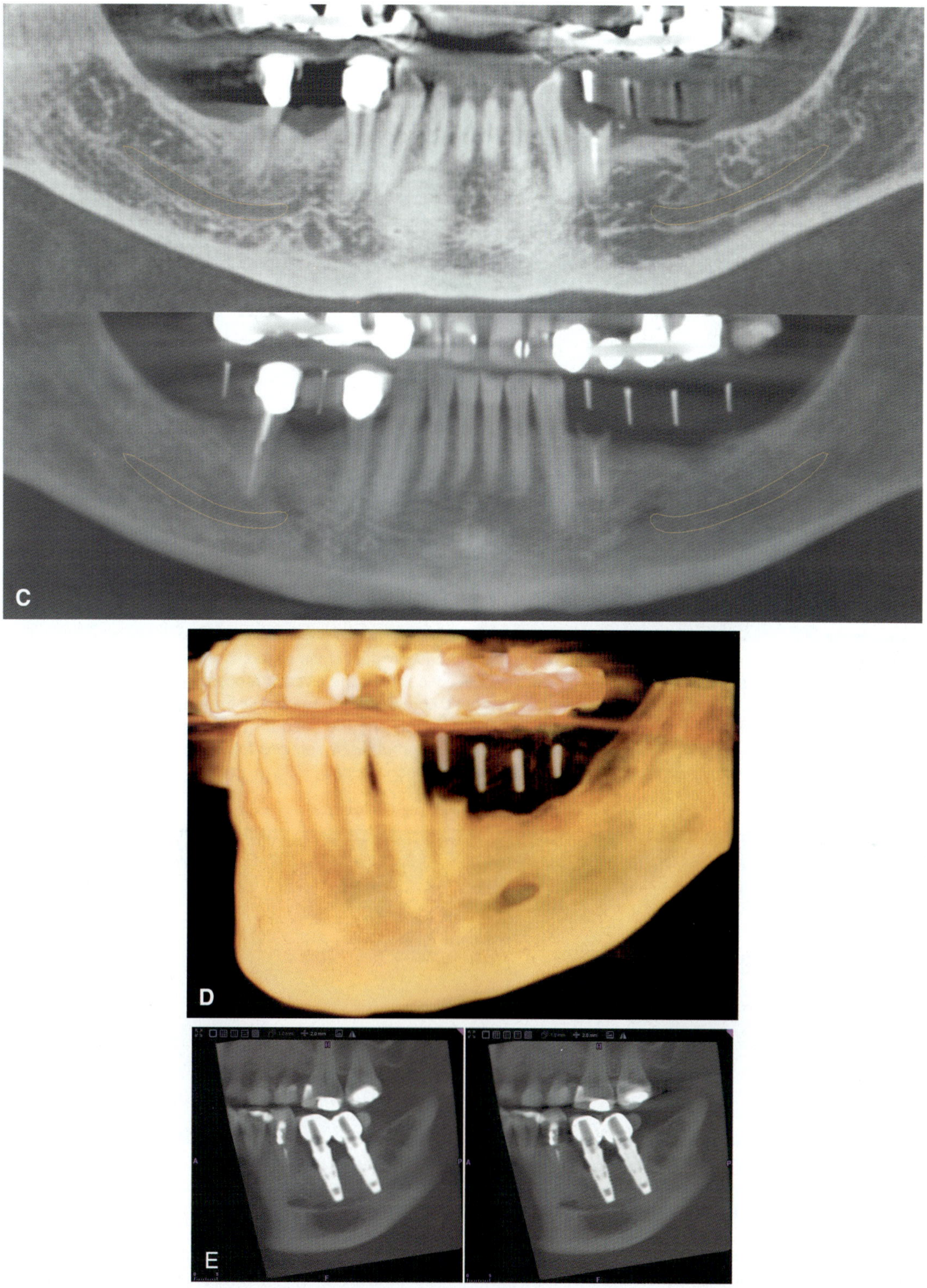

Fig. 31.4, cont'd (C) Pseudopanoramic multiplanar reformat of the mandible with thin (0.2 mm, *top*) and thick slice thicknesses (40 mm, *bottom*). (D) Three-dimensional volume rendering of the edentulous posterior left mandible. (E) Side-by-side comparison of the same mesiodistal view (2-mm thickness) of two dental implants derived from a CBCT study using a metal reduction algorithm *(left)* and without the metal reduction algorithm *(right)*. Note the lack of streaking artifacts around the highly attenuating restorations in the *left* panel due to the reduction algorithm, but also the observation of artifactual thin and dark linings around the dental implants, which are not apparent in the native scan in the *right* panel.

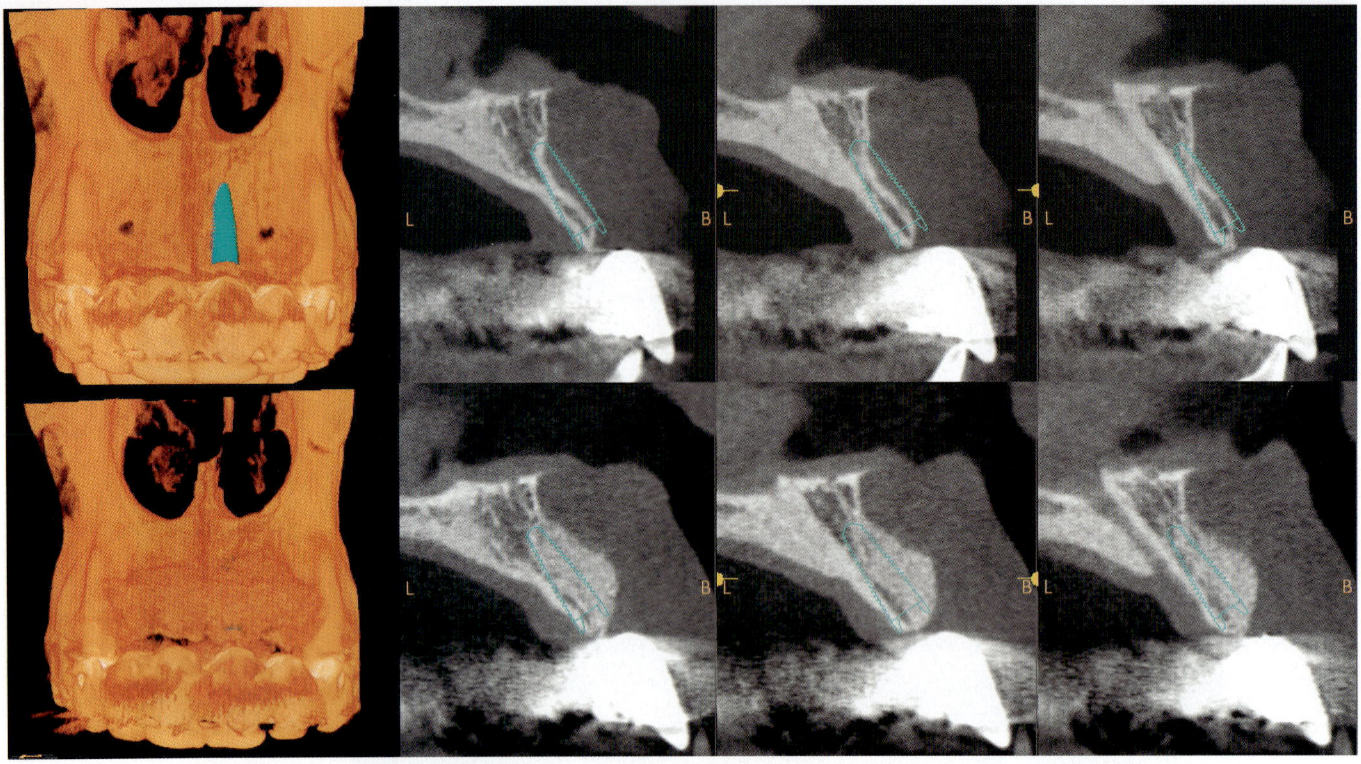

Fig. 31.5 *Top:* Three-dimensional volume rendering and buccolingual cross sections of an edentulous maxillary left central incisor site. Note the prominent buccal concavity of the alveolar process, which prevents the desired implant to be placed without significant esthetic compromises. The virtual implant shows extensive buccal thread exposure if placed in the ideal inclination, identifying the need for buccal bone augmentation prior to implant placement. *Bottom:* Cone beam computed tomography sections following buccal bone grafting. Note how the desired implant size is now fully embedded in bone.

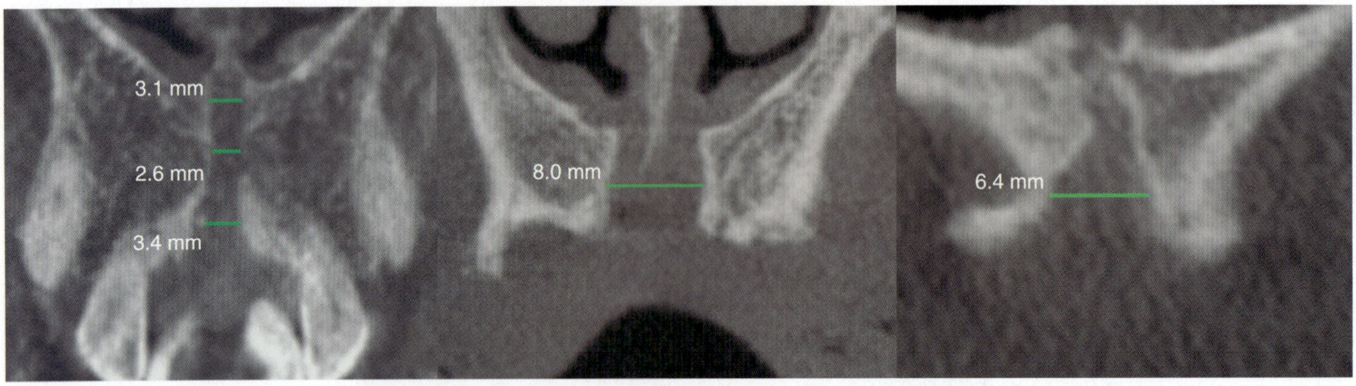

Fig. 31.6 Three examples of morphologic variation in the nasopalatine canal. Coronal slices depicting a thin, uniform canal *(left);* two wide, converging canals *(middle);* and a funnel-shaped canal *(right).*

imaging (Fig. 31.7). If a sinus lift procedure is planned, CBCT provides crucial preoperative information, such as the presence of transverse septa, inflammatory sinus disease, and prominent branches of the posterosuperior alveolar artery (Fig. 31.8).

In the anterior mandible, the usual limitation to implant placement is a narrow buccolingual bone width secondary to residual ridge atrophy. Although clinical palpation of the residual ridge provides an estimate of the available buccolingual bone, only CT imaging can provide a precise assessment. Importantly, the anterior mandible contains a network of anastomosing lingual vessels that can occasionally be identified as bony canals (the median and lateral lingual foramina) (Fig. 31.9A). The mandibular incisive canal, the anterior continuation of the inferior alveolar canal beyond the mental foramen, is another vital structure that may be radiographically apparent (see Fig. 31.9B). These structures, if breached during implant placement, have occasionally been reported to result in hemorrhage and neurosensory disturbances. CBCT depicts these canals better than two-dimensional radiographs; this may allow for a more predictable treatment outcome even within a region that is traditionally considered as a "safe zone" for implant placement.

Although the inferior alveolar canal is often assumed to be the obvious vertical limitation to implant placement in the posterior mandible, it is important to recognize that the mandibular cross-sectional morphology usually follows a sigmoid shape in the buccolingual plane (Fig. 31.10). The buccal surface of the alveolar process is often more

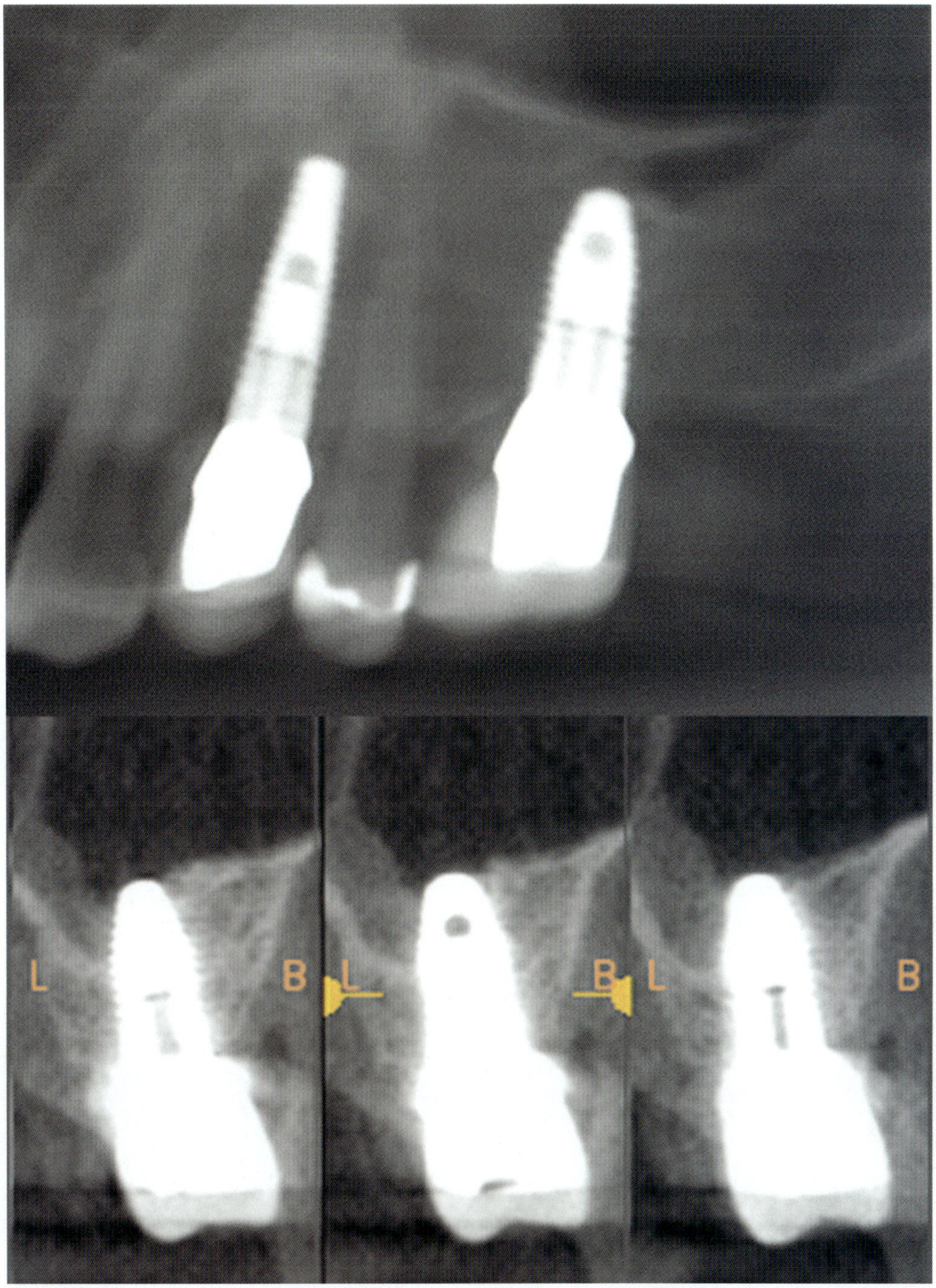

Fig. 31.7 *Top:* A simulated periapical projection reformatted from a cone beam computed tomography study. The position of the maxillary sinus floor relative to the apex of the implant placed at the maxillary left first molar site is difficult to determine due to anatomic superimposition. *Bottom:* These buccolingual cross sections of the same implant demonstrate the irregular pneumatization of the alveolar process, which is difficult to appreciate in a projectional, two-dimensional image. The sinus floor is positioned more superiorly within the buccal aspect of the alveolar process, and more inferiorly positioned in the palatal portion of this site. The apex of this implant is more palatally oriented within the alveolar process, and has been placed beyond the sinus floor.

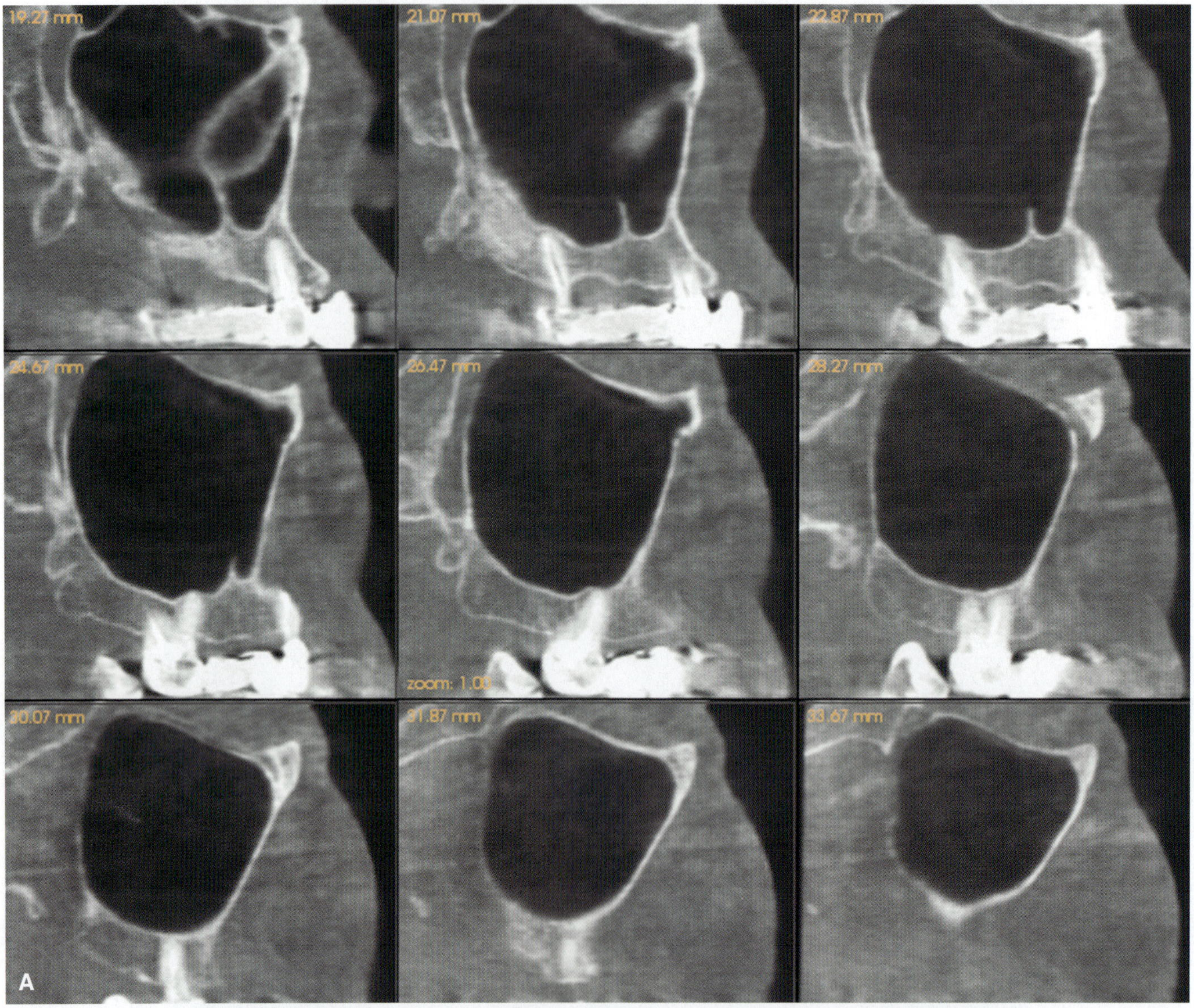

Fig. 31.8 (A) Serial sagittal cross sections of a right maxillary sinus demonstrating a transverse ridge located along the sinus floor apical to the edentulous first molar region, which may complicate a sinus lift procedure. The sinus appears otherwise normal and fully aerated.

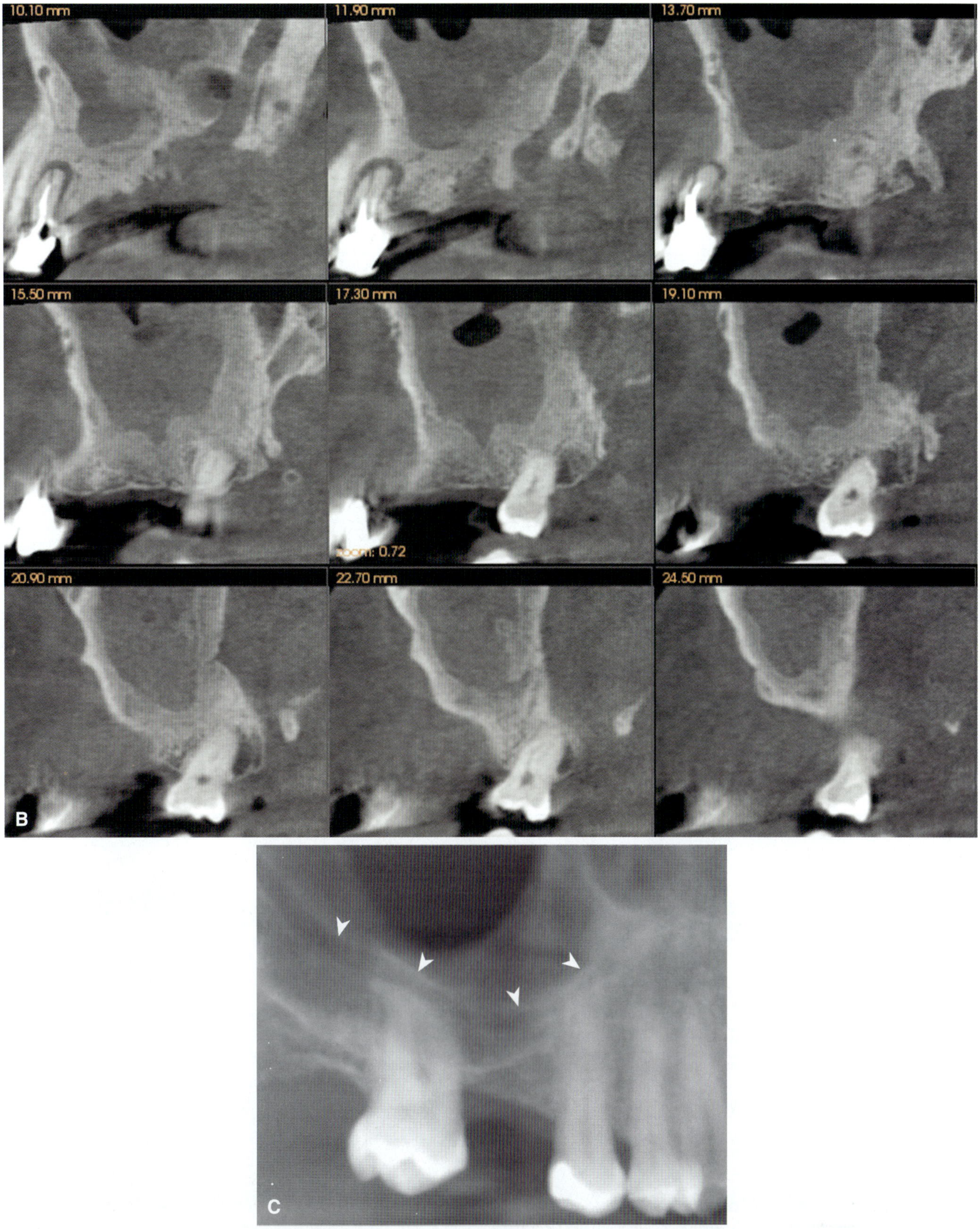

Fig. 31.8, cont'd (B) In contrast to (A), these sagittal cross sections of a left maxillary sinus show that the sinus walls are thickened and sclerotic and that most of the antral space is radiopacified. These findings could imply the possibility of sinusitis, which is a relative contraindication to a sinus lift procedure. (C) Reformatted image from a cone beam computed tomography volume of the right maxilla depicts a prominent branch of the posterior superior alveolar artery *(white arrowheads)*. The three-dimensional location of this vessel can be mapped in preparation for a sinus lift surgery.

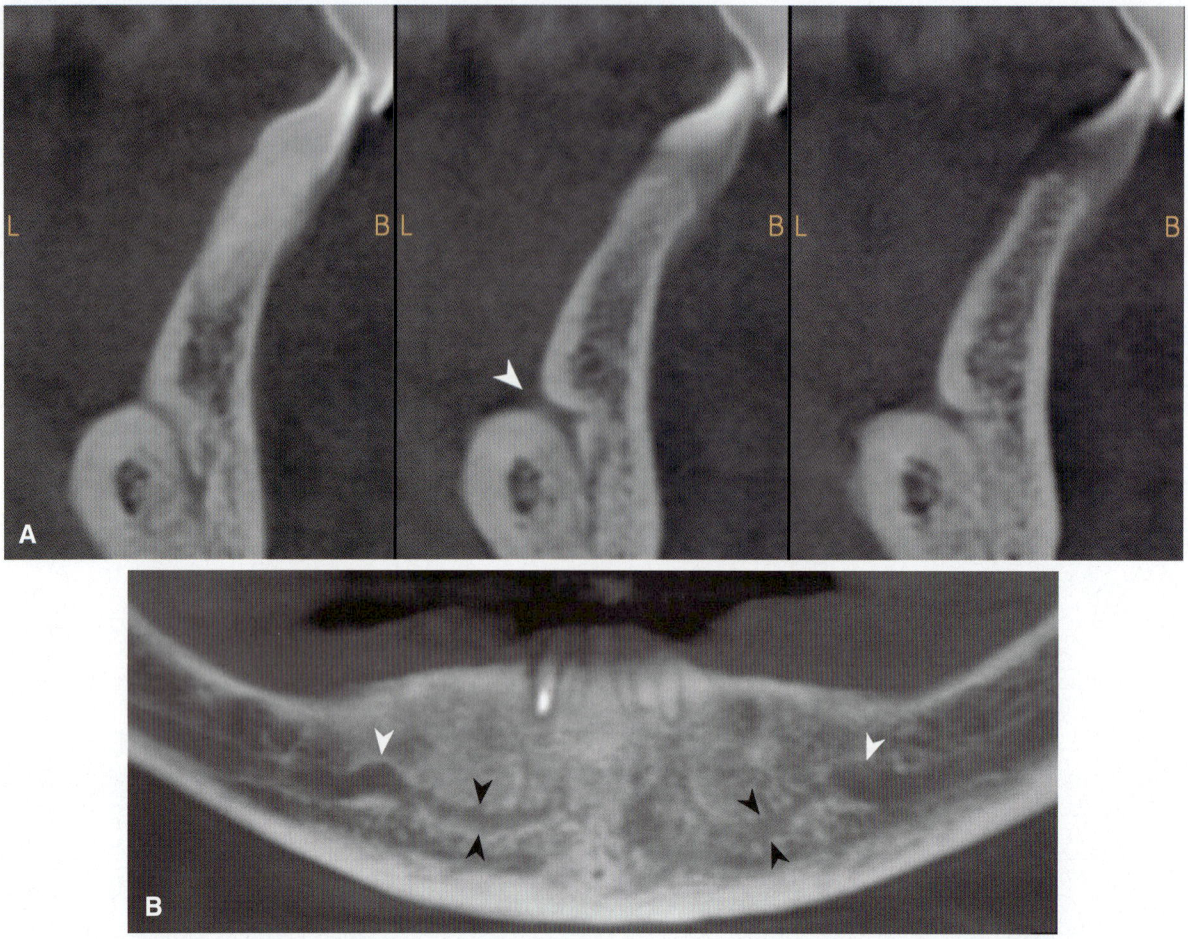

Fig. 31.9 (A) Buccolingual cross-sectional images of the mandibular midline depicting a prominent median lingual foramen *(white arrowhead)*, which could result in hemorrhage if breached during implant placement. (B) Panoramic reformatted image (3-mm slice thickness) demonstrating prominent mandibular incisive canals *(black arrowheads)* coursing anterior to the mental foramina *(white arrowheads)*.

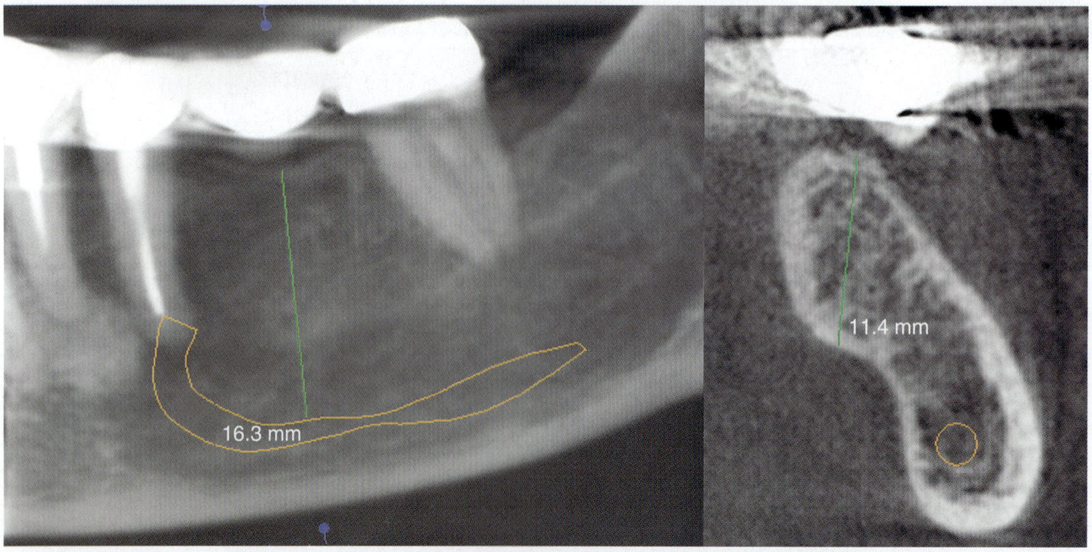

Fig. 31.10 *Left:* Cropped panoramic image reformatted from a cone beam computed tomography study of the site of the mandibular left first molar. The vertical height from the alveolar crest to the left inferior alveolar nerve canal *(outlined in orange)* measures just over 16 mm. *Right:* A cross-sectional slice at the middle of the same site (mandibular left first molar) in the buccolingual plane. A prominent lingual concavity limits implant placement at an optimal angle relative to the pontic restoration and roots of the adjacent teeth. Note that this information cannot be obtained on periapical and panoramic radiographs.

lingually positioned than the underlying mandibular body, and a concavity is present along the lingual surface of the mandible (i.e., the submandibular fossa). This unique morphology is not visualized in periapical and panoramic images, which do not provide information in the buccolingual dimension, and is often undetected during clinical examination because the lingual contours of the mandibular body are difficult to palpate owing to their muscular attachments. Moreover, CBCT has been shown to be superior to panoramic images in identifying the inferior alveolar canal. This, in conjunction with the ability to objectively delineate the buccolingual contours of the mandible, can often result in changes to the size and angulation of the planned implant.

Radiologic Assessment of Bone Quality

Local bone quality is an important factor for implant success. The edentulous bone should provide primary implant stability and a preimplant environment that is conducive to osseointegration. Currently, radiologic assessment of bone quality at the edentulous site is largely a subjective evaluation of the trabecular architecture. Numerous classification systems have been proposed, but few have been validated as practical clinical outcome measures. The classification system proposed by Misch et al. (Table 31.2) is most widely used and describes four categories of bone (D1 to D4) based on the thickness of cortical bone and the density and distribution of trabecular bone (Fig. 31.11). Owing to its ability to clearly visualize the thickness of cortical bone and the organization of trabecular bone, these assessments are better on cross-sectional CT images than on intraoral and panoramic images. However, the distinction between a "thick" or a "thin" cortex and "coarse" or "fine" trabecular bone relies on the subjective thresholds of the observer, which are variable among clinicians.

Objectively, bone density is formally defined as mineral mass per unit volume of bone. When applied to the diagnosis of osteoporosis and assessment of fracture risk, this assessment is typically performed using dual-energy x-ray absorptiometry (DEXA). Crude estimates of bone density obtained from the CT numbers on MDCT images (Hounsfield units, or HU) have been used to predict implant stability. HU ranges for the Misch classification of bone density have been proposed (see Table 31.2). However, owing to their wide beam geometry, increased scatter radiation, and lower contrast resolution, HU measurements from CBCT datasets are unreliable for the prediction of bone density. In general, jaw bone density in the anterior mandible is higher, whereas it is lowest in the posterior maxilla.

Radiologic imaging of proposed implant sites aids in the detection of retained root fragments and foreign bodies and in ruling out residual pathology. Findings that require treatment include inflammatory disease, cysts, and neoplasms, and CBCT imaging provides excellent characterization of their bony extent. Findings that do not require treatment but may still impact implant planning are also occasionally encountered. For example, areas of osteosclerosis are common incidental findings (Fig. 31.12). Although not a direct contraindication to implant placement, the presence of osteosclerosis may cause drill deflection during implant osteotomy. Additionally, osteosclerotic areas have relatively lower vascularity, which can affect healing and osseointegration. Similarly, the presence of periapical osseous dysplasia also complicates implant placement; some case reports have shown that surgical intervention in regions of osseous dysplasia, including implant placement, can result in secondary infection of the dysplastic bone, which can lead to the development of osteomyelitis and bone sequestration (Fig. 31.13).

INTRAOPERATIVE IMAGING

During surgical implant placement, intraoperative imaging is limited to quick, in-office modalities, including digital-based periapical and panoramic radiography. These radiographs confirm appropriate pilot drill position and allow early errors to be identified so that appropriate modifications to the remaining osteotomy steps can be made. Occasionally, surgical accidents may require advanced radiologic imaging in the intraoperative phase—for example, when an implant is displaced into the maxillary sinus (Fig. 31.14A) or placed through the inferior alveolar canal (Fig. 31.14B). In such situations, expedient CBCT imaging will accurately locate the implant or assess the extent of nerve canal encroachment.

IMAGE-GUIDED APPLICATIONS

More recently, advancements in computer technology and stereolithographic prototyping have facilitated image-guided techniques for implant treatment planning and surgical placement. Several implant planning software programs use CBCT datasets to determine the optimal three-dimensional position of a proposed implant. However, the ultimate success of the procedure depends on the successful transfer of the virtual plan to the surgical suite. Various guided surgery techniques have been developed to serve as a physical conduit between the virtual and surgical environments. Such guided surgical approaches are especially helpful in cases where anatomic, functional, or esthetic requirements must be met within a relatively narrow margin of error.

Conventional stereolithographic guides are designed to be supported by one of three tissue types: teeth, mucosa, or bone. In the partially dentate patient, tooth-supported guides are usually preferred,

TABLE 31.2 Misch Classification of Bone Density

Classification Type	Radiographic Appearance	Typical Anatomic Location	MDCT Density Range (HU)
D1	Primarily composed of dense cortical bone Marrow spaces are hardly visible	Occasionally in anterior mandible Rarely in posterior mandible	>1250
D2	Thick outer layer of porous cortical bone Coarse trabecular bone pattern	Commonly in anterior and posterior mandible Occasionally in anterior maxilla	850–1250
D3	Thinner layer of porous cortical bone Fine trabecular bone pattern	Commonly in anterior maxilla, posterior maxilla, and posterior mandible Occasionally in anterior mandible	350–850
D4	Faint to imperceptible outline of thin cortical bone Alveolar process is primarily composed of fine trabecular bone	Commonly in posterior maxilla Rarely in anterior maxilla	150–350

HU, Hounsfield units; *MDCT*, multidetector computed tomography.
Modified from Misch CE. *Contemporary Implant Dentistry*. 3rd ed. Mosby; 2008.

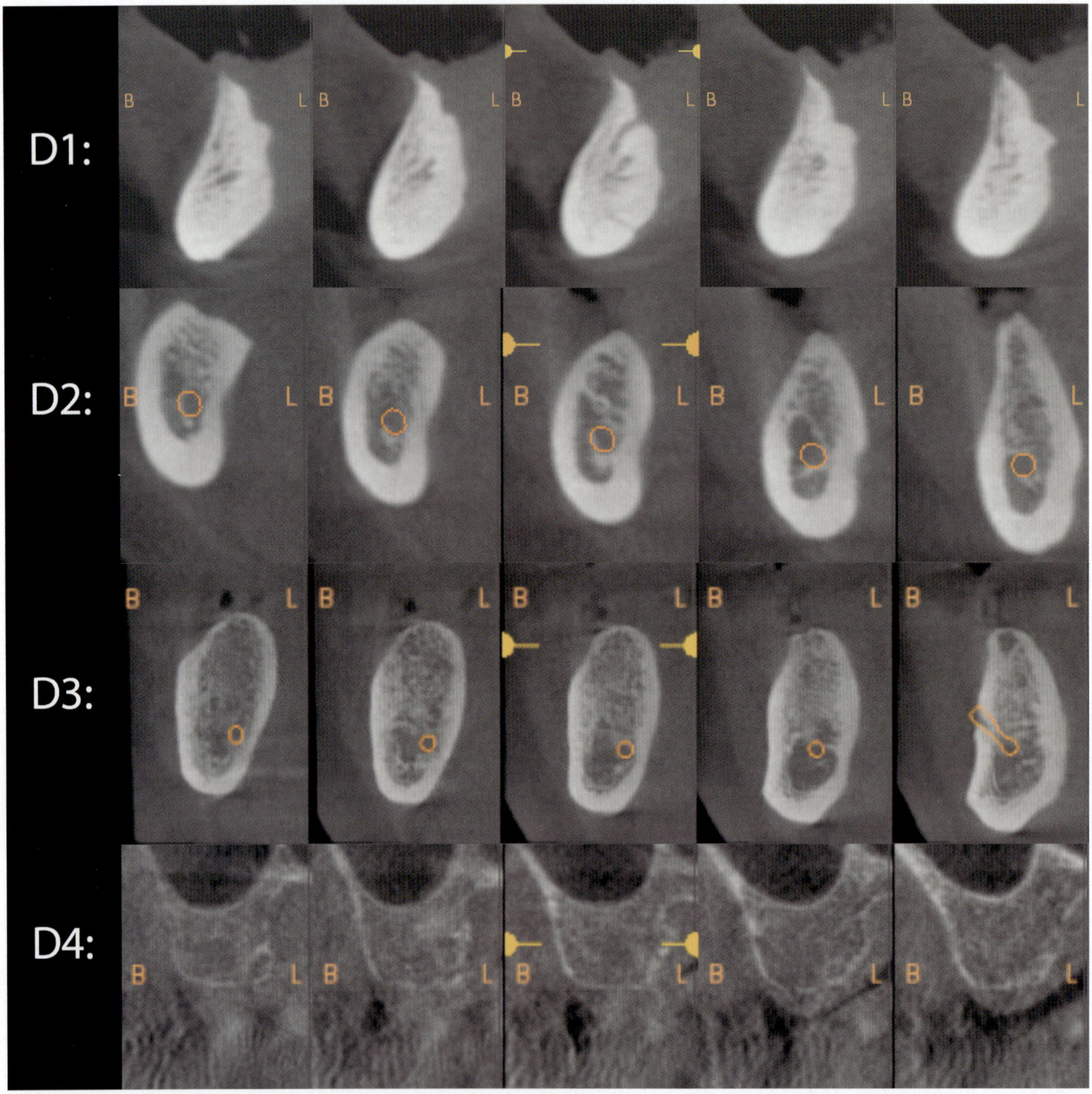

Fig. 31.11 Serial buccolingual cross-sectional images of four different edentulous sites that exemplify the Misch classifications of bone density. Mandibular nerve canals are outlined in *orange*. *First row:* The alveolar process of an edentulous anterior mandible that is primarily composed of dense cortical bone. This is suggestive of a D1 bone density classification. *Second row:* An example of a D2 classification in a posterior right mandible, with coarse trabecular bone surrounded by an outer layer of thick cortical bone. *Third row:* Thin cortical bone lining fine trabecular bone in a posterior right mandible, which is a typical example of a D3 type bone. *Fourth row:* Cross sections of a posterior right maxilla demonstrating a fine trabecular bone pattern covered by a faint lining of cortical bone. This is representative of a D4 bone density classification.

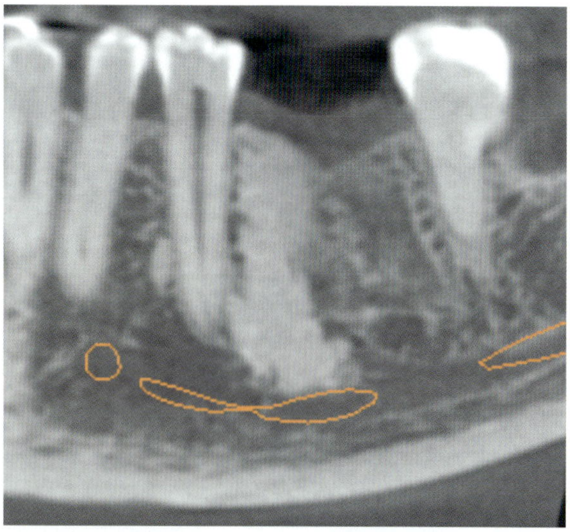

Fig. 31.12 Cone beam computed tomography section through the posterior left mandible demonstrating a large area of osteosclerosis located in the mesial aspect of an edentulous mandibular left first molar site.

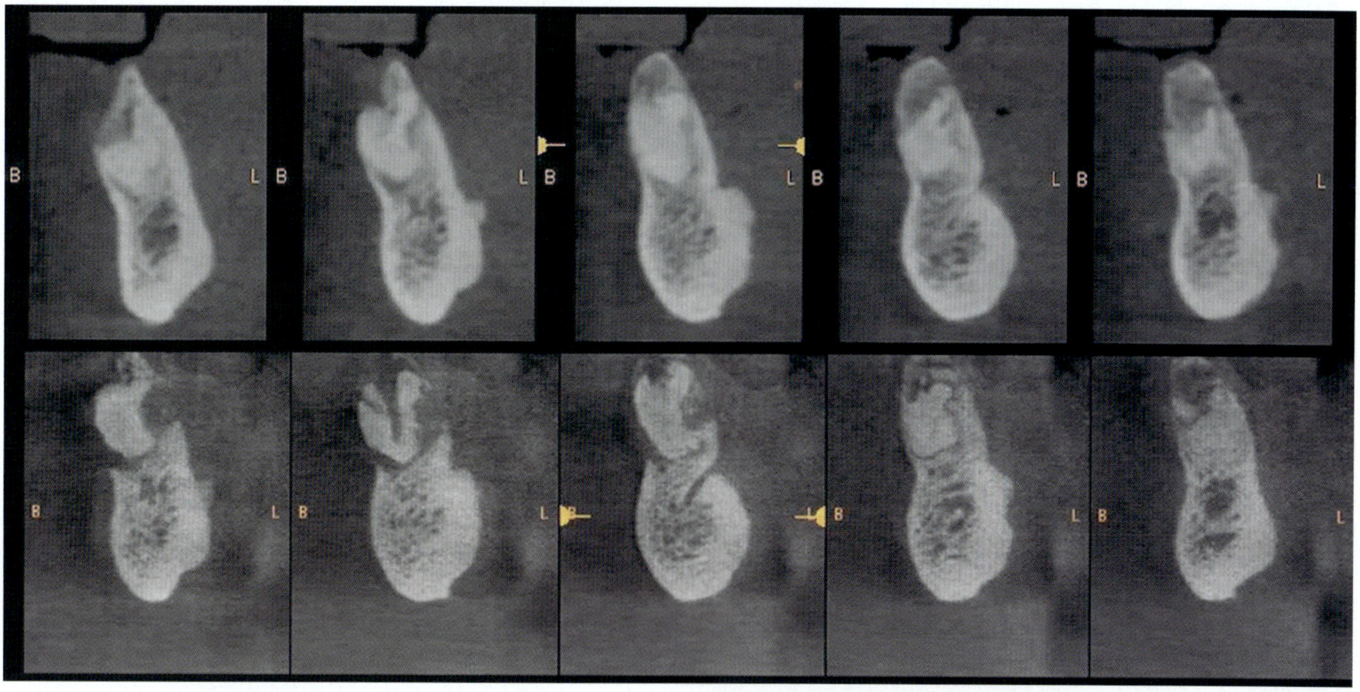

Fig. 31.13 *Top row:* Cone beam computed tomography (CBCT) images of a relatively mature focus of periapical osseous dysplasia in the anterior mandible of a patient evaluated for implant treatment planning. *Bottom row:* Following implant placement, the patient reported pain in the implant area. Two of the implants failed in the immediate postoperative period. Postoperative CBCT sections demonstrate rarefying osteitis around the foci of dysplastic bone and partial loss of the contiguous buccal and lingual cortical plates, suggestive of osteomyelitis.

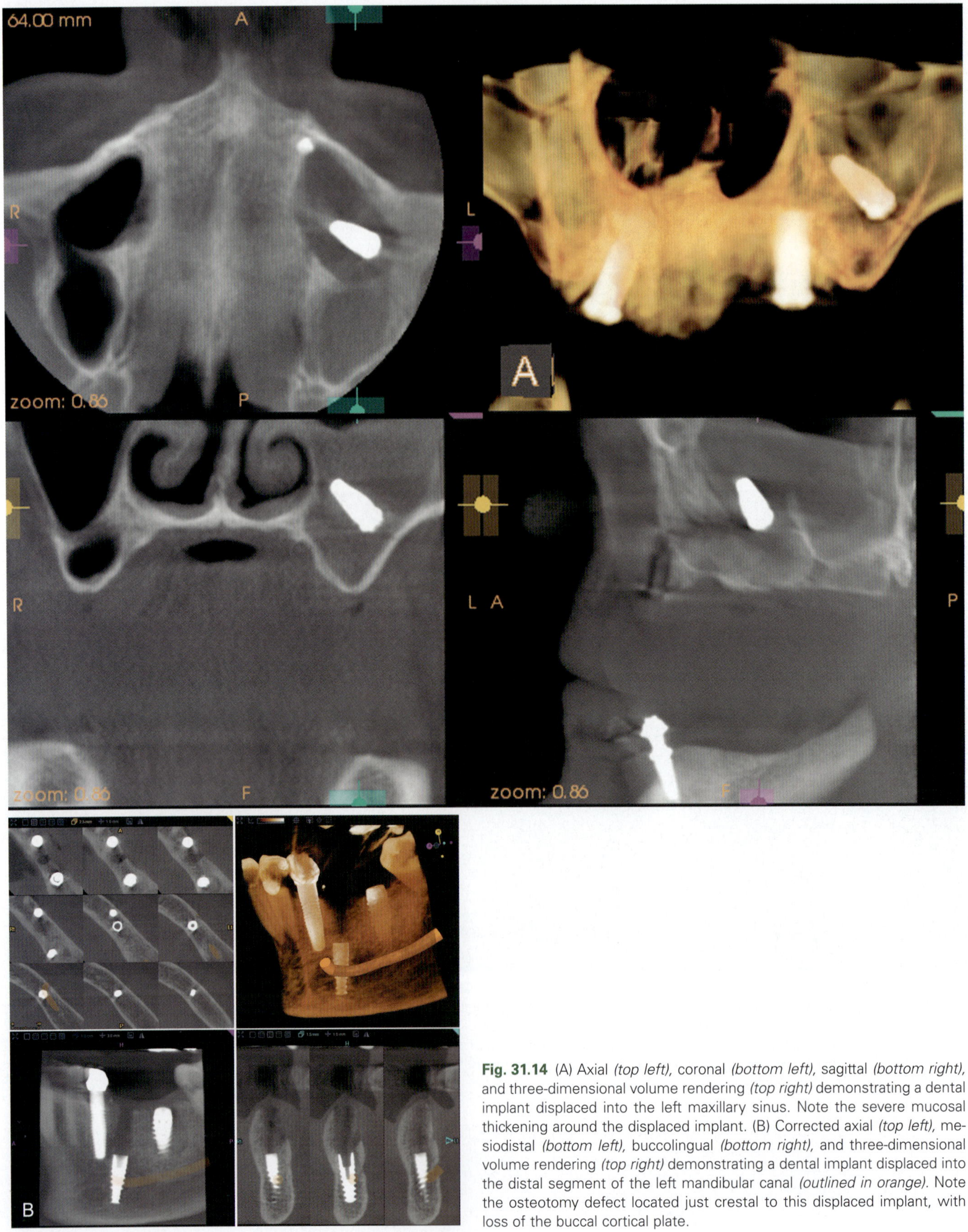

Fig. 31.14 (A) Axial *(top left)*, coronal *(bottom left)*, sagittal *(bottom right)*, and three-dimensional volume rendering *(top right)* demonstrating a dental implant displaced into the left maxillary sinus. Note the severe mucosal thickening around the displaced implant. (B) Corrected axial *(top left)*, mesiodistal *(bottom left)*, buccolingual *(bottom right)*, and three-dimensional volume rendering *(top right)* demonstrating a dental implant displaced into the distal segment of the left mandibular canal *(outlined in orange)*. Note the osteotomy defect located just crestal to this displaced implant, with loss of the buccal cortical plate.

as they allow flapless surgery to be performed while maintaining guide stability without the use of fixation pins (Fig. 31.15). This technique requires at least two or three nonmobile teeth in the arch, and the contours of these teeth can be digitally captured using three-dimensional surface optical scanning of stone models or directly via a specialized intraoral optical scanning camera. This surface model is subsequently superimposed over the CBCT dataset, which allows for accurate profiling of the tooth crowns that would otherwise be obscured by beam hardening artifacts from restorations. Current literature suggests that tooth-supported guides are more accurate than mucosa- and bone-supported guides.

In the edentulous patient, the surgical guide can be supported only by mucosa or bone. A mucosa-supported guide will still allow a flapless surgical approach, but the accuracy of the guide depends on mucosal resilience and the use of fixation pins (Fig. 31.16). Alternatively, a bone-supported guide rests entirely on bone, but the surgeon must first raise an extensive flap to seat the guide (Fig. 31.17). The primary advantage of a bone-supported system is that it confers greater visualization of the surgical field, which allows early detection of positional errors through direct visualization and tactile sensation. However, the need to raise a flap increases patient discomfort and recovery time and may result in postoperative complications such as swelling and bleeding. Some studies have suggested that mucosa-supported guides confer greater clinical accuracy than bone-supported guides.

In addition to static surgical templates, more recent approaches of surgical guidance allow for a more dynamic approach. As with static planning approaches, the position and inclination of the putative implant are planned based on a preoperative CT examination. However, for implant placement in the jaw, these systems employ sophisticated intraoperative navigation technology that provides live feedback on the location and angulation of the surgical handpiece relative to the in silico planned implant position. This is typically achieved using fiducial markers registered with the CT images, positional sensors attached to the patient's stent and the handpiece, and an external digital display depicting the real-time position of the drill head in relation to the virtual planning data (Fig. 31.18). The main advantage of this approach over static surgical templates is that it allows the surgeon to make real-time modifications to the predetermined implant position while still retaining the benefits of CT guidance. However, the additional hardware and software necessary to operate these systems reduces their accessibility compared with static guides, and the added steps of tracking and displaying the surgical instrument introduce potential sources of error.

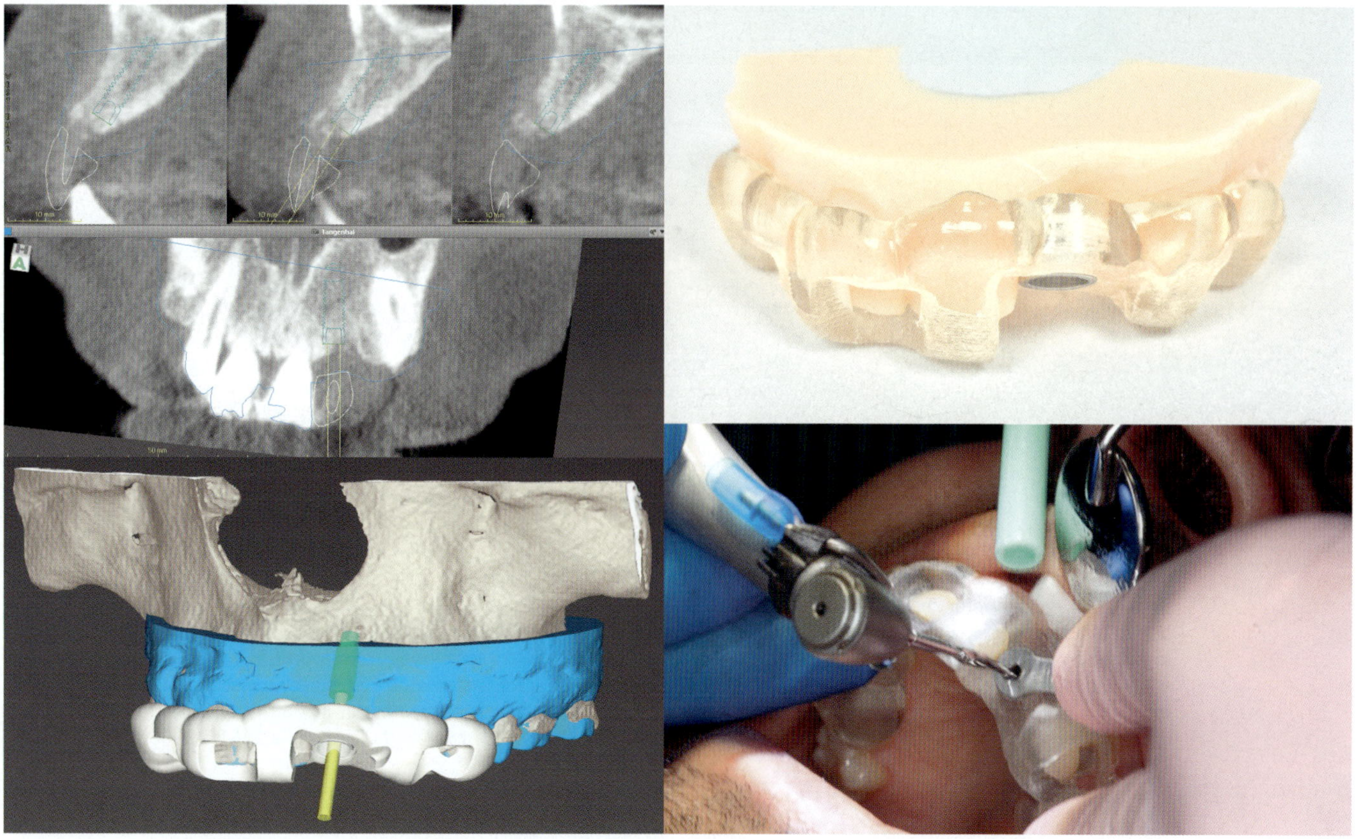

Fig. 31.15 *Top left:* Buccolingual and mesiodistal cross sections of a cone beam computed tomography (CBCT) scan acquired for implant planning at the site of an edentulous maxillary left lateral incisor. Given that the remaining teeth are present, a tooth-supported guide was planned to aid in implant placement. A stone model of the patient's arch was digitally scanned and registered with the CBCT data, which is outlined in *dark blue.* Based on the amount of available bone and the desired position of the prosthetic crown, the ideal position of the virtual implant was determined *(outlined in light blue). Bottom left:* Three-dimensional surface models of the maxillae *(gray),* the maxillary stone model *(dark blue),* and the digitally designed surgical stent *(white). Top right:* The final surgical stent printed through a rapid prototyping technique, securely seated atop a duplicate of the patient's stone model. *Bottom right:* Clinical photograph of the seated surgical stent guiding the implant osteotomy. (Courtesy Canaray: Specialists in Oral Radiology, Toronto, ON, and Dr. G. McLachlin, Calgary, AB.)

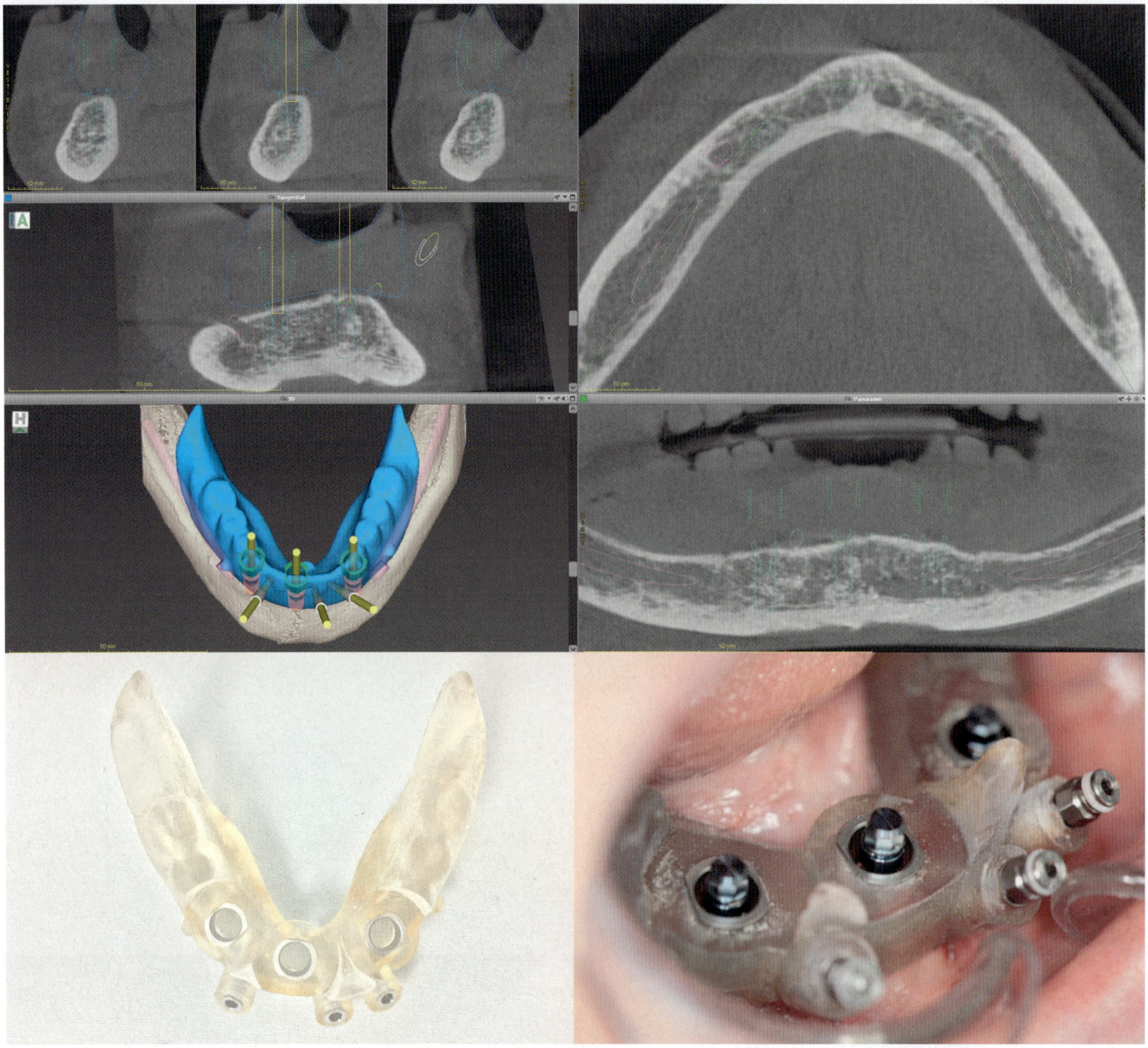

Fig. 31.16 *Top:* Cone beam computed tomography scan of the edentulous mandible coupled with a digitized model of the patient's existing complete lower denture *(dark blue)*. Three vertically oriented implants are planned in the interforaminal region of the mandible to support a fixed, implant-retained prosthesis *(light blue)*. A flapless approach was desired in this case, and a mucosa-supported guide was chosen, which was stabilized by three fixation pins positioned between these implants (also *light blue*). *Bottom left:* The final, printed mucosa-supported guide. Note the additional sleeves to allow for the insertion of fixation pins. *Bottom right:* Clinical photograph of the seated guide with the fixation pins and implants in place. (Courtesy Canaray: Specialists in Oral Radiology, Toronto, ON, Dr. J. Mahn, Paris, ON, and Ms. N. Tomkins and Ms. S. Goergen, Brantford, ON.)

While guided implant placement is an evolving practice, current literature supports relatively high rates of implant survival (96.6%–100%) after using a guided approach over both short- and medium-term observation intervals (ranging from 1 to 5 years), with accurate seating of the guide at the beginning of surgery being a key factor to success. Nonetheless, it is important to recognize that image-guided surgical adjuncts cannot replace sound clinical skill and acumen, and it is naive to consider such a technique as a novice-friendly approach to implant placement. The surgeon must be prepared for all potential intra- and postoperative complications, including the ability to deviate from surgical guidance when unexpected situations arise, such as the need to reflect a flap and perform additional bone augmentation.

POSTOPERATIVE IMAGING AND MONITORING

Immediately following implant placement, a periapical image should be acquired to serve as a baseline image for future comparisons. If multiple implants have been placed, a panoramic image may be

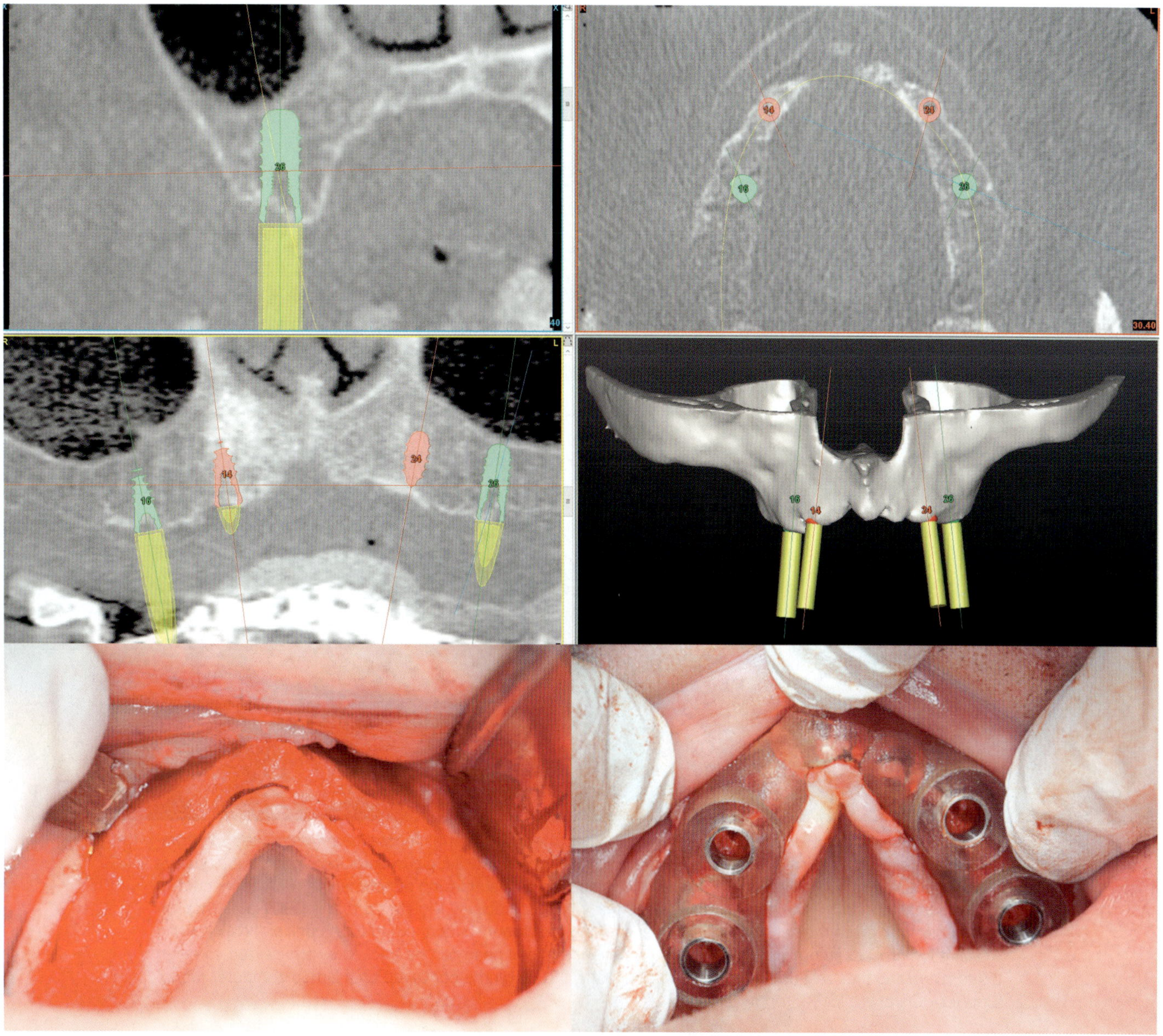

Fig. 31.17 *Top:* Cone beam computed tomography scan of the edentulous maxillae for a removable implant-supported prosthesis. Four implants were planned in the first premolar *(red)* and molar *(green)* regions, to be placed with the aid of a bone-supported guide. *Bottom:* Clinical photographs demonstrating the crestal incision made for a full mucoperiosteal flap *(left)* and the surgical guide fully seated on bone *(right)*. (Courtesy Canaray: Specialists in Oral Radiology, Toronto, ON, and Dr. J. Mahn, Paris, ON.)

appropriate. During the prosthetic phase of treatment, periapical or bite-wing images may be made to ensure complete seating of the implant abutment and restoration. When such images are made, it is important to position the central beam as perpendicular to the longitudinal axis of the implant fixture as possible. Small angular deviations may result in overlapping of the implant threads and allow small gaps between the fixture and prosthesis to go unnoticed (Fig. 31.19).

In the maintenance phase, annual recall imaging through the first 4 years of follow-up has been recommended for asymptomatic patients. This is particularly important in the first year of functional loading, when marginal bone loss and implant failure are most likely to occur. The most reliable indicators of implant success are clinical stability and radiographic evidence of bone adjacent to the implant body. Because of its superior resolution and ready accessibility, periapical imaging is recommended as the first-line modality to monitor implant osseointegration. When the instrument is ideally positioned, the image should demonstrate the apposition of normal bone around the implant threads and the reestablishment of the overlying alveolar crest (Fig. 31.20). To keep interval comparison objective, recall images should strive to maintain the same projection geometry and exposure parameters as the immediate postoperative baseline image. Considering the radiation dose, cost, and its susceptibility to beam-hardening artifacts, CBCT imaging is not recommended for asymptomatic recall patients.

If the patient becomes symptomatic following implant placement, clinical examination and radiologic correlation are indicated. Implant mobility can arise from peri-implant bone loss subsequent to peri-implantitis, failure of the implant to osseointegrate, a loose abutment

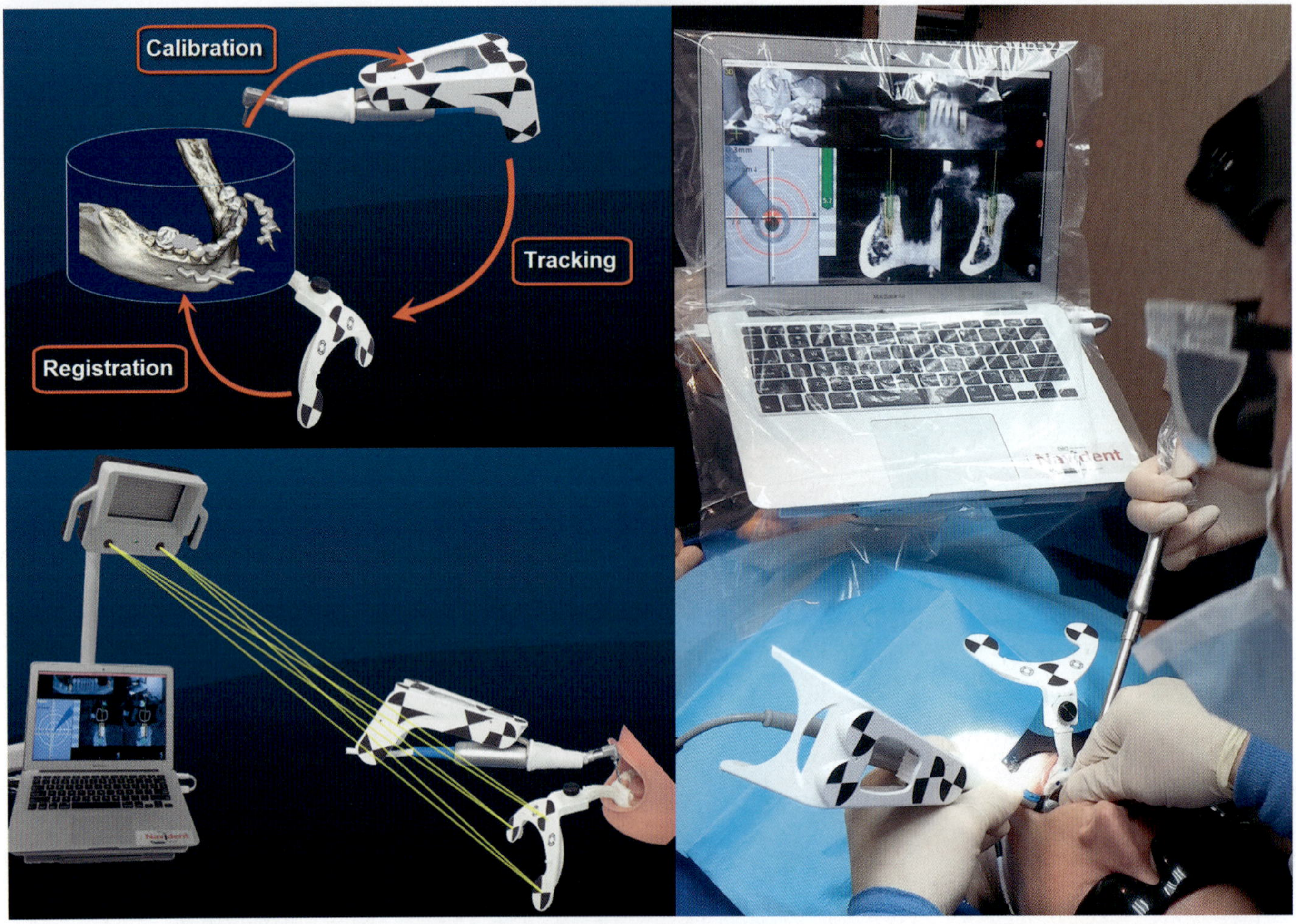

Fig. 31.18 An example of a dynamic surgical guidance system (Navident). A cone beam computed tomography (CBCT) scan is acquired with the patient wearing a specialized fiducial marker *(zig-zagging radiopaque shapes)* attached to an intraoral stent *(top left)*. A patterned optical tracking attachment is then connected to the intraoral stent during the surgery, the position of which is precisely registered to the CBCT data through the fiducial markers in the scan. Another similar tracking attachment is connected to the drill piece. Following a calibration process, the exact positions of the patient and drill head can be tracked by specialized cameras *(bottom left)* and their real-time positions relative to the CBCT volume conveyed on a laptop computer *(right)*. (Courtesy ClaroNav, Inc., Toronto, ON.)

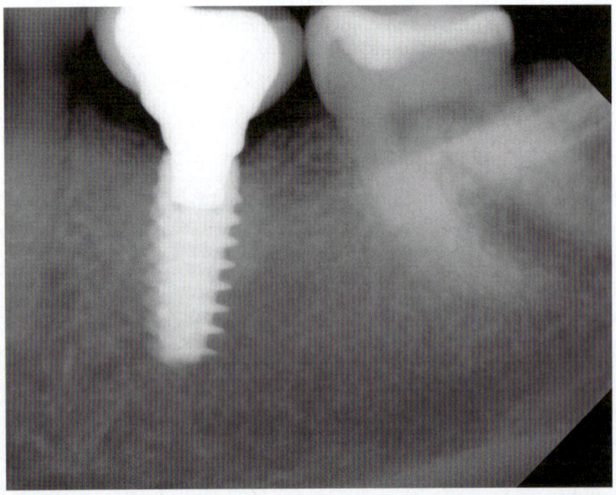

Fig. 31.19 A periapical radiograph that was acquired with an inferiorly positioned central ray, resulting in a diffuse appearance of the implant threads. The junction between the implant fixture and the restorative abutment is also poorly visualized.

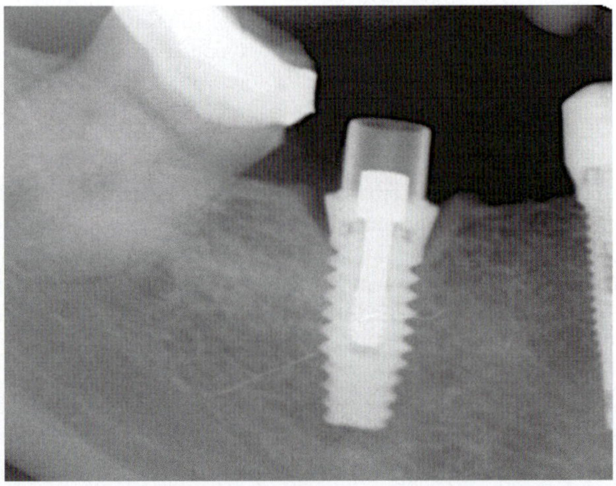

Fig. 31.20 Periapical image of a recently placed implant demonstrating the presence of normal bone adjacent to the implant threads. The overlying alveolar crest has been reestablished. These findings in conjunction with clinical immobility suggest successful implant integration.

or restoration, or a fractured fixture. Similar to periodontal disease, marginal peri-implantitis usually manifests as crestal bone loss with progressive apical migration (Fig. 31.21A), and may be attributed to a combination of poor plaque control, adverse loading, and systemic factors. This condition can be detected by both clinical probing and radiographic examination. Rarely, peri-implantitis may also manifest as bone loss around the apical portion of an implant while its coronal portion remains embedded in bone, which is termed *apical-peri-implantitis* or *retrograde peri-implantitis*. This is thought to arise from persistent disease at the implant site, secondary infection from the adjacent teeth, and/or trauma during implant placement (such as overheating or compression of bone), and its detection relies on radiographic assessment and patient symptoms (Fig. 31.21B). An implant that fails to osseointegrate will reveal a uniform radiolucent junction between the implant fixture and the surrounding bone (Fig. 31.22). When such problems are identified, a CBCT examination may be prescribed to objectively characterize the extent of bone loss, particularly in the buccolingual dimension, and to assess the integrity of the adjacent cortices. These findings may be helpful in planning corrective bone augmentation procedures or the complete removal and replacement of an implant.

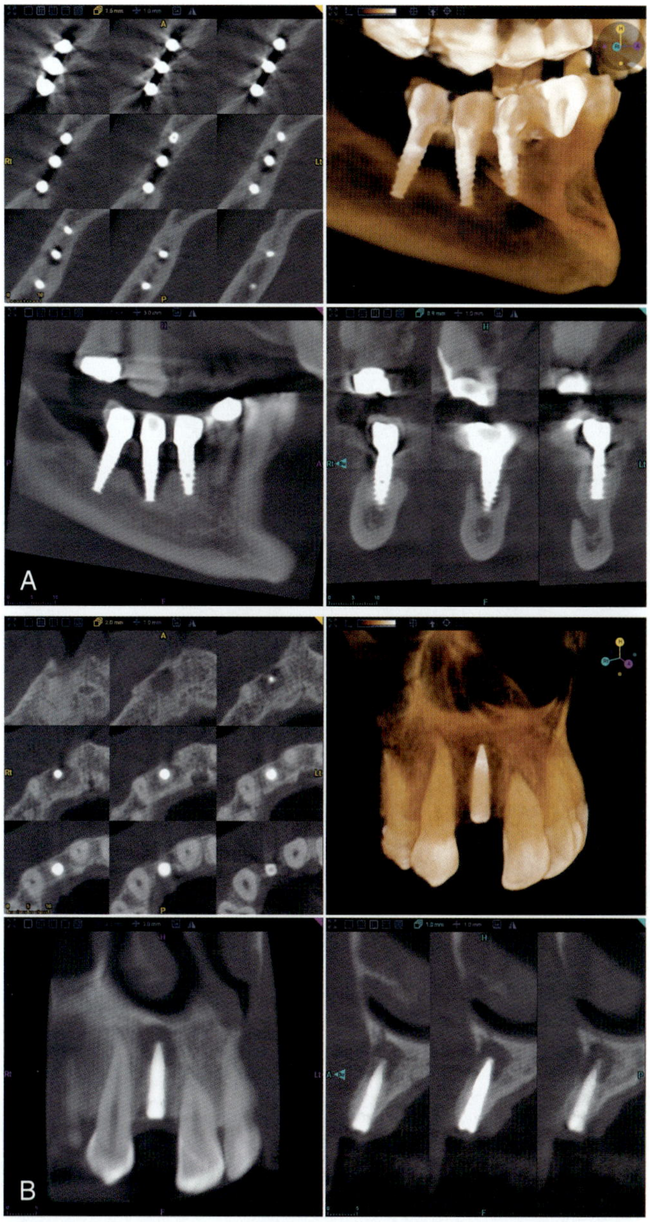

Fig. 31.21 (A) Corrected axial *(top left)*, mesiodistal *(bottom left)*, buccolingual *(bottom right)*, and three-dimensional volume rendering *(top right)* demonstrating mild, moderate, and severe marginal peri-implantitis around the implants placed at the mandibular right second premolar, second molar, and first molar sites (respectively). (B) Corrected axial *(top left)*, mesiodistal *(bottom left)*, buccolingual *(bottom right)*, and three-dimensional volume rendering *(top right)* demonstrating retrograde/apical peri-implantitis around the apical third of the implant placed at the maxillary right lateral incisor site. Note the presence of intact bone surrounding the coronal segment of this implant.

An implant that is placed beyond its local anatomic confines often causes symptoms. In the anterior maxilla and mandible, the presence of a prominent buccal concavity and a relatively thin buccal cortex may result in cortical perforation and thread exposure (Fig. 31.23). This can lead to inflammation of the overlying soft tissue, with symptoms of pain, bleeding, and suppuration. In the posterior maxilla, implants are occasionally placed beyond the maxillary sinus floor, which may result in significant antral mucosal inflammation and the development of sinusitis (Fig. 31.24). In the posterior mandible, implants may extend into the lumen of the inferior alveolar canal, which can lead to altered sensation or numbness (Fig. 31.25). When improperly angled, implants may encroach on roots of adjacent teeth, which may lead to pulp necrosis, often manifesting with nonspecific symptoms (Fig. 31.26). In these situations, CBCT examination may offer valuable insight to elucidate the etiology of the symptoms and to guide management.

In summary, diagnostic imaging is essential for the preoperative planning of dental implants, intraoperative assessment, surgical guidance during implant placement, and the postoperative evaluation of recall and symptomatic patients. With continued scientific and technologic advancements, the practice of dental implantation will likely continue to evolve at a rapid pace. Clinicians will need to remain current with scientific literature and apply appropriate evidence-based treatment decisions that balance diagnostic efficacy, potential radiation risks, and health care costs.

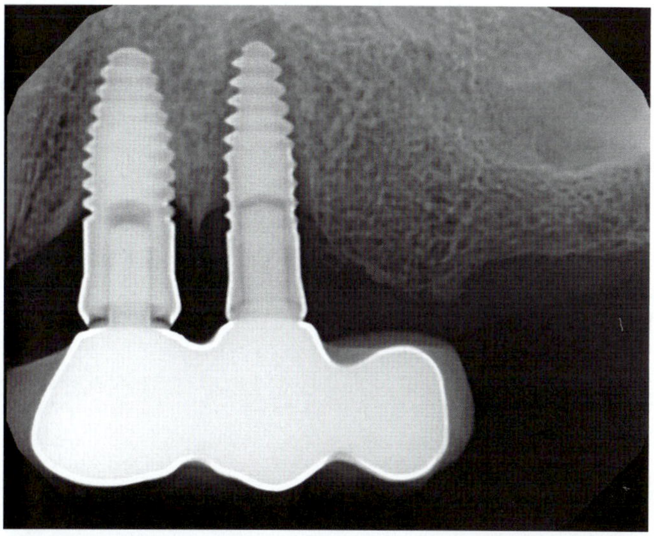

Fig. 31.22 Periapical image of the posterior left maxilla demonstrate a uniform radiolucent lining around the implant placed at the edentulous second premolar site. This could imply the presence of a soft tissue junction, indicating failed osseointegration. Mild crestal bone loss is observed around the adjacent implant at the site of the edentulous first premolar, but the remainder of this implant appears to be embedded in bone.

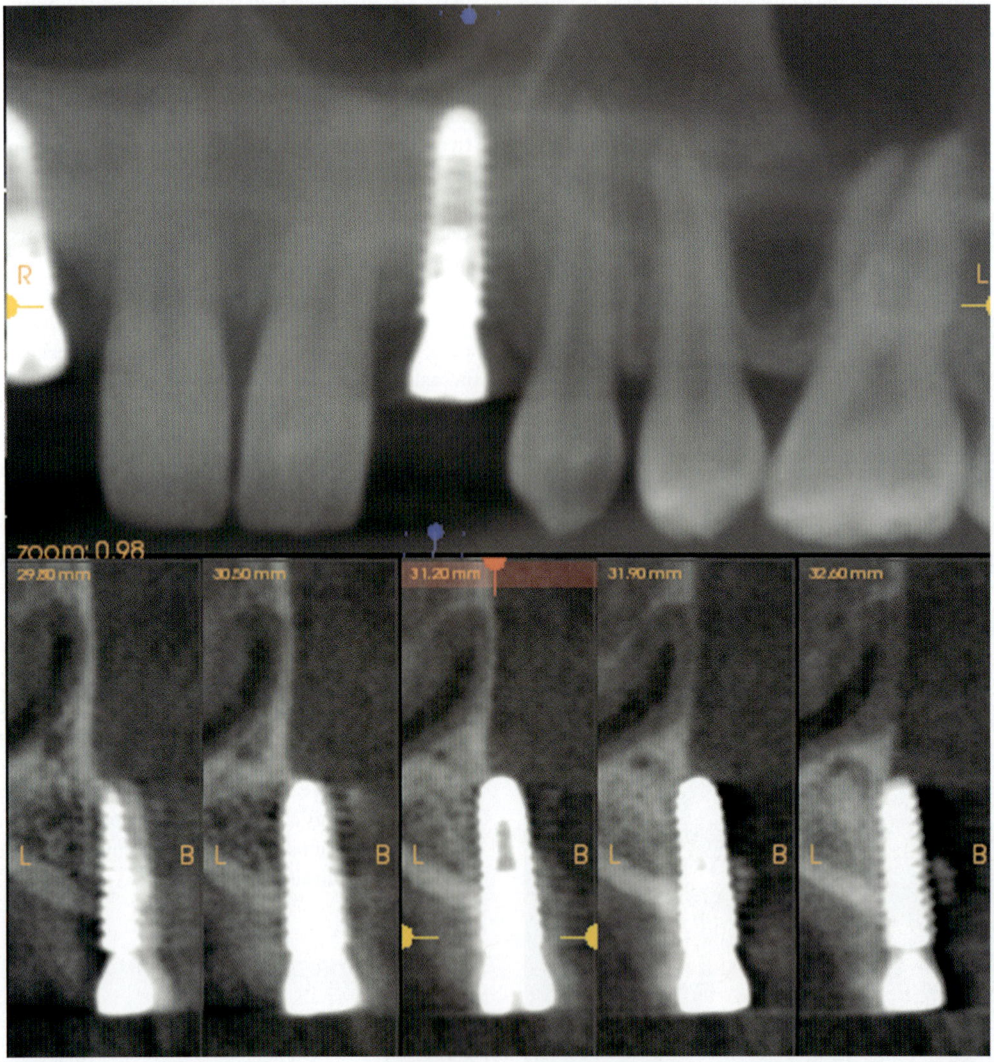

Fig. 31.23 *Top:* Cropped panoramic reformatted image of an implant placed at the site of the edentulous maxillary left lateral incisor. In this view, the implant appears to be embedded in bone. *Bottom:* Buccolingual cross-sectional images of the same implant showing that the buccal threads are exposed through a prominent buccal concavity.

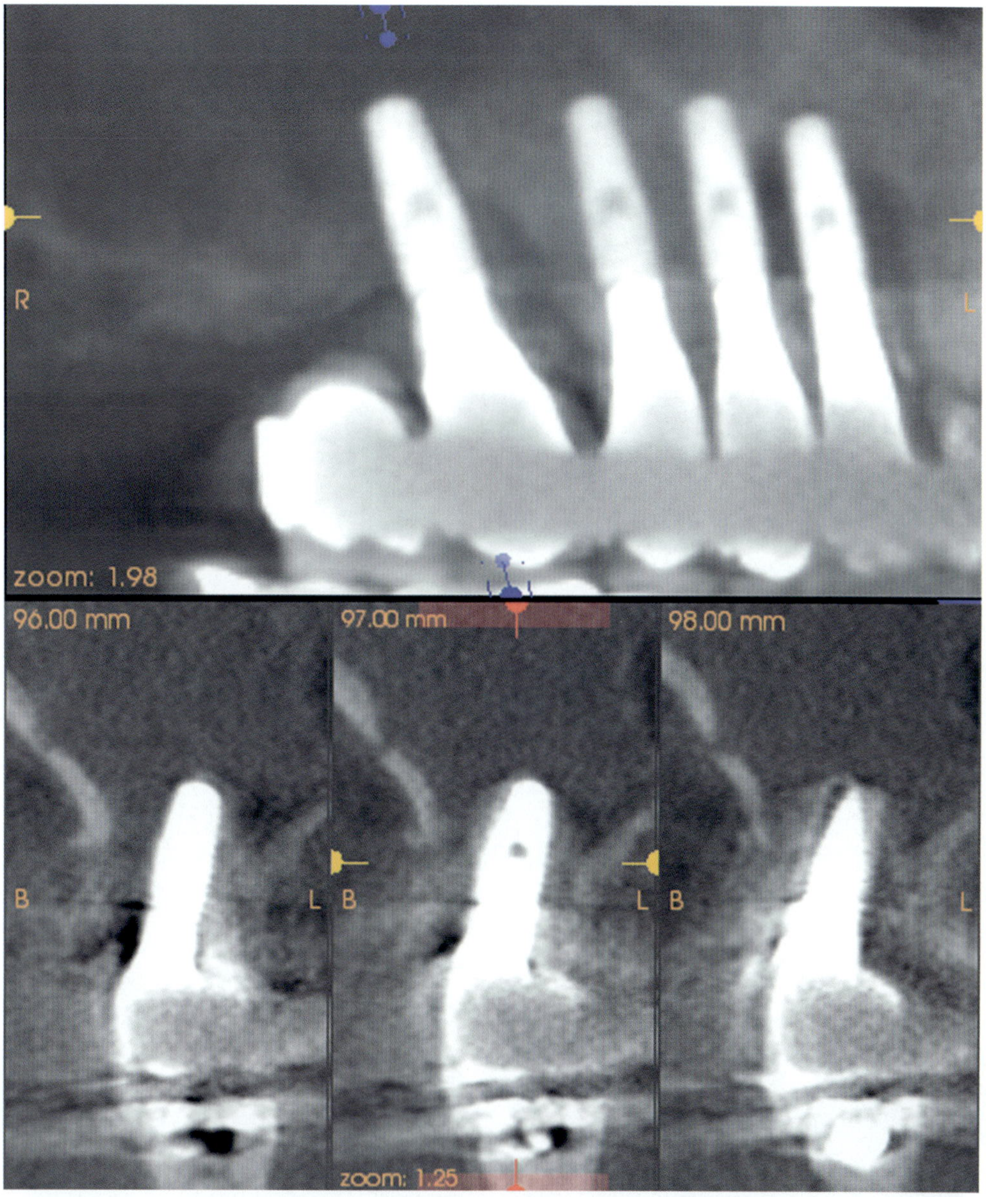

Fig. 31.24 *Top:* Cropped panoramic reformatted image of an implant placed at the site of an edentulous maxillary right first molar. *Bottom:* Buccolingual cross-sectional images of the same implant demonstrating that it has been placed through the floor of the right maxillary sinus. The right antral space is opacified and the sinus walls appear sclerotic, which could suggest the presence of sinusitis.

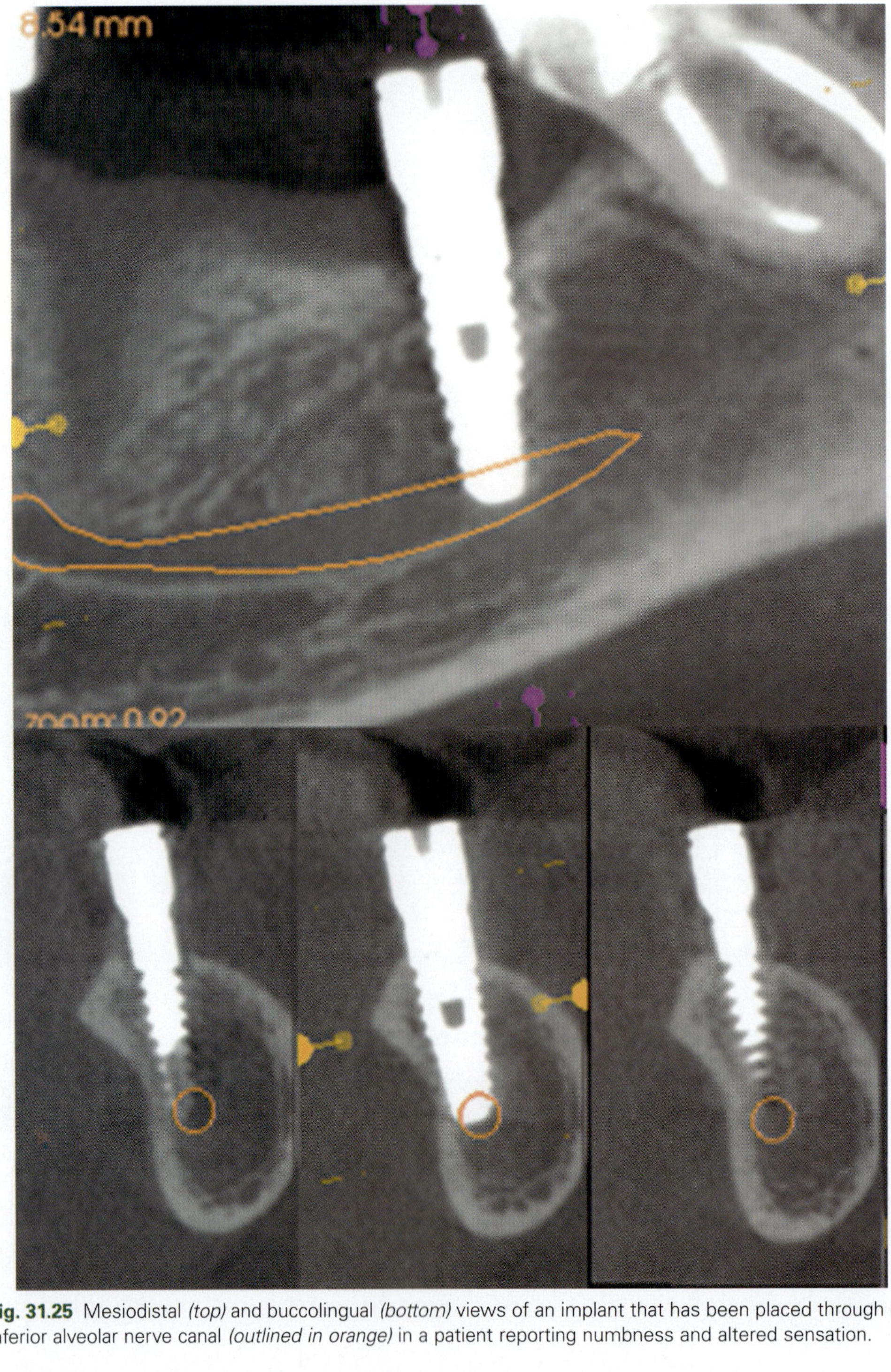

Fig. 31.25 Mesiodistal *(top)* and buccolingual *(bottom)* views of an implant that has been placed through left inferior alveolar nerve canal *(outlined in orange)* in a patient reporting numbness and altered sensation.

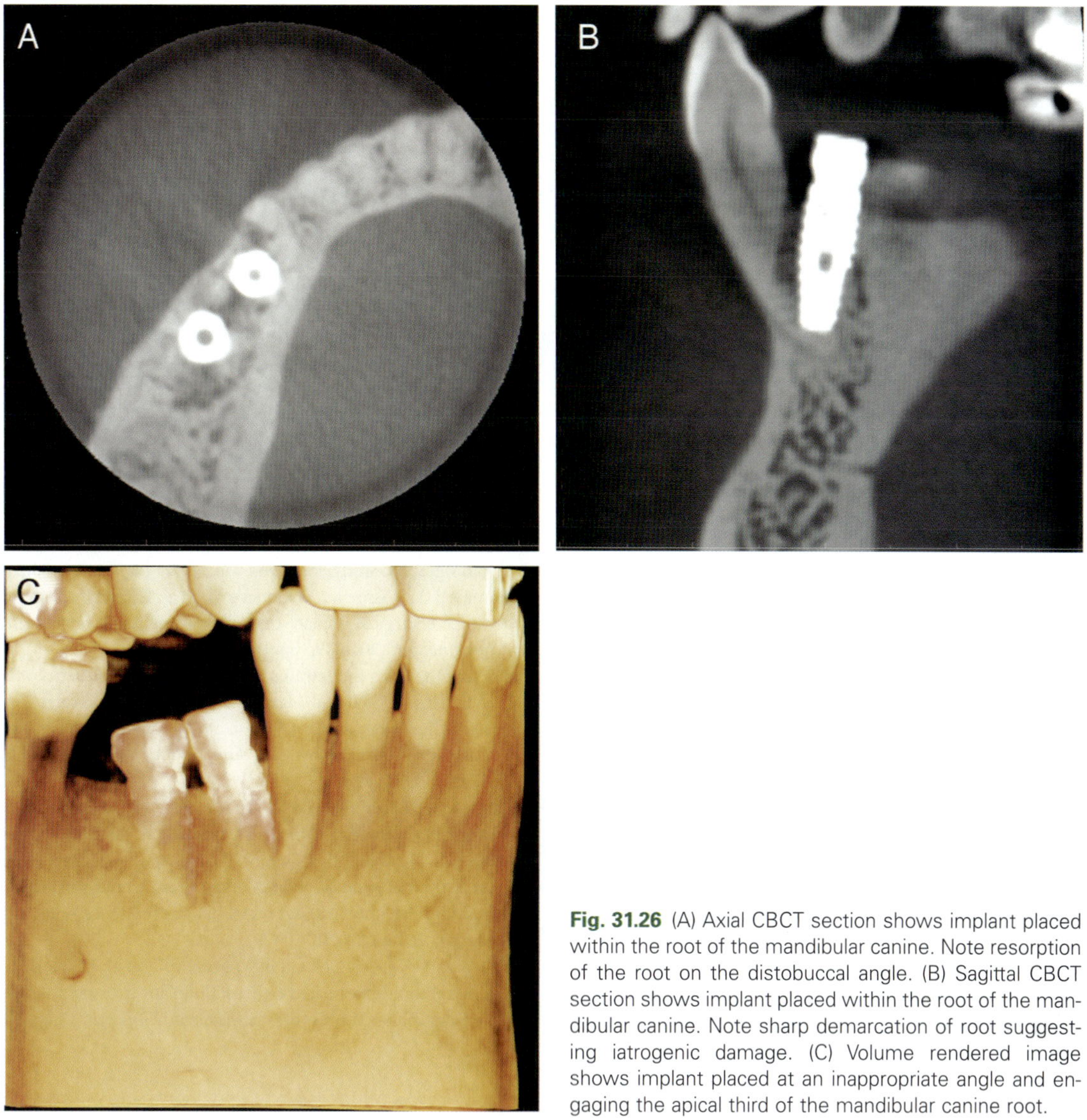

Fig. 31.26 (A) Axial CBCT section shows implant placed within the root of the mandibular canine. Note resorption of the root on the distobuccal angle. (B) Sagittal CBCT section shows implant placed within the root of the mandibular canine. Note sharp demarcation of root suggesting iatrogenic damage. (C) Volume rendered image shows implant placed at an inappropriate angle and engaging the apical third of the mandibular canine root.

BIBLIOGRAPHY

Aguiar MF, Marques AP, Carvalho AC, et al. Accuracy of magnetic resonance imaging compared with computed tomography for implant planning. *Clin Oral Implants Res.* 2008;19(4):362-365.

Angelopoulos C, Thomas SL, Hechler S, et al. Comparison between digital panoramic radiography and cone-beam computed tomography for the identification of the mandibular canal as part of presurgical dental implant assessment. *J Oral Maxillofac Surg.* 2008;66(10):2130-2135.

Arisan V, Karabuda CZ, Ozdemir T. Implant surgery using bone- and mucosa-supported stereolithographic guides in totally edentulous jaws: surgical and post-operative outcomes of computer-aided vs. standard techniques. *Clin Oral Implants Res.* 2010;21(9):980-988.

Arisan V, Karabuda ZC, Ozdemir T. Accuracy of two stereolithographic guide systems for computer-aided implant placement: a computed tomography-based clinical comparative study. *J Periodontol.* 2010;81(1):43-51.

Bencharit S, Schardt-Sacco D, Zuninga JR, et al. Surgical and prosthodontic rehabilitation for patient with agressive florid cemento-osseous dysplasia. A clinical report. *J Prosthet Dent.* 2003;90:220-224.

Bornstein MM, Al-Nawas B, Kuchler U, et al. Consensus statements and recommended clinical procedures regarding contemporary surgical and radiographic techniques in implant dentistry. *Int J Oral Maxillofac Implants.* 2014;29:78-82.

Correa LR, Spin-Neto R, Stavropoulos A, et al. Planning of dental implant size with digital panoramic radiographs, CBCT-generated panoramic images, and CBCT cross-sectional images. *Clin Oral Implants Res.* 2014;25(6):690-695.

Di Giacomo GA, da Silva JV, da Silva AM, et al. Accuracy and complications of computer-designed selective laser sintering surgical guides for flapless dental implant placement and immediate definitive prosthesis installation. *J Periodontol.* 2012;83(4):410-419.

Dioguardi M, Spirito F, Quarta C, et al. Guided Dental Implant Surgery: systematic Review. *J Clin Med.* 2023;12(4):1490.

Ersoy AE, Turkyilmaz I, Ozan O, et al. Reliability of implant placement with stereolithographic surgical guides generated from computed tomography: clinical data from 94 implants. *J Periodontol.* 2008;79(8):1339-1345.

Fortin T, Bosson JL, Isidori M, et al. Effect of flapless surgery on pain experienced in implant placement using an image-guided system. *Int J Oral Maxillofac Implants.* 2006;2:298-304.

Friedrich RE, Laumann F, Zrnc T, et al. The nasopalatine canal in adults on cone beam computed tomograms a clinical study and review of the literature. *In Vivo.* 2015;29(4):467-486.

Gerlach RC, Dixon DR, Goksel T, et al. Case presentation of florid cemento-osseous dysplasia with concomitant cemento-ossifying fibroma discovered during implant explantation. *Oral Surg Oral Med Oral Pathol Oral Radiol.* 2013;115(3):e44-e52.

Gröndahl K, Lekholm U. The predictive value of radiographic diagnosis of implant instability. *Int J Oral Maxillofac Implants.* 1997;12(1):59-64.

Hämmerle CH, Stone P, Jung RE, et al. Consensus statements and recommended clinical procedures regarding computer-assisted implant dentistry. *Int J Oral Maxillofac Implants.* 2009;24(suppl):126-131.

Horner K, Islam M, Flygare L, et al. Basic principles for use of dental cone beam computed tomography: consensus guidelines of the European Academy of Dental and Maxillofacial Radiology. *Dentomaxillofac Radiol.* 2009;38:187-195.

Jung RE, Schneider D, Ganeles J, et al. Computer technology applications in surgical implant dentistry: a systematic review. *Int J Oral Maxillofac Implants.* 2009;24(suppl):92-109.

Kawai T, Hiranuma H, Kishino M, et al. Cemento-osseous dysplasia of the jaws in 54 japanese patients. A radiographic study. *Oral Surg Oral Med Oral Pathol Oral Radiol Endod.* 1999;87:107-114.

Kim YK, Park JY, Kim SG, et al. Magnification rate of digital panoramic radiographs and its effectiveness for pre-operative assessment of dental implants. *Dentomaxillofac Radiol.* 2011;40(2):76-83.

Kusum CK, Mody PV, Indrajeet, et al. Interforaminal hemorrhage during anterior mandibular implant placement: an overview. *Dent Res J (Isfahan).* 2015;12(4):291-300.

Kütük N, Demirbaş AE, Gönen ZB, et al. Anterior mandibular zone safe for implants. *J Craniofac Surg.* 2013;24(4):e405-e408.

Loubele M, Bogaerts R, Van Dijck E, et al. Comparison between effective radiation dose of CBCT and MSCT scanners for dentomaxillofacial applications. *Eur J Radiol.* 2009;71:461-468.

Ludlow JB, Timothy R, Walker C, et al. Effective dose of dental CBCT-a meta analysis of published data and additional data for nine CBCT units. *Dentomaxillofac Radiol.* 2015;44(1):20140197.

Misch CE. Contemporary Implant Dentistry. 3rd ed. Mosby; 2008.

Oliveira MTF, Cardoso SV, Silva CJ, et al. Failure of dental implants in cemento-osseous dysplasia: a critical analysis of a case. *Rev Odontol UNESP.* 2014;43(3):223-227.

Ozan O, Turkyilmaz I, Ersoy AE, et al. Clinical accuracy of 3 different types of computed tomography-derived stereolithographic surgical guides in implant placement. *J Oral Maxillofac Surg.* 2009;67(2):394-401.

Pereira-Maciel P, Tavares-de-Sousa E, Oliveira-Sales MA. The mandibular incisive canal and its anatomical relationships: a cone beam computed tomography study. *Med Oral Patol Oral Cir Bucal.* 2015;20(6):e723-e728.

Raico Gallardo YN, da Silva-Olivio IR, Mukai E, et al. Accuracy comparison of guided surgery for dental implants according to the tissue of support: a systematic review and meta-analysis. *Clin Oral Implants Res.* 2017;28(5):602-612.

Ramanauskaite A, Juodzbalys G, Tözüm TF. Apical/retrograde periimplantitis/implant periapical lesion: etiology, risk factors, and treatment options: a systematic review. *Implant Dent.* 2016;25(5):684-697.

Resnik RR, Kircos LT, Misch CE. Diagnostic imaging and techniques. In: Misch CE, eds. *Contemporary Implant Dentistry.* 3rd ed. Mosby; 2008:38-67.

Ribeiro-Rotta RF, Lindh C, Pereira AC, et al. Ambiguity in bone tissue characteristics as presented in studies on dental implant planning and placement: a systematic review. *Clin Oral Implants Res.* 2011;22(8):789-801.

Rosenfeld AL, Mandelaris GA, Tardieu PB. Prosthetically directed implant placement using computer software to ensure precise placement and predictable prosthetic outcomes. Part 2: rapid-prototype medical modeling and stereolithographic drilling guides requiring bone exposure. *Int J Periodontics Restorative Dent.* 2006;26(4):347-353.

Schneider D, Marquardt P, Zwahlen M, et al. A systematic review on the accuracy and the clinical outcome of computer-guided template-based implant dentistry. *Clin Oral Implants Res.* 2009;20(suppl 4):73-86.

Sharan A, Madjar D. Maxillary sinus pneumatization following extractions: a radiographic study. *Int J Oral Maxillofac Implants.* 2008;23(1):48-56.

Tahmaseb A, Wismeijer D, Coucke W, et al. Computer technology applications in surgical implant dentistry: a systematic review. *Int J Oral Maxillofac Implants.* 2014;29(suppl):25-42.

Tyndall DA, Price JB, Tetradis S, et al. Position statement of the American Academy of Oral and Maxillofacial Radiology on selection criteria for the use of radiology in dental implantology with emphasis on cone beam computed tomography. *Oral Surg Oral Med Oral Pathol Oral Radiol.* 2012;113:817-826.

Van Assche N, Vercruyssen M, Coucke W, et al. Accuracy of computer-aided implant placement. *Clin Oral Implants Res.* 2012;23(suppl 6):112-123.

Vazquez L, Nizamaldin Y, Combescure C, et al. Accuracy of vertical height measurements on direct digital panoramic radiographs using posterior mandibular implants and metal balls as reference objects. *Dentomaxillofac Radiol.* 2013;42(2):20110429.

Yildirim YD, Güncü GN, Galindo-Moreno P, et al. Evaluation of mandibular lingual foramina related to dental implant treatment with computerized tomography: a multicenter clinical study. *Implant Dent.* 2014;23(1):57-63.

Beyond Three-Dimensional Imaging

Kumar C. Shah and Sanjay M. Mallya

Over the past decade, technological advances in three-dimensional (3D) imaging with computed tomography (CT) have enhanced dento-maxillofacial diagnosis and treatment planning. In parallel to the growth of cone beam CT (CBCT), there is an increasing number of digital technologies that are being applied in dentistry. Such technologies are diverse in nature with applications in electronic health record documentation and communication, computer-aided design (CAD), computer-aided manufacturing (CAM), and, more recently, machine learning and artificial intelligence. The ability to integrate digital information from different sources has yielded innovative approaches to treatment planning, fabrication of dental appliances and restorations, and monitoring of treatment. This chapter provides an overview of contemporary technologies that maximize the information provided by CBCT imaging to augment diagnosis and treatment planning.

ARTIFICIAL INTELLIGENCE

Dictionary definitions of intelligence include "the ability to learn or understand or to deal with new or trying situations"; "the ability to learn, understand, and make judgments or have opinions that are based on reason"; "the capacity, especially of a particular person or animal, for learning, reasoning, understanding, and similar forms of mental activity; relative aptitude in grasping truths, relationships, meanings"; and "the ability to think, reason, and understand instead of doing things automatically or by instinct."

The common theme from these definitions is the requirement for a logical approach to problem solving. Applying this to the practice of radiology, intelligence in radiodiagnosis is manifested through pattern recognition and analyzing those findings within an appropriate clinical context.

The term *artificial intelligence* (AI) was first introduced by computer scientist John McCarthy in 1955. In broad terms, it refers to machines performing tasks that typically require human intelligence. Such tasks include learning, sensing the environment, and adapting accordingly. *Augmented intelligence* refers to using technology to enhance or amplify human tasks.

Machine learning (ML) is a subset of AI. In this approach, the computer is not explicitly programmed to perform a task. Rather, computer algorithms provide a set of rules to learn from data, including images, and to make inferences and decisions from these data. Consider the task of radiographic caries detection. A traditional, explicit detection program would define rules based on the radiographic appearance of caries—a radiolucent area within enamel. Explicit program rules would define thresholds for pixel intensity (how radiolucent) and its shape. Defining these rules requires a detailed understanding of the features of dental caries. In the ML approach, an algorithm is trained to generate patterns and rules from existing data, and to apply those rules to new data. ML approaches include:

1. *Supervised learning:* In this approach, a labeled data set is used to train an algorithm. The data labels correspond to specific outputs, and the model learns to map inputs to appropriate outputs, and generalizes these training experiences to unseen data.
2. *Unsupervised learning:* In this approach, the data set is not labeled. Rather, the algorithm finds structure or patterns within the training data used to train an algorithm. Clustering techniques group data into "clusters," based on similarities—data points within the cluster are more similar to each other than to data in other clusters. Dimensionality reduction techniques reduce the number of identifying features without degrading the informational content so that the data set is manageable for analysis and modeling. The goal is to capture the variations that are significant for decision making, and eliminate noise from information that is less relevant to the task.
3. *Semi-supervised learning:* This approach uses labeled and unlabeled data to train an algorithm.
4. *Reinforced learning:* These algorithms learn through interaction and human feedback and learn optimal task-based decisions over time.
5. *Deep learning algorithms:* This subset of ML algorithms uses neural networks with multiple layers and are often used to train algorithms to identify complex features.

Neural networks are ML models that seek to mimic human decision making. The basic processing unit of a neural network is a neuron—it receives input that represents data attributes. The input is weighted and used to produce an output. For example, in image analysis, the input may represent pixel intensity. Neural networks are organized as layers—an input layer, a hidden layer that processes the information, and an output layer that provides the decision or result. In networks that have multiple layers, the input may be derived from the output of a previous layer. This process allows the network to capture categorized relationships. The network models include weights and biases—mathematical modulators of the algorithm that provide flexibility. Convolutional neural networks (CNNs) are best suited to manage image data, including categorization, detection of objects and pathoses (teeth, caries, etc.) and segmentation of images. *Deep learning* involves the use of neural networks with multiple layers, often referred to as deep neural networks, and can learn hierarchical data representation, where combinations of lower level data attributes are grouped into higher levels. This allows the network to extract features from the raw input data. Deep learning models have been successful for image analyses. However, these models require large labeled data sets for meaningful training of the model.

Development Cycle of an Artificial Intelligence Program

1. *Define the problem:* Identify the precise problem(s) or task(s) that the AI program will address. For example, detect caries, measure alveolar crest height, or detect apical periodontitis.
2. *Training data set:* The training data set teaches the AI algorithm to recognize patterns and relationships and to make predictions or classifications of data based on those patterns and relationships. The training data set includes labeled examples that define an input

(e.g., radiolucency on proximal surface of crown not extending into dentin) with an appropriate output decision (e.g., E1 or E2 caries). A large data set is necessary to capture pattern variability for better general application.

3. *Validation data set:* The validation data set examines the model's performance during the training. It includes labeled input, but is smaller in size than the training data set and comprises cases discrete from the training data set. The validation process allows fine-tuning of the algorithm.
4. *Test data set:* This data set can be used to measure the model's performance after the algorithm has been trained and fine-tuned.
5. *Performance measures:* These measures allow the user to determine whether an AI algorithm is suitable for a specific task. Measures used include:
    a. *Accuracy:* Proportion of correctly categorized cases overall.
    b. *Precision:* Proportion of true positive predictions among all positive predictions.
    c. *Sensitivity:* Proportion of true positive predictions among all positive cases in the training, validation, or test data set.
    d. *F1 score:* It measures the harmonic mean of sensitivity and precision and considers false positive and false negative assessments. The F1 score is calculated as:
    $F1 = 2 \times (Precision \times Sensitivity)/(Precision + Sensitivity)$
    e. *Specificity:* Proportion of true negative predictions among all negative cases in the training, validation, or test data set.

A

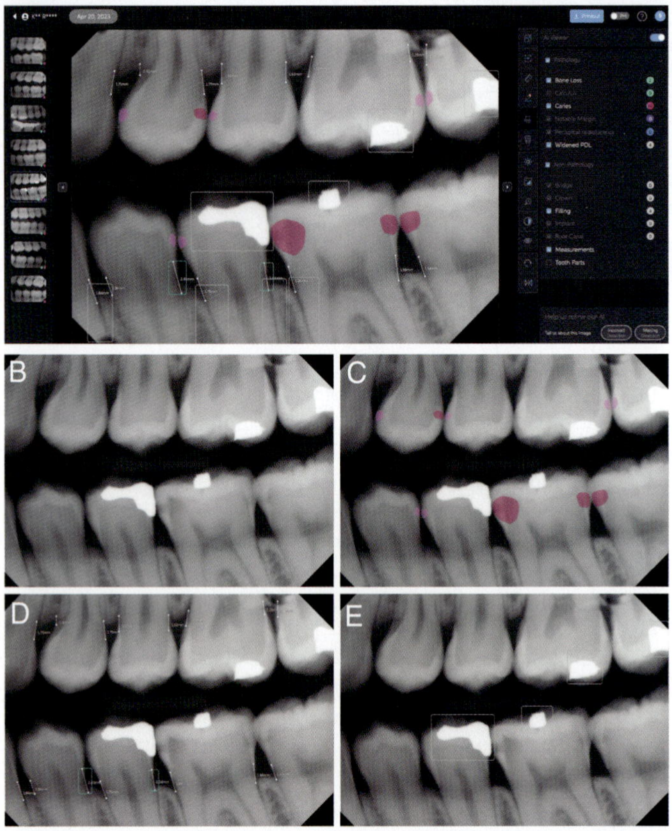

Fig. 32.1 Artificial intelligence-based analyses of dental radiographs. (A) Web-based interface of an AI program for radiologic analyses *(Second Opinion, Pearl, W. Hollywood, CA)*. To facilitate augmented analyses, the user can highlight or hide detected pathoses and other annotations. The user can also print a report that summarizes the AI detections and annotations. (B) Bitewing radiograph, without annotations. (C) Automated caries detection, with caries lesions highlighted in *pink*. Note that the system outlines presumed borders of the caries and its extent into dentin. Caries limited to enamel are shaded differently. (D) Automated periodontal bone measurement, with distances at interproximal bone height measured. (E) Identification of restorations in teeth.

Application of Artificial Intelligence in Oral and Maxillofacial Radiology

AI-based software programs for automated analyses of dental radiographs are commercially available (Fig. 32.1). These products are approved as diagnostic aids, not stand-alone diagnostic devices, and require human intervention to accept or reject the AI assessment. AI can be directed to several different tasks as follows.

- *Caries detection:* Identify presence of caries and segment its extent into enamel and dentin.
- *Periodontal bone loss:* Measure the distance from the alveolar crest to the cementoenamel junction and categorize as bone loss versus normal.
- *Periodontal ligament widening:* Detect wide periodontal ligament space at the apex and along the length of the root.
- *Calculus deposits:* Identify and outline areas where calculus is present on teeth.
- *Restorations and margins:* Identify prosthesis and restorations.
- *Detect pathoses in the jaws:* Identify incidental findings of relevance.
- *Segment the image:* Segment images to identify erupted, unerupted or impacted, and missing teeth. CBCT automatically segmented to provide a 3D view of the anatomy and to allow easy identification of teeth and bones.
- *Cephalometric analyses:* Identify anatomic landmarks and perform analyses.

Potentially, AI-based radiographic analysis can help increase accuracy, efficiency, and consistency of radiologic determinations, and initial results have been promising. Applications of AI-based radiographic analysis in clinical practice is in a nascent stage and its impact on quality care remains to be explored.

COMPUTER-GUIDED TREATMENT PLANNING

Three-dimensional CT data are valuable for presurgical assessment of the maxillofacial anatomy (e.g., to plan reconstructive maxillofacial surgery for cosmetic, functional, and prosthetic indications or to plan placement of dental implants). Several commercial software applications can use CT volumetric data for computer-aided surgical planning. Some vendors offer these advanced functions as modules that can be added to the standard CBCT analysis suite, facilitating their application to clinical practice. The application of CAD/CAM to maxillofacial surgical interventions is expected to increase. Typically, surgical planning software applications use CBCT Digital Imaging and Communication in Medicine (DICOM) data and provide 3D visualization by surface segmentation and volumetric rendering of the anatomic area imaged. The region of interest (ROI) may be a potential implant site, a pathosis in the jaw, a surgical defect, a maxillofacial developmental aberration, or the site of orthognathic surgery. Via an interactive interface, the user manipulates the CT data and simulates surgical procedures (e.g., implant placement or jaw repositioning). The simulated surgical changes are then exported in digital format and a CAD/CAM-generated tangible object such as a stent or surgical guide is made to transfer the in silico plan to the patient's anatomy during surgery.

Dental implant planning: Computer-aided implant planning is widely used in standard clinical practice. The goal of dental implant treatment is functional and esthetic restoration of the patient's dentition. CT imaging provides essential diagnostic information to evaluate the morphology of the edentulous site, the bone quality at the proposed implant site, and the relationships to the adjacent vital structures and teeth. For accurate and predictable outcomes, dental implant placement should be prosthetically driven. There are several commercial software applications for computer-guided planning and placement of dental implants (see Chapter 31).

In general, proprietary implant treatment planning software programs import CBCT data in DICOM format, allowing for a relatively easy transfer of the digital CBCT data to treatment planning software applications. The treatment planning software includes an "implant library"—customized overlays corresponding to the shape and size of individual implant types. Within the planning software, the clinician can virtually place the implant overlays, with consideration to individual anatomic and functional factors, implant parallelism, and the design of the prosthetic restoration. These include the local availability of bone volume, angulation relative to the adjacent teeth, and the proximity to vital structures. The virtually placed implants can be angled and repositioned to simulate the final desired treatment plan (Fig. 32.2A). Virtual implant treatment planning allows the clinician to assess the need for bone augmentation and whether such augmentation could be accomplished at the time of implant placement (see Fig. 32.2B).

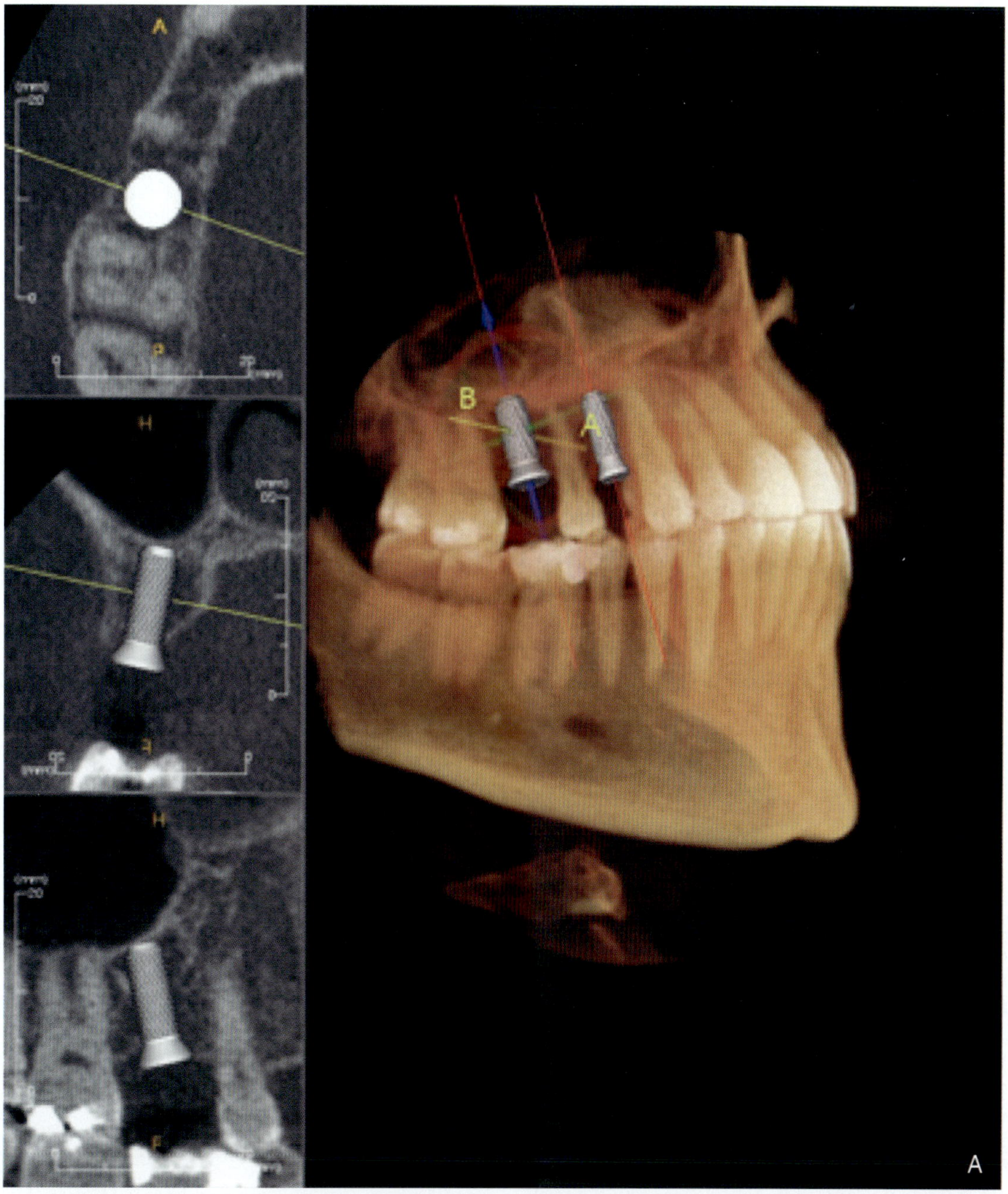

Fig. 32.2 In silico implant planning. (A) Virtual implants are placed in the right maxilla. The three-dimensional volume rendered image shows virtual implants at the first premolar and first molar regions. Axial, coronal, and sagittal sections through the virtual molar implant are shown. The virtual implant is seated between the buccal and palatal cortices and engages the floor of the right maxillary sinus.

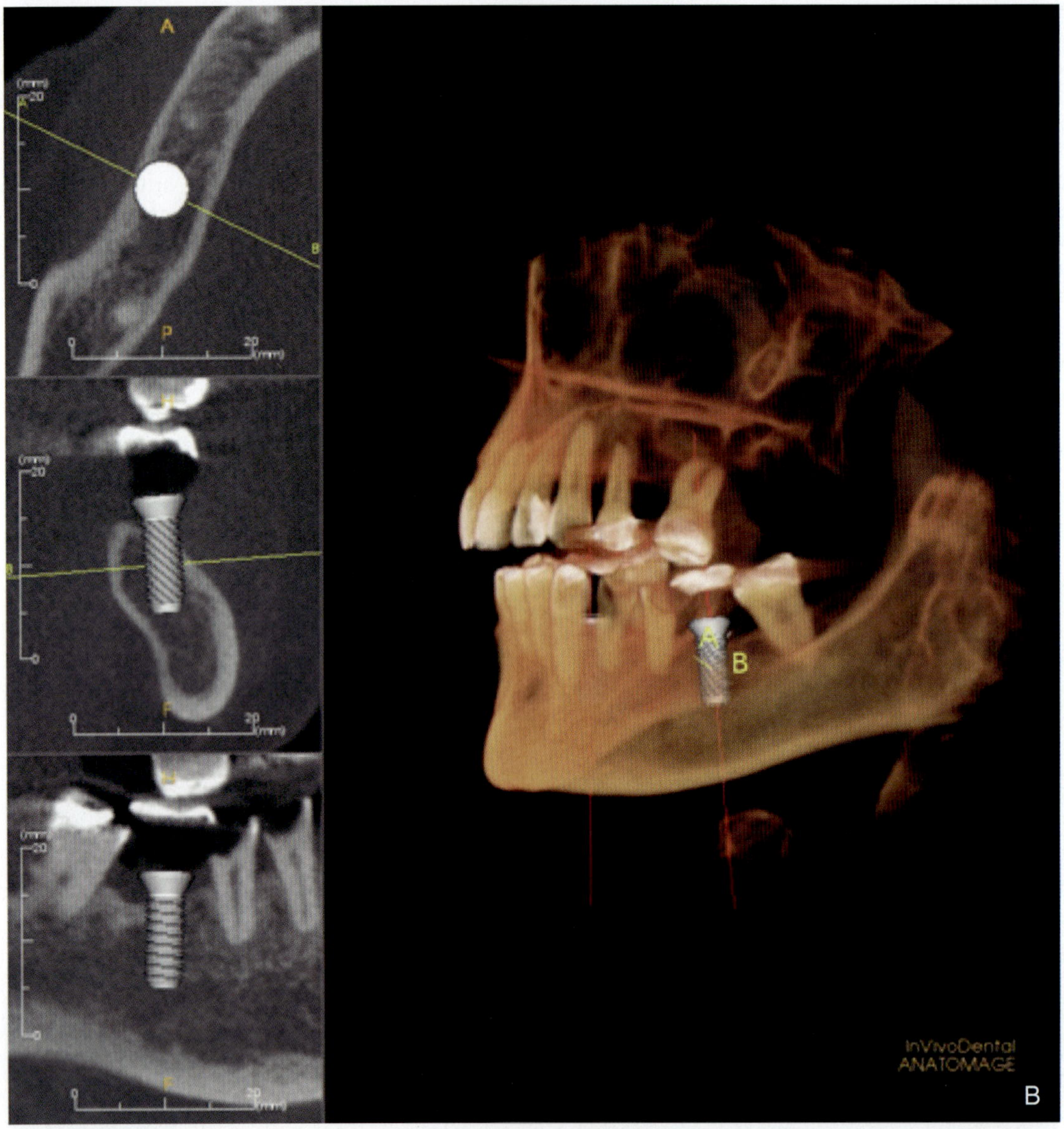

Fig. 32.2, cont'd (B) A virtual implant is positioned in the left mandibular first molar region. The location and angulation of the implant are guided by the radiopaque imaging stent. Axial, coronal, and sagittal sections through the virtual molar implant show exposure of the implant threads, indicating the need for bone augmentation.

The virtual treatment plan directs fabrication of a CAD/CAM-designed surgical guide (Fig. 32.3). The use of surgical guides allows predictable implant placement with decreased intraoperative time. These guides may be mucosa, bone, or tooth supported. Many software applications allow the user to combine data from an optical intraoral scan of the dentition for better identification of the anatomic boundaries of the teeth and edentulous site mucosa to enhance the accuracy of the surgical guide. Clinicians must be aware that computer-guided dental implant placement is not 100% accurate. Even with the use of a CAD/CAM-fabricated surgical guide, there are deviations in the positions of the final placed implants, relative to the planning. Thus the clinician should incorporate appropriate safety zones into the treatment planning process to ensure that implant placement does not compromise adjacent vital structures and teeth or other implants.

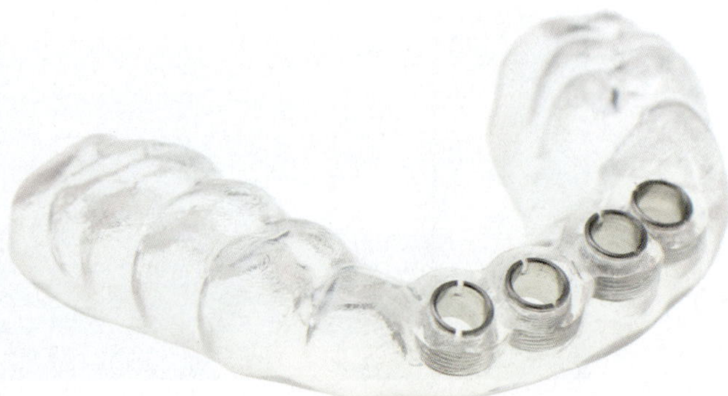

Fig. 32.3 A tooth-supported surgical guide. (Image courtesy Osteoid Inc., Santa Clara, CA.)

Orthognathic surgery: Conventional approaches to planning orthognathic surgery include cephalometric analysis and mock surgery on stone dental models. Virtual planning has been used to plan these surgical approaches, especially in patients with complex craniofacial deformities. Virtual planning with 3D CT data provides several advantages over conventional techniques. Treatment planning software programs can integrate digital data from CT, optical scans of the dental arch, and soft tissues to provide the clinician with a combined interactive virtual model. This is especially valuable in patients with asymmetric malocclusion and facial asymmetry. Easy communication of the virtual plan facilitates collaboration between the treatment team. Importantly, this approach can decrease the operating room time and decrease surgical complications, thereby decreasing costs and improving patient outcomes. Studies have shown that computer-assisted surgical planning has high accuracy, with average errors of less than 2 mm for linear dimensions and approximately 1.2 degrees for angular measurements. Several commercial software packages are available for virtual maxillofacial surgical planning. These include Dolphin (Dolphin Imaging, Chatsworth, CA), InVivo (Osteoid Inc., Santa Clara, CA), Maxilim (Mechelen, Belgium), and MIMICS, and Proplan CMF (Materialise, Belgium). However, these software applications are expensive, and the process of virtual planning requires expertise and is time intensive. Many maxillofacial surgeons use third-party services for the initial planning, software manipulation, and stent construction.

Virtual orthognathic treatment planning involves several steps and starts by combining anatomic data. The skeletal anatomy is provided by CT imaging, either multidetector CT (MDCT) or CBCT. The dental anatomy is captured by optical scanning of the dentition or by digitization of conventional stone models. In addition, the natural head position and the intercuspal occlusal relationships are registered. Three-dimensional photographs provide facial soft-tissue surface information. Fiducial markers may be used to facilitate image data registration and subsequent superimposition of the these anatomic DICOM data sets. Often, these patients may have fixed orthodontic appliances, which cause considerable artifacts on the CT image. Tools in the software application allow removal of these artifactual areas. Using software tools, the surgeon then performs virtual osteotomy, mimicking surgical cuts and repositioning the virtual fragments (Fig. 32.4). The morphology of the jaws and location of vital structures guide the position of the osteotomy and the virtual placement of fixation devices. The planning software also predicts changes in the soft tissue with varying movements of the skeletal fragments. To translate the virtual plan to the operation room, a CAD/CAM-fabricated interocclusal splint is fabricated to guide fragment repositioning during the actual surgery. Custom cutting plates and fixation devices can also be fabricated and printed (Fig. 32.5).

Custom implants for facial augmentation and to restore maxillofacial defects: Proprietary software programs can design and print custom implants for facial augmentation (e.g., to augment the chin, zygomatic bones, and mandible). Similarly, maxillofacial defects from trauma or radical surgery can be restored by designing a custom implant–supported prosthesis. Custom implants provide several advantages over commercial stock implants. Custom implants have a more precise fit and are adapted to the underlying bone contours. When restoring unilateral aberrations, the unaffected side can be mirrored. Custom implants require minimal surgical alteration of the bony anatomy prior to implant placement. This reduces surgical time and cost.

THREE-DIMENSIONAL PRINTING

Three-dimensional printing, also referred to as additive manufacturing or rapid prototyping, is growing technology with increasing applications in health care. Initially developed to produce scale models and prototypes in the engineering industry, this technology has now grown to produce quality parts and objects in small numbers and at a lower cost. In medicine and dentistry, 3D-printed models of a patient's anatomy can be created for presurgical treatment planning, and creation of surgical templates and dental prosthesis. This technology also holds promise to print biologic tissues that may be used to print human organs and tissues.

This technology is of particular relevance to radiologic imaging, which most often provides the anatomic information that forms the basis for CAD/CAM design. In dentistry, many applications of 3D

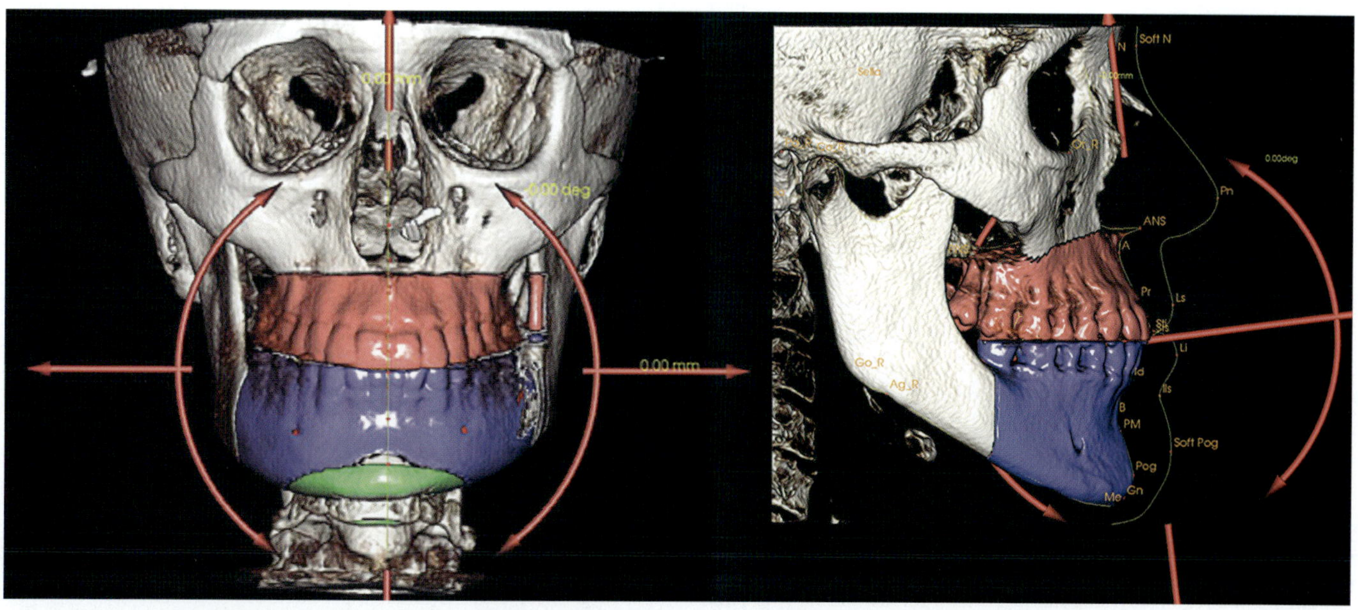

Fig. 32.4 Computer-assisted surgical planning. The osteotomy segments of the maxilla and mandible can be repositioned in any plane. (Images courtesy Osteoid Inc., Santa Clara, CA.)

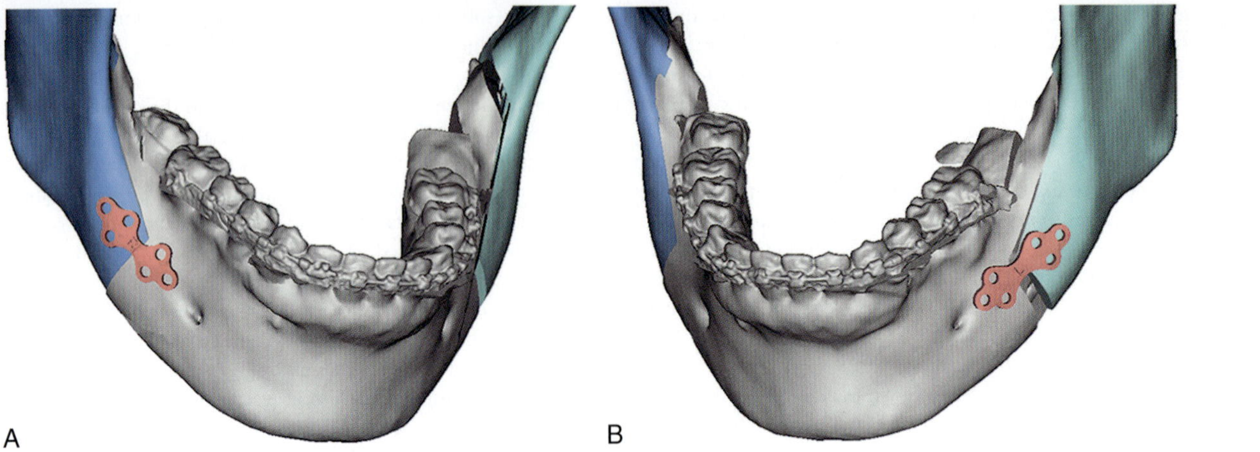

Fig. 32.5 (A and B) Computer-aided design of custom titanium plates to stabilize mandibular segments after a bilateral sagittal split osteotomy. (Modified from Li B, Shen S, Jiang W, et al. A new approach of splint-less orthognathic surgery using a personalized orthognathic surgical guide system: a preliminary study. *Int J Oral Maxillofac Surg.* 2017;46:1298-1305.)

printing are based on skeletal and dental anatomy, acquired via MDCT or CBCT. Anatomic information from CT images support a wide range of 3D printing applications. CT images provide excellent contrast to differentiate between bone and soft tissue, which facilitates postprocessing. The basic steps for generation of a 3D model from CT data are described.

- *CT acquisition and reconstruction:* CT data sets should be reconstructed with isotropic voxels to maintain anatomic truth without loss of information. MDCT examinations should be reconstructed using bone kernels (see Chapter 9). The thickness of the reconstructed sections impacts the accuracy of the printed models. For most applications, reconstruction thickness should be at least 1.25 mm. Thin sections require considerable segmentation which may be time intensive, whereas thicker sections could compromise the accuracy of the printed model. Anatomic areas such as the orbital floor, lamina papyracea, and anterior wall of the maxillary sinus consist of thin bone and require thin sections for accuracy.
- *Image segmentation:* DICOM data from the CT examination are imported into specialized software programs that segment the ROI. For example, if the task is to create a model of the mandible, voxels that represent the mandible have to be partitioned from the remainder of the imaged structures. On CT images, this may be accomplished initially by *thresholding*, to identify pixels in the range of bone CT numbers (see Chapter 9). However, thresholding will delineate pixels based on their gray values but not on spatial location. To isolate pixels that comprise an ROI, region growing segmentation algorithms can be applied. The operator initially selects one or more "seeds" within the anatomic region to be segmented. The computer algorithm compares the gray values of the neighboring pixels and, when similar, adds those pixels to expand the seed. The process is iterative and continues until no more pixels can be added. Operator input may be required to manually add in pixels, modify boundaries, or erase regions. Imperfections in the segmentation manifest as inaccuracies in the 3D-printed model.
- *Create a standard tessellation language (STL) file:* The most widely used file format for 3D printing is STL. The term *tessellation* refers to tiling shapes of different geometry onto a flat surface without any overlaps or gaps. Likewise, an STL file represents the surface of the segmented region as triangular facets. Polygon file format (PLY) and object file format (OBJ) are other formats used in digital dentistry.
- *Creating the 3D-printed model:* The term *3D printing* or *additive manufacturing* encompasses seven categories of technologies used to create models, devices, or implants. The five technologies used in health care are described as follows:
  - *Vat photopolymerization:* Also referred to as *stereolithography,* this process uses a photo-curable liquid resin that solidifies on exposure to an intense light source. A laser beam is used to illuminate only the ROI cross section and cure the resin, producing a 2D cross-section layer of the model. The resin-containing vat is successively lowered (or raised for bottom-up printers) until all sections of the ROI have been printed. The model is then cured using an ultraviolet light source. The final model may require finishing to smooth edges. Small desktop devices are available for in-office use and can be used to fabricate implant guides and models of the jaws and teeth. Resins may be opaque or may be clear to demonstrate internal segmented structures such as neurovascular canals or lesions.
  - *Material jetting:* This process is similar to inkjet printers. A nozzle moves horizontally across and jets the photopolymer onto a build platform. The layer of material is cured by ultraviolet light, and the nozzle continues to build the next layer on top of this layer, printing successive layers of the model. This process allows for multiple materials or multiple colors to be used. Materials used include polymethyl methacrylate, polystyrene, polypropylene, acrylonitrile butadiene styrene, polycarbonate, high-impact polystyrene, and high-density polyethylene. This method has been used to print dental models and implant guides.
  - *Binder jetting:* This process is similar to material jetting. The build material is a powder with a liquid binder that acts as an adhesive. The print nozzle moves horizontally to deposit layers of the powder followed by the liquid binder. The printed object is then lowered, and layers of powder and binder are deposited to successively build the model. Postprocessing includes vacuuming to remove residual powder and infiltrating the model with a resin or elastomer.
  - *Material extrusion:* Also termed *fuse deposition modeling,* this process is widely used for medical and nonmedical applications due to its low cost. The build material is heated in a nozzle and deposited onto a platform, where it cools and hardens. Materials used are plastics and polymers. The resolution of this technique is lower, and the finished products are less accurate.
  - *Powder bed fusion:* Technologies in this category include direct metal laser sintering, electron beam melting, selective heat sintering, selective laser melting, and selective laser sintering. A layer of

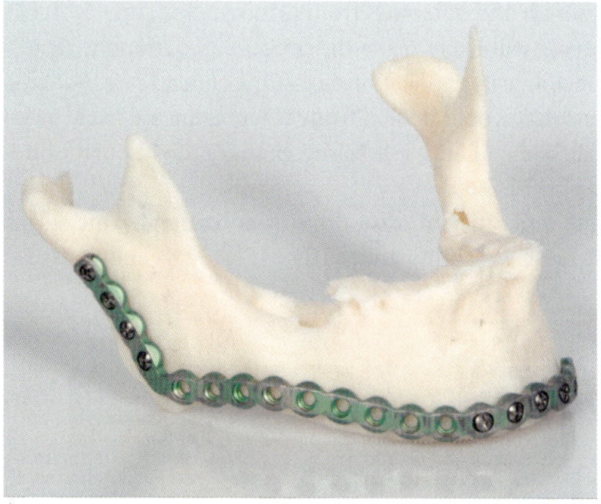

Fig. 32.6 A reconstruction plate is prebent on a 3D-printed model of the patient's mandible. Preparing reconstruction plates prior to surgery decreases operative time and improves patient outcomes. (Image modified from Kuehle R, et al. The value of prebent reconstruction plates and in-house 3D printing. *J Stomatol Oral Maxillofac Surg.* 2023;124:101381.)

powder is deposited onto a build platform, and a laser or electron beam is used to melt and fuse particles within the ROI. Successive layers of the model are built as with previous techniques. Materials used include plastics, polymers, and metals, including biocompatible materials for long-term use.

Clinical Applications of Three-Dimensional Printing

- *Craniofacial trauma and reconstruction:* 3D-printed models aid the surgeon to view complex trauma, in particular the location and the direction of fractures, and dislocation of the fractured segments. This information is essential to plan treatment to avoid damage to vital structures. The models can be used to bend plates and recontour bars prior to surgery (Fig. 32.6) or create custom cutting guides and fixation devices (see Fig. 32.5), decreasing intraoperative time. Mock surgery can be performed on the models, allowing the surgeon to anticipate potential issues that may be encountered at the time of surgery.
- *Implant surgical guides:* Following virtual implant planning, 3D-printed surgical guides may be fabricated to facilitate implant placement (see Fig. 32.3).
- *Maxillofacial prosthesis:* 3D printing can be used to generate CAD-designed prosthesis to restore surgical defects following radical surgery or trauma-related disfigurement.
- *Treatment planning and patient education:* 3D-printed models can be used to perform mock surgical procedures (e.g., orthognathic surgery or graft harvesting for bone augmentation). When vital structures such as neurovascular canals are also segmented in the model, the clinician can anticipate potential intraoperative limitations and better assess the risk to these structures from the surgical procedure.

FOUR-DIMENSIONAL IMAGING

Diagnostic imaging is often performed to assess temporal changes (e.g., to monitor disease progression or recurrence) or to evaluate outcomes of treatment. For the most part, this is typically accomplished by a subjective visual comparison of the regions of interest on two radiographic examinations that were acquired at different times. Special software applications can merge digital information from these two images to identify interval changes that are not easily perceptible by visual evaluation. These applications typically create and display a composite image to provide a visual, interactive interface to facilitate subjective and quantitative evaluation of disease- or treatment-related changes.

Previously, such comparative techniques were used to assess dental caries, periodontal disease, and healing of apical periodontal lesions on conventional two-dimensional (2D) intraoral radiographs. These techniques applied subtraction radiography, a computer-based approach, to merge information from temporally separated digital images and "subtract" the common information to portray the interval change. However, this approach is significantly limited by the 2D nature of periapical and bite-wing radiographs. Small changes in the relationships between the x-ray beam, receptor, and the patient cause perceptible changes in the projected radiographic image and yield artifacts on subtraction images, decreasing the technique's specificity. Thus subtraction radiography using intraoral images has not translated into a routine clinical practice. However, the 3D nature of CBCT images overcomes the limitations of 2D projection geometry. Several software applications have been developed for CBCT image superimposition and quantitative analysis of changes. Some commercial CBCT analysis software suites (e.g., InVivo [Anatomage, San Jose, CA] and OnDemand 3D [Cybermed Inc., Seoul, Korea]) incorporate such modules to facilitate comparison of serial imaging.

Four-dimensional (4D) CBCT imaging, also referred to as image superimposition, uses two CBCT volumes of the same patient acquired at different time points. It is imperative that these two CBCT examinations are reconstructed with the same voxel size. The first step is *image registration*—a process to spatially align the two CBCT volumes. This process establishes spatial correspondence between voxels of the two image data sets. The second step is *image transformation*—where computer algorithms identify corresponding points or regions within the two CBCT data sets and calculate the volume rotations that must be applied to maximize the alignment of corresponding points and regions. Such "rigid body" transformations change only the position and orientation of the scan volume and do not alter the shape or size of the individual CBCT volume. Image registration may be facilitated by providing external markers (e.g., placed on the patient's skin or incorporated into a custom imaging stent). However, this is seldom done in routine clinical practice. Most image registration approaches use the patient anatomy as "markers" for registration. Approaches to image registration are listed as follows:

- *Landmark-based registration:* In this procedure, corresponding anatomic landmark points are identified to serve as spatial location markers on each CBCT volume. These points are recorded via user interaction by manual selection of points on surface segmented images of the two CBCT volumes. Theoretically, three landmark points are sufficient for rigid body transformation of the maxillofacial structures. In practice, more than three points are used. The registration algorithm computes a "centroid"—an average location of the selected points on each image volume. Differences in the 3D spatial location of the two centroids are used to compute the volume rotations that must be applied until distances between corresponding point pairs are minimized.
- *Segmentation-based registration:* Surfaces of the maxillofacial skeleton or skin are identified by segmentation, and the computer algorithm transforms one image volume until the average distance between two corresponding surfaces is minimized. Segmentation is easily accomplished and is computationally less demanding, and the registration can be rapid and automated.
- *Voxel-based registration:* Spatial correspondence is achieved by matching the gray values of individual voxels. The registration algorithm may use the voxels from the entire CBCT volume or from a predefined region selected by the operator. Typically, these methods are fully automated and minimize operator-associated variations in landmark identification. For most maxillofacial applications, the base of the skull has been shown to be a reliable stable region for voxel matching. Voxel-based methods of image registration have been shown to be reliable and reproducible, with registration errors of 0.5 mm or less.

Clinical Applications

The ability to superimpose 3D CBCT volumes facilitates subjective and quantitative evaluations of temporal changes. Some commercial CBCT analysis software suites provide these features, allowing users to apply this technique to clinical practice situations. With software programs that use voxel-based registration, the process of image superimposition is typically automated, reducing operator time and variability. Several research groups have investigated the applicability and reliability of this technique to assess growth and outcomes from orthognathic surgery. Technological enhancements will likely make the process user friendly, rapid, and reliable, and facilitate its application to routine clinical care. Potential clinical applications that would benefit from 4D imaging are listed as follows:

- Evaluate skeletal and soft-tissue changes during orthodontic treatment (Fig. 32.7).
- Evaluate outcomes of orthodontic and orthognathic surgical treatment to assess stability and relapse (Fig. 32.8) and to assess changes to the airway.

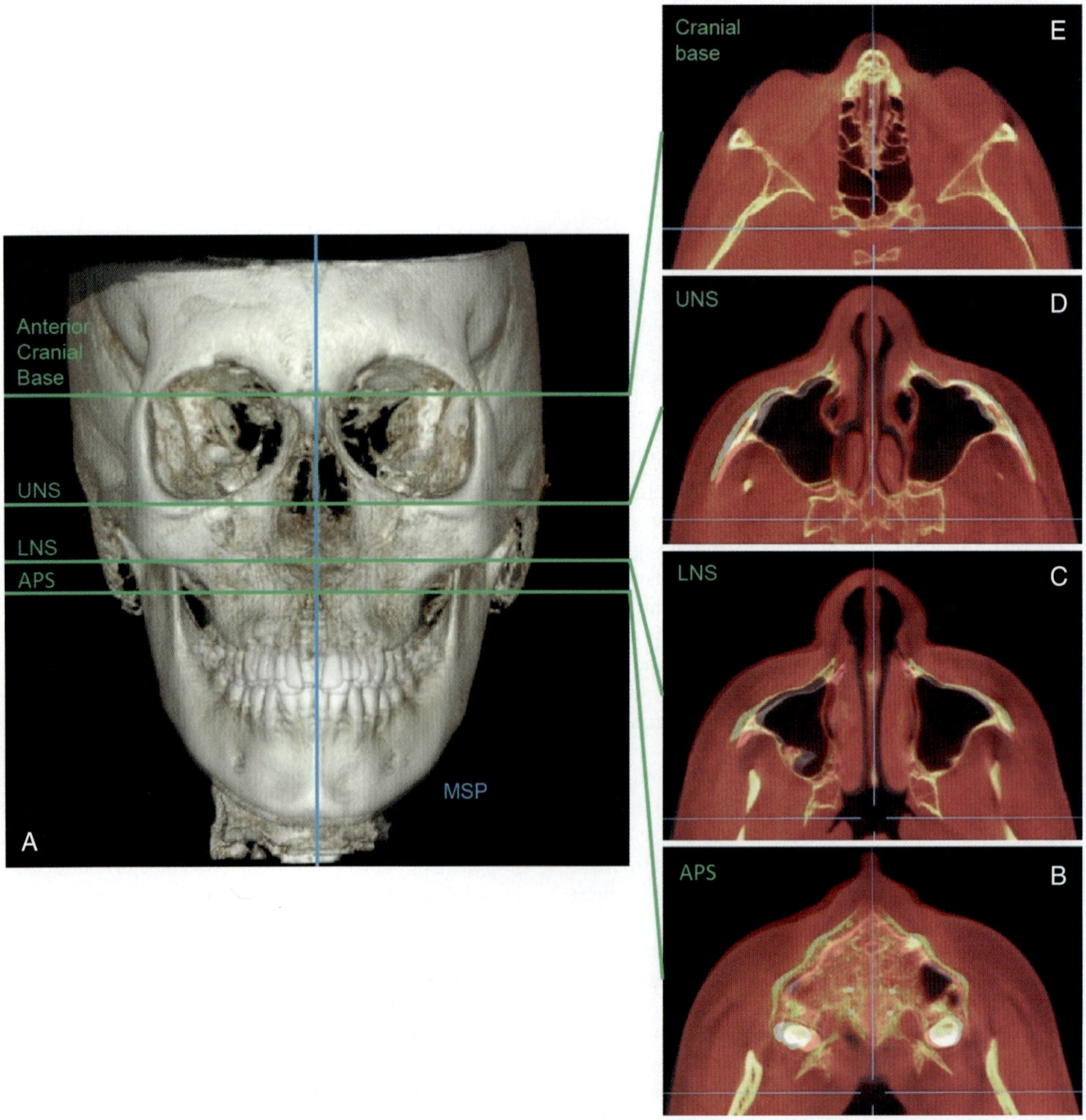

Fig. 32.7 Evaluation of skeletal changes caused by rapid palatal expansion. The maxillary skeletal expander is an implant-assisted device for palatal expansion. In this appliance, four microimplants provide anchorage for forces applied to expand the maxilla. The implants flank the midpalatal suture and engage the cortices of the palate and the nasal floor. Pretreatment and posttreatment cone beam computed tomography scans were registered using automated voxel-based registration (OnDemand 3D, Cybermed Inc., Seoul, South Korea), using the region of the anterior cranial base for spatial correlation. Fused images were analyzed to assess treatment-induced changes in the maxilla and midfacial skeleton. Selected fused sections at axial planes through the palate (B) and the upper and lower regions of the nasal cavity (C and D) demonstrate appliance-induced changes in the maxilla, with separation of the midpalatal suture. There is excellent alignment of the osseous anatomy at the region of the anterior cranial base (E), confirming stability of this region which is unaffected by the palatal expansion device. *APS*, Axial palatal section; *LNS*, lower nasal section; *MSP*, maxillary sagittal plane; *UNS*, upper nasal section. (Image courtesy Dr. Daniele Cantarella and Dr. Won Moon, UCLA School of Dentistry. From Cantarella D, Dominguez-Mompell R, Mallya SM, et al. Changes in the midpalatal and pterygopalatine sutures induced by micro-implant-supported skeletal expander, analyzed with a novel 3D method based on CBCT imaging. *Prog Orthod.* 2017;18:34.)

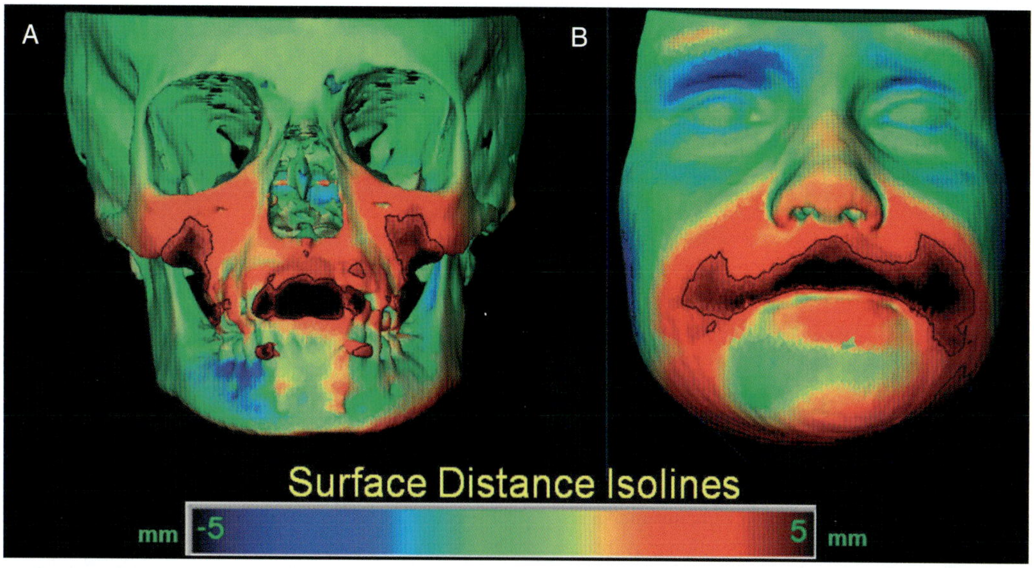

Fig. 32.8 Treatment-related skeletal and soft-tissue changes. Fusion images demonstrate a graphical and quantitative evaluation of changes. The color scale bar at the bottom of the images depicts the magnitude and direction of the changes (*blue* = inward, *red* = outward). Three-dimensional surface model demonstrates changes in (A) the zygomatic processes of the maxilla, and (B) the soft tissue of the upper lip. (Modified from Cevidanes LH, Motta A, Proffit WR, et al. Cranial base superimposition for 3-dimensional evaluation of soft-tissue changes. *Am J Orthod Dentofacial Orthoped.* 137[4 suppl 1]:S120-S129.)

- Assess growth-associated changes in the maxillofacial skeleton.
- Monitor adaptive changes and disease patterns in the temporomandibular joint after orthodontic and maxillofacial surgical treatments.
- Evaluate osseous healing and success of bone grafts placed for ridge augmentation or surgical reconstruction.
- Monitor stability and recurrence of intraosseous pathologic lesions.

BIBLIOGRAPHY

Artificial Intelligence

Dentistry: Overview of Artificial Intelligence and Augmented Intelligence Uses in Dentistry. SCDI White Paper no. 1106. American Dental Association. https://www.ada.org/-/media/project/ada-organization/ada/ada-org/files/resources/practice/dental-standards/ada_1106_2022.pdf?rev=6597958fb295462492935589971e27c3.

Brady AP, Allen B, Chong J, et al. Developing, purchasing, implementing and monitoring AI tools in radiology: Practical considerations. A multi-society statement from the ACR, CAR, ESR, RANZCR & RSNA. *J Med Imaging Radiat Oncol.* 2024;68(1):7-26.

Computer-Guided Treatment Planning

Bornstein MM, Al-Nawas B, Kuchler U, et al. Consensus statements and recommended clinical procedures regarding contemporary surgical and radiographic techniques in implant dentistry. *Int J Oral Maxillofac Implants.* 2014;29(suppl):78-82.

Bengtsson M, Wall G, Greiff L, et al. Treatment outcome in orthognathic surgery—A prospective randomized blinded case-controlled comparison of planning accuracy in computer-assisted two- and three-dimensional planning techniques (part II). *J Craniomaxillofac Surg.* 2017;45(9):1419-1424.

De Riu G, Virdis PI, Meloni SM, et al. Accuracy of computer-assisted orthognathic surgery. *J Craniomaxillofac Surg.* 2018;46(2):293-298.

Li B, Shen S, Jiang W, et al. A new approach of splint-less orthognathic surgery using a personalized orthognathic surgical guide system: a preliminary study. *Int J Oral Maxillofac Surg.* 2017;46(10):1298-1305.

Xia JJ, Shevchenko L, Gateno J, et al. Outcome study of computer-aided surgical simulation in the treatment of patients with craniomaxillofacial deformities. *J Oral Maxillofac Surg.* 2011;69(7):2014-2024.

3D Printing

Marro A, Bandukwala T, Mak W. Three-dimensional printing and medical imaging: a review of the methods and applications. *Curr Probl Diagn Radiol.* 2016;45(1):2-9.

Mitsouras D, Liacouras P, Imanzadeh A, et al. Medical 3D printing for the radiologist. *Radiographics.* 2015;35(7):1965-1988.

Chepelev L, Wake N, Ryan J, et al. Radiological Society of North America (RSNA) 3D printing Special Interest Group (SIG): guidelines for medical 3D printing and appropriateness for clinical scenarios. *3D Print Med.* 2018;4(1):11. https://doi.org/10.1186/s41205-018-0030-y.

Four-Dimensional Imaging

Cevidanes LH, Styner MA, Proffit WR. Image analysis and superimposition of 3-dimensional cone-beam computed tomography models. *Am J Orthod Dentofacial Orthop.* 2006;129(5):611-618.

Cevidanes LH, Hajati AK, Paniagua B, et al. Quantification of condylar resorption in temporomandibular joint osteoarthritis. *Oral Surg Oral Med Oral Pathol Oral Radiol Endod.* 2010;110(1):110-117.

Cevidanes LH, Motta A, Proffit WR, et al. Cranial base superimposition for 3-dimensional evaluation of soft-tissue changes. *Am J Orthod Dentofacial Orthop.* 2010;137(suppl 4):S120-S129.

Koerich L, Weissheimer A, de Menezes LM, et al. Rapid 3D mandibular superimposition for growing patients. *Angle Orthod.* 2017;87(3):473-479.

Nada RM, Maal TJ, Breuning KH, et al. Accuracy and reproducibility of voxel based superimposition of cone beam computed tomography models on the anterior cranial base and the zygomatic arches. *PLoS One.* 2011;6(2):e16520.

Ponce-Garcia C, Lagravere-Vich M, Cevidanes LHS, et al. Reliability of three-dimensional anterior cranial base superimposition methods for assessment of overall hard tissue changes: a systematic review. *Angle Orthod.* 2018;88(2):233-245.

33

Forensics

Robert E. Wood

SCOPE OF FORENSICS IN DENTISTRY

The scope of forensics in dentistry (also called forensic dentistry or odontology) includes the identification of human remains and its associated legal responsibilities. Dental forensic investigation may involve the identification of a single individual cataloguing dental information from unsolved or "cold" cases or, in some instances identification of multiple individuals, as in cases of mass disaster. In the latter example, the task would be conducted by a team including forensic dentists, forensic anthropologists, and forensic pathologists for biologic profiling and population stratification; the sorting of individuals based on gender, age, and, to a lesser extent, racial or ethnic background.

Multiple-fatality stratification is used to identify previously unidentified human remains. This process increases the probability of making a positive identification between an individual and the dental records of a missing person. If an identification is not possible, at the very least an assessment of the developmental age of an individual's dentition using diagnostic imaging may allow the forensic dentist to estimate chronological age. This determination involves a process where the developmental age of the dentition is compared with the corresponding dental developmental ages of a standard population to arrive at an estimate of chronological age. This process can also be performed on living individuals; for example, in identifying individuals to confirm age of majority. There are other methods (not included in this chapter) besides the developmental age of teeth to determine chronologic age, such as determining the developmental age of the bones of the wrist and hand, assessment of the spheno-occipital synchondrosis and maturation of the clavicle.

All age determinations have an associated error rate. According to Saks in his publication, "The Coming Paradigm Shift in Forensic Identification Science," quantification of error rates in the comparative forensic sciences has been problematic. For this reason, it is imperative that the forensic dentist understand the inherent sources of scientific error, and be circumspect in selecting language used in the statement of official opinions.

Forensic dentists also contribute to cases involving bite-mark injuries, including the recognition, documentation, and analysis of injuries. Analysis may involve comparison of a known dentition with a bite mark in a substance, that may include human skin. Such cases may assist a dental regulatory authority or involve civil litigation. Oral and maxillofacial radiology often provides objective data that are useful in supporting the opinions of the forensic dentist. This chapter focuses primarily on the role of the forensic dentist in identifying human remains.

NEED FOR IDENTIFICATION OF HUMAN REMAINS

Human remains are identified for personal, legal, and societal reasons. People place great importance on the verification of the identity of a deceased person from a personal perspective because doing so gives a measure of closure to loved ones, permits appropriate funerary rites, and allows appropriate religious ceremonies to be undertaken. In the absence of knowing for certain that a loved one has died, the grieving process may be delayed or interrupted.

From a legal perspective, certification of death is required before payment of life insurance, settling of wills and estates, dissolution of business partnerships, contracts, marriage, and settling of debts. Just as important from a legal perspective is the commencement of a suspicious death investigation. Knowing the identity of a person who has died under suspicious circumstances may instigate an investigation. Also, fulfillment of the legal requirements for the identification of an individual has importance for society as a whole. A competent forensic death investigation of human remains has four goals: determination of the means, manner, and cause of death, and identification of the remains.

METHODS OF BODY IDENTIFICATION

The primary methods used in body identification are performed visually, by fingerprint, the use of DNA, the presence of unique skeletal or medical devices, and the dentition. Visual identification, although the most common method, is unpleasant and unreliable, given that identification is conducted at a time of high stress and under difficult circumstances. Errors in visual identification are well documented and continue to occur. Fingerprint identification is common but requires the deceased individual to have had fingerprints recorded before death (e.g., criminal record, military or police service), and for the cadaveric fingerprints to remain intact after death. The fingerprints may not be intact in cases where the body has undergone decomposition, maceration, or incineration. Fingerprint identification is impossible with skeletonized remains. DNA identification, accomplished by comparing an *antemortem* (before death) sample with an unknown set of human remains, provides confident identification except between identical twins, who have the same DNA. In addition to comparative identification, DNA analysis can be used to verify a DNA trait, which may indicate the race or ethnicity of a deceased individual. Identification by skeletal or medical devices can be made if these devices have serial numbers or are unusual in form (Fig. 33.1). Additionally, frontal sinus morphology given its variability across the population has also been used, and may be used to *compare antemortem* and *postmortem* (after death) diagnostic images for the purpose of identification but presently has little empirical research backing it. Dental identification has many advantages over the other techniques. Empirical testing has demonstrated that it is reliable and straightforward when *antemortem* images are available; it is also readily accepted by courts of law, is understandable to a jury, and is quick and inexpensive.

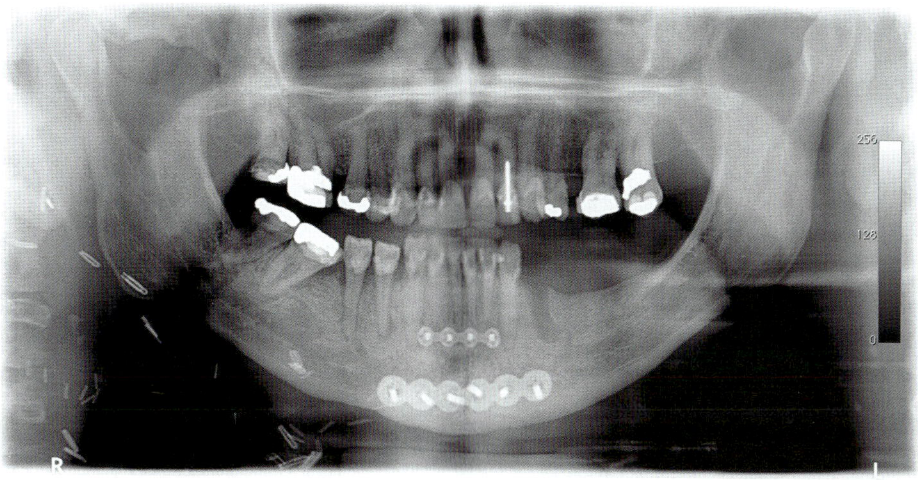

Fig. 33.1 Panoramic image revealing two fixation plates with 10 intraosseous screws placed in the anterior mandible after a mandibulotomy procedure. The shape and position of the plates and orientation of individual fixation screws provide unique information that may be used for identification.

UTILITY OF ORAL AND MAXILLOFACIAL RADIOLOGY FOR BODY IDENTIFICATION

Diagnostic images are used in dental identification because they provide objective evidence of the *antemortem* and *postmortem* conditions. Film-based and digital images are a permanent record of the *antemortem* condition at the time they were made, and they are difficult to misinterpret. In contrast, dental charting by one dentist may not be directly comparable to dental charting of the same patient made by a second dentist. Despite the forensic utility of *antemortem* intraoral images, dentists who practice evidence-based care do not acquire intraoral images routinely at each appointment. Consequently, *antemortem* images should be analyzed in conjunction with the *antemortem* dental chart. *Antemortem* images should never be acquired for the purpose of providing a record for later comparison, even in high-risk groups such as convicted criminals or sex-trade workers. The use of the dental chart and *antemortem* images of known date allows the forensic dentist to produce an *antemortem* odontogram, a record of the patient's dentition, which can be compared with the *postmortem* conditions for the purposes of identification.

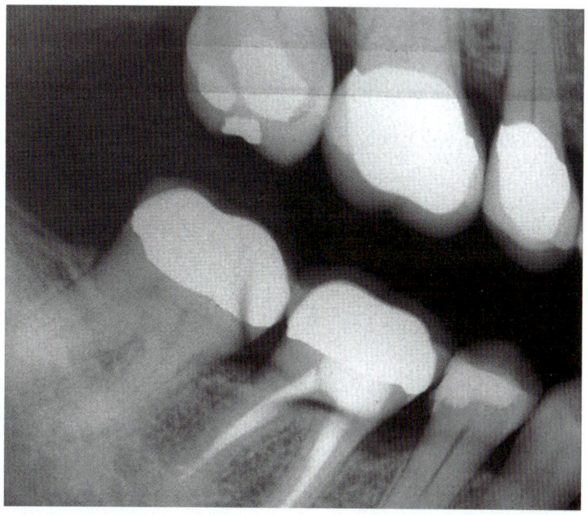

Fig. 33.2 *Antemortem* bitewing image providing potential concordant points because of the presence and unique shape of the restorations and root canal filling material.

IDENTIFICATION OF A SINGLE BODY

The process of body identification using dental criteria is relatively straightforward and is outlined by the American Society of Forensic Odontology. Using diagnostic images, the forensic dentist identifies points of agreement (concordance) between the *antemortem* and *postmortem* images and lists them numerically in a report. There is no set number of points needed for an identification to be made. A deceased person (decedent) who was edentulous before death may not have 32 concordant dental points with other edentulous candidates. However, if teeth are present with restorations, this may provide enough unique information to eliminate all other possible candidates and provide a match for only one putative decedent (Fig. 33.2). Useful concordant points may include the specific teeth present, unique features such as the shapes of the crown and roots, and the presence of restorations, including the materials used including endodontic material, and the unique shapes of the restorations.

Discordant points are also listed in the report. Such points include explainable discrepancies (e.g., points that do not match based on explainable circumstances, such as a restoration being placed after the *antemortem* images were exposed) and unexplainable discrepancies, where the findings cannot be explained without further investigation. An example of an unexplainable discrepancy would be a tooth missing on an *antemortem* examination but present on a *postmortem* examination. Unexplainable discrepancies, if they remain unaccounted for, preclude a positive identification using dental means. Fig. 33.3 shows *antemortem* and *postmortem* bitewing images used in the identification of an individual. After comparing images for concordant points, one may be able to determine whether this is a positive identification.

RADIOLOGIC TECHNIQUES IN BODY IDENTIFICATION

Either film-based or digital images, or *postmortem* multidetector computed tomography may be used in single-person or multiple-fatality dental forensics. Using film in *postmortem* examinations requires the film to be processed on site. The result is a slight delay compared with

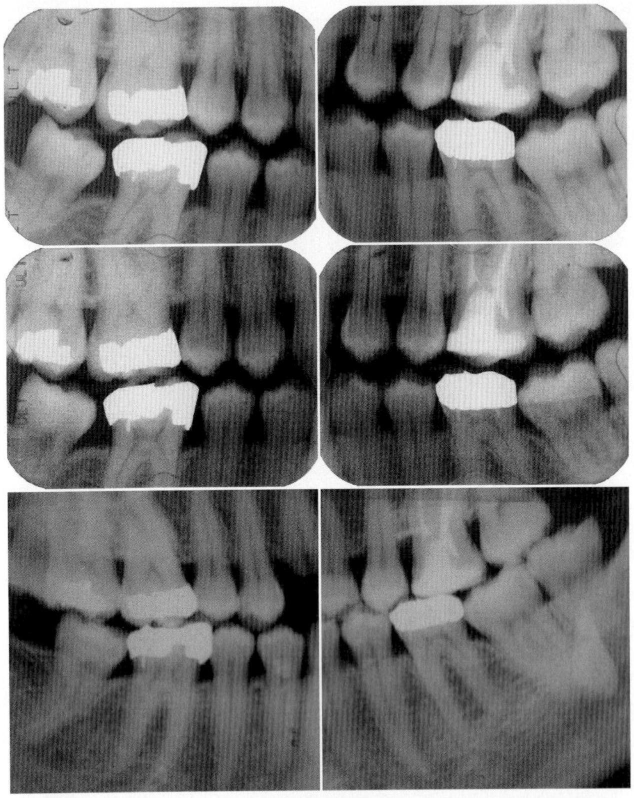

Fig. 33.3 Four *antemortem* film-based bitewing images *(top)* and two *postmortem* bitewing images *(bottom)*. A positive match can be made using the teeth present and the morphology of the teeth, such as root structure and pulp chambers, number and shape of metallic restorations, and endodontic filling material.

using solid state digital sensors. However, film-based images provide the flexibility of using various sizes of image receptors. For example, occlusal size (American National Standards Institute [ANSI] size 4) film can be used for bitewing images (Fig. 33.4). Furthermore, using larger image receptors such as this may permit imaging of the entire dentition with six exposures (Fig. 33.5). In cases where the remains are decomposed, receptors or specimens can readily be wrapped in polyethylene stock bags to prevent contamination (Fig. 33.6). A further advantage of using film is that the wider receptor latitude (compared with a solid state sensor) results in images of diagnostic quality in cases ranging from extremely bloated remains with soft tissue thicknesses up to five times normal, to skeletonized remains, and burned and partly carbonized remains resulting from fire.

Most forensic dentists use digital imaging systems. The advantages of digital systems include the ability to make multiple images in a short period of time by modifying the angle of the incident x-ray beam to replicate the *antemortem* images or to augment the examination instantly, thus improving the speed of identification. However, there are some limitations to the use of digital systems. Occasionally, where there has been considerable loss of tooth structure or soft tissue coverage, the wider latitude of film is superior for imaging small amounts of remaining material (Fig. 33.7). Presently there is a move to use conventional medical-grade multidetector CT scans examined with commercial cone beam CT viewing software. This allows the body to remain in the body bag avoiding contamination. Moreover, the process is rapid, and the volume is readily converted to both 2D images or 3D volumetric images that allow rapid age stratification and identification (Fig. 33.8).

For samples lacking soft tissue coverage, Lucite sheets can be used to attenuate the incoming x-radiation. Otherwise, kVp and mA settings can be reduced, or the x-ray target-to-object distance can be increased. However, in some cases there is so little tissue left that these measures may still not result in more acceptable images. Also, digital

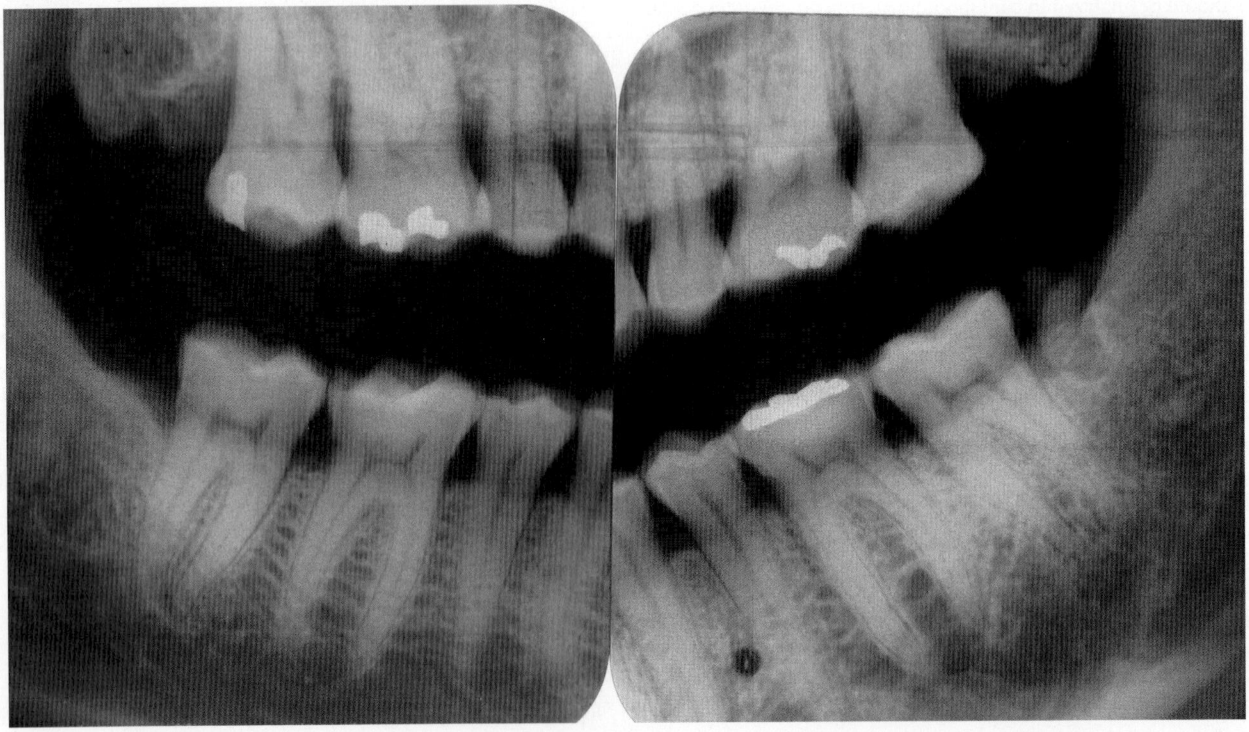

Fig. 33.4 The use of two film-based occlusal size receptors for bitewing imaging allows for a greater amount of tissue to be imaged than if the smaller American National Standards Institute Number 2 receptors had been used.

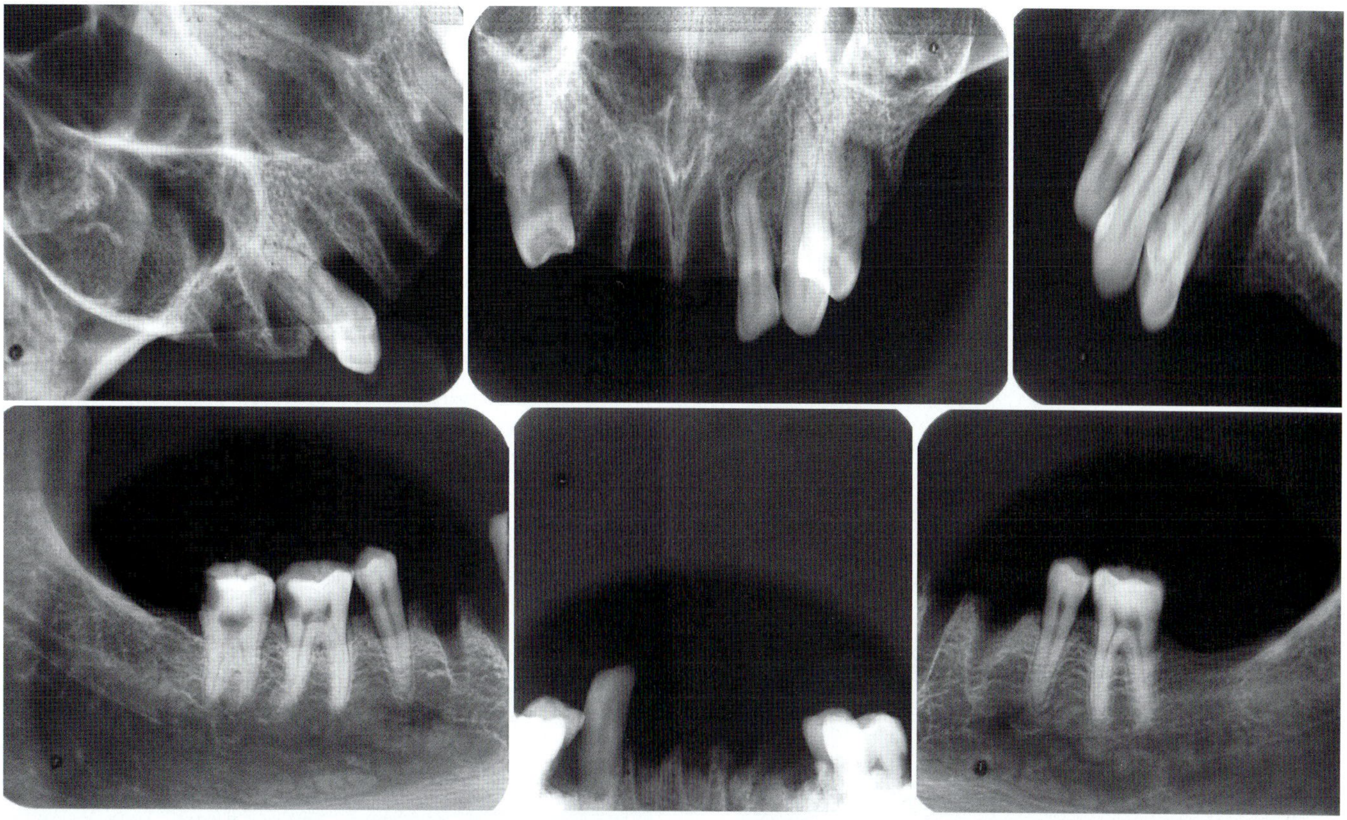

Fig. 33.5 Example of the use of occlusal images to obtain full imaging of the jaws with only six exposures.

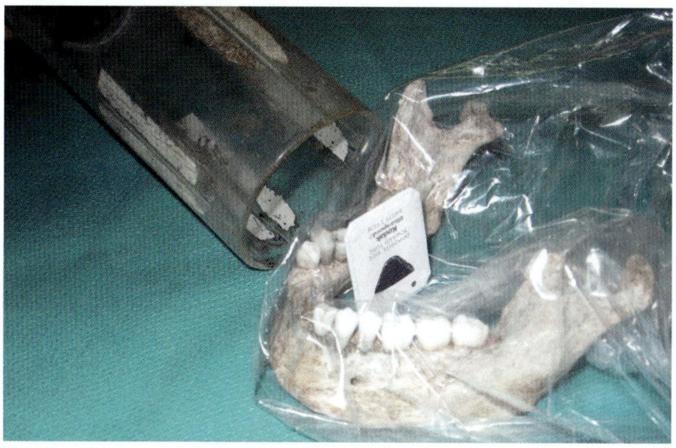

Fig. 33.6 A polyethylene stock bag is used to wrap the specimen for conventional radiographic imaging to protect the forensic dentist and others handling the material.

systems can be expensive, and the image receptor and the length of the attached cord of solid-state receptors must be thoroughly protected lest they become contaminated by the human remains.

Regardless of which image receptor type is selected, it is imperative for the forensic dentist to operate safely by practicing body-substance precautions and radiation safety. With respect to precautions from the body being examined, it is prudent to wrap equipment in impermeable membranes to avoid contamination, and to drape bodies with disposable covers so that all government-mandated laws on the handling of body substances are obeyed.

Where available, handheld dental x-ray generators should be considered mandatory for dental forensics. These devices are highly portable

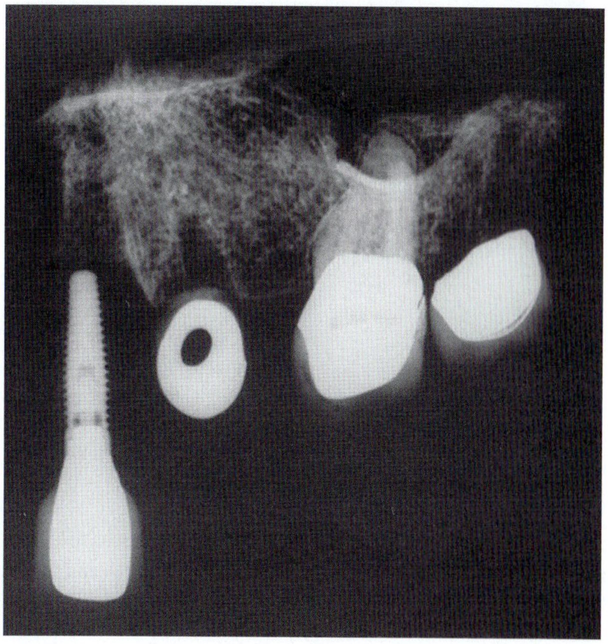

Fig. 33.7 This dark image demonstrates the difficulty of obtaining images with acceptable density when one is dealing with very small amounts of tissue.

and allow battery packs to be exchanged in cases of heavy use. Moreover, they are compatible with either film or digital receptor systems.

Finally, with regard to forensics, it is better to make too many images than too few. There is no concern with radiation dose to the deceased, so the entire tooth-bearing areas of the jaws should be imaged.

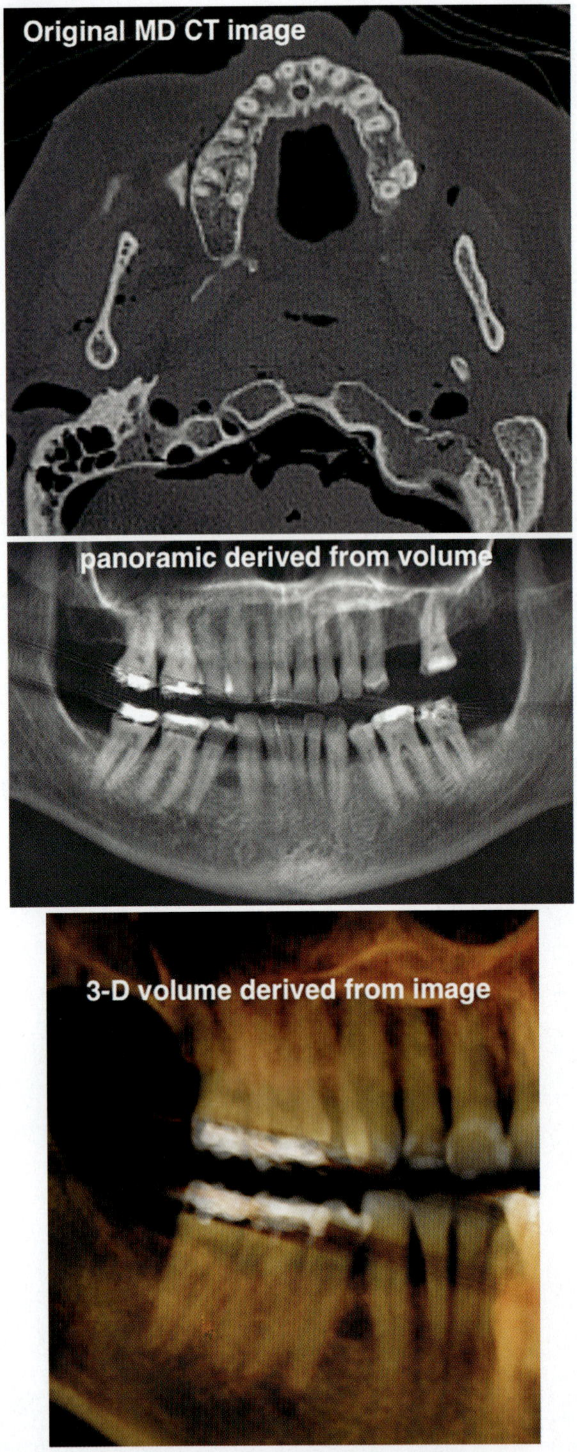

Fig. 33.8 Reconstituted images of the dentition and adjacent anatomy derived from a multidetector computed tomographic volume using cone beam computed tomography viewing software.

Equally important, the forensic dentist or forensic radiographer should keep in mind the goal of *postmortem* imaging, which is to provide images of high quality for forensic comparison with *antemortem* images. Diagnosis of disease is not the goal of forensic imaging. *Postmortem* images may be made in advance of receipt of any *antemortem* records; therefore, with respect to this use of radiologic imaging, the maxim "when in doubt, max out" is operative. Finally, in situations where the case is being entered into a "found-human-remains/missing persons" database such as the National Missing and Unidentified Persons System (NamUs), National Crime Information Center (NCIC), International Police Organization (INTERPOL), or others, the body may be buried or otherwise irretrievable by the time any *antemortem-postmortem* comparisons are performed.

FORENSIC DENTAL IDENTIFICATION REPORT

After the examination is conducted, the forensic dentist writes a report for the coroner or medical examiner. Box 33.1 shows the items that should appear in the report regardless of the style of report employed.

Style of Reporting Concordant Points

It is recommended that the name of each tooth be spelled out rather than using a tooth numbering system. This procedure reduces the chance of error in the event that the report is read by persons not accustomed to using either the World Dental Federation (FDI) tooth-numbering system or the Universal (US) numbering system. For example, the report may include the following statement: "*The maxillary right third molar is present and malformed with especially stunted roots on both antemortem and postmortem radiographic examinations.*"

Materials Used in a Report

The forensic dentist must keep materials used in the examination in a secure place while they are in use. After the examination has been completed and the report submitted, it is recommended that a copy of

BOX 33.1 Forensic Dental Identification Report

What Must Be in a Report

- Title of the report
- Name of the coroner or medical examiner
- Name of the pathologist
- Autopsy number or case agency number assigned to the deceased
- Name of the putative deceased person whose records are compared with the records of the remains
- Date of the *postmortem* examination
- Date of the report
- Brief description of the materials provided to you (e.g., radiographs, charts)
- Brief description of how the *postmortem* examination was conducted
- Points of concordance between the *antemortem* and *postmortem* materials
- Points of discordance between the *antemortem* and *postmortem* materials
- Results of your comparison
- Your name and signature but without your address, phone number, or other contact information

What Should Be in a Report

- Where the examination took place
- What the examination consisted of in detail (e.g., *postmortem* images exposed)
- Who provided materials (e.g., radiographs, charts) not generated by yourself and how they came to be in your possession
- Means of your comparison
- Points of identification listed and individually numbered
- Points of discordance listed and individually numbered
- Statement saying that your report is based only on the materials available to you, such as, "This report is based on the materials provided to me at the time of the comparison. If new evidence is made available, the author of this report reserves the right to amend or change this report."
- Statement that your report was returned to the authorizing agency along with materials provided and the date this was done

the report be retained and all materials be returned to the coroner or medical examiner. This practice places the onus for safe, secure, and permanent storage of all materials on the coroner or medical examiner so that the chain of custody is maintained.

APPLICATIONS OF RADIOLOGIC IMAGING IN MASS DISASTERS

Forensic dental identification is very useful in multiple-fatality incidents that result in a large number of human remains that may be commingled, macerated, burnt, or otherwise damaged. If the multiple-fatality event is small and can be managed by local providers, it may be simply a matter of undertaking multiple single identifications. However, if the incident is too large for local authorities to manage with confidence, it may be necessary to call on trained and experienced teams of forensic dentists from outside the local jurisdiction. Such situations are not the place for a well-meaning dentist lacking training, or even dentists with extensive case experience. Most people underestimate the stress involved with these situations, even on a seasoned practitioner.

The process of identification of remains in multiple-fatality situations is the same as the individual identification except for the organization. Normally, three teams are formed: (1) an *antemortem* team that collects, organizes, and collates incoming data obtained by investigators; (2) a *postmortem* team that examines, images, and charts the remains; and (3) a comparison team that makes identifications. In all cases, it is imperative to work with at least two members in each team so that errors can be identified.

In situations where the number of remains is large or fragmentation of the remains occurs, the comparisons become especially complex. Numerous computer software programs are available that can aid in the comparison (for websites, see bibliography section at the end of this chapter). These programs rank possible matches and mismatches using simple algorithms. However, all final identifications are made individually by human experts.

APPLICATION OF RADIOLOGIC IMAGING TO LONG-TERM UNIDENTIFIED REMAINS

Methods of identification of long-term unidentified remains are limited to situations where there are *antemortem* records of acceptable quality for comparison with *postmortem* records. In the United States, there are approximately 100,000 active missing-persons cases and 40,000 sets of human remains contained in repositories at any given time. This situation has been termed a silent, slow, mass disaster. In many instances, radiologic examinations of human remains can identify potential objective points of concordance and, with some degree of age stratification, can suggest a possible match of this set of human remains to a missing person. Many agencies attempt to provide this service, including NamUS, NCIC, and INTERPOL. These agencies use methods of coding the features of the dentition that facilitate the comparison process. In most cases, this comparison process is ongoing and updated at regular intervals. Once the information for a set of remains has been entered into one or more databases, it remains there until an identification is made. Similarly, *antemortem* records remain on the database until the person returns (in the case of a missing person) or until a match to *postmortem* remains is made. The information in some of these programs is available for public viewing on websites, whereas other programs keep the information exclusively for law enforcement. Generally, the wider the dissemination of this information, the greater the benefit. Also, and perhaps counterintuitively, for best results, the less dental minutiae entered into the coding system, the better. The presence of excessive detail increases the chance of false rejection of a match.

BIBLIOGRAPHY

Adams BJ. The diversity of adult dental patterns in the United States and the implications for personal identification. *J Forensic Sci.* 2003;48:497-503.

American Board of Forensic Odontology. http://www.abfo.org/.

Kirk NJ, Wood RE, Goldstein M. Skeletal identification using the frontal sinus region: a retrospective study of 39 cases. *J Forensic Sci.* 2002;47:318-323.

National Institute of Justice (U.S.). Missing persons and unidentified remains: the nation's silent mass disaster. https://nij.ojp.gov/topics/articles/missing-persons-and-unidentified-remains-nations-silent-mass-disaster.

National Research Council. *Strengthening Forensic Science in the United States: A Path Forward.* 2009. http://www.nap.edu/catalog.php?record_id=12589.

Saks MJ, Koehler JJ. The coming paradigm shift in forensic identification science. *Science.* 2005;309:892-895.

Wood RE, Kirk NJ, Sweet DJ. Digital dental radiographic identification in the pediatric, mixed and permanent dentitions. *J Forensic Sci.* 1999;44: 910-916.

Dental Identification Websites

DVI guide. https://www.interpol.int/en/How-we-work/Forensics/Disaster-Victim-Identification-DVI.

WinID3. https://abfo.org/winid/.

Missing Persons Websites

British Columbia. Ministry of Public Safety and Solicitor General, Unidentified Human Remains in B.C. https://governmentofbc.maps.arcgis.com/apps/webappviewer/index.html?id=1a60c24b82ed41699d8a55338fb11076&extent=-13708798.5797%2C6308623.5721%2C-13705741.0985%2C6309925.3902%2C102100.

FBI. NCIC Missing Person and Unidentified Person Statistics for 2010. http://www.fbi.gov/about-us/cjis/ncic/ncic-missing-person-and-unidentified-person-statistics-for-2010.

National Missing and Unidentified Persons System (NamUs). https://www.namus.gov/MissingPersons/Search.

Royal Canadian Mounted Police. National Centre for Missing Persons and Unidentified Remains (NCMPUR). https://www.rcmp-grc.gc.ca/en/national-centre-missing-persons-and-unidentified-remains-ncmpur.

INDEX

Note: Page numbers followed by "f" indicate figures, "t" indicate tables, and "b" indicate boxes.

D

P